5425

J. Roger de Lange, Jr. A.H.S.

January 23, 1992

TEXTBOOK OF
DENTAL RADIOLOGY

SECOND EDITION
TEXTBOOK OF DENTAL RADIOLOGY

By

OLAF E. LANGLAND, D.D.S., M.S., F.A.C.D.

Diplomate, American Board of Oral and Maxillofacial Radiology
Professor and Director of Oral and Maxillofacial Radiology
Department of Dental Diagnostic Science
The University of Texas Health Science Center
San Antonio Dental School
San Antonio, Texas

FRANCIS H. SIPPY, B.S., M.Ed.

Assistant Professor, Director of Dental Radiology Clinic
Department of Oral Pathology and Diagnosis
College of Dentistry, University of Iowa
Iowa City, Iowa

ROBERT P. LANGLAIS, D.D.S., M.S.

Diplomate, American Board of Oral and Maxillofacial Radiology
Diplomate, American Board of Oral Medicine
Professor and Director of Graduate Program in Diagnostic Science
Department of Dental Diagnostic Science
The University of Texas Health Science Center
San Antonio Dental School
San Antonio, Texas

With Additional Contributors

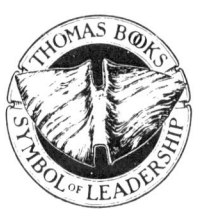

CHARLES C THOMAS • PUBLISHER
Springfield • Illinois • U.S.A.

Published and Distributed Throughout the World by
CHARLES C THOMAS • PUBLISHER
2600 South First Street
Springfield, Illinois 62717

This book is protected by copyright. No part of it
may be reproduced in any manner without written
permission from the publisher.

© *1973 and 1984 by* CHARLES C THOMAS • PUBLISHER
ISBN 0-398-04910-6
Library of Congress Catalog Card Number: 83-17908

First Edition, First Printing, 1973
Revised Second Printing, 1977
First Edition, Third Printing, 1981
Second Edition, 1984

With THOMAS BOOKS *careful attention is given to all details of manufacturing and design. It is the Publisher's desire to present books that are satisfactory as to their physical qualities and artistic possibilities and appropriate for their particular use.* THOMAS BOOKS *will be true to those laws of quality that assure a good name and good will.*

Printed in the United States of America
Q-R-3

Library of Congress Cataloging in Publication Data
Langland, Olaf E.
  Textbook of dental radiology.

  Rev. ed. of: Textbook of dental radiography. c1973.
  Includes bibliographies and index.
  1. Teeth—Radiography. I. Sippy, Francis H. II. Langlais, Robert P. III. Langland, Olaf E. Textbook of dental radiography. IV. Title.
  [DNLM: 1. Radiography, Dental. WN 230 L282t]
  RK309.L36 1984   617.6'07572   83-17908
  ISBN 0-398-04910-6

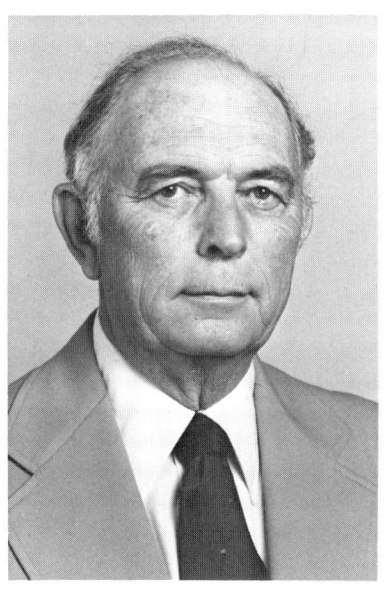

THIS TEXTBOOK IS DEDICATED TO:

CHARLES R. MORRIS, D.D.S., F.A.C.D.

Diplomate, American Board of Oral and Maxillofacial Surgery;

Diplomate, American Board of Oral and Maxillofacial Radiology;

Professor and Chairman, Department of Dental Diagnostic Science, The University of Texas Health Science Center at San Antonio, San Antonio, Texas

SURGEON, RADIOLOGIST, TEACHER, INVENTOR, FRIEND

CONTRIBUTORS

WILLIAM DOSS McDAVID, Ph.D.

Assistant Professor, Department of Dental
Diagnostic Science, The University of Texas
Health Science Center at San Antonio,
San Antonio, Texas

JOHN W. PREECE, D.D.S., M.S.D.

Diplomate, American Board of Oral and
Maxillofacial Radiology; Professor,
Department of Dental Diagnostic Science,
The University of Texas Health Science
Center at San Antonio, San Antonio, Texas

EMILY E. TAYLOR, Radiologic Technologist II

Department of Dental Diagnostic Science,
The University of Texas Health Science Center
at San Antonio Dental School, San Antonio,
Texas

PREFACE TO THE SECOND EDITION

THE purpose of this edition is the same as that which is stated in the Preface of the first edition. Dental radiology is a clinical subject, and in this book it emphasizes the use of the radiograph in the competent practice of dentistry.

All chapters have been revised and up-dated with new subject material. There are six new chapters: Radiation Biology, Quality Assurance, Principles of Interpretation, Normal Anatomy, Developmental Anomalies, and Dental Disease Interpretation.

This textbook was written to serve four purposes:

First, to serve as a reinforcement of the learning acquired in lectures in dental radiology;

Second, to serve as a reference guide for the clinical application of the radiographic procedures learned in lectures in dental radiography;

Third, to serve as a reference after completion of courses in dental radiology;

Fourth, to serve as a source of information for the dental assistant, dental hygienist, radiology technologist, and dentist.

Specifically, it is hoped that this textbook will aid the student in dental radiology to develop competence in the skills and understandings of dental radiography; provide an orderly progression of learning for the student of dental radiography; arouse the spirit of curiosity in the student of dental radiography; stimulate the student of dental radiology to become more responsive to the changing needs of dental radiology and to promote the dentist's awareness of his responsibility to his patient to use dental radiographic procedures intelligently.

This textbook represents a compilation of information based for the most part on publications of our contemporaries and predecessors.

In order to present the material in an informal manner, continuous references to these sources have been deleted. However, the reader will find a list of suggested references at the end of each chapter. We realize that this textbook could not have been written without the ideas, data, observations and conclusions of others. Therefore, this textbook is dedicated to our contemporaries and predecessors who have made this textbook a reality.

O. E. L.
F. H. S.
R. P. L.

ACKNOWLEDGMENTS TO THE SECOND EDITION

THE authors wish to express their appreciation to their many colleagues who generously and willingly gave permission to use illustrative material and diagrams from their published works. A special thanks to the Eastman Kodak Company for their permission to use many of their fine illustrative materials. Without the kind assistance of these people, this book would not have been completed.

We wish to give our gratitude to unnamed friends, advisors, students, and technologists who may recognize in this book the results of their help. Please acknowledge our indebtedness to you.

We are especially grateful to W. Doss McDavid and Emily E. Taylor for the truly masterful job they did in writing and illustrating Chapter 10 on Quality Assurance and to W. Doss McDavid for writing Chapter 16 on Panoramic Radiography; and to John W. Preece who wrote Chapter 5 on Radiation Biology and Chapter 6 on Hazards and Protection.

We wish to acknowledge Ray Aldrete, J. Louie Vazquez, and Dieter F. Karkut, photographers at UTHSCSA, Department of Education Resources, for their excellent work.

The illustrations and diagrams were skillfully prepared by Nancy O. Reid and Carolyn Wittlif, medical illustrators of the UTHSCSA, Department of Education Resources. Their work speaks for itself.

We are especially grateful for the tireless efforts, patience, sound advice, and cooperation given to use by the dental x-ray technologists of the Department of Dental Diagnostic Science, University of Texas Dental School at San Antonio: Leo Bedock, Felix Cordero, Joan Pluchinsky, and Emily Taylor.

We would like to thank our secretaries Pat Brownlow and Rebecca Cox, who contributed unselfishly of their time, skillfully typing each chapter many times and carefully collecting illustrative material in the preparation of this manuscript.

We wish to express our sincere appreciation to our colleagues at the Department of Dental Diagnostic Science, The University of Texas Dental School at San Antonio, who gave us helpful suggestions, time, assistance, encouragement, and cases.

We are particularly grateful for the encouragement, guidance, and assistance given us by Payne Thomas of Charles C Thomas, Publisher. His understanding, support, and gentle urging were most helpful.

We wish to recognize our wives, Ruth, Rose Ann, and Denyse, whose encouragement, understanding support, and patience were deeply appreciated.

Finally, we want to recognize Charles R. Morris, for his support, advise, and encouragement, and to whom we dedicate this book.

Olaf E. Langland
Francis H. Sippy
Robert P. Langlais

ACKNOWLEDGMENTS TO THE FIRST EDITION

IT is difficult to acknowledge every individual and manufacturer who has assisted us in the writing of this textbook.

We are indebted to our administrators of the University of Iowa and Louisiana State University for providing the facilities and opportunity to complete this project. Special appreciation is due Dean Edmund E. Jeansonne of Louisiana State University, School of Dentistry.

We are particularly grateful to Mr. Raymond Calvert, L.S.U. Dental Illustrator, for his excellent art work; Mr. William Stallworth, L.S.U. Photographer, for his excellent photography; and Mr. Claude Mahaffey, R.T., L.S.U. School of Dentistry, for his skillful radiography.

We are indebted to several of our colleagues and predecessors for their publications, which served as a valuable source of reference. Included in this group are Professor Albert Richards of the University of Michigan; Dr. J. Meschan of Bowman Gray School of Medicine; Mr. William Bloom of General Electric; Dr. William Updegrave of Temple University; Dr. Lincoln Manson-Hing of the University of Alabama; Dr. Harrison Berry, Jr. of the University of Pennsylvania; Arthur Fuchs (deceased) of Rochester, New York; Dr. Michel Ter-Pogossian of Washington University (St. Louis); Mr. F. Jaundrell-Thompson of London, England; and Mr. Herman Seeman of Rochester, New York.

Special mention should be made of the following publishers and manufacturers for permission to use illustrations and to quote from articles in which these illustrations appeared: W. B. Saunders Company; C. V. Mosby Company; Charles C Thomas, Publisher; General Electric Medical Systems; B. F. Wehmer Company; Eastman Kodak Company; Rinn Corporation; Pennwalt Corporation; and Siemens Medical of America.

We are very grateful to our associates who in our discussions gave us pertinent advice concerning the manuscript: Dr. Robert Fleming, the University of Iowa; Dr. A. Peter Fortier of L.S.U.; Dr. Charles H. Boozer, L.S.U.; and Dr. Ronald Barrett of L.S.U.

It is with sincere appreciation that we acknowledge the superb secretarial work of Mrs. Judy Carriere, Miss Carol Pagragan, and Miss Linda Lotz in the preparation of the manuscript. Their loyalty and patience is without peer.

We are indebted to Mr. Payne Thomas for his encouragement, guidance, and patience. He is truly an understanding and astute editor.

O. E. L.
F. H. S.

CONTENTS

Page

Contributors vii
Preface ix
Acknowledgments to the Second Edition xi
Acknowledgments to the First Edition xiii

Chapter

1	Introduction and History of Dental Radiology	3
2	X-rays, Their Production, and the X-ray Beam	43
3	Attenuation and Recording the Radiographic Image	88
4	Diagnostic Quality of Dental Radiographs	130
5	Radiation Biology (by John W. Preece)	153
6	Radiation Hazards and Prevention (by John W. Preece)	181
7	Intraoral Radiographic Techniques	206
8	Film Processing and Duplication	281
9	Analysis of Errors and Artifacts	322
10	Quality Assurance (by W. Doss McDavid and Emily E. Taylor)	352
11	Principles of Interpretation of Pathologic Conditions	367
12	Normal Radiographic Anatomy	380
13	Developmental and Acquired Anomalies of Teeth and Jaws	412
14	Radiologic Interpretation of Dental Disease	432
15	Atlas of Special Techniques in Dental Radiology	504
16	Rotational Panoramic Radiography (by W. Doss McDavid)	619
17	Legal Aspects and Future of Dental Radiology	636

Index 653

TEXTBOOK OF DENTAL RADIOLOGY

Chapter 1

INTRODUCTION AND HISTORY OF DENTAL RADIOLOGY

INTRODUCTION

RADIOGRAPHIC examination is as essential for diagnostic purposes in dentistry as it is in medicine. A clinical examination of the oral cavity without the aid of radiographs is restricted to the exposed surfaces of the teeth and associated soft tissues. Therefore, dental radiology offers the only preoperative means of inspecting the hidden structures of the oral cavity, namely, the roots and internal structures of the teeth, the approximal surfaces of the teeth and the surrounding alveolar bone. It is obvious, then, that a general radiographic examination of the oral structures is essential to the diagnosis of dental and oral conditions.

Kurt H. Thoma,* well-known authority in medicine and dentistry, had this to say concerning dental radiographic examination.

> "Radiographic examination is useful to discover, to confirm, to classify, to define, and to localize a lesion. It is helpful in establishing an early diagnosis, in finding the origin of symptoms and cause of disease, and in discovering the extent of tissue involvement. It is of great value in establishing a differential diagnosis between inflammatory processes and benign and infiltrating tumors. Finally, radiographic examination is a valuable aid in checking the progress of treatment."

The purpose of dental radiography is to provide the dentist with a radiograph of the best diagnostic quality. The requisites of any good diagnostic radiograph, regardless of technic used, are (1) proper contrast and density of the tissues radiographed, (2) maximal definition and minimal distortion of the anatomical structures involved, (3) anatomical accuracy, and (4) coverage of the boundaries of the anatomical region under consideration. Of course, to attain these requisites, every step in the radiographic procedure must be thoroughly understood and carried out. The equipment must be adequate; the projection, exposure, and processing technics must be correct; and the operator must be completely competent.

Although radiography is defined as the art and practice of making radiographs, it is much more than a series of procedures — it is both a **science** and an

---
*Thoma, Kurt H.: *Oral and Dental Diagnosis,* 3rd edition. Philadelphia, W. B. Saunders Co., 1949.

art. It is a **science** in that it embodies the sciences of physics, mathematics, and chemistry; it is an **art** in that it requires practice, study, experience, and judgment to attain the desired skill.

Those that desire to become competent in dental radiology must possess the following abilities:

1. understand the scientific principles that govern radiographic technics;
2. understand the means by which those principles are applied;
3. be able to produce an acceptable diagnostic radiograph consistently;
4. determine common radiographic errors that cause poor radiographs and be able to correct these errors;
5. appreciate and guard against the dangers of x-radiation;
6. manage dental patients correctly under difficult situations.
7. Interpret radiographs accurately and competently.

It is important to remember that the slightest inaccuracy in a dental radiograph may nullify its possible assistance in oral diagnosis. Any misconception of the images on the radiograph by the dentist may cause an interpretative error that in turn may cause the dentist to arrive at an incorrect diagnosis. Thus, the ability to master dental radiology is of equal importance as the ability to interpret the radiograph. These abilities go "hand-in-hand" because a poor radiograph could not be accurately read by the best dental diagnostician, and a quality radiograph is useless unless read properly.

HISTORICAL BACKGROUND OF DENTAL RADIOLOGY

The Discovery of X-Rays

X-rays were discovered on Friday afternoon, November 8, 1895 by Wilhelm Conrad Roentgen (pronounced Renken), Professor of Physics and Director of the Physical Institute of the University of Wurzburg in Bavaria (Germany). X-rays rank with anesthesia as the two greatest discoveries that have revolutionized the medical and dental professions. Today, it is extremely difficult to imagine practicing either profession without the aid of these discoveries.

One must remember that the apparatus used by Roentgen in his discovery represented the labor of many ingenious investigators. Various European investigators twenty-five years before the discovery of x-rays began intensive experimentation with glass tubes and the production of fluorescence. The first glass tubes used were called Geissler tubes after Heinrich Geissler, a glassblower from the University of Bonn (Germany) (1885). He had built a mercury vacuum pump that he used to evacuate part of the gases from sealed glass tubes. Geissler demonstrated beautiful colorful effects when high tension discharges were passed through them. Later, the tubes were called by the names of investigators that modified the original Geissler tubes (for example, the Lenard, Hittorf, and Crookes tubes).

During the years between 1859 and 1895 Julius Plucker, Wilhelm Hittorf, Heinrich Hertz, and Philip Lenard of Germany, Sir William Crookes of England, and others had revealed many new and interesting phenomena concerning the production of fluorescence in sealed glass tubes. Fluorescence is the instantaneous emission of light by a substance caused by varying kinds of stimuli (e.g. light, chemicals, electrons, and ionizing radiation).

In 1870 Wilhelm Hittorf of Germany used a partially evacuated glass tube and observed that light rays left the negative electrode in straight lines, produced heat, and caused a greenish yellow fluorescence on the glass where the light rays struck. These early so-called vacuum tubes depended on the incomplete evacuation of air to provide the cathode with negatively charged particles or ions, which were then directed with the aid of high voltage current (30–50 kV) against the anode. When these negatively charged particles struck the glass wall, it produced a greenish yellow fluorescence.

It was Goldstein of Germany who first called these negatively charged particles (ions) **cathode rays,** which were later called electrons.

In 1894, Philip Lenard, a student of Heinrich Hertz, of Bonn University in Germany, discovered that cathode rays (electrons) could penetrate through a special thin aluminum foil window built into the walls of glass discharge tubes. The cathode rays would penetrate the aluminum window and cause the air outside the tube to become electrically conductive and glow, but the cathode rays (electrons) would be absorbed by 5 cm or less of free air. He also found that cathode rays would cause fluorescence in certain fluorescent screen salts. (Fluorescent screens contain crystals of various organic salts called phosphors, which emit light when excited by various forms of radiant energy.)

Lenard might have been the discoverer of the x-ray had it not been for an unfortunate chain of events. First, Lenard was using a fairly insensitive fluorescence screen, which contained a material called keton. He was a student and was not permitted access to Dr. Hertz's supply of plantinocyanide screens, which were much more sensitive to x-rays. His insensitive keton screen would not fluoresce for distances greater than 8 cm from the tube. Second, Lenard's research was disrupted when he moved from Bonn, Germany, to Breslau (Wroclaw), Poland.

In May 1894, Wilhelm Conrad Roentgen set about the task of repeating Lenard's experiments with cathode rays. Previously, he had purchased a Lenard-type discharge tube for $8.70 from Müller-Unkel, a glassblowing firm, and Lenard had contributed a set of his own aluminum foils for the experiments. This "set the stage" for one of the most important scientific discoveries in the history of medicine and dentistry.

Wilhelm Roentgen did not have a supply of keton on hand, but he had some barium platinocyanide, which he knew would fluoresce in ultraviolet light. He reasoned that the barium platinocyanide could serve as a temporary substitute until his supply of keton arrived from a Dr. Krafft in Heidelberg.

Roentgen found that the barium platinocyanide screen fluoresced brightly only when it was placed fairly close to the aluminum foil window of the Lenard tube. Then he placed the barium platinocyanide screen in front of a Hittorf-Crookes tube without the aluminum foil window and found that this tube also caused fluorescence. The thicker-walled, windowless Hittorf-Crookes tube was known from previous experiments to absorb all of the cathode rays (Fig. 1-1). At first, he thought that the fluorescence caused by the Hittorf-Crookes tube was something intrinsic to the tube. To eliminate this factor, he placed some heavy black cardboard around the Hittorf tube so that none of the light produced within the tube could penetrate the light-proof jacket.

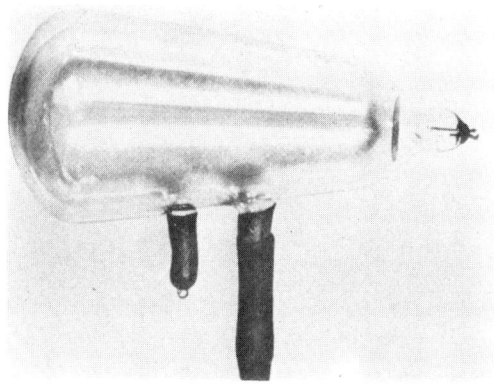

Figure 1-1. Roentgen's Hittorf-Crookes tube used by him to make the first radiograph. (Photograph courtesy of A. Haupt and Cie, Wurzburg, Germany.)

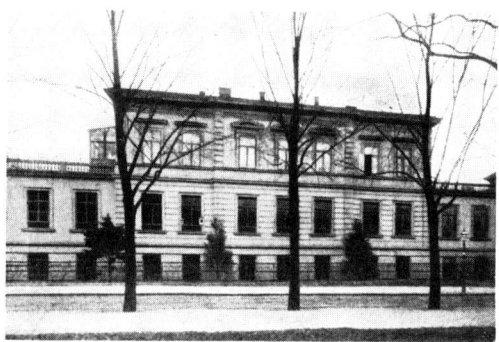

Figure 1-2. Photograph of the Physical Institute of University of Wurzburg, made in 1896. The upper story was Roentgen's private residence. Roentgen's laboratory was on floor just below his private residence.

the table near the tube. He thought at first his slight color-blindness (that made green difficult to distinguish) was playing tricks on him. Not believing what was happening, he repeated the experiment exactly. He noted the same greenish fluorescence. He lit a match and discovered the glowing object to be the coated barium platinocyanide screen he had used in his previous experiments (Fig. 1-3).

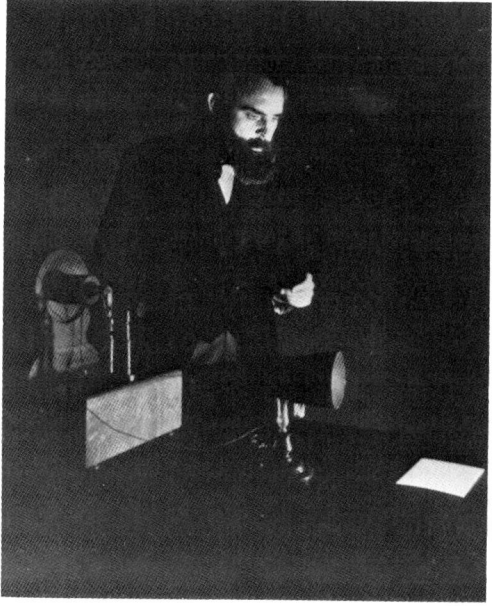

Figure 1-3. A staged version of Roentgen's discovery of x-rays. (From Glasser, Otto: 50 years of roentgen rays, *Dent Radiogr Photogr,* 19(1):1-5, 1946. Copyright Eastman Kodak Company, Rochester, New York. Reprinted by permission.)

In a darkened room in his laboratory in the Physical Institute of the University of Wurzburg (Fig. 1-2), late in the afternoon of November 8, 1895, Roentgen passed a discharge through the light-proof Hittorf-Crookes tube. To his satisfaction, he found that none of the light inside the tube penetrated the black cardboard cover. However, to his surprise, he noticed a faint greenish glowing object coming from

Cathode rays had never been known to span anywhere as great a distance as he now observed (approximately one yard away).

The fluorescence of the barium platinocyanide screen that great a distance from the Hittorf-Crookes tube, he reasoned, must be due to some powerful unknown ray that penetrated both the thick glass and the thick black paper. The rays could not be cathode rays or light rays.

In the next eight weeks Roentgen tested and examined this new kind of ray in every detail. During this time he did not divulge any information concerning his discovery to anyone, including his wife or colleagues at the University (Wurzburg). When asked by a close friend why his whole personal behavior with everyone had changed, he evasively said "I have discovered something interesting, but I don't know whether or not my observations are correct."

He first placed a book in the path of the rays and found the fluorescence persistent but somewhat diminished. By replacing the book with heavier materials such as metals he discovered that the radiation was absorbed in varying degrees. He determined that lead was the only material that stopped the rays completely.

Next, Roentgen (Röntgen) replaced the absorbing materials by his own hand. He was the first to see a living hand projected on a fluorescent screen. The screen revealed the denser shadows of the bones within the outlines of the flesh.

Since the photographic plate was a part of the general armamentarium in the research of cathode rays in these days, it was a natural step to replace the fluorescence screen with a photographic plate.

One evening after dinner (December 22, 1895), Roentgen asked Bertha, his wife, to come downstairs to the laboratory with him. He placed her hand on a cassette loaded with an unexposed photographic plate and directed the rays from the tube on it for fifteen minutes. When he developed the plate, it revealed an outline of the bones of her hand, which appeared light, and dark shadows of the surrounding flesh. This was the first radiograph ever taken of the human body (Fig. 1-4).

It was during this period that Roentgen determined that the new kind of ray could not be deflected in a strong magnetic field. It was a well-known fact that cathode rays could be deflected by magnets. Also, through further experimentation, he determined that the new radiation was produced in the glass wall of the Hittorf-Crookes tube (Fig. 1-5) and in the aluminum foil window of the Lenard tube.

Roentgen's x-ray apparatus consisted of a rather large Ruhmkorff induction coil machine, which was able to produce sparks from four to six inches in length, and was equipped with a Deprez mercury interrupter to generate potentials of 40 – 70 kV. He used a Hittorf-Crookes "fixed vacuum" tube (Fig. 1-6).

The Ruhmkorff induction coil was operated by five small storage batteries. The coil consisted of a primary or inner coil containing a few turns of coarse wire wrapped around a core of soft iron (magnetic core). The outer or secondary coil was made up of many turns of insulated fine wire.

Since a transformer (coil) cannot change low voltage current into high voltage current from a direct current (DC) source, Roentgen used an interrupter to change direct current into alternating current. Roentgen's interrupter was a mercury type interrupter that utilized an electric motor to dip a platinum tipped rod in and out of a container of mercury. The purpose of the interrupter was to interrupt rapidly the current going into the primary coil. By doing so the magnetic field surrounding the primary coil would collapse, which in turn induced a very high voltage current within the secondary coil. This high voltage was necessary to excite the Hittorf-Crookes tube. Roentgen's apparatus produced a potential difference of about 50 kV and a current with a fraction of an mA.

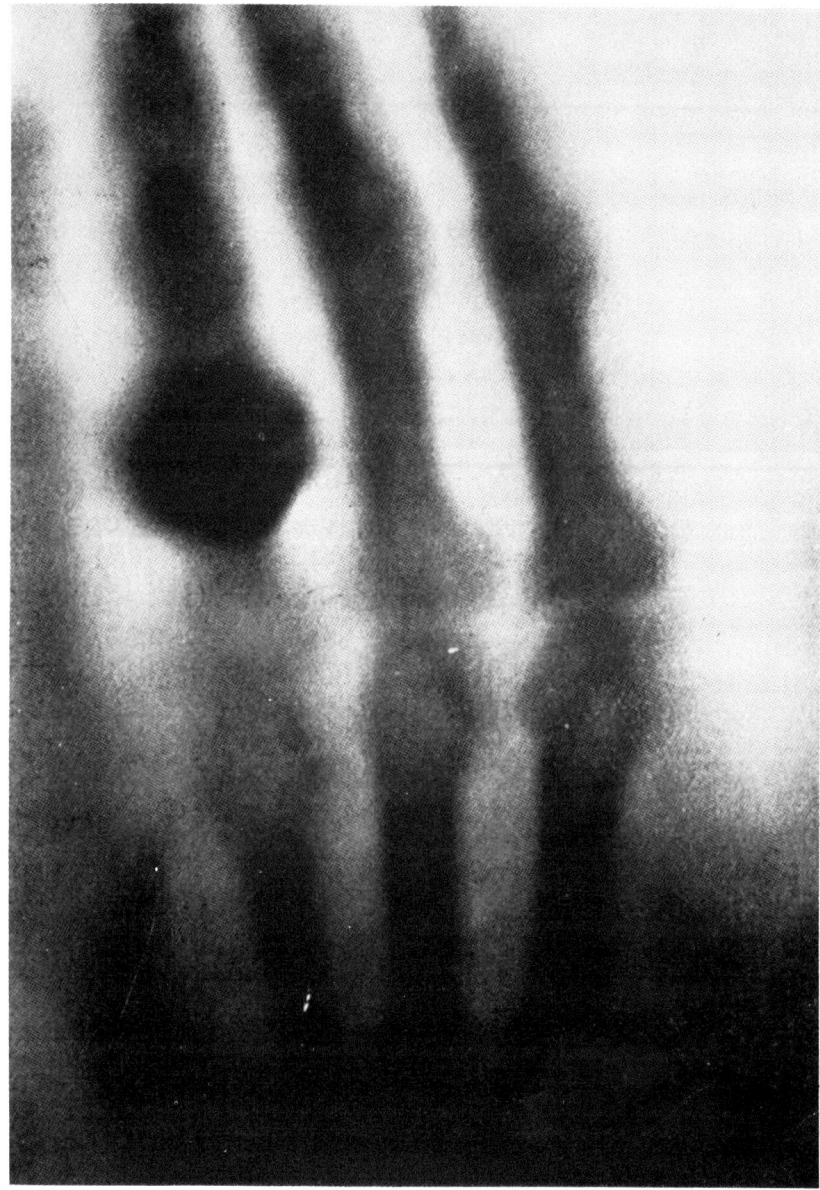

Figure 1-4. This is a photograph of the first radiograph ever taken (December 22, 1895). It is of Mrs. (Bertha) Roentgen's hand. Note that when a "positive" paper print is made of a negative X-Ray film, the values are reversed. The radiopaque (white) areas become "black," and the radiolucent (dark) areas become "white." (From Glasser, Otto: *Wilhelm Conrad Roentgen,* 1934. Courtesy of Charles C Thomas, Publisher, Springfield, Illinois.)

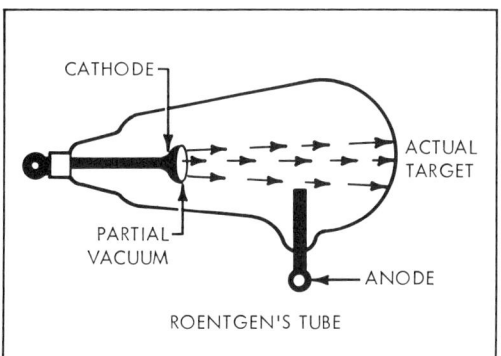

Figure 1-5. Hittorf-Crookes tube. X-rays were produced when the cathode rays (electrons) hit the side of the thick glass tube.

On December 28, 1895, Roentgen handed the manuscript of his preliminary report of his discovery to Professor Karl Lehmann, President of the Physical Medical Society of Wurzberg. It was printed as a preliminary communication in the "Annals of the Society," since no meetings had taken place during the Christmas vacation. It was rushed to the printers and his "Preliminary Communication on a New Kind of Ray" was published almost immediately.

On New Year's Day in 1896, Roentgen addressed copies of reprints of his Preliminary Communication and some prints of x-ray pictures he had later taken of his wife's hand to F. Exner, a friend and physicist in Vienna, and to certain other physicists in various other experimental centers throughout Europe.

Exner showed the prints to a group of friends and colleagues. One of Exner's friends, without Exner's consent, had the story published on January 6, 1896 in the *Wiener* (Vienna) *Press*. The news was cabled to London the same day. The report was copied by newspapers throughout the world, and the news spread like "wildfire."

The American announcement of the discovery appeared in the *New York Herald,* January 7, 1896, as the news was sent by cable from London. A translation of Roentgen's original paper appeared in *Nature* (London) on January 23, 1896, and was reprinted in *Science* (New York) February 14, 1896.

Humorists had a field day. In fact, their claims for the new rays were so nonsensical that the press found it necessary to print a qualifying statement to their readers stating "there is no joke or humbug in the matter. It is a serious discovery by a serious German professor."

Roentgen's first lecture demonstration on the "X rays" (his term, X meaning unknown quantity) was made before the Physical-Medical Society of Wurzburg on January 23, 1896. This was probably the only public lecture he ever gave on the subject. At this meeting Roentgen demonstrated numerous successful experiments with the x-rays and exhibited various x-ray pictures; they, of course, excited the greatest interest. After the lecture and demonstration, Albert Von Kölliker, great anatomist, suggested that the new rays be called "Roentgen Rays."

Professor Roentgen published two subsequent scientific papers on the x-rays. In his second communication on March 9, 1896, he reported on the ionization effects of x-rays. His third and last paper on the subject was printed in May, 1897. In these three papers Roentgen described thoroughly the various properties and characteristics of x-rays.

As one of his colleagues later observed, "Roentgen was a genius of interpretation of phenomena, had a keen sense of observation, and unexhaustible thoroughness of critical judgment, combined with brilliant experimental skill" (Fig. 1-7).

In 1900, Roentgen became professor of physics at the University of Munich (Germany). He died February 10, 1923 in

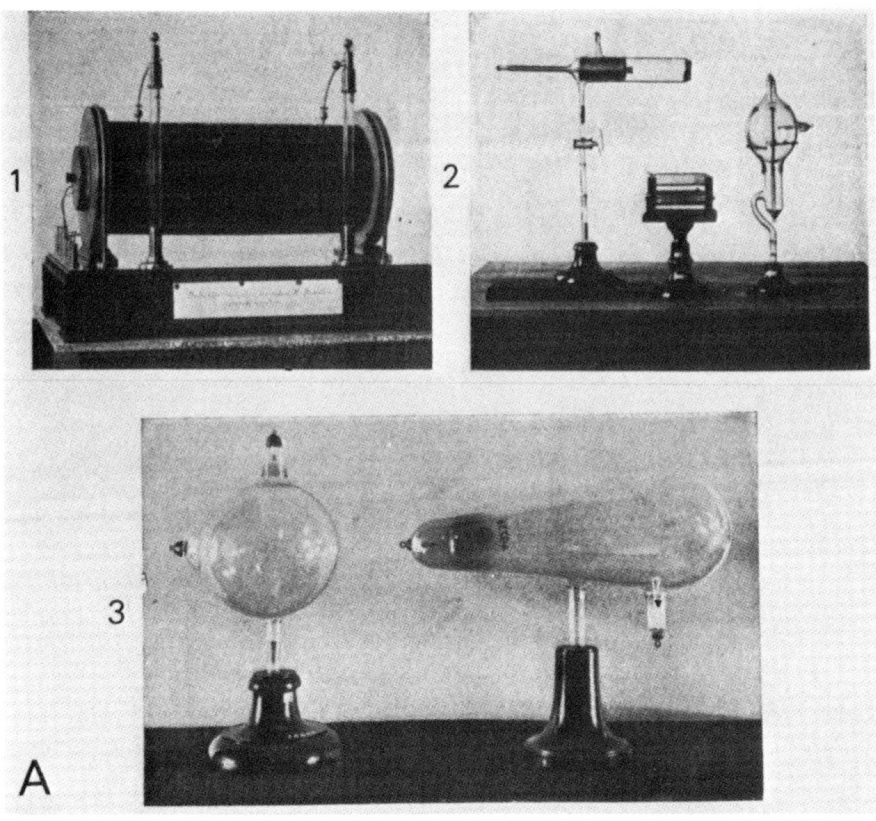
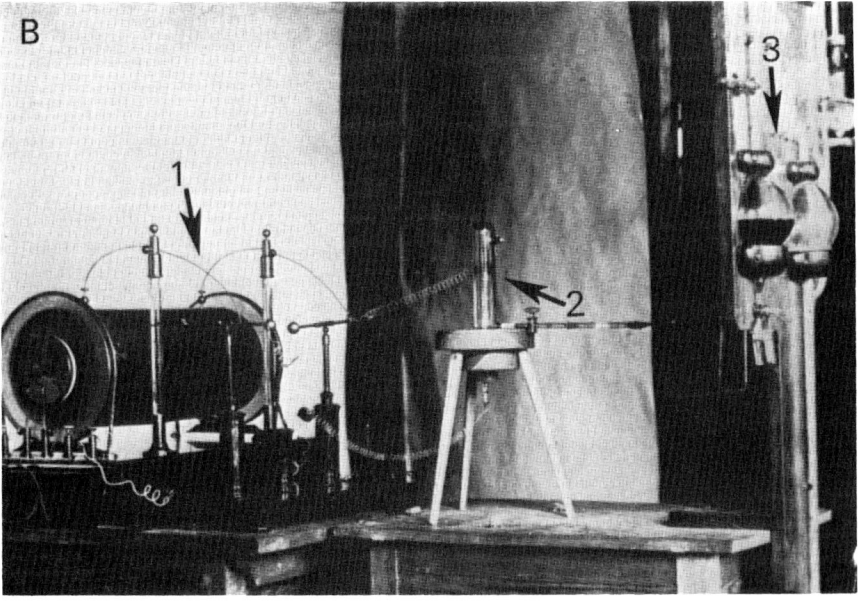

Figure 1-6. **(A)** Equipment used by Roentgen when he discovered x-rays. (1) Ruhmkorff-conductive coil. (2) Lenard Tubes. (3) Hittorf-Crookes tubes. (From Glasser, Otto: *Wilhelm Conrad Rontgen*, 1934, Courtesy of Charles C Thomas, Publisher, Springfield, Illinois.) **(B)** Photograph of equipment used by Roentgen. It was found among his property at his death. (1) Ruhmkorff coil. (2) Lenard tube. (3) Duprez mercury interrupter. (From Ernst Streller: The German Roentgen Museum, SRW News #22, Siemens Co., 1963.)

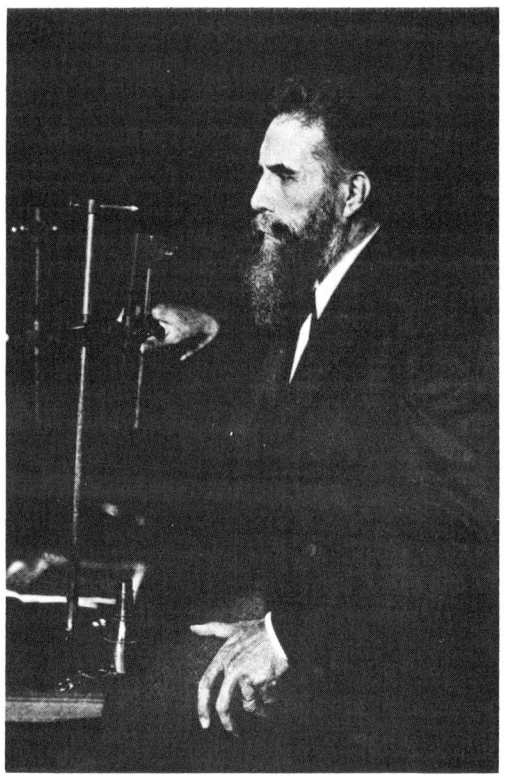

Figure 1-7. Wilhelm Conrad Rontgen. (Original photograph by Nicola Perscheid, Hofphotograph, Berlin, 1906, Courtesy of Deutsches Rontgen Museum at Remsheid-Lennep, Germany.)

Munich and was buried at Giessen, Germany (Fig. 1-8).

All through his life, Roentgen carefully avoided exposing himself to acclaim, but overreacted greatly to criticism. Only a few of the honors traditionally given to great men were received by Roentgen personally. One of these that he did receive personally was the first Nobel prize ever awarded in physics, for which he traveled to Stockholm in 1901. He refused to give a Nobel Prize lecture for personal reasons.

Although most scientists gave Roentgen full credit for the discovery of x-rays, there were attempts by a few to credit one of his assistants for the first crucial observation of the fluorescence of the screen. These absurd rumors persisted throughout Roentgen's life and deeply hurt him. With advancing years, he retired behind a protective screen and eventually became very bitter. He refused to publish anything further on x-rays after his three original communications, and in his will he stipulated that all correspondence concerning the discovery of x-rays written between 1895 and 1900 be burned unopened at his death. One of the few letters of correspondence written during this crucial period (1895 – 1900) has been preserved and is shown in Figure 1-9.

At the time of the discovery of x-rays, the essential equipment for producing x-rays was available in every well-established laboratory of physics. It consisted of either a Ruhmkorff coil, a Telsa coil, or a static machine to produce the necessary high-tension current. The second essential was the Hittorf-Crookes tube. Therefore, very quickly scientists throughout the world began duplicating Roentgen's discovery and producing all kinds of useful and important new data on x-rays.

Dental Diagnosis

Probably the first person to speak on the "usefulness of radiation to dental diagnosis" was M. Jastrowitz. He spoke on this subject on January 6, 1896 before the Berlinger Gesellschaft für Innere Medizin. His paper was published in a dental journal, *Zahnärztliches Wochenslatt,* Nr. 450, February 15, 1896.

Supposedly, the first dental radiograph ever made was completed by Otto Walkhoff of Braunshweig, Germany, on January 14, 1896, fourteen days after the announcement of the discovery of x-rays by Roentgen. He made the first dental radiograph by placing in his own mouth a

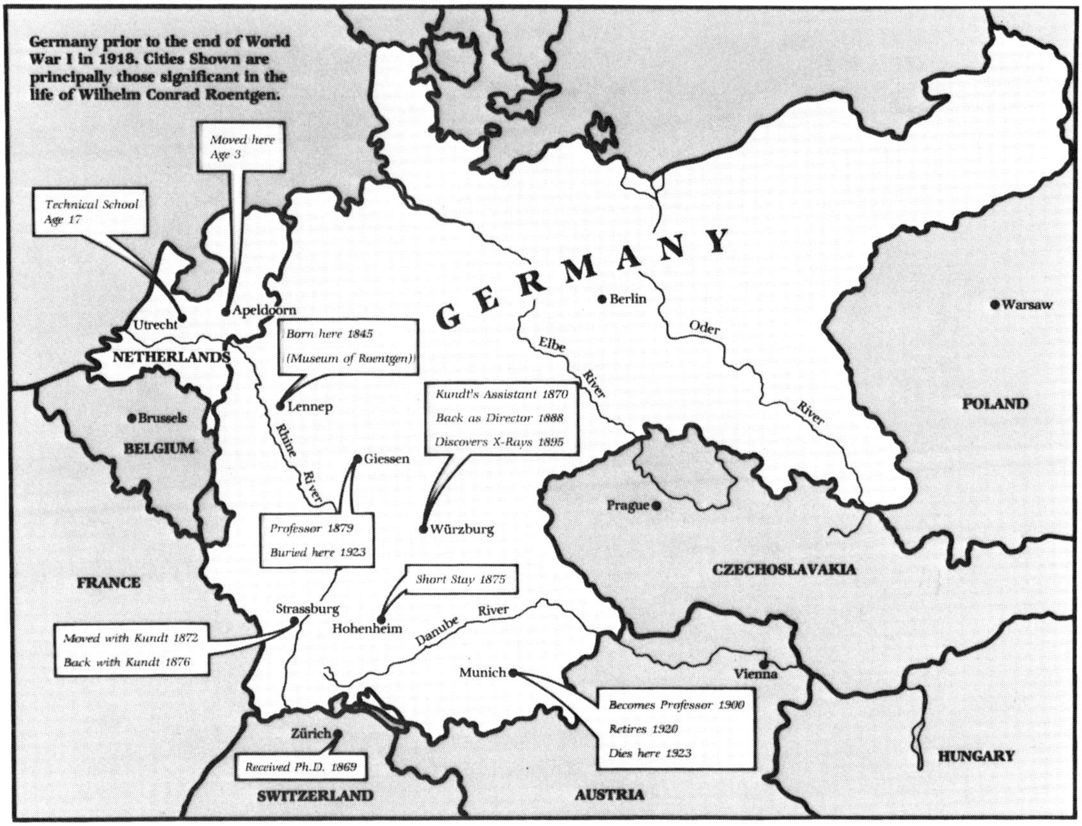

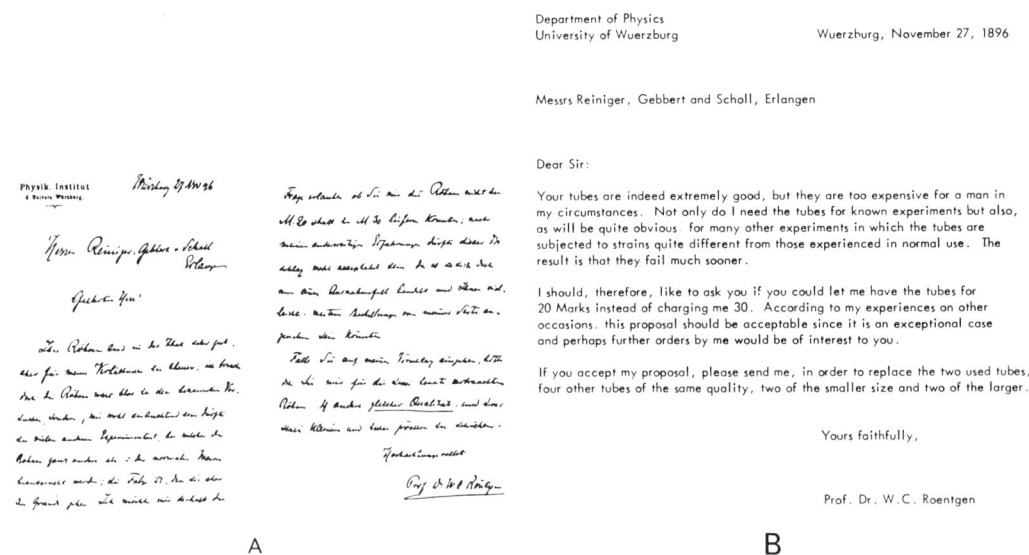

Figure 1-8. Pre-World War II (1918) map of Germany showing principal cities in the life of Roentgen.

Department of Physics
University of Wuerzburg

Wuerzburg, November 27, 1896

Messrs Reiniger, Gebbert and Scholl, Erlangen

Dear Sir:

Your tubes are indeed extremely good, but they are too expensive for a man in my circumstances. Not only do I need the tubes for known experiments but also, as will be quite obvious, for many other experiments in which the tubes are subjected to strains quite different from those experienced in normal use. The result is that they fail much sooner.

I should, therefore, like to ask you if you could let me have the tubes for 20 Marks instead of charging me 30. According to my experiences on other occasions, this proposal should be acceptable since it is an exceptional case and perhaps further orders by me would be of interest to you.

If you accept my proposal, please send me, in order to replace the two used tubes, four other tubes of the same quality, two of the smaller size and two of the larger.

Yours faithfully,

Prof. Dr. W.C. Roentgen

A   B

Figure 1-9. (A) This is a letter written in W. C. Roentgen's own handwriting in 1896 asking for a reduction in price of x-ray tubes sold by a company in Erlanger, Germany, which was the forerunner of the Siemens Corp., Erlanger, West Germany. (B) Translation of letter in (A). (Courtesy of Siemens Corp., Erlanger, West Germany)

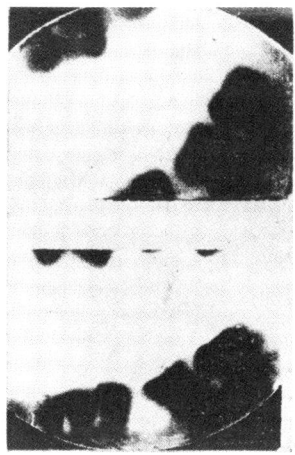

Erste Zahnaufnahme vom Lebenden angefertigt 14 Tage nach der Veröffentlichung Röntgens im December 1895 auf einer zu- geschnittenen photographischen Glasplatte von Dr. Walkhoff Zahnarzt in Braunschweig.

Figure 1-10. The first dental radiograph was taken on approximately January 14, 1896 by Otto Walkhoff of Baunschwerg. The exposure was 25 minutes. (From L. Ennis, H. M. Berry, and J. E. Phillips: *Dental Roentgenology,* 6th Edition, 1967. Courtesy of Lea & Febiger, Philadelphia.)

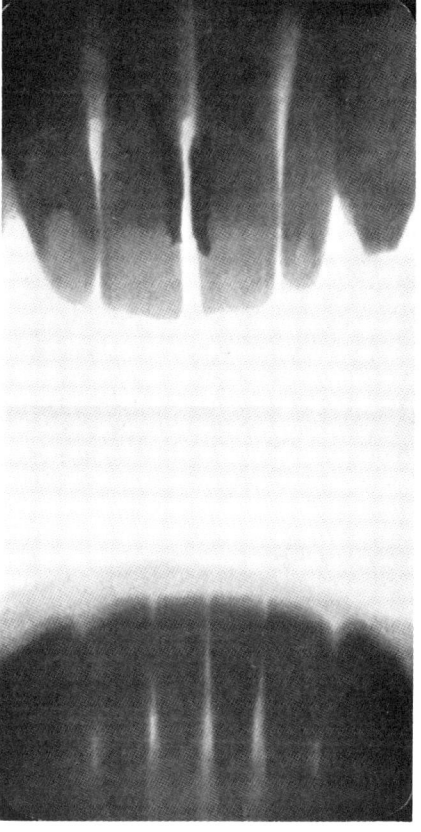

Figure 1-11. Reproduction of one of the earliest dental radiographs taken by W. Konig of Frankfort, Germany, in February 1896.

glass photographic plate wrapped in black paper, covered with a rubber dam, and submitted himself to twenty-five minutes of x-ray exposure (Fig. 1-10). This dangerous experiment indicated the reckless ignorance of some of the early pioneers in the use of radiation.

P. Hauser of Franfort University (1966) believes the first intraoral radiograph was taken by a physicist, Dr. Walter Konig, of Frankfort, Germany, later professor at Giessen, on February 1, 1896 (Fig. 1-11). Konig's fourteen intraoral radiographs were published by Johann Ambrosius Barth in March 1896.

Some few weeks after Roentgen's discovery, Professor Salvioni of Perugia, Italy, announced that he had arrived (apparently independently) at the property of the platinocyanides to fluoresce under the influence of x-rays. He had put this property to practical use by constructing an instrument called a "cryptoscope," which was a type of cassette that held the photographic film against a platinocyanide intensifying screen.

In many other laboratories, scientists worked on improving the principle of fluorescence. Dr. Michael I. Pupin of Columbia College in New York was one of the first to use intensifying screens in the United States and took x-ray photographs

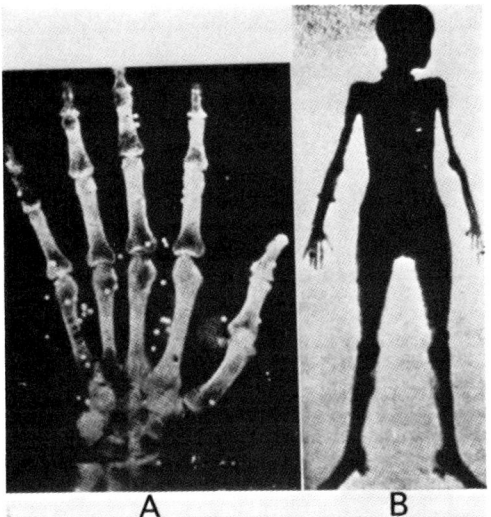

Figure 1-12. (A) Radiograph taken by Michael Pupin of New York in January 1896, of Mr. Butler Hall, a well-known attorney from New York, who accidently had discharged a shot gun into his hand while hunting in England. (B) Dr. William J. Morton's whole body radiograph of thirty-year-old female taken in 1897. Exposure time thirty minutes. Film was 3 × 6 foot in size. (From E. R. N. Grigg: *The Trail of Invisible Light,* 1965, pp. 30, 79. Courtesy of Charles C Thomas, Publisher, Springfield, Illinois.)

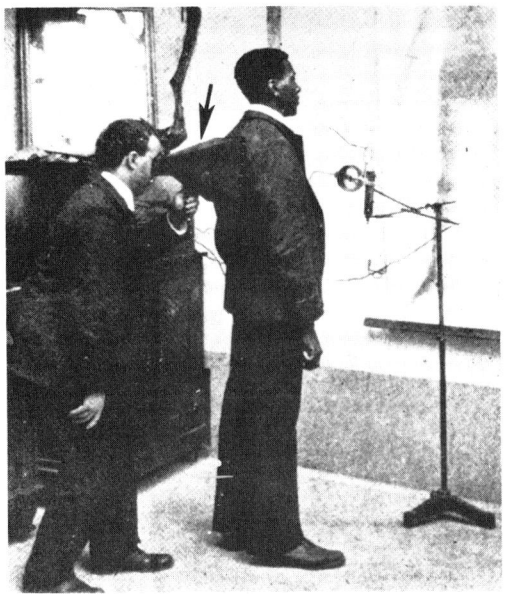

Figure 1-13. Equipment and type of tube used at the Medicochirugical College, Philadelphia, 1900. Dr. M. K. Kassabran is using hand fluoroscope (see arrow) with no protection to patient or physician. Dr. Kassabran later died from carcinoma secondary to radiation effects. (From G. E. Phafler: The development of roentgen therapy during fifty years. *Radiology, 45:*59, November 1945. Courtesy of the Radiological Society of North America, Inc., Oak Brook, Illinois.)

as early as 1896. He used a platinocyanide fluorescent screen placed behind a photographic plate within a lighttight cassette — the precursor of the intensifying screen. One of Pupin's early roentgen pictures (February 1896) was widely circulated and wellknown. It was used to locate foreign bodies in a patient's hand (Fig. 1-12A).

Thomas A. Edison also devoted himself and his well-organized staff at Menlo Park, New Jersey, to experimentation with x-rays and fluorescent screens. Edison invented a fluoroscope, which was displayed at the Edison Exhibit in New York City in May, 1896. Roentgen described Edison's fluoroscope in his third communication as "a box similar to a stereoscope which can be held lighttight against the head of the observer and whose cardboard end is coated with calcium tungstate" (Fig. 1-13). When an object was placed next to the screen and it was bombarded with x-rays, an image was produced. Edison's selection of calcium tungstate, from 8,500 fluorescent materials, was of prime importance in the development of the radiographic intensifying screen. The photographic plate emulsion was more sensitive to the fluorescent light waves emitted by calcium tungstate than any of the others.

It is tragic to recall that Mr. Dally, one of Edison's assistants in his experiments involving the fluoroscope, contracted severe radiation burns, which eventually caused Dally's death in 1904. This sad event could have been one of the reasons why Edison discontinued his experiments with x-rays.

One of the earliest x-ray photographs taken of a pathological condition in the Western hemisphere was taken by Professor Edwin B. Frost of Dartmouth College on February 3, 1896. It was taken of a young male with a fractured radius and ulna. Professor Frost used a special Crookes tube called a Puluj tube, energized with an induction coil and Grove batteries. The fractured arm was placed on a photographic plate holder containing the photographic film. The length of exposure was fifteen to twenty minutes (Fig. 1-14).

We will probably never know who made the first dental radiograph in the Western hemisphere. It was either William James Morton, M.D., of New York; C. Edmund Kells, D.D.S., of New Orleans; or William Herbert Rollins, D.D.S., M.D., of Boston, Massachusetts.

W. J. Morton

W. J. Morton, M.D., of New York made dental x-ray pictures very early and gave a lecture on April 24, 1896 before the New York Odontological Society in which he called attention to the possible usefulness of roentgen rays in dental practice. The lecture was illustrated by many roentgen pictures of the teeth, among which one was especially illustrative. It revealed an impacted tooth, which was otherwise invisible.

In his April 24, 1896 lecture, Morton discussed the gagging patient, and the technic he used to place the film in the mouth of a living patient.

He folded small cut pieces of rolled photographic film into three layers of paper, which were placed into a gutta-percha packet in the darkroom. Morton then adjusted the packet to the patient's mouth and took the exposure. If the patient gagged too much a cocaine spray was used.

One of Dr. Morton's more ambitious experiments in radiography was making the first whole body radiograph in 1897. This was accomplished on a thirty-year-old female using a three by six foot sheet of film. The exposure time was thirty minutes! The fate of the young girl was not recorded (*see* Fig. 1-12B).

C. E. Kells

Most people, however, claim that the first dental radiograph taken in this country of a living subject was by C. Edmund Kells of New Orleans (Fig. 1-15). Morton was a physician and his interest in dentistry was purely academic; it was Kells who first put the radiograph to practical use in dentistry.

Dr. Kells became interested in x-rays soon after the announcement of Roentgen's discovery, when he attended a public lecture and demonstration of x-rays given by Professor Brown Ayres, Dean of the Scientific Department, Tulane University (New Orleans). Professor Ayres took an x-ray picture of the human hand, which required a twenty minute exposure. Kells reasoned that if the bones of the hand could be shown by this method, it might work to reveal the roots of the teeth in bone. After consulting with Professor Ayres after the demonstration, he purchased a Telsa coil and a modified Crookes tube to pursue the task of taking a dental radiograph (Fig. 1-16).

He discovered at once that his first x-ray patient could not hold the film in the mouth for long periods of time without moving. To overcome this difficulty he constructed a film holder, made from a

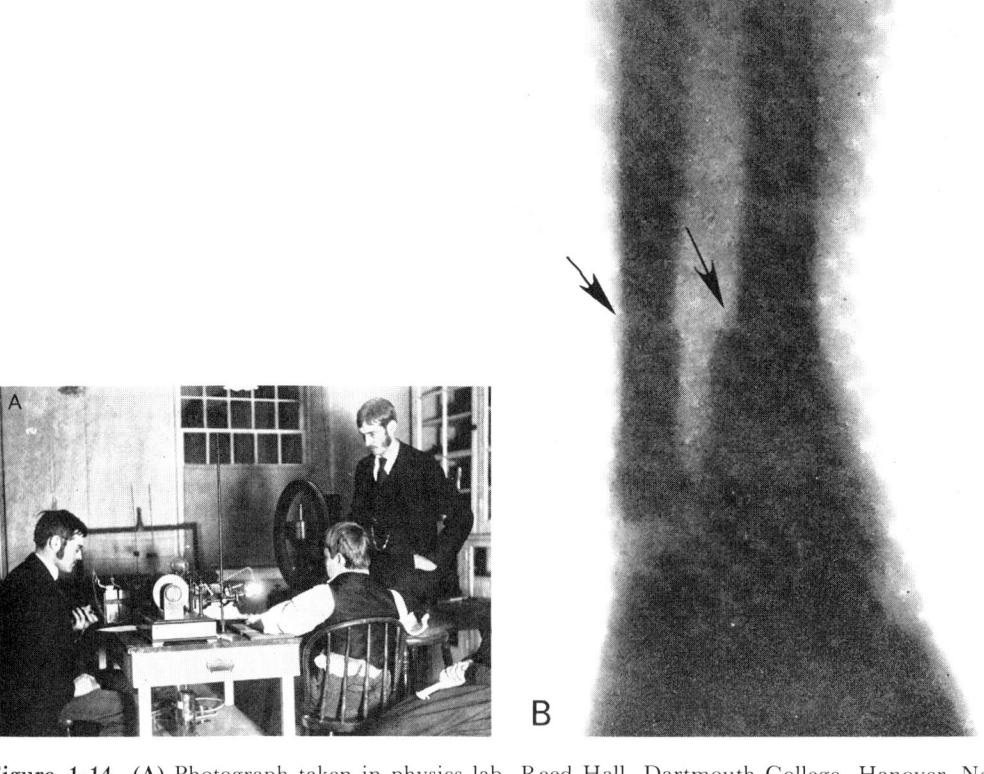

Figure 1-14. (A) Photograph taken in physics lab, Reed Hall, Dartmouth College, Hanover, New Hampshire, on February 3, 1896. Professor Edwin B. Frost is sitting with watch in hand on the left. The patient, Edward McCarthy, is seated at right of table. Dr. Gilman Frost is standing at right. (B) The first radiograph of a pathological condition taken in America, February 3, 1896. The fracture lines of the radius and the ulna are distinctly shown. (From A. C. Cipollardo: The earliest demonstration of a pathological lesion in America. *Radiology, 45:*557, November 1945. Courtesy of The Radiological Society of North America, Inc., Oak Brook, Illinois.)

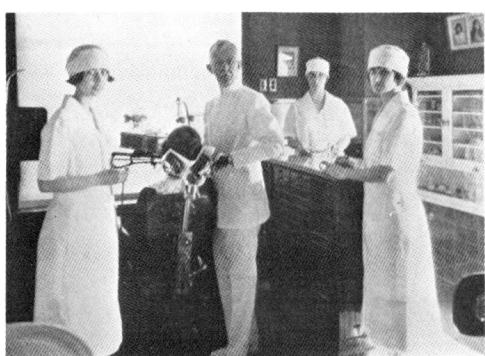

Figure 1-15. C. Edmund Kells, DDS, New Orleans, Louisiana. (From Kells, C. Edmund: *The Dentist's Own Book,* St. Louis, C. V. Mosby Co., 1925.)

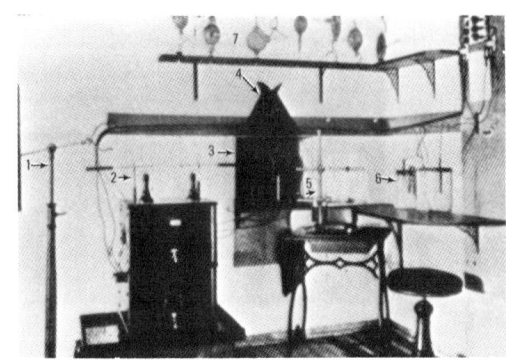

Figure 1-16. Dr. Kells x-ray laboratory, 1896: 1, the adjustable tube stand; 2, Telsa coil; 3, rheostat; 4, fluoroscope; 5, grounded aluminum shield; 6, electrolyte interrupter; 7, tube rack. (From Kells, C. Edmund: *Three Score Years and Nine.* New Orleans, C. E. Kells, Publ., 1926.)

thin aluminum plate and gutta percha, which allowed the patient to bite into occlusion thereby holding the film in place during swallowing. The patient was one of his assistants, who was seated in a chair with the film holder and film held into position with the mouth closed. The head was placed against the side of a thick fixed board positioned between the tube and the patient's face. Kells had unknowingly prevented the patient's face from receiving an erythematous (burn) dose of radiation by using this thin board. The exposure time for Kells' first radiograph was fifteen minutes. Supposedly, this radiograph was taken in April of 1896.

By July 1896, Kells felt experienced enough in the use of the x-ray to bring his equipment to the twenty-seventh annual meeting of the Southern Dental Association in Asheville, North Carolina. The demonstration clinic he presented was acknowledged to be the first clinic on the use of x-rays in dentistry held in this country.

He brought with him his Telsa coil, tubes, fluoroscope, film, and developing solutions. Kells even brought his own patient with him with a previously prepared film holder to demonstrate taking a radiograph, as he would not have time to make a custom-made film holder for a new patient at the meeting. At the Battery Park Hotel, where the meeting was held, Kells also improvised a dark room in which he would develop the films he would take. All these preparations went for naught because the demonstration had to be held in the evening, the only time in which the electric current was available. A society ball was scheduled in the hotel that same evening (July 29, 1896), but when it was rumored that an x-ray machine was being demonstrated in the same hotel, those attending the ball, as well as others in the hotel, swarmed into the clinic room. Everybody wanted to see the bones in their hands, especially the women.

The fluoroscope was all they wanted to see demonstrated. The spectators did not give Kells time to take a radiograph of his patient's teeth and develop it, as the electricity was turned off at midnight.

He did, however, demonstrate to the Association members his method of taking skiagraphs ("ski," Greek word for shadow) as he called them, and presented several skiagraphs he brought with him, taken in five to fifteen minutes, showing the perfect outlines of teeth in bone of living subjects. Kells explained to the group that since these pictures were shadowgraphs it was essential that the film plate be placed as close as possible to the object and at the same time parallel to their plane surfaces to prevent distortion.

C. Edmund Kells was the first to use a diagnostic wire, which is indispensible in endodontics. According to his records it was on May 10, 1899, while he was attempting to fill a root canal of a fractured upper central incisor for a young boy. Although the end of the tooth was fully formed, the canal was quite large in diameter, which presented a problem in filling the canal to the exact end of the tooth. In those days Kells was using lead wires with zinc oxychloride or chloropercha to fill large canals. It occurred to him that if he placed a lead wire in the root canal and took a radiograph of the tooth, he would be able to determine whether the lead wire extended to the end of the root canal or not. Of course, the lead wire was quite visible on the radiograph he took and this began the universal practice of using diagnostic wires in endodontic procedures.

In 1910, Sir William Hunter, M.D., of England (Fig. 1-17) read a paper before the Faculty of Medicine of McGill University at Montreal criticizing "American dentistry" and referring to dental bridges

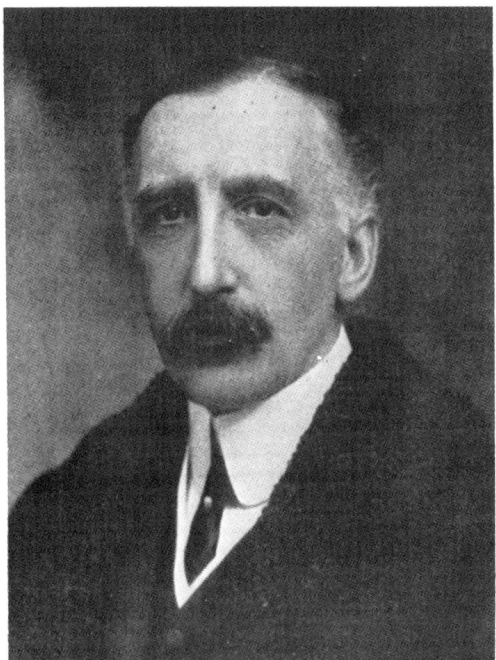

Figure 1-17. Sir Wilhelm Hunter, MD, FRCP, of England, in 1910, delivered an address entitled "The Role of Sepsis and of Antisepsis in Medicine," at McGill University, Montreal, Canada. His address almost completely demoralized and threatened to change the whole complexion of dental practice.

as "mausoleums of gold over a mass of sepsis." According to Hunter, causes of anemia, colitis, arthritis, kidney disease, and many other diseases could be traced to infection around teeth. He cited a number of case histories of patients who had been ill, some even bedridden for months and years, who had recovered entirely or had been very much improved as the result of the removal of artificial restorations and the teeth that carried them. The physicians of the United States responded almost immediately to Dr. Hunter's advice. People, young and old, had their teeth removed on prescription of their physicians. Many had their mouths wrecked and their faces disfigured without apparent improvement in their health.

It was Kells who fought against the majority of his colleagues at this time by calling for "the preservation of every tooth, whether vital or pulpless, just as long as it can be made to function properly and was not a menace to the patient's health." While dentists across the country (even of the famed Mayo Clinic) were routinely extracting good pulpless teeth, Kells advocated the treatment of abscessed teeth with root canal fillings, followed by periodic monitoring of these treatments with radiographs. Needless to say, time proved Kells was right. Nowadays, the dentist with the aid of the radiograph can determine which teeth must be removed and which teeth may be left in the mouth with safety.

During the first ten years after the discovery of x-rays, dependence was placed upon the larger Rukmkorff or Telsa coils and the larger static machines to produce the great volume of high tension current to produce x-rays. Later, the static machines were discarded because the atmospheric conditions caused much trouble with them (Fig. 1-18).

The x-ray tubes used by Hittorf, Crookes, Lenard, and Roentgen were of the fixed or stationary type, meaning that the vacuum could not be altered during the life of the tube. Also, Kells and other pioneers used these "fixed or incomplete vacuum" tubes. Actually, the air left in the tube provided a source of electrons at the cathode, which were then directed by a high voltage current against the anode or sides of the glass to produce x-rays. The vacuums in these early manufactured tubes were quite variable, which affected the quality of the x-ray beam produced.

Therefore, each tube had to be tested first for its penetrating qualities before it could be used on a patient. A low vacuum tube (low penetrating) would produce a

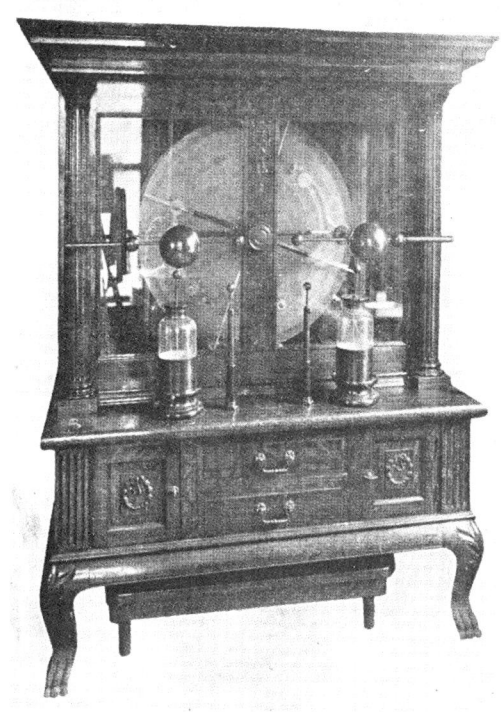

Figure 1-18. Static Machine. (From Raper, Howard: *Elementary and Dental Radiography.* London, Claudius Ash, Sons & Co., Ltd., 1913.)

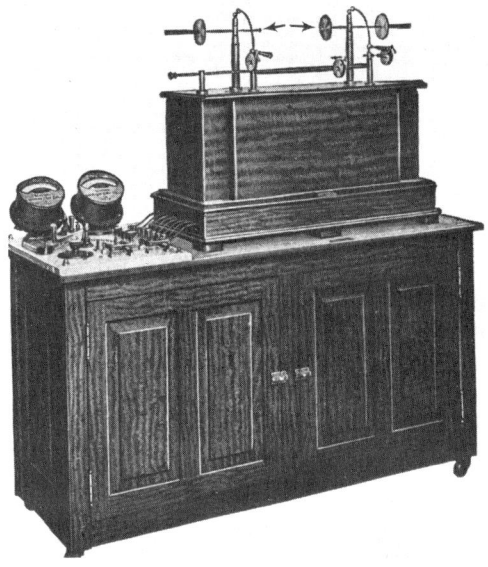

Figure 1-19. Ruhmkorff Coil. Voltage was estimated by the length of the point to point parallel spark-gap of the coil (see arrows). (From Raper, Howard: *Elementary and Dental Radiography,* London, Claudius Ash, Sons & Co., Ltd. 1913.)

dark blue area extending from the cathode to anode. A higher vacuum tube (more penetrating rays) would produce the characteristic **yellow or apple green color.**

In those days there were no voltmeters or milliampere meters. The voltage was estimated by the length of the point-to-point spark-gap of the coil (Fig. 1-19).

Coils were rated and designed according to the maximum number of inches of atmosphere the secondary current was made to jump. When the current jumped from one terminal to the other of the secondary winding, a spark occurred, due to the resistance of the atmosphere to the flow of current. The voltage was estimated by the number of inches required to jump one inch of atmosphere (approximately 1 inch equalled 10,000 volts); therefore, a six-inch coil in full operation would supply a current with a potential of 60,000 volts.

The milliamperage of the secondary current of the induction coil varied according to the resistance through which the current was forced. The milliamperage could be increased or decreased by lengthening or shortening the spark gap. By shortening the length of the spark gap, the operator could increase the milliamperage. The milliamperage strength was roughly estimated by the appearance of the spark: a thin blue spark indicated low amperage; a fat, fuzzy spark indicated high milliamperage. A coil that could give at least six inches of fat, fuzzy spark was imperative in dental radiographic work. The patients probably thought they were in Frankenstein's laboratory. One of Kells' dental assistants said she would hold a large palmetto fan over the patient's head so they couldn't see the bright colored light from the tube or the coil. Also, the operator had to be extremely careful to keep the tubes and their attached wires at least twelve to fourteen inches away from the patient.

If by chance the patient got his head or hand too close to the tube or wires (6-7 inches) during the exposure, the whole current output of the machine could jump the wire to the patient. The patient then would receive a severe shock. Although it usually was not a fatal shock, it would be a stunning shock (Fig. 1-20).

Early pioneers in dental radiography suspended the X-Ray tube stand from the ceiling or from between two clamps, one on either side of the bulb. The tube stands had limited mobility but Dr. William R. Rollins of Massachusetts, in 1896, probably invented the first X-Ray arm and bracket specifically for use in the dental office. Later Dr. Kells of New Orleans and Dr. Blum of New York invented adjustable tube holders for dental use (Fig. 1-21).

Unfortunately, the early methods of observing the appearance of the discharging tube and spark-gap were not reliable in the determination of the penetrating qualities of the beam.

Since Edison had invented his fluoroscope only a few month after Roentgen's discovery, it was only natural for the early pioneers to use it determining the quality and quantity of the beam. The accepted method for "setting the tube" as they called it was to take the fluoroscope in their right hand and place the left hand in front of it between the tube and the fluoroscope (Fig. 1-22). The X-Ray machine was started, the rheostat was adjusted until the bones in the hands showed clearly. Then, the patient was positioned

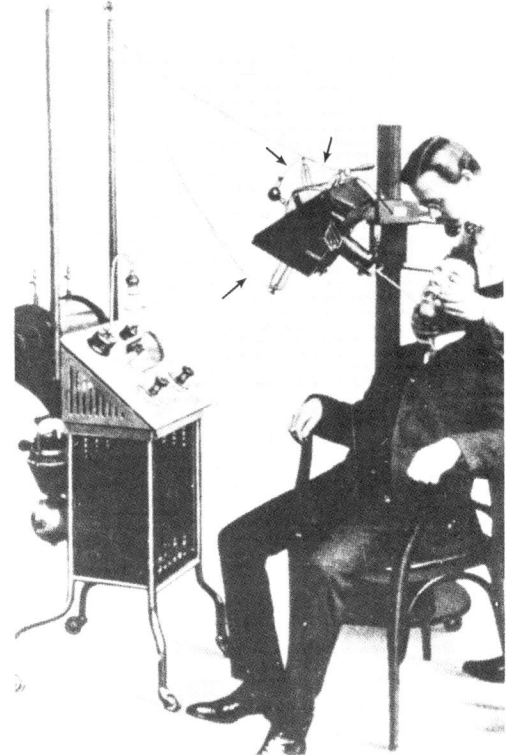

Figure 1-20. A dental X-Ray unit called "The Record." Manufactured by Reiniger-Gebbert and Schall of Germany (later Siemens Corp.) in 1905 and probably was the first commercially manufactured dental X-Ray unit in the world. Notice how close the exposed high-voltage wires are to the patient's head (see arrows). (From Glenner, Richard A.: 80 years of dental radiography, *JADA,* 90:554, March 1975. Copyright by the American Dental Association. Reprinted by permission.)

and the radiograph was taken. This procedure of "setting the tube" was the cause of early deaths of many of the early radiologists.

In due time, Dr. Kells was to pay the penalty for his pioneering work in the unknown world of X-Rays. Ceaselessly he worked to perfect his new technique of X-Ray diagnosis. "I was like a hound dog on the trail of a rabbit," he used to chuckle of

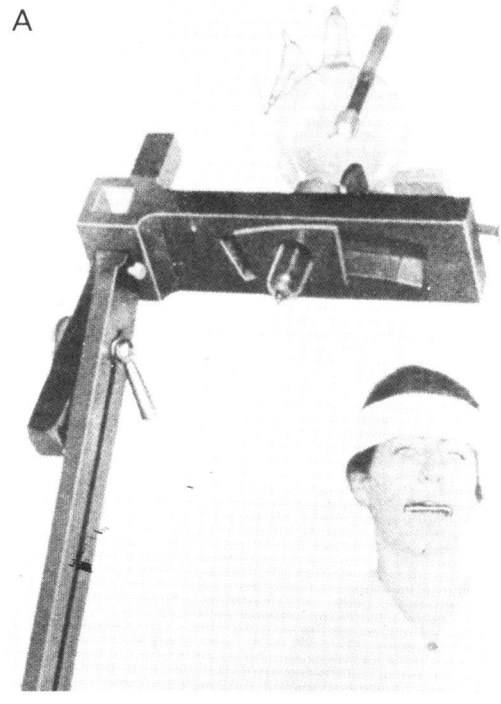

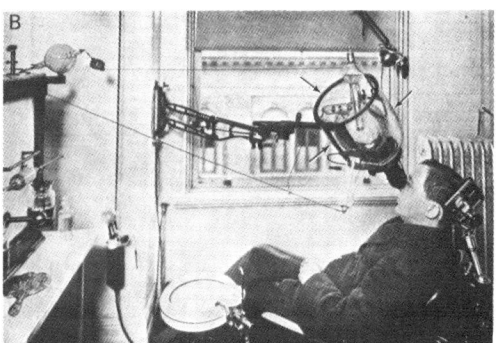

Figure 1-21. (A) this was the X-Ray tube stand used by C. Edmund Kells of New Orleans. In this photograph, the tube has been positioned superiorly to show patient's face and bandage that binds the head to the headrest. The long exposures required immobility of the head. (From C. Edmund Kells: Steroscopic Roentgenology., Stereographs. *Dental Items of Interest, 41*:128, February 1919). (B) Dr. Blum of New York prior to 1913 was using a wall bracket fixture as shown here to support a water-cooled type tube fitting into a lead glass shield (see arrows). (From Raper, Howard R: *Elementary and Dental Radiography.* Consolidated Dental Mfg. Co., New York, 1913, page 62.)

his experiments. Time and time again every day for years his hands were exposed to the X-Rays. He was extremely fascinated by his X-Ray work and took scores of pictures of rats, mice, fish, eels, crabs, and other creatures. Also, since he obtained better results in the early days than any of the other radiologists in New Orleans, he was called upon to take most of the body radiographs for the local surgeons.

On April 10, 1896, three months after Roentgen's announcement of his discovery, J. Daniel of Vanderbilt University reported the loss of hair from the head of a colleague where his skull had been photographed with the X-Rays. On July 22 of the same year, W. Marcuse in Berlin published the first microscopic study of the effect of radiation on tissues. It was a report of a seventeen-year-old male with severe skin reactions including epilation following prolonged and frequent exposures to roentgen rays for public demon-

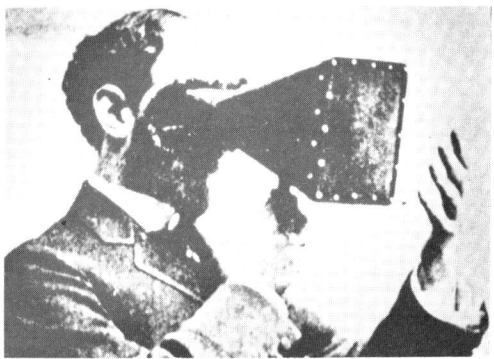

Figure 1-22. Using the fluoroscope to "set the tube." This procedure was the primary factor leading to the death of many of the early radiologists. (From Grigg, E.R.N.: *The Trail of Invisible Light*, 1965, p. 15. Courtesy of Charles C Thomas, Publisher, Springfield, Illinois.)

strations. A bare glass tube was used in the early days with no protection to either the patient or the operator. The volume of the current was very small, so that one heard of exposures of three hours to make a picture of the hip joint or kidney. As a result, there were many serious injuries because the heating of the tube softened the rays and most of them were absorbed in the soft tissues of the patient.

In 1904, Bergonie and Tribondeau of France gave a complete histologic picture of the changes produced by radiation in the rat's testicle, showing the focus of the attack to be on the embryonic structures. They then formulated the law, known by their names, which is the basis of our knowledge of the effect of rays upon all cells and tissues:

> "Immature cells and cells in an active stage of division are more sensitive to radiation than are cells which have already acquired their adult and morphological and physiologic characters."

Early in the history of roentgenology these injurious effects (dermatitis, alopecia, and eye pain) were thought by some, including Telsa, the great American scientist, to be electrical, and he recommended the use of a grounded aluminum screen placed between the tube and the patient to prevent such injuries. Although these screens did not carry away any electrical current in the air, they probably saved many patients from serious injury by filtering out the soft X-Rays in the X-Ray beam.

Ten years after he began experimenting with X-Rays (1906), Kells noticed some keratosis (callus-like) on his hands; they looked a little different than normal but that was all. Two years later (1908), an ulcer about the size of a dime appeared on the back of his left hand. This was cut out and the ulcer healed. During the next fourteen years (1908-1922) ten to twelve ulcers (ulcerative dermatosis) appeared from time to time, but then several epidermoid carcinomas began to grow without any break in the skin. Most of them yielded to simple surgery or radium treatments, with the exception of one on a finger. Surgery and grafts all failed, and the finger was sacrificed to save the cancer from spreading. Presently other lesions appeared on the left hand and would not heal.

Dr. Kells went to Johns Hopkins Hospital in Baltimore about thirty times for finger amputations, skin grafts, and removal of his left axillary lymph nodes. He kept on practicing dentistry and invented dental instruments with attachments so he could use them with what was left of his fingers and the thumb of his left hand. Finally, the surgeons at Johns Hopkins told him that they must take off his left arm to save his life. Dr. Kells' face whitened. "A one-armed dentist!" However, it was too late to stop the progress of the results of the previous X-Ray exposures. In 1926, the surgeons at Johns Hopkins removed his left arm just below the shoulder.

Through it all, he worked as no other man has worked. He completed countless inventions and patented more than thirty of them. One of his inventions was a suction apparatus for the aspiration of fluids and the irrigation of cavities in the human body during surgical operations. This replaced the old technique of mopping the surface with surgical sponges.

Dr. Kells was a true soldier of science, and he looked the part. He was a small man, never weighed more than 100 pounds, but he had a slim, erect, military figure, white hair, sandy moustache, and keen blue eyes. His empty left sleeve represented as much a decoration of valor as any medal bestowed on the field of battle

Introduction and History of Dental Radiology

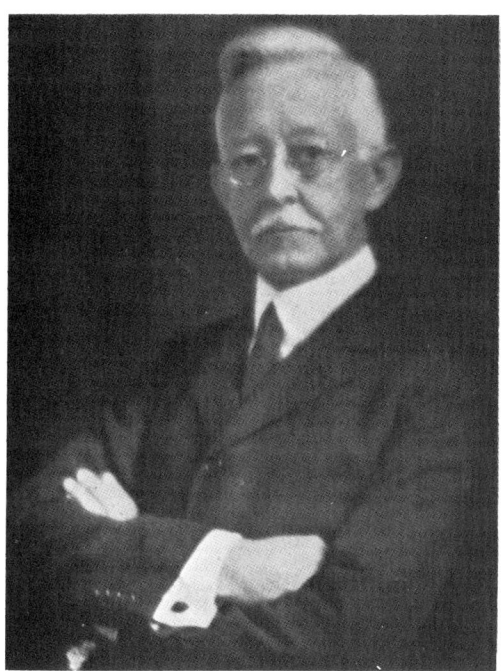

Figure 1-23. C. Edmund Kells, New Orleans (1865-1928). (From Kells, C. Edmund: *The Dentist's Own Book*, St. Louis, C.V. Mosby Co., 1925.)

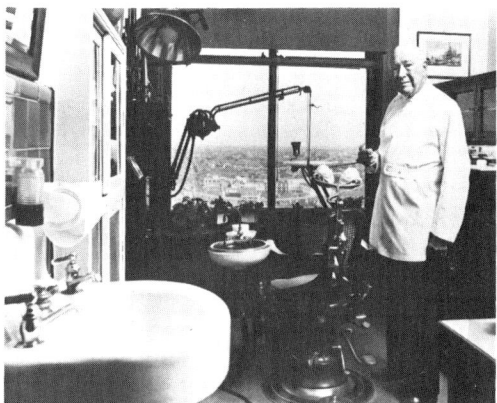

Figure 1-24. Dr. Major Brooks Varnado (1882-1971), associate of Dr. Kells from 1918 to 1928. He practiced in this office, suite 1237 of the Masson Blanche Building in New Orleans, for fifty-three years.

(Fig. 1-23). By 1926 his right hand had become affected with epidermoid carcinomas, and the skin grafts and the finger amputations began all over again. Finally the heart and lungs became affected. This was the end, and he knew it. He had had forty-two operations in all. The intensity of the pain during this period made it difficult for him to think coherently. He refused to take narcotics, according to Dr. Major Brooks Varnado, who became a partner of Kells in 1918 (Fig. 1-24). His eyesight was failing him.

He finished the manuscript of his third book "Conservation of Natural Teeth," which was never published, on almost the same day he died. He dreaded, more than most men, the prospect of being a helpless burden on those he loved. Always a conqueror, Eddie Kells (as his friends called him) could not endure such a humiliating defeat. He was seventy-two years old. On Monday afternoon, May 7, 1928, at 2 PM in his office, proud of spirit, he became the master of his own destiny and placed a bullet in the brain that had done so much to help suffering humanity through the application of electricity and X-Rays.

Those who knew Dr. Eddie Kells intimately never considered his act of suicide an act of cowardice. For twenty years he had suffered pain such as few humans ever knew, and without a whimper. Few people, knowing the truth, can find it in their hearts to say that his last act on earth represented anything but the highest courage and the deepest consideration for others, especially his family.

W.H. Rollins

William Herbert Rollins, D.D.S., M.D., is called by many "dentistry's

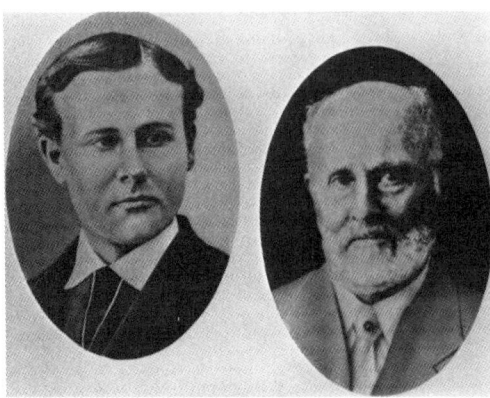

Figure 1-25. William Herbert Rollins, DDS, MD (1852-1929). Rollins as a young man on left and on the right as an older man. (From Sweet, Porter S.: William Herbert Rollins, DDS, MD, Dentistry's Forgotten Man. *Dent Radiogr Photogr,* 33(1):3, 1960. Courtesy of Eastman Kodak Company, Rochester, N.Y. Reprinted by permission.)

forgotten man" because, although he did so much for dentistry, he was such a shy moderate man, and exceedingly retiring by nature, that few people knew of his accomplishments (Fig. 1-25). Rollins may have been the first person to make a dental radiograph on a live patient in the Western hemisphere. He invented, made, used, and published a description of an intraoral cassette and an oral fluoroscope by July, 1896, less than seven months after the first American announcement of the discovery of X-Rays. Also, during 1896, he invented an X-Ray tube arm and bracket for use in the dental office, which was undoubtedly the first of its kind. Probably William H. Rollins' greatest contribution to science passed unnoticed. Early X-Ray workers like Rollins observed that burns occurred when the X-Ray tube was discharged. At that time Rollins believed, as did others, that their burns were caused by electricity coming from the excited X-Ray tube, but he decided to investigate.

As early as February 14, 1901, he made an announcement that, had it been acted upon, could have saved some of the early X-Ray workers' lives. His research findings were based on the use of guinea pigs that were exposed to "X Light" (name he gave to X-Rays).

He published a simple letter to the editor of a Boston medical journal entitled "X Light Kills." This letter fell on deaf ears. He kept up his research and persistently warned physicians and dentists of the dangers involved in using X-Rays. He was one of the first persons to use a protective screen and an adjustable diaphragm to prevent unnecessary radiation to the patient.

By 1914 the dental profession became well aware of the dangers of X-radiation and started doing something about it, but by then nobody remembered what had been said by a shy unknown dentist in Boston in 1901. His research and subsequent protective measures did some good as it prolonged his own life and that of his brother-in-law, F.H. Williams, M.D. Dr. Rollins died in 1929 at age 77. Dr. Williams lived to be 84 years old.

Other Pioneers

Two other dental X-Ray pioneers should be mentioned: Frank Van Woert, of New York City, and Weston A. Price, of Cleveland, Ohio. Dr. Van Woert gave a practical demonstration of radiography before the New York Odontological Society in 1897 (Fig. 1-26). He was one of the first to appreciate the advantage of film over photographic glass plates and to use film in intraoral radiography.

Early dental radiographers used ordinary photographic glass plates. To adapt them for the intraoral radiography, they were cut into small pieces in the darkroom and doubly wrapped in black paper and rubber dam material for pro-

daylight processing of dental X-Ray film.

Dr. Weston A. Price of Cleveland, Ohio, was one of the early pioneers in dental radiography. He advocated the use of a thick celluloid type film cut to size for the mouth, enclosed in an unvulcanized black rubber covering for intraoral radiography, as early as May, 1899. He was one of the first to write on the subject of dental radiographic interpretation; this was in August, 1900. In 1904, Weston Price first proposed an X-Ray projection technique based on the age-old "rule of isometry," later called the "bisection of the angle" technique.

The Development of the Dental X-Ray Machine

At the turn of the century X-Ray pictures were still taken with very long exposure times (1-5 minutes for a single exposure). Why were such long exposure times necessary? There were three reasons: (1) direct current was the only available source of power (AC power was not yet in universal use); (2) the gas tubes had poor efficiency; and (3) the film used had extreme lack of emulsion sensitivity.

A transformer cannot transform low-voltage current into high-voltage current from a direct current source. To overcome this obstacle, the early X-Ray pioneers used mechanical or electolytic interrupters to change direct current into alternating current. The problem with these interrupters was that they had limited current capacity, which made for long X-Ray exposures. Also, they were unpredictable.

X-Rays were produced in the gas tube used by Roentgen (see Fig. 1-5) by the bombardment of the glass by electrons produced by ionizations of the residual gas in the tube. Later, a target of metal was inserted into the tube to replace the

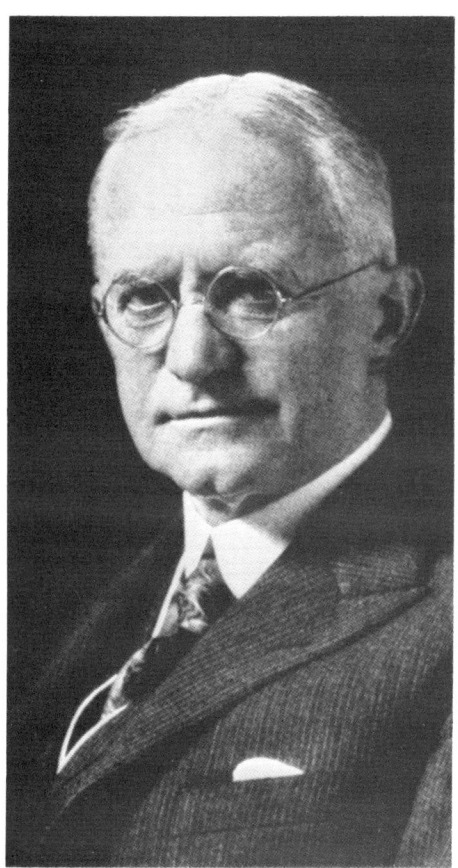

Figure 1-26. Dr. Frank Van Woert of New York City. One of the first to appreciate the advantage of the use of film rather than photographic glass plates in intraoral radiography. (From Sweet, Porter S.: Frank Van Woert. *Dent Radiogr Photogr,* 21(1):1, 1948. Courtesy of Eastman Kodak Company. Rochester, N.Y. Reprinted by permission.)

tection against white light and moisture. Van Woert was one of the first to use Kodak® roll film cut into small pieces for intraoral radiography. He held the film in place using impression compound similar to the way Kells did. Other contributions included a metal film holder, an improved angulator for bisecting technique, an automatic time switch, and a tank for

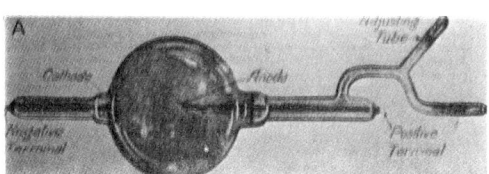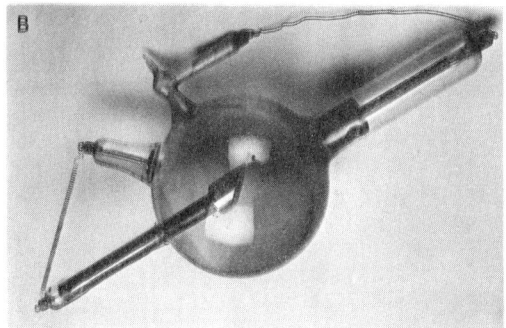

Figure 1-27. (A) & (B) These are later model GE low-vacuum tubes with vacuum regulators attached. The early types of X-Ray tubes all contained gases and were extremely temperamental. The tubes demanded a continued effort on the part of the operator to maintain the proper vacuum. (From Glenner, Richard A.: 80 years of dental radiography. *JADA, 90:*557, March 1975.) Copyright by the American Dental Association. Reprinted by permission.

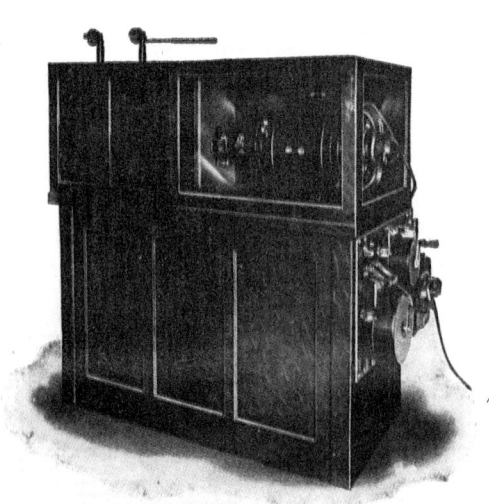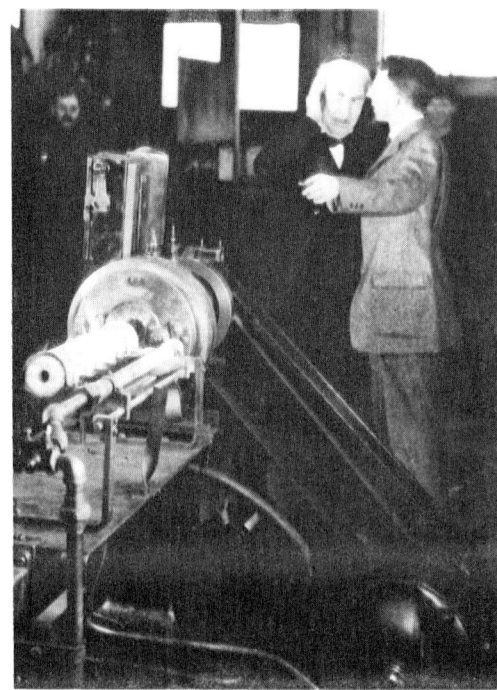

Figure 1-28. *Interrupterless coil* (transformer) X-Ray machine consisted of a *rotary converter* in the DC machine, or *synchronous motor* in the AC machine, a step-up transformer, and a rectifier switch. It could be operated on DC or AC current. (From Raper, Howard R.: *Elementary and Dental Radiography.* New York, Consolidated Dental Mfg. Co., 1913, page 18.)

Figure 1-29. During a visit by Thomas A. Edison (age 67 at the time) to the GE Research Laboratory in Schenectady, New York, in 1914, Dr. William D. Coolidge (age 41), assistant director, explains how tungsten is made ductile by means of the apparatus in the foreground. Edison, partly deaf, cups hand over ear to aid in hearing. (Courtesy of General Electric Research and Development Center, Schenectady, NY.)

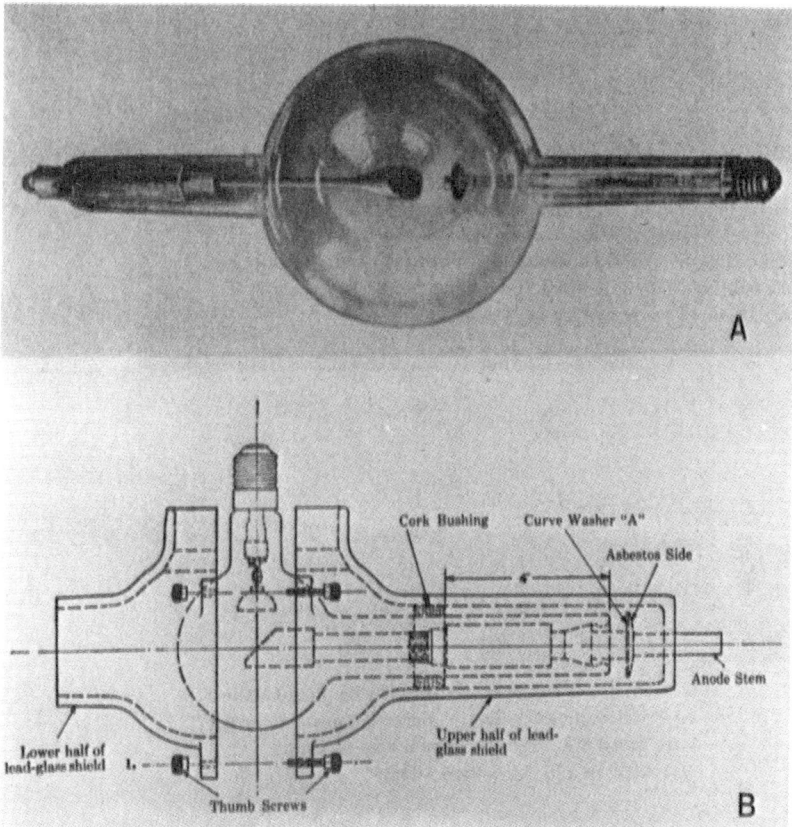

Figure 1-30. (A) This is the hot-cathode high vacuum tube developed by William D. Coolidge in 1913. It had a stable reproducible output and independent control of radiation quality and quantity. (B) This tube was designed especially for dental application in early 1920's by G.E. (From Glenner, Richard A.: 80 years of dental radiography. *JADA*, 90:557, March 1975. Copyright by the American Dental Association. Reprinted by permission.)

glass as an area of electron bombardment (Fig. 1-27). Focusing structures within the tube served to focus the electrons on the target. The real obstacle to duplication of results was the variability of the vacuum within the tube. Under continued use, the vacuum changed and hence the number of electrons available to produce X-Rays. Early X-Ray workers had a whole series of gas tubes to "fit" the occasion. All sorts of pressure regulators were devised to regulate the vacuum in the tube. This variability of the vacuum tube made for long exposure times.

This was the state of affairs when Clyde Snook became interested in X-Rays in 1903. Alternating current was just becoming available in some cities and even where direct current was in use, AC current could be produced by means of a converter. Two years later, in 1905, Snook produced a combination of the closed-core AC transformer with a motor-driven centrifugal switch or rectifier. It did away with the unpredictable interrupter, and in the radiologist's eyes this was a giant step

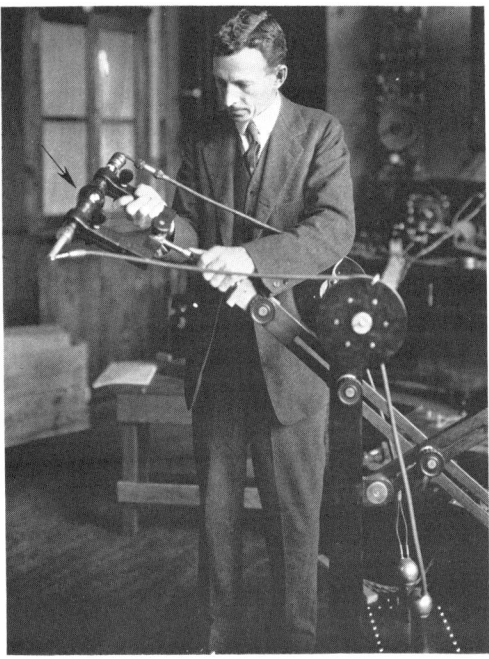

Figure 1-31. William Coolidge, age 46, in 1919, working on an early portable X-Ray tube and machine he designed for the U.S. Army in World War I. (Courtesy of General Electric Research and Development Center, Schenectady, N.Y.)

forward. Instead of calling it the straightforward name "mechanical rectifier," they hailed the machine as the "interrupterless coil" (Fig. 1-28).

This machine solved the problem of the high voltage source needed in the production of X-Rays, but the gas tube still needed much improvement. About this time, in 1907, Dr. W.D. Coolidge of General Electric Research Laboratory in Schenectady, New York, produced the first ductile (plastic) tungsten. By mechanically hot-working bulk tungsten, he was able to draw the metal into fine wires as strong as steel, thin enough to be used as lamp filaments, even down to one-sixth the diameter of human hair (Fig. 1-29).

After the ductile tungsten process had been developed sufficiently for the needs of the incandescent lamp manufacture in 1911, Coolidge turned his research efforts towards the invention of a new type of X-Ray tube.

After Dr. Irving Langmuir, a Nobel laureate working at General Electric, found that electron emission not only persisted in a high vacuum but favored it by getting rid of the last traces of gas, Coolidge developed an X-Ray tube with the highest attainable vacuum in 1913. He replaced the cold aluminum cathode of the old gas tube with a hot tungsten filament that supplied the electrons and substituted ductile tungsten for the platinum anode targets previously used in the old cathode tubes. Also, by vacuum casting copper around a ductile tungsten disc, he increased the target's (1) heat conductivity to absorb more heat energy (copper) and (2) capability to produce more X-Rays (tungsten) (Fig. 1-30).

The output of the hot cathode or Coolidge tube could be predetermined and accurately controlled. The Coolidge tube was patented in 1916 and quickly superceded previous gas models, becoming the prototype of all modern X-Ray tubes used in medicine and dentistry.

World War I presented new X-Ray challenges. A portable X-Ray unit was needed near the front in France, and Coolidge was given the task of developing an X-Ray generator (transformer) for the equipment. By developing a self-rectifying tube, one which allows the current to pass through it in only one direction from the filament (cathode) to the target (anode), he made obsolete the commonly used "interrupterless coil" or mechanical rectifier, which was bulky and noisy (Fig. 1-31).

There were cooling problems with these early hot-cathode tubes. Heat was dissipated from the tungsten target via the

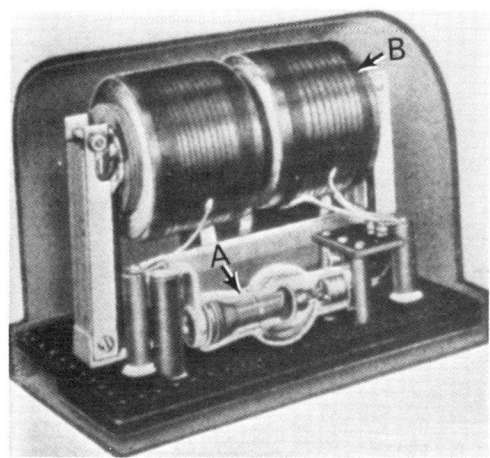

Figure 1-32. This is an interior view of the first "shockproof" X-Ray tubehead, which was patented by Coolidge in 1919. A small Coolidge tube (A) and the transformers (B) immersed in oil (From Glenner, Richard A.: 80 years of dental radiography, *JADA, 90*:March, 1975. Copyright by the American Dental Association. Reprinted by permission.)

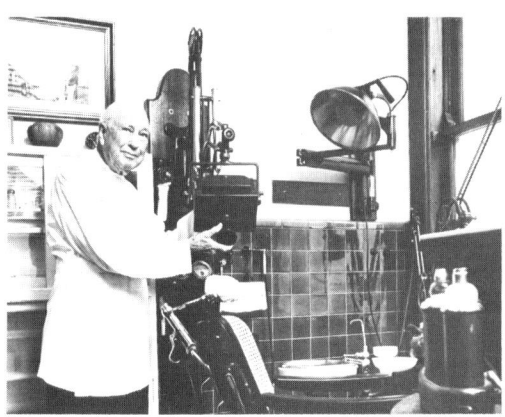

Figure 1-33. Dr. Major Brooks Varnado, a former associate of Dr. C. Edmund Kells, holds a tube head of one of the original Victor CDX wall-mounted models (circa 1923), which was still in use when this photograph was taken in 1971. Dr. Varnardo was 89 years of age at the time.

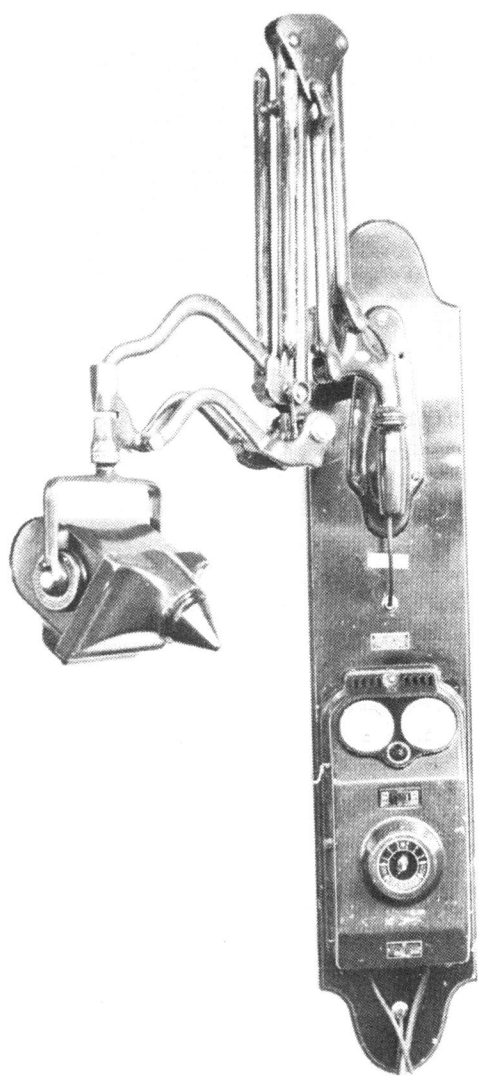

Figure 1-34. In 1933, ten years after the original Victor CDX was introduced to the dental profession, General Electric introduced a new CDX, model E, which included many new features (From Glenner, Richard A.: 80 years of dental radiography. *JADA, 90*:559, March 1975. copyright by the American Dental Association. Reprinted by permission.)

copper metal to either air or water cooling devices, which were far from satisfactory.

In 1919 William Coolidge modified his portable army unit for peacetime purposes. He achieved maximum portability, safety, and convenience by designing a small, self-rectifying tube that, with its 63,000 volt supply transformer, was enclosed in an oil-filled metal case. The oil served as an electrical insulation for the tube and transformer and also aided in cooling the tube. This was the first shockproof X-Ray unit (Fig. 1-32).

The Victor X-Ray Company of Chicago was the first to introduce (1923) a dental X-Ray machine with this Coolidge shockproof tube head principle of immersing the transformer and hot-cathode tube in a metal container. They called this X-Ray unit the CDX, which became a workhorse for the dental profession for many years. The new principle permitted the use of much smaller high voltage transformers and the use of an "autotransformer," which replaced the old rheostat. The Victor X-Ray company in a few years became a subsidiary of the General Electric Corporation (Fig. 1-33).

In 1933, ten years after the original Victor CDX X-Ray machine was introduced, General Electric introduced a new CDX, Model E, which retained the oil-immersed Coolidge tube and transformers but included several new features (Fig. 1-34). The Ritter Corporation manufactured an open-tube machine with a Coolidge tube until 1930. These X-Ray machines were not shockproof and the dentist or patient received an occasional shock from them if they got too close to the high tension wires (Fig. 1-35).

Coolidge's name became inseparably linked with the hot-cathode tube that he invented. His "Coolidge tube" unveiled in 1913 completely revolutionized the generation of X-Rays and remains to this day the model upon which all X-Ray tubes for medical and dental X-Ray machines are patterned. Dr. William D. Coolidge retired as director of General Electric Research in 1944 at the age of 71. He died February 4, 1975 at the age of 101 (Fig. 1-36).

Dental X-Ray machine design changed little until General Electric introduced a variable kilovoltage machine in 1957; in 1966, XRM (now SS WHITE) introduced a recessed long-beam tube head, an invention of A.G. Richards of University of Michigan. Dental X-Ray machines currently exist that employ constant po-

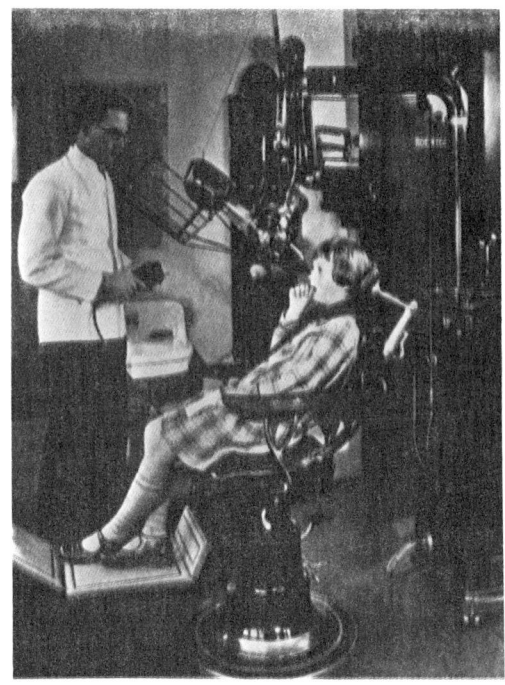

Figure 1-35. Ritter open-tube dental X-Ray machine, with cage surrounding the tube to protect patient and operator from high tension wires. (From Pammenter, Elmer J.: Value of X-Ray and photographic work in children's dentistry. *Dent Radiogr Photogr*, 2(3):May 15, 1929. Copyright Eastman Kodak Co., Rochester, NY. Reprinted by permission.)

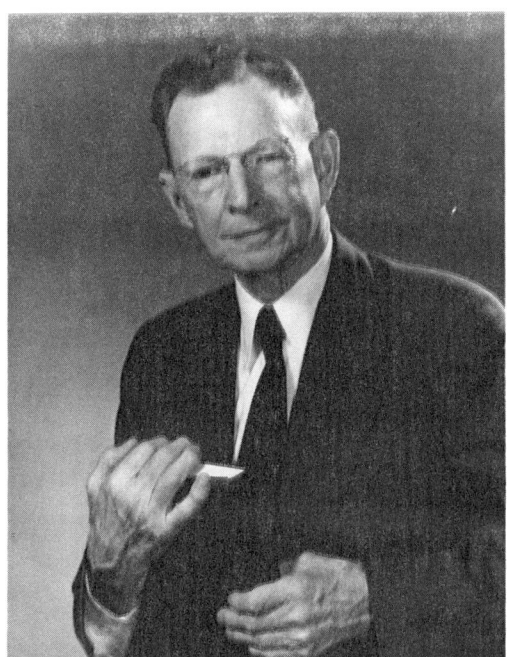

Figure 1-36. William D. Coolidge (1874-1975). Photograph was taken in 1954 when he was 81, ten years after he had retired as director of General Electric Research and Development Center in 1944. He died at the age of 101 in 1975. (Courtesy of General Electric Research and Development, Schenectady, N.Y.)

tential across the X-Ray tube. The combined effects of constant potential and an increased thickness of aluminum filtration or rare-earth filtration make possible the production of radiographs with lower radiation doses without a significant reduction in radiographic information.

History of Dental X-Ray Film

Between 1896 and 1913 the first X-Ray packets consisted of photographic emulsion glass plates or Kodak roll film cut into small pieces and wrapped by the radiographer in black paper and rubber dam.

In 1913 the first hand-wrapped dental X-Ray film packets made by Eastman became commercially available. They were cellulose nitrate base films with single emulsions and were highly flammable because of the combination of nitrate and cellulose.

The next improvement in films was what was known as *dupli-tized* film, which was produced in 1918. It could be purchased in five by seven inch sizes, as well as larger sizes. Some dentists cut these films to dental size and hand-wrapped them. These films had emulsions on both sides of the base for greater speed and contrast.

In 1920 the first machine-made periapical film packet was made. This marked the first step in the production of a film packet that would not cause the patient discomfort.

In 1924, Dr. Howard R. Raper of Albuquerque, New Mexico, in collaboration with the Eastman Kodak Company, designed and introduced the "Bite-Wing" film packet for the purpose of detecting caries in the interproximal surfaces of the teeth. The procedure is still widely used today. Dr. Raper was a 1906 graduate of Indiana University and served on their faculty until 1917. He is credited with being the first person to introduce dental roentgenology into the dental school curriculum in 1910 at Indiana University. It was his constant pressure on the *Institute of Dental Pedogogies* that finally resulted in the teaching of dental radiology in every dental school in America today. Also, Raper wrote the first book on dental roentgenology in 1913 (Fig. 1-37).

In 1925 dental films with a safety (cellulose acetate) base were introduced. The cellulose acetate base was safer because the acetate was slow-burning.

In 1929, the all-white film packets were introduced; and in 1930 small periapical films for children and adults with narrow arches were developed. The earlier dental films had the emulsion coat on

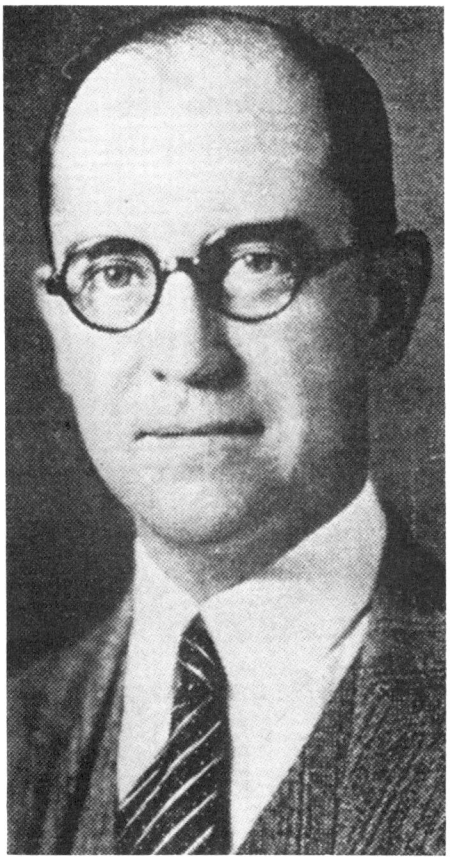

Figure 1-37. Dr. Howard Riley Raper (1887-1978). He was the first to introduce dental radiology in the dental school curriculum; first to write a textbook on the subject; and inventor of the bite wing radiograph.

one side only. It was placed in the mouth with the emulsion side toward the region being radiographed, and it was read from the shiny or noncoated side.

The one-sided emulsion films were slow-speed films and were superseded by the faster double-coated emulsion films.

The present day Kodak Ultra-Speed and Ekta-Speed films have emulsions on both sides of the base and have very sensitive film emulsions. They are a great improvement over the slower speed films of the past. The exposure time can be greatly decreased, which in turn reduces radiation exposure to both the operator and the patient.

History of Intraoral Radiographic Technics

Radiographers discovered early that X-Rays were very similar to light rays in the production of images on film. Since both types of rays were divergent rather than parallel to each other, inherent distortions resulted in images produced by them. To minimize these distortions in intraoral radiography, two different projection technics emerged. One was called the "bisection-of-the-angle" technic, the other the "paralleling or right angle" technic.

Although it is difficult to determine who first devised the bisection-of-the-angle projection technic, it was probably Weston Price of Cleveland, Ohio, in 1904. The technic is based on the geometric "rule of isometry," which states that "if two triangles have two equal angles and a common side, the two triangles are equal." Price reasoned that if the radiologist projected the central ray of the X-Ray beam perpendicular to a line bisecting the angle formed by the mean plane of the tooth and the film, the resultant image of the tooth projected onto the film would not be distorted.

The "bisection of angle" technic has been the technic of choice by the dental profession for many years. The paralleling technic is gaining in popularity now because of its advantage in producing a more diagnostic radiograph.

Dr. Raper of Indiana University (1907-1917) refined the original bisecting angle technic by the introduction of average projection angles for the different regions of the dental arches. Dr. Clarence O. Simpson, of Washington University at St. Louis, later modified these original

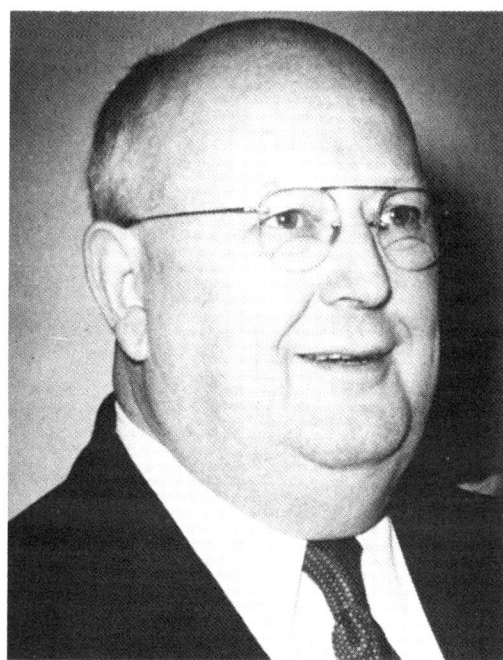

Figure 1-38. Dr. LeRoy M. Ennis (1893-1978). A pioneer in the field of dental radiology, he organized the department of oral roentgenology at Pennsylvania University in 1919 and was author of one of the most popular textbooks in the field.

Dental Association in Asheville, North Carolina, July 29, 1896. At this meeting Kells gave a clinic on his method of taking skiagraphs (shadowgraphs, as he called them) of the roots of teeth in living subjects. He explained that these X-Ray pictures were similar to shadowgraphs as produced by light rays. Therefore, it was essential for the film to be as close to the teeth as possible, and at the same time parallel to the teeth to prevent distortion.

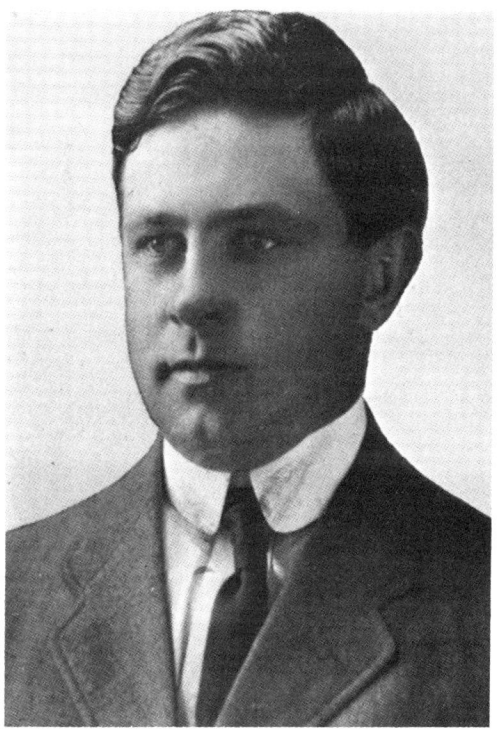

Figure 1-39. Franklin W. McCormack. First to put the paralleling principle of X-Ray projection to practical use in dental radiology.

angles proposed by Raper. Probably the greatest advocate of the "bisecting angle" technic was Dr. LeRoy M. Ennis of the University of Pennsylvania. He began teaching dental roentgenology at Pennsylvania in 1919, organized a department of oral roentgenology, and was its chairman until his retirement in 1963 (Fig. 1-38). Dr. Ennis coauthored with Robert H. Ivy one of the first dental roentgenology books, published in 1923, and in 1931 published his own textbook *Dental Roentgenology*, which became one of the most widely used texts on the subject and has gone through seven editions.

Probably the first advocate of the paralleling projection technic in intraoral radiography was C. Edmund Kells of New Orleans at a meeting of the Southern

However, it was a medical X-Ray machine salesman by the name of Franklin W. McCormack who first put the paralleling principle to practical use in dental radiography (Fig. 1-39). In 1911 he opened one of the first dental X-Ray laboratories

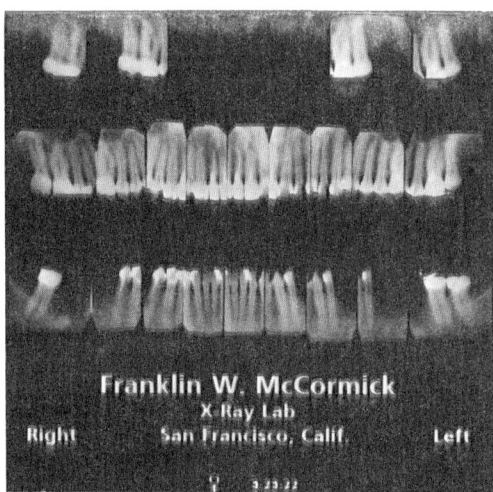

Figure 1-40. A sample of the complete periapical survey taken by the Franklin W. McCormack laboratories in San Francisco using the paralleling technique with patient in the recumbent position. Note name is spelled *McCormick* rather than correct spelling *McCormack*. (Courtesy of Dr. Gordon Fitzgerald, San Francisco, California.)

in San Francisco, California. He hand-wrapped his dental films in black paper, adding a flat metal plate to give the film rigidity, then wrapped both in waxed paper for use in the patient's mouth.

McCormack placed his patient prone on a paddled table. The patient held the wrapped film parallel to the teeth and at right angles to the X-Ray beam. The film was hand-held at first and in about 1935 he began using a hemostat and wooden bite-blocks. He utilized a Coolidge "universal" X-Ray tube and twenty-four to forty inch source-film distances. He referred to his technique as the "McCormack Long Distance Technique" and described his method in a talk before the Missouri State Dental Association at its 55th annual meeting in Kansas City, April 12, 1920. This lecture was published in the *Journal of Dental Research* in September 1920, giving him the distinct honor of becoming the first layman

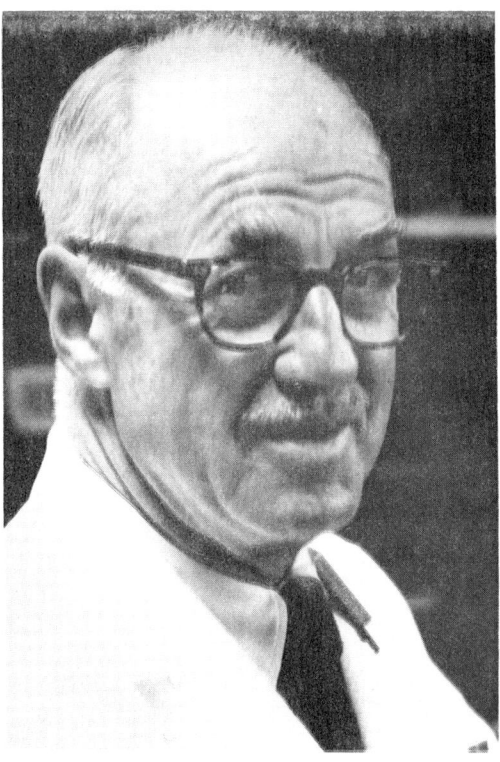

Figure 1-41. Dr. Gordon M. Fitzgerald (1907-1981), San Francisco, CA (taken May, 1969 at age of 62). One of the first to teach the paralleling X-Ray technique in a dental school. One of the founding fathers of the American Academy of Dental Radiology and the Western Roentgenology Workshop. (Courtesy of Mrs. Pat Worthington, Carlsbad, CA.)

to have his research published in a dental research journal. A sample of the type of complete mouth film survey as taken by the Franklin McCormack laboratories is shown in Figure 1-40.

Dr. Gordon Fitzgerald, son-in-law to Franklin McCormack, began as a dental technician in one of McCormack's X-Ray laboratories. In the mid-thirties he attended the dental school at the University of California at San Francisco, and upon graduation, Gordon Fitzgerald began teaching oral roentgenology at his alma mater in 1938. He converted McCor-

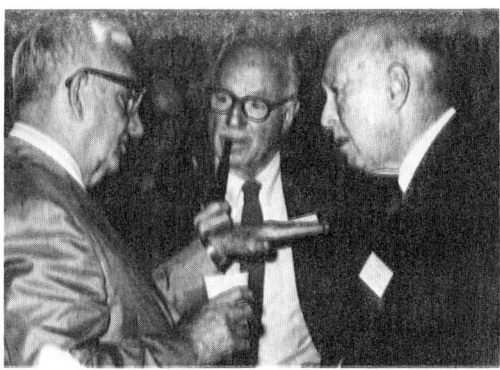

Figure 1-42. A photograph of three dental radiology pioneers taken at the Eastern Radiology Workshop at New Orleans in 1971. From left to right: Dr. Colin McHardy, former student of Dr. C. Edmund Kells and member of Louisiana State Board of Dental Examiners; Dr. Gordon Fitzgerald, former dental laboratory X-Ray technician for Franklin McCormack; and Dr. Major B. Varnado, associate of Dr. C. Edmund Kells.

mack's tabletop, long distance technic to the dental chair, so the dentist could use it in his office. After a brief tour in the Navy during World War II, he returned to teach oral roentgenology at the University of California until his retirement in 1972 (Fig. 1-41). Gordon Fitzgerald liked to teach good radiographic technic, and dentists from around the world came to learn of his paralleling technic methods. He was an excellent interpreter of dental radiographs and spent many hours of his time traveling throughout the United States teaching interpretation (Fig. 1-42).

Dr. Gordon Fitzgerald wrote four classic articles on his "long cone paralleling technique" in the *Journal of the American Dental Association* between 1947 and 1950. From this beginning, dental radiology teachers such as Dr. Donald T. Waggener of the University of Nebraska, Dr. William J. Updegrave of Temple University, and Dr. Art H. Wuehrmann of Alabama University began teaching the long cone paralleling technique in their dental schools. At present it is taught in almost all the dental schools throughout America.

Dr. Gordon M. Fitzgerald was one of the founding members of the American Academy of Oral Roentgenology (now called American Academy of Dental Radiology) in 1949, along with such persons as Henry Cline Fixott, Sr., of Portland, Oregon; Leroy M. Ennis of the University of Pennsylvania; Edward Stafne of the Mayo Clinic; and Leroy Main of St. Louis University. The first meeting of the Academy of Oral Roentgenology was held in Atlantic City, New Jersey in 1950. This book is dedicated to a past President of the American Academy of Dental Radiology (1981), Dr. Charles R. Morris of the University of Texas Dental School at San Antonio.

Within the past twenty-five years the development of a dental X-Ray machine that can take a single radiograph of the entire upper and lower jaws with one continuous exposure has become a reality. They are called panoramic X-Ray machines. The machines utilize either an intraoral or an extraoral source of radiation. The units that use an extraoral source are called rotational panoramic machines and are the most popular. Although panoramic radiography does not give the excellent definition that conventional intraoral dental radiography does, the technique is quite popular when used as an adjunct to conventional dental radiography because of its better radiographic coverage of the jaws, and the convenience of the technique. The father of panoramic radiography was Dr. Y. Paatero of Finland, who worked twenty years in the field to perfect a practical X-Ray machine to use in dental offices. He called his machine the Orthopantomograph. Colonel Donald Hudson of the United States Air

Force, working with John Kumpula of the National Bureau of Standards in Washington, D.C. in the 1950s, invented a panoramic machine now marketed as the Panorex by S.S. White (Pennwalt). Later, General Electric engineers at Milwaukee, Wisconsin, introduced to the market in the late 1960s a machine called the Panelipse, utilizing a slightly different rotational method than the others. In the 1970s several new panoramic machines were introduced to the market. Japan exports several machines that are marketed by American dental equipment manufacturers and supply companies. In Chapter 16, panoramic radiography will be discussed in further detail.

Photographs of some of the various modern dental X-Ray machines are shown in Figure 1-43.

The Development of Dental Radiology

The development of dental radiology to its present important position in dentistry may be attributed to the research and investigation by hundreds of dental researchers, practitioners, and teachers.

The dental profession owes a lasting debt to these pioneers who by their accomplishments distinguished themselves as benefactors of the dental profession. The following is a partial list of the outstanding members of the dental profession and allied professions who have shared in the establishment of dental radiology as an indispensable branch of dental science.

Dr. Holly Broadbent – Western Reserve University
Dr. William D. Coolidge – Schenectady, New York
Dr. LeRoy M. Ennis – University of Pennsylvania
Dr. Gordon M. Fitzgerald – University of California
Dr. Henry Cline Fixott, Sr. – Portland, Oregon
Dr. Donald C. Hudson – San Antonio, Texas
Dr. C. Edmund Kells – New Orleans, Louisiana
John W. Kumpula – Nashwauk, Minnesota
Dr. Leroy Main – St. Louis University
Dr. John McCall – New York University
Franklin W. McCormack – San Francisco, California
Dr. James McCoy – University of Southern California
Dr. W. James Morton – New York City
Dr. Robert T. Nelsen – Washington, D.C.
Dr. H. Numata – Tokyo, Japan
Dr. R. Ottolenqui – Buffalo, New York
Dr. Yrjo V. Paatero – Turku, Finland
Dr. Weston A. Price – Cleveland, Ohio
Dr. Guy Poyton – Toronto, Canada
Dr. Howard Raper – Indiana University and Albuquerque, N.M.
Prof. Albert G. Richards – Michigan University
Dr. William Rollins – Boston, Massachusetts
Dr. F.L. Satterlee – New York City
Dr. Clarence O. Simpson – Washington University at St. Louis
Dr. Edward Stafne – Mayo Clinic, Rochester, Minnesota
Dr. A. Porter Sweet – Rochester, New York
Dr. Kurt Thoma – Boston, Massachusetts
Dr. Walter Thompson – University of Southern California
Dr. William J. Updegrave – Temple University
Dr. Frank V. Van Woert – New York City
Dr. Donald T. Waggener – University of Nebraska
Dr. Sam Wald – New York University
Dr. H.M. Worth – Guy's Hospital, London, England
Dr. Arthur H. Wuehrmann – University of Alabama

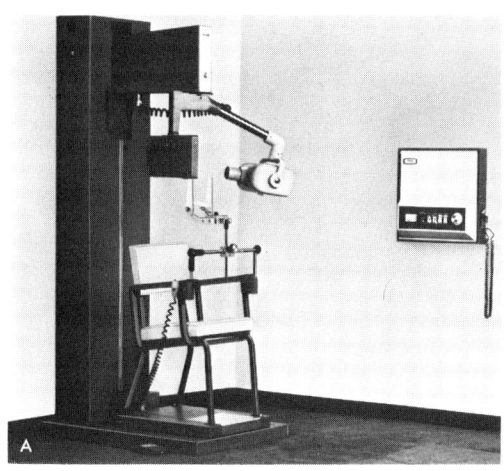
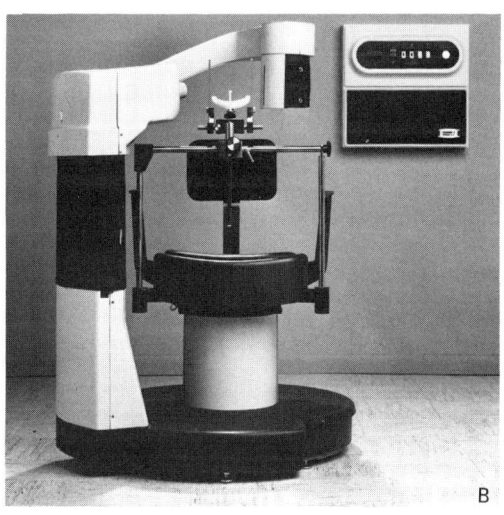

Figure 1-43. Modern panoramic dental X-Ray machines. **(A)** Panorex I-(S.S. White/Pennwalt) Panoramic machine. (Courtesy of Pennwalt Corp., Philadelphia, PA.)

(B) Panorex II (S.S. White/Penwalt) Panoramic machine. (Courtesy of Pennwalt Corp., Philadelphia, PA.)

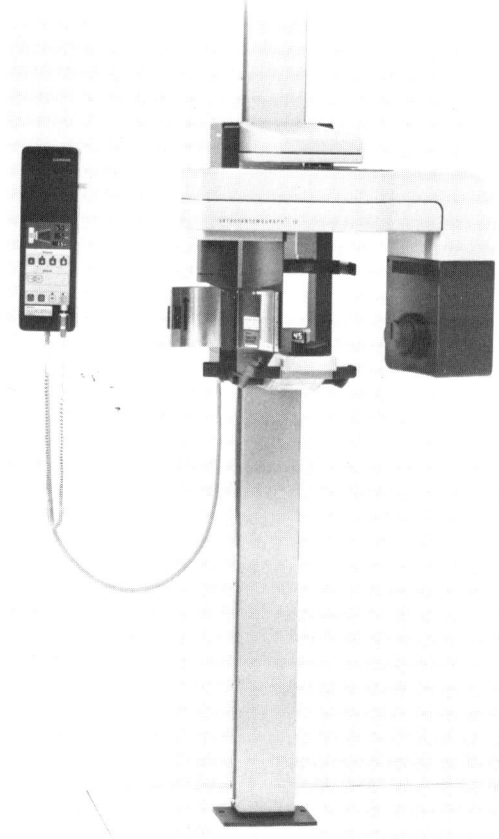
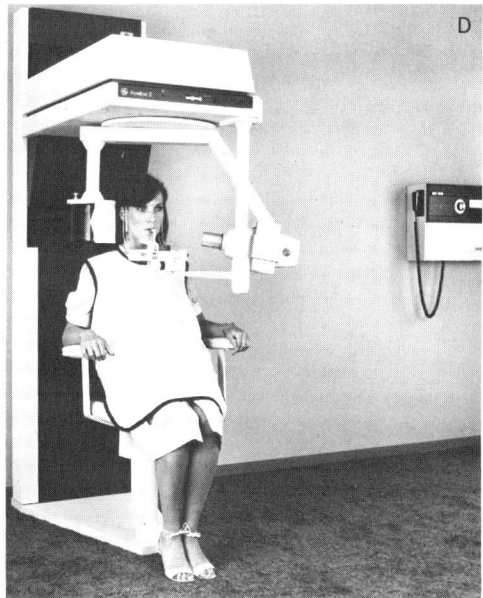

(C) Orthopantomograph OP10 Panoramic machine (Palomex/Siemens). Has multipulse high frequency current, rare earth screens, and narrowed V-shaped collimator. (Courtesy of Siemens Corp., Dental Division, Iselm, N.J.)

(D) Panelipse II Panoramic machine (General Electric) (courtesy of General Electric Co., Medical Systems Division, Milwaukee, WI.)

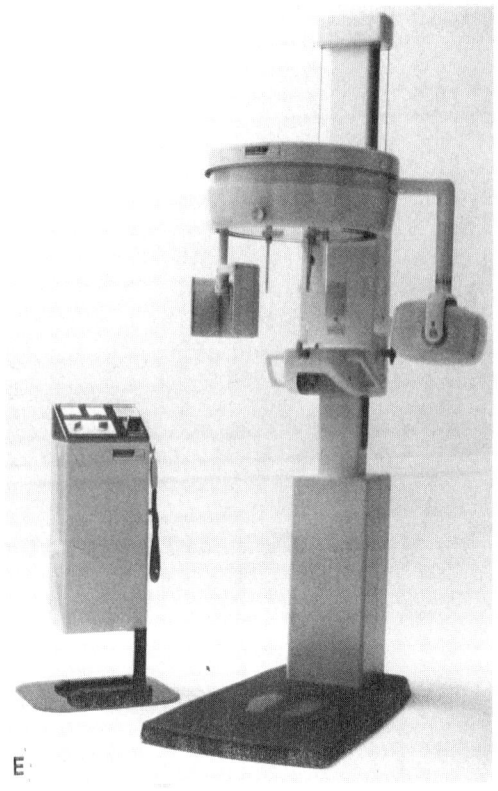

(E) Panoral panoramic machine (Ritter/Sybron). (Courtesy of Sybron Corp., Dental Products Division, Romulus, Michigan.)

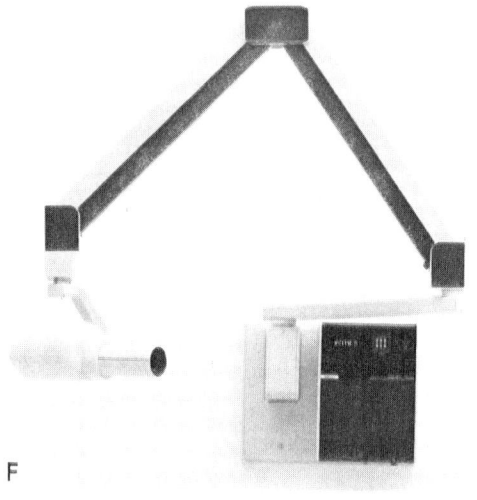

(F) Intrex 70 kVp intraoral X-Ray machine (S.S. White/Pennwalt). (Courtesy of Pennwalt Corp., Philadelphia, PA.)

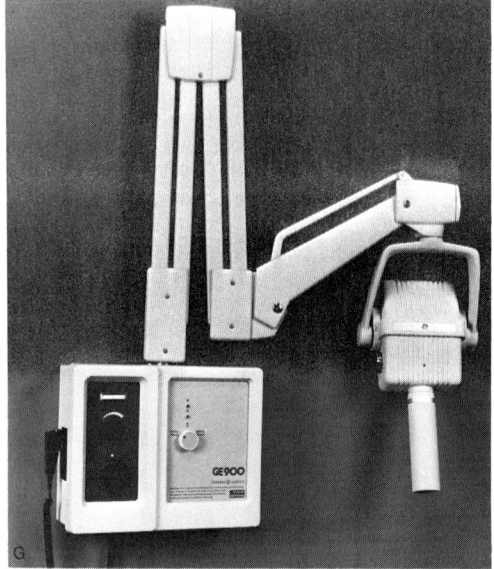

(G) GE 900 intraoral X-Ray machine, 70/90 kVp fixed settings at 15 mA. (Courtesy of General Electric Co., Medical Systems Division, Milwaukee, WI.)

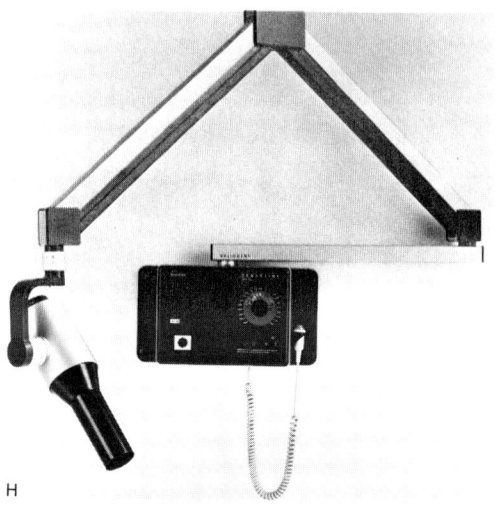

(H) Heliodent intraoral X-Ray machine 70 kVp (Siemens Corp). (Courtesy of Siemens Corp., Dental Division, Iselm, N.J.)

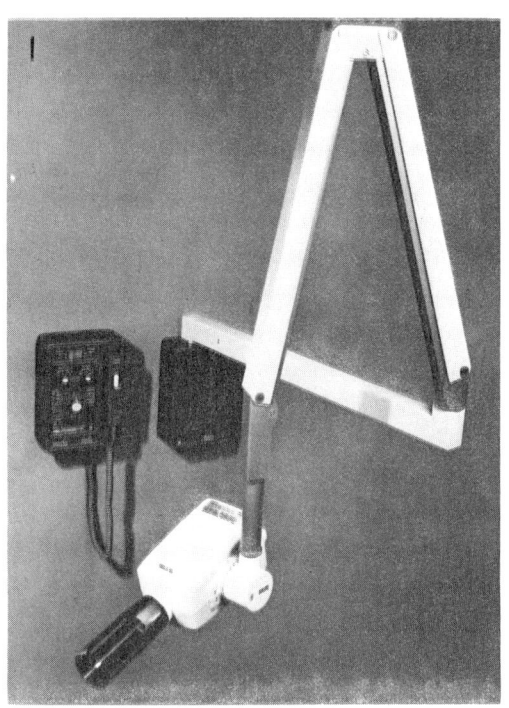

(I) Philips Oralix 65 wall model. (Courtesy of Philips Corp., Netherlands.)

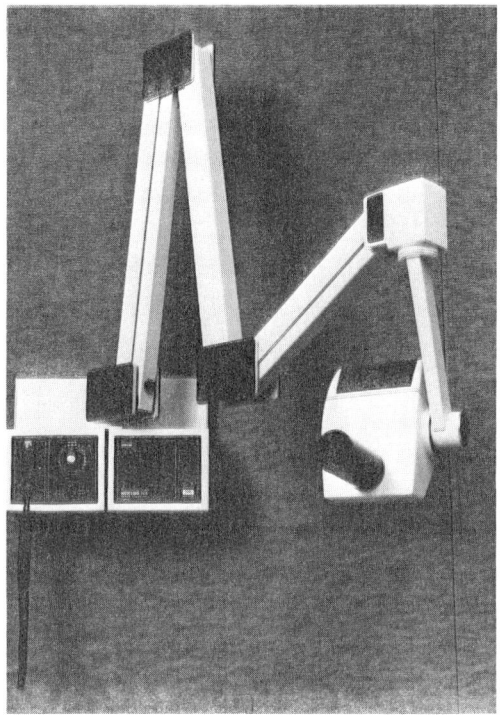

(J) Raflex 70, wall model. (Courtesy of MDT Corp., Torrance, CA.)

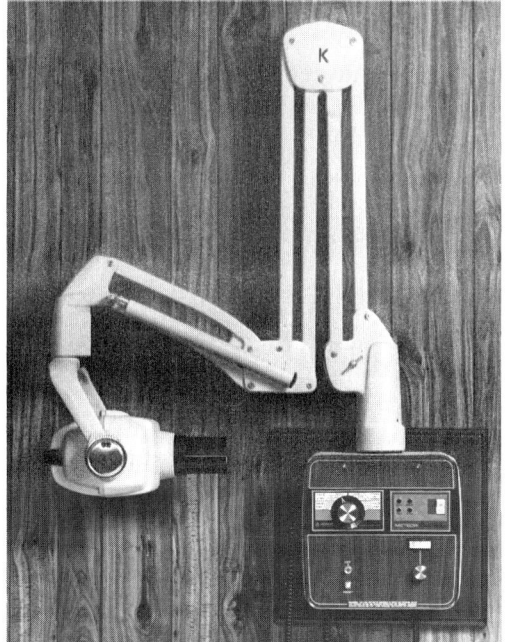

(K) Ritter Meteor II Model R-1A System. (Courtesy of Sybron/Ritter Corp., Rochester, NY.)

Bibliography

ADA Newsletter, November 1980 (Malvina Cueria, Kells' Dental Assistant).

Andrews, C.: Half a century of shadows. Radiography, 22:250-254, 1956.

Beck, C.: Roentgen Ray Diagnosis and Therapy. New York, D. Appleton, 1904, p. 75.

Bergonie, J.; and Tribondeau, L.: Action de rayons X sur le testicule du rat blanc. Compt rend soc de biol, 57:400, 1904.

Bremner, M.K.K.: The Story of Dentistry, 3rd ed. Brooklyn, Dental Items of Interest, 1959, pp. 298-304.

Brown, P.: American Martyrs to Science Through the Roentgen Rays. Springfield, Charles C Thomas, 1936.

Chenitz, P.: To the memory of C.Edmund Kells, at the third anniversary of his death. Dental Items of Interest, 53:307-311, 1931.

Christie, A.C.: A Manual of X-Ray Technic. Philadelphia, Lippincott, 1913.

Christie, A.C.: The American Roentgen Ray Society: Historic sketch "Lest We Forget," AJR, 76:1-6, 1956.

Clark, G.L.: Contributions of a quarter century of electron physics to roentgen-ray science. AJR, 26:528-539, 1931.

Coolidge, W.D.: The development of modern roentgen-ray generating apparatus. AJR, 24:605-620, 1930.

Coolidge, W.D.: Oil-immersed X-Ray generating outfits. AJR, 7:181-189, 1920.

Coolidge, W.D.; and Carlton, E.E.: Roentgen ray tubes. Radiology, 45:449-466, 1945.

Crane, A.W.: The research trail of the X ray. Radiology, 23:131-148, 1934.

Cryer, M.H.: Some uses of the roentgen rays in studies of the internal anatomy of the face. Dental Cosmos, 47:1-17, 60-63.

Daniel, J.: The X rays. Science, 3:566, April 10, 1896.

Dennis, J.: The roentgen energy today. Dental Cosmos, 41:853-857, 911-914, 1899.

Dewing, S.B.: Modern Radiology in Historical Perspective. Springfield, Charles C Thomas, 1962.

Ennis, L.; and Berry, H.M., Jr.: Dental Roentgenology, 5th ed., Philadelphia, Lea & Febiger, 1959, pp. 11-15.

Ennis, L.M.: A resumé of roentgenology. Oral Surg, 15:680-692, June 1962.

Ennis, L.M.: Dental Roentgenology. Philadelphia, Lea & Febiger, 1931.

Etter, L.E.: Some historical data relating to the discovery of the roentgen rays. AJR, 56:220-231, 1946.

Farman, A.G.; and Shawkat, A.H.: Survey of radiographic requirements and techniques. J Detn Educ, 45(9):581-588, 1981.

Fitzgerald, G.M.: Dental roentgenography I. Control of geometric unsharpness. J Am Dent Assoc, 34:1-20, January 1947.

Fitzgerald, G.M.: Dental Roentgenography II. Vertical Angulation. J Am Dent Assoc, 34:160-170, February 1947.

Fitzgerald, G.M.: Dental roentgenography III. Upper molar region. J Am Dent Assoc, 38:293-303, March 1949.

Fitzgerald, G.M.: Dental roentgenography IV. Voltage factor. J Am Dent Assoc, 41:19-28, July 1950.

Fixott, H.C.: Dental radiography. Northwest J Dent, 5:14-19, 1917.

Fixott, H.C.: What should a radiogram possessing diagnostic value show? Northwest J Dent, 10:19-21, 1922.

Glasser, O.: Strange repercussion of Roentgen's discovery of the X rays. Radiology, 45:425-427, November 1945.

Glasser, O.: The Science of Radiology. Springfield, Charles C Thomas, 1933, pp 1-14.

Glasser, O.: Wilhelm Conrad Roentgen. Springfield, Charles C Thomas, 1934.

Glasser, O.: Fifty years of roentgen rays. Dent Radiogr Photogr, 19, No. 1, 1946.

Glasser, O.: W.C. Roentgen and the discovery of the Roentgen rays. AJR, 25:437-450, 1931.

Glenner, R.A.: 80 years of dental radiography. J Am Dent Assoc, 90:549-563, March 1975.

Grigg, E.R.N.: The Trail of Invisible LIght. Springfield, Charles C Thomas, 1965.

Hauser, P.: Proceedings of the Twentieth Internaitonal Congress of the History of Medicine. Berlin, 1966.

Herschfeld, J.J.: Dr. C. Edmund Kells — Pioneer in the field of dental radiology. Bull Hist Dentistry, 25:105-108, October 1977.

Hickey, P.M.: The first decade of American roentgenology. AJR, 20:249-256, 1928.

Hickey, P.M.: The Caldwell lecture, 1928. AJR, 25:177-195, 1931.

Imboden, H.M.: Progress in the development of the roentgen-ray apparatus. AJR, 25:4378-450, 1931.

Jauncy, G.M.E.: The birth and early infancy of X rays. Am J Physiol, 13:1-21, 1945.

Jerman, E.C.: Protection from an X-Ray standpoint. Int J Orthod, 11:1061-1066, 1925.

Kassabian, M.K.: Roentgen Rays and Electrotherapeutics. Philadelphia, Lippincott, 1907, pp 170-196.

Kells, C.E.: Transactions of southern Dental Association Meeting, July 28-30, 1896,

Asheville, N.C. *Dental Cosmos, 38*:850-1013, December 1896.

Kells, C.E.: Roentgen rays. *Dental Cosmos, 41*:1014-1029, 1899.

Kells, C.E.: Plea for a standardized technic for oral radiography. *J Dent Res, 2*:551-555, 1920.

Kells, C.E.: Protection for the roentgen ray. *Dental Items of Interest, 24*:805, 1912.

Kells, C.E.: *Three Score Years and Nine.* New Orleans, C. Edmund Kells, 1926, p. 404.

Kells, C.E.: Stereoscopic roentgenographs, stereographs. *Dental Items of Interest, 41*:120-139, February 1919.

Kells, C.E.: Dental stereographs. *Dental Items of Interest, 42*:189-192, 1920.

Kells, C.E.: The X-Ray in dental practice; The crime of the age. *J Am Dent Assoc, 7*:241-272, March 1920.

Kells, C.E.: Thirty years experience in the field of radiography. *J Am Dent Assoc, 13*:693-711, June 1926.

Kells, C.E.: Roentgen ray burns. *J Am Dent Assoc, 14*:235-243, 1927.

Kells, C.E.: The limitations of the roentgen ray in dental practice. *J Am Dent Assoc, 12*:1078-1083, September 1925.

Langland, O.E.; and Fortier, A.P.: C. Edmund Kells. *Oral Surg, 34*:680-689, October 1972.

Langland, O.E.; and Fortier, A.P.: The contributions of Dr. C. Edmund Kells: A bibliography. *Bull Hist Dentistry, 19*:34-43, December 1971.

Langland, O.E.; Langlais, R.P.; and Morris, C.R.: *Principles and Practice of Panoramic Radiography.* Philadelphia, Saunders, 1982.

Leach, F.D.: Symposium on dental radiographic technique. *Int J Orthod, 2*:467-469, 1916.

MacKee, G.M.; and Remer, J.: Radiation measurement. *Dental Cosmos, 56*:35-42, 1914.

Marcuse, W.: Dermatitis und alopecia nach Durchlenchlungoversuchen mit. *Rontgenstrahlen Deutsche Med Wehnschi, 22*:481, 1896.

Martin F.C.; and Fuschs, A.W.: Historical evolution of roentgen ray plates and films. *AJR, 26*:540-548, 1931.

Matas, R.: Delayed or remote appearance of X-Ray burns after long periods of latency. *Trans Am surg Assoc,* pp. 462-467, 1923.

Mazzola, P.V.: Early reports of X-Ray dangers. *Bull Hist Dentistry, 22*:1, June 1974.

McCall, J.O.; and Wald, S.S.: *Clinical Dental Roentgenology,* 4th ed. Philadelphia, Saunders, 1957, pp. 1-4, 35-38, and 82.

McCormack, F.W.: A plea for standardized oral radiography. *Br Dent J, 41*:1162, 1920; abstracted *J Dent Res, 11*:496, September 1920.

McCormack, D.W.: Dental roentgenology: A technical procedure for furthering the advancement toward anatomical accuracy. *J Calif State Dent Assoc,* pp 89-116, May June 1937.

McCormack, D.W.: Mechanical aids for obtaining accuracy in dental roentgenology. *J Am Denta Assoc, 40*:144-153, February 1950.

McCoy, J.D.: *Dental and Oral Radiography.* St. Louis, Mosby, 1925, pp 17-22.

McCoy, J.D.: Suggestions in X-Ray technique for the orthodontist. *Int J Orthod, 2*:1-13, 1916.

McCoy, J.D.: The interpretatin of dental and oral radiographs. *Int J Orthod, 2*:285-294, 1916.

McCoy, J.D.: The nature of the X ray and its discovery. *Int J Orthod, 2*:385-390, 1916.

McCoy, J.D.: X-Ray machines. *Int J Orthod, 3*:111-127, 1917.

Morton, W.J.: The X ray and its application in dentistry. *Dental Cosmos, 38*:478-86, July 1896.

Nitske, W.R.: *The Life of Wilhelm Conrad Roentgen.* Tucson, Arizona, U of Ariz Pr, 1971.

Peterson, S.: *Clinical Dental Hygiene,* St. Louis, Mosby, 1959, pp. 199-200.

Pfahler, G.E.: The development of roentgen therapy during fifty years. *Radiology, 45*:503-521, November 1945.

Pollio, J.A.: Fundamental principles of alveolodental radiography. *Dental Items of Interest, 47*:405, 1925.

Preece, J.W.: Roentgen alchemy, Part I and Part II. *Oral Surg, 28*:680, November 1969; *28*:830, December 1969.

Price, W.A.: The technique necessary for making good dental skiagraphs. *Dental Items of Interest, 26*:161-171, 1904.

Price, W.A.: The science of dental radiography. *Tr Third Intl Dent Congress, 11*:245-370, 1900.

Pursey, A.; and Caldwell, E.W.: *The Practical application of Roentgen Rays in Therapeutics and Diagnosis.* Philadelphia, Saunders, 1903.

Raper, H.: *Radiodontia.* Brookly, Dental Items of Interest Publishing, 1925, pp. 17-18.

Raper, H.: Critical analysis of three radiodontic technics introduction. *Dent Surv,* p. 731, June, 1955.

Raper, H.: Mathematical angulation technic. *Dent Surv,* p. 863, July 1955.

Raper, H.: Criticism of mathematical angulation technic. *Dent Surv,* p. 986, August 1955.

Raper, H.: Advantages and disadvantages of

three radiodontic technics. *Dent Surv*, p. 1404, November 1955.

Raper, H.: A new kind of X-Ray examination for preventive dentistry. *Int J Orthod, 11*:173-181, 275-179, 370-374, 470-477, 575-577, 678-683, 764-771, 1925.

Raper, H.: *Elementary and Dental Radiography.* New York, Consolidated Dent Mfg Co., 1913.

Raper, H.: The teaching of dental radiography. *Minutes Inst Dent Pedagogies*, pp. 80-87, 97-96, 1913.

Rollins, W.: An oral camera (cassette) for rontgen photography. *Boston Med Surg J, 135*:90, July 23, 1896.

Rollins, W.: A roentgen ray converter for internal use. *Int Dent J, 17*:445-446, July 1896.

Rollins, W.: Dental uses for rontgen's discovery—support tube. *Int Dent J, 17*:559-560, 1896.

Rollins, W.: Notes on X-light. Letter to editor. *Boston Med Surg J, 144*:317, February 23, 1901.

Rollins, W.: Notes on X-light: the control of guinea pigs. *Boston Med Surg J, 144*:317, March 28, 1901.

Rollins, W.: Notes on X-light: vacuum tube burns. *Boston Med Surg J, 146*:39-40, January 9, 1902.

Rollins, W.: *Notes on X-light.* Boston, University Press, 1903.

Röntgen, W.C.: Über eine neue Art von Straklen. Vorläufige Mitteitung. *Sitzgber. Physik-Med Ges Wurburg*, pp. 1132-141, December 28, 1895. (Roentgen's first article on X rays called "On a New Kind of Rays, Preliminary Communication,"Published by Wurzburg Physical Medical Society.)

Röntgen, W.C.: Uber eine neue Art von Straklen. II Mitteilung. *Sitzgber. Physik-Med Ges Wurzburg*, pp. 11-16, March 9, 1896. ("On a New Kind of Rays, Second Communication," published by Wurzburg Physical Medical Society.)

Röntgen, W.C.: Weiter Beobachtungen über die Eigensnaften der X-strahlen. *Sitzgber. Preuss Akad Wiss, Physik-Math Kl*, p. 392, 1897 ("Further Observations on the Properties of X ray," published by Academy of Sciences in Berlin.)

Satterlee, F.L.: *Dental Radiology.* New York, Swenarton Stationery, 1914.

Shearer, J.S.: Electrical dangers in X-Ray laboratories. *Int J Orthod, 2*:857-866, 1925.

Simpson, C.O.: *Advanced Radiodontic Interpretation*, 34d ed., St. Louis, Mosby, 1947.

Skinner, E.H.: Early American roentgeniana. *AJR, 26*:549-555, 1931.

Skinner, E.H.: A pioneer roentgenologist— Eugene Rollin Corson. *AJR, 26*:759-764, 1931.

Smyth, H.D.: X rays to nuclear fission. *Am Sci, 35*:485-501, 1947.

Squire, Lucy Frank: *Fundamentals of Roentgenology.* Cambridge, Mass., Harvard U Pr, 1964.

Sweet, A.P.: William Hebert Rollins, DDS, MD: Dentistry's forgotten man. *Dent Radiogr Photogr, 33*:3, 1960.

Sweet, A.P.: Some historical aspects of radiodontics. *Dent Radiogr Photogr, 15*:9-11, 1942.

Thoma, K.H.: *Oral Roentgenology.* boston, Ritter, 1917, pp. 11-15.

Thoma, K.H.: *Oral and Dental Diagnosis*, 3rd ed. Philadelphia, Saunders, 1949, p. ix.

Thoma, K.H.: Differential radiographic diagnosis in oral lesions. *J Dent Res, 13*:1-19, 19-24, 1933.

Thompson, J.R.: A cephalometric study of the movements of the mandible. *J Am Dent Assoc, 28*:750-761, 1941.

Thompson, W.S.: *Operative and Interpretive Radiodontia.* Philadelphia, Lea & Febiger, 1936, pp. 2-20.

Trout, E.D.; and Kelley, J.: The evolution of equipment for dental radiography. *J Ontario Dent Assoc, 35*:10-18, September 1958.

Van Woert, F.V.: X rays. *Trans New York Odont Soc*, p. 121, 1897.

Varnado, M.B.: Dr. C. Edmund Kells: As I remember him. *Bull Hist Dentistry, 19*:26-33, December 1971.

Wantz, J.B.: A consideration of some phases of X-Ray machine construction from an engineering standpoint. *Int J Orthod, 3*:234-237, 1917.

Watson, W.: 1895 and all that. *Radiography, 27*:305-315, 1961.

Wuehrmann, a.: The long cone technic. *Prac Dent Monogr*, pp 3-4, July 1957.

Chapter 2

X-RAYS, THEIR PRODUCTION, AND THE X-RAY BEAM

X-RAYS

WHEN Wilhelm Conrad Roentgen announced to the world the discovery of a new kind of ray, he called it the X-ray" after the algebraic symbol for unknown quantity. The scientific world for the most part called it the "roentgen ray" in honor of the discoverer.

Radiology: The science of ionizing radiations, encompassing radium and other radioactive materials as well as x-rays. *Radi* means radiation and *ology* means the study of or science of. It is a branch of the medical sciences that deals with the use of X-rays and nuclear medicines for diagnosis and treatment of disease.

Roentgenology: A science of roentgen rays (or x-rays) solely; includes the taking of x-ray pictures, their interpretation, and the use of x-rays in the treatment of disease (therapeutic use).

Radiograph: It is the visible photographic record on film produced by the passage of x-rays through an object or body. It makes it possible to study the inner structures of the human body and aid in diagnosis. The word can be used as a verb or a noun. Some of the synonyms used for the word "radiograph" are roentgenograph, roentgenogram, radiogram, skiagraph, skiagram, shadowgram. The authors prefer the term "radiograph" because it has more common usage and is less cumbersome than "roentgenogram."

Radiography: It is the use of ionizing radiation (usually x-rays or gamma rays) to produce a transmission image of an object on a photosensitive material (usually film). Synonyms used for "radiography" are actinography, roentgenography, and skiagraphy. The authors prefer the words "radiography" and "radiographic" rather than "roentgenography" and "roentgenographic" for the same reasons as given above.

Dental Radiography: Dental radiography, for the most part, deals with projection, exposure, and processing technics. These technics are based on the knowledge on the knowledge of the fundamentals of ionizing radiation, its production, and the potential hazards involved. Therefore, it is important that the student of dental radiograpy be familiar with the nature of x-rays, their production, and methods for protection in order to enable himself to operate and maintain dental x-ray equipment with precision, safety, and confidence. In this way, the student will better prepare himself to produce quality radiographs routinely.

The Structure of the Atom

In order to understand the nature of x-rays, it is important to be familiar with the structure of the atom.

Matter is defined as a physical manifestation possessing mass (occupies space and has weight). All matter is composed of atoms. There are at present 105 known types of atoms. The structure of the atom can be described as a miniature solar system. Each atom consists of a small dense *nucleus*, which has a positive electric charge, and a number of lighter particles with negative charges called *electrons* moving around the nucleus in definite orbits.

The atom is said to be neutral when the net number of positive charges of the nucleus (protons) equals the negative charges of the orbital electrons. The electrons are kept in their orbits by the balance between (1) the electrostatic attraction of unlike charges and (2) the centrifugal forces of the fast-moving electrons.

Nuclear Composition

The nucleus is composed of protons and neutrons. These particles are called nucleons. Protons carry a positive charge, which is equal in magnitude but opposite in size to the charge carried by the electrons. The neurtrons carry no electrical charge (Fig. 2-1).

Atoms differ from one another in the constitution of their nuclei and in the number and arrangement of their electrons. The atomic number, Z, is the number of protons in the nucleus as well as the number of electrons outside the nucleus. Z ranges from one for the simplest atom (hydrogen) to 105 for the most complex yet discovered (Hahnium). The chemical properties of an atom are determined by the atomic number.

A second important characteristic is

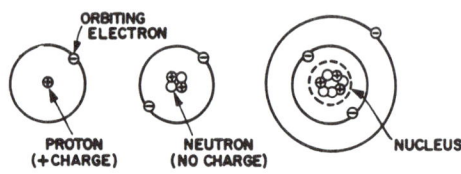

Figure 2-1. Structure of the first three atoms of the periodic table. A neutral atom has the same number of protons in the nucleus as the number of negatively charged orbitory electrons.

mass number, or atomic weight. The mass of the atom is derived mainly from the nucleons. The mass of a proton or a neutron is approximately 1,840 times that of an electron. Although the electrons have very little mass, they do occupy a great deal of space within the atom. For example, if the atom was increased to the size of a convention hall, the nucleus in the center of the hall and would be the size of a pinhead. The atom is composed mostly of empty space. For instance, the uranium nucleus contains 99.998 percent of the entire mass of the atom. The mass number is the sum of the weights of the protons and neutrons in the nucleus of a given atom and is represented by the letter "A." Hydrogen always has a Z of 1 (protons), while A may be either 1, 2, or 3 depending on the number of neutrons present in the nucleus. Helium is located next to hydrogen in the atomic table. It has an atomic number (Z) of 2, since the nucleus has two protons, but may have a mass number of 3 or 4 depending whether there are one or two neutrons present in the nucleus.

The mass number A is placed as a superscript to the left of the chemical symbol, and the atomic number Z is placed as a subscript tot he left. Thus, hydrogen with atomic number of 1 and mass number of 2 is written as ^2_1H. In present practice the element in question is written either ^1H, ^2H, or ^3H.

If two atoms have the same number of protons (Z) but differ in mass number (A), they are called isotopes. They are two forms of the same element and have the same chemical properties.

Chemical elements isolated from natural sources are often a mixture of isotopes. Tin has the largest number of naturally occurring isotopes: it has an atomic number (**Z**) of 50 (protons) and is found in nature with mass number of 112, 114, 115, 117, 118, 119, 120, 122, and 124 (neutrons vary from 62 to 74). Each of these various isotopes of tin behaves chemically in the same way.

If two atoms have the same number of neutrons (**N**) they are called **isotones,** and if they have the same number of nucleons (protons plus neutrons), then they have the same mass number **A** and are called **isobars.** (Fig. 2-2.)

varying distances from the nucleus. The arrangement of the electrons around the nucleus determines the way atoms interact with each other. A maximum number of seven potential electron-containing shells exist. No known atom contains more than seven shells. These seven shells are designated as K, L, M, N, O, P, Q in order of increasing distance from the nucleus. Each orbit or shell can contain only a certain maximum number of electrons (Fig. 2-3).

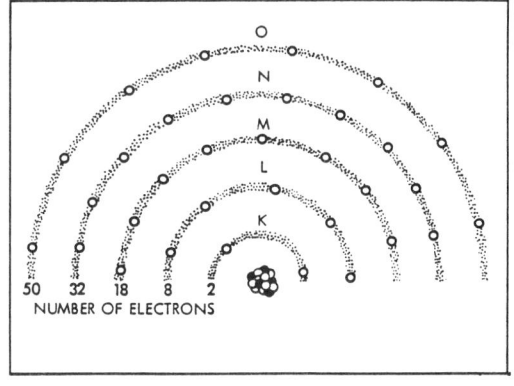

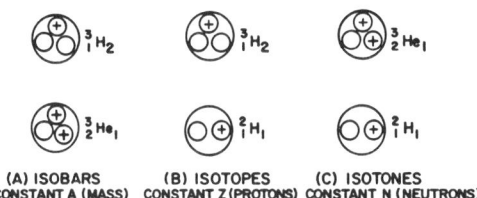

(A) ISOBARS (B) ISOTOPES (C) ISOTONES
CONSTANT A (MASS) CONSTANT Z (PROTONS) CONSTANT N (NEUTRONS)

Figure 2-2. The (+) circles represent protons and the clear circles represent neutrons. Only the nuclei of the atoms are illustrated. (**A**) *Isobars:* atoms with same mass number. (Hydrogen 3 and Helium 3 are isobars.) (**B**) *Isotopes:* atoms with same Z number (protons) but different N numbers (neutrons). (Hydrogen 3 and Hydrogen 2 are isotopes.) (**C**) *Isotones:* atoms with same N numbers (neutrons) but differen Z numbers (protons). (Helium 3 and Hydrogen 2 are isotones.)

Figure 2-3. The maximum number of electrons that can exist in each shell. Schematic representation of a tungsten atom. (Courtesy of Dr. Michel Ter-Pogssian.)

K-shell (No. 1)	2 electrons
L-shell (No. 2)	8 electrons
M-shell (No. 3)	18 electrons
N-shell (No. 4)	32 electrons
O-shell (No. 5)	50 electrons
P-shell (No. 6)	72 electrons
Q-shell (No. 7)	98 electrons

Orbital Electrons

Electrons are very small particles carrying one unit of negative charge, and they revolve around the nucleus in well-defined shells or specific areas that exist at

These numbers for each shell need not be memorized, because in atomic theory each of these shells is characterized by the number in the **principal of quantum**

number that has the values of 1, 2, 3, and 4 and so forth beginning with the K shell outward. The maximum number of electrons that can occupy each shell follows the formula ($2m^2$) where **m** equals the number of the shell. In addition to the limitation on the maximum number of shells allowed in each shell, the outermost shell of an atom, no matter what shell it is in, never contains more than eight electrons. Electrons in the outermost shell are termed valence electrons and determine for the most part the chemical properties of the atom (Fig. 2-4).

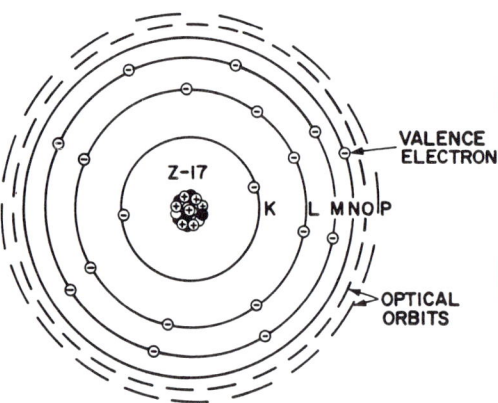

Figure 2-4. Electron orbits of potassium (Z = 17). For x-ray purposes one is interested in the motion of the tightly bound K, L, and M shells, while the motion of the outer electrons is of importance in determining the optical spectrum of the material.

Ionization

In their normal state, atoms are electrically neutral: the electrical charge is 0 because the number of protons in the nucleus equals the number of orbital electrons. When an atom loses or gains an electron it is said to be ionized. An ionized atom (called an ion) is not electrically neutral but carries a charge equal to the difference between the number of protons and electrons.

Many of the elements have incompletely filled outer shells, which tend to capture electrons quite readily from adjacent atoms. Of course, when this ocurs, the atom has more electrons than it should, and it becomes a **negative** atom. When atoms lose electrons, they become deficient in negative charges and, therefore, will behave as a positively charges and, therefore, will behave as a positively charged atom. An atom that is not electrically balanced is called an ion.

In any ionization process, ion pairs are formed, and it is this process that elicits chemical changes in matter.

X-rays are a form of energy that can form ion pairs in atoms. When an x-ray transfers its energy to an orbital electron, it ejects it from the atom, and an ion pair is formed. The atom becomes a positive ion (+1 charge) because it has lost an electron, and the ejected electron has a negative charge (−1). Thus, an ion pair has been formed (Fig. 2-5).

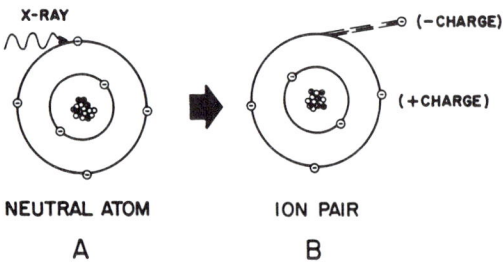

Figure 2-5. Ionization of a neutral atom by x-rays. **(A)** Neutral atom with x-ray ejecting an orbital electron. **(B)** Ion pair formed by ejected electron (− charge) and the ionized atom with more protons than electrons (+ charge).

Molecular Structure and Bonds

Atoms combine to form molecules by sharing their outer valence electrons so that the other shells of all the atoms involved tend to be filled.

Atoms are held together to form molecules by three important types of bonds: **the ionic bond, the covalent bond,** and **the hydrogen bond. The hydrogen bond** is one of the weaker bonds and is commonly found in protein molecules, which are prone to disassociation.

In the **ionic bond,** the single valence electron of sodium is transferred to the chlorine atom to fill the hole in its M shell forming a sodium (+) ion and a chlorine (−) ion (Fig. 2-6A). **Covalent bonds** are bonds formed between two hydrogen atoms and one oxygen atom (Fig. 2-6B) it is accomplished by sharing electrons 1, 2, 3, and 4 to form H-O-H (water). The

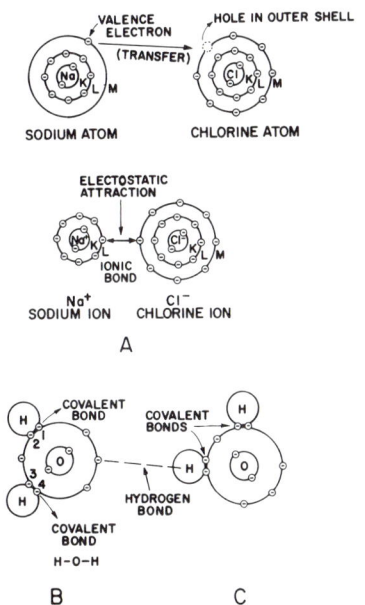

Figure 2-6. Molecular bonds. **(A)** Ionic Bond: ions held together by electrostatic attraction. **(B)** Covalent Bond: two atoms sharing electrons, which produces an attraction or bond. **(C)** Hydrogen Bond: In water, a hydrogen atom can share two neighboring oxygen atoms forming a bond. Hydrogen has a slightly positive charge and oxygen is slightly electronegative.

electrons 1, 2, 3, and 4 are shared by hydrogen and oxygen and will spend part of their time in each orbit. However, the electrons will spend slightly more time in the oxygen orbit because oxygen tends to attract electrons since it is electronegative.

In the **hydrogen bond** (Fig. 2-6C) two molecules are held together by hydrogen of one of the molecules. It is a weak bond compared to the others and in this illustration, (Fig. 2-6C), hydrogen of one molecule of water is attracted to an atom of oxygen of another molecule of water. Hydrogen has a slightly positive charge and oxygen has a slightly negative charge. The hydrogen bond exists in nitrogen compounds, which include proteins and DNA molecules.

Atom Energy Levels

The electrons in an atom do not spontaneously fly off from the nucleus by centripetal force or, on the other hand, drop into the nucleus by electrostatic attraction (unlike charges attract), because in the normal atom there is a balance between centripetal force and electrostatic force. This balance results in a definite electron path or orbit for each electron around the nucleus. These orbits are called shells. Each shell has a different energy level, which is dependent upon the atomic number of the atom and the distance the electron if from the nucleus. For each element, these orbital energy levels are different and characteristic. The attractive force between the positively charged nucleus and the negatively charged electrons is the force that keeps the electron in the atom. This is called the binding force of the electron. This force or energy is a negative energy. In other words, to remove an electron from an atom its energy value must be raised to 0 or to a positive value. Kinetic energy is always a positive value. The energy to raise the energy value to zero is called the binding energy of the electron. It is also the energy value designated for the atomic shell that holds the electron. The binding energy is greatest near the nucleus and diminishes with increasing distance from the nucleus (Fig. 2-7).

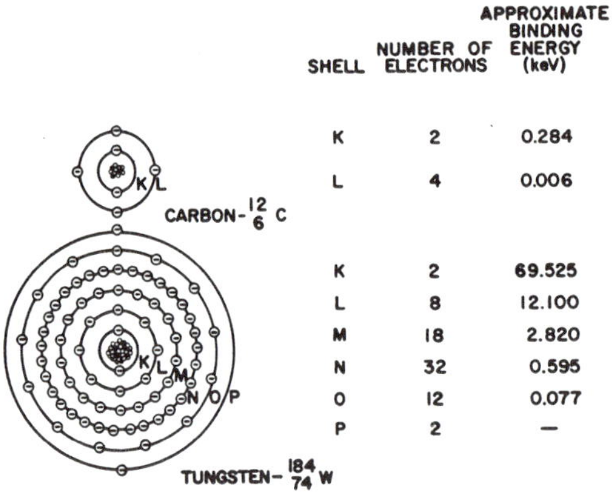

Figure 2-7. The approximate binding energies for two important elements in radiology — carbon and tungsten. Notice that binding energies are greater for each element for the inner-shell electrons. Also, tungsten a more complex element than carbon has higher binding energies in each shell than carbon. (Adapted from Bushong, Stewart: *Radiologic Science for Technologists.* St. Louis, C. V. Mosby, 1975.)

Carbon - $^{12}_{6}$C

SHELL	NUMBER OF ELECTRONS	APPROXIMATE BINDING ENERGY (keV)
K	2	0.284
L	4	0.006

Tungsten - $^{184}_{74}$W

SHELL	NUMBER OF ELECTRONS	APPROXIMATE BINDING ENERGY (keV)
K	2	69.525
L	8	12.100
M	18	2.820
N	32	0.595
O	12	0.077
P	2	—

Energy is measured by the amount of work done or the amount of work capable of being done. The most useful unit of energy for our purposes is the **electron-volt.** It is the kinetic energy of an electron accelerated through a potential difference of 1 volt. Larger multiple units of the electron-volt are frequently used: keV or 1,000 or kilo-electron-volts; MeV for 1 million or mega-electron-volts*.

---

*An electron has a charged of 1.60×10^{-19} coulombs; therefore, 1 electron volt (eV) = 1.00 volt × 1.60×10^{-19} coulombs = 1.60×10^{-19} joules. The joule (newton-meter) is the SI (Système International d'Unités) unit for work and energy and is equal to 1 newton (0.225 lbs) expended along a distance of 1 meter. By 1984 the International Commission on Radiation Units and Measurements (ICRU) has urged that SI units, the meter-kilogram-sec (MKS) system, be used completely instead of older centimeter-gram-sec units (CGS system) (Table 2-I).

Table 2-I

METRIC UNIT SYSTEMS

Physical Quantity	cgs		SI (mks)	
	Unit Name	Symbol	Unit Name	Symbol
Length	centimeter	cm	meter	m
Mass	gram	g	kilogram	kg
Time	sec	s	sec	s
Charge	electrostatic unit	esu	coulomb	C
Energy	erg;electron volt	erg; eV	joule	J
Exposure	roentgen	R	—	C/kg
Absorbed dose	rad	rad	gray	Gy
Radioactivity	curie	Ci	becquerel	Bq

For example the binding energies of the K, L, and M shells of tungsten are 70 keV, 12 keV, and 3 keV respectfully. To remove a K shell electron from tungsten would require an energy of 70 keV (Fig. 2-7).

Since the electrons in the inner shells have greater binding energies, it takes x-rays, gamma rays, or high-energy particles to remove electrons from these shells. Electrons in the outer shells are not held so tightly to the nucleus and, therefore, can be affected by lesser energies, such as visible light rays and ultraviolet rays.

Radioactivity

There are strong and opposing forces present within the atomic nucleus. While powerful forces tend to tear the nucleus apart, there is a strong binding force tending to hold the nucleus together. In most cases, the forces holding the nucleus together are successful and the atom is **stable.** Elements composed of atoms of this group are called **stable isotope** nuclides.

Many factors affect nuclear stability, but the neutron/proton ratio perhaps is the most important. When the atomic nucleus has either too few or too many neutrons, the atom spontaneously emits particles and energy and transforms itself into another atom. this process is called radioactive decay or radioactive disintegration, and the nucleus will continue to eject particles or energy until a stable isotope is reached.

These unstable isotopes are **radioactive** and are called **radioactive isotopes.** In recent years the terms isotope and radioisotope have been replaced by the terms nuclide and radionuclide, respectively. The term nuclide is more precise than isotope because it means any individual nuclear species plus its orbital electrons. The term isotope refers to two or more forms of the same element. The correct usage of radioactive isotopes would be to say that ^{197}Hg and ^{203}Hg are radioisotopes because they are two forms of the same element. However, ^{197}Hg and ^{131}I are **not** radioisotopes but are radioactive nuclides (radionuclides) because they are two different elements.

A few of the stable and unstable radioisotopes of some of the lighter elements are given in Table 2-II.

Notice that hydrogen has an atomic number (Z) of 1 and two stable isotopes with mass numbers (A) or 1 and 2, but an unstable isotope (radioisotope) with a mass number (A) of 3 called tritium (extra heavy hydrogen).

Radioisotopes of an element are usually produced in machines such as particle accelerators or nuclear reactors. A few of the elements have naturally occuring radioisotopes as well. There are two sources of these naturally occurring radioisotopes. They were either formed at the time of earth's formation (e.g. ^{238}U series) or they are formed in the upper atmosphere by action of cosmic radiation (e.g. ^{226}Ra, ^{228}Ra).

The original radionuclide in any method of decay is called a parent, and the nuclide to which it decays, is called a daughter, which may be stable or unstable. If the daughter is unstable, a new method of decay is started that may be altogether different from the parent.

There are basically three emissions

Table 2-II*

ATOMIC NUMBERS, ATOMIC WEIGHTS AND MASS NUMBERS
OF A FEW OF THE LIGHTER ELEMENTS

Element	Symbol	Atomic Number (Z)	Atomic Weight (A)	Mass Numbers of Stable Isotopes (A)	Mass Numbers Of Unstable Isotopes (A)
Hydrogen	H	1	1.0080	1, 2	3
Helium	He	2	4.003	3, 4	5, 6, 8
Lithium	Li	3	6.940	6, 7	5, 8, 9
Beryllium	Be	4	9.02	9	6, 7, 8, 10, 11, 12
Boron	B	5	10.82	10, 11	8, 9, 12, 13
Carbon	C	6	12.010	12, 13	9, 10, 11, 14, 15, 16
Nitrogen	N	7	14.008	14, 15	12, 13, 16, 17, 18
Oxygen	O	8	16.0000	16, 17, 18	13, 14, 15, 19, 20

*From H. Johns and J. Cunningham: *Physics of Radiology,* 3rd ed, 1978. Courtesy of Charles C Thomas, Publisher, Springfield, Illinois

from radionuclides by which they decay to stability. They are by alpha and beta particles and gamma rays.

Types of Ionizing Radiation

Radiation is a process in which energy is emitted from an object as particles or waves. Ionizing radiation is a form of radiation that makes an electrically neutral atom (the total number of electrons in the orbital shells equals the number of protons in the nucleus) unbalanced electrically by removing or adding an electron to the atom. Ionizing radiation can knock an electron out of an electrically neutral atom, which results in an atom having one more proton (+) than the residual number of electrons. This makes it a positive ion. The ejected electron and ionized positive ion makes an ion pair. The ejected electron may exist awhile as a free electron (negative charge), but it will eventually do one of two things: it may attach itself to a neutral atom and form a **negative ion** (see Fig. 2-5), or it may attach itself to a positive ion and form a **neutral atom.**

There are two forms of ionizing radiation:
(1) corpuscular or particulate radiation and (2) electromagnetic radiations (Table 2-III).

Particulate Radiation

Particulate radiations are actually minute particles of matter that travel in straight lines at high speeds from their sources. Although incredibly small, they possess mass. All are charged electrically, except the neutrons, and they all move extremely fast, in fact, sometimes almost as fast as light. Examples of particulate radiation follow:

Alpha Particles

Alpha particles are composed of a combination of two protons and two neutrons. It is the helium nucleus (Z = 2, A = 4) without orbital electrons. Alpha particles are emitted only from the nuclei of heavy metals. As compared to the other particles, the **alpha particle** is enormous and exerts an large electrostatic attraction. They have little ability to penetrate tissues, and give up their large energies within a very short distance in air (5 cm) and in soft tissue (100 microns).

Electron

Electrons have a very small mass when compared to protons. Electrons abound in nature. We are interested in the following two:

Beta particle (negatron): They are emitted from the nucleus of radioactive atoms and possess one unit of negative charge. They have very small atomic masses. Beta particles (negatrons) are more penetrating than alpha particles and may penetrate 10-100 cm of air and approximately 1-2 cm of soft tissue.

Cathode Rays (electrons): They are streams of electrons passing from the hot filament of the cathode to the target of the anode in an x-ray tube. They differ from

Table 2-III

IONIZING RADIATION CLASSIFICATION

Radiation Type	Mass Units	Charge	Origin
Particulate			
Alpha particle	4.003*	+2	Nucleus
Beta particle	0.000548	-1	Nucleus
Cathode rays	0.000548	-1	Filament of x-ray tube
Protons	1.007597	+1	Nucleus
Neutrons	1.008986	0	Nucleus
Electromagnetic			
Gamma rays	0	0	Nucleus
X-rays	0	0	Electron orbital system of atom

*Chemical atomic weight of helium

beta particles in their place of origin. Beta particles come from the nucleus of radioactive atoms while the cathode rays originate from orbital electrons of the atoms of the filament material of an x-ray tube.

Protons

Protons are accelerated hydrogen nuclei. They are approximately 2,000 times the mass of the electron. Since protons are heavy, charged particles, they lose kinetic energy rapidly as they penetrate matter.

Neutron

It carries no electric charge and has nearly the same mass as a proton. The characteristic of being electrically neutral has proved of great importance in nuclear physics, since such a particle can penetrate into the nucleus of an atom without being subjected to the enormous forces of repulsion that resist the entrance of a positively charged particle.

Electromagnetic Radiation

X-rays and gamma rays belong to a group of radiations called electromagnetic radiations. Electromagnetic radiation is the propagation of energy through space accompanied by electric and magnetic force fields (hence the name electromagnetic radiation).

X-rays and gamma rays are identical except for their origin. X-rays are produced outside the nucleus in the electron orbital system. Gamma rays are emitted from the nucleus of a radionuclide and are usually associated with alpha and beta emission (Fig. 2-8).

Ionization Rate

When ionizing radiation passes through any material, it leaves a "track" of excited and ionized atoms and molecules.

An average **alpha particle** because of its enormous mass and charge will ionize approximately **40,000 atoms** for every centimeter of travel through air. This is called the **specific ionization,** and it is usually specified in ion pairs per centimeter of air or per micron of water. X-rays and gamma rays produce approximately **100 ion pairs** per cm, which is about equal to that of **beta particles.**

The alpha particle has a very short distance range through matter because it quickly dissipates all of its kinetic energies in ion pair production. Another unit used to describe this phenomenon is **linear energy transfer (L.E.T.)** It is the amount of energy deposited per unit length of travel expressed in keV per micron. A particle with a higher mass but with the same energy as another particle will de-

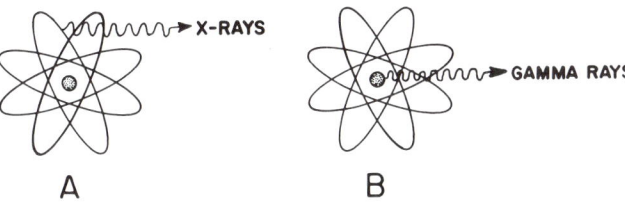

Figure 2-8. (A) X-rays are produced outside the nucleus of stable atoms. (B) Gamma rays are emitted from the nucleus of radioactive atoms. (Adapted from Bushong, Stewart: *Radiologic Science for Technologists* St. Louis, C. V. Mosby, 1975.)

posit more energy per unit length of travel and so it has a higher L.E.T. radiation.

External sources of alpha radiation are nearly harmless because alpha particles can only travel 5 cm through air, and 100 microns in soft tissue. However, an internal source of alpha particles is the exact opposite. Alpha-emitting radionuclides within the body can severely irradiate local tissue. As soon as an alpha particle loses all its kinetic energy it will come to rest, attract two electrons, and become a helium atom.

The **beta particle,** which has very little mass compared to the **alpha particle,** has a much longer range of penetration through matter. An average **beta particle** will penetrate about 10-100 cm of air and 1-2 cm of soft tissue. As soon as a beta particle loses all its kinetic energy, it will come to rest and attach itself to an atom that needs an electron.

Although the specific ionization of gamma rays and x-rays are approximately the same as for beta particles, they have an unlimited range in penetrating matter when compared to particulate radiation (Table 2-IV).

In nuclear medicine technology, alpha particles, beta particles, and gamma rays are of prime importance. In diagnostic radiology, x-rays are of prime importance because they have low specific ionization of matter and penetrate tissues for long distances (Fig. 2-9).

The Nature of X-Rays

As we have learned previously, x-rays are a form of electromagnetic radiation. In order to understand the production of a radiograph, we must first understand the nature of x-rays.

The interactions of electromagnetic radiations are difficult to understand. Some interactions are best explained by the theories of wave propagation, while other interactions are only explained if they are assumed to be particles or bundles of energy called quanta or photons. It is necessary to discuss electromagnetic radiations as if they were both waves and particles. That x-rays have the aspects of both waves and photons does not mean

Table 2-IV

CHARACTERISTICS OF SEVERAL TYPES OF IONIZING RADIATION

Type of radiation	Approximate energy	Specific ionization (ip/cm of air)	Aproximate range		Origin
			In air	In soft tissue	
Particulate					
Alpha particles	4-7 MeV	20,000-60,000	1-10 cm	Up to 0.1 mm	Heavy radioactive nuclei
Beta particles	0-3 MeV	100-400	0-1 m	0-2 cm	Radioactive nuclei
Electromagnetic					
X-rays	0-10 MeV	Up to 500	0-100 m	0-30 cm	Electron cloud
Gamma Rays	0-5 MeV	Up to 500	0-100 m	0-30 cm	Radioactive nuclei

From Bushong, Stewart: *Radiologic Science for Technologists*, ed. 2, 1980. Courtesy of C. V. Mosby Co., St. Louis.

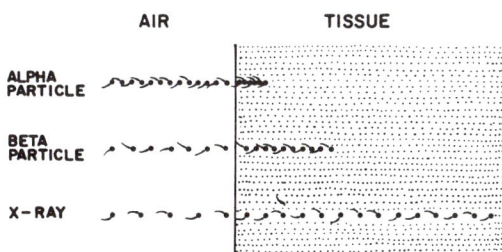

Figure 2-9. Various types of ionizing radiatio ionize matter differently. Alpha particles have large masses and charges ionize matter rapidly and have very short ranges in matter. Beta particles do not ionize matter as readily as alpha particles and, therefore, penetrate matter farther than alpha particles. The low specific ionization of x-rays allows x-rays to penetrate matter for long distances. (From Bushong, Stewart: Radiologic Science for Technologists. St. Louis, C. V. Mosby, 1975.)

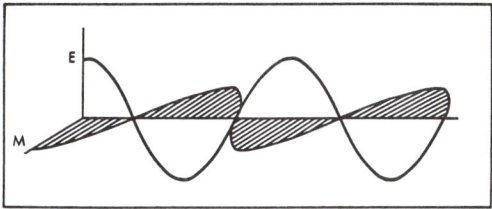

Figure 2-10. Simplified diagram of electromagnetic waves. The elctric (**E**) and magnetic (**M**) force fields are at right angles to each other and perpendicular to the direction of the wave propagations. (Courtesy of Dr. William Hendee.)

that a beam of radiation changes irratically from waves to photons and back again. Instead, other factors, such as the method used to detect it or the way x-rays are being used, determine which aspect (waves or photons) is the more useful concept.

Wave Concept of Electromagnetic Radiation

Electromagnetic radiation is the propagation of wavelike energy through space or mass at the speed of light (186,000 miles per second or 3×10^8 m/sec). A wave can be defined as a variation or disturbance that transfers radiant energy progressively from point to point in a medium. (Energy is the capacity to perform work.)

It is called electromagnetic radiation because the energy that is radiated is accompanied by oscillating electric and magnetic fields.

Each field is in phase with and perpendicular to each other and perpendicular to the direction of wave propagations (Fig. 2-10).

Examples of electromagnetic radiation are —

1. the radio waves that we hear;
2. the light waves we see;
3. the infrared waves that can take pictures in the dark;
4. the ultraviolet rays that cause sunburn;
5. the x-rays that you will be studying;
6. the gamma rays of the atomic bomb;
7. the cosmic rays, which hinder our travel in space.

The waves we are familiar with (waves traveling down a stretched rope when one end of the rope is moved up and down in rhythmic motion, waves traveling in water, or sound waves traveling in air) must be propagated in a medium. Electromagnetic waves need no such medium, as they can be propagated through a vacuum.

All waves have an associated wavelength and frequency. The wavelength of a wave is the distance between two successive crests, or valleys, and is given the symbol λ (the Greek letter *lambda*, the symbol for length) (Fig. 2-11).

The number of waves passing a particular point of time is called the frequency and is given the symbol ν (the Greek letter *nu*, the symbol for number). It is usually

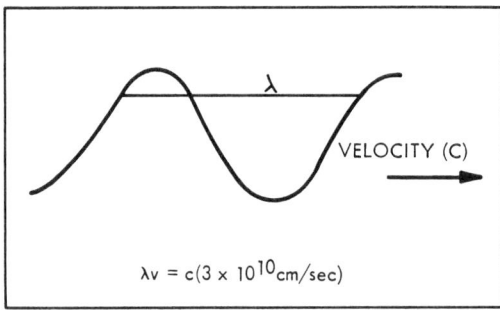

Figure 2-11. Diagram of a wave illustrating the wavelength, and the formula representing the relationship between velocity, frequency, and wavelength.

ν = frequency per second (Hz)

Since the velocity is always known, the wavelength of the radiation can be determined if the frequency is known, and conversely, the frequency if the wavelength is known. Also, it holds true that if the frequency of the wave is high, the wavelength will be short, and if the frequency is low the wavelength will have to be long.

All the forms of electromagnetic radiation are grouped according to their wavelengths in what is called the *electromagnetic spectrum* (Fig. 2-13).

identified as oscillations per second or cycles per second. The unit of measurement is the **hertz** (Hz). One hertz equals one cycle per second (Fig. 2-12).

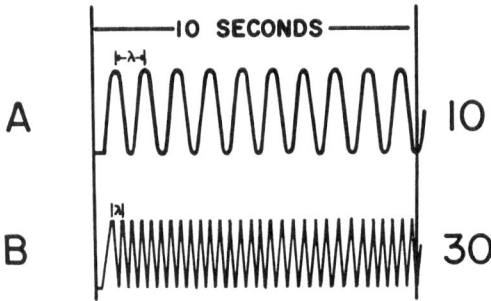

Figure 2-12. Two energies with different wave lengths. The shorter the wavelength the higher the frequency. **(A)** ten frequencies or cycles in 10 seconds equals 1 hertz. **(B)** thirty frequencies or cycles in 10 seconds equals 3 hertz.

Electromagnetic radiations travel at the speed of light (3×10^8 meters per second) in a vacuum. The velocity of light is given the symbol c. The relationship between velocity, frequency, and wavelength can be expressed as (*see* Fig. 2-11):

$$c = \lambda\nu$$

where c = velocity of light (m/sec)
λ = wavelength in meters

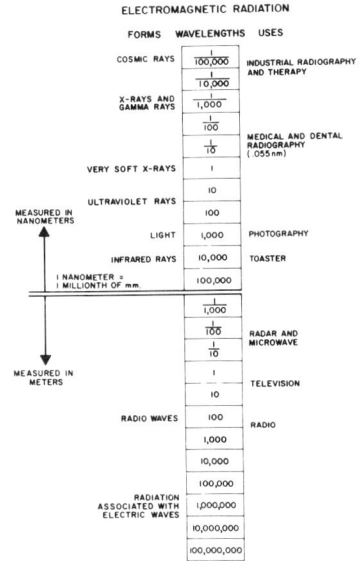

Figure 2-13. Diagram of the spectrum of electromagnetic radiatio. (Copyright Eastman Kodak Company Rochester, NY. Reprinted by permission.)

All of the energies of the electromagnetic spectrum possess certain properties in common:

1. They have no mass (weight) or electrical charge (neutral polarity).
2. They travel with the speed or velocity of light waves in a vacuum (186,000 miles/second, or 3×10^{10} centimeters/

second).
3. They all travel with wave motion.
4. As they travel through space, they propagate an electric field at right angles to their path of travel. At right angles to this electric field, a magnetic field is formed; hence the name — electromagnetic wave.

When the wavelengths change, the properties change. For example, the length of electromagnetic waves generated by 60 hertz (cycles per second) alternating current is about the distance from coast to coast of the United States. The wavelength of the standard broadcast portion of radio waves are as long as a football field and the wavelengths used in television are about equal to the height of an average man. Visible light has wavelengths measured in microns, and x-rays used in making radiographs are only about 1/10,000 the wavelength of visible light. This is approximately one-billionth of an inch. X-rays are usually measured in nanometers (abbreviated nm), one of which is equal to one-millionth of a millimeter.

The useful range in medical and dental radiography is approximately 0.01- 0.05 nm (0.1- 0.5 angstrom units). In previous years, wavelengths for electromagnetic radiation were often given in angstrom units (abbreviated Å). One angstrom unit is equal to 10^{-8} cm or 1/10 nanometer. All electromagnetic wavelengths longer than that of x-rays interact with matter primarily as a wave phenomenon.

The wave concept of electromagnetic radiations explains why these radiations may be reflected, refracted, diffracted, and polarized. However, there are some phenomenon that cannot be explained by the wave concept.

Particle Concept of Electromagnetic Radiation

X-rays behave sometimes as a wave and other times as if they consisted of small particles.

A particle is a discrete bundle of energy called *quantum* or *photon*. These photons travel at the speed of light. The dual nature (waves and particles) is inseparable. For instance, the amount of energy carried by each quantum or photon depends on the frequency (ν) of the radiation. If the frequency (vibrations per second) is doubled, the energy of the photon is doubled.

In 1901, Max Planck, a German physicist, found that a quantum of energy carried by a single photon (photon energy) is directly proportional to the electromagnetic radiation, according to his equation:

$$E = h\nu$$

where E = photon energy
h = Planck's constant
ν = frequency of radiation in question

Although Planck's constant is fundamental in nature, it is not completely understood. The constant has been determined experimentally to be 4.13×10^{-18} keV sec (cgs system) and 6.61×10^{-34} joule* sec (mks system). It is an exceedingly small number.

The electron volt is the preferred unit to measure the energy of x-ray photons. An electron volt is the amount of energy that an electron gains as it is accelerated by a potential difference of one volt. X-ray energies are usually measured in terms of kilo-electron-volts. X-rays are usually discussed in terms of energy rather than their wavelengths; however, the two are related as follows:

$$c = \lambda\nu \text{ or } \nu = c/\lambda$$

and
$$E = h\nu$$

Substituting c/λ for ν:
$$E = hc/\lambda$$

---

*The joule is the unit of work and energy equal to one newton expended along a distance of one meter (a newton is a unit of force that when applied to a mass of 1 kilogram will accelerate it one meter per second per second).

When the unit of energy (E) is in keV and the wavelength λ is in angstrom units, the product of Planck's constant (h) and the velocity of light (c) is equal to 12.4. The final equation showing the relationship between energy and wavelength is —

$$E = 12.4/\lambda$$

where E = energy in keV
λ = wavelengths in angstrom (Å) units

Table 2-V shows the relationship between wavelength of x-rays and its energy.

Table 2-V

RELATIONSHIP BETWEEN WAVELENGTH AND ENERGY

Wavelength (Å)	Energy (keV)
.0005	24,800
.08	155
.10	124
	(x-rays)
1.24	10
100	.124
4000	.003
	(Ultraviolet light)

Adapted from Table 1-1, Christensen, E.E., et al.: *An Introduction to the Physics of Diagnostic Radiology*. Philadelphia, Lea & Febiger, 1978.

It takes fifteen or more electron-volts of energy for a photon to be capable of ionizing atoms and molecules. X-rays, gamma rays, and some ultraviolet rays have photon energies high enough to be called ionizing radiations.

What Are X-Rays?

X-rays are weightless packages of pure energy (photons), are without electrical charge, and travel in waves with specific frequency at a speed of 3×10^{10} cm/sec. Their energies depend upon the frequency of their wavelengths. The greater the frequency of the wavelength, the greater will be the energy of the photon.

Properties of X-Rays

To gain more understanding of x-rays, it is necessary for you to know a little more of how they act and what they do. Fundamentally, x-rays obey all of the laws of light, but among their special properties some are of interest to the student of dental radiography.

1. X-rays are invisible and weightless. You cannot see, hear, feel, or smell them.
2. X-rays travel in straight lines. They can be deflected from their original direction, but the new trajectory is linear.
3. X-rays travel at the speed of light (3×10^8 m/sec). 186,000 miles/second
4. X-rays have a wide range of wavelengths, 0.1 A- 0.5A, or 0.01- 0.05 mm, in length.
5. X-rays cannot be focused to a point.
6. Because of their extremely short wavelength, they are able to penetrate materials that absorb or reflect visible light.
7. X-rays are differentially absorbed by matter. This absorption depends on the atomic structure of the matter and the wavelength of the x-rays. It is this property that produces an image on a photographic film, which in turn can be made visible by chemical development.
8. They cause certain substances to fluoresce, that is, to emit radiation of longer wavelength (for example, visible and ultraviolet radiation). It is this property that makes it possible to use intensifying screens in radiography.
9. They produce biologic changes valuable in radiation therapy, but necessitating caution in the use of

x-radiation.
10. They can ionize gases, that is, remove electrons from atoms to form ions, which can be used for measuring and controlling exposure (ionization chambers).

These special properties have application in dental, medical, and industrial radiography, raidation therapy, and research.

PRODUCTION OF X-RAYS

X-rays are generated when fast-moving electrons (small particles, each bearing a negative electrical charge) collide with matter in any form (Fig. 2-14). X-ray production is a process of energy conversion when electrons are suddenly decelerated in the target of the x-ray tube.

The x-ray machine contains three important parts: the **x-ray tube,** the **generator,** and the **exposure timer.**

X-Ray Tube

The x-ray tube used in dental radiography is called the "hot cathode" or Coolidge tube. The tube is sealed in a lead glass envelope, from which air has been pumped, and which contains two important parts — the cathode and the anode (Fig. 2-15). The air is removed

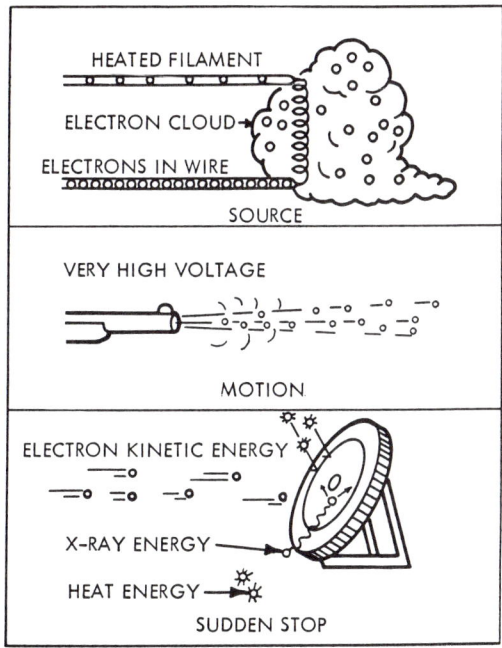

Figure 2-14. the sudden decelaration or stoppage of rapidly moving electrons forms heat energy and x-ray energy. Three things are needed to produce x-rays: (1) source of electrons, (2) high voltage potential, and (3) a target of high atomic number for electrons to strike.

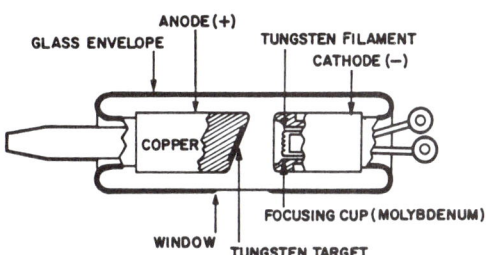

Figure 2-15. Simple stationary-anode x-ray tube. Diagram shows the relation of the anode (target) and the cathode (filament) to each other.

from the tube to prevent ionization of gas molecules, wich would reduce the speed of the electron movement toward the tungsten target. The basic principles of the "hot cathode" tube are as follows:

1. The filament must be heated for a source of electrons. The higher the temperature, the more electrons are freed by **thermionic** emission

(Fig. 2-16), which may be defined as the emmission of electrons resulting from the absorption of thermal energy. A pure tungsten filament must be heated to a temperature of at least 2200°C to emit a useful number of electrons.

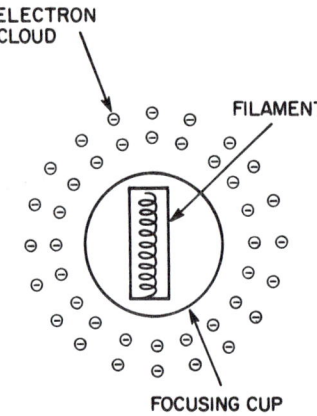

Figure 2-16. Electrons emitted from the tungsten filament form a small cloud in the immediate vicinity of the filament.

2. When the kilovoltage is applied, electrons are driven from the filament (cathode) to the targed (anode).
3. If the kilovoltage supplies the electrons with enough speed, x-rays will be produced when the electrons hit the target.

Cathode

The cathode of the x-ray tube is the negative terminal of the tube and consists of a tungsten wire (filament) wound in the form of a spiral set in a molybdenum cup-shaped holder (called a focusing cup) (*see* Fig. 2-15).

Tungsten is used for the filament because it has a high melting point (3370°C) and can be drawn into a thin wire (0.2 mm in diameter) and still remain quite strong. When the filament is heated to a "glowing hot" temperature (at least 2200°C), some of the outer shell electrons of the atoms of the tungsten acquire enough thermal energy to move a short distance from the surface of the wire. Their escape is referred to as the phenomenon of **thermionic emission (therm** standing for heat, **ionic** for ionized atoms of the filament, and **emission** for discharge of electrons from the surface of the filament).

The electrons emitted or "boiled off" from the tungsten filament form a small **electron cloud** or **space charge** in the immediate space surrounding the filament.

If a large potential difference (for example, 90 kVp) is applied across the tube, giving the filament a 45 kVp negative charge and the anode target an equal 45 kVp positive charge, the resulting strong electron field would cause the "electron cloud" electrons to accelerate at very high speeds (approximately half the speed of light) across a 1-3 cm gap to the target of the anode. Electron current across an x-ray tube is always in one direction only (cathode to anode). The number of x-rays (quantity) that will eventually be produced depends on the number of elecrtrons that flow from the filament to the target of the anode.

Dental x-ray machines utilize either 10 mA or 15 mA current. The higher the mA the more electrons that will be available, and of course, the more x-rays produced in a unit of time.

Cathode Focusing Cup

The cathode focusing cup is needed to focus the electrons to an acceptable area on the target of a required shape and size. If the focusing cup was not used, the electron stream because of the forces of mutual repulsion and the great numbers of electrons involved (10mA = 10^{16} electrons) would bombard an unacceptable large area of the anode of the x-ray tube. The focusing cup is usually made of molybdenum, and it is designed to direct the electrons to a certain area on the target of the anode. It has a negative potential (the same as the filament) when the electron current is flowing from the cathode to the anode (Fig. 2-17).

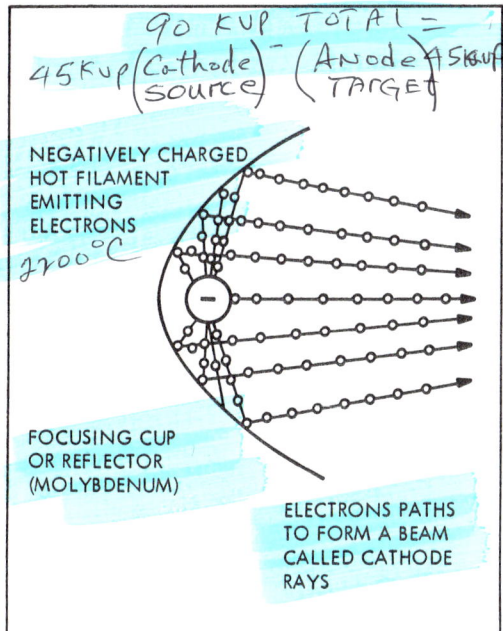

Figure 2-17. the focusing of the electron stream by the molybdenum focusing cup of the cathode. it is negatively charged when the electrons are flowing and is designed to direct the electrons to an acceptable spot on the target of the anode. (Courtesy of General Electric Company.)

Anode

The anode is the positive side of the x-ray tube. There are two types of anodes — the stationary anode used in dental x-ray machines and the rotating anode used in the larger medical x-ray machines.

The Stationary Anode

The stationary anode usually consists of a small tungsten plate, 2-3 mm thick, embedded in a mass of the copper. The tungsten plate is either square or rectangular in shape with each side greater than 1 cm; it is called the target of the anode. Tungsten is chosen for the target because it has a high atomic number (74), which makes it more efficient in the production of X-Rays, and it has a high melting point (3370°C) to withstand the high temperature produced. It also provides a reasonably good metal for the absorption of heat and the rapid loss of heat from the target area.

The small area of the target that most of the electrons strike is called the **focal spot** and is the source of the x-radiaton. The size of the focal spot has a very important effect upon the sharpness of the x-ray film image. The smaller the focal spot, the sharper the x-ray image. However, the smaller the focal spot becomes the less heat the focal spot will be able to absorb at one time. Some method had to be found to obtain a practical size of the focal spot that would provide image detail. The **Benson line focus** principle developed in 1918 is such a method and is employed in the stationary anode tubes (Fig. 2-18).

The target face is made at an angle of 15-20 degrees to the cathode as shown in the diagram. As the angle of the anode is made smaller, the projected focal spot also becomes smaller. When the rectangular focal spot is viewed from below — in the position of the film — it appears more nearly square. This is called the "effective focal spot." Thus, the projected focus or "effective focal spot" is only a fraction of the size of the actual focal spot. By using x-rays that emerge at this angle, **radiographic definition** is improved while the **heat capacity** of the anode is increased because the electron stream is spread over a greater area. The "effective focal spot" of most dental x-ray tubes measures approximately 0.8-1.5 sq. mm depending upon the manufacturer.

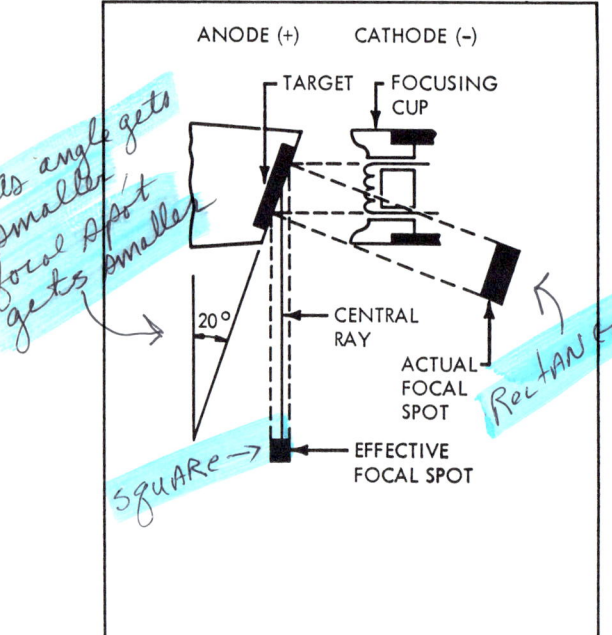

Figure 2-18. Diagram showing how use of the line focus principle and a 20 degree angle f the target face of thea node provides a small effective focal spot. (Copyright Eastman Kodak Company, Rochester, NY. Reprinted by permission.)

Rotating Anode

As larger x-ray machines were built, the limiting factor became the x-ray tube itself. The stationary x-ray anode could only withstand a certain amount of heat, so the rotating anode principle was developed to produce anodes capable of withstanding the heat generated by large electron exposures.

This type of anode has the tungsten target rotating at approximately 3,000 rpm during the bombardment of the electrons. In this way the electrons are still focused to a certain small area, but the surface that they are striking is always new. Because of this the heat is not concentrated in one particular area but is spread over a much larger area.

The tungsten disc is beveled at an angle of 6-20 degrees. The bevel is used to take advantage of the line focus principle (Fig. 2-19).

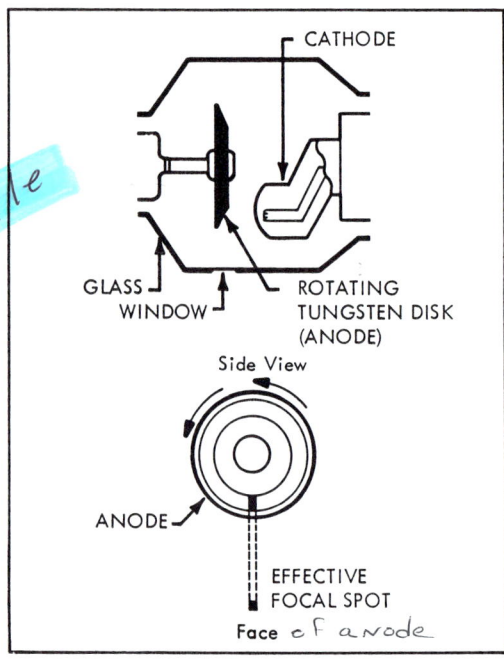

Figure 2-19. Diagram of side view (upper) and face of rotating anode (bottom). (Copyright Eastman Kodak company, Rochester, NY. Reprinted by permission.)

X-ray Generator

The x-ray generator of the x-ray machine supplies the electrical power to the x-ray tube. The x-ray generator begins with an electrical source of energy (usually 110 or 220 volts and 60 Hz alternating current) and then modifies it to supply the needs of the x-ray tube.

In order to understand how the generator works, we should first review some basic electrical physics because x-rays are produced by the use of electricity.

Electricity

Electric current or electricity is the flow of electrons through an electric conductor very much like water flowing through a pipe. If the electrons are made to flow in one direction along a conductor, the electrical current is called direct current or DC (Fig. 20). Most applications of electricity in radiology require the electrons to flow first in one direction and then in the opposite direction. Current in which electrons oscillate back and forth is called alternating current or AC (Fig. 2-21).

The term "cycle" in AC refers to the curve above and below the horizontal line. The number of cycles per second is called the frequency of AC. Each cycle consists of two alternations; that is, the voltage starts at 0, rises gradually to the maximum in one direction called the kV peak, and finally returns to 0. These are 120 alternations per second with 60 cycle current. However, only 60 alternations per second are useable in the self-rectified x-ray tubes. This is because only half of the available cycle is used to produce x-rays (Fig. 2-22). Rectification, which is a

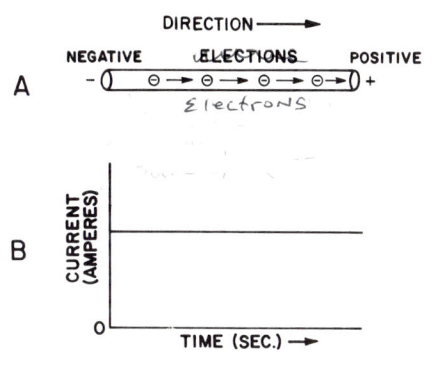

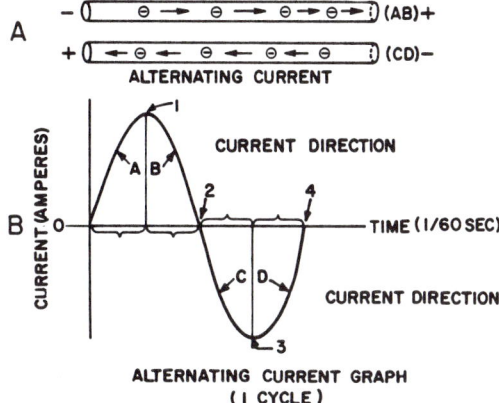

Figure 2-20. (A) In direct current (DC), electrons flow in one direction only. (B) Graph of associated wave form of direct current. The distance between the horizontal line and the time axis represents the magnitude or velocity of the electrons. (Adapted from Bushong, Stewart: *Radiologic Science for Technologists.* St. Louis, C.F. Mosby, 1975).

Figure 2-21. Alternating current (AC). (A) Electrons flow in one direction and alternately in the opposite direction, always from the negative to the positive pole. (B) Example of a sine wave of alternating current. Note that electrons flow first in positive direction and then in a negative direction (below the 0 axis). At point 0 the electrons are at rest and increase in velocity during segment A. When they reach maximum velocity they are at point 1, where the electrons begin to slow down in segment B. They come to rest again at point 2, they then reverse motion, and flow of the electrons begins again in a negative direction. At point 4 the cycle ends, which takes 1/60 second in 60 hetz (cycles/sec) current.

process of changing alternating current into direct current, will be covered more fully when we discuss the production of x-rays.

There are three factors that characterize a simple electrical circuit. These are **potential difference, current, and resistance. Potential difference** may be defined as a difference in electrical potential energy between two points in an electric current due to excess of electrons at one point relative to the other. The unit of potential difference or electrical pressure is the **volt,** which is defined as the **potential difference** that will cause a current of one ampere to flow in a circuit where **resistance** is one ohm. The kilovolt (kV) is equal to 1,000 volts.

The second factor in an electrical circuit is **current,** which is defined

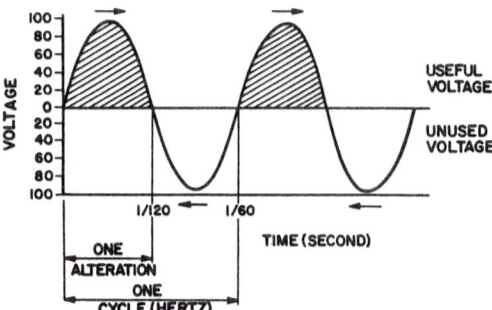

Figure 2-22. Self-rectified current used in dental radiography. Alternating current is a 60-cycle current — it flows first in one direction and then it flows in the opposite direction, changing directions every 1/120 second. It makes a complete cycle every 1/60 second. In the dental x-ray tube, the anode is first positive and then negative with respect to the cathode during each half-cycle (1/120 sec). When anode is positive, the electrons flow by attraction to anode; when the anode is negative, the electrons are not attracted to the node, hence, no current flows in the tube.

as the amount of electricity (electrons) flowing per second through a conductor (wire). In a water pipe, this would be the amount of water flowing past a given point in one second. The unit of current is the **ampere,** which may be defined as the quantity of electrons representing 6.3×10^{18} free electrons flowing through a conductor in one second. The number of electrons involved is enormous. A milliampere is equal to 1/1000 of an ampere.

The third factor of the electrical circuit is **resistance** and is a property of the materials of the circuit itself. Electrical resistance is that property of a circuit that opposes or hinders the flow of an electrical current (electrons). The unit of electrical resistance is the **ohm,** defined as the resistance of a standard volume of mercury under standard conditions.

There is a definite relationship between potential difference (volts), current (amperes), and resistance (ohms) when a steady direct current is flowing in an electrical circuit. The relationship is expressed in Ohm's Law (named after the German physicist, Georg Ohm) which is represented by the following formula:

$$I = V/R \text{ or } V = IR$$

where I = current in amperes
V = potential difference in volts
R = resistance in ohms

The x-ray tube requires electrical energy for two purposes: (1) to boil electrons from the x-ray filament and (2) to accelerate and direct these electrons from the cathode to the anode. The x-ray generator has a separate current for each of these functions, which will be referred to as (1) the filament circuit and (2) the high voltage circuit.

The third circuit of the x-ray generator is the timer mechanism, which regulates the length of exposure, which we will discuss later in this chapter. These three circuits are interrelated.

The x-ray generator is contained in two separate compartments: the control panel (box) and the tube head assembly. The control panel contains the main off-and-on switch, the exposure button, mA selector control, kVp selector control, time selector, x-ray emission light, and pilot light (see Fig. 2-53A and 2-53C).

The tube head assembly of the x-ray generator contains a low-voltage transformer, high voltage transformer, and x-ray tube (see Fig. 2-53B and 2-53D). Since the potential difference in these circuits may be as high as 100,000 volts, the transformers and x-ray tube are emersed in oil. The oil functions as an insulator and prevents sparking from one electrical component to another in the tube head.

Transformer

By definition a transformer is an electromagnetic device that changes an alternating current from low voltage to high voltage or from high voltage to low voltage without loss of appreciable amount of energy (less than 10%).

The flow of electrons represents a current, and it is produced by potential difference. The terms potential difference and voltage are synonyms and are used interchangeably.

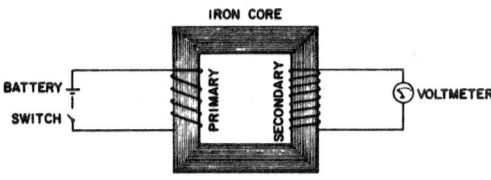

Figure 2-23. A closed core step-up transformer. Current is induced in the secondary coil by rapidly increasing or decreasing the magnetic field created by the current in the primary coil.

A transformer is composed of two wire coils wrapped around the opposite ends of an iron core (Fig. 2-23). The first coil circuit is called the primary circuit or input side, and the second coil circuit is called the secondary circuit or output side. When current flows through the primary circuit and coil, it produces a magnetic field within the magnetic core, and the magnetic field induces a current in the secondary coil and circuit. However, current will not flow in the secondary or output circuit unless the magnetic field is changing (either decreasing or increasing); the current will **not** flow if the magnetic field is in a stable state.

Alternating current is used for transformers because in alternating current the voltage changes continuously so it produces a continuously changing magnetic field. Therefore, this change in the potential difference in magnitude and polarity of the alternating current in the primary coil induces an alternating current in the secondary coil (*see* Fig. 2-22).

Laws of Transformers

There are two laws that govern the actions of transformers. They are as follows:

1. The voltage induced in the secondary coil is to the voltage in the primary coil as the number of turns in the secondary coil is to the number of turns in the primary coil. It is expressed as shown below:

$$\frac{Vs}{Vp} = \frac{Ns}{Np}$$

where Vs = voltage in secondary coil
Vp = voltage in primary coil
Ns = number of turns in the secondary coil
Np = number of turns in primary coil

This means that if the number of turns in the secondary coil is twice the number in the primary coil, then the voltage in the secondary coil will be twice the voltage in the primary. A **step-up** transformer has more turn in the secondary coil than the primary coil (Figs. 2-23 and 2-24). A transformer with fewer turns in the secondary coil than in the primary coil decreases the voltage and is called a **step-down** transformer (Fig. 2-25).

2. The second law of transformers states that the product of the voltage and the current in the two circuits must be equal. According to the law of conservation of energy, there can be no more energy coming out of the

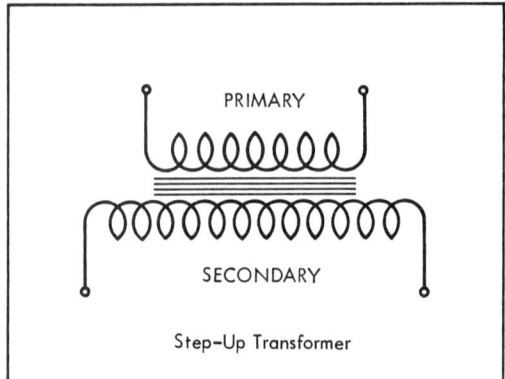

Figure 2-24. Step-up transformer. (Courtesy of General Electric Company.)

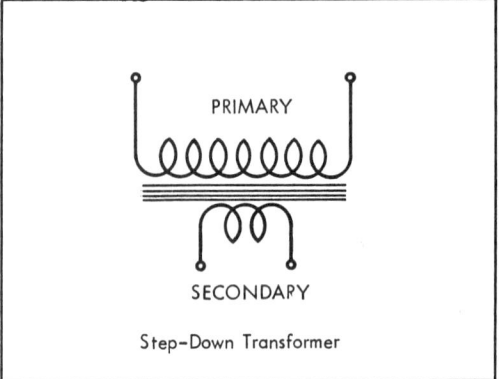

Figure 2-25. Step-down transformer. (Courtesy of General Electric Company.)

transformer than the amount of energy that entered the transformer in the first place.

The second law of transformers is represented by this formula:

$$IsVs = IpVp$$

where Is = current in amperes in the secondary coil
Ip = current in amperes in the primary coil
Vs = voltage in the secondary coil
Vp = voltage in the primary coil

Thus, in dental x-ray equipment, the step-up transformer takes 110 or 120 voltage current and increases this voltage to 65,000 to 100,000 volts (60 × 100 kVp) thereby providing the high voltage necessary to drive the electrons to the x-ray tube at speed. At the same time it must decrease the current to 10 to 15 thousandths of an ampere (milliampere) to follow the law of conservation of energy.

Example of Step-up Transformer in High Voltage Circuit

Primary
150 volts ×
9 amperes =

Secondary
90,000 volts ×
.015 amperes =
90 kVp × 15 mA

Example of Step-down Transformer in Filament Circuit

Primary
150 volts ×
.20 amperes
(200 mA) =

Secondary
10 volts ×
3 amperes

These two laws of transformers assume 100 percent efficiency; however, in practice the efficiency is more likely to be 90-95 percent with about 5-10 percent less power output (product of voltage and current in watts) than power input, the loss appearing as heat.

As stated previously, there are two electrical circuits necessary in the x-ray machine to produce x-rays in the x-ray tube. the first is the **filament circuit,** which provides a source of electrons by heating the filament to incandescence to "boil off" the electrons from the filament of the cathode. The second circuit is the **high voltage** necessary to accelerate the electrons from the cathode to the anode at high speeds.

The Filament Circuit

The filament circuit regulates the current flow to the filament of the x-ray tube.

The filament is a thin coiled wire. The filament circuit contains a variable resistor (rheostat) and a step-down transformer. (Fig. 2-26). The variable resistor is in the primary circuit of the step-down transformer and is the mA selector of x-ray exposure. It controls the amount of current that flows through the x-ray filament (Fig. 2-27). If the variable resistance is increased, the current in the filament circuit decreases so there is less heating of the filament, a smaller electron emission, which results in a much smaller tube current.

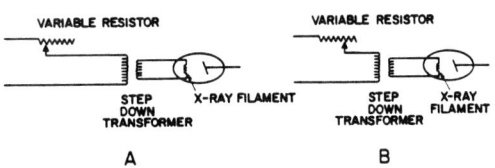

Figure 2-27. Diagram of filament circuit where resistance setting in A filament of a circuit is smaller value than in the B filament circuit. In the A filament circuit a larger current flows, resulting in higher heating of the filament and a larger electron cloud; in turn, more electrons are emitted from the filament which results in more x-rays.

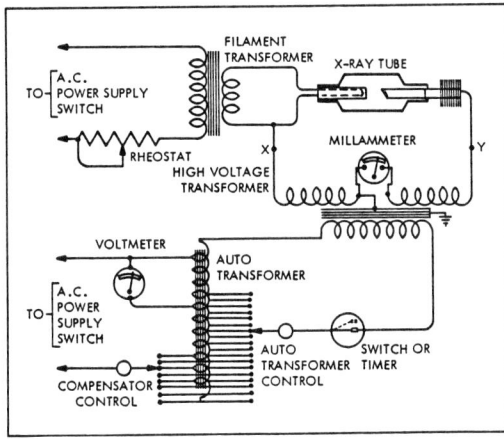

Figure 2-26. Schematic drawing of a dental self-rectified x-ray current showing filament and high voltage circuits.

The step-down transformer in the filament circuit reduces the potential different (110 or 220 volts) in the primary coil to 8-12 volts in the secondary coil, which results in a high current of 3-6 amperes to heat the current.

Although the current (amperes) in the filament circuit only heats the filament and does not represent the current (mA) across the x-ray tube, it actually increases the x-ray tube current (cathode to anode electrons) by increasing the filament temperature. A hotter filament emits more electrons, and electrons represent the current (mA) through the tube.

High Voltage Circuit

The high voltage circuit has two transformers: an autotransformer and a step-up transformer.

As you remember, the step-up transformer has a fixed ratio of voltage output to voltage input. Therefore, because the voltage input is fixed at 110 or 220 volts depending on the power supply and type of equipment, only a fixed single kilovoltage output would be available to the dentist, which would seriously limit the higher range of dental radiographic techniques, since various kilovoltages are necessary to obtain beams with a variety of penetrating abilities. Although in dental radiography you will find x-ray machines with fixed kVp such as 65 or 70 kVp, it is an advantage to have an x-ray machine in which you can vary the kilovoltage.

The kilovoltage can be varied by the use of an autotransformer. The autotransformer is an electromagnetic device that operates on the principle of self-induction. A single coil of insulated wire is wound around a large iron core, which serves as both the primary and secondary coil, the number of turns being adjustable.

At regular intervals along the coil, the insulation is interrupted and the bare points connected or tapped to metal buttons. By moving a metal conductor to various metal taps on the wire, the number of turns included in the secondary circuit of the autotransformer is varied, which in turn varies the output voltage. Therefore, the autotransformer serves as a kVp selector because it varies the kVp available to the primary coil of the step-up transformer (Fig. 2-28).

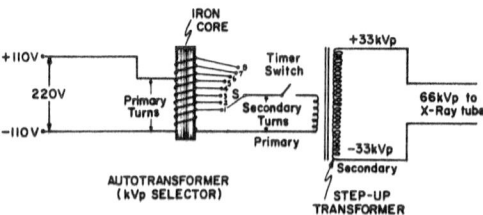

Figure 2-28. Diagram of the high voltage circuit. In the autotransformer only a single coil is used. If the kVp selector (S) is placed at 1 as shown, the autotransformer has a 7/3 ratio, that is, the voltage is being stepped down. If S is turned to 6, the ratio now becomes 7/8 and the voltage is stepped up. By varying the voltage input into the primary coil of the step-up transformer, the kVp of the x-ray machine can also be varied.

The step-up (high voltage) transformer has many more turns in the secondary coil than the primary coil, and it increases the voltage to a factor as high as approximately 450 with a potential difference as high as 100,000 volts in some x-ray machines. This is why it is important to imerse the transformer assembly in oil for maximum insulation. The switch that controls the high voltage circuit is located between the autotransformer and the high voltage transformer (see Fig. 2-28). This switch begins and ends the x-ray exposure. The switch is operated by a timing mechanism, which will be discussed later in this chapter.

Rectification

Although transformers operate on alternating current, the x-ray tube requires direct current. Rectification is the process of converting alternating voltage into direct voltage, or therefore alternating current into direct current. The device that produces the change is called a rectifier.

Although the current is still alternating, the electrical circuits that we have been describing can produce x-rays by a process called self-rectification. The x-ray tube acts as the rectifier and changes AC to DC. Self-rectification is used in dental x-ray units and small, mobile medical x-ray units, but even these are now being replaced with more sophisticated methods of rectification.

In self-rectified circuits, the potential between the cathode and anode changes back and forth from positive to negative sixty times each second or one cycle every 1/60 second. During the positive half cycle of the AC curve when the cathode is negative and the anode is positive, electrons flow between the two, and x-rays are produced. During the negative half cycle, when the anode is negative and the cathode (filament) is positive and despite the presence of high voltage, the current will not flow from the anode to the cathode, in the wrong direction, because no electron cloud exists about the anode. Therefore, by blocking the current in the negative half cycle of AC, and x-ray tube changes AC into DC, so in effect it is a rectifier.

When only half of the electrical wave is used to produce x-rays, this wave-form is called half-wave rectification (see Fig. 2-22).

Diode Rectification

As it becomes necessary for x-ray tubes to carry more power, as in the larger medical x-ray units, it is desirable to prevent them from operating as self-rectifiers and to find some means of preventing the inverse voltage from being applied to the x-ray tube. This is accomplished by introducing diodes into the high-voltage circuit. This results in maximum efficiency of the equipment. Of course, the AC must be rectified in the secondary circuit of the step-up transformer because a transformer will not function with direct current in the primary circuit. Until recently, all diode (two electrodes) rectifiers were valve tubes, very similar to x-ray tubes. The cathode and anode in valve tube rectifiers are constructed differently so x-rays are not emitted. Recently the valve-tube has been replaced in x-ray machines by solid-state silicon rectifiers. They have several advantages over valve-tubes. They are smaller than valve-tubes and do not require a heated filament, which prolongs the life of the rectifier.

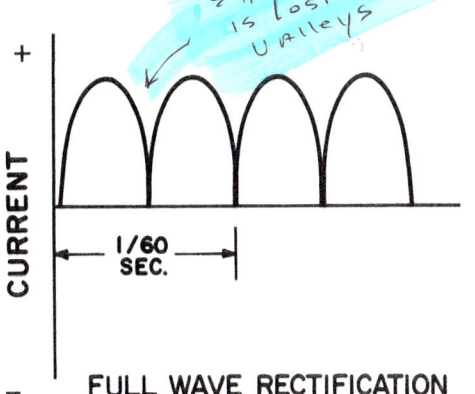

Figure 2-29. Electrical waves formed from full-wave rectification. The pulsed x-ray output of a full-wave rectified x-ray unit occures 120 times each second instead of 60 times per second as with half-wave rectification.

Full-wave Rectification

Full-wave rectification is employed in all modern medical x-ray machines because it utilizes the full potential of the electrical supply. In full-wave rectification, both halves of the alternating voltage are used to produce x-rays, which allows for a greater x-ray output per unit of time. It is twice as large as with half-wave rectification (Fig. 2-29). In full-wave rectification at least four diodes are used: two diodes conduct current during the positive half cycle and two diodes conduct current during the negative half cycle. The cathode is always negative and the anode always positive even though the induced voltage of the step-up transformer secondary circuit alternates between positive and negative. The major disadvantage of pulsed full-wave rectification is that exposure time is lost in the valley between the two pulses.

Half-wave and full-wave forms are produced by single-phase electric power, and it results in a pulsating x-ray beam. One method to overcome this discrepancy is to generate three simultaneous voltage wave forms out of step with each other. Thus a three-phase generator will produce voltage across the x-ray tube in a nearly constant exposure. There will be no deep valley between pulses. Three-phase power is becoming more popular in both angiography and routine medical radiography (Fig. 2-30).

Exposure Timers

X-ray exposure timers have gone through a series of improvements during the years. All the various types of exposure timers are still in use from the simple mechanical timers to the highly complicated automatic electronic timers, so we will discuss each of them briefly.

Mechanical Timer. The simple mechanical timer is the hand-held timer found on the older dental x-ray units. When the button is pushed, it closes the circuit and allows the current to flow. When the exposure time is expended, the circuit is broken. These timers are usually inaccurate for exposure times of less than one second.

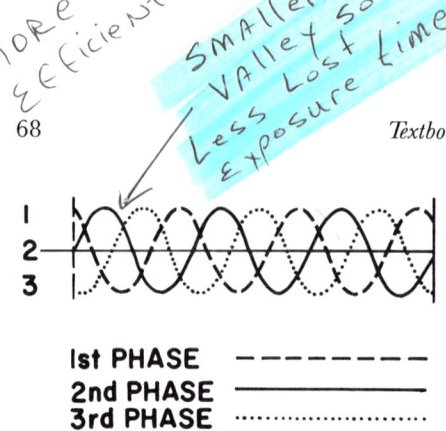

1st PHASE ---------
2nd PHASE ————
3rd PHASE ....

THREE-PHASE ALTERNATING WAVE-FORM

Figure 2-30. Three-phase power is a more efficient way to produce x-rays than single phase power because the effective voltage is almost constant as shown in the above waveform.

timer uses a synchronous motor. It is called a synchronous timer because the motor that runs it must rotate at the same speed as the alternating current or generator that supplies the power. It is limited because of this fact and cannot be faster than the generator running it. These are accurate to 0.1 second.

Electronic Timers. As more powerful generators were developed, the exposure times became too short to be controlled by synchronous timers. Electronic timers were developed to meet this need. Electronic timers are capable of delivering extremely accurate x-ray exposures as short as 1 millisecond (1/1000 sec). Electronic timers can be placed within either the primary or the secondary circuit of the high voltage transformer circuit.

Synchronous Timer. The synchronous

ELECTRON INTERACTIONS AT THE ANODE TUNGSTEN TARGET

X-rays are produced when fast moving electrons from the filament of the x-ray tube interact with the tungsten target of the anode and convert their kinetic energy into x-rays. Kinetic energy is the energy of motion.

The kinetic energy (KE) of an electron flowing from the cathode to the anode is determined by its electronic charge (e) and the voltage (v) or potential difference across the x-ray tube. It can be expressed by —

$$\text{Kinetic energy} = e \times \text{volts}$$
$$\text{(kiloelectron volts)} \quad \text{(charge)} \quad \text{(kilovolts)}$$

Since the electronic charge (e) of the electron does not change (e = 1.6×10^{-19} coulombs), it is obvious that changing the voltage (kilovolts) will change the kinetic energy (kiloelectron volts) of the electron. Voltage in an x-ray machine is expressed in kilovoltage peak (kVp). At this time we must make the distinction between kVp and keV (kiloelectron-volts). For instance, 100 kVp means that the maximum voltage causing the acceleration of electrons across the tube is 100,000 volts (100 kVp = 100,000 peak volts).

A kiloelectron-volt signifies the amount of kinetic energy of any one electron in the beam (100 keV = 100,000 electron volts). When operating the x-ray tube at 100 kVp, very few of the electrons acquire the kinetic energy of 100 keV, because the voltage applied pulsates from a lower value to the selected kVp (*see* Fig. 2-22). The kinetic energy of the electron will depend upon the voltage being applied to the tube at that instance. In a single phase, half-wave self-rectified circuit, the useful voltage will vary from 0 to the maximum kVp and back to 0 at the rate of 60 times per second. Therefore, the high-speed electrons striking the target do not have the same kinetic energies because the voltage (v) across the tube that provides the potential to accelerate the electrons is variable. In other words, the energy (eV) of the electrons that encounter the target (anode) covers a broad range of energies.

When the electrons impinge upon the heavy tungsten atoms of the target, they interact with these atoms and transfer their kinetic energy to the target metal. These interactions occur within a very small depth of penetration of the target metal. As the kinetic energy of each electron becomes expended, they slow down and nearly come to rest, at which time they can be conducted through the x-ray anode assembly and out into the associated circuits.

The electron interacts either with the orbital electrons or the nuclei of the tungsten atoms. These interactions result in conversion of kinetic energy into thermal energy and electromagnetic energy in the form of x-radiation. Nearly all of the kinetic energy of the impinging electrons in converted into heat.

The impinging electrons interact with the outer shell electrons of the tungsten atoms, but they do not transfer enough energy to these outer shell electrons to ionize them (eject electron from its orbit). Actually, the outer shell electrons are simply raised to an excited or higher energy level, then they immediately drop back to their normal energy state with the emission of heat (infrared radiation). This constant **excitation** and restabilization of the outer shell electrons of the tungsten atoms generates an enormous amount of heat in the anode of the x-ray tube (Fig. 2-31).

The efficiency of x-ray production of the modern x-ray tube is very low. At 80 kV only about 0.6 percent of this energy is converted to x-rays while the remaining 99.4 percent appears as heat; besides this, only 1/1000 of the kinetic energy of the projected electrons eventually result in useful radiation because x-rays are emitted in all directions from the target; only a small part of these x-rays leave the window of the x-ray tube and become the useful x-ray beam (Fig. 2-32).

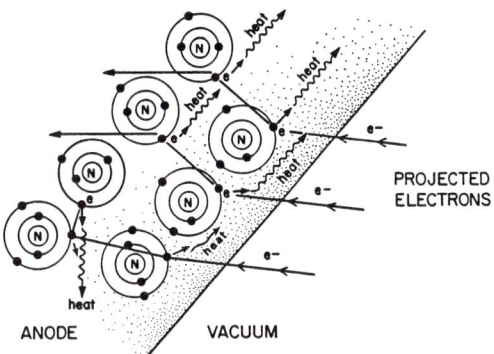

Figure 2-31. Almost all the kinetic energy of the projected electrons is converted into infrared radiation (heat). These interactions are primarily an excitation interaction rather than ionization interaction.

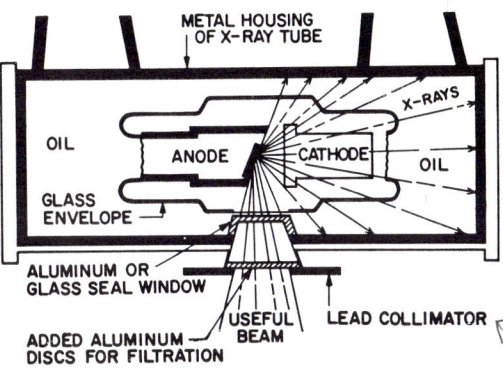

Figure 2-32. Since x-rays radiate in straight lines in all directions from the source, there is a need for a metal housing for the tube. Approximately 1/1000 of the kinetic energy converted into x-rays comprises the useful beam emitted frm the window of the x-ray tube. The added aluminum serves to filter out the long wavelength is used to limit the beam size to reduce patient x-rays exposure.

The efficiency of x-ray production is

independent of tube current (mA) but will increase by increasing the voltage, which will increase the energy of the projected electrons. At 60 kVp only 0.5 percent of the electron kinetic energy is converted to x-rays, at 80 kVp it is 0.6 percent, and at 20 MeV (large medical therapy machines) it is 70 percent.

Electron Interactions with Anode Tungsten Target Atom to Produce X-rays

When high speed electrons lose their energy in the target of the anode, x-rays are produced by two different processes.

The first process involves interaction of the projected electrons with the nucleus of the tungsten atoms producing x-rays that are called **general radiation** or **bremsstrahlung** (Brems radiation).

The other process involves the collision of one of the high-speed electrons and the electrons of the inner shell (K or L shells) of the tungsten atoms producing x-rays called **characteristic radiation**. It is called characteristic radiation because the energy of the x-rays produced are characteristic of the target element (tungsten) and the involved shells (K or L shells).

General Radiation (Bremsstrahlung)

Most of the x-rays produced by the dental x-ray machine are called **bremsstrahlung, brems, white,** or **general radiation**. Bremsstrahlung is derived from two German words: **bremse** meaning "brake" and **strahl** meaning "ray." It is called "braking radiation" because the radiation is produced by "braking" or deceleration of high-speed electrons. A projected electron that completely avoids the orbital electrons of an atom of the tungsten target may come sufficiently close to the nucleus to become under its influence. Since the electron is negatively charged and the nucleus positively charged, there is an electrostatic attraction between them. As the electron approaches the nucleus it is influenced by a nuclear force, which is stronger than the electrostatic attraction of the electron and the nucleus. Thus, the electron slows down and is deflected from its original course, thereby losing some of its kinetic energy (Fig. 2-33a). The kinetic energy lost by the electron is limited directly in the form of photon raidation (x-radiation).

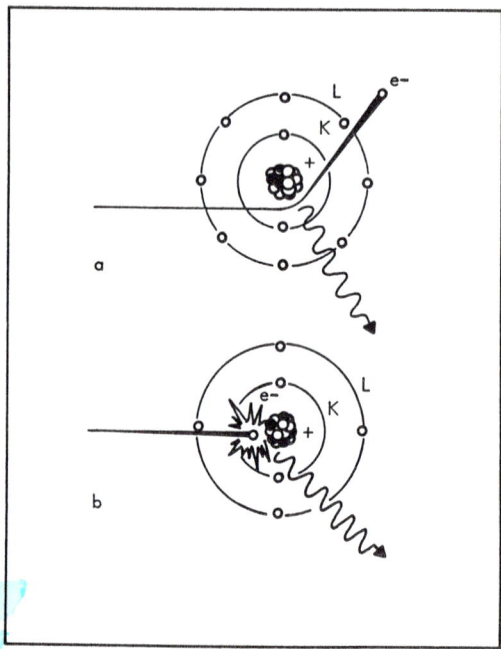

Figure 2-33. Generation of general or white radiation (Bramsstrahlung) produced by interaction of an electron with a tungsten atom nucleus: **(A)** impinging electron deflected and decelerated by nucleons, **(B)** occasionally total kinetic energy of impinging electron is converted into x-radiation. (Courtesy of Dr. Michel Ter-Pogassian.)

Most of the electrons that strike the target will give up their energy by reactions with many atoms before coming to rest. Each time an electron is decelerated, it give only a part of its energy. The electron will penetrate many layers of atoms of the target material before giving up all its energy. Therefore, not all of the x-rays are produced on the surface of the target. A fraction of the electrons approach the nucleus head-on and are completely stopped by the electrostatic field. In this collision all the energy of the electron appears as a single x-ray photon (Fig. 2-33b).

Brems radiation is heterogeneous or polyenergetic, that is, **not** uniform in energy and wavelength. There are two factors that produce this wide distribution in the energy of radiation produced by the "braking" phenomenon. **First** the electrons in a majority of the cases will undergo many reactions before coming to rest. With each deceleration a corresponding amount of kinetic energy is converted in photons of equivalent energy. As the deceleration or "braking" varies, so does the energy of the photons of x-radiation. The **second factor** is that the impinging electrons have widely different energies. As the applied kV varies, so will the energy of the impinging electrons. In a self-rectified half-wave 60 cycle alternating current operated at 100 kVp, very few of the electrons will acquire the kinetic energy of 100 keV because the voltage pulsates from a low value to the peak value of 100 kVp. The energy of the electron will depend upon the voltage being applied at that particular instance (Fig. 2-34).

In review, the energies emitted from x-ray photons from the "braking" of electrons in an electric field varies. The variation is produced because the impinging electrons that reach the target have different energies, and also because most of these impinging electrons give up their kinetic energies in stages. The highest energy photons are dictated by the kilovoltage peak used. The lower energy

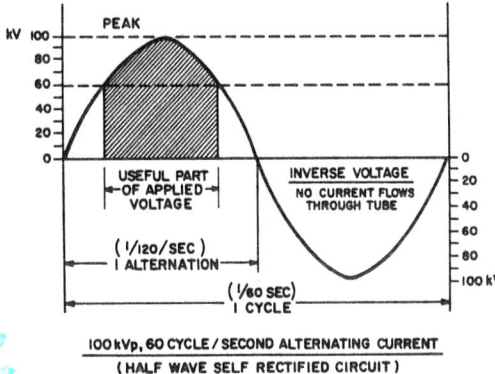

100 kVp, 60 CYCLE/SECOND ALTERNATING CURRENT
(HALF WAVE SELF RECTIFIED CIRCUIT)

Figure 2-34. Voltage during the useful voltage of aalteration of each cycle will vary from a low value to a peak value. The energy of the impinging electrons will vary according to the voltage applied at the instance the electrons are projected toward the target of the anode.

(long wavelengths) photons produced will probably never reach the patient because they will either be filtered out within the x-ray tubehead (target material, glass, and oil insulation) or by the added aluminum filter placed outside the tubehead exit window. Figure 2-35 is a graph

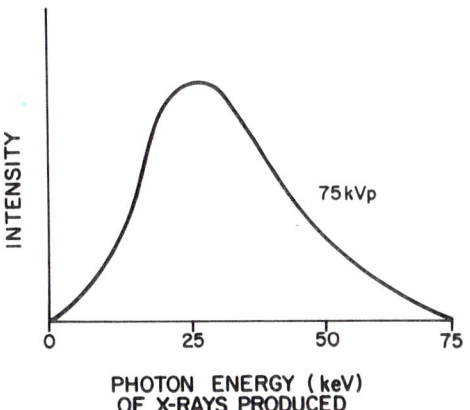

Figure 2-35. The continuous spectrum of x-rays produced by Bremsstrahlung using 75 kVp current. The spectrum extends from 0 to the maximum number of x-rays produced with about 1/3 the photon energy being at the 25 keV level.

of the bremsstrahlung distribution spectrum. It compares the intensity (number of x-rays) with the photon energy of the x-rays produced at a particular kilovoltage. Then, Brems radiation, which makes up the majority of the x-ray beam, is heterogenous, meaning it is comprised of photons of various energies (wavelengths) (Fig. 2-36).

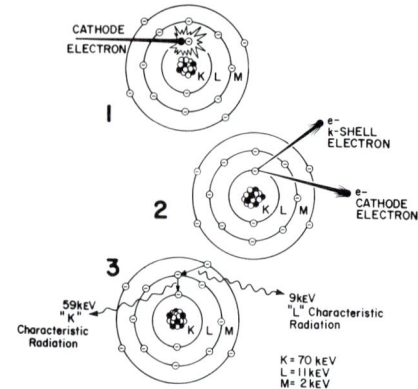

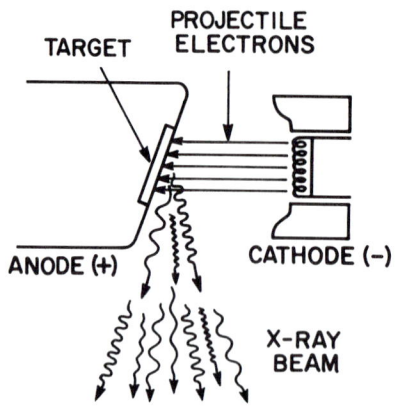

Figure 2-36. Heterogenous beam is composed of photons of various energies (wavelengths).

2nd Type of radiation

Characteristic Radiation

The other process by which X-rays can be produced in an x-ray tube is when the projectile electron has sufficient energy to ionize a target tungsten atom by ejecting an inner orbital electron (example, in K or L shell). To free a K shell electron, work has to be done to overcome the attractive force of the nucleus. The binding energy of an electron in the K shell of tungsten is about 70 keV. Therefore, the projectile electron must have energy of more than 70 keV to eject the K shell electron. Both the K shell electron and the projectile electron leave the atom (Fig. 2-37). A 60 kVp electron will not contain any electrons that will eject a K shell electron from tungsten.

The "hole" or space vacated by the electron is immediately filled by a replacement electron from one of the outer shells of the atom. Usually the "hole" is filled with an electron from the L shell; however, they may come from any of the outer shells.

Figure 2-37. Production of Characteristics x-rays. (1)The incoming cathode electron collides with a K-shell electron of tungsten. (2) Both cathode electron and K-shell electron leave the atom. The atom is now in an "excited" state. (3) An electron from the L-shell jumps from L-shell into K-shell giving the off K characteristics radiation with photon energy of 59 keV. The space left in L-shell is filled by the M-shell electron and L characteristic radiation with photon energy of 9 keV is emitted.

Remember the binding energy of an atomic shell is a negative value; it is the energy that an electron in a shell must be given to raise the energy value to zero. To free a K electron from tungsten, the electron must be given 70 keV of energy, while only 11 keV are required to free an L electron.

When the L electron moves into the space vacated by the K shell electron that was ejected, it results in the emission of energy equal to the difference in the binding energy between the two shells. In tungsten, the binding energy difference between the K shell (70 keV) and L shell (11 keV) is 59 keV. This photon energy emitted is called **characteristic x-rays** because its energy is characteristic of the target material (tungsten) and the involved shells. In fact, when the L shell electron moves into the K shell a vacancy is created that, in turn, must be filled by an electron from still a higher level or shell, and another x-ray photon will be produced. The energy of the radiation produced on the outer electron shell transitions are small and produce mostly heat or x-rays, which are absorbed by the glass walls of the glass tube (Fig. 2-37).

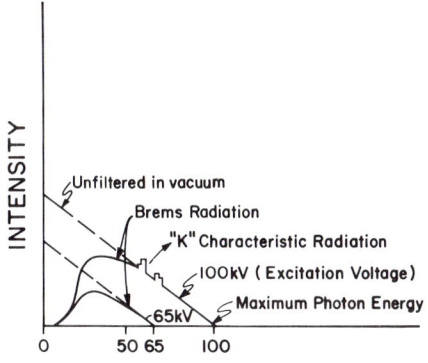

Figure 2-38. The spectrum of bremsstrahlung and K-characteristic radiation. K-characteristic radiation will not be produced unless the projectile electrons have energies of at least 70 keV.

In review, Bremsstrahlung or general radiation is heterogenous radiation with a continuous range of energies (and wavelengths) due to the "braking" or deceleration of x-rays by a strongly positive electron field of the tungsten atoms of the target. Brems radiation constitutes 85-90 percent of the emitted x-rays when 80-100 kVp is appled to the tube and 100 percent of radiation below 70 kVp. Characteristic radiation consists of a limited, discrete number of photons, consisting of about 10-15 percent of the emitted x-rays when the tube voltage is in the range from 80 to 100 kVp. Below 70 kVp there is no K shell characteristic radiation produced in a tungsten atom because it takes a cathode electron with a least 70 keV to remove an electron from the K shell (Fig. 2-38).

Intensity of the X-ray Beam

Since the x-ray beam is composed of photons with many energies (heterogenous), it is common to speak of quality and quantity of a beam of photons. **Quality** refers to the energy of particular photons, and **quantity** refers to the number of photons in the beam each with a particular energy. Quality and quantity are described together in a concept known as **intensity,** defined as the total energy contained in the beam (quality times quantity) per unit area per unit time.

$$\text{Intensity} = \frac{(\text{\# of photons in beam}) \times (\text{energy of each photon})}{(\text{area}) \times (\text{exposure rate})}$$

The area referred to is the cross-sectional area of the beam at a particular point in space. Since most photons spread out as they move away from the source, it is important to specify where the intensity is being calculated (distance from source).

The intensity of the x-ray beam varies with the target material, the mA (current), exposure time (rate), distance of film from source (inverse square law), and filtration. Actually, in the use of modern dental x-ray units, the only variables over which the operator has control are the **kVp, mA, exposure time, and source-to-film distance.** The target material and filtation are already placed properly in the machine when the x-ray machine is purchased from the manufacturer.

X-ray Emission Spectrum

Since the ordinary x-ray beam is heterogenous in wavelength and energy, a particular x-ray beam can be specified to a high degree of precision by sorting out the x-rays by wavelength, or its photons according to energy. This can be done by a special distribution curve or spectrum of x-rays of various wavelengths or photon energies. Graphically, the general shape of the x-ray emission spectrum is the same for all dental x-ray machines, but the relative position of the axis can change. The farther to the right the spectrum is the higher the effective energy of the photons, or **quality** of the x-ray beam. The greater the area of the curve the higher the intensity of the x-ray beam.

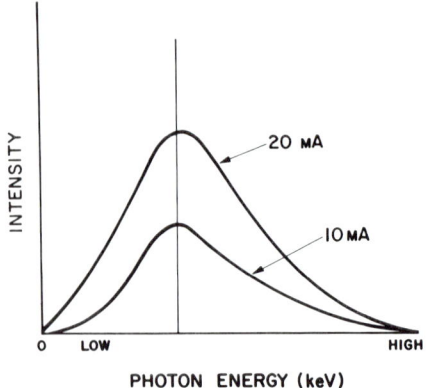

Figure 2-39. A change in the mA makes a comparable change in the intensity of the x-ray beam at all photon energies.

Influence of x-ray Tube Current (mA) on Intensity

The number of x-rays produced naturally depends on the number of electrons emitted by the cathode filament.

The number of electrons emitted by the cathode filament depends directly on the tube current or mA used. If the operator changes the mA on the control panel from 10 mA to 20 mA, while other factors remain constant, twice as many electrons will flow from cathode to anode. A change in the mA will make a proportionate area change in the x-ray emission spectrum (change in intensity of x-ray beam) (Fig. 2-39).

Influence of Exposure Time on Intensity

Exposure time is the interval during which x-rays are being produced. The more exposure time used, the more x-rays produced. In dental radiography, the exposure time is the factor that is most commonly used to compensate for anatomic variables of patients. It is the most easily understood by the operator and the most easily changed. Most of the dental exposure technics use a fixed kVp-mA technic and vary only the exposure time.

In medical radiography the mA and exposure time is fixed and the kVp is varied accordig to the differences in the thickness of the patient's body structure. This is called the varied kVp technic and is used by some dental schools, one being the University of Texas Dental School at San Antonio.

Traditionally, timer intervals in dentistry have been in fractions and whole numbers of a second such as 1/4, 1/2, 3/4, 1, and 2. The new *American National Standard for Exposure Time Designations under 1 second for Timers of X-Ray Machines* calls for timer **impulse** intervals, of 1, 2, 3, 4, 5, 8, 10, 12, 15, 19, 24, 30, 38, 48, 60, 75, 96, and 120. With a 60 Hertz (cycle) alternating current and a half-wave self-rectified dental x-ray tube, there are 60 impulses per second of electrical energy. Therefore, 1 impulse equals 1/60 of a second. Any number over 60 is designated in seconds (for example 120/60 = 2 seconds). Manufacturers are asked to comply with this standard but are not obligated to do so.

The **mA** and the **exposure time** have a direct effect on the quantity or number of photons produced in an x-ray beam. When these two factors (mA and seconds) are multiplied together it forms a common factor, mAs. In the future this common factor will be called mAi (milliampere-impulses). Milliampere-seconds or milliampere-impulses determine the total number of photons produced in the beam, but it does not indicate the energy of each photon in the beam. The effective energy of the photons in the beam depends upon the kVp applied across the cathode to the anode.

mAs Rule: The milliamperage required for a given exposure time is **inversely proportional** to the exposure time. That is, the higher the milliamperage the shorter the exposure time. Some examples of mAs and mAi are given to show how the factors may be varied without influencing the quantity of radiation produced.

```
mA × sec = mAs      mA × imp = mAi
10 × 1/2  = 5       10 × 30  = 300
15 × 1/3  = 5       15 × 20  = 300
```

Since the mAs and mAi in the above examples remain the same, the quantity of the radiation produced remains the same. The following formula can be used to change the mA or time in either seconds or impulses while keeping the radiation produced the same.

Original mA × Original Time =
    (A)   (B)

New mA × New Time
  (C)   (D)

mAs Example: Suppose the original milliamperage and exposure time to expose the mandibular incisors was 10 mA at 3/4 seconds. What would be the new exposure time if you keep all the factors the same, but changed the milliamperage setting to 15 mA?

Solution: D = $\frac{A \times B}{C}$

         = $\frac{10 \times 3/4}{15}$

         = .5 or 1/2 sec.

Influence of Tube Potential (kVp) on Intensity

Unlike mA, a change in kVp affects both the amplitude (area under the distribution curve) and the position of the x-ray emission spectrum.

The higher kVp techniques will (1) increase the amount of radiation produced (quantity) and will (2) determine the maximum energy (quality) of the x-rays produced. Kilovoltage controls the speed (kinetic energy) of each electron, which in turn has important effects on the photon energy of the x-rays produced. As kVp is increased, the area under the distribution curve increases, and the position of the x-ray emission spectrum shifts to the right to include more of the higher x-rays energies (Fig. 2-40).

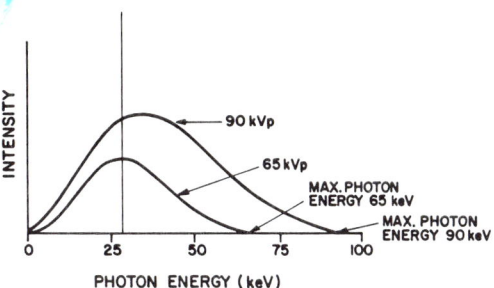

Figure 2-40. A change in kVp changes the amplitude of the x-ray spectrum and shifts the spectrum to the right toward the high energy side. Therefore, an increase in kVp increases the amount of radiation as well as the amount of higher energy photons produced.

Radiation produced in the higher kilovoltage range (85-100 kVp) has greater energy, higher frequency, and shorter wavelengths; such x-rays are much more penetrating and are called "hard" x-rays. Radiation produced in the lower kilovoltage range (55-65 kVp) has less energy, lower frequency, and longer wavelengths; such x-rays are less penetrating and are called "soft" x-rays (Fig. 2-41).

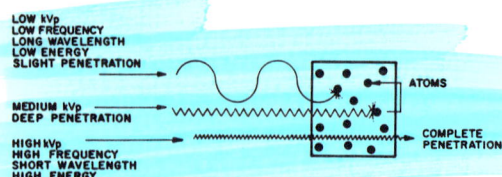

Figure 2-41. Penetrating power (quality) of x-rays dependent upon the kVp or potential produced by the x-ray tube. The extent whether x-rays will penetrate a structure depends on the photon energy of the x-rays, and the thickness, density (mass/unit volume), and atomic number of the structure.

Half-Value Layer

In radiology, the quality or penetrating power of the x-ray beam is measured by its **half-value layer** (HVL). The HVL of an x-ray beam is the thickness of absorbing material (usually Al or Cu) necessary to reduce the x-ray intensity to one-half its original value. A diagnostic x-ray beam usually has an HVL in the range of 1-5 mm of aluminum. The higher the HVL the more penetrating the beam.

Besides controlling the penetrating power (quality) of the x-ray beam, kilovoltage also influences x-ray quantity. The change in quantity is proportional to the square of the change in kVp. If the kVp were doubled from 50 kVp to 100 kVp, the x-ray intensity increases by a factor of four. In practice, this situation does not prevail, because as kVp is increased the quality (penetrability) of the x-rays is increased and fewer x-rays are absorbed by the patient and therfore **more** x-rays interact with the film. This will increase the darkness (density) on the film with much less increase in kVp than indicated. Actually to double the x-ray intensity by kVp manipulation alone you would only have to increase the kVp by 41 percent. This helps to explain the x-ray "rule of the thumb" used by x-ray technologists to relate kVp and mAs changes to produce constant density (darkness) on the film. The rule states that "an increase of 15 percent in kVp should be accompanied by a reduction of one-half in mAs." In dentistry, usually an increase of 15 kVp requires halving the exposure time, and a decrease of 15 kVp would necessitate doubling the exposure time.

Example: What would be the new exposure time if changing from a 60 kVp, 10 mA, 1 second technique to a 75 kVp, 10 mA technique? (All other factors remain the same, such as type of film, distance, and filatration.)

SOLUTION: Increasing the x-ray technique by 15 kVp requires halving the previous 1 second exposure time to 1/2 second to maintain the same density (darkness) on the film. (The mA remained the same.)

Influence of Anode Target (source)-Film Distance on Intensity

Primary Beam

X-rays as they are created at the focal spot of the tungsten target of the anode of the x-ray tube are emitted in all directions (see Fig. 2-32). They act like visible light waves in that they radiate from the source in all directions unless stopped by an absorber. For this reason the x-ray tube is enclosed in a heavy metal housing that absorbs most of the x-radiation — only the **useful rays** are permitted to leave the metal housing through an aperture or **window.** Some radiation may leak through the metal housing, and this is called "leakage radiation." The useful rays that pass through the window of the metal housing are called the **primary beam.** The pencil of radiation at the center of the primary beam is called the **central ray.** The aperture in the metal housing that the primary beam passes through is covered by a permanent seal, usually of aluminum or glass, to seal in the insulating oil that surrounds the tube.

Inverse Square Law: The x-rays of the primary beam emerge from the protective housing not as parallel waves but as divergent rays. The **primary beam**, then, is shaped very much like a cone. Therefore, the intensity of the beam decreases as the distance from the source increases since the same amount of radiation covers a larger area at longer distances. You can prove this to yourself by a simple demonstration. In a darkened room, move a single light nearer to and farther away from a printed page. As you move the lamp away from the page, the light falling on it is less and less bright. Exactly the same thing happens with x-rays — as the distance from the object to the source of radiation is decreased, the x-ray intensity at the object increases; as the distance is increased, the radiation intensity at the object decreases. This relation between distance and intensity of radiation is called the **inverse square law**, because the intensity of radiation varies inversely as the square of the source-film distance (Fig. 2-42).

A practical formula to use in adjusting the exposure factor is as follows:

$$\frac{\text{Original mAs}}{\text{New mAs}} = \frac{\text{Original SFD}^2}{\text{New SFD}^2}$$

where SFD = source-film distance
mAs = milliampere/seconds

Example: When the SFD distance is changed from 8 to 16 inches or twice the distance, the mAs value will have to be increased four times.

Original SFD = 8 inches
Original mAs = 2.5 (1/4 second at 10 mA) 0.25
New SFD = 16 inches

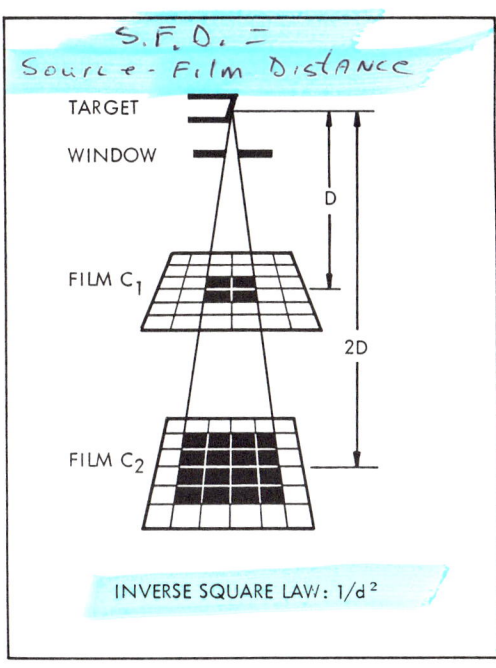

S.F.D. = Source-Film Distance

Figure 2-42. Diagram showing how the x-ray intensity is altered by changing the source-film distance. (Copyright Eastman Kodak Company, Rochester, NY. Reprinted by permission.)

SOLUTION:

$$\frac{2.5}{X} = \frac{8^2}{16^2}$$

$$64X = 640$$
$$X = 10 \text{ (1 sec at 10 mA)}$$

Many times the kVp and mA will be fixed or constant in dentistry, and you may want to change from a short cone to a long cone technique, perhaps from 8 inch SFD to 16 inch SFD. This is doubling the SFD distance, so you will have to increase the exposure time by the square of the distance or by factor of 4 to maintain the same density (darkness) on the film. The intensity of the beam at 16 inch SFD would be one-fourth the intensity as that at 8 inch SFD. Since the photons spread out as they move away from the source, the source-film distance is an important factor in determining the intensity of the beam, because it determines the cross-sectional area of the beam at a particular distance from the source. As th SFD is increased the cross-sectional area of the beam becomes larger so that the x-radiation is spread out over a larger area, which, in turn, decreases the intensity of any given point in the beam.

Influence of Filtration on Intensity

Filtration is the process of increasing the effective or mean energy of heterogeneous or polychromatic radiation by passing it through an absorber. The x-ray beam is composed of all kinds of photon energies. The mean or average energy is from one-third to one-half of the peak energy applied, thus many of the photon energies fall in the lower energy range. The mean energy of a 90 keV peak energy unfiltered beam is 30-45 keV photon energy. As a polychromatic x-ray beam passes through a patient, only the higher energy radiation penetrates the patient to form the image on the film. The lower energy photons of the beam are absorbed in the first few centimeters of the patient's skin tissue, and the patient receives much more radiation than is necessary. The patient can be protected from this unnecessary low-energy x-radiation by placing a filter material between the patient and the x-ray tube (*see* Fig. 2-32).

Sheets of aluminum (Z = 13) are usually used because they are excellent absorbers of low-energy radiation. The next step is to select the appropriate thickness for the filter. Two millimeters of aluminum absorb virtually all photons with energies less than 20 keV; a filter of 3 mm of aluminum offers no advantage because the quality (penetrability) of the beam is not significantly altered and the intensity is greatly diminished.

During a radiographic exposure the x-ray beam is filtered by absorbers at three different levels:

1. the x-ray tube and its housing (inherent filtration);
2. sheets of aluminum placed in the path of the beam (added filtration);
3. the patient.

Inherent filtration is the filtration afforded by the x-ray tube and its housing through which the beam must pass after leaving the target. In fact, a few of the lower energy x-ray photons are absorbed by the target of the anode if they are produced deeply within the tungsten. The materials responsible for inherent filtration are the anode target metal, the glass envelope of the tube, the insulating oil surrounding the tube, and the aperture window material of the metal housing. The glass envelope of the x-ray tube produces by far the most inherent filtration. The inherent filtration is usually expressed in equivalent thickness of aluminum and varies between 0.5 and 1.0 mm for a typical x-ray machine.

Added filtration is the result of sheets of aluminum placed in the path of the beam. The total filtration of an x-ray beam represents the sum of the inherent filtration and the added filtration.

The National Council on Radiation Protection and Measurement (*NCRR Report No. 35 on Dental X-ray Protection*) recommends that the total filtration of the useful beam should **not** be less than that stated below:

Operating Potential	Minimum Total Filtration
Below 50 kVp	0.5 mm aluminum
50-70 kVp	1.5 mm aluminum
Above 70 kVp	2.5 mm aluminum

Adding filtration to a dental x-ray machine has an effect on the x-ray emission spectrum similar to increasing the kVp (Fig. 2-43). Also, filtration reduces the intensity in the beam by decreasing the

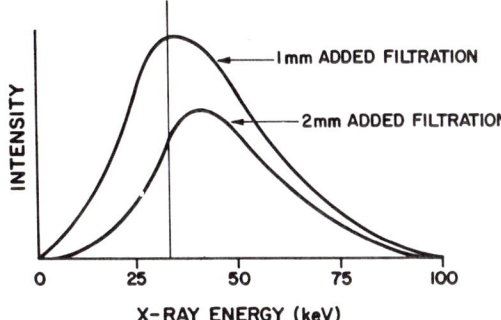

Figure 2-43. By adding filtration, the mean photon energy increases (axis shifts to right), but the amount of photons decreases (area under the curve). Most of the photons that are removed from the beam are low energy photons. The same mAs and kVp was used to produce this distribution curve, only the filtration was changed.

amount of photons absorbed by the filter already in the beam. Most of the photons are low energy unnecessary photons; however, some of the higher energy useful photons are absorbed by the filtration. This requires an increase in the exposure time of up to 50 percent in some cases to compensate for the loss in intensity of the beam. Although the use of filtration does require an increase in exposure time, it has been demonstrated that filters can reduce patient skin exposure by as much as 80 percent.

Aother advantage in the use of filtration is that it increases the average penetrating ability (quality) of the beam, or in other words, it increases the half-value layer of the beam.

Scatter and Secondary Radiation

When x-ray photons arrive at the patient with energies produced by dental x-ray machines, three things can happen: (1) x-rays can pass through the patient without interacting with the tissue atoms, (2) some of the x-ray photons are absorbed completely in the patient, and (3) some are merely scattered. When the x-ray photons are transmitted through the patient without an interaction, they produce densities (blackness) on the film. The photons that are absorbed are completely removed from the x-ray beam and cease to exist. When the x-rays are scattered, they are deflected to all directions and therfore contribute no useful information to the film.

These scattered x-rays add to the overall blackness on the film and it interferes with film image quality. Scattered radiation on the film is called **film fog** and can completely obscure the film image. There are two ways in which the photons can be scattered: (1) by coherent or unmodified scattering and (2) by Compton scattering.

Unmodified (Coherent) Scattering

Coherent or classical scattering is when low energy x-rays (below 10 keV) interact with matter and the x-rays undergo a change in direction **without** a change in wavelength. For this reason the name **unmodified** is sometimes used. In this type of interaction between x-rays and matter, no energy is transferred and no ionization occurs. Its only effect is to change the direction of the incident radiation (Fig. 2-44).

Most **coherent scattering** is in a forward direction. It is of little importance in dental radiography because it primarily involves low-energy x-rays that contribute little to the radiograph anyway. However, there is some coherent scattering throughout all the ranges of energies in the beam. At 70 kVp, perhaps less than 5 percent of the radiation undergoes coherent scattering, which contributes only slightly to film fog. It is too small to be of any importance in diagnostic radiology.

Compton (Incoherent) Scattering

Almost all of the scatter radiation in dental radiography comes from **Compton**

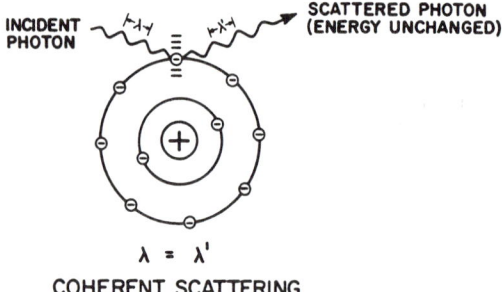

COHERENT SCATTERING

Figure 2-44. Coherent or unmodified scattering. An incident photon (usually of low energy) interacts with one of the outermost electrons. they are essentially free because they are so loosely bound. The electron starts to vibrate at the frequency of the incident photon. Since the electron is charged particle, it emits radiation with the same frequency of the incident radiation and the atom returns to its stable state again.

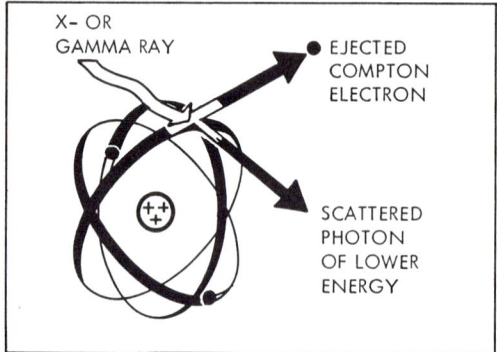

Figure 2-45. Compton scattering results in ionization of the atom and change in direction and reduction in energy of the incident x-ray photon.

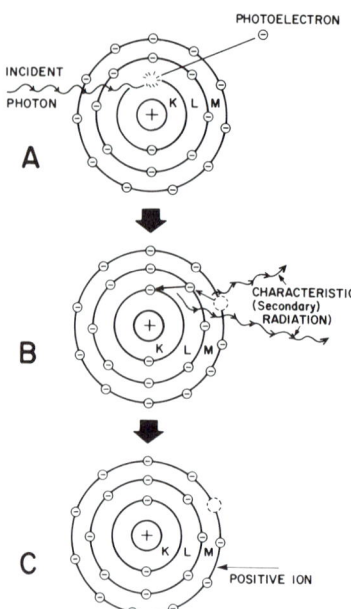

Figure 2-46. Photoelectric effect. (**A**) Photon with energy a little higher than binding energy of K-shell electron knocks electron out of atom. Ejected electron is called photoelectron. (**B**) L-shell electron drops into K-shell vacancy, M-shell electron drops into L-shell vacancy giving off K-shell and L-shell characteristic radiation. (**C**) Atom is now a positive ion.

scattering. An x-ray with relatively moderate to high energy strikes a loosely bound (free) outer-shell electron, ejecting it from its orbit. the incident photon is scattered in a new direction (including backwards) and retains most of its original energy. This reaction ionizes the atom producing an ion pair, a positive atom and a negative electron, called a **Compton electron** or **recoil electron**. The interaction was first described by A.H. Compton in 1923 (Fig. 2-45).

Both the scattered x-ray photon and the Compton electron may have sufficient energy to undergo many more ionizing interactions before losing all of their energy.

Finally, the incident x-ray photon in the Compton reaction will be absorbed by a **photoelectric reaction** (Fig. 2-46) and The original Compton (recoil) electron will drop into an atomic shell vacant hole created previously by another ionization event. Compton electrons that are scattered at narrow angles have an excellent chance of reaching the x-ray film and producing film fog. Compton scatter is also a safety hazard to the patient, as well as to the dentist and other personnel using dental x-ray equipment. In fluoroscopy, it is a real safety hazard because the scatter radiation from the patient is almost as energetic as the primary beam.

Secondary Radiation

Secondary radiation (characteristic) is produced during ionized interactions of x-rays in the diagnostic energy range, when inner-shell electrons (usually the K shell) of atoms and the x-ray photons are **not** scattered but completely absorbed. The K shell electron is ejected from its orbit by the incident photon, which must have a little more energy than the binding energy of the K shell electron. The photon disappears completely, giving up all its energy to the electron. The ejected electron flys out into space and is called a **photoelectron.** It is a negatively charged particle and almost immediately is absorbed by another atom because it has little penetrating power. The remaining atom is now a positive ion as it has an electron void in the K shell orbit. This is an unnatural state and is instantly corrected by an outer shell electron (usually the L shell) from the same atom, which drops into the vacancy. When the L-shell electron drops into the vacancy, it gives up energy in the form of an x-ray photon equal to the difference in the binding energies of the K shell and the L shell. These are **characteristic x-rays** and are called **secondary radiation,** and they behave in the same manner as scattered x-rays. They are very similar to scatter x-rays in that a photon is deflected from its original path. Secondary radiation contributes nothing of diagnostic value, and they occur with very small intensities. Calcium, which as the highest atomic number of any element found in the jaws, emit a 4 keV maximal energy characteristic photon (when an outer shell electron moves into the K shell void), which is very little energy by x-ray standards. This type of secondary radiation is absorbed within a few millimeters of its origin. Barium and iodine found in contrast agents used in medical radiology are the only elements that emit characteristic (secondary) radiation with enough energy to leave the patient and fog an x-ray film (Fig. 2-46).

The probability of a given x-ray photon undergoing a photoelectric interaction is a function of both the photon energy and the atomic number of the absorber. The photon must have a greater energy than binding energy of the inner shell electron, but the photoelectric reaction will more likely occur when the electron binding energy and photon energy are nearly the same. Photoelectric reaction (absorption) is good in that it enhances film contrast (differences in the densities on the radiograph) without producing a significant number of scatter x-rays. However, photoelectric interaction will produce more patient exposure to radiation than the other types of interactions discussed (Compton and coherent scattering interactions).

In summary, in dental radiography, x-ray photons that arrive at the patient may interact in many ways with the tissue of the patient. There are x-rays that are transmitted though the patient without interacting. Other x-ray photons are absorbed by the tissue by photoelectric interaction (absorption) while still other x-ray photons are scattered away from the film or scattered toward the film by Compton and coherent (unmodified) scattering interactions (Fig. 2-47).

Beam-Restricting Devices

Beam restrictors have two functions: (1) protect the patient and (2) decrease scatter radiation. Beam restrictors protect the patient by decreasing the x-ray field; the smaller the x-ray field, the smaller the volume of the patient irradiated. The ideal shape for an intraoral radiographic field for maximal patient protection is rectangular because dental x-ray films are

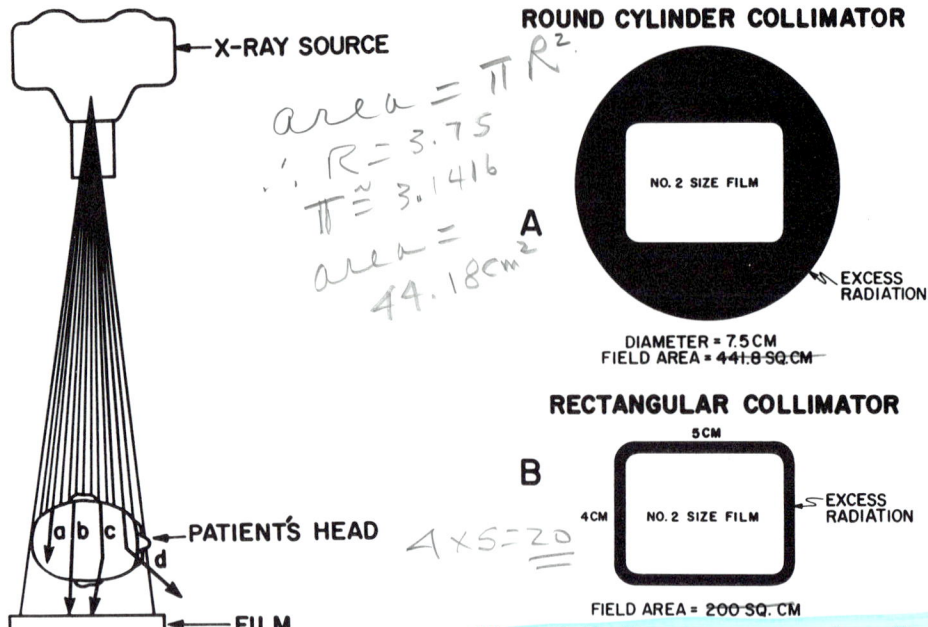

Figure 2-47. Radiation interactions with patient. a: X-ray photon is absorbed by photoelectric reaction. b: X-ray photon is transmitted through patient without an interaction. c: X-ray photon scattered onto film. d: X-ray photon scattered away from film. X-rays of types b and c are called remnant radiation because they are x-rays that have passed through patient and will strike the film.

Figure 2-48. By using a rectangular collimator (A) instead of a round cylinder beam restrictor (B) the area irradiated by the patient has been decreased by 50 percent.

rectangular in shape. Round fields expose portions of the patient unnecessarily (Fig. 2-48). There are times, however, when a round field is better than a rectangular or square field, such as when taking a radiograph of the paranasal sinuses or round anatomical objects, or when dental filmholders with alignment devices are difficult to use properly.

The second function of beam restrictors is to reduce the amount of scatter radiation. As the number of scatter x-rays increases, image clarity decreases. The radiography loses contrast (differences between densities) and looks dull and foggy. The imaged anatomic structures appear blurred and are difficult to visualize.

Grids are sometimes used in dentistry to decrease scatter radiation in skull radiographic techniques. They will be discussed in Chapter 15.

There are basically three beam-restricting devices used in dentistry: (1) the aperture diaphragm, (2) position-indicating devices (PID), and (3) variable aperture collimaters.

Aperture Diaphragm. The simplest of all beam restriction devices is the aperture diaphragm. It basically consists of a sheet of lead with an opening in the center. The opening in the diaphragm is usually designed to cover precisely the size and shape of the film used in a particular examination. The lead is usually soft, made of 4 pound lead, meaning four pounds to the square foot, and is approximately 1/16 inch thick. In dental radiography, the routine source-film distance eight inches or sixteen inches. The diaphragm aperture

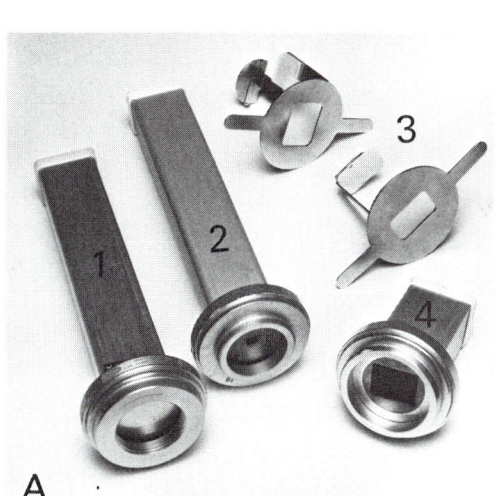
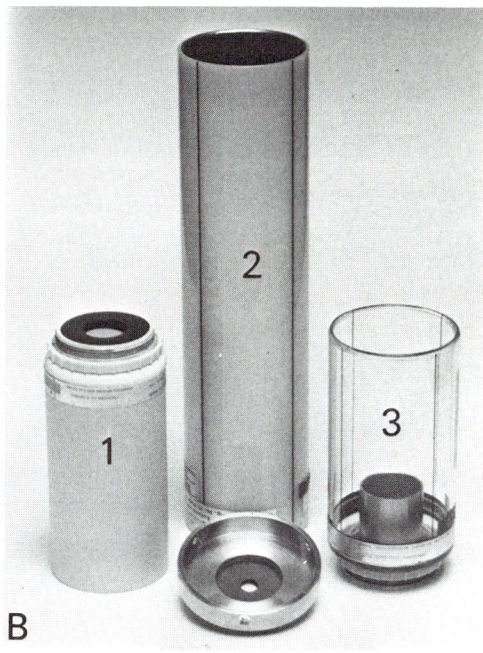

Figure 2-49. Types of dental x-ray collimation. **(A)** Rectangular collimation. 1, Weber long rectangular P.I.D. 2, GE long P.I.D. 3, Precision (Masel) film holders. 4: S.S. White (Pennwalt) recessed anode P.I.D. **(B)** Round collimation. 1, GE short lead-lined cone. 2, GE long round lead-lined cone. 3, GE short round plastic cone with extended metal collimator.

usually employed in these techniques is a round diaphragm aperture that is typically 18-25 mm in diameter for 8 inches SFD and 9-10 mm in diameter for 16 inches SFD. Rectangular collimation (which requires precise alignment and positioning of the x-ray beam, the patient, and the film) is recommended because it reduces scatter radiation (improves quality) and reduces patient exposure (surface/volume exposure). When using rectangular collimation in dentistry, it requires the use of a film and x-ray tube alignment device to prevent "cone-cutting" (partial images.) The rectangular diaphragm aperture opening in dental x-ray machines for 16 inch SFD is approximately 6 mm by 8 mm.

Position (Beam) Indicating Devices. Position (beam) indicating devices can be considered modifications of the aperture diaphragm. There are three basic types: conical, cylindrical, and rectangular in shape (Fig. 2-49). The cone is flare-shaped with a flare of the cone usually greater than the flare of the x-ray beam. When used it is little more than the aperture, not a collimator. It is **not** used in dentistry anymore.

Beam restriction with a cylinder takes place at the end of the cylinder, so there is less penumbra than with the cone. The cylinder is usually lead-lined to restrict the beam from unnecessary scatter radiation. Several modifications of the cylinder P.I.D. have been made—one of them is the recessed-anode, which was an innovation of Professor Albert G. Richards of Michigan University (now retired) (Fig. 2-50). It has the appearance of a short P.I.D. but actually has an extended source-film distance. The rectangular

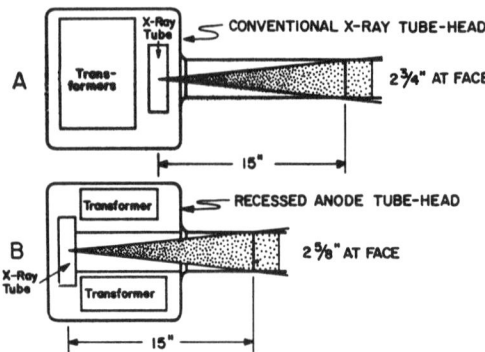

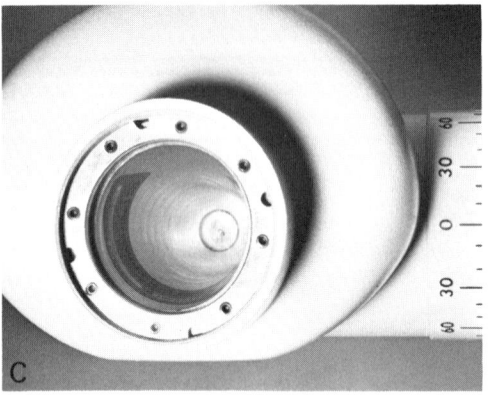

inch thick. they work in pairs and are independently controlled, producing a square or rectangular field. Light localization is used with these collimators. (Fig. 2-51).

In cephalometric radiography, it is prudent to use a rectangular collimator placed at the tube head to restrict the beam so it will cover the size of the cassette and no more (Fig. 2-52A).

In rotational panoramic radiography, the x-ray beam is collimated (restricted) at the tube head and also between the patient and the film cassette. Besides preventing undue scatter radiation to the film, the slit collimators produce a narrow, limited beam of x-rays necessary in the rotational x-ray technique as described in Chapter 16 (Fig. 2-52B, C, D).

In summary, the dental x-ray machine is composed of the **tube head,** which contains the x-ray tube and transformers and the **control panel,** which contains the autotransformer (kV selector), rheostat (mA selector), and exposure button. A schematic drawing of this circuitry is shown in Figure 2-53.

Figure 2-50. (A) conventional x-ray tube head. (B) The Richards' recessed-anode extended source-skin distance tube without the use of the external cone. (Courtesy of Professor albert richards.) (C) Recessed-anode of Intrex (SS White/Pennwalt) x-ray machine. X-ray P.I.D. appears short; however, SFD is long because anode is recessed into tubehead.

P.I.D. is made of metal; the dimensions are slightly larger than a No. 2 regular dental film (*see* Fig. 2-49).

Variable-aperture collimator. The variable aperture collimator is probably the most common beam-restricting device used in medical radiology. The collimator shutter leaves are usually lead, at least 1/8

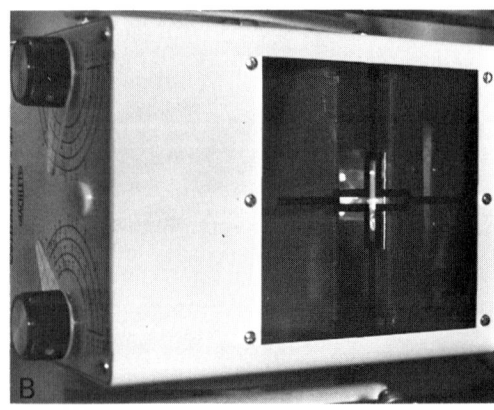

Figure 2-51. Machlett variable aperture collimator used with Franklin Head-holder in skull radiography.

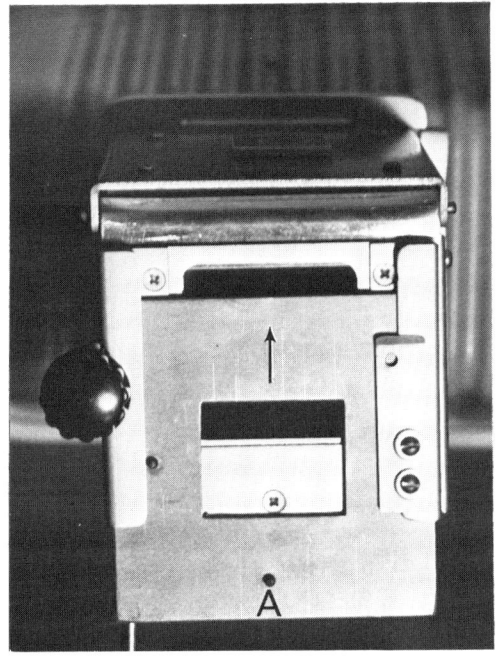
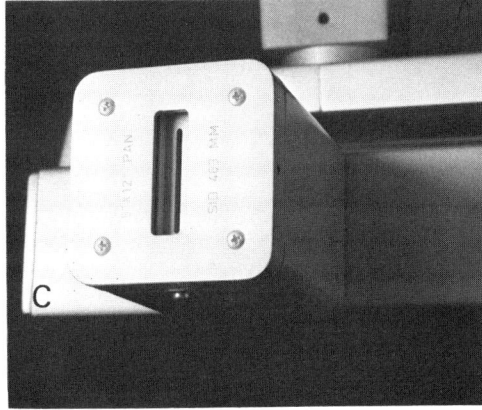
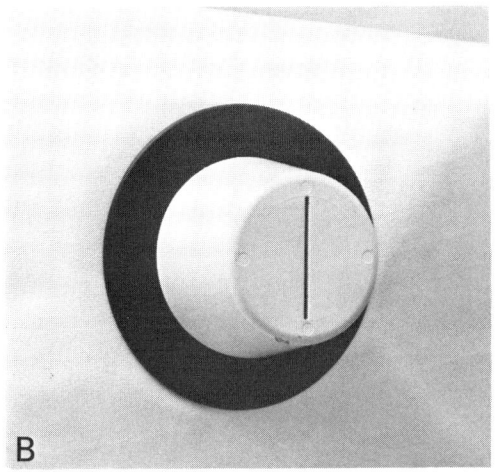
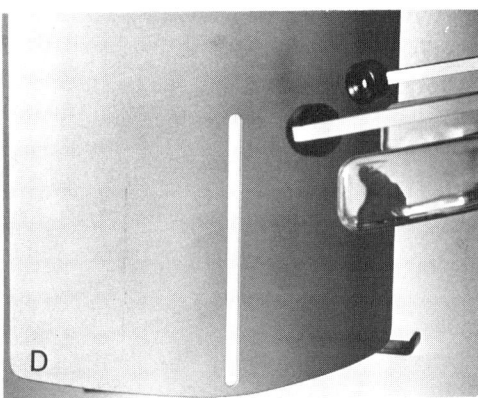

Figure 2-52. **(A)** Rectangular collimator being placed at cephalometric x-ray tube. **(B)Slit-beam collimator at tube head of Panorex II (SS. White/Pennawalt) x-ray machine.** **(C)** Slit-beam collimator at tube head of Orthopantomograph x-ray machine (Siemens). **(D)** Slit-beam collimator between patient and film cassette or Orthopantomograph x-ray machine (Siemens).

86 Textbook of Dental Radiology

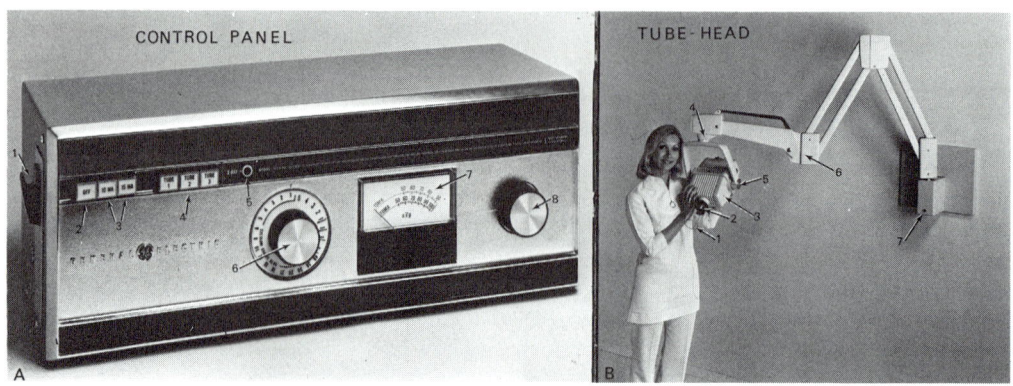

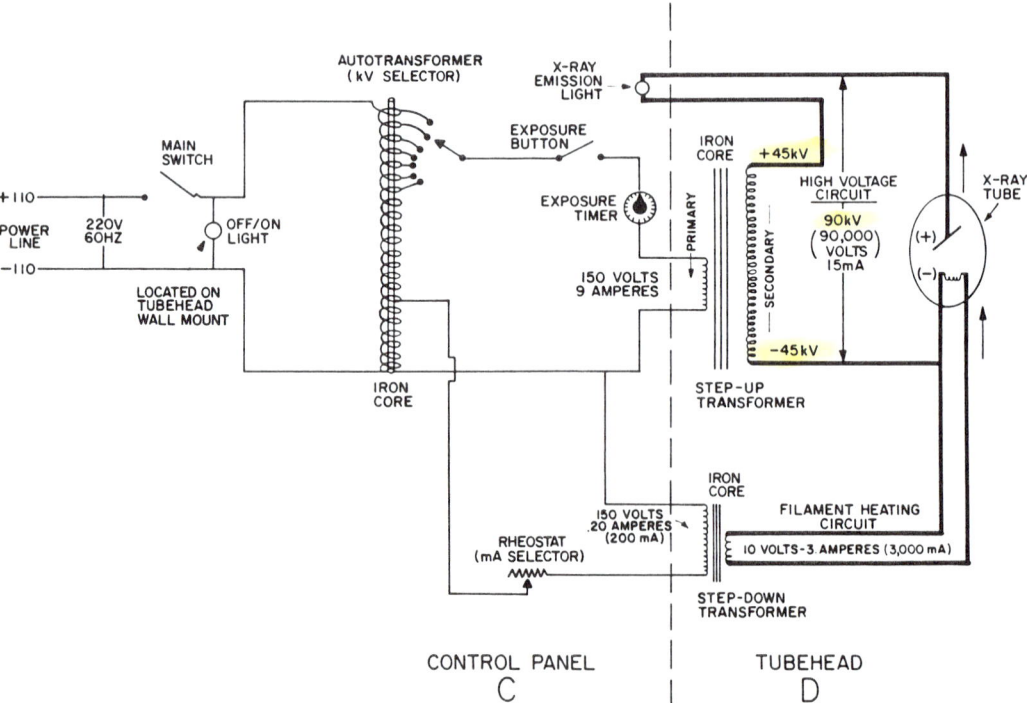

Figure 2-53. Schematic circuitry of typical dental x-ray unit. **(A)** Control panel of GE dental x-ray unit: 1, holder for exposure button; 2, main switch; 3, variable resistor (mA selector); 4, x-ray tube selector; 5, x-ray emission light; 6, exposure timer, 7, kVp-mA dial; 8, autotransformer kVp selector. **(B)** X-ray tube and extension arm of wall model GE x-ray machine: 1, short round cone; 2, collimator; 3, tube head (includes transformers and x-ray tube); 4, horizontal rotation; 5, vertical rotation; 6, extension arm; 7, off/on light. **(C)** Schematic drawing of control panel. **(D)** Schematic drawing of tube head.

Bibliography

Beck, James O.: *Syllabus of Oral Radiology.* University of Minnesota, School of Dentistry, 1970.

Bushong, S.C.: *Radiologic Science for Technologists: Physics, Biology and Protection.* St. Louis, Mosby, 1975.

Christensen, E. E.; curry, T. S.; and Dowdey, J. E.: *An Introduction tot he Pysics of Diagnostic Radiology.* Philadelphia, Lea & Febiger, 1978.

Fundamentals of Radiography, 12th ed. Rochester, N.Y., Eastman Kodak Co., 1980.

Goodwin, P. N.; Quimby, E. H.; and Morgan, R. H.: *Physical Foundatios of Radiology,* 4th ed. New York, Har-row 1970.

Heidersdorf, S. D.: X-ray fundamentals. *Dental Radiological Health Course Manual.* Cincinnati, Robert A. Taft Sanitary Engineering Center, U. S. Dept. of Health, Eduction and Welfare, January, 1961.

Hendee, W. R.: *Medical radiation Physics.* Chicago, year BK Med. 1970.

Herz, R. H.: *The Photographic Action of Ionizing Radiations.* New York, Wil, 1969.

Hodges, F. J.; Lampe, I.; and Holt, J. F.: *Radiology for Medical Students,* 3rd ed. Chicago, Year Med, 1961.

Johns, H. E.; and Cunningham, J. R.: *The Physics of Radiology,* 3rd ed. Springfield, Charles C Thomas, 1969.

Manson-Hing, L. R: *Fundamentals of Dental Radiography.* Philadelphia, Lea & Febiger, 1961.

Muncheryan, H. M.: *Modern Physics of Roentgenology.* Los Angeles, Wetzel, 1940.

Noz, Marilyn; and McGuire, G. Q.: *Radiation Protection in the Radiologic and Health Sciences.* Philadelphia, Lea & Febiger, 1979.

Peterson, S.: *Clinical Dental Hygiene.* St. Louis, Mosby, 1972.

Principles of Dental Radiography. Milwaukee General Electric X-ray Department.

Radiology Specialist. Washington, D. C., Department of the Air Force, 1958.

Seemann, H.: *Physical and Photographic Principles of Medical Radiology.* New York, Wiley, 1968.

Selman, J.: *The Fundamentals of X-ray and Radium Physics,* 6th ed. Springfield, Charles C Thomas, 1977.

Stewart, O. M.: *Physics.* Chicago, Ginn and Co., 1931.

Ter-Pogossian, M. M.: *The Physical Aspects of Diagnostic Radiology.* New York, Har-Row, Hoeber Medical Div., 1967.

Thompson, Jaundrell F.: *X Ray Physics and Equipment,* 2nd ed. Philadelphia, Davis Co., 1970.

X Rays in Dentistry. Rochester, N.Y., Eastman Kodak Co., 1977.

Chapter 3

ATTENUATION AND RECORDING THE RADIOGRAPHIC IMAGE

ATTENUATION

As we have learned previously, an x-ray beam is composed of many energies. Therefore, it is common to speak of quality and quantity of a beam of photons. Remember, **quality** refers to the energy of particular photons, and **quantity** refers to the number of photons that have a specific energy. The **intensity** of the beam is defined as the product of the quantity (number of photons) and quality (energy of the photons) per unit area (distance from source) per unit time of exposure (impulses or seconds). A beam with an average of 40 keV photons has a greater intensity than a beam made up of a comparable number of photons with an average keV of 20 when both beams are measured at 15 inches from the source, at half second exposure times.

Attenuation is the reduction in the intensity of an x-ray beam as it traverses matter by either absorption (photoelectric effect) or deflection (Compton effect) of photons from the beam.

There are three types of x-rays that are important in making a radiographic image on a recording film (Fig. 3-1):

1. those scattered by Compton interaction;
2. those absorbed by the photoelectric effect;
3. those x-rays transmitted through the body without interacting.

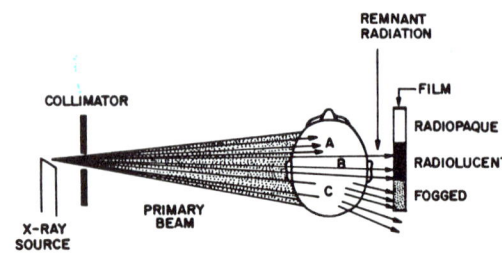

Figure 3-1. (A) X-rays absorbed completely by photoelectric effect. (B) X-rays transmitted to film without interaction. (C) X-rays scattered by Compton interaction.

The Compton scattered x-rays contribute no useful information to the film; they tend to blur the film and obscure the radiographic image. These scattered x-rays result in film fog and give a generalized dulling of the x-ray image by producing film densities that do not represent diagnostic information. Scatter radiation can be decreased by using **collimators** to reduce the x-ray field and **grids** to reduce the number of scattered x-rays that reach the x-ray film.

X-rays that undergo photoelectric absorption produce diagnostic information in a negative sense. Since these x-rays do not reach the film, they represent structures that have high absorption characteristics and result in clear, white areas on the film. These white or bright areas, which usually represent cortical bone, enamel, or metallic restorations, are called radiopaque structures or materials.

There are other x-rays that penetrate the jaws and are transmitted with no interaction whatsoever. They result in dark (high density) areas on the radiograph. These areas are called radiolucent because structures such as soft tissue, pulp, and periodontal ligament are easily penetrated by the x-radiation.

Basically, since Compton scatter adds nothing to the diagnostic information of the radiographic image, the x-ray image results from the difference between those x-rays absorbed by the photoelectric effect and those not absorbed at all. This characteristic of making a radiographic image is called differential absorption or differential attenuation. As the photons of the beam enter the patient, they have a uniform distribution, but they emerge with a specific pattern of distribution. The transmitted photons carry the x-ray image, but their pattern of distribution also carries a memory of the absorbed photons. The transmitted and absorbed photons are equally important. If all the x-rays were transmitted, the radiograph would be all black (radiolucent); if all the x-rays were absorbed, the radiograph would be all white (radiopaque). A radiographic image would not be produced in either case. Therefore, radiographic image formation depends on differential absorption. There are some tissues that absorb more x-ray photons than other tissues, and the size of the differential absorption determines the amount of contrast between tissues (subject contrast). The relationship among x-ray intensities in different parts of the remnant radiation that leaves the patient (aerial image) is called "subject contrast" (Fig. 3-2).

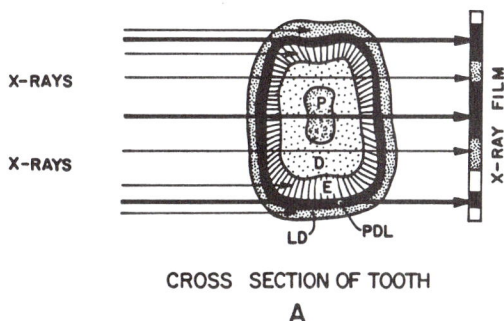

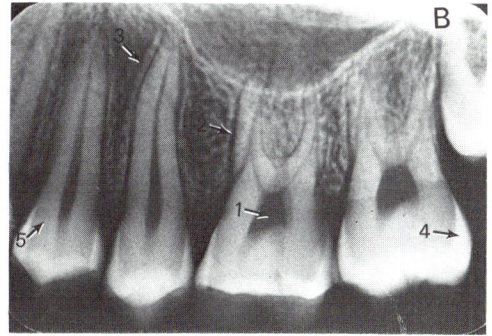

Figure 3-2. Differential absorption. **(A)** Cross-section of tooth: LD, lamina dura; PDL, periodontal ligament space; E, enamel; D, dentin; P, pulp. The enamel and lamina dura completely absorb radiation; dentine partially absorbs radiation; pulp and periodontal ligament transmit most of the radiation because those tissues absorb very little radiation. **(B)** Radiograph of maxillary premolar and molar region: 1, pulp; 2, periodontal ligament space are black (radiolucent); 3, lamina dura, and 4, enamel are white (radiopaque); and 5, dentin is gray.

Factors Affecting X-Ray Absorption

The following are some factors that influence absorption of x-radiation:

Radiation	Matter
1. Energy keV	1. Thickness
	2. Atomic Number
	3. Density

Energy

As a general rule, as the radiation energy (kVp) increases, x-ray transmission through an absorber increases and attenuation (reduction of intensity of beam) decreases. As discussed earlier, at the lower kilovoltages, x-rays with longer wavelengths are absorbed more easily than x-rays of higher energy kilovoltages (those of shorter wavelengths). Therefore, the energies produced by the higher kilovoltages will penetrate materials more readily than energies produced with the lower kilovoltages. The percentage of transmitted photons through a material will increase as the mean energy of the x-ray beam increases (*See* Fig. 2-40).

Relationship of Energy and the Thickness of the Absorber

Remember that an x-ray beam is polychromatic and contains a whole spectrum of photons of various energies. The most energetic photons of the beam are determined by the kilovoltage (kVp) used to generate the beam. As mentioned previously, the mean energy of polychromatic radiation is between one-third (1/3) and one-half (1/2) of its peak energy. A 100 kVp beam has a mean energy of about 40 kV. This will depend on the amount of filtration used.

The relationship of thickness of the absorber to the x-ray beam is rather obvious: a thick piece of any material will absorb more x-ray photons than a thin piece of the same material.

However, as a polychromatic x-ray beam passes through an absorber, the quality (mean kV) of the beam increases because the lower-energy photons are more readily attenuated than the higher-energy photons. The number of the photons decreases because some of the photons are deflected and absorbed out as the beam passes through the various layers of the absorber. Therefore, as the beam passes through an absorber, the quantity (number of photons of the beam) decreases and the quality (mean energy) of the beam increases (Fig. 3-3).

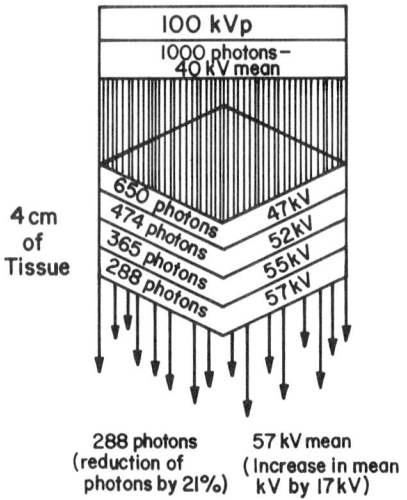

Figure 3-3. Attenuation of polychromatic radiation. As beam penetrates each centimeter of tissue, the number of photons are reduced by the thickness of the material. However, the mean keV of the beam increases because the lower energy photons are readily attenuated out of the beam, leaving a greater percentage of the higher energy photons in the beam. (Adapted from Christensen, Curry and Dowdy: *An Introduction to the Physics of Diagnostic Radiology*. Philadelphia, Lea & Febiger, 1978.)

Atomic Number of the Absorber

Usually a material with a higher atomic number will absorb more x-rays than a material with a lower atomic number. A sheet of aluminum, which has a lower atomic number (13) than lead (82), absorbs a smaller amount of x-rays than a sheet of lead of the same area and weight. This is why lead is used in the tube housing, wall of x-ray rooms, and protective aprons instead of aluminum.

Absorption depends on atomic number in a rather complicated way, which is related to the energy of the incident photons. A photon cannot eject an electron unless it has more energy than the binding energy of its K shell electron. The binding energy of the K shell electron of a material is called the K-edge. Thus, with two materials that are close in atomic number, one may absorb more x-rays than the other for certain energies; however, the situation may be reversed for other energies. It depends upon whether the incident energies are slightly more or less than the K-edge of the absorber. This relationship between atomic number and x-ray energy is a factor that is important in the selection of phosphors for fluorescent intensifying screens. The recent success of rare earth intensifying screens is due in large part to the skillful matching of their K-edges to beam energies. We will discuss this subject more later.

Density of the Absorber

Density is the quantity of matter per unit of matter and usually is defined in units of g/cm^3. It is the compactness of a material or, basically, how tightly the atoms of a substance are packed. When the density of a material is doubled, the chance for x-ray interaction is doubled because there are twice as many electrons available for interaction. Therefore, approximately twice as many x-rays would be absorbed and scattered in bone than soft tissue. Bone has a density of 1.85 g/cm^3, and soft tissue a density of 1.00 g/cm^3. Water and ice are composed of the same amount of atoms, but ice occupies more volume and has a density of 0.919 g/cm^3 as compared to 1.00 g/cm^3 for water. Ice floats in water because it has less density than water.

Differential absorption in air-filled cavities such as the paranasal sinuses is primarily due to density differences. The atomic numbers of air and soft tissue are approximately the same (7.4), but the density of soft tissue is about 773 times that for air for the same thicknesses. Therefore, many more x-rays will be absorbed by the soft tissue than air.

Tissue density is one of the most important factors in x-ray attenuation. The differences in the densities of the tissues of the body is one of the prime reasons we can see an x-ray image on a radiograph.

Differential Absorption

In considering the dental use of x-rays, one must understand that the human jaws are complex structures made up of not only different thicknesses but of materials with different atomic numbers and densities. These structures absorb x-rays in different degrees. That is, metallic restorations such as amalgam and gold absorb more x-rays than enamel does; enamel more than dentin does; dentin more than cementum does; cementum more than cortical bone; cortical bone more than cancellous bone; cancellous bone more than soft tissue such as the periodontal membrane, the pulp, and oral mucosa. Teeth and bone contain large amounts of calcium and phosphorus with atomic numbers of 20 and 15 respectively, whereas, the atomic number of muscle is approximately 7.4. Furthermore, diseased structures often absorb x-rays differently than normal dental structures. Even the age of the patient may have a bearing on absorption — for example, in the elderly, the bones of the jaws many times have less calcium content and, hence, there is less x-ray absorption.

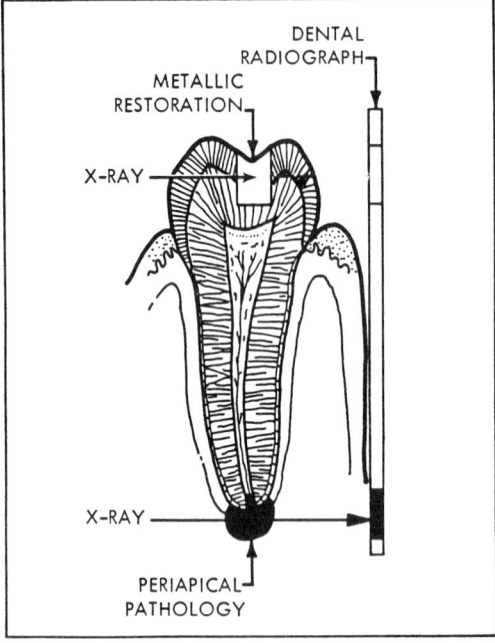

Figure 3-4. Diagram showing the variations of absorption in the human jaws. The metallic restoration absorbs the radiation, resulting in a white or radiopaque area on the radiograph. The periapical pathology is easily penetrated by the x-radiation, resulting in a dark or radiolucent area on the film.

The variations in the intensity transmitted through one part of a subject compared to that through another part is called subject or radiation contrast. If the intensity of the beam transmitted through soft tissue alone is three times as great as the intensity of the area transmitted through the bone, the subject contrast would be 3. Subject contrast is the result of the attenuation of the x-ray beam of the patient and depends, as stated previously, upon the nature of the subject (thickness, Z number, and density) and upon the kVp used.

Materials that absorb or resist the passage of x-radiation to a large degree are considered **radiopaque** and appear within the range of light gray or white when recorded on a radiograph. This means that most of the energy of the x-rays have been absorbed and very little if any x-radiation has reached the surface of the radiograph. Radiopaque objects in the dental radiograph are metallic restorations, enamel, dentin, and compact or cortical bone.

Materials that are freely penetrated by the x-rays are called **radiolucent**, and appear within the range of dark gray to black on the radiograph. This means that the objects do not resist the passage of or absorb the x-radiation to any great extent and that most of the energy of the radiation freely passes through the object to the recording surface of the radiograph (Fig. 3-4).

Recording the Radiographic Image

After interaction of the x-ray beam with the anatomic structures of the patient, the exit beam or beam of **remnant** x-rays consists of a pattern in which different areas have different numbers of photons corresponding to the pattern of thicknesses, atomic numbers, and densities through which the beam has passed. We are unable to make direct use of this information (an aerial image) and must transfer it to a recording medium suitable to viewing by the eye. The most important method to decode this information carried by the attenuated beam is by means of photographic film. The film may be exposed by the direct action of the

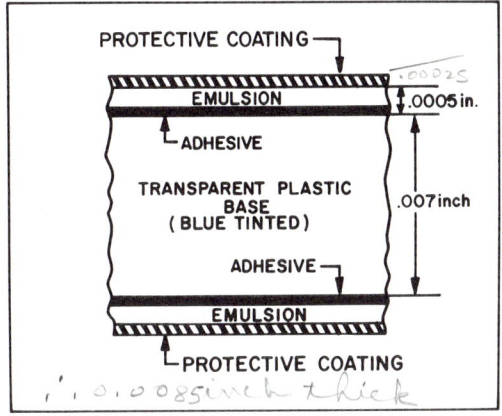

Figure 3-5. Cross-section of x-ray film showing its components. (Courtesy Eastman Kodak Company, Rochester, NY. Reprinted by permission.)

x-rays as is done in intraoral radiography in dentistry, or the energy of the x-ray beam may be converted into light by intensifying screens, and this light in turn is used to expose the film. This latter method is used in extraoral radiography.

X-Ray Film

Radiographic film is composed of a radiation sensitive or photographically active emulsion, usually coated on both sides of a transparent sheet of plastic called the base. The emulsion layers are attached to the base by a thin layer of adhesive. The delicate emulsions are covered by a supercoating of gelatin, which protects the emulsion from rough handling prior to exposure, scratching, pressure, and contamination during processing.

The emulsion is coated on both sides of the base (called double-emulsion films) to provide increased speed to the film. This increased speed also means less radiation for both the patient and the operator because of less radiation and fewer retakes as a result of movement during exposure (Fig. 3-5).

Base

The base is composed of a thin clear plastic, usually either of triacetate or polyester. A blue tint is added providing a film that is easier to view and that prevents eyestrain. Polyester is more resistant to warping with age and stronger than triacetate. Therefore, polyester bases can be made thinner than triacetate bases, but just as strong. Polyester is the film base of choice by almost all the manufacturers of radiographic film.

Emulsion

The emulsion consists of a homogeneous mixture of gelatin and silver halide. The gelatin is similar to that used in salads but is of much higher quality. It is made from cattle bone. The gelatin is clear, so that it will transmit light, and is sufficiently porous for the processing chemicals (developer and fixer) to penetrate it to gain access to silver halide crystals rapidly without destroying its strength or performance.

Silver Halide

The active ingredient of the radiographic emulsion is the silver halide crystal. In the typical emulsion, 80-99 percent of the silver halide is silver bromide and about 1-10 percent silver iodide. The presence of AgI gives the emulsion a higher sensitivity than a pure AgBr emulsion. These atoms have relatively high atomic numbers (I = 53, Br = 35, Ag = 47) compared to the gelatin and base, both of which are about 7. The interaction of the x-ray photons or light photons with these atoms results in the formation of a latent image, which cannot be detected by ordinary physical methods.

However, when the exposed film is processed in a solution called a developer, a chemical reaction takes place reducing the exposed silver iodo-bromide crystals to tiny masses of black metallic silver and leaving the unexposed crystals essentially unaffected. The silver, suspended in the gelatin, is the visible image on the radiograph.

Formation of the Latent Image

The latent image is defined as that invisible image produced in the film emulsion by light or x-rays that is converted to a visible image upon development. We will now examine what happens when light or x-rays strike a silver iodo-bromide crystal, which averages 1.0-1.5 microns (1 micron = .001 millimeter) in diameter and about 6.3×10^9 grains per cubic centimeter of emulsion. Each grain or crystal contains approximately 1 million to 10 million silver ions.

The silver iodo-bromide grain is flat and triangular in shape and the arrangement of the atoms in the crystal is cubical (Fig. 3-6). The lattice of the silver iodo-bromide crystal contains silver, bromine, and iodine atoms held together by electrovalence forces. Silver is a positive ion (an atom that has too few electrons); bromine and iodine are negative ions (atoms with too many electrons). An ion is not electrically neutral. When the silver iodo-bromide crystal is formed, the silver atoms each release an outer shell electron, and the electrons become attached to either a bromine or iodine atom. The silver atom is now missing an electron and is a positively charged ion, identified as Ag^+. The iodine and bromine atoms each have one extra electron and, therefore, are negatively charged ions, now defined as Br^- and I^- (Fig. 3-7).

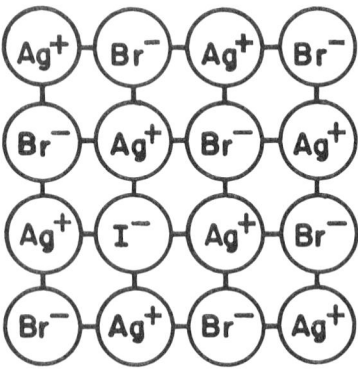

Figure 3-7. Latice diagram of silver iodo-bromide (AgIB) crystal. The straight lines joining the circles represent the electrovalence forces holding the ions together in the crystal.

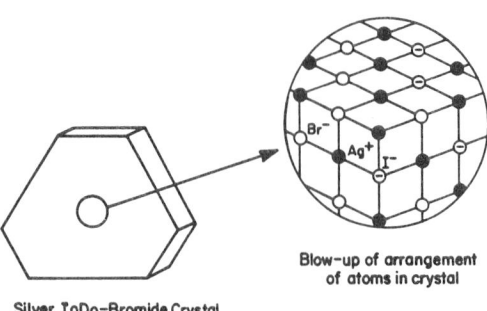

Figure 3-6. Silver iodo-bromide crystal is triangular in shape, but latice arrangement of atoms in the crystal is cubical. (Adapted from Bushong, S.C.: *Radiologic Science for Technologists*. St. Louis, C V Mosby Company, 1975.)

The silver iodo-bromide crystal is not rigid as are some crystals (diamond crystals are very rigid), and there are some conditions where the ions drift freely through the crystal lattice. Bromine and iodine are generally concentrated along the surface of the crystal giving it a negative charge. This is matched by the positive charge of the Ag^+ ions inside the crystal.

The silver iodo-bromide grain or crystal is not perfect, and some of the imperfections are thought to result in the imaging sensitivities of the crystals. The imperfection thought to be responsible is a chemical contaminant added to the emulsion. The chemical commonly used is a sulfur-containing compound called allylthiourea, which reacts with the silver halide to form silver sulfide. The silver sulfide is usually located on or near the surface of the crystal and is called the **sensitivity speck**. The sensitivity speck entraps electrons to begin the formation of the **latent image centers** (Fig. 3-8).

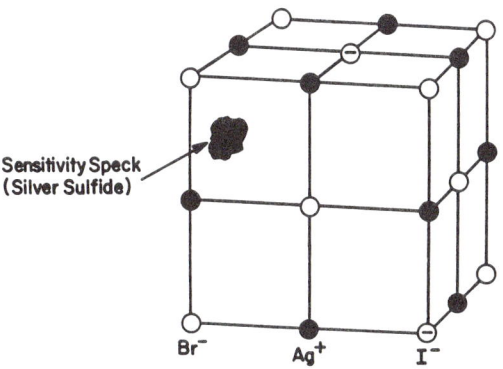

Figure 3-8. The sensitivity speck (silver sulfide) makes the crystal very sensitive to x-rays and light. (Adapted from Selman, J.: *The Fundamentals of X-Ray and Radium Physics*, 6th ed., Springfield, IL, Charles C Thomas, 1978.)

The differences in speed, resolution, contrast, and latitude of various films are controlled by the manufacturers by changing such things as the concentration of the crystals in the emulsion, the number of sensitivity specks per crystal, and the size and distribution of the crystals in the emulsion. The composition of a manufacturer's radiographic emulsion is usually a closely guarded secret.

The description of the formation of the latent image on a film is explained primarily from the **Gurney-Mott hypothesis**, named after the two scientists who proposed it. This hypothesis is being modified by continuing research, but it provides a simple method to explain many photographic and radiographic phenomena.

When an x-ray photon interacts with the Ag, Br, and I atoms of the silver iodobromide crystal of the emulsion, it may be totally absorbed by photoelectric absorption or partially absorbed by Compton scattering. Nevertheless, in both cases, a secondary or free electron (photoelectric or Compton) is released. These secondary electrons, while traversing the crystal, will have sufficient energy to dislodge additional electrons from other atoms of the crystal lattice. Therefore, as a result of one x-ray photon interaction, a great number of electrons are released and drift about inside the crystal.

The same result occurs when visible light photons from an intensifying screen interact with the Ag, Br, and I atoms of the radiographic film emulsion. However, many more light photons are needed to produce an equal number of drifting electrons because light photons have lower energies than x-ray photons.

In time, these migrating electrons are caught by the sensitivity speck area in the crystal. The "sensitivity specks" are composed of silver sulfide, which was introduced during the emulsion-making process. In any case, the effect is to hold the electron at least temporarily in one place. Most of these trapped electrons come from Br^- and I^- ions because these negative ions have one extra electron.

By the loss of one electron, the negative electrons (Br^-, I^-) are converted into neutral atoms, which results in the deterioration of the crystal lattice. Since the bromine and iodine atoms are no longer bound by ionic forces, they are free to migrate out of the crystal into the gelatin portion of the emulsion.

The concentration of electrons at the sensitivity speck creates an area of negative electrification. As the bromine and iodine atoms migrate away from the crystal, the remaining positive silver ions (Ag^+) are attracted to the sensitivity speck. The Ag^+ ion is an atom that is missing an electron. At the sensitivity speck, the Ag^+ ion gains an electron and becomes a neutral silver atom. In each crystal or grain exposed by x-ray or light photons, only a small number of silver atoms (maybe less than 100) are deposited at the sensitivity speck area. Therefore, the concentration of silver atoms at this area (called the **development center** on the crystal) is not observable, even microscopically (Fig. 3-9). This unobservable image on the exposed film composed of radiation- or light-activated silver halide crystals and non-activated silver halide crystals is called the latent image.

The development of the exposed film by the developer solution starts at the development center (sensitivity speck) of the radiation or light-activated silver halide crystal. The silver there acts as a catalyst, spreading out from it until the whole grain becomes an irregular mass of black silver. Under normal development, the grains that have not absorbed sufficient light or x-ray photons to form development centers will develop into clear, transparent areas on the film.

Types of X-Ray Film

X-ray films used in dentistry can be the intraoral type or the extraoral type.

Dental Intraoral X-Ray Film

Dental x-ray film is individually wrapped in packets of white, pebbled, moisture-resistant paper. Within it, the film is further protected by black interleaving paper and backed by lead foil. The sheet of lead foil placed in back of the film protects it from radiation that may be backscattered by the tissues of the oral cavity during exposure. Also, the lead foil contributes to the rigidity of the packet. The Eastman Kodak Company places a herringbone pattern in the lead foil backing that will appear in the radiographic image if the back of the film packet is placed toward the x-ray tube during exposure (Fig. 3-10).

All of the dental films manufactured at present are double-coated emulsion films. In order to identify the "tube side" of the film, a "raised dot" is placed in the corner of the film. The raised portion of the dot is always toward the x-ray tube, and the

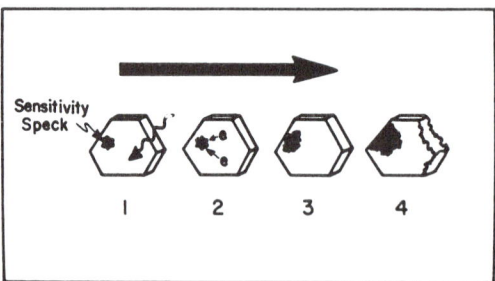

Figure 3-9. Production of the latent image. (1) An x-ray or light photon interacts with an AgIBr crystal to allow an electron to escape from a Br⁻ or I⁻ ion. The Br⁻ or I⁻ ion, which becomes neutral by loss of an electron, migrates from the crystal and is taken up by the gelatin of the emulsion. (2) The free electron is captured and temporarily held at the sensitivity speck in the crystal. (3) The trapped electron attracts a mobile interstitial Ag^+ ion to the sensitivity speck, forming a neutral Ag atom. (4) The first Ag atom acts as an electron trap for a second interstitial Ag^+ ion. The repeated attraction and the neutralizing of interstitial silver ions builds up a clump of silver atoms, called the latent image center in the crystal, which must be present before the developing process will cause visual amounts of metallic Ag to be deposited. (Adapted from Bushong, S.: *Radiologic Science for Technologists.* St. Louis, C V Mosby Company, 1975.)

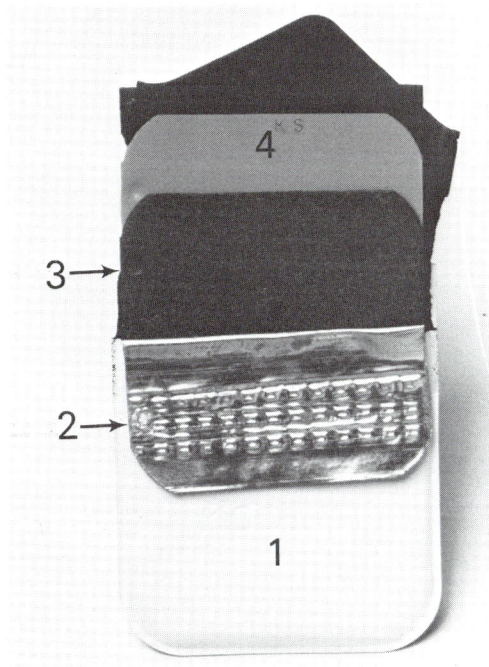

Figure 3-10. Photograph of components of dental x-ray intraoral film packet. Note the **(1)** white moisture-resistant outer covering, **(2)** sheet of lead foil to protect the film from radiation backscatter, **(3)** black interleaving paper, **(4)** double emulsion film.

depressed side of the dot is toward the tongue. A black dot on the printed label of the film packet locates the position of the "raised dot" on the x-ray film.

The older, slower films were coated with a single emulsion on one side of the film base (similar to photographic film). The emulsion side of the film (dull to reflected light) was always placed toward the x-ray tube and the nonemulsion side (shiny side) was always placed toward the tongue. When the film was developed and dried, it was read from the shiny or noncoated side, as if you were inside the patient's mouth looking out. This is why many dentists today mount and read their films as if they were inside the patient's mouth looking out.

There are three types of intraoral dental film:

1. periapical film;
2. bite-wing film;
3. occlusal film.

Periapical Film: As the name suggests, the objective of the periapical film is to show the apex of the tooth and surrounding bone, but it should show the entire crown also. There are three sizes of periapical film: the No. 0 or No. 00 child film, the No. 1 (narrow) adult anterior film, and the No. 2 (standard) adult film.

Bite-wing Film: The bite-wing packet has a wing, or tab, attached or placed on the side that the patient bites on. The posterior bite-wing film shows the crowns of the maxillary and mandibular posterior teeth and their interproximal alveolar crests on one film. The adult No. 3 posterior bite-wing film is longer and narrower than the No. 2 standard film. A bite-tab attached to the No. 2 periapical film converts it to a bite-wing film. In nine- to twelve-year-old children, a No. 2 standard film on each side of the arch is sufficient, but two No. 2 standard films on each side of the arch are usually necessary for adults. A bite-wing film can be made for five- to nine-year-old children by placing a tab on a No. 1 film, and one for children under five years of age by placing a tab on a No. 0 periapical film packet.

Occlusal Film: The occlusal film is considerably larger than the periapical film and is so named because the patient bites upon the entire film. The objective of the occlusal film is to show large segments of the maxillary and mandibular arches and the floor of the mouth.

The Size and Speed of Intraoral Film

Dental intraoral film sizes and speed have been standardized by the American

Table 3-I

SIZES OF INTRAORAL FILM

TYPE-SIZE NUMBER*	DIMENSIONS	
	MILLIMETERS	INCHES
Periapical		
1.00	21 × 32	4/5 × 1 1/4
1.0	22 × 35	7/8 × 1 3/8
1.1	24 × 40	15/16 × 1 9/16
1.2	31 × 41	1 1/4 × 1 5/8
Bite-wing (Interproximal)		
2.00	21 × 32	4/5 × 1 1/4
2.0	22 × 35	7/8 × 1 3/8
2.1	24 × 40	15/16 × 1 9/16
2.2	31 × 41	1 1/4 × 1 5/8
2.3	27 × 54	1 1/16 × 2
Occlusal		
3.4	57 × 76	2 1/4 × 3

* The digit at the left of the decimal point represents the use of the film (periapical, bite-wing, or occlusal). The digits on the right indicate the size of the film (00, 0, 1, 2, 3, or 4).

Dental Association. The standard was originally developed by the American National Standards Institute (ANSI) Committee PH6 (Table 3-I).

The comparative sizes of the intraoral films used in dentistry are shown in Figure 3-11.

The efficiency with which a film responds to x-ray exposure is known as **film sensitivity** or — more commonly — "speed." X-ray films that require very little exposure to x-radiation to produce a radiograph are said to be very sensitive, or very fast, or possess high speed. Then, exposure time and film speed vary inversely.

A high speed film requires a lower mAs factor to produce comparable densities (blackness) on a film than a slower

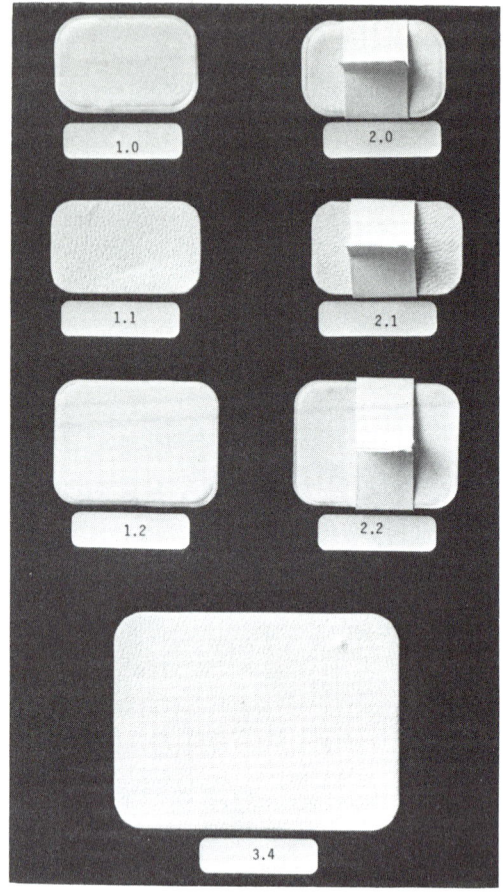

Figure 3-11. Types of intraoral film: 1.0 periapical No. 0 children's film, 1.1 periapical No. 1 narrow-anterior size film, 1.2 periapical No. 2 regular adult size film, 2.0 interproximal No. 0 children's (5 years old and under) size film, 2.1 interproximal No.1 (6-9 years) size film, 2.2 interproximal No. 2 adult size film, 3.4 occlusal film.

speed film. The speed of the film is dependent upon the sensitivity of the emulsion and is governed by the manufacturer. This is accomplished in several ways:

1. Special x-ray film emulsion dyes sensitize the silver bromide crystals to become more radiosensitive.
2. In the film "ripening" process, the

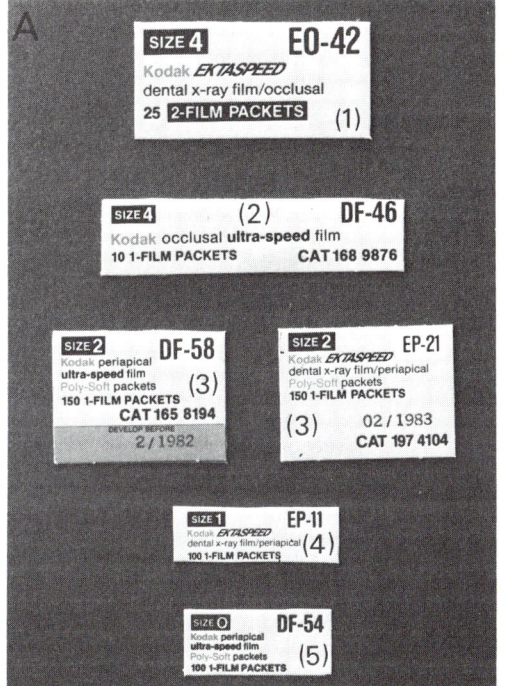
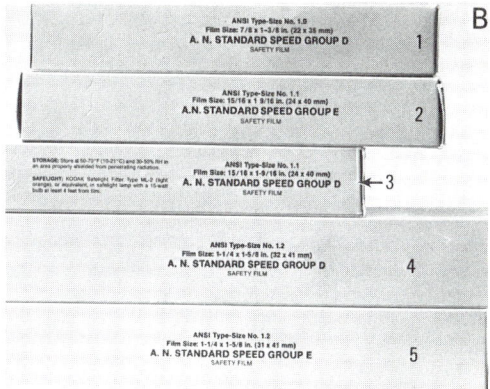

Figure 3-12. Examples of how x-ray film boxes are labeled according to speed and expiration date. (A) 1, (front view) occlusal film size 4, Kodak EKTASPEED, Speed E; 2, (side view) occlusal film, size 4 Kodak Ultra-speed, Speed D; 3, left, D speed, No. 2 size film, note expiration date; right, E speed film, No. 2 size film, note expiration date; 4, size 1 film, E speed film; 5, size 0 film, D speed film. (B) Types and speed of film is imprinted on intraoral film boxes. 1, size 1.0 film (periapical child film speed D film; 2, Size 1.1 film (anterior periapical) speed E film; 3, Size 1.1 film (anterior periapical) speed D film; 4, Size 1.2 film (regular periapical) speed D film; 5, Size 1.2 film (regular periapical) speed E film.

emulsion granules are maintained more constant in size and rendered more sensitive by bringing the silver emulsion up to a temperature of approximately 100°C and keeping it there for a few minutes.
3. Covering the base on both sides with emulsion will increase the speed of the film.
4. The thicker the emulsion and the larger the silver iodo-bromide grain size, the faster the speed of the film.

At the present time, manufacturers of dental film record the film speed on the outside of the packet in an alphabetical classification with the expiration date (Fig. 3-12).

Intraoral film speeds have been standardized on an alphabetical basis according to a speed range recorded in "reciprocal roentgens" (Table 3-II).

X-ray films are compared by determining their relative sensitivity. This is actually measured by determining the amount of x-radiation necessary to produce a certain density (or "blackness") in the emulsion that has been processed in a rigidly controlled manner. For example, if Film E requires half as much x-radiation as Film D to produce the same blackness in the emulsion, Film E is said to be twice as fast as Film D. The film emulsion is

Handwritten note at top: Each film speed is 2× faster than the one preceding ∴ Radiation can be reduced 50% by 1 step (D to E) in film speed.

Table 3-II
SPEED CLASSIFICATION OF INTRAORAL FILM

Speed Group[*]		Speed Range In Reciprocal Roentgens[†]
A *NA*	SLOWEST	1.5- 3.0
B *NA*		3.0- 6.0
C *NA*		6.0-12.0
D		12.0-24.0
E		24.0-48.0
F *NA*	FASTEST	48.0-96.0

[*] No films are sold in speed groups A, B, C, and F. Examples of films sold in groups D and E are Kodak Ultra-Speed in Group D and Kodak Ekta-speed in Group E.

[†] A roentgen is a measure of radiation exposure or quantity. A reciprocal roentgen is $1/R$ or one over the amount of exposure in roentgens to achieve a certain density (blackness) on a film.

sensitive to a number of conditions. Some of these conditions are heat, light, x-rays, fumes, bending, and pressure. The high-speed emulsions are even more sensitive to these conditions.

Film Fog

All unexposed films show a certain amount of density (blackness) after processing. This is called the **base density** of the film. It is a constant factor and is caused by the absorption of a small quantity of light during the manufacture of the film base.

Fog is defined as the density (blackness) of the film due to the development of unexposed silver iodo-bromide grains. A film may also become fogged by the accidental exposure of the film to radiant energy in the form of x-rays or light. Fogging will give the radiograph a hazy appearance.

To determine whether films are fogged or not, compare the density difference between an unexposed film that has been fully processed with one that has only been fixed, washed, and dried. Fogging of a film interferes with contrast by increasing the density (blackness).

Fogging of films can be caused by several conditions:

1. **Age of film**: Age fog is the result of using outdated film. All films have an expiration date because fog increases with time (do not use films past the expiration date).
2. **High temperature and high humidity storage**: High temperatures and humidity increase the production of fog. Ideal storage conditions are temperatures of 50°-70° F and 40-60 percent relative humidity.
3. **Excessive time and/or temperature development**: Processing solutions are chemicals that when applied to the invisible latent image of the exposed x-ray film produce a visible and permanent radiographic image. Radiographic density increases with the time of development and with the temperature of the developing solutions. For optimum results, the time and temperature method of development as recommended by the manufacturer is important. Excessive developing time will increase the density of the radiograph, while excessive fixing time will decrease the density.
4. **Inadequate protection of stored films from x-rays**: Do not store film adjacent to the x-ray machine in unprotected containers.
5. **Darkroom safelight too bright**: A 15 watt bulb used at a minimum of 4 feet above the working surface is the recommended intensity for direct illumination.
6. **Wrong filter in safelight**: The Kodak Morlite® filter is designed for use with

intraoral film only. Extraoral screen-type films should be used with Kodak GBX filters or their equivalent and **not** with Morlite filters.

7. **Too long exposure to safelight**: Fogging of films will take place if unwrapped films are left under the safelight for periods of time that are excessive for the safelight conditions.

8. **Light leaks in the darkroom**: As mentioned previously, the higher speed films are more sensitive to light as well as x-rays.

Extraoral Films

There are two main groups of extraoral films: no-screen and screen film.

No-Screen Film

Those extra-oral films with emulsions that are sensitive to direct exposure of x-rays are called **no-screen films**. They have a double emulsion and a thickness greater than intraoral films. It takes four to five times the exposure time with no-screen film when compared to screen film. This is why the no-screen film (5 × 7 inches or 8 × 10 inches) is recommended only to radiograph the thinner portions of the body such as the hands, feet, and jaws. No-screen film has a high silver content and therefore has a higher inherent contrast (differences between densities) than screen film. It has a thicker emulsion than screen film, requiring it to be processed 50 percent longer when manually processing films. Also, no-screen film cannot be used in the automatic processors unless the roller spaces are adjusted. In the past, no-screen film has been used with a cardboard holder composed of two pieces of x-ray transparent paper board hinged together with binding cloth (Fig. 3-13); however, it is now sold in expensive prepackaged cassettes (readypacs). Because of the many disadvantages in the use of no-screen film, it is thought that in the future a rare earth system similar to Kodak's Min-R® cassette with a single Lanex screen used with Min-R or Ortho M film will replace no-screen film for recording the extremities of the body when high quality images are a priority.

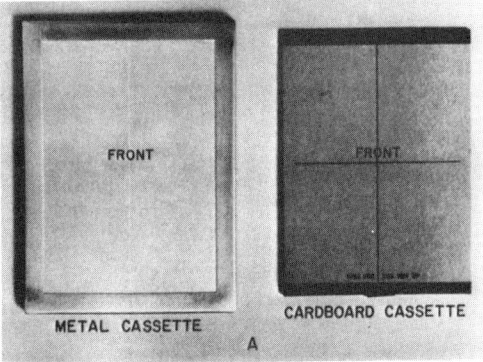

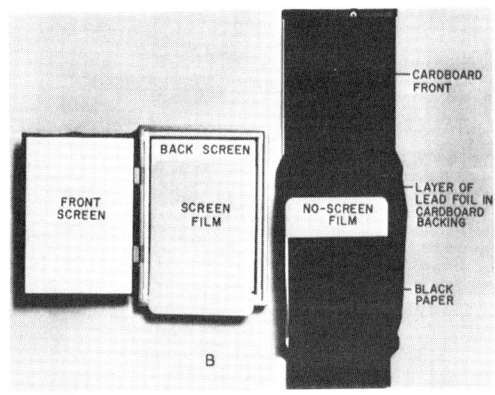

Figure 3-13. Screen and nonscreen cassettes. (**A**) Screen cassettes opened. (**B**) Nonscreen cassette opened. (This cassette is becoming obsolete because most of the nonscreen film at present is sold in prepackaged cassettes.)

Screen Films

Screen type film is film that is sensitive to the fluorescent light of intensifying screens. The visible fluorescent light from the intensifying screen is amplified by the direct action of x-ray photons. For dental use the following sizes are available: 5 × 7 inches, 5 × 12 inches (panoramic), 6 × 12 inches (panoramic), 8 × 10 inches, and 10 × 12 inches.

The very thing that makes x-rays useful, their penetrating power, also makes them difficult to record. The sensitivity of film to direct x-ray exposure is low; for example, of the intensity of the radiation in the beam emerging from the patient, only 1-2 percent is absorbed by the x-ray film emulsion, and 98 percent of it is wasted. Early in the history of dental radiology the need to use more of the wasted x-ray energy was recognized. This led to the introduction of fluorescent intensifying screens.

Intensifying Screens

An intensifying screen is a device that transfers the energy of the x-ray beam into visible light. The visible light produced can then interact with the x-ray film emulsion, forming the latent image on the film.

Light is a form of energy that is more readily absorbed by photographic film than are x-rays. Therefore, light generated by the absorption of x-rays by the screen has a greater effect than x-rays alone. The screen intensifies the effect of x-rays on the film, hence the name. In fact, as much as 98 percent of the recorded density (blackness) on the film exposed by intensifying screen may be due to the light emitted by the screens, and the remaining 2 percent from direct x-ray exposure. This lowers the radiation dose to the patient considerably; however, it does cause some loss in image clarity, which is not serious due to quality of the modern intensifying screens.

Film-Screen Combinations

A characteristic of x-rays is that they cause certain materials to fluoresce, that is, give off ultraviolet and/or visible radiation. Such fluorescent materials are called "phosphors." The ability of phosphors to fluoresce when excited by x-rays makes the intensifying screen possible. Fluorescence is a form of luminescence, which refers to the emission of light by a substance caused by various kinds of stimuli such as light, chemical reactions, and ionizing radiation. **Fluorescence** is produced when light is emitted instantaneously (within 10^{-8} seconds of the stimulation). It is sometimes confused with **phosphorescence** (also called afterglow), which is a form of luminescence applied to the emission of light delayed beyond 10^{-8} seconds in time. Phosphorescence is practically nil in intensifying screens but is strong in fluoroscopic screens. The intensifying

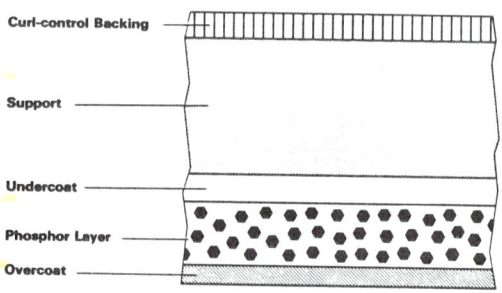

Figure 3-14. Physical characteristics of intensifying screen. Curl control backing: prevents warping or distortion of screen. Support layer: made of paper, plastic, or cardboard to impart required stiffness to screen. Phosphor layer: consists of tiny phosphor crystals embedded in binder. Undercoat may be light-reflective, light absorptive, or simply transparent layer depending on desired performance characteristics of screen. Using the undercoat as a reflector of light will increase the speed of the screen. Overcoat: plastic protective coat. (Copyright Eastman Kodak Company, Rochester, NY. Reprinted by permission.)

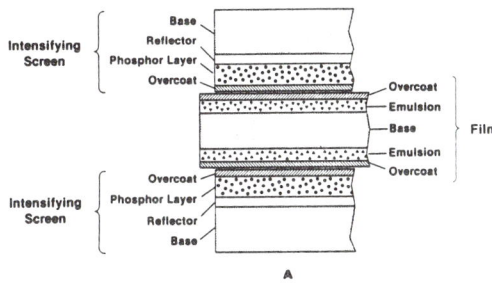

The radiographic film used with intensifying screens has photosensitive emulsion (screen film) on both sides. The film is sandwiched between two intensifying screens in a cassette, so the film emulsion is exposed to the light from its most adjacent screen (light from either of the screens will be almost completely absorbed by the film emulsion nearest it) (Fig. 3-15).

Cassette

The cassette is the rigid holder that contains the screens and the film. The front surfaces, the side facing the tube, should be made of material containing elements with low atomic numbers, such as in plastics, cardboard, or Bakelite®, and should be as thin as practical.

Attached to each cover is an intensifying screen, and the radiographic film is loaded between them. Between each screen is a compression device, such as felt or rubber, which maintains close film contact when the cassette is closed and latched. The back cover is usually made of heavy metal (aluminum, lead lined) in order to minimize backscatter. The hinges and hold-down clamps are usually made of stainless steel (Fig. 3-16).

A high quality screen film radiograph depends upon intimate contact maintained between the film and intensifying screen. If there is any space between the screen and the film, a loss of sharpness of the outline of the radiographic images will incur. Poor contact can be attributed to several factors:

1. air trapped in cassette between screens and film;
2. damaged cassette frames;
3. foreign objects on the screen;
4. damaged latches;
5. improperly mounted screens.

Some of the newer cassettes such as the Kodak X-Omatic® cassette feature a

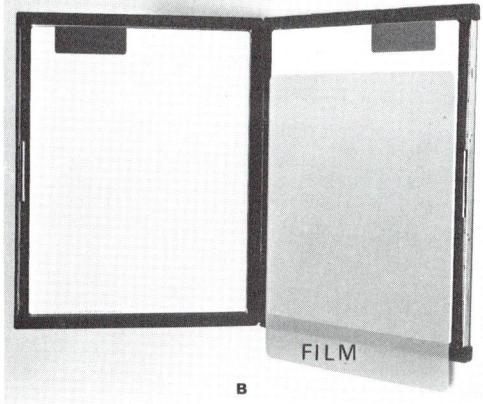

Figure 3-15. (A) Illustration shows the double-coated film sandwiched between two intensifying screens. All components of film-screen combination are shown but not drawn to scale. For example, the thickness of the phosphor layer of the top screen may differ from that of the lower screen. (Copyright Eastman Kodak Company, Rochester, NY. Reprinted by permission.) (B) Photograph of an 8 × 10 inch cassette. Note the two white intensifying screens. The film will be placed between them in the darkroom and the cassette closed tightly to hold film between the two intensifying screens during exposure.

screen is built up in layers (Fig. 3-14). The typical total thickness of the average intensifying screen is approximately 15-16 mils (1 mil = .001 inch). The thickness of the phosphor layer is about 4 mils for par-speed (medium speed) screens and is increased by 1-2 mils for the high speed screens. The thickness is decreased slightly in the detail (slow-speed) screens.

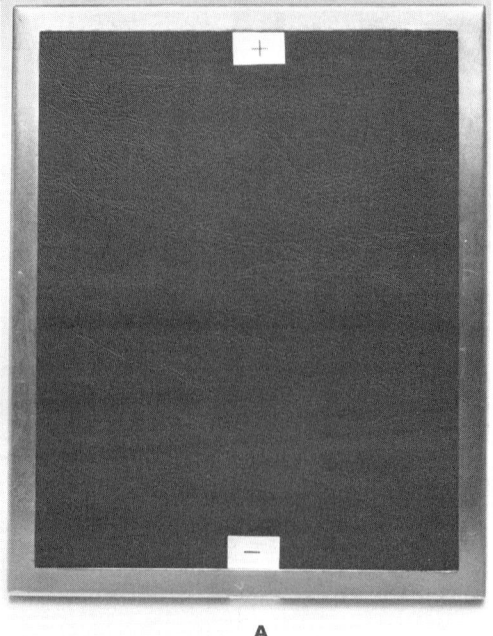

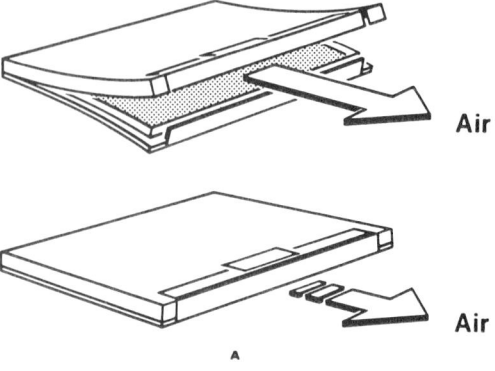

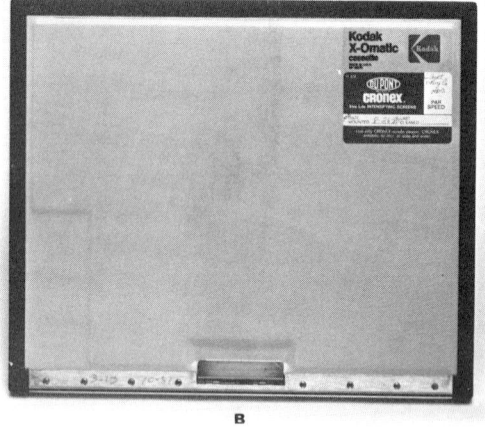

Figure 3-17. (A) Kodak X-Omatic Cassette with curved construction for more efficient expulsion of trapped air and better maintenance of contact without springs. (B) Front of Kodak X-Omatic Cassette. (Copyright Eastman Kodak Company, Rochester, NY. Reprinted by permission.)

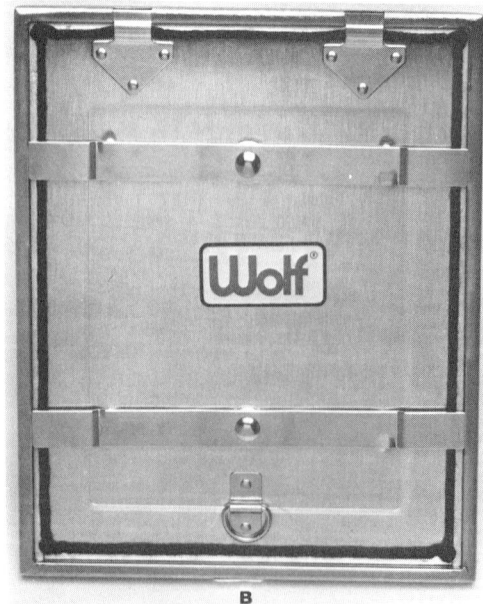

Figure 3-16. Stainless steel cassette with (A) bakelite front and (B) (back) aluminum lead-lined door, stainless steel hinges, and cross bars.

curved construction for more efficient expulsion of trapped air (Fig. 3-17).

Phosphors

The phosphor of the intensifying screen has one purpose: the conversion of the x-ray beam into visible light. This action of the phosphor can be viewed by opening a cassette in a darkened room and, while standing behind a protective barrier, exposing the intensifying screen to x-radiation. The screen will glow brightly. Depending upon the phosphor selected and its treatment during manufacture, light of almost any desired color may be obtained.

The original phosphor used in x-ray intensifying screens was calcium tungstate ($CaWO_4$). It was chosen because its emission is in the ultraviolet and blue regions of the spectrum where the natural sensitivity of the silver halide emulsions used in x-ray films is high.

Since 1970, there have been a whole host of new screens introduced with their corresponding films to increase screen speed over that available with calcium tungstate. However, since calcium tungstate has been the most widely used and accepted intensifying screen material in radiography for the past many years, we will discuss calcium tungstate screens first.

Shortly after Roentgen's discovery of the x-ray in 1895, Thomas Edison and his investigators at Menlo Park in New York concluded that calcium tungstate ($CaWO_4$) was the best phosphor available for both fluoroscopic screens and intensifying screens.

The first commercial calcium tungstate screens were made in Europe in 1896, and in the United States in 1912. However, screen/film combinations did not come into common use until about the time of World War I (1914-1918).

Calcium tungstate is well suited for use in intensifying screens because it meets many of the requisites of a good intensifying screen:

High X-Ray Absorption. Calcium tungstate ($CaWO_4$) has a high atomic number and it responds well to the kV range ordinarily used in diagnostic radiography. This makes for relatively high x-ray absorption by the $CaWO_4$ phosphor.

At diagnostic x-ray energies (80-150 kVp), absorption is almost entirely due to the **photoelectric effect**, which is most likely to occur (1) in elements with high atomic numbers (tungsten 74) and (2) when the x-ray photon (energy) and the binding energy of the K-shell electron (69.5 keV) are almost the same. The fraction of the x-ray beam absorbed by a pair of par-speed $CaWO_4$ screens is about 20 percent and with high speed $CaWO_4$ screens it is about 40 percent. The increased absorption in the faster $CaWO_4$ screens occurs because a thicker screen is used.

Relative High Conversion Efficiency. The ratio of the light energy emitted by the screen to the x-ray energy absorbed in it is referred to as the **screen conversion efficiency** or "amplification." Screen conversion efficiency should not be confused with **intrinsic efficiency of the phosphor**, which is the efficiency with which the phosphor converts x-rays to light. The intrinsic efficiency with which x-ray energy is converted to light differs from phosphor to phosphor. The intrinsic efficiency of calcium tungsten is about 5 percent. **Screen conversion efficiency** depends on the ability of the light emitted by the phosphor to escape from the screen and expose the film. For the typical screen, about half the generated light gets to the film; the rest is absorbed or wasted. Therefore, the screen conversion efficiency is **usually only one-half** the intrinsic efficiency of the phosphor.

Emits Blue Light. Calcium tungstate emits a blue and violet light to which ordinary x-ray film is particularly sensitive. Photographic films are selective in their response to light of various wavelengths. When a certain type of film is exposed to light of various wavelengths, its speed varies. It is said that film is more sensitive to one part of the spectrum than to another. A film's response to various wavelengths (color) is referred to as its **spectral sensitivity**. Calcium tungstate produces light primarily in the blue region of the visible spectrum (Fig. 3-18), with a wavelength range of 3500-5800 Å (1 angstrom = .0001 microns = .00000001 cm), with a peak wavelength of about 4300 angstrom units or 430 nanometers, which is seen by the eye as a violet (bluish green) color. As shown in Figure 3-18, the film does not show a photosensitivity to red light, so red light can be used in the darkroom without producing any photographic effect on the film. The panoramic screens used in dentistry use calcium tungstate phosphors so the darkroom should be equipped with a Kodak GBX (red) safelight.

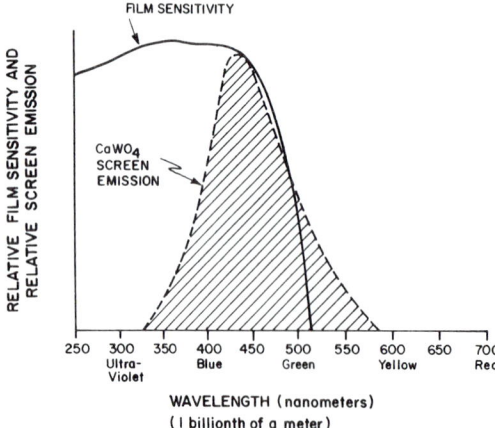

Figure 3-18. The spectral sensitivity curve for this type of film compares favorably to the spectral emission of calcium tungstate. This film is most sensitive to the ultraviolet and blue region of the spectrum, and calcium tungstate emits light primarily in the blue region.

The Kodak Morlite (ML-2) filter (light orange) used with intraoral films is **not** recommended when panoramic or extraoral screen films are developed in the darkroom. As shown in Figure 3-18, the film sensitivity of the screen film used with calcium tungstate screens is too close to the yellow wavelengths in the color spectrum and would fog the panoramic or extraoral film.

Stability. The calcium tungstate phosphor does not deteriorate with use or with age. It has the ability to withstand a variety of ambient conditions such as tropical heat and humidity.

Uniform quality. The calcium tungstate phosphor can be used to manufacture screens of uniform quality.

No phosphorescence. The calcium tungstate phosphor does not have significant afterglow or phosphorescence. This is the tendency of the phosphor to continue to give off light after the x-ray exposure has stopped. It could affect the appearance of radiographs made at short exposures, as in rapid serial film changers used in medical radiography.

Screen Speed

An intensifying screen is defined as being fast or having high speed when a relatively small x-ray exposure produces a given output of light and causes a certain degree of blackening on the film. A screen is said to be slow when a relatively large light exposure is required for a given amount of film blackening. The speed or the **intensifying factor** of a screen is the ratio of the x-ray exposure required to produce the same density (blackness) on a film with and without the screen.

$$\text{Intensifying Factor (speed)} = \frac{\text{exposure without screens}}{\text{exposure with screens}}$$

The denominator will always be larger than the numerator because the exposure with screens is always less than that without screens for the same amount of film blackening. Conventional calcium tungstate screens are available in five speed categories shown in Table 3-III, each followed by its approximate intensifying factor at 70 kV.

Table 3-III
CLASSIFICATION OF CALCIUM TUNGSTATE SCREENS

Ultra Speed	200
High Speed	
(300 microns thick)	100
Par Speed or Medium Speed	50
Detail or Slow	
(50 microns thick)	35
Ultra Detail	15

This means that a high speed screen with an intensifying factor (speed) of 100 takes 1/100 of the exposure to obtain the same film blackening as it would require without screens.

Speed of Calcium Tungstate Intensifying Screens

The following is a summary of some of the factors that influence the light emission or speed of calcium tungstate intensifying screens:
1. Screen absorption
   a. phosphor type
   b. quality of x-ray beam
   c. thickness of phosphor layer
   d. concentration of phosphor crystals in phosphor layer
2. Particle size
3. Presence or absence of light absorbing pigments or dyes in phosphor layer.

Speed Factors Influence Sharpness

Of course, a faster screen is desirable because it decreases patient x-ray exposure, but unfortunately, there is a price to pay for speed. The higher speed calcium tungstate screens record less detail on the radiograph.

When x-rays interact with a screen phosphor, a larger area of the film emulsion is activated by the emitted light than would be activated by the direct exposure of x-rays, which results in a radiographic image that becomes more blurred (less sharp).

Generally, factors that increase the speed of the screen will also increase the blurring or unsharpness of the radiographic image. Sharpness of the image produced by intensifying screens depends for the most part on how faithfully the light image from each individual phosphor is reproduced on the film. The ideal situation would be that the light output of each phosphor would appear as an extremely small clearly defined point of density (blackness) on the film; however, in reality, the image of each crystal appears as a small disc. The blurring of the screen image results from the diffusion or spreading of light as it travels through the screen from the phosphor crystal in which it originates to the film where it is recorded. The larger the size of the disc image (light spread) produced on the film, the less sharp or more blurred will the images appear on the radiograph.

Speed and Absorption Factors of Calcium Tungstate Screens

The first function of the screen is to absorb x-rays. When x-rays are absorbed, fluorescence occurs. The x-ray absorption of a phosphor is a measure of the phosphor to absorb x-rays. In general, the more x-rays absorbed by the calcium tungstate screen, the greater the fluorescence of the screen or the speed of the screen. There are several factors that influence screen absorption: type of phosphor, quality of the beam (keV), thickness of phosphor layer, and concentration of the phosphor in the phosphor layer.

Type of Phosphor. Phosphors differ in their x-ray absorption characteristics. Calcium tungstate has the physical requirements for chemical compounds making up a highly absorbing phosphor: high atomic number (probability of interaction high), high density (mass per unit volume), and responds well to kV range used in radiography (K edge position).

Quality of Beam. As the kV is increased, the intensification factor also increases. Remember, the intensification factor is the ratio of the x-ray absorption in a screen-film combination to x-ray absorption in the radiographic film alone. Thus, at 70 kV the intensification factor with par (medium) speed screens is about 50, whereas at 80 kV it increases to about 75.

Thickness of Phosphor Layer. A screen with a thicker phosphor layer will have a faster speed because the thick layer will absorb more x-rays than a screen with a thin phosphor layer. Although the thicker screens will be faster, the screen thickness has an opposite effect on sharpness. If all factors remain equal, a thin screen will produce a sharper image than that produced by a thicker phosphor layer. The primary reason for the reduction in image sharpness produced by a thick screen can be explained by the geometry of the thick screen construction (Fig. 3-19). A thin screen produces radiographic images that are more sharp because the light photons are produced closer to the film.

Concentration of Phosphor Crystals in Phosphor Layer. The higher the crystal concentration, the higher the screen speed. It is measured in grams per cubic centimeter (gm/cm³). A fast calcium tungstate screen has a packing density of approximately 6.1.

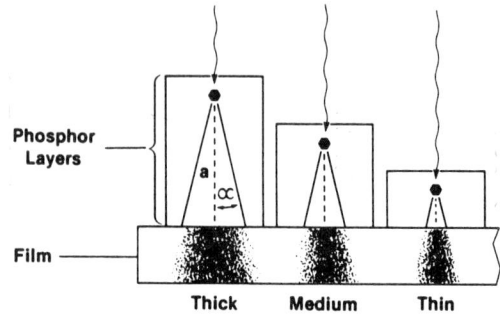

Figure 3-19. Effect of screen thickness on image sharpness. Geometrically the cones are similar. Cone angle α is the same for all three cones, but the altitude (a) varies. Notice then the area of the base varies, and it varies directly with changes in altitude. The taller the cone, the larger the area of the circle. The larger the light cone, the larger the disc image. Therefore, the thicker screen produces larger maximum disc sizes. The conclusion is that a thick screen produces greater light output, but sacrifices sharpness in doing so. (Copyright Eastman Kodak Company, Rochester, NY. Reprinted by permission.)

Phosphor Particle Size

If other factors remain unchanged, increasing the size of phosphor crystals tends to increase the intensity of screen light emitted (speed). You would expect that the larger the phosphor particle, the greater its fluorescent emission, which would, in turn, reduce radiographic sharpness (Fig. 3-20). However, in actual practice, this turns out to be rather unimportant because the crystals are so extremely small, averaging approximately 5 micrometers (10^{-6} meters), with a range of 4 micrometers for the slow screens to 8 micrometers for the fast screens. This range of phosphor crystal size is so small it has very little effect on radiographic image sharpness.

screens regularly to keep them free of dirt and foreign material. Such material can interfere with the diagnosis by casting an artifact on the film, which confuses the image or causes blurring of the image by interfering with screen-film contact. Screens may be washed with cotton and bland soap, rinsed with cotton moistened with water; and then dried by cotton. Screens should be further dried by standing the half opened cassette on its side for about one-half hour in a dust-free room. Screens can also be cleaned with a commercial solution containing an antistatic compound and a detergent.

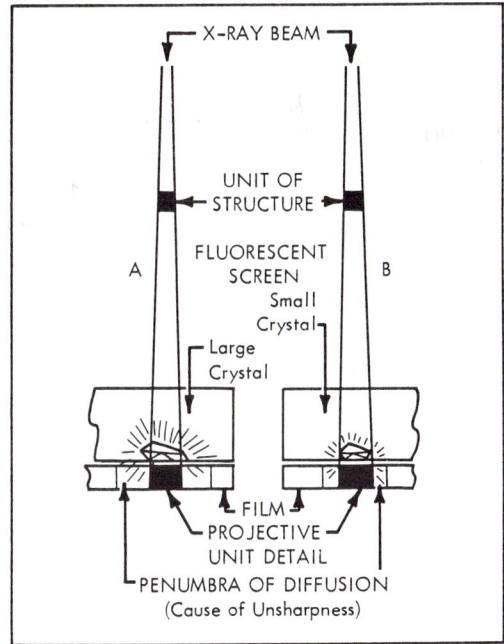

Figure 3-20. Effect of crystal size on the sharpness of the radiographic image. (A) Screen with large crystals. (B) Screen with small crystals. (Redrawn from Fuchs, Arthur W.: *Principles of Radiographic Exposure and Processing*, 2nd ed., Springfield, IL, Charles C Thomas, Publisher, 1958.)

Presence or Absence of Light-Absorbing Pigments or Dyes

A light-absorbing dye or pigment is incorporated in the binder of the phosphor layer of some screens. This is done to reduce the lateral light emission spreading and thereby decrease the blurring of the screen image. It should be noted that the sharpness gained by the use of light-absorbing dye in the binder is achieved at a sacrifice to speed, because it reduces the light intensity emitted by the screen. Such screens may have a gray, pink, or yellow tint, depending upon the absorbing material used (Fig. 3-21).

Care of Screens

It is important to inspect and clean the

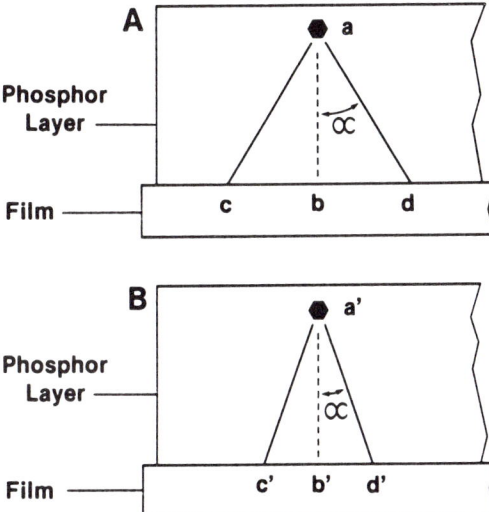

Figure 3-21. The effect of using a light absorbing dye in screen to increase radiographic sharpness. All conditions are the same between phosphor layers A and B except example B contains a light absorbing dye. Although the screen thicknesses are the same in A and B, the dye in the binder reduces the spread of light in B, producing a sharper radiographic image. However, the dye in the binder B effectively shields some of the light energy away from the film and thus reduces the light output from the screen. Therefore, the speed of screen B has been reduced. (Copyright Eastman Kodak Company, Rochester, NY. Reprinted by permission.)

Newer Phosphors

By the early 1970s it was usually agreed that the maximum useful speed of calcium tungstate screens had been achieved. About 1973, newer screen phosphors became available that permitted greater speed than calcium tungstate screens. Some of these newer phosphor screens were rare earth screens. The periodic table is divided by chemists into four basic groups: alkaline earths, rare earths, transition elements, and nonmetals. The term rare earth started because these elements are difficult and expensive to separate from earth and each other, not because the elements are scarce. The rare earth group consists of elements between lanthanum ($Z = 57$) through lutetium ($Z = 71$), which includes gadolinium ($Z = 64$) and europium ($Z = 63$). Since lanthanum is the first element in the rare earth group, the group is also known as the lanthanide series. Lanthanum (La) and gadolinium (Gd) are used as rare earth phosphors. A related phosphor, yttrium (Y) with atomic number of 39, is not a rare earth but has some properties similar to the rare earths.

The rare earths used as phosphors are produced as crystalline powders of terbium-activated gadolinium oxysulfide (Gd_2O_2S:Tb) and terbium-activated lanthanum oxysulfide (La_2O_2S:Tb) Unlike calcium tungstate ($CaWO_4$), the rare earths do not fluoresce properly in the pure state.

The terbium-activated oxysulfide compounds of gadolinium and lanthanum emit approximately 60 percent in the green (544 nm) and 25 percent in the ultraviolet and blue portion (430 nm) of the spectrum. The remainder of the light emitted from these screens is in the yellow—red portion of the spectrum. Therefore, when the blue-sensitive films developed for the calcium tungstate screens were combined with lan-

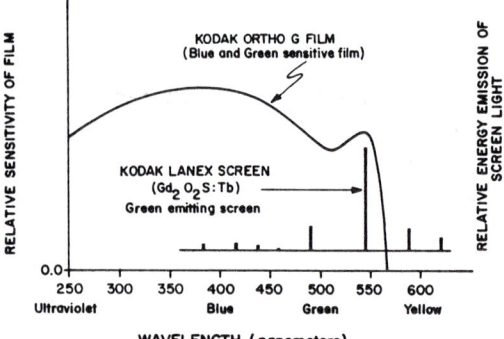

Figure 3-22. Approximate spectral emission spectrum of Kodak Lanex Regular Screens superimposed on graph showing spectral sensitivity of Kodak Ortho G Film, which is sensitive to green light as well as to ultraviolet and blue light. The spectral emission of the rare earth phosphors is produced by the terbium ion. The terbium emission is not a continuous spectrum (as $CaWO_4$) but is concentrated in narrow lines with a strong peak at 544 nm, which is the green light part of the spectrum. The vertical lines represent Lanex screen emission, and height of the lines represent the relative energy in the spectral emission bands from the screens. (From *Medical Radiography and Photography*, 53 (1): 1977, published by Health Sciences Markets Division, Eastman Kodak Company, Rochester, NY. Courtesy of Daniel J. Lawrence.)

thanum and gadolinium oxysulfide screens, there was no large increase in speed relative to that of calcium tungstate screens. As a result, orthochromatic films (such as Kodak Ortho G or L films and 3M Trimax type XD or XM films) with a sensitivity to green as well as blue light were designed for use with these primarily green emitting phosphors (Fig. 3-22). With the green-sensitive film, the usual amber (6B) safelight filter previously used with blue-sensitive film has to be changed to a filter shifted more toward the red portion of the spectrum. Such a filter was developed by Kodak and is called the GBX filter (red). The GBX filter can be used satisfactorily with both blue-sensitive and green-sensitive films.

There are some newer phosphors designed to be used with ultraviolet and blue-sensitive films. They are terbium and thulium-activated lanthanum oxybromide (LaOBr:Tb, LaOBr:Tm) such as General Electric Blue Max I and II screens, europium-activated barium fluorochloride (BaFCl:Eu) such as DuPont Quanta II screens, and europium-activated barium strontium sulfate such as Kodak X-Omatic regular screens. Although barium fluorochloride and barium strontium sulfate are not rare earths (except for a minute amount of activator) they both emit primarily ultraviolet light.

Some of the screen and film combinations presently available are listed in Table 3-IV. The screens in the first group yield about the same speed of a reference film DuPont Cronex 4 or Kodak X-Omat RP film, XRP, and a pair of DuPont Cronex par speed screens (calcium tungstate). The film/screen combinations in the second group yield about two times the speed of the reference film/screen combinations. The third group has a speed of about four times that of the reference system.

The film/screen combinations in the third group have about the same **resolution** (ability to record separate images of small objects placed very close together) as the high-speed calcium tungstate screen/medium blue film combinations of the second group (Soila et al., 1977).

The Kodak Lanex (rare earth) film/screen systems are compared to conventional Kodak film/screen systems in Table 3-V.

Crossover Reduction

A characteristic of conventional silver halide emulsions is that they absorb more ultraviolet than visible light. For this reason, intensifying screens that feature ultraviolet-emitting phosphors can offer a reduction of **crossover**. The degradation of a radiographic image by the escape of light from one film emulsion layer to the other is called crossover. Ideally, each emulsion layer would be exposed only by light from the screen with which it is in contact. Unfortunately, this is seldom the way it happens. In actual practice, some light from the upper screen is transmitted by the upper film emulsion. The escaped light traverses the film base and some of it exposes the lower emulsion. In the same way, the light from the lower screen escapes and exposes the upper emulsion. This is crossover (Fig. 3-23).

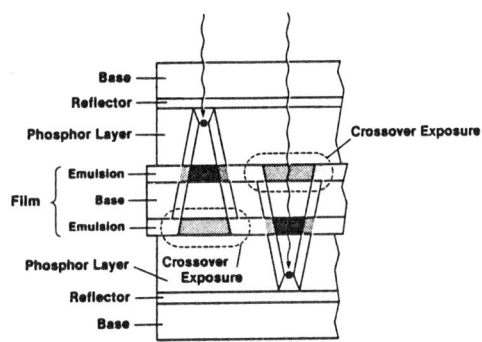

Figure 3-23. This illustrates the effect of crossover. Light emitted from opposite screen (not adjacent to a film emulsion) exposes the emulsion to additional light, which produces an image that is not as sharp as the image obtained when exposure is by the screen adjacent to it. (Copyright Eastman Kodak Company, Rochester, NY. Reprinted by permission.)

Barium strontium sulfate (Kodak X-Omatic regular) and barium fluorochloride (DuPont Quanta II), which have spectral emission peak wavelengths of 380 nm and 390 nm respectively, absorb more of the ultraviolet radiation available and allow less of the ultraviolet light to pass through. Both of these phosphors produce less crossover when compared with

Table 3-IV

TYPICAL SCREEN/FILM COMBINATION*

SPEED FACTOR	FILM†	SCREENS	SCREEN PHOSPHOR	COLOR EMITTED
1	Medium blue	DuPont Cronex Par-speed	$CaWO_4$	Blue
1	Slow green	Gafmed Rarex BG Detail	$Gd_2O_2S:Tb/Y_2O_2S:Tb$	Blue-green
1	Slow green	Kodak Lanex Fine	$Gd_2O_2S:Tb$	Green
1	Slow blue	Kodak X-Omatic Regular Intensifying	$BaSO_4:Sr,Eu$	Ultra-violet
1	Medium blue	Siemens Titan D	$LaOBr:Tb$	Blue
1	Slow green	3M Trimax 2	$Gd_2O_2S:Tb$	Green
2	Medium blue	DuPont Cronex Hi-Plus	$CaWO_4$	Blue
2	Slow green	Gafmed Rarex BG Mid-speed	$Gd_2O_2S:Tb/Y_2O_2S:Tb$	Blue-green
2	Slow green	Kodak Lanex Medium	$Gd_2O_2S:Tb$	Green
2	Medium blue	Siemens Titan U	$LaOBr:Tb$	Blue
2	Slow green	3M Trimax 4	$Gd_2O_2S:Tb$	Green
4	Medium blue	DuPont Cronex Lightning Plus	$CaWO_4$	Blue
4	Slow blue	DuPont Cronex Quanta II	$BaFCl:Eu$	Ultra-violet
4	Slow blue	DuPont Cronex Quanta III	$LaOBr:Tm$	Blue
4	Slow green	Gafmed Rarex BG High Speed	$Gd_2O_2S:Tb/Y_2O_2S:Tb$	Blue-green
4	Slow green	Kodak Lanex Regular	$Gd_2O_2S:Tb$	Green
4	Medium blue	Siemens Titan HS	$LaOBr:Tb$	Blue
4	Slow green	3M Trimax 8	$Gd_2O_2S:Tb$	Green
6	Slow green	3M Trimax 12	$Gd_2O_2S:Tb$	Green
6	Medium blue	Agfa-Gevaert MR 600	$LaOBr:Tb$	Blue
8	Medium blue	DuPont Cronex Quanta III	$LaOBr:Tm$	Blue
8	Medium green	Kodak Lanex Regular	$Gd_2O_2S:Tb$	Green
8	Medium green	3M Trimax 8	$Gd_2O_2S:Tb$	Green

* Adapted from J. Skucas and J. Gorski: Application of Modern Screens in Diagnostic Radiology. *Med Radiogr Photogr, 56* (2):25, 1980.

† *Film Types* (Examples): *Slow blue*: Kodak X-Omat G (XG) and DuPont Cronex 7. *Medium blue*: Kodak X-Omat RP (XRP) and DuPont Cronex 4. *Slow green*: Kodak Ortho G (OG), Kodak Ortho L (OL), and 3M Trimax XD. *Medium green*: Kodak Ortho H (OH) and 3M Trimax XM.

$CaWO_4$ (18% versus 32% are typical values) (Fig. 3-24).

Evaluation of Screen/Film Combinations

In evaluating screen/film combinations, there are specific properties that should be taken under consideration. They are speed, image contrast, and image quality (sharpness, resolution, and radiographic noise); these factors are all interrelated.

Speed

The speed of a screen/film combination is the reciprocal of the exposure required to yield a given density (blackness). The speed of a system depends on a number of factors:

1. absorption efficiency;

Table 3-V

KODAK SCREEN/FILM COMBINATIONS

Relative Film Speeds with Various Screens

Film	Film Characteristics	Lanex Fine	Medium Speed $CaWO_4$	Lanex Medium	High Speed $CaWO_4$	X-Omatic Regular	Lanex Regular
X-Omat RP	High contrast Medium speed Automated & Manual Blue sensitive	—	100	—	250	200	250
Blue Brand	High contrast Medium speed Manual & Long-cycle automated Blue sensitive	—	120	—	250	200	250
X-Omat G	High contrast Automated & Manual Blue sensitive Responds well to ultraviolet = emitting screens	—	60	—	120	100	120
Ortho G	High contrast Automated & Manual Orthochromatic sensitivity	100	—	250	—	—	400
Ortho L	Wide latitude Automated & Manual Orthochromatic sensitivity	100	—	250	—	—	400
Ortho H	Medium contrast Automated & Manual 2 × speed of Ortho G Orthochromatic sensitivity	200	—	500	—	—	800
Min-R	Wide latitude Automated & Manual Singe Coated To be used with Single Lanex fine screen Orthochromatic sensitivity	Single Screen Extremity 20	—	Single Screen Extremity 40	—	—	—
Ortho M	Automated & Manual Approx 2 × speed of Min-R To be used with Singe Lanex fine screen Orthochromatic sensitivity	Single Screen Extremity 40	—	Single Screen Extremity 80	—	—	—

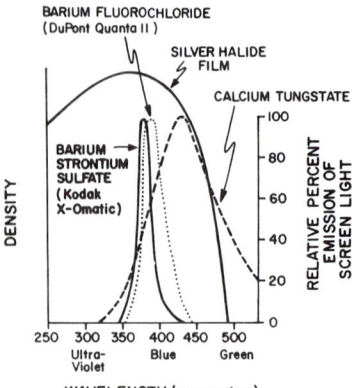

Figure 3-24. Approximate spectral emission of calcium tungstate, barium strontum sulfate, and barium fluorochloride, compared to natural sensitivity of conventional silver halide film. There is less crossover with the barium screens than the calcium tungstate screens because the barium screens absorb more of the ultraviolet radiation available and allow less of the ultraviolet light to pass through. (Copyright Eastman Kodak Company, Rochester, NY. Reprinted by permission.)

2. screen conversion efficiency;
3. response to kilovoltage;
4. screen spectral emission matched to film spectral sensitivity (discussed previously);
5. inherent film speed (discussed previously).

Since there are so many variables involved, most clinicians do not measure the speed of screen/film combinations in absolute values—they normalize it to clinically realistic exposure factors. Usually a pair of par-speed screens and Kodak X-Omatic RP film is taken as a reference point to which all other screen/film systems are compared.

Most rare earth phosphors are faster than calcium tungstate ($CaWO_4$) for two reasons: higher absorption efficiency and greater conversion efficiency.

High Absorption Efficiency

Calcium tungstate when compared with such rare earth phosphors as gadolinium oxysulfide and lanthanum oxybromide has less absorption efficiency of x-ray photons in the energy range used in diagnostic radiology (Table 3-VI).

Table 3-VI

ABSORPTION EFFICIENCY OF SCREENS COMPOSED OF 100 MG/CM² PHOSPHORS

PHOSPHOR	ABSORPTION (%) (at 80 kV, Filtered Source)
LaOBr:Tm or Tb	41.5%
BaFCl:Eu	39.7%
Gd_2O_2S:Tb	37.7%
Y_2O_2S:Tb	27.0%
$CaWO_4$	26.7%

*Adapted from H. W. Venema: X-ray absorption, speed, and luminescent efficiency of rare earth and intensifying screens. Radiology, 130:767-771, March, 1979.

Thus, the rare earth and barium screens waste fewer of the x-ray photons available. The light output with gadolinium or lanthanum phosphors can be increased considerably without significant loss of image quality because more x-ray photons are absorbed.

The x-ray absorption efficiency of a phosphor increases sharply at the K-edge of the prominent heavy metal present. The K-edge (K-shell binding energy) of Ba, La, and Gd correspond closely to the maximum intensity of x-rays in the primary x-ray beam. Thus, these phosphors have higher absorption of x-rays (photoelectric effect) used in diagnostic radiology as compared with $CaWO_4$, even though the atomic number (Z) of tungsten (74) is higher than barium (56), Lanthanum (57), or gadolinium (64). Up to 50 keV, Gd_2O_2S:Tb and $CaWO_4$ absorb about the same; at 50.2 keV, the K-shell

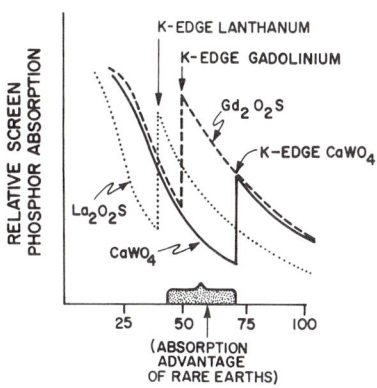

Figure 3-25. Approximate absorption curves of GdO₂S, La₂O₂S, and CaWO₄. The rare earths have absorption advantage over CaWO₄ between 39 keV (lanthanum) to 70 keV range.

Table 3-VII

CONVERSION EFFICIENCY

*Y₂O₂S:Tb	18%	(Yttrium)
GdO₂S:Tb	18%	(Gadolinium)
La₂O₂S:Tb	13%	(Lanthanum)
CaWO₄	3-5%	(Tungsten)

*The absorption of yttrium (39) is the same as tungsten (74) from 17 and 70 keV, but yttrium is faster because of higher conversion efficiency.

binding energy of Gd, there develops an advantage of four to five times for Gd₂O₂S over CaWO₄ that will persist until the 69.5 keV K-edge of tungsten is reached. Lanthanum (La) has a K-shell binding energy of 38.9 keV, which effectively shuts out any absorption advantage of CaWO₄ over the two rare earths, lanthanum and gadolinium, in the 39-70 keV range (Fig. 3-25).

Screen Conversion Efficiency

The rare earths have a second advantage over calcium tungstate in that the rare earth phosphors produce more light photons for each x-ray photon absorbed. Thus, they have a higher "amplification" or greater x-ray to light conversion efficiency than calcium tungstate. Some of the conversion efficiency figures quoted in the literature are shown in Table 3-VII.

Barium fluorochloride (europium activated) (DuPont Quanta II) owes much of its increased speed to a more efficient conversion of x-ray energy to light. It is faster than DuPont Lightening Fast, DuPont's fastest calcium tungstate screen.

Response to Kilovoltage

The kilovoltage response of CaWO₄ screens to kVp for all practical purposes is linear; an increase in kVp will make a corresponding increase in speed in the screen. The kilovoltage response of rare earth and barium screens is **not** linear. These screens show a maximum speed at about 80 kVp, with slightly less speed at 50-65 kVp and slightly higher speeds over 100 kVp. With the rare earth and barium screens, it is advisable to use a **variable mAs-fixed kVp exposure technic,** which is opposite to the variable kVp-fixed mAs technic used with calcium tungstate screens.

Image Contrast

Radiographic contrast refers to the difference in the density (blackness) between areas in the radiograph. The difference in degrees of blacks, grays, and whites on the film, or contrast, allows the clinician to see the diagnostic information on the film. It depends primarily on **subject contrast** (type of object being radiographed and kVp used), **film contrast** (type of film used and processing conditions) and **fog** and **scatter** radiation. It depends secondarily on screen characteristics.

Rare Earth Phosphor Screens Produce

Higher Contrast Films. With higher kVp techniques and conditions of high scatter (patient body part), calcium tungstate screens will yield a **lower contrast** than rare earth screens. Scattered x-ray photons are lower in energy than the primary beam x-ray photons. Rare earth screens lose their speed advantage over calcium tungstate screens at lower energy ranges, and therefore, they are less sensitive to scattered photons. This is why rare earth screens will exhibit **higher contrast** than calcium tungstate screens during those exposure techniques in which there is considerable scattered radiation present.

Image Quality

Image quality is defined as the ability of a film to record each point in the object as a point on the film.

In the use of intensifying screens in extraoral radiography, the point-to-point reproduction is never perfect because of the diffusion of light by the screens. Image quality is determined by **sharpness, resolution,** and **radiographic noise.**

Radiographic Sharpness

Sharpness (detail or definition) is the ability of the x-ray film to define an edge. It is related to the abruptness of the density change across a boundary. Good definition or sharpness permits the detection of minimal changes in structure.

Sharpness is related to contrast in that if the contrast is high the abruptness of change can easily be seen, while if the contrast is low the abruptness in change is poorly visible (Fig. 3-26).

Radiographic contrast was previously discussed. It is the density difference between the structure of interest and its surroundings. As you remember, radiographic contrast is the product of **subject contrast** and **film contrast.**

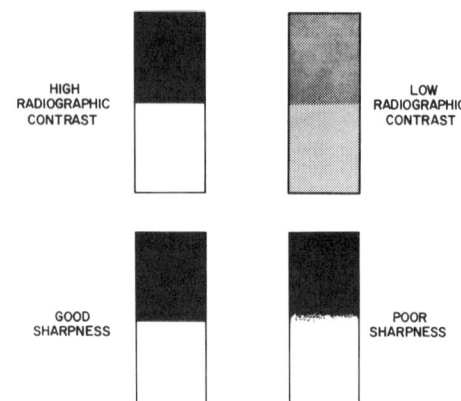

Figure 3-26. *Top:* Radiographic contrast in combination of subject contrast and film contrast that results in density differences between adjacent areas on the radiograph. *Bottom:* Sharpness is the abrupt change in going from one density to another on a radiograph.

Radiographic blurring (unsharpness) is the width of the density change across a boundary, that is, the distance in the radiograph over which the density changes between the structure of interest and its surroundings. The blurring (unsharpness) of a radiographic image is influenced by geometric and screen-film factors.

The geometric factors are focal spot size, source-object distance, subject-film distance, and motion. Blurring or penumbra size (unsharpness) is decreased by using the smallest focal spot size possible, a source-object distance as long as possible, a subject-film distance as short as possible, and the reduction of motion of the patient.

Blurring in screen/film combinations can be reduced by decreasing the lateral spread of light in screens during exposure. This can be done by reducing the screen thickness, using light absorbing dyes and pigments in the binder, reducing the size of the phosphor, and using good screen-film contact.

Rare earth systems can obtain approximately twice the speed with little or no loss in sharpness compared with conventional calcium tungstate screens. Also, if the same speed is maintained, the rare earth systems improve sharpness, because a pair of screens composed of a rare-earth phosphor can be thinner than a pair of calcium tungstate screens and still maintain similar absorption characteristics, resulting in the same speed for both systems, but with improved sharpness for the rare earth system.

For instance, Kodak Lanex medium screens (rare earth screens) and Kodak Ortho (OG) film (slow green) have essentially the same speed but improved sharpness when compared with a HiPlus calcium tungstate screen/film system.

Resolution

Resolution is defined as the ability of an imaging system to produce images of closely spaced objects (Fig. 3-27). Although sharpness and resolution are different entities, they are governed by similar factors such as geometry, light diffusion in screens, and motion. Therefore, sharpness and resolution are often used interchangeably; however, the two terms are different. An imaging system may be able to record sharp edges (sharpness) but be unable to resolve fine details (resolution). On the other hand, another system may yield blurred, unsharp edges (unsharpness) but still be able to reveal fine detail (resolution).

Sharpness and resolution can be defined separately, but their complex interrelationship ultimately aids in the determination of image quality.

An objective measurement of the combined effects of sharpness and resolution has been formulated, and the concept is called modulation transfer function (MTF). Basically, MTF is derived from

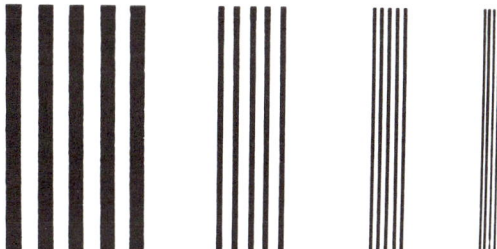

Figure 3-27. Parallel line test pattern for measuring resolution of intensifying screens. (Resolution is defined as the ability of an imaging system to produce images of closely spaced objects.)

what is known as line spread function (LSF). If we expose directly (without screens) a film to an extremely narrow beam (usually 10 microns), a sharp line image would be obtained. It is so severely collimated it is called a "line source" x-ray beam. When a film-screen combination is exposed by the same line source x-ray beam, the line image produced will have blurred edges due to diffusion of light in the phosphor layer of the screen. The LSF represents the measurement of the width of the line imaged; a microdensitometer, which reads density of an extremely small area, is used to make this measurement. By a complex process known as Fourier analysis, LSF can be converted to MTF. At present, MTF is the best measure to evaluate the combined performance of contrast, sharpness, and resolution of an imaging system. The physics and mathematics involved in MTF is highly complex and will not be discussed here. There are some excellent articles that describe LSF and MTF concepts in detail in the references at the end of the chapter.

Radiographic Noise

Radiographic noise is the third major component of image quality. It is the unwanted fluctuation in radiographic density. It may seem strange to refer to **noise**

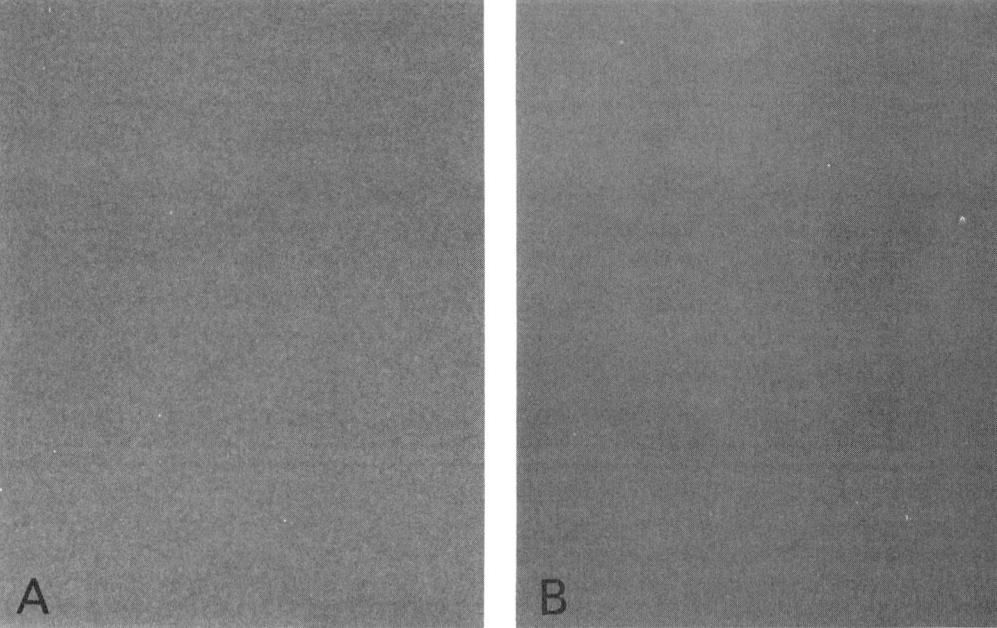

Figure 3-28. Radiographic mottle. **(A)** This image was produced by a screen-film combination that was given an x-ray exposure. The irregular density pattern is due to quantum mottle. **(B)** This film was produced by uniform exposure of the film alone (without intensifying screens). (From Figure 43, page 60, *The Fundamentals of Radiography*, 12th ed. Courtesy Health Sciences Markets Division, Eastman Kodak Company, Rochester, NY. Reprinted by permission.)

as something **seen** rather than **heard**. The term has been borrowed from the field of electrical engineering along with various other mathematical tools that have been useful in understanding of radiographic imaging. "Noise" as we will use it refers to density variations that obscure the radiographic image much in the same manner that static interferes with our ability to hear a radio broadcast.

There are two factors that govern radiographic noise: artifacts and radiographic mottle.

Artifacts. Artifacts are unwanted density variations that are blemishes on the radiograph, caused by common errors in handling, processing, exposure, and darkroom procedures. We will discuss artifacts in a later chapter. They are preventable and not difficult to recognize.

Radiographic Mottle. Radiographic mottle is defined as the density variation in a radiograph made with intensifying screens that have been given a uniform x-ray exposure. It has three components: screen structure mottle, film graininess, and quantum mottle. The first two are unimportant in diagnostic radiology.

Quantum Mottle. Quantum refers to a distinct packet of energy carried by one x-ray photon. An x-ray beam contains a certain number of "bundles" or "packets" of energy referred to as quanta or x-ray photons.

Mottle refers to a pattern of nonuniform density of the x-ray film. Quantum mottle is defined as the variation in density of a uniformly exposed radiograph that results from the random spatial distribution of the x-ray quanta absorbed in the screen (Fig. 3-28).

This means that the x-ray beam is not uniform because the number of quanta in a cross-section of the x-ray beam (before it reaches the patient) is randomly different from one area to another. If the number of quanta or photons were counted in each square millimeter of a cross-section of the beam, it would be unlikely that any two square millimeters would contain the same number of quanta or photons. This is because the emission of x-ray photons from the x-ray source is a random event, and the actual number of photons per square millimeter in a given cross-section of the beam follows the law of probability.

The random distribution of quanta within the x-ray beam produces a random pattern of x-ray absorption in the phosphor layer of the screens.

The pattern of light emitted by the phosphors produces a density pattern on the radiograph corresponding to the random location of the x-ray photons absorbed by the screens. These density variations in the radiograph are quantum mottle.

The fewer the number of x-ray photons used in image formation, the greater the quantum mottle, because quantum mottle is caused by the statistical fluctuation in the number of quanta per unit area absorbed by the intensifying screen.

In statistics, the law of probability states that the percent fluctuation from the actual number becomes greater as the average number becomes smaller.

For instance, let us compare two hypothetical screen-film combinations, one requiring an average of 10,000 photons per mm^2 to produce a density of 1.0 on a radiograph and one requiring only an average of 100 photons per mm^2 to produce the same density. The **law of probability** states that the **variance of fluctuation** from the average is equal to plus or minus the square root of the average number. Therefore, in the film-screen combination requiring an average of 10,000 photons per mm^2 to produce the density of 1.0 on the radiograph, approximately 68 percent will receive between 9,900 and 10,100 photons per mm^2 (10,000 $\pm \sqrt{10,000}$ or 10,000 $\pm$ 100). For 68 percent of the mm^2, the number of photons will be within 1 percent 100/10,000 or 1% fluctuation from the average value. For the film-screen combination requiring only an average of 100 photons per mm^2 to produce a density of 1.0 on the radiograph, approximately 68 percent of the mm^2 will have received from 90 to 110 (100 $\pm \sqrt{100}$ or 100 $\pm$ 10) photons for each mm^2 for a relative deviation of $\pm$ 10 or a 10 percent (10/100) fluctuation from the average value.

Although the film-screen combination requiring an average of only 100 photons per mm^2 would be a much faster combination than the first one, the radiograph produced would have greater quantum mottle because of the higher fluctuation percent (10% as compared to 1%).

Factors Affecting the Appearance of Quantum Mottle

Quantum mottle (noise) is dependent on several factors: film speed, film contrast, screen conversion efficiency, screen absorption, and kVp.

Film Speed and Quantum Mottle. If speed of a screen-film combination is increased by using a faster film, quantum mottle will increase because fewer quanta are required to form an image of a given density. On the other hand, a slower film offers a way to decrease quantum mottle.

Film Contrast and Quantum Mottle. As film contrast increases, quantum mottle increases. A film with high contrast will produce more quantum mottle than a

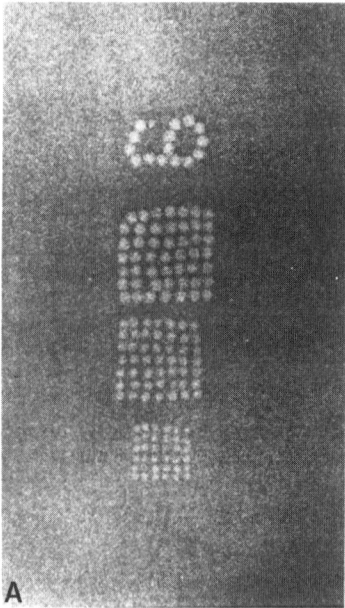 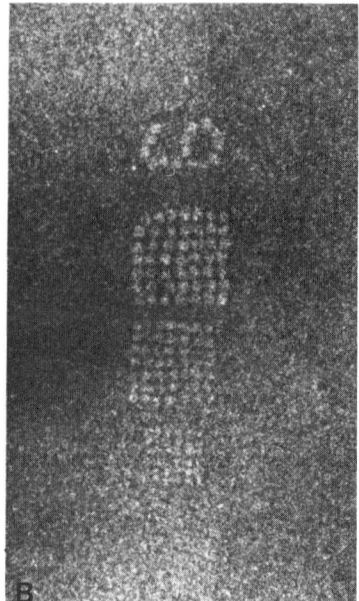

Figure 3-29. Illustration of how quantum mottle affects perceptibility of low-contrast structures, such as acetate beads. **(A)** Slower film-screen combination using many x-ray photons to produce the image. **(B)** Radiograph produced using a fast film-screen combination with relatively few x-ray photons. (From Figure 45, *The Fundamentals of Radiography*, 12th edition. Courtesy of Health Sciences Markets Division, Eastman Kodak Company, 1980.)

low contrast film because of its greater enhancement of the brightness differences in the emission patterns of the phosphors of the intensifying screens. Also, quantum mottle is difficult to see unless a high quality radiograph is produced. Quantum mottle will **not** be visible on radiographs produced with poor contrast and quality.

Screen Conversion Efficiency and Quantum Mottle. As screen conversion efficiency increases, so does quantum mottle because fewer x-ray photons are required to produce an image (Fig. 3-29). The newer rare earth screens are faster than calcium tungstate screens because they have an increased absorption efficiency (no change in mottle) and a higher efficiency in converting x-ray energy to light (with an increase in mottle). The increase in quantum mottle produced by rare-earth screens can be compensated for by use of slower films with these screens.

Screen Absorption and Quantum Mottle. We can increase the speed of a screen without increasing quantum mottle by increasing the absorption of the x-ray quanta in the screen. Screen absorption can be increased in two ways: changing the thickness of the phosphor layer or using a phosphor with a high absorption efficiency for x-rays (rare earths).

By increasing the thickness of the phosphor layer of a screen, the thicker screens will absorb a higher percentage of the x-ray beam and therefore increase the speed of the screen without changing the quantum mottle (Fig. 3-30).

Another method to increase the number of photons used by the screen is to increase the absorption efficiency of the phosphor used. One of the reasons the newer rare earth screens are faster than the calcium tungstate screens is that they absorb (use) a larger percentage of the x-ray beam. A more absorbing phosphor will waste fewer x-ray quanta in producing a radiograph of a given density, and it does it without increasing quantum mottle (noise).

Radiation Quality (kVp) and Quantum Mottle. When the average energy of the x-ray beam is increased by raising the kilovoltage, the average energy of the x-ray quanta absorbed by the screen is usually increased. The greater the energy of each incident photon, the brighter the light emitted, on the average, when the x-ray photon is absorbed. The brighter the light emitted, the fewer number of incident x-ray photons required to produce a given density.

It is for this reason that the use of higher kilovoltages is thought to increase quantum mottle somewhat. In the range of energies used in extraoral radiography in dentistry, the effect of kVp on quantum mottle is very small.

Reduction of Scattered Radiation by Use of Grids

A heavier part of the body such as the skull will produce a much higher proportion of scattered radiation than a thinner part such as the mandible. A method of controlling scatter radiation, besides the use of collimation, is a **grid.** A radiographic grid is a device composed of alternating strips of lead and spacer materials. A spacer material (fiber or aluminum) is chosen that has a low x-ray absorption. The lead strips absorb a considerable amount of the oblique scattered radiation, that is, the rays not traveling in the direction of the primary beam (Fig. 3-31). The transparent spacers allow most of the primary rays to pass through to the film. This technique for reducing the amount of scatter radiation reaching the

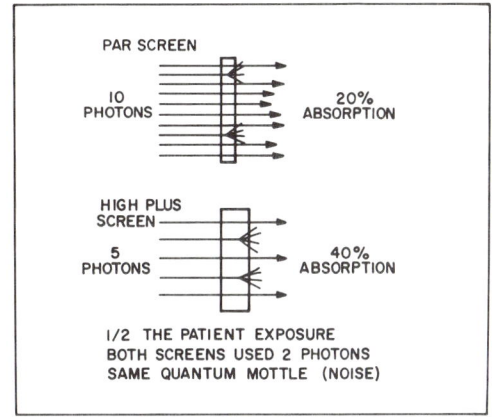

Figure 3-30. Increasing speed of CaWO$_4$ screens by increasing thickness of phosphor layer without increasing quantum mottle. (Adapted from Christensen, E. E.; Curry, T. S.; and Dowdey, J. E.: *An Introduction to the Physics of Diagnostic Radiology.* Philadelphia, Lea & Febiger, 1978, 2nd edition.)

film was first demonstrated by Dr. Gustave Bucky in 1913.

The **grid ratio** is the relation of the height of the lead strips to the width of the radiotransparent spacers.

$$\text{Grid ratio} = \frac{\text{Height of lead strips}}{\text{Thickness of interspacers}}$$

For example, if the height of the lead strip is 8 times the width of the interspace, the grid ratio is 8:1; if the height is 16 times the width, the ratio is 16:1. Everything being equal, the greater the ratio, the more efficiently the grid absorbs radiation. A 5:1 ratio grid will clean approximately 85 percent of the scatter radiation, while a 16:1 ratio may clean 97 percent of the scatter radiation. Usually a 8:1 ratio grid will give adequate results for general diagnostic radiography below 90 kVp. Above 90 kVp, a 12:1 ratio grid is preferred. Since the grid absorbs a large amount of scattered radiation as well as some of the primary radiation, the x-ray exposure must be increased to compensate for this loss if the same density of the

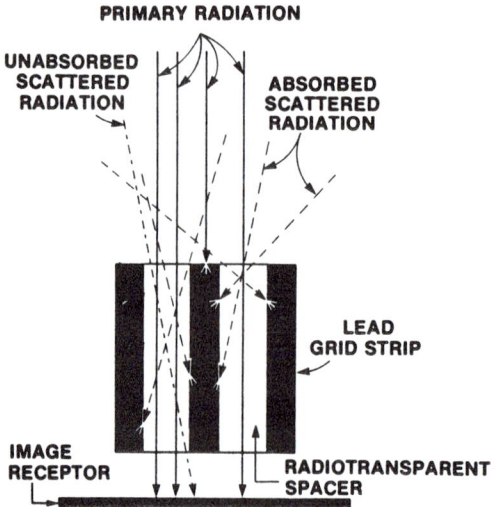

Figure 3-31. Cross section of a grid. Diagram illustrates how a great proportion of the scattered radiation is absorbed and image-forming primary radiation passes through to the film. (From Figure 23, page 28, *The Fundamentals of Radiography,* 12th Edition. Copyright Health Sciences Markets Division, Eastman Kodak Company, Rochester, NY. Reprinted by permission.)

radiograph is to be maintained. The more efficient the grid (higher the grid ratio), the greater the exposure increase must be.

Types of Grids

There are four basic types of grids: linear, crossed, focused, and moving. The first three grids are called stationary grids.

Linear Grids. In a linear grid, the lead strips are parallel to each other in their longitudinal axes. The disadvantage of linear parallel grids is the undesirable absorption of primary x-rays in the grid called **grid cutoff.** Grid cutoff may be partial or incomplete and may result in reduced density or total absence of film exposure. Grid "cutoff" may occur with any type of grid used or if the grid is improperly positioned, but it is more common with linear parallel grids (Fig. 3-32).

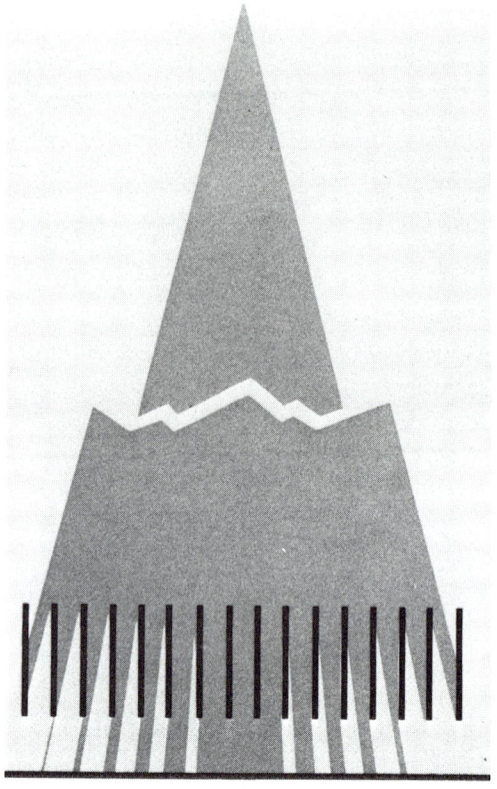

Figure 3-32. Linear parallel grid. Notice the grid cut-off at the periphery of the grid. To avoid grid cut-off with parallel grids, long source-film distances are recommended with beam restricting devices to collimate the beam to the central portion of grid.

Crossed Grid. A crossed grid is made up of two superimposed linear grids with lead strips running parallel to the long and short anex of the grid. Crossed grids are much more efficient than linear grids in cleaning up scatter. Actually, a crossed grid has a higher contrast improvement factor than a grid of twice the grid ratio. For instance, a 6:1 crossed grid will clean up more scatter than a 12:1 linear parallel grid. There are two serious disadvantages of crossed grids: (1) grid positioning is critical and (2) oblique projections are not

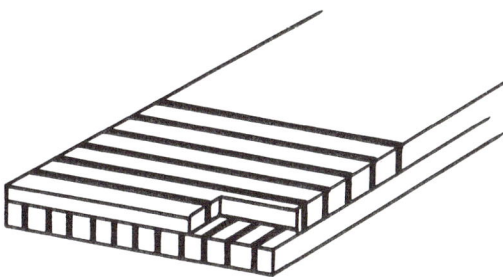

Figure 3-33. Crossed grids made by sandwiching two linear parallel grids together with their grid lead strips perpendicular to each other. (Adapted from Bushong, S.: *Radiologic Science for Technologists.* St. Louis, C. V. Mosby Co., 1975.)

possible (Fig. 3-33).

Focused Grid. A focused grid has lead strips progressively angled so that lines extended from each strip converge to a point. The distance from this point of convergence, or focal point, to the grid is called its focal distance or radius (Fig. 3-34). The main disadvantage of linear parallel and crossed grids is grid cut-off. The focused grid is designed to minimize this tendency. Every focused grid is marked with its recommended focal-grid distance. If the recommendations are not followed, grid cutoff will occur. Usually there is sufficient latitude to produce acceptable radiographs when used at a SFD between 36 and 44 inches. High-ratio grids have less positioning latitude than low-ratio grids.

Moving Grids. An obvious annoying disadvantage of stationary grids is that they produce grid lines on the radiograph. They are line images made when the primary beam x-rays are absorbed by the grid lead strips. Even though the grid lines are very small, their images can still be seen.

In 1920 Dr. Hollis E. Potter invented a major improvement in grid design. The Potter-Bucky grid is moving as the exposure is made and the motion blurs the grid

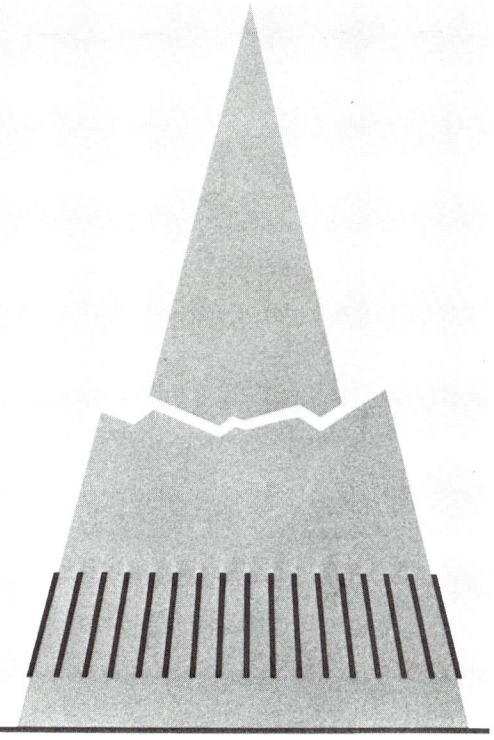

Figure 3-34. *Focused Grid.* Notice there is no grid cut-off. The source-grid distance falls within the focal range recommended by the manufacturer. (From Figure 24, Page 29, *The Fundamentals of Radiography,* 12th edition. Copyright Health Sciences Markets Division, Eastman Kodak Company, Rochester, NY. Reprinted by permission.)

lines and makes them indistinguishable. The device comprising the grid and the mechanism for moving it is called a Potter-Bucky diaphragm or simply a "Bucky." There are three types of Bucky grids: single stroke, reciprocating, and oscillating. Reciprocating mechanisms that move back and forth are usually used. The length of travel must be restricted so the grid will not exceed its range of motion and produce cutoff. The motion of the lead strips must be synchronized with the impulses of the x-ray machine, and the exposure time must be long enough to avoid producing a striped pattern or irregular densities on the film.

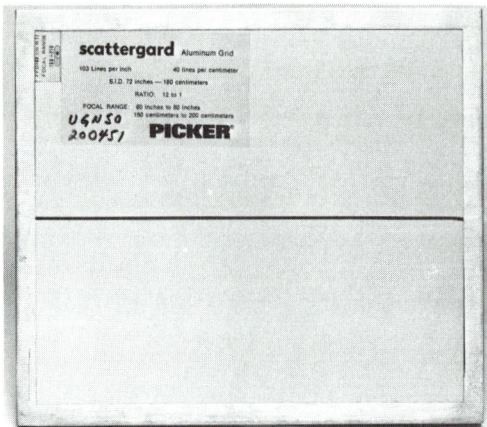

Figure 3-35. Grid-front cassette, focused cassette, recommended SFD range 60-80 inches with 103 lines per inch. Grid ratio 12:1.

Line Spacing of Grids

Another factor that affects the efficiency of a grid is the number of lead strips (lines) per cm or inch. This number may vary from 20 to 40 or more lines per cm (50 to 100 or more lines per inch). As the number of strips per inch is increased, the absorption of both scatter and primary radiation is increased for a given lead thickness. Thus, a compromise has to be made between contrast needed and patient exposure. Grids with thin lead strips of 100 or more per inch are often chosen for stationary use because thinner strips are less visible on the radiograph.

A grid (grid-front) cassette is a special x-ray cassette, usually used in skull radiography, with a grid built into the front of the cassette. Most grid-front cassettes have focused grids and have a medium grid ratio of 8:1 to 12:1 (Fig. 3-35).

Exposure Factors in Dental Radiographic Procedures

It is important for the dental radiographer to understand the relationship between exposure a film receives and the way the film responds to the exposure. The proper selection of exposure factors and type of film is essential in producing a radiograph with the highest quality.

Exposure of film or a film/screen combination is proportional to the product of milliamperes and time (impulses or seconds). For instance, using 15 mA for 2 seconds would be an exposure of 30 milliampere-seconds, usually written as 30 mAs. Exposure (mAs) of a radiographic film produces density (blackening) of a film. The quality of the beam (kVp) produces some effect on blackening or density, but its main effect is upon image contrast (differences in density or variations in blackness).

Most dental x-ray machines operate at 10 and/or 15 mA. If 15 mA is used instead of 10 mA, it usually requires the operator to reduce the exposure time by approximately 30 percent. The exposure time in modern dental x-ray machines is given in impulses. There are 60 impulses per second, therefore, 30 impulses would be the same as ½ second ($^{30}/_{60}$). Milliampere-impulses (mAi) is the product of milliamperage times the impulses of energy. For instance, 10 mA × ½ second = 5 mAs, which is equivalent to 300 mAi (10 mA × 30 impulses).

In determining the proper exposure technique, there are several factors to take into consideration. These are film speed, screen speed, filtration, collimation, size and age of patient, anatomic region, use of grids, source-film distance, kilovoltage, and processing.

Film and Screen Speed

This subject has been discussed previously in this chapter. Both film and screen speed must be taken into consideration when preparing an exposure technique chart for a particular x-ray examination.

Filters

As previously mentioned, filters are thin pieces of aluminum, which are placed in the x-ray beam to absorb the unnecessary low photon energies. This will **increase** the penetrability of the x-ray beam. However, added filtration also absorbs some of the useful higher photon energies of the beam at the same time, which **reduces** the total quantity of the primary beam. This tends to reduce radiographic contrast and density. In order to compensate for this reduction, the mAs must be increased.

Collimation

This is restricting or limiting the primary beam of radiation by use of a collimator or diaphragm. The collimator is usually composed of a sheet of lead in which an aperture has been cut of a size to permit x-ray coverage of a desired film area. It is located between the x-ray tube and the cone. Decreasing the size of the aperture decreases the production of scatter radiation, which is produced when the primary radiation strikes the soft tissue of the patient. Scatter radiation increases the overall density of the radiograph and tends to decrease the contrast. Therefore, if the collimation is increased too much, the mAs may have to be increased.

Size of Patient

The size of a patient varies greatly and exposure time for any patient, regardless of age, should be adjusted according to the patient's size. For the larger than average patient, increase the mAs by 25-50 percent. For the smaller than average patient, decrease the mAs by 25 percent or more.

Thin patients: These people will usually require less exposure time to maintain the desired density.

Patients with "fat cheeks" (obese individuals): This will require more exposure time in order to avoid low density films.

People with ruddy, red complexions: These patients have more blood in the surface tissues and may require more exposure time in order to avoid low density films.

Age of Patient

There are also some modifications to be made according to the patient's age.

The recommended exposures are based on requirements for adults twenty to fifty years of age, average build, and with teeth present.

For children under twelve years of age, reduce the exposure time about one-third to one-fourth. For patients over fifty years of age with teeth, the exposure time may have to be increased to maintain the desired film density—the pulps of these teeth have reduced in size considerably. However, many elderly individuals have a condition called osteoporosis of the bone. In this condition, the cortex of the bone becomes thin and the trabeculae of the cancellous bone becomes reduced in number. Naturally, the exposure time should be reduced in a patient with this condition.

In edentulous areas reduce the exposure time approximately 25 percent.

Anatomic Region Being Recorded

Several starting exposure techniques for intraoral radiography exist. They all use the mandibular molar region as the baseline. The average exposure times for the various anatomic regions are given as percentages of the recommended exposure times for the mandibular molar

Table 3-VIII

RECOMMENDED AVERAGE EXPOSURES GIVEN AS PERCENTAGES OF INCREASE OR DECREASE OF AVERAGE MANDIBULAR MOLAR EXPOSURE TIME

Anatomic Area	Exposure Percentage (Fixed kV Technic)	
Maxillary molar	+50	+33
Maxillary premolar	0	0
Maxillary cuspid	0	0
Maxillary incisor	0	+16
Mandibular molar	0	0
Mandibular premolar	-25	-16
Mandibular cuspid	-25	-33
Mandibular incisor	-25	-50
Posterior bitewings	0	0

region.

An exposure variation is recommended for the different areas of the oral cavity in order to compensate for the differences in the quantity of the hard and soft structures encountered. Greater amounts of exposure are required to penetrate areas that have thicker amounts of tissue.

In Table 3-VIII, two different fixed kV technics are given where the mAs is the exposure factor of change.

Although fixed voltage technics are used almost universally in dental radiography, it is possible to use a variable kilovoltage technic (Table 3-IX). In this technic, the kilovoltage is varied according to the difference in the anatomic region, and the mAs is fixed. The variable kilovoltage technic will tend to produce a complete radiographic survey that is without density variations between the different anatomic regions.

Use of the Grid

When thicker body parts are radiographed, grids are placed between the patient and the film to absorb the emerging scatter radiation, which tends to interfere with the definition of the radiograph. Although grids are used primarily in medical radiography, they have a place in dental radiography, when the dentist is taking skull radiographs.

When grids are used, the mAs factor must be increased.

Table 3-IX

A TYPICAL VARIABLE kVp TECHNIC
Type of Film: Eastman Kodak® Ultra-Speed
(D Speed Film)
mAs: 10 mA at ¾ sec.
Source-Film Distance: 16 inches

	Male	Female
Maxilla		
Central-Lateral	78 kV	72 kV
Canines	80 kV	74 kV
Premolars	86 kV	80 kV
Molars	90 kV	84 kV
Mandible		
Central-Lateral	74 kV	68 kV
Canines	76 kV	70 kV
Premolars	78 kV	72 kV
Molars	81 kV	75 kV
Posterior Bitewings		
Premolars	65 kV at 1¾ sec	65 kV at 1¾ sec
Molars	90 kV	90 kV

According to Dr. Don Wagner of the University of Nebraska.

Source-Film Distance

When source-film distance is changed, the total amount of x-rays must be increased or decreased in order to give a comparable exposure when using a new distance. The inverse square law states that the intensity of the x-ray beam varies inversely as the square of the distance. Therefore, to produce a given density at a different distance, it is necessary to vary the exposure directly to the square of the distance.

For instance, the exposure time must be increased for an increase in distance, and decreased for a decrease in distance.

The formula for time-distance relations is as follows:

$$\frac{\text{New Time}}{\text{Original Time}} = \frac{(\text{New Distance})^2}{(\text{Original Distance})^2}$$

Or

$$NT = \frac{(OT) \cdot (ND)^2}{(OD)^2}$$

For example, doubling the source-film distance would **decrease** the intensity of the beam by one-fourth its original intensity. Therefore, to maintain the density by doubling the SFD, multiply the old exposure by four.

Kilovoltage Changes

Conditions often arise that require a change in kilovoltage. The relation between kilovoltage and exposure is complex. When kilovoltage is raised, all wavelengths present in the lower kilovoltage beam are present in the higher one, but at greater intensity, along with new, shorter wavelengths not present previously. The effect of kilovoltage changes depends on such factors as type of x-ray examination, patient size and age, and x-ray machine used. Although the exposure time varies inversely to the kilovoltage, no definite mathematical relationship exists between the two. Changes in exposure conditions to compensate for kilovoltage changes have to be determined through practical experience. See Figure 3-36 for an approximate relationship table between kilovoltage and time.

A rule of thumb to use in changing from one kVp to another states that a 15 kVp increase will double the radiation output. For example, if the kVp is changed from 65 kVp to 80 kVp (15 kVp), the exposure time should be decreased by 50 percent or one-half of the original time.

Example Problem: If the present exposure factors are 8 inch SFD, 60 kVp, 10 mA, $^{48}/_{60}$ sec, what is the new exposure time for this machine set with a 16 inch SFD, 15 mA, and 90 kVp?

SOLUTION:

Step 1. By changing from an 8 inch SFD to a 16 inch SFD, the intensity decreases to one-fourth the original intensity; therefore, we must increase exposure by 4 to $^{192}/_{60}$ sec to maintain film density.

Step 2. By changing 10 mA to 15 mA, we need a 30 percent reduction in exposure time or $^{143}/_{60}$ sec.

Step 3. By changing 60 kVp to 90 kVp (30 kVp change), there is a fourfold increase in radiation output; therefore, reduce exposure time by one-fourth to $^{36}/_{60}$ sec. (Each 15 kVp change doubles the exposure change.)

The answer is $^{36}/_{60}$ **seconds or 36 impulses.**

Processing

The objective of any exposure technic should be to provide the minimum amount of radiation to a patient and still produce a radiograph that has maximum diagnostic quality. The film developing process can provide a valuable test in determining whether a film has been exposed to the proper amount of radiation. Develop an exposed sample film for 8-9 minutes (5 minutes is recommended) at 70° temperature, fix, and dry. This is overdevelopment; however, it is practically impossible to overdevelop properly exposed or underexposed film. If the film

DECREASE IN EXPOSURE TIME	INCREASE IN KILOVOLTAGE		INCREASE IN EXPOSURE TIME	DECREASE IN KILOVOLTAGE	
	With Medium Speed Screens	Without Screens		With Medium Speed Screens	Without Screens
25%	7%	15%	25%	5%	10%
50%	20%	40%	50%	10%	18%
75%	50%	100%	75%	13%	25%
			100%	16%	30%

Figure 3-36. Approximate kilovoltage-time relationship. (Copyright Eastman Kodak Company. Reprinted by permission.)

is dark, the film has been overexposed. If the film has the proper density, expose another film and develop this film at the recommended 5 minutes at 70°, fix, and dry. If this film has a low density (light), the film has been underexposed. However, if the film is of the optimal density, the film has been properly exposed.

Bibliography

Arnold, B.A.; Eisenberg, H.,; and Bjarngard, B.E.: The LSF and MTF of rare-earth oxysulfide intensifying screens. *Radiology, 121*:473, November 1976.

Buchanan, R.A.; Finkelstein, S.I.; and Wichersheim, K.A.: X-ray exposure reduction using rare-earth oxysulfide intensifying screens. *Radiology, 105*:185, 1972.

Bushong, S.C.: *Radiologic Science for Technologists. Physics, Biology, and Protection.* St. Louis, Mosby, 1975.

Characteristics and Applications of X-ray Grids, ref. ed. Cincinnati, Liebel Flarsheim Co., 1968.

Christensen, E.E.; Curry III, T.S.; and Dowdey, J.E.: *An Introduction to the Physics of Diagnostic Radiology,* 2nd ed. Philadelphia, Lea & Febiger, 1978.

Cleare, H.M.; Splettstosser, H.E.; and Seemann, H.E.: An experimental study of the mottle produced by x-ray intensifying screens. *AJR, 88*:168, July 1962.

Coltman, J.W.; Ebbinghausen, E.G.; and Alter, W.: Physical properties of calcium tungstate x-ray screens. *J Appl Physics, 18*:530, 1947.

Doi, K.; and Rossmann, K.: Measurements of optical and noise properties of screen-film systems in radiology. *SPIE Medical X-ray Photo-Optical Systems Evaluation, 56*:45, 1975.

Etter, L.E.: *Glossary of Words and Phrases Used in Radiology, Nuclear Medicine, and Fundamentals of Radiography,* 12th ed. Rochester, N.Y., Eastman Kodak Co., 1980.

Fuchs, A.W.: *Principles of Radiographic Exposure and Processing,* 2nd ed. Springfield, Charles C Thomas, 1969.

Goodwin, P.N.; Quimby, E..H.; and Morgan, R.: *Physical Foundations of Radiology,* 4th ed. New York, Har-Row, 1970.

Green, F.; Costa, L.F.; and Donovan, J.L.: Measured light emission efficiency and quantum yield for x-ray screens and phosphors. *J Opt Soc Am, 59*:848, July 1969.

Guide to Dental Materials and Devices, 4th ed. American Dental Association, 1968.

Hendee, W.R.: *Medical Radiation Physics.* Chicago, Year Bk Med, 1970.

Herz, R.H.: *The Photographic Action of Ionizing Radiation.* New York, Wiley, 1969.

James, T.H. (Ed.): *The Theory of the Photographic Process.* New York, Macmillan, 1977.

Jaundrell-Thompson, F.; and Ashworth, W.J.: *X-ray Physics and Equipment,* 2nd ed. Springfield, Charles C Thomas, 1970.

Johns, H.E.; and Cunningham, J.R.: *The Physics of Radiology.* 3rd ed. Springfield, Charles C Thomas, 1969.

Lawrence, D.J.: *Kodak X-Omatic and Lanex Screens and Kodak Films for Medical Radiography.* Radiography Markets Division, Eastman Kodak Co., File No. 5.03, June 1976.

Lawrence, D.J.: Kodak X-Omatic and Lanex screens and Kodak films for medical radiography. *Med Radiogr Photogr, 53*:2-10, No. 1, 1977.

Ludwig, G.W.; and Prener, J.S.: Evaluation of Gd_2O_2S:Tb as a phosphor for the input screen of X-ray image intensifiers. *IEEE Trans Nucl Sci, NS-19*:3, August 1972.

Mattsson, O.: Aspects of the interpretation of contrast and detail in radiographs. *Acta Radiol, 38*:477, December 1952.

Meredith, W.J.; and Massey, J.B.: *Fundamental Physics of Radiology.* Baltimore, Williams & Wilkens, 1968.

Morgan, R.H.: Characteristics of X-ray films and screens. *Radiology, 49*:90, 1947.

Neblette, C.B.: *Photograph, Its Material and Processes,* 6th ed. New York, Van Nostrand, 1962. (Gurney-Mott hypothesis of latent image formation.)

Patterson, C.V.S.: Roentgenography: fluoroscopic & intensifying screens. In Glasser, O. (Ed.): *Medical Physics,* Vol. 3. Chicago, Year Bk Med, 1960.

Rao, G.U.V.; Fatouros, P.P.; and James, A.E.: Physical characteristics of modern radiographic screen-film systems. *Invest Radiol, 13*:460, Sept-Oct 1978.

Rao, G.U.V.; and Fatouros, P.P.: The relationship between resolution and speed of x-ray intensifying screens. *Med Phys, 5*:205, May-June 1978.

Reynolds, J.; Skucas, J.; and Gorski, J.: An evaluation of screen/film speed characteristics. *Radiology, 118*:711-713, March 1976.

Rossi, R.P.; Hendee, W.R.; and Ahnens, C.R.: An evaluation of rare earth screen/film combinations. *Radiology, 121*:465, November 1976.

Rossmann, K.: *Image Quality—Physics of Diagnostic Radiology.* USDHEW Pub # (FDA) 74-8006, November 1973.

Rossmann, K.: Modulation transfer function of radiographic systems using fluorescent screens. *J Opt Soc Am, 52*:774, July 1962.

Rossmann, K.; and Lubberts, G.: Some characteristics of the line spread-function and modulation transfer function of radiographic films and screen-film systems. *Radiology, 86*:235, 1966.

Rossmann, K.: Point spread function, line spread function, and modulation transfer function. *Radiology, 93*:257, 1969.

Seeman, H.E.: *Physical and Photographic Principles of Medical Radiography.* New York, Wiley, 1968.

Sensitometric Properties of X-ray Films. Rochester, N.Y., Radiography Markets Division, Eastman Kodak Company.

Skucas, J.; and Gorski, J.: Application of modern screens in diagnostic radiology. *Med Radiogr Photogr, 56*(2):25, 1980.

Sprawls, P.: *The Physical Principles of Diagnostic Radiology.* Baltimore, Md., The University Park Press, 1977.

Stevels, A.L.N.: New phosphors for x-ray screens. *Medicamundi, 20*:12, 1975.

Soila, P.; Edgren, J.; Landtman, M.; and Laasonen, L.: Test of rare earth oxysulphide intensifying screens. *Br J Radiol, 50*:205-207, March 1977.

Swank, R.K.: Calculation of modulation transfer functions of x-ray fluorescent screens. *Appl Opt, 12*:1865, August, 1973.

Ter-Pogossian, M.M.: *The Physical Aspects of Diagnostic Radiology.* New York, Har-Row, 1967.

Thompson, T.T.; Radford, E.L.; and Kirby, C.C.: A look at rare-earth and high-speed intensifying screens. *Appl Radiol, 6*:71, 1977.

Trout, E.D.; Kelley, J.P.; and Cathey, G.A.: The use of filters to control radiation exposure to the patient in diagnostic roentgenology. *AJR, 67*:942, 1952.

Venema, H.W.: X-ray absorption, speed and luminescent efficiency of rare earth and other intensifying screens. *Radiology, 130*:765, March 1979.

Chapter 4

DIAGNOSTIC QUALITY OF DENTAL RADIOGRAPHS

DIAGNOSIS IS THE ART of distinguishing one disease from another. In order to use the dental radiograph as an aid in the diagnosis of dental disease, it is important that the dentist have a radiograph that provides the maximum possible information concerning a particular anatomic region. In other words, the dentist must have a radiograph that has the highest possible quality. Radiographic quality refers to the fidelity (exactness in detail) with which an anatomic structure is represented on the radiograph and denotes the visibility and definition of the images of structural details. Definition (sharpness) refers to the distinctness and sharp demarcation of all elements in the dental film. Detail is the point-by-point delineation of the minute structural elements of the object in the images formed in the dental film.

Radiographic images of the smallest structures are many times called **details** or simply **detail**. In other words, the dental X-Ray operator must always attempt to obtain a radiograph that has the greatest amount of detail or information possible.

The diagnostic quality of a dental radiograph is dependent upon four conditions:

1. **Proper Visual Characteristics of Radiograph**
   a. Density
   b. Contrast
2. **Minimal Geometric Characteristics of Radiograph**
   a. Radiographic image unsharpness
      1. Geometric unsharpness
      2. Motion unsharpness
      3. Screen unsharpness
   b. Magnification
   c. Distortion
3. **Anatomical Accuracy of Radiographic Images**
4. **Adequate Coverage of Anatomic Region of Interest**

A clear understanding of the effects and significance of each factor will aid the operator in the routine production of radiographs of diagnostic quality.

VISUAL CHARACTERISTICS

The diagnostic quality of the radiograph is directly influenced by two visual characteristics of the radiographic image called **density** and **contrast**.

Radiographic Density

Radiographic density refers to the degree or gradation of "blackness" on a radiographic film. It depends on the amount of radiation reaching a particular area on the film and the resulting mass of metallic silver per unit area. As you recall, the silver halides of the emulsion that have been sensitized by radiation are changed by the developing agents into particles of metallic silver, which appear black because of their finely divided state. The greater the amount of X-Ray energy that reaches the film, the greater the degree of blackening on that area of the film. In areas where relatively few or no X-Ray photons reach the film, these areas on the film will appear gray or translucent on the processed radiograph.

After the exposed film is processed, the film is viewed by placing it in front of an illuminator. It is the variation in the amount of light through the film that identifies the image seen by the eyes. The heavier the deposit of black silver masses, the greater the quantity of light absorbed (and not transmitted), and the darker the area appears. The darker areas on the film are regions of the anatomical part of the body that freely let the X-Rays pass through to expose the film and are called **radiolucencies**. A high degree of radiographic density gives a **dark** film; a **light** film has a thin or low degree of radiographic density.

Radiographic density is measured by an instrument called a **densitometer**, which indicates the relationship between the intensity of light beam of an illuminator as it strikes one side of a given area of a radiograph (called incident light intensity) as compared to the light transmitted through the radiograph (transmitted light intensity).

Density is expressed mathematically as a logarithm,* using the common base 10. It is defined by the following equation (see Fig. 4-1):

$$\text{Density} = \frac{\text{Incident light intensity (I)}}{\text{Transmitted light intensity (T)}}$$

Example. When the silver allows 1/10 of the illuminator or incident light through the radiograph, the ratio is 10/1, which is equal to 10. The common logarithm of 10 is 1, and therefore, the density of the film is equal to 1. Again, if the silver allows only 1/100 of the light to pass through the radiograph, the ratio is equal to 100/1 or 100. The common logarithm of 100 is 2, and the density of the film is equal to 2.

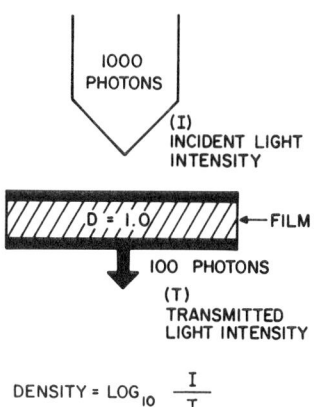

Figure 4-1. Radiographic density: The reduction in intensity or the ability of the film to stop light in this instance is 1000/100 or 10, or one-tenth of the light is transmitted through the film. The log of 10 is 1. Thus the density of this radiograph is 1.0.

---

*The power of a number is the product obtained when it is multiplied by itself a given number of times. Thus, $10^3 = 10 \cdot 10 \cdot 10 = 1,000$. The figure 3 is the *exponent*. The exponent used in raising 10 to a given power is called the *common logarithm* of the value. For example, the relation $1,000 = 10^3$ then will result in the statement "the common logarithm of 1,000 is 3." In symbols, this is usually written as $\log_{10} 1,000 = 3$. ($10^1 = 10$; $10^2 = 100$; $10^3 = 1,000$; $10^4 = 10,000$; $10^5 = 100,000$.)

The dental radiograph obviously contains a great many different densities in the various areas that comprise the image. These densities range from 0.4 in the relatively clear radiopaque areas (metallic restorations), to 3.0 in the blackest radiolucent areas. That is, the silver content allows approximately 1/2 of the light to pass through the radiopaque areas (density of 0.3), and only 1/100 of the light to pass through the blackest radiolucent areas (density of 3.0) (Table 4-I). Useful densities in diagnostic radiography are in the range between 0.5 and 2.5.

TABLE 4-I

COMMON VALUES OF I/T (ABILITY OF FILM TO STOP LIGHT), DENSITY (LOG$_{10}$), AND PERCENT OF LIGHT TRANSMISSION

Ability of film to stop light (I/T)	Density (Log$_{10}$ I/T)	Percent of Light Transmitted
1	0	100 (transparent)
2	0.3	50
4	0.6	25
8	0.9	10
10	1.0	10
30	1.5	3.2
100	2	1 (black)
1,000	3	0.1

Density is expressed as a logarithm because logarithms allow for wide differences in numbers on a small scale. Radiographic densities contain densities ranging from 0 to 4 (clear to black). A density of 4 means only 1/10,000 of the light photons are capable of penetrating the processed film, while a density of 1 means that 1/10 of the light photons are allowed to pass through the film. Actually, one does not have to know logarithms to use a densitometer, since it is calibrated to read density directly.

If an unexposed film were processed, it would have a density of approximately 0.12 or 76 percent light transmission. This density consists of base density and fog density. **Base density** usually has an average density of approximately 0.07. It is due to the plastic base material, which absorbs some light, and also to the blue dye, which is added to the base to make the film more desirable for viewing.

Fog density is due to the inadvertent development of some silver halide grains in the X-Ray film emulsion during the manufacture of the film. Film fog averages about 0.05 in fresh film.

Characteristic Curve

It is important to understand the relationship between the amount of exposure a film receives and degree of blackness on the film (density) produced by the exposure. The study of quantitative relationships of exposure and density is called **sensitometry**.

The principal measurements involved in sensitometry—density and exposure—can be plotted as a curve, known as the H & D characteristic curve (after F. Hurter and V.C. Duffield who first published such a curve in 1890). Characteristic curves are constructed by taking a series of exposures of a certain film type, developing the film, reading the density by use of a **densitometer**, and plotting the density readings against a known exposure. A typical H & D characteristic curve is shown in Figure 4-2. There are great variations in exposure at the high and low levels of exposure, which results in very small changes in density. These low and high levels of the curve are called the toe (low density) and the shoulder (high densities), respectively. In the intermediate portion of the curve, small changes in exposure result in large changes in density. This is called the straight-line portion of the curve and is the area of proper exposure.

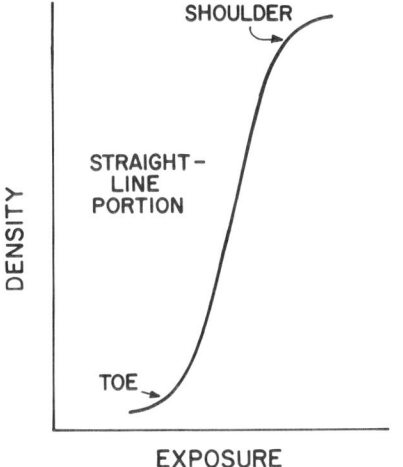

Figure 4-2. The typical characteristic curve of a radiographic film, which graphically shows the relationship between exposure and density.

Since radiographic film is sensitive over a wide range of exposures, the exposure values are presented in logarithmic fashion, which allows for a wide range of exposures to be presented in a compact graph. Also, the use of a log relative exposure makes for easier analysis of the characteristic curve.

By use of the log relative exposure scale, two exposures with a constant proportion to each other (for instance, one twice the other) will be separated by the same distance on the exposure scale. The log relative exposure scale is divided into segments of 0.3 because the log of 2 is 0.3. Therefore, increase in the log relative exposure of 0.3 will always represent the doubling of the exposure (mAs) (Fig. 4-3).

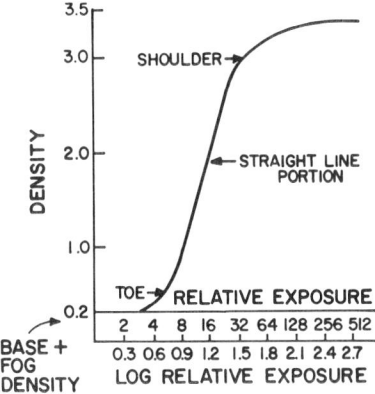

Figure 4-3. Characteristic curve: The relationship between relative exposure and log relative exposure. An increase in the log relative exposure by 0.3 always represents a doubling of the relative exposure. The density (darkened area) below 0.2 represents fog and base density.

The characteristic curve will give useful information concerning the contrast, speed (sensitivity), and latitude of the film.

Exposure Factors that Control Density

Listed below are the three important exposure factors that control density of a radiograph. In dental radiography, the first factor mentioned (mAs) is generally the factor of choice.

Milliampere-Seconds. The density or blackness of the radiograph varies directly and proportionately as the milliamperage (tube current) and the exposure time. Therefore, exposure time and milliamperage are interchangeable and considered as a **single** factor (mAs). For instance, the density of a radiographic image produced by a direct exposure of 2 seconds at 10 milliamperes is identical to the density of the image produced by an exposure time of 4 seconds at 5 milliamperes. The product of mA and exposure time is equal to 20 mAs in each instance. The higher the mAs, the more X-Rays that will strike the film and the greater the quantity of metallic silver deposited in the film emulsion. The quantity (or mAs) of the X-Ray beam is usually measured by the use of a **roentgen meter**.

Kilovoltage. Kilovoltage is referred to as the "penetrating power" of the X-Ray beam and influences density. (See Figure 3-36 for a table giving the approximate exposure relationship for various changes in kilovoltage.) As the kilovoltage becomes greater, and the effective wave lengths of the X-Ray beam become shorter, the penetration of the X-Ray beam becomes greater. Therefore, a greater amount of x-radiation will strike the film emulsion, which, in turn, will cause more metallic silver to be deposited in the emulsion. This will result in a higher radiographic density if all other factors remain constant.

Source-Film Distance. Since the intensity of an X-Ray beam varies **inversely** as the square of the source-film distance (inverse square law), the time of exposure necessary to maintain a constant density in a radiograph varies **directly** as the square of the focal-film distance. The smaller the distance between the focal spot and the film, the more X-Rays that strike the film, and therefore, the **higher** the density. **Example**: Doubling the distance gives one-fourth the density; halving the distance gives four times the density.

Secondary factors that affect density are as follows.

Patient Thickness. Body parts that are thicker require more mAs or kVp in order to maintain a constant density.

Development Conditions. The radiograph may be darker or lighter depending on whether the films are under- or overdeveloped. However, it is difficult to overdevelop a film that has been properly exposed.

Type of Film. High speed films require less mAs in order to cause a density change.

Screens. High-speed screens require less mAs in order to lower the density in the radiograph.

Grids. The use of grids requires more mAs in order to keep a constant density.

What Degree of Radiographic Density is Most Desirable?

The desirable degree of radiographic density cannot be fixed as a permanent thing because one dentist may prefer a certain degree of density while another may prefer a greater or lesser density for the same region. The degree of radiographic density may be considered to be largely a matter of individual preference. Of course, you do not want a film that is too dark or too light — you need the right amount of density to visualize the anatomic structures accurately.

In dental radiographs of correct density, the dentist should be able to see a

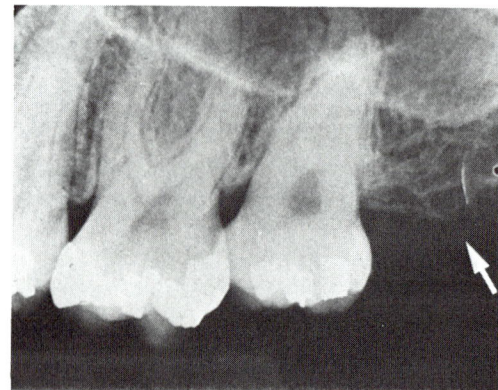

Figure 4-4. Radiograph of maxillary molar region. Notice thin shadow of soft tissue over bone in tuberosity area distal to maxillary second molar.

faint outline of the soft tissues in edentulous spaces or distal to the molar teeth when the radiographs are examined in the manner habitually employed (Fig. 4-4).

Contrast

Contrast is the difference in densities visualized on radiographs. On the radiograph you will see variations in "blackness." Some areas will be black (radiolucent), other areas will be gray, and other areas white (radiopaque). In the black areas a great many of the X-Rays reached the film, while in the white areas, very few of the X-Rays penetrated the object.

As you will remember from previous chapters, radiographic contrast depends upon subject contrast and film contrast. Subject contrast is determined by differential attenuation as the X-Ray beam passes through the patient. The controlling factors of subject contrast are thickness, density, and atomic differences of the tissues of the patient; the kVp used; and scatter radiation. The correct kVp is very important in producing the proper subject contrast. This relationship will be discussed later.

Film Contrast and the Characteristic Curve

Film contrast is influenced by three factors: (1) characteristic curve of the film, (2) film density, and (3) film processing.

Film Contrast

Film contrast is inherent in the type of film being employed. By analysis of the characteristic curve, one can determine readily the degree of contrast for a particular film. The film with the steepest slope of the straight line portion of the characteristic curve will have the highest film contrast (Fig. 4-5).

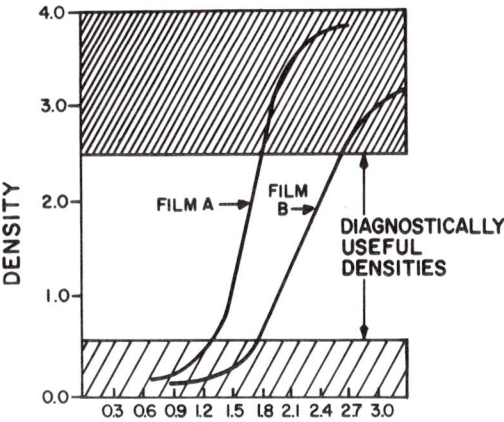

Figure 4-5. Film A has a higher contrast than Film B because the slope of the straight portion of the characteristic curve is steeper. Also, Film A is faster in speed than Film B because Film A requires less exposure than Film B to produce any density.

There is no simple method to define film contrast. The most often employed method is the average gradient or slope of the useful straight line portion of the characteristic curve. The average gradient is the steepness of the slope of a straight line joining two points on the characteristic curve at density levels of 0.25 and 2.0 above the combined base and fog densities. The equation for the average gradient is as follows:

$$\text{Average Gradient} = \frac{D_2 - D_1}{\text{Log RE}_1 - \text{RE}_2}$$

D_1 is always 0.25 plus the base and fog density, and D_2 is 2.0 plus the base and fog density; therefore, $D_2 - D_1$ is always 1.75. Most average gradients of radiographic films are above 1, usually in the range of 2.5 to 3.5 (Fig. 4-6).

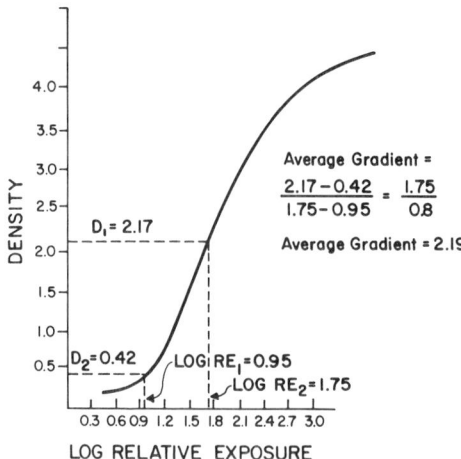

Figure 4-6. The average gradient of an X-Ray film. Average gradient of characteristic curve shown here is 2.19. (Base density = .06; fog density = 0.11.)

$$D_1 = 2.0 + 0.6 + 0.11;$$
$$D_2 = 0.25 + .06 + 0.11.$$

Film Contrast and Film Density

The slope of the characteristic curve (contrast) changes with film density, especially in the toe and shoulder regions. The diagnostically useful range of densities apparently lies in the range 0.5 to 2.5, and when the exposure of the radiograph results in densities outside this range, film contrast is lost. A radiograph with a density level of 3 (0.1% of light transmitted) will result in less visible film contrast under normal viewing conditions.

The human eye cannot distinguish film contrast well at low brightness levels, which is why the spotlight is useful in viewing films with high film densities. Also, an underexposed film will result in low film density and poor film contrast, which will be difficult to interpret adequately. Thus, it is important to expose the film properly so the film densities fall in the range between 0.5 and 2.5 and not in the toe and shoulder regions of the characteristic curve. Otherwise, film contrast will be reduced considerably.

Film Contrast and Film Processing

It is important to follow the manufacturer's instructions in processing film. Increasing the time and/or temperature of development will—

1. increase film contrast;
2. increase film speed (increase density for given exposure);
3. increase film fog (decrease film contrast).

Also, decreasing the development time will reduce film contrast and film speed. Automatic processing has eliminated some of the problems concerning the standardization of the time of development of films and the temperature of processing solutions.

Subject Contrast (Radiation Contrast)

Subject contrast depends primarily on **kilovoltage**; however, it is also dependent upon the **thickness, density (mass/volume), and atomic number** of the tissue of the patient irradiated.

An increase in kVp increases the penetrating ability of the X-Ray beam because the beam will have a higher percentage of X-Ray photons with greater energy (shorter wavelengths). If the kilovoltage is high (90 kVp), a greater percentage of the wavelengths of the beam will be shorter, the penetration of the X-Rays through the tissue will be greater, the density differences of adjacent areas are small, and the film will have what is called **long-scale contrast**. There will be a long-scale of grays between the black and white portions of the radiographic image. If the kilovoltage is low (65 kVp) a greater percentage of the wavelengths of the beam will be longer, and the amount of penetra tion will be less. The density differences between adjacent areas will be great, and the film will have **short-scale contrast**. There will be fewer shades of gray between the lighter and darker areas of the radiographic image.

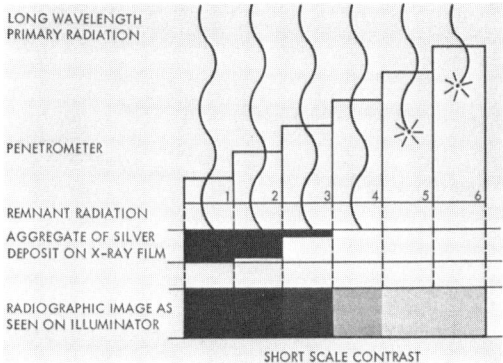

Figure 4-7. Short-scale contrast. (Redrawn from Fuchs, Arthur W.: Principles of Radiographic Exposure and Processing, 2nd ed. Springfield, Il. Charles C Thomas, Publisher, 1958.)

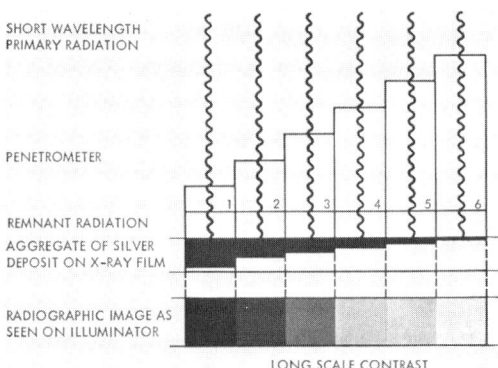

Figure 4-8. Long-scale contrast. (Redrawn from Fuchs, Arthur W.: Principles of Radiographic Exposure and Processing, 2nd ed. Springfield, Il. Charles C Thomas, Publisher, 1958.)

Long- and short-scale contrast can be illustrated by means of a **penetrometer**. The quality of an X-Ray beam or its wavelength is usually measured by determining the rate of absorption in some material. A penetrometer is a radiographic testing device made of aluminum and built up in steps of varying thicknesses. Figures 4-7 and 4-8 show an aluminum penetrometer or step-wedge being irradiated by X-Rays; the exposed X-Ray film in enlarged cross section is shown beneath the step-wedge or penetrometer; the resulting radiographic image as it appears when viewed on the illuminator is depicted below the film cross section in both illustrations. The penetrometer demonstrates how long-scale contrast compares with short-scale contrast (Fig. 4-9).

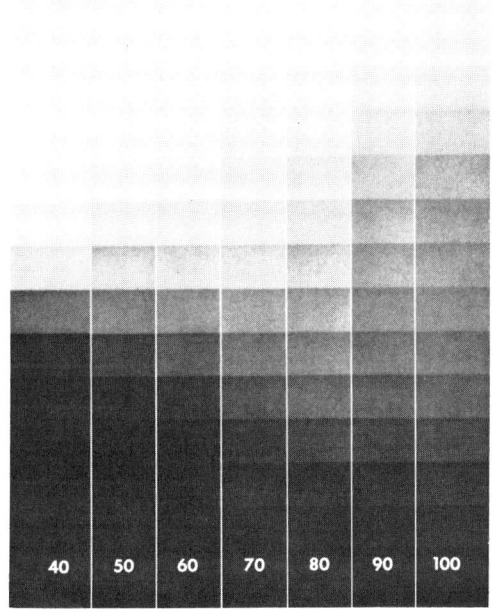

Figure 4-9. Comparison of long-scale contrast and short-scale contrast using a penetrometer.

Relationship Between Contrast, Density, and Exposure

When the contrast is changed, the radiographic density of the film will be altered. However, when radiographic density is altered by itself, there will be no obvious change in the contrast. Why is this true?

A change in kilovoltage will produce a change in contrast. The higher the kilovoltage, the less will be the contrast. However, since kilovoltage is also a controlling factor in radiographic density, an increase in kilovoltage will also increase the radiographic density. Therefore, when the kilovoltage is **increased**, the milliampere-seconds (a controlling factor in radiographic density) must be **decreased** in order to maintain the previous radiographic density. To ilustrate this concept, examine the exposure table in Figure 4-10 for the maxillary molar region using D speed film and a 16 inch target-film distance. Notice that the mAs using the 90-15 technic is 7.5, as compared with the 10 mAs for the 65-10 technic (Fig. 4-10).

DENSITY	CONTRAST	KVP	MA	SECONDS	MAS
Same	Less or Long-scale	90	15	.5	7.5
Same	Greater or Short-scale	65	10	2	20.0

Figure 4-10. The relationship between contrast, density, and exposure.

Contrast cannot be varied by a change in milliamperage unless a variation in voltage is made to compensate for the milliamperage variation. The higher the mA, and the lower the voltage, the greater will be the contrast.

Density can be altered without changing the contrast. How is this accomplished? Milliampere-seconds is the prime factor in controlling radiographic density, but it is not a controlling factor in contrast. Therefore, a change in mAs will produce a change in radiographic density but not a noticeable change in contrast.

Example. Two radiographs of the same region can be made, one of greater density (higher mAs), and one of lesser density (lower mAs) with the kVp remaining constant in both radiographs. These two films will have differences in overall blackness but the extreme blacks and whites of both films will remain the same.

Latitude

There are two types of latitude: (1) film latitude, and (2) exposure latitude.

Film Latitude

On the characteristic curve, film latitude refers to the range of log relative exposures (mAs) to which an X-Ray film

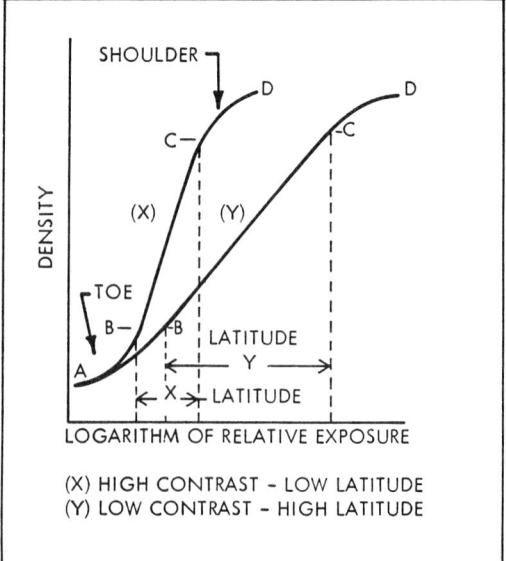

Figure 4-11. Characteristic curve for films X and Y showing the differences in speed, contrast, and latitude. Film X has faster speed, higher contrast, and lower latitude than film Y. (Adapted from Bloom, W.L., Jr.; Hollenbach, J.L.; and Morgan, J.A.: *Medical Radiographic Technic*, 3rd ed. Springfield, Il., Charles C Thomas, Publisher, 1965.)

will respond with densities within the accepted range for diagnostic radiology (usually considered to be a density range from 0.5 to 2.5). Figure 4-11 shows two films with different latitudes. Notice film (Y) has a greater latitude but less film contrast than film (X). Generally speaking, film latitude varies with the reciprocal of film contrast. In other words, the greater the film latitude, the lower the film contrast.

Conversely, a film with high contrast (short scale contrast) will have narrow latitude.

Exposure Latitude

Exposure latitude is the range of exposures of an X-Ray film permissible for a good diagnostic result. The greater the exposure "error" that can be tolerated, the greater is the latitude of the radiographic exposure technic. Exposure latitude improves when the kVp is increased, and the film contrast decreases.

In practice, a high kVp technic has more room for error in choice of exposure time (fixed mA) because the exposure latitude is greater. At lower kilovoltage, the latitude is less, and the mAs must be carefully selected.

GEOMETRIC CHARACTERISTICS

The formation of an accurate radiographic image is dependent upon minimizing certain geometric characteristics that are present to a certain degree in every radiograph. There are three geometric characteristics:

1. **radiographic image unsharpness** (diffusion of detail). This fuzzy, unsharp margin that surrounds the radiographic image is called the **penumbra** (from Latin **pene** for almost, and **umbra** for shadow).
2. **Magnification** or enlargement of the radiographic image.
3. **Distortion** in shape of the radiographic image (unequal enlargement).

There will always be a certain amount of unsharpness, magnification, and shape distortion of the radiographic image for three reasons:

1. X-Rays originate from a definite area rather than a point source. It is impossible to have a point source of X-Rays because of the limited heating capacity of X-Ray tubes. The source of radiation in modern dental X-Ray machines varies from 0.8 to 1.5 mm^2, depending upon the mA and kVp used.
2. X-Rays travel in diverging straight lines as they radiate from their source of origin. This divergent quality of ionizing radiation is an important source of magnification.
3. The structures of the human jaws have depth as well as length and width. Therefore, in dental radiography, a three-dimensional object is recorded upon the two-dimensional surface of a film. This results in unequal magnification of different parts of an object because of varying distances of these parts from the film. In dental radiography, the lingual cusps of the posterior teeth are magnified less than the buccal cusps because the lingual cusps are nearer the film (Fig. 4-12B).

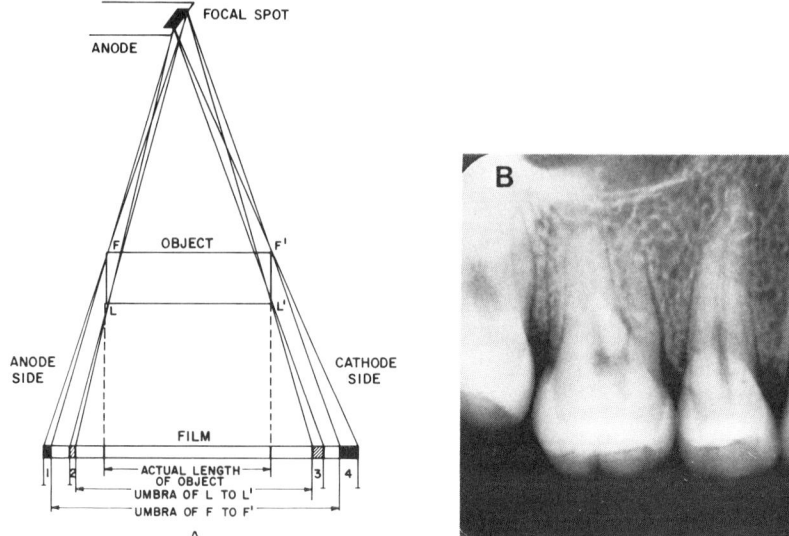

Figure 4-12. **(A)** Diagram illustrating why there is always some degree of unsharpness (penumbra formation), magnification (equal enlargement) and shape distortion (unequal enlargement). 1 and 4 are the penumbras of facial (F) portion of object, and 2 and 3 are penumbras of lingual (L) portion of object. Facial portion of object is more magnified and has more unsharpness than lingual portion of object. **(B)** The lingual cusps (1) are less magnified and are more defined than (2) buccal cusps of premolars and molars.

In Figure 4-12A, areas 1 and 4 are penumbras of points F and F¹ corresponding to facial surface points of a tooth. Areas 2 and 3 are penumbras of points L and L¹ corresponding to lingual surface points of a tooth. Notice that penumbra 2 is smaller than 1 and penumbra 3 is smaller than 4. This is because points L and L¹ are closer to the film than points F and F¹. Also, note that penumbra 1 on the anode side is smaller than penumbra 4 on the cathode side. Maximum sharpness is always achieved on the anode side of the X-Ray tube. The umbra of F-F¹ is longer than L-L¹. The surface closer to the film is always magnified. The **umbra** is the region of the object that is imaged on the film and means **shadow**. The **penumbra** is the zone of **geometric unsharpness** (blurring) that surrounds the umbra (complete shadow).

To understand how these geometric characteristics can interfere with radiographic image accuracy, we will first investigate how these same geometric characteristics are produced by light waves. After all, X-Rays are no more than very short invisible light waves.

In order to demonstrate shadow formation by light, obtain a small light source (7 1/2 watt bulb). Place your hand approximately an inch from the wall with the small light source positioned three feet from the wall. The shadow produced will be nearly the same size as your hand with its edges clear and well-defined. If you move your hand toward the light source, you will notice the shadow of your hand will enlarge and its edges wil become fuzzy and indistinct.

Next, substitute a large frosted bulb or a flashlight for the light source. You will notice this time that the hand shadow will have fuzzy edges even with your hand close to the wall. This fuzziness at the edges is caused by the large light source. The fuzzy portion of the shadow around the umbra (shadow) is called the **penumbra** or the **area of unsharpness**. In order to minimize the **unsharpness** of the light shadow, the **penumbra** must be reduced.

You can also distort your hand image by placing the light source in such a manner that the light waves strike your hand in an oblique direction rather than perpendicularly. This is called shape distortion.

In order to avoid confusion in comparing light waves and X-Rays, remember that light waves produce shadows by reflecting light from an opaque object. X-Rays will penetrate this same object and will not produce a true shadow because details of the object will be visible in the processed film. Therefore, X-Rays produce images rather than shadows.

Nevertheless, the same laws that apply to the shadow at the edge of the object (penumbra) apply to the details of the internal structures of the object. The five rules for accurate shadow casting by light waves are also applicable to X-Rays in the formation of an accurate radiographic image.

Five Rules for Accurate Image Formation

1. The X-Rays should proceed from as small a focal spot as conditions will allow.
2. The distance between the focal spot (source) and the object to be examined should always be as long as is practical.
3. The film should be as close as possible to the object being radiographed.
4. Generally speaking, the central ray should be as nearly perpendicular to the film as possible to record the adjacent structures in their true spatial relationships.
5. As far as is practical, the long axis of the object should be parallel to the film.

By following the above five rules, measures can be taken to minimize the inherent geometric characteristics found in every radiograph. The effects produced when these five rules are followed are diagrammatically represented in Figures 4-13 and 4-14.

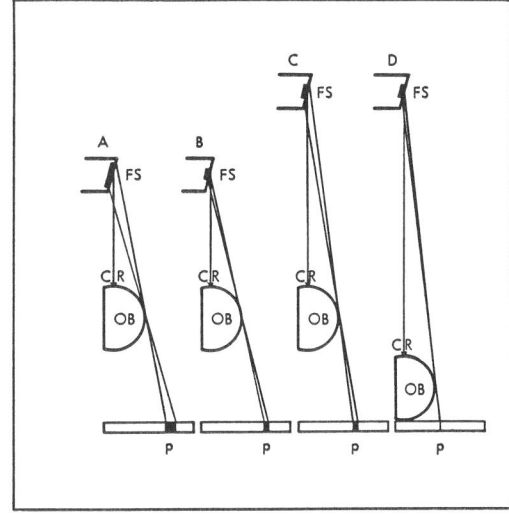

Figure 4-13. Diagrams illustrating how the accuracy of the radiographic image can be improved by decreasing the size of the penumbra (P). The penumbra affects image unsharpness and magnification. Notice the changes in size of the penumbra (P): from A to B by decreasing the size of the focal spot of the anode; from B to C by increasing the distance between the focal spot and the film; from C to D by decreasing the distance between (OB) and the film. (Redrawn from Fuchs, Arthur W.: *Principles of Radiographic Exposure and Processing*, 2nd ed. Springfield, Il., Charles C Thomas, Publisher, 1958.)

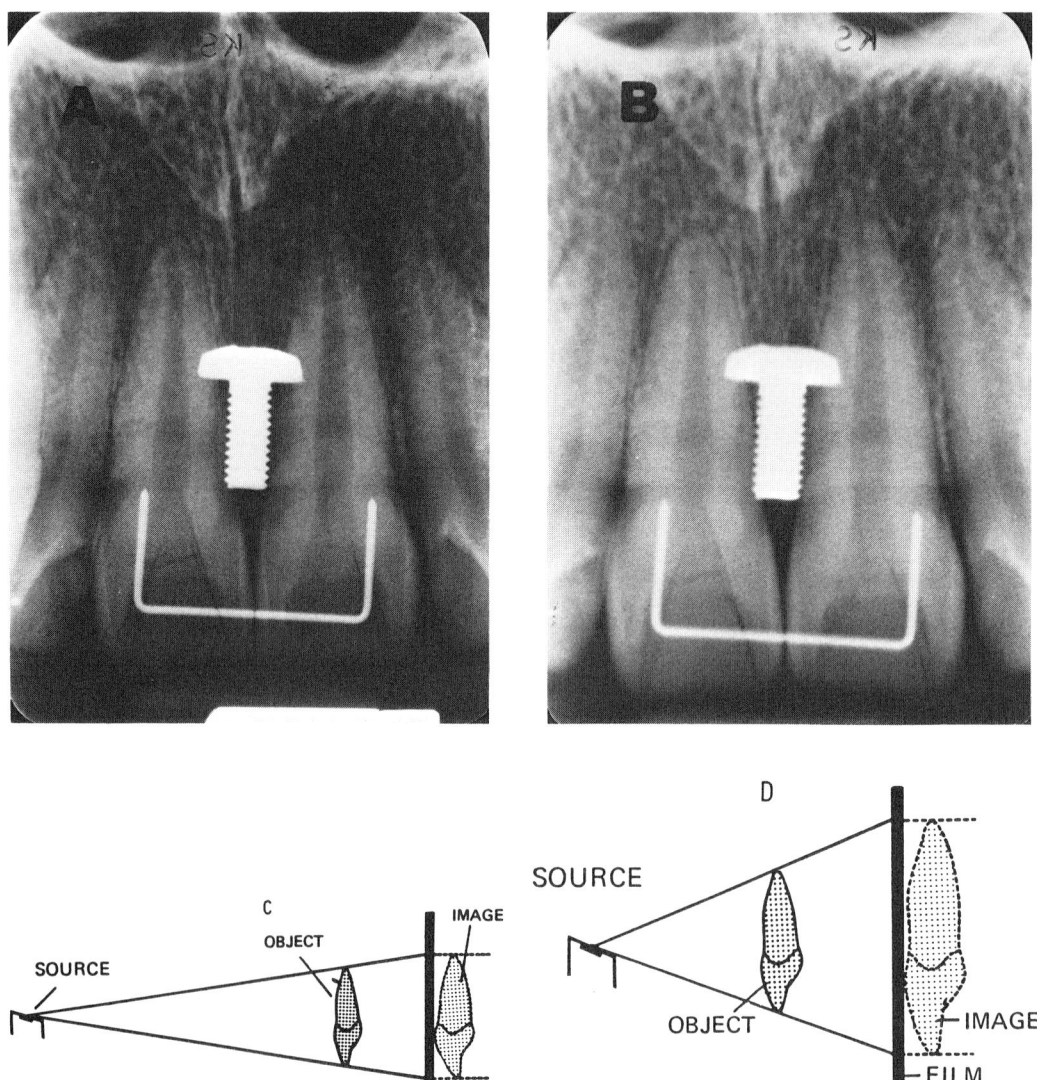

Figure 4-14. Radiograph (A) was taken with distance factors shown in diagram (C). Radiograph (B) was taken with distance factors shown in diagram (D). The object-film distance was the same in both cases; only the source-film distances were different. Notice the sharpness (less penumbra) of outline of the screw in radiograph (A) taken with the longer source-film distance as compared to radiograph (B) taken with the shorter source-film distance.

Factors that Influence Geometric Characteristics of the Radiographic Image

Radiographic Image Unsharpness

Radiographic image unsharpness is the fuzzy area surrounding the contour lines of the teeth and osseous tissues of the radiograph. Considering the relatively small size of the dental structures and tissues, it is very important to minimize these areas of fuzziness or unsharpness in the dental radiograph. A dental radiograph must have maximum definition of detail, and the contour lines of the teeth and the osseous tissues must be clearly defined and distinct.

There are three types of radiographic image unsharpness (diffusion of detail by penumbra formation) found in the dental radiograph, all of which influence definition:

1. geometric unsharpness;
2. motion unsharpness;
3. screen unsharpness.

Geometric Unsharpness

Geometric unsharpness is the fuzzy outline of the radiographic image which is called the **penumbra**, or sometimes the **edge gradient**. The penumbra is influenced by the size of the focal spot, the source-object, and the object-film distance.

The smaller the size of the focal spot, the smaller the penumbra and, consequently, the sharper the definition of the radiographic image (Fig. 4-13 A,B). When the focal spot is relatively small (0.8-1.5 mm), as in dental X-Ray tubes, the radiographic image is influenced very little by magnification.

The width of the zone of geometric unsharpness or penumbra can be illustrated by the following equation:

$$U_g = F \cdot \frac{d}{D}$$

where U_g = penumbra size (mm)
F = focal spot size (mm)
d = object-film distance in inches
D = source-object distance in inches

Example. From the above formula, calculate and compare the penumbra widths of the following two radiographic techniques:

Technique A: Focal spot width = 1 mm
Object-film distance = 1 inch
Focal spot-object distance = 15 inches

Technique B: Focal spot width = 1.5 mm
Object-film distance = 1 inch
Focal spot-object distance = 7 inches

Calculation

Technique A:

$$p = \frac{1 \times 1}{15} = .07 \text{ mm}$$

Technique B:

$$p = \frac{1 \times 1.5}{15} = .21 \text{ mm}$$

In all situations, sharpness is improved when the source-object distance is increased (Fig. 4-13 B,C).

The longer the object-film distance the greater the **unsharpness**. In the dental radiograph, the portion of the dental structure closest to the film will have the greatest sharpness. Therefore, the lingual cusp and the lingual root of a tooth will have more sharpness on the radiograph than the buccal cusp and the buccal root

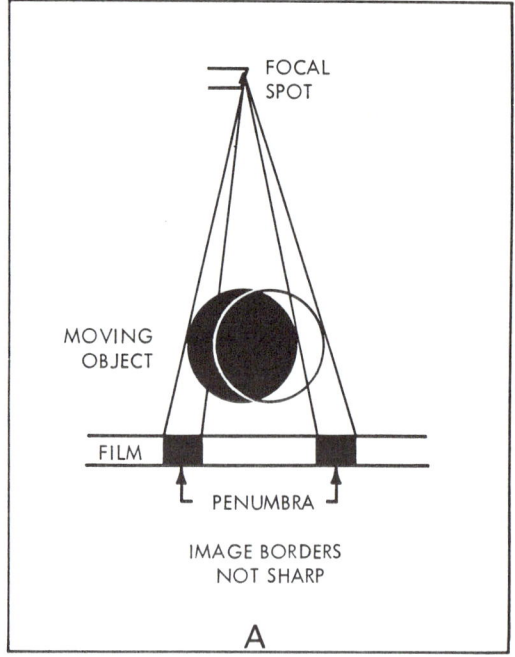 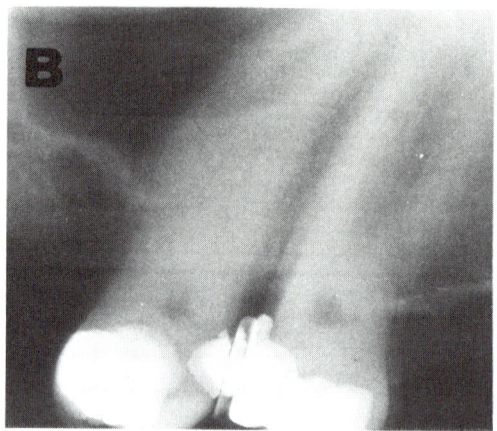

Figure 4-15. (A) Diagram illustrating the influence of motion in producing image unsharpness. (Redrawn from Fuchs, Arthur W.: *Principles of Radiographic Exposure and Processing*, 2nd. ed. Springfield, Il., Charles C Thomas, Publisher, 1958.) (B) Radiograph of gagging patient who had moved during exposure of radiograph. Notice that image is elongated from film bending and the image outline is blurred from penumbra formation.

or roots, because they are closer to the film (Fig. 4-13, C, D).

In summary then, geometric unsharpness can be minimized by reducing the width of the focal spot, reducing the object-film distance, and increasing the source-object distance (Fig. 4-14).

Motion Unsharpness

Motion by the patient, motion of the film, and/or motion of the tube directly influences sharpness of the image definition. Even a slight motion of the film may cause **motion unsharpness** in the radiographic image. Any motion of the tube may cause vibration of the focal spot, which increases the size of the focal spot, thereby causing an increase in image unsharpness of the resulting images in the radiograph. The influence of patient movement on the definition of the radiographic image is illustrated in Figure 4-15.

The movement of the film without patient movement during exposure will cause the greatest amount of motion unsharpness on the film.

Screen Unsharpness

Screen unsharpness is introduced to the radiograph when intensifying screens are used in extraoral radiography. The amount of unsharpness is dependent on several factors, which have been discussed in Chapter 3.

Magnification

Magnification is the equal enlargement of the actual size of the object upon the projection of the radiographic image. The factors that influence magnification are the same factors that influence geometric unsharpness; however, the distance factors (source-film distance and object-film distance) have more influence than the focal spot size.

Since the focal spot size is controlled by the manufacturer, the two distance factors are the only factors that can be controlled by the operator. It is possible to minimize magnification (enlargement) of the dental structures by increasing the source-film distance and reducing object-film distance to practical distances.

The relationship between the X-Ray beam, the object being radiographed, and the image of the object being projected on the film can be shown in a simple drawing (Fig. 4-16).

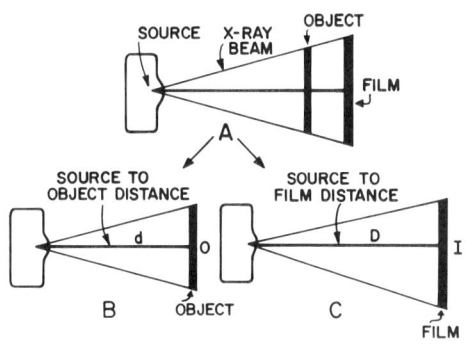

$$\frac{d}{D} = \frac{\text{Object size}}{\text{Image size}} \quad \left(\text{Object size} = \frac{(S-O-D)(\text{Image size})}{S-F-D}\right)$$

Figure 4-16. (A) Drawing shows the relationship between the source of X-Ray, the X-Ray beam, the object being radiographed, and the image of the object on the film. (B) and (C) two similar triangles formed from triangle (A) showing proportional relationship of two triangles.

Since X-Rays are emitted from the focal spot of the anode in diverging straight lines, a triangle can be formed using either the object or the image of the object as the base of the triangle. The vertex of the triangle is the source of the X-Ray beam at the anode, and the central ray of the X-Ray beam drawn perpendicular to the object base or image base represents the altitude (Fig. 16A). This type of drawing will produce two triangles, one with the object as the base and the other with the object image on the film as the base.

Although these triangles are of different sizes, they are known as **similar triangles** because their angles are equal. This results in their corresponding sides and altitudes being proportional to each other (Fig. 4-16B,C).

This means that—

$$\frac{d(\text{source-object distance})}{D \text{ (source-film distance)}} = \frac{(O) \text{ object size}}{(I) \text{ image size}}$$

From the above proportional relationship, the true size of the object can be calculated because d, D, and I can be measured directly.

Example. What is the true size of a tooth when the source-to-film distance is 16 inches, the source-to-object distance is 15 inches, and the tooth image length measured on the radiograph is 28 mm?
SOLUTION.

$$\frac{15(d)}{16(D)} = \frac{(O)}{28(I)}$$

$$(O) \text{ object size} = \frac{15}{16} \cdot 28 = 26.3 \text{ mm}$$

The percent of magnification is calculated by the following formula:

$$\text{Percent of Magnification} = \frac{\text{size of image}}{\text{size of object}} - 1.00$$

In the above example the percent of

magnification is calculated as follows:

$$\% \text{ Magnification} = \frac{28}{26.3} - 1$$

$$= 1.0646 - 1.00$$

$$= .064 \text{ or } 6.5\%$$

The graph in Figure 4-17 depicts the effect of source-film, object-film relationship or percentage of image enlargement or magnification.

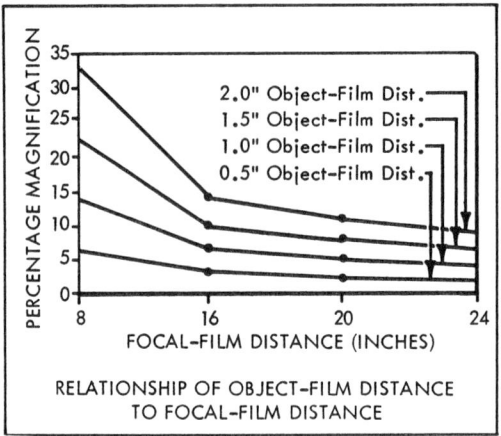

Figure 4-17. Relationship of the source-film distance to the object-film distance. (Courtesy of Dr. William Updegrave.)

In summary, magnification depends on two factors: (1) source-film distance, and (2) object-film distance.

Magnification of the radiographic image of an object can be kept at a minimum by keeping the object as close as possible to the film and the source-film distance as long as possible or practical. In Figure 4-14, radiograph (A) taken with the long source-film distance reveals teeth that are less magnified than the teeth in radiograph (B) taken with a shorter source-film distance. The width of the staple measured 2.0 mm longer in radiograph (B) taken with the shorter source-film distance.

Dimensional Distortion

Dimensional distortion of the radiographic image is a variation from the true shape of the anatomical structure radiographed. It is unequal magnification of different parts of the same structure.

Dimensional distortion results from improper alignment of the object, the film, and the projected beam of radiation. It can be minimized by placing the film parallel to the major planes of the object and directing the central ray of the X-Ray beam perpendicular to the major planes of the object and the film.

Dimensional distortion occurs when an angular relationship is created between the object and film or the beam of radiation with the film. The parts of the object farther away from the film will be projected in an incorrect relationship to the parts closer to the film and will result in the image not accurately representing the object. When an oblique angle radiographic technique is used in the maxillary molar region, the buccal roots are projected proportionately lower on the film than the lingual root; hence, there is an abnormally foreshortened appearance of the buccal roots (Fig. 4-18).

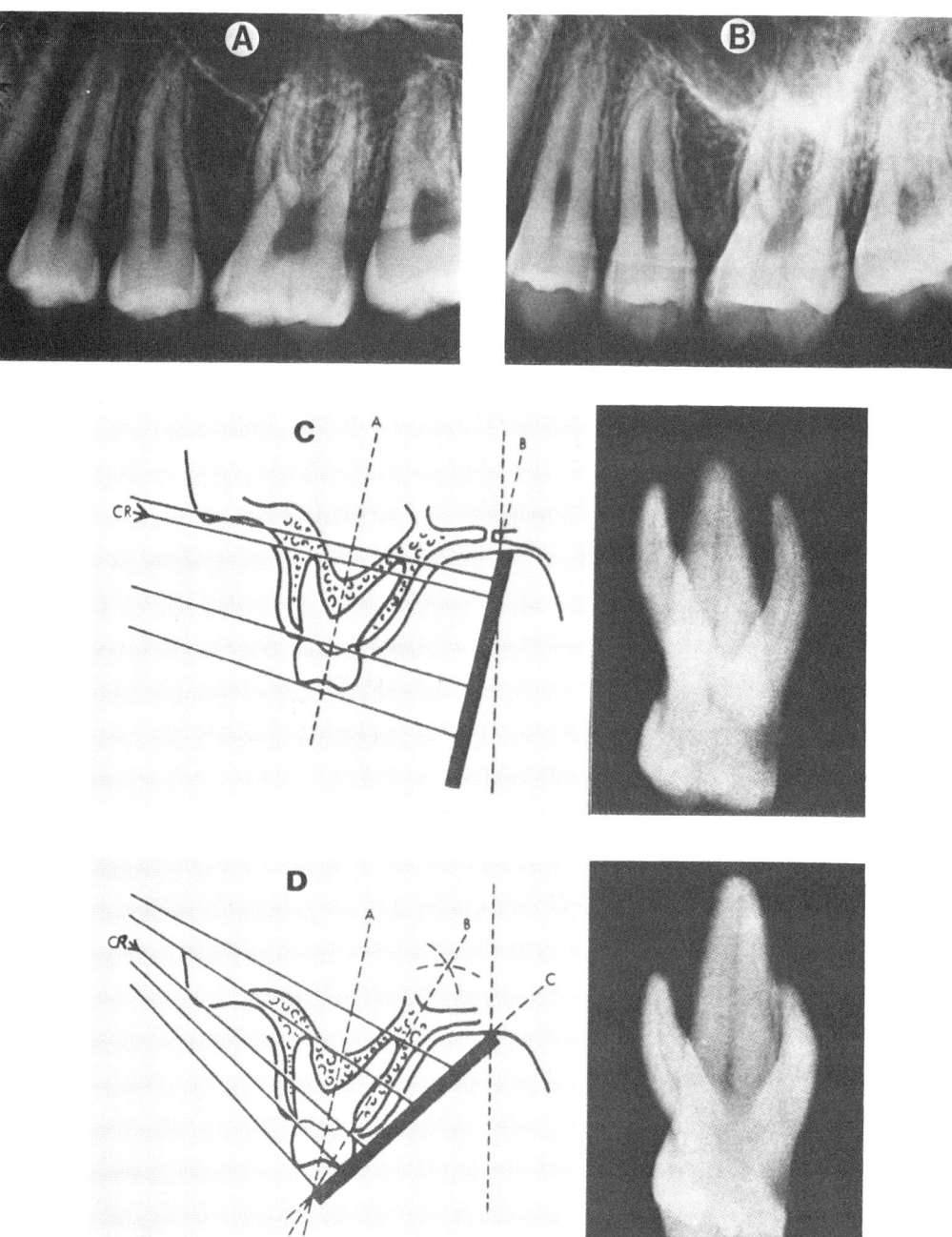

Figure 4-18. Radiograph (A) was taken with a paralleling technique as shown in diagram (C). Radiograph (B) was taken with the bisecting angle technique shown in diagram (D), which is an oblique angle technique. Notice the amount of foreshortening of the buccal roots of the maxillary molar shown in (D) when compared to the buccal roots of maxillary molar shown in (C) taken with the paralleling technic. Compare radiograph (A) with radiograph (B) for anatomical accuracy. Both radiograph (A) and (B) were taken of the left maxillary molar region of the same patient.

ANATOMICAL ACCURACY

Anatomical acccuracy occurs when the anatomic structures are reproduced on the film in the true spatial relationship as they normally appear.

Shape distortion will interfere with anatomic accuracy because it changes the resulting radiographic images so they no longer represent the true shape of the object being radiographed. If the object itself is **actually rectangular**, it is a definite disadvantage interpretively to project its image so that it **looks square**. A distortion of this kind can be avoided and anatomic accuracy obtained when the film is placed parallel to the long axis of the teeth and the radiation beam directed perpendicular to both.

A radiograph is said to have anatomic accuracy when—

1. the labial and lingual cementoenamel junctions of the anterior teeth are superimposed;
2. the buccal and lingual cusps of the posterior teeth (especially the molars) are superimposed;
3. the contacts of the teeth are opened in at least one of the projections of a given area;
4. the buccal portion of the alveolar crest is superimposed over the lingual portion of the alveolar crest (posterior teeth); and
5. there is no superimposition of the zygomatic arch over the roots of the maxillary molar teeth.

In Figure 4-18 compare radiograph (A) taken with the paralleling technique (film and tooth long axes parallel to each other and X-Ray beam directed perpendicular to both) and radiograph (B) taken with the bisecting angle technique (X-Ray directed perpendicular to a line bisecting the angle formed by long axes of tooth and film).

The long-cone paralleling technic radiograph has greater anatomic accuracy than the short-cone bisecting technic radiograph because the paralleling long-cone technic radiograph reveals the following:

a. better superimposition of buccal and lingual cusps (better caries detection);
b. better superimposition of buccal portion of alveolar crest over the lingual portion of alveolar crest (better interpretation of crestal alveolar bone height);
c. least superimposition of zygomatic arch over roots of maxillary molars (better for interpreting periapical pathology);
d. better definition and less magnification (better film for overall interpretation); and
e. minimal foreshortening of buccal roots of molars (better for endodontic preoperative and postoperative radiographs).

RADIOGRAPHIC COVERAGE

It is important that the area of interest is well covered in the radiograph. In the periapical radiograph, an adequate amount of bone surrounding the apices of the teeth should be revealed on the radiograph (Fig. 4-19A,B).

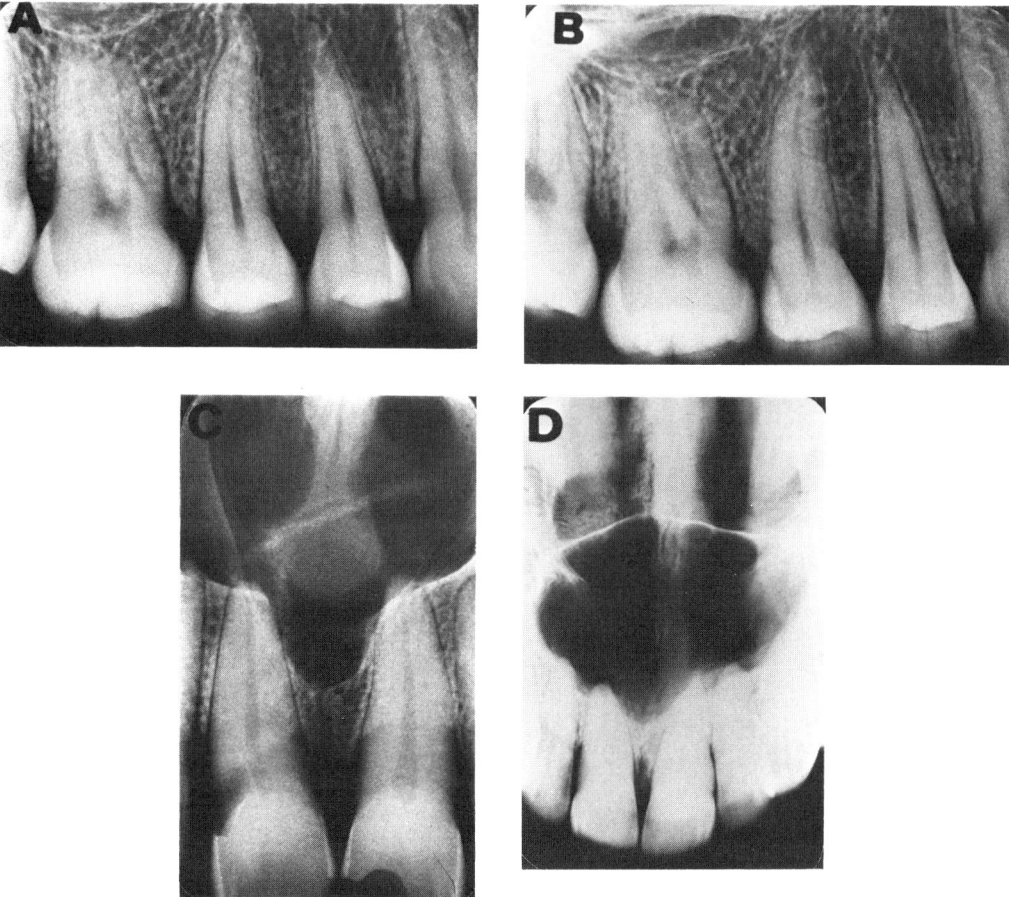

Figure 4-19. (A) Radiograph of maxillary premolar region without adequate periapical coverage. (B) Radiograph of maxillary premolar region of same patient, but with adequate periapical coverage. (C) Periapical radiograph of maxillary central incisor region showing large radiolucency. (D) Occlusal radiograph of same patient in (C) showing complete outline of large radiolucency in palate.

Supplemental films taken at right angles to each other may be mandatory at times in order to localize the area of interest (Fig. 4-19C,D and 4-20). Adequate coverage of the area of interest depends upon several factors:

1. proper alignment of film and the radiation beam to area of interest;
2. proper selection of film types; and
3. proper selection of film projection technics.

SUMMARY

The diagnostic quality of the radiographic film is dependent upon the proper utilization of several factors. The functions of these factors are given below:

1. *Focal spot size* influences unsharpness and magnification of radiographic im-

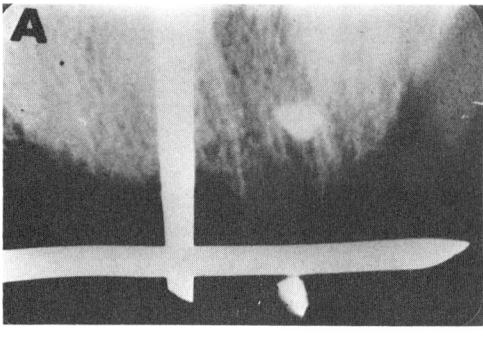
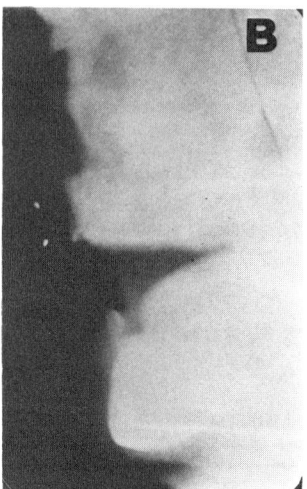
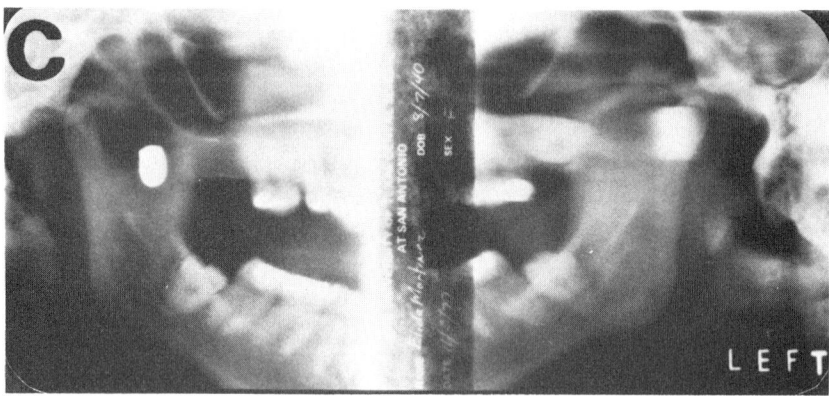
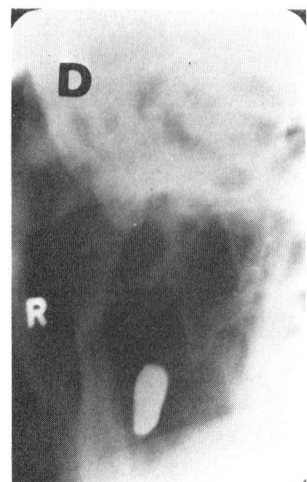

Figure 4-20. (A) Occlusal radiograph of patient with seemingly a metal fragment in the maxillary palate and one in the lip. (B) Anterior profile radiograph of same patient in (A) locating both metal fragments in the lip. (C) Special TMJ panoramic (SSW Panorex) radiograph revealing bullet in area of mandibular (sigmoid) notch of ramus of mandible. (D) AP radiograph of mandibular condyle of same patient revealing bullet is medially placed to right mandibular ramus.

age.
2. *Source-film and object-film distances* influences density, unsharpness, and magnification of radiographic image.
3. *Alignment of film and beam of radiation to object* influences anatomic accuracy, distortion, and coverage of radiograph.
4. *Kilovoltage*—
   a. regulates degree of penetration of tissues;
   b. influences scatter radiation fog;
   c. regulates contrast scale;
   d. determines exposure latitude;
   e. influences density of radiograph.
5. *Milliampere-seconds (mAs)* regulates density of radiograph.

Therefore, if all other exposure factors remain constant, the factors listed in Figure 4-21 will influence the X-Ray image characteristics of density, contrast, geometric unsharpness, magnification, and shape distortion in various ways.

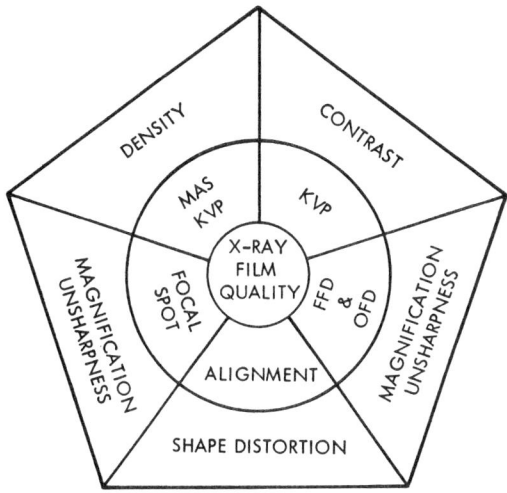

Figure 4-21. Summary of controlling factors of density, contrast, geometric unsharpness, magnification, and distortion.

Bibliography

Beck, J: *Syllabus of Dental Radiology*. University of Minnesota School of Dentistry, 1970.

Bloom, W.J.; Hollenbach, J.L.; and Morgan, J.A.: *Medical Radiographic Technic*, 3rd ed., Springfield, Charles C Thomas, 1969.

Bushong, S.C.: *Radiologic Science for Technologists*. St. Louis, Mosby, 1975, pp. 218-250.

Christensen, E.E.; Curry, T.S.; and Dowdey, J.E.: *An Introduction to the Physics of Diagnostic Radiology*, 2nd ed. Philadelphia, Lea & Febiger, 1978, pp. 137-184.

Ennis, L.; Berry, H.: and Phillips, J.E.: *Dental Roentgenology*, 6th ed. Philadelphia, Lea & Febiger, 1967.

Files, G.W.: The relation, radiographically, of kilovolts peak to time of exposure. *Radiology*, 7:255, 1926.

Fitzgerald, G.M.: An investigation in adumbration, or the factors that control geometric unsharpness. *J Am Dent Assoc, 34*:5, 1947.

Fitzgerald, G.M.: Dental roentgenographic IV. The voltage factor. *J Am Dent Assoc, 41*:19-28, July 1950.

Fitzgerald, G.M.: *Ginns' Review of Dentistry*. St. Louis, Mosby, 1949.

Fitzgerald, G.M.: Dental roentgenography I: An investigation in adumbration, or the factors that control geometric unsharpness. *J Am Dent Assoc, 34*:1-20, January 1947.

Fitzgerald, G.M.: Roentgenologic rebuttal. *Oral Surg, 13*:1218, October, 1960.

Franklin, J.B.: The effect of aluminum filter disks in roentgenocephalometry. *Angle Orthod, 32*:252, October, 1962.

Fuchs, A.: *Principles of Radiographic Exposure and Processing*, 2nd ed. Springfield, Charles C Thomas, 1971.

Hendee, W.R.: *Medical Radiation Physics*. Chicago, Year Bk Med, 1970.

Intraoral Radiography With Rinn XCP-BAI Instruments. Elgin, Ill., Rinn Corp., 1980.

Jaundrell-Thompson, J.; and Ashworth, W.J.: *X-Ray Physics and Equipment*, 2nd ed. Philadelphia, Davis Co, 1970.

Jacobi, C.A.; and Paris, D.Q.: *Textbook of Radiology Technology*, 5th ed. St. Louis, Mosby, 1972.

Johns, H.; and Cunningham, J.: *The Physics of Radiology*, 3rd ed. Springfield, Charles C Thomas, 1969.

Langland, O.E.; and Sippy, F.H.: A study of radiographic longitudinal distortion of anterior teeth using the paralleling technique. *Oral Surg, 22*:737, December 1966.

Mattson, O.: Practical photographic problems in radiography with special reference to high voltage technic. *Acta Radiol [Supp] 20*, 1955.

McCormack, D.: Dental roentgenology: A technical procedure for furthering the advancement toward anatomical accuracy. *J Calif State Dent Assoc*, May-June 1937.

McCormack, F.W.: A plea for standardized technique for oral radiography. *J Dent Res, 2*, 1920.

Meredith, W.J.; and Massey, J.B.: *Fundamental Physics of Radiology*. Baltimore, Williams & Wilkins, 1972.

Muncheryan, H.M.: *Modern Physics of Roentgenology*. Los Angeles, Wetzel, 1940.

Radiology Specialist. Washington, D.C., Department of the Air Force, March 1958.

Richards, A.G.: Technical factors that control radiographic density. *Dent Clin North Am*, 371-377, July 1961.

Rossman, K.: Image quality. *Radiol Clin North Am, 7*:419, 1969.

Seeman, H.E.: *Physical and Photographic Principles of Medical Radiography*. New York, Wiley, 1968.

Selman, J.: *The Fundamentals of X-Ray and Radium Physics*, 6th ed. Springfield, Charles C Thomas, 1978.

Sweet, A.P.: Dental seminar: radiographic density. *Dent Radiogr Photogr, 4*, 1949.

Sweet, A.P.: Peripheral geometry. *Dent Radiogr Photogr, 25*, 1952.

Ter-Pogossian, M.M.: *The Physical Aspects of Diagnostic Radiology*. New York, Hoeber Medical, 1967.

The Fundamentals of Radiography, 12th ed. Rochester, N.Y. Eastman Kodak Co., 1980.

TM-8-280, *Military Roentgenology*. Washington, D.C., U.S. Government Printing Office, 1944.

Updegrave, W.: Simplifying and improving intraoral dental roentgenography. *Oral Surg, 12*:704-716, June 1959.

Updegrave, W.: High or low kilovoltage. *Dent Radiogr Photogr, 4*, 1960.

Updegrave, W.: Higher fidelity in intraoral roentgenography. *J Am Dent Assoc, 62*:3, 1961.

Waggener, D.T.: The right-angle technique using the extension cone. *Dent Clin North Am*, 783-788, November 1960.

Wuehrmann, D.T.: The long cone technic. *Prac Dent Monogr*, 3-30, July 1957.

Wuehrmann, A.; and Manson-Hing, L.: *Dental Radiology*. St. Louis, Mosby, 1965.

Wuehrmann, A.; and Monacelli, C.J.: Selection of optimum kilovoltage for dental radiography. *Radiology, 57*:240, August 1951.

Wuehrmann, A.; and Curby, W.A.: Radiopacity of oral structures as a basis for selecting optimum kilovoltage for intraoral roentgenograms. *J Dent Res, 31*:27, February 1952.

X-Ray Generation and Radiographic Principles in Dentistry. Milwaukee, X-Ray Department, General Electric Co.

X-rays in Dentistry. Eastman Kodak Co., Radiography Markets Division, Rochester, N.Y., 1977.

Chapter 5

RADIATION BIOLOGY

John W. Preece

ABSORPTION OF RADIATION

Temporal Sequence

X-RAYS are generated within the head of the x-ray machine when a stream of high speed electrons possessing a large amount of kinetic energy strikes the target of the anode. The kinetic energy of the colliding high speed electrons is converted primarily into heat; a small quantity is converted into x-ray photons. These photons of x-radiation are tiny packets of pure energy without mass and are capable of penetrating tissues and producing an effect upon a film emulsion. As x-ray photons travel through the tissues, some of their energy is transferred to atoms and molecules forming the tissue, the intensity of the beam diminishes, and biologic changes are initiated. It is the attenuation of the beam of radiation by tissues of different density that ultimately results in the production of the radiographic image; additionally, the transfer of energy to various tissues of the body initiates a series of complex events that form the basis for the science known as radiation biology.

As x-ray photons enter the body and begin to lose their energy, various biologic effects may be produced. The biologic effects of any type of ionizing radiation, whether corpuscular or noncorpuscular, stems from the transfer of energy to the electrons of the absorbing biological material. During this transfer or absorption of energy, the electrons of the absorbing tissue are converted into moving electrons possessing kinetic energy, which is subsequently dissipated through numerous interactions with other atoms within the absorbing tissue. When the energy imparted to the tissue is expressed per unit of tissue mass, it is called absorbed dose.

As the photons of x-radiation enter a biologic system, a primary interaction occurs in which a tissue electron is set in motion to produce the series of events diagrammatically represented in Figure 5-1. The approximate energy of x-ray photons used in dentistry is in the range of 35 keV; multiple interactions of the type illustrated will be required to completely absorb the energy of one incident x-ray photon.

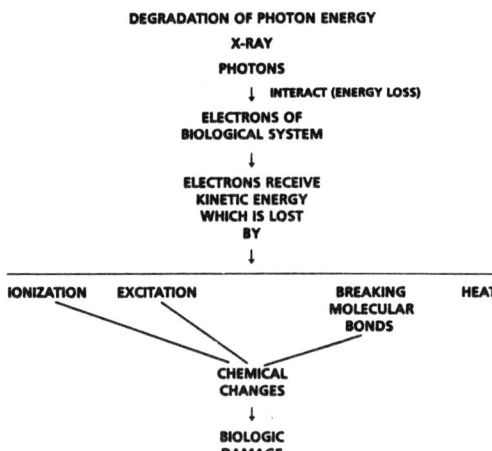

Figure 5-1. Temporal sequence of radiation absorption. (Modified from Johns, H. E., and Cunningham, J.: *The Physics of Radiology*, 3rd ed. Springfield, Il., Charles C Thomas Publisher. 1969, p. 136.)

Linear Energy Transfer (LET)

LET is a measure of the energy deposited (or ion pairs produced) by an ionizing particle per micron of particle track length. As the ionizing particle or photon travels through the tissue, it randomly transfers some of its energy through a number of interactions with tissue electrons. This process of transferring energy from x-radiation to tissue electrons is known as ionization and excitation. Ionization results in the formation of a positively charged tissue atom and a negatively charged electron with kinetic energy called an ion pair. Excitation is a transfer of energy to the tissue electron that raises the electron to a higher energy level but does not knock it out of the atom or molecule. At each interaction the electron loses some of its energy and may be scattered in a slightly different direction. The track followed by the primary ionizing particle or photon is termed the primary track. In some interactions a large amount of energy may be transferred to a tissue electron and this electron may produce a track of ionized particles of its own in a direction different from the primary ionizing photon or particle track; this secondary track is known as a delta ray.

Just prior to coming to a complete stop, there is a rapid increase in the amount of energy transferred and the separation between ionizing events decreases rapidly until all of the kinetic energy of the moving electron is dissipated (Figure 5-2).

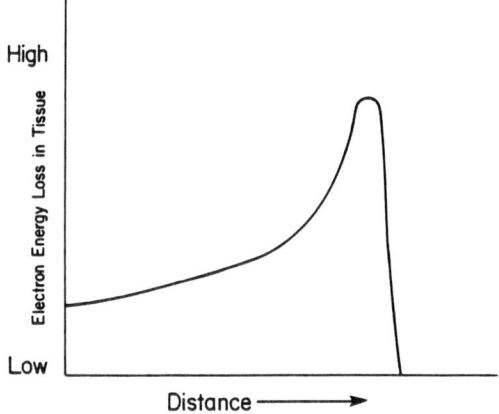

Figure 5-2. Electron energy loss in tissues; energy transfer from the moving electron increases rapidly as the velocity of the moving electron decreases and is maximum prior to coming to a complete stop.

LET is therefore a measure of the energy transferred by the primary ionizing particle or x-ray photon as it travels through tissue, forming ion pairs or excited molecules; it is usually expressed in units of kilo-electron-volts (keV) per micron of track length. LET values vary depending upon the type of ionizing radiation. The higher the LET value the greater is the possible biologic effect upon the tissue being irradiated, since more energy is transferred to the tissue per unit of track length. For example, the LET of cobalt 60 is 0.25 keV per micron. Thus 250 electron-volts of energy are transferred to the tissue per micron of track. In contrast, larger, slower moving particles of corpuscular radiation such as alpha particles may have an LET value of 250 keV per micron; thus alpha particles would transfer approximately 1000 times more energy per micron of track length. (Figure 5-3).

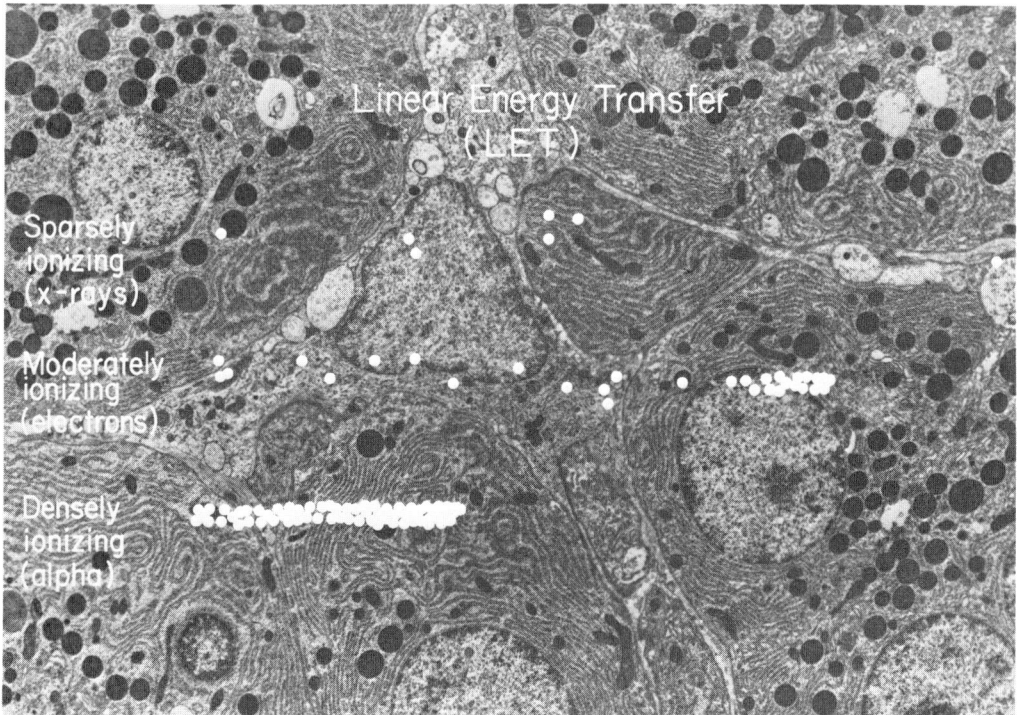

Figure 5-3. Representation of linear energy transfer for various types of ionizing radiations within a tissue.

Ionizing particles of larger size encounter more friction as they pass between the atoms and they will lose their energy more rapidly per unit track length compared to electrons and photons. Examples of some LETs are shown in Table 5-I.

Because of differences in energy transfer, different amounts of different types of ionizing radiation will be necessary to produce the same amount and type of biologic effect. For example, it may take 100 units of electron or x-radiation to produce a particular biologic effect, and it may only require 20 units of proton irradiation to produce the same biologic effect; thus proton radiation is considered to be about five times more efficient in producing a particular biologic effect. This difference between radiation amounts necessary to produce a particular biologic effect is referred to as the quality factor (QF) or radiobiological equivalent (RBE).

Quality factor is a LET-dependent factor used for radiation protection purposes. Examples of quality factors are shown in Table 5-II.

Table 5-I

IONIZING PARTICLES OF RADIOBIOLOGICAL INTEREST

Particle	Charge	Energy (MeV)	LET (keV/μ)
Electron	−1	0.001	12.3
		0.010	2.30
		0.100	0.42
		1.00	0.25
		200 kvp x-rays	0.4-36
		Cobalt 60 γ-rays	0.2-2
Proton	+1	small	92
		2	16
		5	8
		10	4
Alpha	+2	small	260
		5	95
Neutron	(62) 0	2.5	15-80 (peak at 20)
		14.1	3-30 (peak at 7)

From H. E. Johns and J. R. Cunningham: *The Physics of Radiology.*, 1969. Courtesy of Charles C Thomas, Publisher, Springfield, Il.

Table 5-II

QUALITY FACTORS

LET keV/micron	QF	Types of Radiation
3.5 or less	1	x to β rays; β > .03 MeV
7	2	β < .03 MeV
23	5	slow neutrons
53	10	neutrons and protons to 10 MeV, α particles
175	20	heavy recoil nuclei (nuclear fission fragments)

Modified from H. E. Johns and J. R. Cunningham: *The Physics of Radiology.* Springfield, Il., Charles C Thomas, Publisher, 1969.

The radiobiological equivalent or the relative biological effectiveness (RBE) is an experimentally determined value used primarily in radiobiology to compare the dose of two types of radiation to produce the same biologic effect. RBE values are relative and will vary depending on the specific effect to be produced and the types of radiation under comparison. For this type of comparative evaluation, a "standard" radiation quality has been defined (200 kVp x-rays with a HVL of 1.5 mm copper) and its biologic effect is compared to the "test" radiation according to the equation:

$$RBE = \frac{\text{Dose of standard radiation to produce specified biologic effect}}{\text{Dose of test radiation to produce specified biological effect}}$$

For most types of ionizing radiation, RBE and QF are similar. For x-rays, QF and RBE are both equal to 1.

Theories of Radiation Action

The effect of energy absorption is to produce excitations and ionizations in molecules of the medium. Chemical changes follow these, leading ultimately to the observed effects. However, the quantitative yield of each of the possible ionizations and excitations is proportional to the energy absorbed almost irrespective of the type and velocity of the charged particle; therefore, the biological response per unit energy absorbed is an appropriate method for determining the potential biologic effect of various types of ionizing radiation. One of the key methods of evaluating the biologic effect of radiation on a system is through the development of a dose response curve.

The dose response curve is one of the most important diagrams in radiation biology because greatly differing biologic effects may be used for evaluating the actions of radiation; for example, the formation of free radicals, enzyme inactivation, loss of DNA activity, induction of specific mutations, killing effects on cells or organisms. In most cases, the surviving fraction, such as enzyme activity or living cells, is plotted against dose. Such curves are called "dose response," "dose ef-

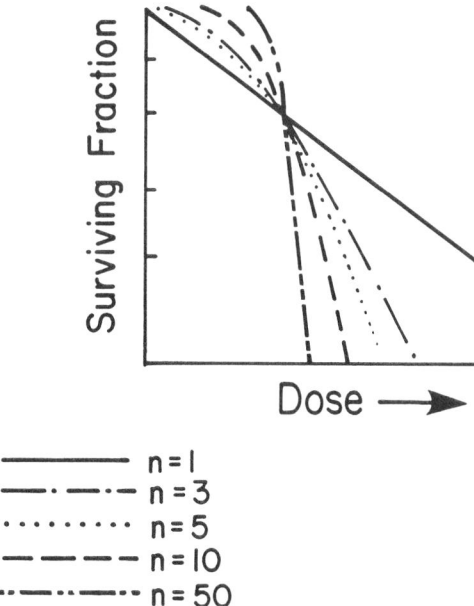

―――――― n = 1
―・―・― n = 3
・・・・・・・・・ n = 5
― ― ― ― n = 10
・・―・・―・・― n = 50

Figure 5-4. Dose response curves for number of hits on a biologic target.

fect," or "survival" curves. It is through the use of these curves that the complexities of radiation biology may be broken down into their known physical and chemical processes.

Historically, early radiation biologists attempted to interpret the biologic effects of radiation described by various dose response curves in terms of the amount of energy required to produce a specific effect. One of the earliest theories was known as the "Hit Theory." The goals of the hit theory were to provide a mathematical description of dose response curves and to permit the determination of characteristic parameters such as hit and target numbers from a given curve. Typical curves are illustrated in Figure 5-4.

Determination of the target volume (cm^3) multiplied by the dose represented the mean number of hits (ionizing events) occurring within the volume after the specified dose; the probability of exactly (N) hits occurring within this volume could be determined by statistical methods. According to this postulate, if "N" hits are required for inactivation, then any object receiving N-1 or fewer hits will survive.

The hit theory correctly explained certain data, but it was incapable of explaining all variations in biologic response. The basic premise, however, concerning the existence of biologic targets and hits is clearly correct; the main criticism of the theory is that it forces one to postulate (for biologic effects requiring multiple hit action) that only the (Nth) hit causes the test effect, and all other hits had no effect. Because of this limitation, the theory could not explain "sublethal" effects on complex structures such as cells, bacteria, and fungi.

Target Theory and Action Cross Section

A more acceptable method of describing the physical process of biologic effects has been developed, called the target theory. Basically, the theory attempts to determine the number of hits per unit volume and to derive from this the volume of the target and therefore, the size of the radiation sensitive substructures within the biological system. In the case of ionizing radiation, a "hit" depends on the transfer of a certain minimum amount of energy, the magnitude of which depends on the kind of damage and the system irradiated. The test effect, therefore, occurs when a certain minimum amount of energy is transferred by the passage of an ionizing particle (secondary electrons) through a sensitive region. The target theory assumes that the test effect occurs once a minimum amount of energy is deposited by an ionizing particle. If this minimum loss of energy is not transferred, no biological response occurs. In the target theory, therefore, it is not necessary to assume an accumulation of prior energy loss events. With this theory, not all energy loss events will be effective since there is a minimum amount of energy required to produce the test effect, and this is taken into consideration by introducing the concept of "action cross-section."

The action cross-section is LET-dependent since the statistical probability that a given amount of energy will be deposited per unit length of a particle track increases with increasing LET. The occurrence of a target hit, therefore, can be correlated to the passage of a charged particle through a formally defined cross-section called the "action cross-section." Applying this theory to cellular radiobiology, a concept develops in which minimal energy absorption in a critical volume or target might be necessary to cause a specified effect.

Unfortunately, the concept of a target or action cross-section does not make any allowance for damage from "outside" the radiation sensitive structure being transferred to or affecting the biologically sensitive elements, which is the rule rather than the exception. The possibility that energy can be transferred from outside the sensitive structure (target) to initiate a biological change in the structure has lead to developing the concepts of the direct and indirect effects of radiation.

Direct and Indirect Effects

The classification of biologic effects as being either direct or indirect is particularly meaningful at the molecular level. If absorption of radiation occurs in the molecule in which the lesion appears, this is the direct action of radiation. With indirect action, the absorption of radiation energy and the response to this energy occurs in different molecules, e.g. irradiated water molecules may disassociate to form free radicals in which new chemical groups may be added to a sensitive target molecule; in addition, an intermolecular transfer of energy from one molecule to an adjacent molecule may also be included as a part of this phenomenon. Intramolecular energy transfer or the transfer of energy from one portion of a large biologically active molecule to another more sensitive area within the same molecule would be considered a direct effect. The temporal stages of radiation action for direct and indirect effects of radiation at a molecular level are illustrated in Figure 5-5. Direct and indirect effects will be further discussed under cellular effects.

Radiation Chemistry

Radiation chemistry or molecular radiobiology concerns itself with the molecular events resulting from the interaction of radiation with biomolecules. Its primary goal is to define the molecular sequences that follow the absorption of radiation energy. These molecular disturbances initiate complex chains of biochemical and physiological reactions, which ultimately lead to observable damage in subcellular organelles and subsequently in living cells and systems.

Electromagnetic radiation when absorbed by molecules leads to the production of excited and/or ionized molecular states. Excited molecules can respond in several ways by ionizing various atomic

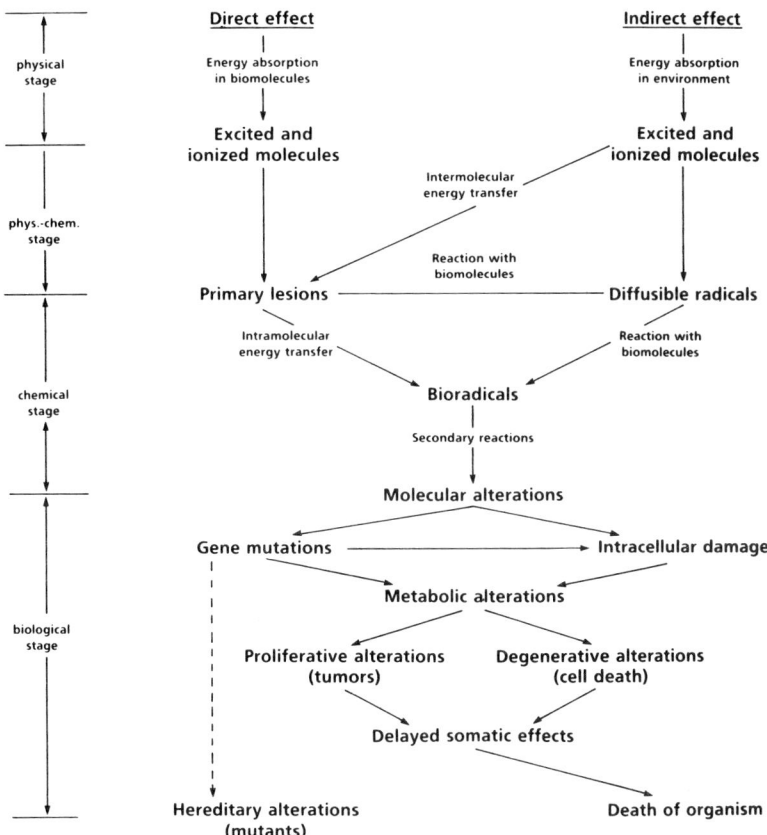

Figure 5-5. Temporal stages of radiation action for direct and indirect effects of radiation at a molecular level. (Modified from Dertinger, H., and Jung, H.: *Molecular Radiation Biology,* New York, Springer Verlag, 1970.)

bonds, which may result in breaking up the original molecule or the elevation of electrons into higher energy levels with the release of this excess energy through the emission of light or through electronic vibrational or thermal losses. The last two processes (light and heat loss) lead to molecules in their original state, whereas the other processes lead to the formation of new molecules with different chemical characteristics.

Ionization

When atom A is ionized, a negatively charged electron is knocked out of an atomic orbital to travel along a track and interact with other atoms; the remainder of the atom becomes a positively charged ion: $A \rightsquigarrow A^+ + e^-$ The electron cannot stay free for long and it will be rapidly captured by another molecule to yield a negative ion: $e^- + B = B^-$

A second possible reaction will occur if the original ionized molecule A^+ (positive ion) recaptures the electron before it leaves the molecule. This process is called **charge neutralization.** The molecule formed by the capture of the electron has appreciably more energy than the normal molecule and dissociates immediately to form a very reactive free radical, e.g. A^+

$+ e^- \to A^* \to C^0 + D^0$. A **free radical** is an electrically neutral molecule or atom having an unpaired electron; it is chemically extremely reactive. Free radicals are almost always intermediaries between ion pairs and the final chemical products. Thus, the absorption of radiation along the track taken by the ionizing particle may lead to the production of ion pairs, excited molecules, and free radicals.

Free radical combinations

Recombination, with no change in molecule: $RH \leadsto R^0 + H^0 \to RH$

They can join with other formerly unassociated radicals: $R^0 + S^0 \to RS$ (radical combination). This newly formed compound may significantly alter the system under investigation, e.g. genetic changes.

Radicals can also react with ordinary molecules, for example, O_2 to form a peroxyl radical: $R^0 + O_2 \to RO_2^0$, which thus becomes a new, very reactive molecule in the system capable of initiating widespread changes.

Irradiation of Water

Roughly 80 percent of biological structures are water. $H_2O \leadsto H^0 + OH^0$. Various recombinations can occur between this and other ionized water molecules to form H_2O, H_2O_2, H_2, O_2. Hydrogen peroxide formation is not particularly harmful in biological systems containing peroxide-destroying enzymes such as catalase and peroxidases. However, it can serve as a prototype reaction for the formation of organic peroxides, which may have greater biologic importance.

If oxygen is added to irradiated water, the oxygen combines with the hydrogen radical to form a peroxyl radical: $H^0 + O_2 \to HO_2^0$. This molecule is less reactive in terms of its oxidizing ability, but its longer life span permits it to diffuse farther from its site of formation to undergo further reactions.

In dilute aqueous solution, the vast majority of molecules are water; thus, most of the ionizations will occur in water molecules and the effect on the biologically active chemicals will be primarily "indirect" and mediated through changes occurring in the water molecules.

The OH^0 and HO_2^0 radicals and H_2O_2 are all oxidizing agents; that is, they are capable of removing an electron from another molecule to pair with its unpaired electron. Hydroxyl radicals can initiate polymerization, add to organic compounds at their double bonds, reduce powerful oxidizing agents, and remove hydrogen atoms from organic molecules.

In the reaction $RH + OH^0 \to R^0 + H_2O$, the organic molecule becomes a free radical capable of a variety of reactions that could lead to the formation of *new* molecules with altered biologic effect.

The HO_2^0 radical can oxidize substances and remove hydrogen atoms from organic substances. It can also donate an oxygen atom to a molecule, leading to the formation of different molecules with unknown biologic response. The hydrogen (H^0) radical is a powerful reducing agent that readily gives up its unpaired electron. The H^0 radical can initiate polymerization and remove H atoms from organic molecules.

When more than one type of solute molecule is present in a solution, the free radicals will react most readily with those that are largest in size, most numerous, and those that are most reactive.

One of the characteristics of the indirect effect of radiation is a **linear** relationship between dose and effect, which is independent of the concentration (above a certain critical value). This is because as the dose doubles, the number of ion pairs formed doubles, the number of free radicals formed doubles, and the number of solute molecules also doubles.

Macromolecular Effects

As a result of the chemical processes discussed, very large molecules common to biological systems may undergo a variety of structural changes that lead to altered function or molecular "death": (1) macromolecules may be degraded, or broken down into smaller components; (2) intramolecular cross-linking may occur in long molecules with a flexible structure; and (3) intermolecular cross-linking may occur between different molecules. All of these make the macromolecule incapable of its normal function. In addition, cross-linking may alter solubility and the resulting gel would produce a different physical-chemical state than the original. Many macromolecules are normally held in rigid complex three-dimensional configurations by intramolecular cross-linking bonds, most of which are hydrogen bonds. These bonds are easily broken and the resulting structural alteration can severely alter the biochemical properties of the molecule.

Proteins

Proteins compose the structural elements of the cell as well as enzymes that catalyze essential chemical reactions, hormones, antibodies, etc. Many of these proteins have primary, secondary, and teriary structures resulting in complex, three-dimensional structures. In proteins, side chains are more radiosensitive than the primary protein structure. Most proteins can be inactivated by 50-200 eV deposited directly in the molecule or it can be inactivated by the indirect action of 10-200 OH^0 radicals formed from irradiating water next to the molecule. Radiation can produce a variety of other effects on proteins such as increasing or decreasing viscosity, changes in refractive index, optical rotation, and electrical conductivity. Irradiation effects on enzymes result in inactivation of the enzyme.

Nucleic Acids — DNA, RNA

The action of radiation on nucleic acids may result in alterations in base sequence, changing the genetic code and leading to gross biochemical or physical alterations within the cell or organism. Single/double strand breaks result in a variety of chromosomal aberrations.

Lipids

Lipids — fats and waxes — are important to the cells as nutrients and as structural elements. The effect of radiation on these substances results in formation of organic peroxides, which can alter other molecules greatly.

Carbohydrates

The primary radiation effect on carbohydrates is degradation of polysaccharide chains.

Effects of Radiation on Chromosomes

The Cell. Most mammalian cells have certain common features of internal organization grossly subdivided into the nucleus and the cytoplasm with its various subcellular organelles.

Cell Division

Many mammalian tissues and organs do not divide regularly, and the average period between divisions is measured in years, except for blood-forming tissues, male germinal epithelium, female generative organs in cyclic changes, G.I. tract epithelium, and the epidermis. Typically, cell division involves a division of nuclear material (karyokinesis) followed by cytoplasmic or cell division (cytokinesis).

Mitosis. Mitosis is the process by which two daughter cells receive identical chromosome complements. This process is artificially divided for convenience into a series of histologically observable stages. The majority of the cell's cycle is spent in **interphase.** During interphase the individual chromosomes are indistinguishable, the nucleus less chromatic, and the nucleolus visible. This phase of the cell cycle is divided into three periods: (1) a postmitotic nonsynthetic period (G_1) in which the synthesis of proteins and enzymes required for DNA synthesis occurs, (2) a synthetic period (S) during which active synthesis and duplication of DNA occurs, and (3) a premitotic nonsynthetic period (G_2) in which there is an active synthesis of proteins necessary for mitosis. Following the premitotic nonsynthetic period (G_2), the cell moves rapidly through the stages of mitosis: prophase, metaphase, anaphase, and telophase, as illustrated in Figure 5-6.

In general, the active synthesis of DNA occurs only during the synthetic period of the interphase cycle, while RNA and protein synthesis occurs throughout the cell cycle. The relationship between intracellular damage to DNA and the subsequent response of the cell is one of the fundamental problems of molecular radiobiology. Since the sequence of bases forming the DNA molecule is so unique and crucial for cell function and the overall concentration is so small relative to other proteins and macromolecules within the cell, damage to DNA molecules is presumed to be the main cause of lethality in cells following relatively high doses of radiation. Of the various nucleic acids found within the cell, DNA is the most sensitive to radiation effects, followed by

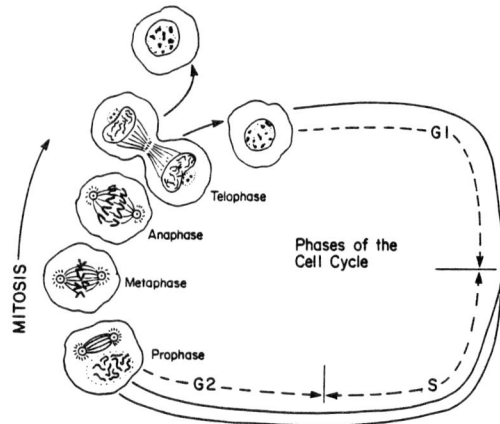

Figure 5-6. Phases of the cell cycle.

messenger RNA, ribosomal RNA, and transfer RNA. Amino acids and proteins are the least radiation sensitive nucleic acid building blocks.

Division Delay

Severe damage to various targets within the cell may lead directly to cell death or a permanent inability of the cell to reproduce itself. Sublethal damage within various targets of the cell may, however, lead to delays in the progression of the cell through the various metabolic pathways inherent in the cell cycle: G_1 to S to G_2 to mitosis, a process known as division delay.

In general, irradiation of the cell during the postmitosis nonsynthetic phase (G_1) leads to relatively little delay in the time of cell division, since only precursors to DNA synthesis are being synthesized. As DNA synthesis begins and DNA molecules accumulate, irradiation during the S phase lengthens the time required for division to occur. Irradiation during the premitotic nonsynthetic phase (G_2) produces even greater delays in cell division because radiation effects on DNA molecules would prevent synthesis of proteins required for mitosis. Should irradiation occur late in G_2 after all or most proteins necessary for mitosis have been synthesized, the cell will divide without significant delay. In general, cell division is delayed least if irradiation occurs during G_1 or S phases, because the cell has ample time to repair damage or synthesize new proteins prior to the end of the cycle.

Chromosomal Changes

Chromosomal damage can occur at any stage of the mitosis cycle; the changes are most easily observed in the metaphase or anaphase stages of division. Aberrations are classified as "chromosome-type" when they involve both chromatids of a chromosome at identical loci and act as if it was the result of a single break in the chromosome before replication into chromatids (spiral filaments); in this case, both chromatids would be affected identically and are usually the result of irradiation early in the cell cycle before DNA synthesis and replication occur. "Chromatid type" aberrations appear to be the result of a change within an individual chromatid after replication has taken place; such changes occur by irradiation of the chromosomes while they are visibly separated chromatids; they are formed when cells are irradiated in late prophase or early metaphase.

Chromosomal aberrations produced by one ionizing event of the "single hit" variety tend to increase linearly with dose and are not dependent on dose rate, while "two hit" chromosomal aberrations are dependent upon dose rate. In order for sparsely ionizing radiations to produce two hit type aberrations, the two single breaks usually must occur together spatially and within a certain interval of time. Because of the proximity of ionizing events, densely ionizing radiations produce two hit aberrations in numbers proportional to the dose (Fig. 5-7).

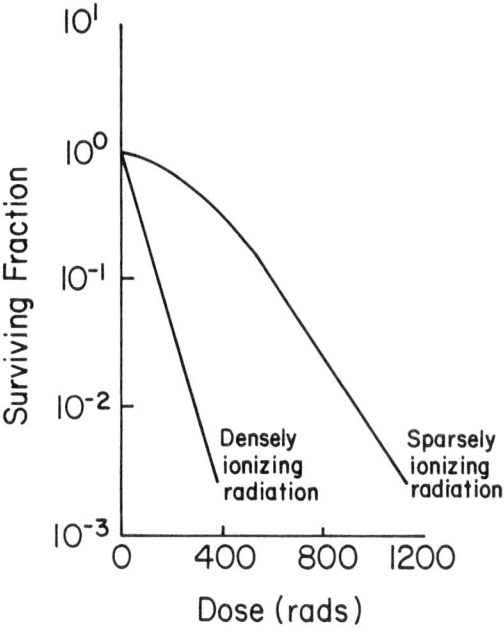

Figure 5-7. Dose response curve demonstrating the difference in biologic response following exposure to different types of ionizing radiations.

THRESHOLD AND NONTHRESHOLD RADIATION EFFECTS

Physical-chemical reactions following the absorption of radiation occur extremely quickly at the molecular/chemical level. However, for these changes to manifest themselves in terms of altered cellular function and ultimately as detectable changes in the physiological function of the irradiated cells, tissues, and organs, varying amounts of time will be required. In general, time permits alterations in biologically active molecules such as DNA, mRNA, tRNA, and subcellular organelles to become fully manifested; the amount of time required will depend on many factors, which will be discussed later.

It is important to recognize that all potential radiation effects do not manifest themselves immediately after irradiation. The time interval between irradiation and development of the observed biologic effect is known as the **latent period.** The latent period may vary from seconds, hours, days, months, to twenty-five or more years depending on the particular biologic manifestation to be observed. Radiation — induced changes are not unique to radiation and mimic other changes produced by toxic chemicals, normal aging processes, and various disease states. A squamous cell carcinoma induced by radiation exposure appears histologically similar to a squamous cell carcinoma in a patient without previous radiation exposure. The only difference between the two cancers is found using an epidemiological/statistical approach with large population groups, where patients having received radiation exposure would show a statistically higher incidence of cancer compared to the nonexposed group.

From a radiobiological perspective, the tissues of the body have been traditionally subdivided into two basic categories depending on their response to radiation injury. The two categories are somatic and genetic tissue. **Somatic tissues** include all tissues of the body except sperm and ovum, which are **genetic tissues** responsible for transmitting species traits from one generation to the next.

When somatic tissues are irradiated, a low level of radiation can be given that will not apparently produce a specified observable effect at any organizational level, i.e. subcellular, cellular, physiological, functional, or clinical. Progressive in-

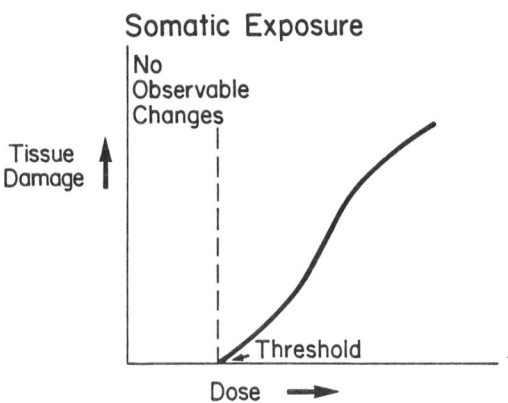

Figure 5-8. Typical dose response curve illustrating a nonthreshold linear type of biologic response.

creases in radiation dose may not produce an observable effect *until* the tissue has received a minimal level of exposure called the **threshold dose** (Fig. 5-8). Once the threshold dose has been exceeded, increasing increments of dose produce a proportional increase in the amount of observable tissue damage. Erythema or reddening of the skin following irradiation is a typical example of a threshold response in humans. At doses below 200 rads few (less than 5 percent) individuals demonstrate a clinically detectable erythema; at 800 rads, about 95 percent of irradiated patients will show erythema. For development of erythema as the specific biologic endpoint in a group of patients, the response is not observable at radiation doses between one and approximately 200 rads; after the threshold of 200 rads has been reached, there is a progressive increase in the number of observable cases with increasing dose.

The most commonly used biologic end point for irradiated genetic tissue is the number of mutations formed. The number of mutations produced during irradiation increases in proportion to the dose of radiation without an apparent threshold dose. Observations of an increased mutation frequency have extended to levels of radiation below normal background radiation levels, indicated by the dotted line in Figure 5-9. The potential significance of the genetic dose response curve is that all genetic exposures, even at very low levels, carry the potential for producing inheritable mutations since there is no apparent "threshold." Of equal importance is the knowledge that the smaller the genetic exposure the smaller the potential for mutation risk, and the smaller the number of mutations formed; the higher the dose the larger the number of mutations produced.

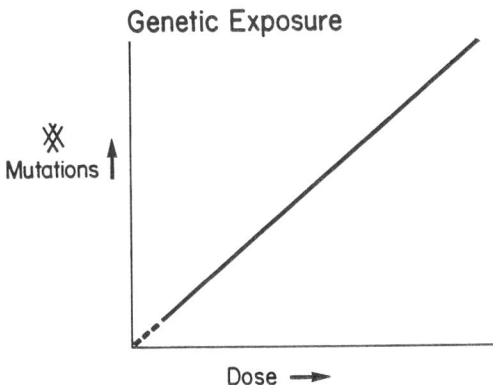

Figure 5-9. Typical dose response curve illustrating a nonthreshold-linear type of biologic response.

The threshold-nonthreshold concept of tissue irradiation is generally applicable for most clinically observable biologic end points, for example, genetic mutations, erythema, cataract formation, epilation (loss of hair), sterility, xerostomia (diminished salivary function), and skin necrosis.

Evidence is accumulating to suggest that radiation-induced carcinogenesis following exposure of somatic tissues (skin, bone marrow, salivary glands, brain, etc.) should not be considered a purely threshold response. However, the potential for carcinogenesis is based on statistical methods requiring for the most part extrapolation of cancer risk known to occur at relatively high levels of radiation exposure to the statistical possibility that lower levels of exposure in the diagnostic x-ray range will also increase the risk of cancer formation above that found normally in the population.

The dose response curves for different types of cancers vary greatly, and for low levels of radiation the estimated potential risk of cancer literally depends on the underlying statistical assumptions. Four statistical models permit equally credible extrapolations of cancer risk but the magnitude of the risk depends on whether one assumes a linear, curvilinear, quadratic, or linear-quadratic relationship between dose and cancer risk. The arguments for and against these statistical approaches are beyond the scope of this chapter.

The Committee on Biologic Effects of Ionizing Radiation (1980, BEIR III Report) choose to utilize the linear-quadratic dose-effect relationship because it was felt to provide a reasonable approximation explaining available radiobiological data for both low and high doses of radiation. Using this relationship to describe carcinogenic effects of radiation assumes that there is no threshold in terms of cancer induction. Such an approach supports the concept that carcinogenesis may result from mutations in somatic tissues that, with time, are manifested through malignant transformation of the irradiated tissue.

Because the difference between somatic threshold and genetic nonthreshold effects are not as clearly definable as once thought, the term **stochastic** has been used to describe radiation effects *whose probability of occurence* in an exposed population is a direct function of dose; they are regarded as having no threshold so that even small doses may produce some statistically observable effect, assuming the exposed population is large enough. Hereditary effects and cancer induction are considered to be stochastic. Typically, stochastic effects measure *incidence in a population group rather than the severity* of the effect in an affected individual. **Nonstochastic** is the term used to describe biologic effects whose *severity* is a function of dose. For these effects, there may be a threshold. Erythema, cataract formation, hematologic deficiencies, impaired fertility, and epilation are all nonstochastic effects, since their severity increases with increasing dose yet there is a level of exposure below which these effects are not observable.

Effects of Radiation on Cells

Cellular Events of Biologic Importance

Some ionizations produced within cells by the passage of an ionizing particle may have little or no biologic importance since the primary or secondary chemical alterations they cause may not alter sensitive molecules or vital organelles. In addition, ionization may affect only a small proportion of plentiful molecules or organelles contained by the cell, i.e. mitochondria. In contrast, some other ionizing events may have a profound effect on cells when the resulting primary or secondary chemical alterations involve a change in highly specific or unique molecules or structures of great importance to cell function and viability, e.g. DNA.

Cellular effects of ionizing radiation may result from either the direct deposition of energy within the cell or through mechanisms working outside the cell to damage it. At the molecular level it was relatively simple to discuss the direct and indirect effects of radiation on a molecule; however, because cells and tissues represent a more complicated organizational pattern, the action of radiation on these structures is usually discussed in terms of being relatively direct or relatively indirect.

Relatively direct effect is a term used for radiation effects seemingly caused by mechanisms contained within the structure specified as being affected. **Relatively indirect effect** is a term used for effects apparently caused at least in part by mechanisms not contained within the structure specified as affected.

For example, irradiation of an organ may result in atrophy of the organ — a direct effect. However, the actual cause of the atrophy may be a direct effect resulting from energy absorption by the parenchyma, producing both direct and indirect changes in molecules or organelles within the cell leading to destruction of the tissue. Atrophy of the organ may also occur secondary to an increase in the histohematic barrier due to impairment of blood circulating within the organ and the concomitant starvation of the parenchymal tissue through hypoxia and malnutrition. It is important to understand that irradiated cells may be damaged both by mechanisms contained within themselves and by various events triggered at the time of irradiation operating at a distance. Such effects may occur a long time after irradiation. Cells of different nature, types, and degrees of activity will take different amounts of time to manifest fully the effects of radiation absorbed within them. In addition, various relatively indirect mechanisms also require different amounts of time to develop and may affect different types of cells in different ways.

Relative Radiation Sensitivity of Cells

All mammalian cells can be altered in

various ways by ionizing radiation; however, the dose required to produce a specific cytopathologic end point varies greatly. Thus, the concepts of **radiation sensitivity** and **radiation resistance** are relative terms and are concerned with differences in degree of responsiveness.

Essential radiosensitivity is based on the cells' inherent constitution within a normal environment.

Conditional radiosensitivity is based on changes in cell constitution due to changes in the normal environment or to other factors that may alter the cells' relative sensitivity to limited degrees.

Conditional effects may be produced by the following: (1) For low LET radiations, cells under high oxygen tension will be more sentitive to radiation effects than when irradiated under anoxic conditions. High LET radiations (alpha, neutrons, slow electrons) do not demonstrate as pronounced an oxygen effect. (2) Poor blood circulation reduces the sensitivity of cells while an abundant circulation increases sensitivity. (3) Hydration enhances conditional radiation sensitivity while dessication decreases it. (4) Increased temperature increases cellular sensitivity, while a decrease in temperature reduces cellular sensitivity.

Law of Bergonie and Tribondeau

Two investigators, Bergone and Tribondeau, evaluated the effect of irradiation on testes and found (1) that when cell death was used as a biologic end point, actively proliferating cells were most sensitive to radiation and (2) that their radiation sensitivity varied inversely with the degree of cellular differentiation. In other words, cells that divide frequently and are more primitive (less differentiated) are more sensitive to radiation effects than those cells that do not divide and are very specialized (well differentiated) in function. Since their observations were generally applicable to many cell types, it became known as the Law of Bergonie and Tribondeu.

Since 1906 the basic principles of their observation have been demonstrated to be accurate but there are presently many exceptions and contradictions to the "law." For example, small lymphocytes do not divide yet are extremely sensitive to radiation; in terms of cell death, not all proliferating cells are relatively radiosensitive, and some primitive cells have been shown to be more radioresistant than their more differentiated forms.

Classification of Cells According to Relative Sensitivities

Relative radiosensitivity of a cell depends on many factors: cells cycle (G_1, S, G_2, etc.), cytopathologic end point to be observed, cell type, length of interphase, frequency of division, dose rate, conditions of irradiation (in vivo/in vitro), RBE, LET, radiation type, etc. However, it is important to realize that the radiation sensitivity of any cell or tissue is relative to the specific biologic end point evaluated. As a result, the relative rank order of a particular cell may change if the end point changes. The following classification utilizes cell death as the measure of cell sensitivity; if functional alterations were selected as a biologic end point, then the relative sensitivity of the cells would change.

Class I — Vegatitive Intermitotic Cells. Cells in this category are most sensitive to radiation and tend to be short-lived, to be primitive, to divide regularly, and to produce daughter cells that may or may not differentiate. Example: stem cells of hematopoietic tissues (hemocytoblasts, lymphoblasts, erythroblasts, myeloblasts), intestinal glands (crypts of Lieberkuhn), spermatogonia, granulosa cells of ovarian follicles, basal epidermal and gastric gland cells, holocrine glands (sebacious), large and medium sized lymphocytes. *Exception:* small lymphocytes do not divide as such but are among the highly radiosensitive cell types.

Class II — Differentiating Intermitotic Cells. Cells in this category are relatively radiosensitive but less than the above type and are short-lived as individuals. They normally divide for a limited number of divisions, and they differentiate between divisions. The more differentiated the stage, the less sensitive they become. Examples: hematopoietic series for granulocytic and erythrocytic bone marrow series, spermatocytes, ovocytes.

Class III — Multipotential Connective Tissue Cells. Cells in this category have an intermediate sensitivity. They divide irregularly or sporadically in response to special stimuli and may undergo transitions from one to another morphologic and functional form. Individual cell life span in variable. Examples: endothelial cells, fibroblasts, mesenchymal cells.

Class IV — Reverting Postmitotic Cells. Cells in this category are relatively radioresistant and possess long cell lives; they do not undergo regular or periodic division in the adult and do not divide except under abnormal conditions (damage, destruction, or loss of large cell numbers). Some have highly specialized functions, others do not. Examples: epithelial parenchymal cells and salivary gland duct cells, liver, kidney, pancreas; basal and parenchymal cells of merocrine glands (sweat glands) and endocrine glands such as adrenal, thyroid, parathyroid and pituitary; interstitial cells of the gonads, corpora lutea, sertoli cells, septal cells of the lung, fixed stem cells (reticulum cells).

Class V — Fixed postmitotic cells. Highly radioresistant, do not divide, highly differentiated morphologically and functionally. Some have very long lives, all undergo progressive aging until death. Examples: neurons, some muscle, polymorphonuclear granulocytes, erythrocytes, spermatids, spermatozoa.

Effects of Radiation on Tissue

Tissue effects of radiation, like cellular effects, may be either essential or conditional; they are relative values that depend upon the specific criteria or effect serving as the biologic end point. The criterion commonly used is direct loss of the parenchymal cells of the tissue (hypoplasia) with resulting atrophy of the tissue. Direct effects of radiation are typically brought about by mechanisms entirely contained within the affected tissue.

The mechanisms for direct radiation-induced hypoplasia and atrophy of rapidly or continually self-repopulating tissues includes inhibition of mitosis, normal and precocious maturation, loss of cells without replacement, and mitosis-linked death. Thus, tissues composed of vegetative or differentiating intermitotic cells will tend to be highly radiosensitive with respect to effect associated with mitosis. In contrast, tissues composed of cell types that rarely divide, ie. reverting postmitotic cells, require large doses of radiation to produce direct radiation-induced hypoplasia and atrophy through the mechanism of interphase death; these tissues are radioresistant.

Relative radiosensitivity of a tissue depends on —
1. relative sensitivity of its parenchymal cells;
2. the relative radiosensitivity of the most radiosensitive cell in a cell line;
3. limited conditional factors: local fine vasculature, blood supply, tissue fluid, connective tissue; and
4. indirect effects: arising from

changes in vasculature and connective tissues as a result of irradiation.

Radiation can cause early or acute lesions in vegetative or differentiating intermitotic type cells through direct mechanisms without mediation of the effect through damage to the fine vasculature and interstitial connective tissue.

In more radioresistant tissues composed of reverting or fixed postmitotic parenchymal cells, acute early lesions resulting from direct effects of radiation are produced by very high radiation levels. At doses of radiation less than necessary to produce interphase death, direct effects are mediated through changes in the fine vasculature and connective tissues rather than as a direct effect of radiation on the parenchymal cells (Table 5-III).

Table 5-III

TISSUE AND ORGAN SENSITIVITY

Tissue/Organ	Relative Radiosensitivity
Lymphoid; hematopoietic spermatogenic, ovarian follicular epithelium; intestinal epithelium	High
Skin and other organs and tissues with epidermoid linings include cornea, oral cavity, esophagus, bladder, lens, stomach	Fairly High
Connective tissue, fine vasculature, growing cartilage and bone	Medium
Mature cartilage and bone, salivary gland, kidney, liver, thyroid, respiratory endocrine glands	Fairly Low
Nerve muscle, spinal cord	Low

Modified from A. P. Cassaret: *Radiation Biology*. Englewood Cliffs, NJ, Prentice Hall, 1968.

Effects of Radiation on Small Blood Vessels

Necrosis of endothelial cells permits contact between blood and damaged cells or subendothelial connective tissue promoting thrombus formation, which occludes the small lumens. In addition, overly exuberant repair mechanisms may cause endothelial cells to proliferate — occluding lumens, forming tortuous pathways, or shortening the normal vascular course.

In response to radiation damage to endothelial or parenchymal cells, hyperemia occurs. Along with the increased congestion of blood cells in the area, the permeability of the cells increases and blood fluid leaks into the surrounding connective tissue. Swelling of the endothelial cell occurs through direct/indirect damage to the cell, and the bulging endothelium narrows and constricts the lumen, impending circulation.

Following the preceeding relatively rapid changes in the vascular tissues, other connective tissue changes begin to occur slowly. Perivascular edema may result in increased interstitial colloid formation in the affected region and may serve as sites for fibroblastic proliferation and scar formation. Even though scar formation is a secondary repair process, it nonetheless leads to progressively increased damage that is self-perpetuating. The fibrous reaction becomes progressively more severe as the radiation dose increases.

Early changes in the fine vasculature are subtle and relatively inconspicuous, especially after moderate amounts of radiation (typically 500-1000 rads) where the changes are spotty in distribution along the course of a vessel and not continuous or uniform. With progression of the vascular damage, more and more points along the course of the affected blood vessel may show degenerative or fibrotic change. Ultimately, marked changes may be induced in the parenchymal tissues dependent upon the affected capillary network. The end result is that the affected tissue is deprived of nutrition and oxygen, a gradual atrophy occurs, and the tissue's ability to resist further injury, stress, or functional demands is comprised long after irradiation.

Infection or diffuse trauma of irradiated organs in which the fine vasculature has been reduced and in which regeneration of the fine vasculature is inhibited by an increase in the histohematic fibrous barrier is often a precipitating factor in delayed radionecrosis of the organ.

Recovery and Repair Processes

Recovery is the degree to which a tissue or organ has returned toward normal or preirradiation function and morphological integrity. Repair processes are the means by which tissues or organs recover from radiation effects. They are of two types:

1. **Primary** (typical) **repair** processes include repair of intracellular damage and the recovery and regeneration of cells killed by irradiation by replacement with their own cell type, i.e. homeotypic regeneration — repopulation of a tissue by division of skin cells. Heterotypic regeneration involves the formation of specialized stem cells from undifferentiated cells not regularly engaged in producing cells of the kinds lost, ie. reticulum cells can be induced to produce bone marrow stem cells.
2. **Secondary** (atypical) **repair** processes are those by which tissue cells killed by irradiation are replaced by cells and matricies of a different kind, usually fibrous tissue replacement. Such repair processes may also include replacement by cells with a lower level of specialization. Fibrous replacement usually involves a decrease in the original functional capacity and resilience.

Residual damage is a term denoting the extent and nature of the deficit in recovery from radiation damage at a particular time. **Permanent residual damage** refers to the deficit in recovery *after maximal recovery* from radiation damage has taken place and only includes permanent defects. Permanent residual damage includes: —

1. gene mutations;
2. chromosomal aberrations;
3. intracellular structural/functional changes;
4. defective cell products;
5. reduced regenerative capacity:
   a. permanent hypoplasia
   b. fibroatrophy;
6. asynchronous or atypical repair;
7. degenerative sclerotic changes in fine vasculature; and
8. reduction in reserve functional capacity of tissue.

The condition of a tissue at any particular time after irradiation depends on (a) the type and degree of initial radiation damage, (b) the type of repair that has occurred, (c) the types and degrees of further insult or stress experiences, and (d) the nature and degree of residual damage resulting from the effects of the irradiation and other insulting agents.

Cumulative Effects of X-Radiation

Radiobiologic studies indicate that repair processes exist in humans at all levels of cellular organization from the repair of DNA molecules to cellular repair or replacement. The degree of injury depends upon many factors; at most levels of radiation exposure commonly used for radiobiological studies, there is always a certain amount of permanent residual injury. At high dose levels of radiation, the amount of permanent residual injury will be high and easy to detect; at low levels of radiation exposure, many more difficulties will be encountered in trying to distinguish radiation-induced tissue changes from those produced by normal aging processes. At diagnostic radiography dose levels, permanent residual injury will be virtually impossible to detect because it will be masked by the gradual accumulation of normal aging injury within the tissues. Such changes are illustrated in Figure 5-10.

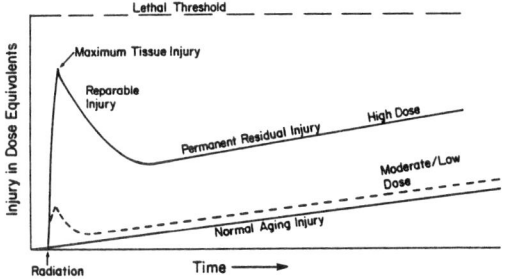

Figure 5-10. Diagramatic representation of radiation injury and repair following exposure to radiation. (Modified from Casarett, A.P.: **Radiation Biology.** Englewood Cliffs, NJ, Prentice Hall Inc., 1968, p. 272.)

When multiple exposures to ionizing radiation occur, there will be a progressive increase in the amount of permanent residual injury acquired by the tissue above normal aging processes. Thus, the effects of radiation are said to be cumulative from the standpoint that cellular repair processes never completely repair all radiation damage and that multiple exposures to ionizing radiation produce an additive effect in terms of accumulating permanent residual injury.

Clinically Significant Changes in Tissues and Organs

In summary, the development of histopathologic effects from subclinical to clinical levels of importance depends on a wide range of factors including: —
1. organ radiosensitivity;
2. dose;
3. time;
4. effects on fine vascularity, recovery, repair, and residual damage;
5. structural nature of the organ related to its function;
6. reserve functional capacity of the organ;
7. function of the organ irradiated;
8. relative functional importance of the organ to the body; and
9. clinical detectability of the related functional changes.

Late Effects of X-Radiation

Normal Tissues

The late effects of radiation changes in normal tissues and organs may be recognized no later than three months after irradiation but many other effects may require a latent period of eight to ten years, or even longer. Late effects are usually manifested as progressive degenerative processes induced by radiation and their incidence increases with time to a maximum, and then declines.

There is an indirect relationship between the degree of early reaction in a tissue and the probability of developing a late reaction, but the pathogenesis of early and late reactions is different. The immediate radiation reaction depends predominantly on the number of parenchymal cells killed by radiation; late radiation effects are associated with ischemia and fibrosis of the tissue organ. Ischemia results from damage to the endothelial cells and walls of the blood vessels. Increased vascular permeability leads to extravasation of protein into the area surrounding the endothelium and parenchymal cells leading to interstitial fibrosis, vascular sclerosis, and endarteritis. Radiation effects will be more severely manifested if the individual irradiated has intercurrent diseases accompanied by generalized endarteritis, such as diabetes mellitus and hypertension from any cause.

Factors Modifying Biologic Effects

Type of Radiation

The biologic effect will depend upon the amount of energy deposited within a tissue, and this is a function of LET. Gamma and x-rays have relatively uniform absorption depending on density and volume of tissue and the inverse square law. Maximum dose occurs close to the surface and diminishes with increasing depth. The attenuation of electrons is variable; initial entry into a system results in relatively little ionization, and most *energy deposition occurs near the end of its track* when the electron's velocity and energy have been degraded. The range for a 5 MeV electron is about 2 mm in tissue, while high energy electron beams from megavoltage betatron's or linear accelerators deposit their energy at an appreciable depth in the irradiated tissue.

Alpha particles are about 8000 times heavier than an electron and are densely ionizing particles but penetrate only a short distance (few hundred microns). Their greatest density of ionization occurs near the end of the alpha ray track.

Neutrons do not disturb charged materials and are effective in producing biologic damage only by undergoing elastic collisions with the nuclei of atoms to produce "recoil protons," which are knocked on and produce ionization similar to alpha particles with a high LET at the end of the proton track.

Oxygen Effect

In general, hypoxic tissues tend to be less radiation sensitive than well-oxygenated tissues. An example of this effect is shown in Figure 5-11, which illustrates the effects of hypoxia of fibroblasts in tissue culture. Large tumor masses are con-

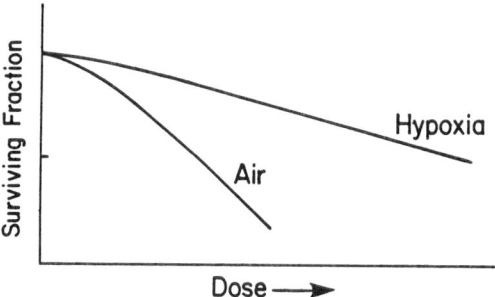

Figure 5-11. Diagramatic dose response curve for x-radiation in air and hypoxia. Hypoxic tissues tend to be more radioresistant than oxygenated tissues.

sidered to be relatively hypoxic relative to the surrounding normal tissues and are thought to be more radioresistant. Radiotherapists may utilize hyperbaric oxygen techniques in an attempt to increase the oxygen concentration within the tumor and hence make it more radiosensitive.

Phase of Cell Cycle

The phase of the cell in its cell cycle will influence its sensitivity to radiation. Cells about to undergo, or undergoing mitosis are the most sensitive. It is important to stress that it is not the whole of a particular phase of the cell cycle that is radioresistant or radiosensitive but that **sensitivity varies throughout the phases of the whole cycle.** One part of one phase may be just as sensitive or resistant as another portion of another phase, e.g. cells completing G_1 and beginning S (transition between phases) or more sensitive than cells actually in G_1 or S alone.

Fractionation of the Dose

Dividing a dose into equal parts delivered over a period of hours or days results in a reduced effectiveness of the total radiation dose, mostly as a result of the cell's ability to recover from radiation damage. The lower the dose and the longer the interval between exposure, the more opportunity the cell has to repair sublethal or potentially lethal damage and hence the smaller the effect on the tissue (Fig. 5-12).

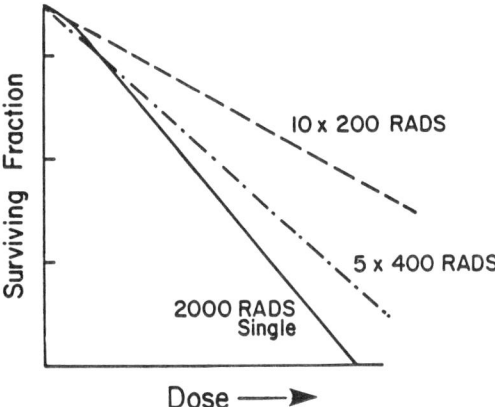

Figure 5-12. Diagramatic dose response curves depicting differences in biologic effect with different dose fractions.

Dose Rate

For sparsely ionizing radiations, the dose rate is a significant factor in determining the biological consequences of a given absorbed dose. In general, as dose rate is lowered the biologic effect of a given dose is reduced.

Acute and chronic exposure. In general, an acute radiation therapy dose rate is considered to be in the range of 100 rads/min (6000 rads/hour) versus a chronic exposure rate of 25 rads/hour. Acute exposures minimize chances for the cell to recover or repair, consequently biologic damage with acute exposure tends to be more severe than when chronic exposures are used. Cell survival at chronic exposure is nearly exponential because cells recover from sublethal damage at a constant rate (Fig. 5-13).

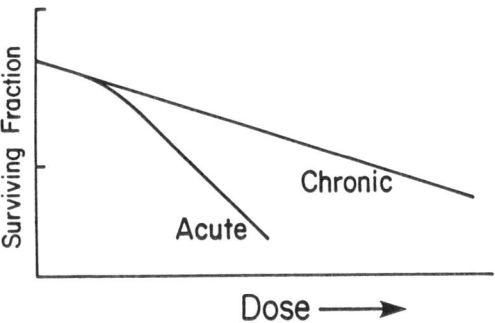

Figure 5-13. Diagramatic dose response curves depicting differences in biologic effect with acute or chronic radiation exposures. Chronic exposure results in reduced biologic effect.

Dental radiographic exposure rates are approximately 333 mrads/sec (assuming 85 kVp, long cone, and "D" speed film), compared to an acute exposure rate of 1700 mrad/sec and a chronic exposure rate of 7 mrads/sec. One would assume, therefore, the potential biologic effects of dental diagnostic x-rays to be intermediate in consequence and potentially less than one-fifth as detrimental as the acute dose rate.

Volume Factor

The clinical and biological response to irradiation is influenced by the volume of tumor and normal tissues irradiated. The effect is mainly due to the degree of cell depletion, which may be modified by vascular damage, persistence of cellular elements to repopulate the area, and toxic products from cell destruction. In general, the larger the volume of normal tissue irradiated, the greater the reaction to a given dose of radiation.

Whole Body versus Local Area Irradiation

The potential biologic effect of a given dose of radiation on the whole organism is influenced significantly by the amount of tissue irradiated at one time. It requires less total radiation to kill an animal if it is administered to the total body. In general, total body irradiation produces more adverse systemic effects than if smaller well-localized areas of the body are irradiated. An example of this effect is observable in the difference between a whole body exposure to 400 rads and a localized head and neck radiation therapy dose of 6000 rads for cancer treatment. The whole body exposure will be a fatal dose for most humans because damage to the hematopoietic system is severe. Local area irradiation of 6000 rads produces very severe localized tissue damage, and patients may be quite debilitated for a time, but this dose is not lethal.

Hyperthermia Effect

Elevated temperatures have a synergistic effect with x-rays in increasing radiation bioeffects. The mechanism is poorly understood, but certain tumors have been shown to be more sensitive to heat treatment than normal cells. This selective effect is more pronounced above 42°C. The combination of heating and x-radiation apparently produces a reduction in the differential radiosensitivity of cells throughout the cell cycle. Recovery from sublethal radiation damage is reduced in heated cells; in addition, hypoxic cells are more sensitive to hyperthermia than well-oxygenated cells.

Chemical Effects

Various chemicals have been shown to increase the radiosensitivity of various tissues and tumors. Drugs may be used in a complementary role to increase local effects of radiation within the treated volume or they may be used as supplementary chemotherapy primarily to destroy disseminated cancer cells outside the volume of irradiation.

Chemotherapeutic agents may influence radiation effects in three ways: additive effects, potentiating effects, or sensitization effects. For **additive effects,** the drug and radiation work independently to produce the lethal effect on cells. Example: alkylating agents. The combined effect of the drug and radiation may be greater than that of the individual treatments, and the radiation effect is **potentiated** by the drug. Examples: 5-fluorouracil, methotrexate, actinomycin D, bleomycin. **Sensitization** occurs when the drug has little or no lethal effect on the cells but influences their response to radiation by augmenting the effect. Example: oxygen is one of the most powerful radiation sensitizers.

Hyperbarric oxygen at 3 atmospheres increases oxygen diffusion distances about tenfold; it is used to saturate tissue and plasma fluids to improve oxygenation of hypoxic tumor cells. Oxygen must be present in the biologic specimen during the radiation exposure in order for the oxygen effect to occur. The presence of increased oxygen concentration just before or just after exposure is not effective. The mechanism for oxygen effect is via free radical formation to produce organic peroxides (RO_2), which is a nonrestorable form of the target material.

Age Effects

Certain radiobiologic effects demonstrate age-dependent effects. For example, cataractogenesis is both a species- and an age-dependent phenomenon. Older animals tend to have a greater radiation effect and a shorter latent period following irradiation.

Tissue Effects

Biologic damage depends on the type of cells or tissues irradiated and has been previously discussed.

Species Differences

Animals differ in their overall sensitivity to whole body exposure to ionizing radiation. The potential lethality of a given dose of radiation may vary significantly for different species of animals and within the same species. For radiobiological purposes, it is convenient to discuss whole body lethality in terms of lethal dose (LD), the dose of radiation that will kill a specified percentage of individuals within a specified period of time. The LD 50/30 is a frequently used lethal end point representing the dose of radiation necessary to kill 50 percent of a population within 30 days. The mean lethal dose in humans ranges from 200-450 rads.

EFFECTS OF RADIATION THERAPY ON THE ORAL CAVITY

Source of Radiation

The type of radiation used and the dose administered will depend upon a variety of factors. Exophytic lesions generally respond better than necrotic infiltrating tumors for radiation therapy alone. Epidermoid carcinoma and Hodgkin's disease respond well to radiation therapy, while spindle cell carcinoma, verrucous carcinoma, and many sarcomas respond poorly. Benign lesions should never be irradiated, since radiatation therapy may stimulate malignant transformation. Additionally, the postirradiation effects are potentially more serious than the consequences of other forms of management of benign disease. Since many oral cancers and Hodgkin's disease limited to neck nodes are surface phenomena, they are particularly susceptible to cobalt 60 therapy, which delivers its maximum dose 5 mm below the skin. At 5 cm the dose is 80 percent of maximum and at 10 cm is 55 percent. Other sources of radiation include super and mega voltage x-rays, which have a maximum dose at 10 cm.

In addition to external sources of radiation, a variety of implants are used. They are usually used in combination with other sources of radiation such as cobalt 60. There are three basic types of implants: needles, wires, and grains. Each of these deliver a dose of 2000-3000 rads in the vicinity of the implant. Radium or cesium needles are used to treat malignancies involving the tongue and floor of the mouth. Iridium wires may be used for tumors of the buccal mucosa and lip. Gold grains are usually deposited in smaller or less accessible areas than those treated by either needles or wires. Needles and wires are removed upon completion of therapy, while gold grains are usually left in place. For palatal lesions, molds or applicators are fabricated so that the prosthesis containing the radioactive implant can deliver the appropriate dose to the tumor. One of the big advantages of using implants is that the radiation is delivered more accurately to the tumor with less damage to unaffected tissues surrounding the lesion. The usual dose of cobalt 60 is 6000 rads delivered in thirty divided doses of 200 rads per day, five days a week. The clinical consequences of radiation therapy to the oral cavity include effects on salivary glands, teeth, the oral mucosa, taste, the jaw bones, the masticatory apparatus, and nutritional problems.

Salivary Glands

The primary consequences of irradiation to the salivary glands is the development of xerostomia. Shannon found that patients treated with cobalt 60 at 225 rads per day for four days lost 60 percent of their salivary flow after the first week of therapy. Weekly flow rate decreased to 40, 19, 24, 19, 9, and 5 percent by the sixth treatment week. Driezens found similar decreases in flow, including a 95 percent loss of salivation persisting three years postirradiation. Although some patients reported a subjective improvement in salivation, flow rates indicated no increase in saliva production. With the decrease in salivary volume, the saliva also tends to be more viscous.

The histologic changes to the salivary glands consist of acute inflammatory changes in the earlier states followed by parenchymal atrophy, replacement fibrosis, and radiation induced endarteritis. These degenerative changes are responsible ultimately for the altered quantity and quality of the saliva once the repair mechanisms have been completed. The most significant result of postirradiated xerostomia is the development of radiation caries in the teeth.

Teeth

When developing teeth fall within the primary beam, tooth development and eruption are delayed. Some teeth may fail to develop completely, while others may be small and malformed. The enamel may be discolored and hypoplastic. Prophylactic restoration of these teeth is important since caries followed by pulpitis may lead to the development of osteoradionecrosis. Although irradiation of developing teeth usually results in delayed eruption, they invariably erupt. The eruption of irradiated developing teeth should be carefully followed radiographically, particularly if hypoplastic enamel changes appear to be present.

It has been clearly shown by a number of investigators that radiation has *no* primary effect on erupted teeth that would make them susceptible to radiation caries. Radiation caries develops both directly and indirectly as a result of the cariogenic environment produced by the altered quality and quantity of the saliva. Some of the protective functions of normal healthy saliva have been postulated as follows:

1. Elements from saliva are absorbed by the surface layers of enamel, particularly upon eruption.
2. The integrity of enamel is maintained by virtue of its content of Ca^+ and PO_4^- ions, thus preventing loss of tooth salts into saliva.
3. Saliva contains a number of antacid buffering systems including bicarbonate, phosphate, and protein systems. The bicarbonate and phosphate systems are important since they operate at a pH of 6-7, while the proteins operate around 3.6.
4. There are a number of antibacterial immune factors in saliva that contribute to the restriction of the microbial substrate.
5. Normal saliva participates directly in the clearance of sugar taken in the diet — with the exception of sugar-containing foods that stick to the

teeth, most sugars are cleared within one hour of ingestion.
6. The posterior direction of flow of saliva in the mouth along with many swallows per day produce a physical flushing action that contributes to the elimination of bacteria.
7. Saliva is capable of participating in the remineralization of decalcified tooth surfaces, thus slowing down and in some cases reversing the early caries process.

In patients with radiation xerostomia, there are significant changes in ionic content including Na^+, Ca^{++}, Mg^{++}, and Cl^-. Additionally, the protein and HCO_3^- content are altered, thus producing decreases in the buffering, remineralization, and immune functions. Additionally, Brown et al. have reported that these patients change their eating pattern to that of a more frequent, nondetergent, high carbohydrate content diet and have noted a decreased sugar clearance function of the saliva in patients with radiation xerostomia. Finally, Brown et al. have demonstrated the emergence of a highly acidogenic microbial population including *Streptococcus mutans, Lactobacilli, Candida*, and *Staphylococci* and decreases in *Sanguis, Neisseria*, and *Fusobacterii*. These changes are the etiologic factors that act in concert to produce radiation caries.

Radiation caries may occur within three months after therapy and typically start at the incisal edges of anterior teeth, the cusp tips of the posterior teeth, and along the lingual surfaces of anterior and posterior teeth. This effect is believed due to the diminished salivary flow eliminating the distinction between "clean and unclean" tooth areas with all tooth surfaces vulnerable to caries induction.

Radiation caries is distinguishable from routine dental caries in that there is widespread massive loss of tooth structure due initially to a generalized demineralization of the enamel with little cavitation. Proteolysis and loss of the organic matrix occurs later, and all teeth including the mandibular anterior teeth become involved. The rapid demineralization of calcified material in advance of proteolysis may leave teeth "rubbery" and flexible.

In many instances, radiation caries is limited to the gingival one-third of the teeth on all surfaces. As this "wrap around" pattern progresses, the teeth fracture off, a process known as amputation caries. Radiation caries occurs in every tooth and on every surface and will develop regardless of the original preirradiation condition of the teeth. Post-irradiation caries induction stems invariably from a failure to comply with daily oral hygiene instructions and 1 percent fluoride gel applications. Radiation caries risk is enormous, omnipresent, and requires life-long patient cooperation and vigilance.

The following daily home-care regimen is suggested for the prevention of radiation caries.

1. Thoroughly remove all plaque: use a properly designed small, soft toothbrush; floss all interproximal surfaces; flush with a high speed water jet; check for plaque using plaque disclosing solutions or tablets, a dental mirror, and adequate lighting; rebrush and recheck until all plaque is removed.
2. Apply sodium fluoride to the teeth: use a custom fabricated tray that closely approximates all teeth such as the soft mouthguard; leave carriers in place for at least five minutes; upon removal of the carrier refloss the interproximal areas to help carry the fluoride to these areas; avoid rinsing or eating for thirty minutes; thoroughly clean and rinse the fluoride

carriers.
3. Follow this procedure meticulously without deviation, daily without exception, for the remainder of the individual's life.

The most significant effect of radiation caries is the development of osteoradionecrosis in the jawbones.

Jawbones

When the jaws have received therapeutic doses of radiation, they are more susceptible to the development of a specific form of osteomyelitis known as osteoradionecrosis. This increased susceptibility is primarily due to radiation fibrosis of the vascular supply. Additionally, the mandible is particularly susceptible due to the relative lack of a collateral blood supply. In order for osteoradionecrosis to develop, the following three etiologic factors must be present: therapeutic doses of radiation, trauma, and infection. Since the increased susceptibility to osteoradionecrosis is permanent and since this condition is extremely difficult to manage once it develops, prevention is to be greatly encouraged. According to Driezens et al., osteoradionecrosis occurs most commonly within the first two years postirradiation. Additionally, they found an overall incidence of 21 percent and and incidence of 27 percent in dentate individuals and 5 percent in edentulous patients. Some suggested treatment planning considerations include —

1. extraction of all teeth prior to the initiation of radiation therapy particularly if any of the following are present: extensive caries, poor oral hygiene, moderate or advanced periodontal disease;
2. removal of all impacted teeth prior to radiation therapy; and
3. removal of all tori and exostosis prior to radiation therapy.

When these surgical procedures are to be performed, the following adjunctive measures should be taken for this group of special patients: antibiotic coverage, extensive alveolectomy if multiple extractions are to be performed, meticulous closure, and careful postoperative follow-up. Ideally, surgery should be completed three weeks prior to the initiation of radiation therapy.

Daly and Drane have described the following features characteristic of the osteoradionecrosis profile:

1. inadequate postsurgical healing prior to the initiation of radiation therapy;
2. irradiation of lesions in close proximity to bone;
3. high-dose irradiation with or without proper fractionation;
4. combination therapy using external radiation sources with intraoral implants;
5. poor oral hygiene and poor patient cooperation;
6. surgery in irradiated areas;
7. trauma from badly designed or poor fitting prostheses, and from other sources; and
8. presence of contributing physical disabilities or nutritional factors.

Thus, even small superficial traumatic ulcers, small carious lesions, and minimal periodontal infections should be treated aggressively but without trauma to the alveolar bone. This will mean the use of antibiotics systemically, local applications of zinc peroxide packs, and the application of 1 percent neomycin solution. Once osteoradionecrosis has involved large areas of bone, hemimandibulectomy may become necessary. In recent years, it has been found that increasing the oxygen content in the tissues greatly enhances healing. This can be accomplished by hydrogen peroxide perfusion of the extremities or the administration of hyperbaric oxygen. Specific effects of hyperbaric oxygen include —

1. enhancement of fibroblast formation;
2. increased blood vessel budding;
3. increased mitoses;
4. stimulation of osteogenesis; and
5. stimulation of osteoclastic resorption of necrotic bone.

Other Oral Consequences of Radiation Therapy

Impairment of tast detection and recognition thresholds may be observed approximately three weeks after the beginning of radiation therapy. Bitter and salt qualities show the earliest and greatest impairment; sweet quality the least. At present, mechanisms of taste impairment are unknown; it is probable that most taste buds are functioning in an abnormal manner while some function in a normal capacity. It is not known whether the taste effects are due to radiation effects on the taste buds or secondary to xerostomia.

Recovery of the sense of taste occurs between twenty and sixty days postirradiation. Although taste usually returns within six months, dysgeusia sometimes persists. For these patients, 110 mg of zinc sulfate with each meal and with a snack at bedtime may produce an enhancement of taste sensation.

The mucosal lining of the oral cavity is affected both on a short-term and long-term basis. In the short-term, there is the development of radiation mucositis. During a full course of therapy, the following sequence of events occur:

First week: (100 rads) A "tumoritis" occurs in which tumor becomes outlined by specked leukoplakia and a pseudomembrane.
Weeks 2-3: (2000-3000 rads) There is mucositis of the soft palate.
Weeks 3-4: (3000-4000 rads) There is mucositis of the pharyngeal wall.
Weeks 4-5: (4000-5000 rads) There is mucositis of the buccal mucosa.
Weeks 5-6: (5000-6000 rads) There is mucositis of the tongue.

Mucositis is characterized by hyperemia, edema, pseudomembrane formation, denudation, and ulceration. This produces pain and difficulty with eating, swallowing, and speaking. Healing usually occurs within two weeks following radiation therapy in the absence of secondary infection.

Radiation mucositis may be palliated by either of the following:

: benadryl elixir and kaopectate solution in equal parts. Hold one tablespoonful in mouth for one minute and expectorate. Repeat every two hours.
: Solution of Tetracycline, 500 mg; Nystatin, 1,200,000 units; Hydrocortisone, 100 mg; Benadryl elixir g.s., 250 ml.

Sig: Swish and hold one tablespoonful as needed or four to six times daily.

Once radiation mucositis has subsided Driezens et al. state that patients with a history of radiation therapy are more susceptible to candidiosis. Candidal infections should be treated immediately upon discovery to prevent hematogenous spread and seeding of the esophagus with swallowed organisms. Nystatin vaginal tablets dissolved as an oral lozenge six times daily for a minimal period of two weeks is recommended. Resistant cases may respond to clotrimazole vaginal tablets or intravenously administered amphotericin B. Should bacterial infections occur in the form of caries or periodontal disease, they should be eliminated for the reasons previously discussed.

Another problem of irradiated patients includes trismus due to radiation fibrosis of the masticatory muscles. This may be relived by asking the patient to open as wide as possible and repeat this twenty times through a minimum of three cycles daily. Custom-tailored prosthetic appliances are available to enhance the exercise program.

Nutritional deficiencies and altered diet and eating pattern contribute both to the development of malnutrition and indirectly to radiation caries. Eating patterns change in patients with xerostomia hypogeusia (diminished taste), trismus, and possibly pain due to radiation caries or osteoradionecrosis. These patients often resort to eating soft foods with inadequate nutritional value; vitamin supplements and nutritional counseling is recommended in these individuals.

Bibliography

Andrews, J.R.: *The Radiobiology of Human Cancer Radiotherapy.* Philadelphia, Saunders, 1968.

Arena, V.: *Ionizing Radiation and Life.* St. Louis, Mosby, 1971.

Bacq, Z.M.; and Alexander, P.: *Fundamentals of Radiobiology,* 2nd ed. New York, Pergamon, 1961.

Casarett, G.: *Radiation Biology.* Englewood, NJ, P-H, 1968.

Dalrymple, G. V.; Gaulden, M. E.; Kollmorgen, G. M.; and Vogel, H. H.: *Medical Radiation Biology.* Philadelphia, Saunders, 1973.

Daly, T. E.; Castro, J. R.; and Boone, M.L.M.: *Management of Dental Problems in Irradiated Patients.* Houston, The University of Texas at Houston, M. D. Anderson Hospital and Tumor Institute and Dental Branch, 1971.

Dertinger, H.; and Jung, H.: *Molecular Radiation Biology.* Berlin, Springer-Verlag, 1970.

Driezens, S.; et al.: *Cancer,* 38(1):273-278, July 1976.

Driezens, S.: *J Dent Res,* 56(2):99-104, Feb. 1977.

Duncan, W.; and Nias, A.H.W.: *Clinical Radiobiology.* Edinburgh, Churchill Livingstone, 1977.

Fabrikont, J. I.: *Radiobiology.* Chicago, Year Bk Med, 1972.

Fajardo, L. F.: *Pathology of Radiation Injury.* New York, Masson Publ, 1982.

Fletcher, G. H.; and MacComb, W. S.: *Radiation Therapy in the Management of Cancers of the Oral Cavity and Oropharynx.* Springfield, Charles C Thomas, 1962.

Fletcher, G. H.: *Textbook of Radiotherapy,* 3rd ed. Philadelphia, Lea & Febiger, 1980.

Hall, E. J.: *Radiobiology for the Radiologist,* 2nd ed. New York, Har-Row, 1978.

Holaender, A.: *Radiation Biology.* New York, McGraw, 1954.

National Academy of Sciences: *Research Needs for Estimating the Biological Hazards of Low Doses of Ionizing Radiation.* Washington, D. C., National Academy of Sciences, 1974.

National Research Council, Advisory Committee on the Biological Effects of Ionizing Radiation (BEIR III): *The Effects on Populations of Exposure to Low Levels of Ionizing Radiation.* Washington, D.C., National Research Council, 1980.

Pizzarello, D.L.; and Witcofskik, R. L.: *Medical Radiation Biology,* 2nd ed. Philadelphia, Lea & Febiger, 1982.

Potten, C. S.; and Hendry, J H.: *Cytotoxic Insult to Tissue.* Edinburgh, Churchill Livingston, 1983.

Powsner, E. R.; and Raeside, D. E.: *Diagnostic Nuclear Medicine.* New York, Grune, 1971.

Prasad, K. N.: *Human Radiation Biology.* New York, Har-row, 1974.

Chapter 6

RADIATION HAZARDS AND PREVENTION

JOHN W. PREECE

Radiation Measurement

THE QUANTITIES associated with units of radiation measurement are defined by convention in much the same way as we measure a pound or a kilogram of rice, a quart or liter of milk, a kilowatt of electricity, or any other quantity. The interaction of X-Ray photons with air molecules results in the formation of ion pairs through the process called ionization. An indirect measure of radiation quantity is to determine the amount of ionization occurring during the complete absorption of X-Ray energy within a specific volume and mass of air. The unit of radiation measurement associated with the ionization of air is the **roentgen**. The roentgen is called the special unit of exposure; it is defined only for electromagnetic ionizing radiations (x and gamma). By definition, an exposure of 1 roentgen (1 R) is the amount of radiation producing an electrical charge of $2.58 \cdot 10^{-4}$ coulombs in a kilogram of air at standard temperature and pressure (approximately $2.08 \cdot 10^9$ ion pairs). The roentgen does not provide an accurate estimate of potential biologic effect; it measures the amount of energy reaching an organism but does not describe the amount of energy actually absorbed or deposited within the irradiated organism and hence provides only a general index of potential biologic damage or the risk of damage to a specific organ or tissue.

To more accurately evaluate the biologic consequences of ionizing radiation, it is necessary to measure the amount of energy deposited within a specific mass of tissue; the unit used to describe this is the **rad.** The rad is defined as the special unit of absorbed dose; a dose of 1 rad is by definition the absorption of 100 ergs of energy per gram of tissue. The physical calculations for interconversion between units of radiation measurement in roentgens and rads is beyond the scope of this text but for purposes of comparison an exposure of 1 roentgen is roughly equivalent to an absorbed dose of 0.87 rads.

The rad as a unit of radiation measurement may be used to describe the energy absorbed by tissues from *all* types of ionizing radiation, alpha, beta, x, gamma, neutrons, and protons. As discussed in Chapter 5, a specific absorbed dose of one type of ionizing radiation may not necessarily produce the same biologic effect as another (different) type of ionizing radiation. The difference in effect is related to the relative biological effectiveness (RBE) or quality factor (QF) of the ionizing radiation. To compare the biologic risk of a specified dose among all types of radiation, a special unit of radiation measurement called the *rem* is used. The rem is called the unit of dose equivalence (DE) and is obtained by multiplying the absorbed dose in rads by either the RBE or QF of the ionizing radiation in use. A dose of 300 rem of any type of ionizing radiation can therefore be expected to produce a similar biologic effect regardless of radiation type.

$$\text{rads} \cdot \text{RBE} = \text{rem}$$

e.g. neutrons: 30 rads · 10 = 300 rem
x-rays: 300 rads · 1 = 300 rem

Table 6-I

SOME RBE VALUES

Radiation	RBE
X-rays, gamma rays, electrons, and beta particles	1.0
Fast neutrons and protons up to 10 MV	10.0
Naturally occurring alpha particles	10.0

With regard to dental radiation exposures, it is acceptable to consider the roentgen, rad, and rem roughly equivalent to each other, even though each term has a very specific definition, and use.

1 R = 1 rad = 1 rem

In July, 1974, the International Commission on Radiation Units and Measurements recommended the adoption of new units of absorbed dose expressed in joules/kilogram (1 rad = 0.01 j/kg). The new unit of measurement is the **gray** (Gy). An absorbed dose of 1 gray is equal to 1 joule/kilogram; therefore an absorbed dose of 1 Gy is equal to 100 rads. The new unit of biologic equivalence is the **sievert** (Sv); 1 Sv = 100 rem. The interconversion of old and new units is depicted in Table 6-II. For most dental dosimetry purposes, roentgens, rads, and rems are large units of measurement and it is more convenient to discuss dental doses in milliroentgens, millirads, or millirems, where 1 milliroentgen is equivalent to 1/1000 of a roentgen.

Radiation Protection Concepts

Historically, ionizing radiation was identified as a potential health risk to patients and operators shortly after its discovery in 1895. As a result, efforts have been made to determine the most appropriate balance between the potential risk to the patient and the obvious benefits of radiation in terms of improved diagnosis and treatment. The efforts to identify this acceptable balance point has resulted in the promulgation of radiation protection standards. Most radiation protection standards utilize the underlying assumption that in estimating the effects of radiation on humans, a linear relationship between dose and effect in low dose regions exists, for which direct observational data are not available. Such an assumption tends to be conservative and estimates the upper limits for any particular effect.

The establishment of an acceptable exposure limit assumes that there is a practical limit of exposure that will make the "risk so small that it is readily acceptable to the average individual." For example, occupationally exposed persons are those individuals who derive the benefits of earning a livelihood from their work; persons requiring the therapeutic application of radiation derive the benefit of a poten-

Table 6-II
UNITS OF RADIATION EQUIVALENCE

Old Terminology					New Terminology			
roentgen* (R)	milliroentgens (mr)	rad/rem	millirad(s)† (mrad)	coulombs/kg (C/kg)	gray (Gy)	sievert (Sv)	Sv or Gy	Sv or Gy
100	100,000	100	100,000	258x10⁻²	1	1	1	1
10	10,000	10	10,000	25.8x10⁻³	0.1	0.1	10⁻¹	1 deci Sv or Gy dSv or dGy
1	1,000	1	1,000	2.58x10⁻⁴	0.01	0.01	10⁻²	1 centi cSv or cGy
0.1	100	0.1	100	2.58x10⁻⁵	0.001	0.001	10⁻³	1 milli- mSv or mGy
0.01	10	0.01	10	2.58x10⁻⁶	0.0001	0.0001	10⁻⁴	.1 milli- or 0.01 micro- mSv or mGy
0.001	1	0.001	1	2.58x10⁻⁷	0.00001	0.00001	10⁻⁵	.01 milli- or 0.1 micro- mSv or mGy
0.0001	0.1	0.0001	0.1	2.58x10⁻⁸	0.000001	0.000001	10⁻⁶	.001 milli- or 1 micro- mSv or mGy μSv
Exposure		Absorbed Dose	Dose Equivalence	Exposure	Absorbed Dose	Dose Equivalence		

*Technically 1R = 0.87 rads or 86 ergs or 0.0086 j/kg; therefore, 1.14R = 1 rad = 100 ergs = 0.01 J/kg in air.
†For X-Rays, millirads and millirem are equivalent.

Roentgen and coulombs/kg are units of radiation exposure.
Rad and gray are units of absorbed dose.
Rem and sievert are units of biologic dose.

tial increase in life span through tumorcidal effects of radiation. As a result acceptable exposure limits may differ markedly for each group and be larger than those appropriate for the general population. For occupationally exposed persons, the exposure limits are established at a level to make the risk essentially the same as that present in ordinary occupations not involving exposure to radiation.

Current exposure limits are expressed in terms of the permissible dose or **maximum permissible dose** (MPD) concept. As defined by the "International Commission on Radiation Protection (ICRP) —

> the permissible dose for an individual is that dose, accumulated over a long period of time or resulting from a single exposure, which in the light of present knowledge, carries a negligible probability of severe somatic or genetic injuries; furthermore, it is such a dose that any effects that ensue more frequently are limited to those of minor nature that would not be considered unacceptable by the exposed individual or by competent medical authorities.

The MPD is therefore the maximum dose that just fulfills the requirements of "permissible dose" and is the highest one permissible under the stipulated conditions of exposure. Present international usage restricts 'maximum permissible dose' to occupational situations; for population exposures (nonoccupational) **dose limit** is preferred. When calculating the MPD or dose limits for occupationally or nonoccupationally exposed persons, radiation received from environmental background sources and diagnostic medical and dental exposures (for the individual's personal health care) are specifically excluded from calculations, primarily because medical and dental exposures are presumed to have a benefit far exceeding potential risk and exposure to environmental background radiation cannot be effectively controlled or limited.

Table 6-III
PERMISSIBLE ANNUAL DOSES*

Organ/tissue	Maximum Permissible Dose[†] (Occupational Exposure)	Dose Limit[‡] (Nonoccupational Exposure)
Whole body/ gonads	5 rem	0.5 rem
Hematopoietic/ lens of eye	5 rem	0.5 rem
Skin of whole body	30 rem	3 rem
Hands/forearm Feet/ankles	75 rem	7.5 rem
Head/neck	75 rem	7.5 rem

*NCRP reports 17,35 also provide maximum limitations on weekly or quarterly exposures based on a 50 week work year.
[†]For pregnant occupationally exposed workers the MPD is 1/10 occupational exposure or 0.5 rem during the pregnancy.
[‡]Dose Limits are assumed to be 1/10 of the occupational exposure.

Currently acceptable permissible annual doses are listed in Table 6-III. Whole body or gonad exposures for occupationally exposed persons are limited to 5 rem/year and 1/10 of the occupational exposure for nonoccupationally exposed persons and pregnant occupationally exposed persons (during pregnancy).

Age Proration Formula

The age proration formula was a permissible exposure concept introduced in 1957 to serve as a guide to limit the accumulated whole body or genetic dose of occupationally exposed persons:

$$\text{MPD} = (N - 18) \times 5 \text{ rem/year}$$

where N = person's age in years
(For occupationally exposed persons below 18 years of age the MPD was to be that of a nonoccupationally exposed person.)

Based on available data at that time, the concept assumed that genetic damage accumulated in direct proportion to accumulated dose, independent of dose delivery pattern. Current data suggests that the cumulative effect of low LET radiation, either genetic or somatic, **is not** strictly proportional to accumulated dose and that for low LET radiation, the effect is minimized if each exposure occurs at both low dose and low dose rates where the effect may be proportional to accumulated dose but where the rate of increase is much less than for higher doses and dose rates. Based on this newer information, the age proration formula no longer serves as an acceptable method for assessing accumulated genetic or somatic damage.

ALARA Concept

Radiation protection concepts involving the establishment of permissible doses and dose limits are still currently in use; however, more recent National Council on Radiation Protection (NCRP) and ICRP recommendations are summarized in the prinicple of ALARA (As Low As Reasonably Achievable). This principle expresses their intent to encourage the implementation of radiation protection practices that are better than any prescribed minimum level could produce. Applying this principle to occupationally and nonoccupationally exposed persons simply means that every available method for reducing exposure to ionizing radiation will be implemented to minimize potential risks and adverse consequences.

The ALARA concept used for the maximum benefit of all persons means that diagnostic radiographic procedures should be conducted using every available dose reducing means possible.

Specific Protection Concepts

Dose limiting recommendations contain a criterion equivalent to requiring "avoidance of appreciable bodily injury." Genetic effects are presumed to be predominantly deleterious and undetectable except by long-range sophisticated statistical studies. For somatic tissues the absence of observable biologic change is not an adequate criterion for determining somatic exposure limits and a more subtle and indirect line of reasoning may be required.

In judging somatic effects of radiation in individuals, the significance of the irradiated structures with regard to the economy of the organism is very important, along with the general interplay between various tissues. As a means of reducing the underlying radiobiologic variables, simplifying assumptions are made that focus attention on various tissues and organs that experience has shown to be particularly vulnerable to developing potential late effects detrimental to the quality of life of the organism. As a result certain organs are considered "critical" from the point of view of protection:

1. **skin** with respect to cancer;
2. **blood-forming organs** (red bone marrow) with respect to leukemia;
3. **gonads** with respect to impairment of fertility and mutations;
4. **eyes** with respect to cataracts;
5. **thyroid** with respect to cancer;
6. **pregnancy** with respect to possible fetal effects; and
7. **breast** with respect to cancer.

With whole body exposures, the

greatest hazard to health will be due to irradiation of particular tissues or organs because the maximum number of cells are irradiated and for a given dose there is a maximum probability that damage may occur to a single cell, or group of cells, resulting in malignancy or other effects. Unequal exposure to body tissues and organs results in the exposed tissue assuming a greater importance in terms of its potential radiobiologic effect on the individual. Thus, there is a broad range of interpretations of what constitutes a "critical" organ: at one end, a critical organ may have high radiosensitivity in terms of cell death or carcinoma induction; at the other end, it may be an organ such as the thyroid whose uptake of radioiodine causes it to reach the highest concentration and absorbed dose (Table 6-IV).

Table 6-IV

CRITICAL ORGANS

Tissue/Organ	Radiation Effect
Hematopoietic	Leukemia
Gonads	Impaired fertility/mutations
Skin	Carcinoma
Eyes	Cataract
Thyroid	Carcinoma
Pregnancy	Fetal effects
Breast	Carcinoma

Assessing Dental Radiation Risks

The harmful effects of low doses of X-Radiation normally associated with dental and medical radiographic procedures cannot be proved scientifically as a directly observable discrete change in a specific individual that can be directly attributed to the diagnostic exposure. The observable deleterious effects of X-Radiation manifest not as specific changes in specific individuals but as statistically demonstrable increases in the frequency of normally occurring disease states among the general population. In other words, a squamous cell carcinoma in an unexposed individual will have the same characteristics as the same type of cancer in an exposed individual; the only difference is that from a statistical perspective, irradiated populations tend to have more of this kind of cancer than nonirradiated populations. The higher the dose, the higher the cancer rate and the easier it is to demonstrate a correlation between irradiation (the cause) and cancer (the effect); on the other hand, at very low doses of radiation it becomes increasingly difficult to demonstrate the cause and effect relationship between radiation and its effect with the results (especially in studies dealing with human beings) highly dependent upon the statistical approach in use. As a result, the literature concerning low dose effects of radiation tends to be highly confusing and frequently contradictory in nature.

One may, therefore, legitimately ask: "What are the potential risks to patients from medical or dental radiographic procedures?" Gregg (1977) estimates that the potential risk of dental radiographic procedures inducing a fatal cancer in a human being is three chances in one million, compared to our "normal" risk of developing cancer, which is approximately 3300 chances in 1 million. Of those 3300 individuals who develop cancer, 1760 per million population will die as a direct consequence of their disease. It is estimated that a single dose of 10 rads

(10,000 mrads) of whole body exposure will increase an individual's cancer mortality risk 0.5-1.4 percent above the normal rate of 15 percent. Without some other point of comparison, this may seem unreasonably high; consideration should be given to the fact that the cancer mortality risk of smokers is 50-70 percent higher than for nonsmokers and that the annual projected mortality as a consequence of coal combustion in the United States is approximately 37,000 deaths per year.

In any discussion of the potential harmful effects of radiation, it is necessary to emphasize that dental radiographic procedures irradiate a small, well-localized area of the human anatomy and do not irradiate the entire (whole) organism. Studies indicate that an organism can tolerate and survive relatively large doses of radiation to a small localized area of the body (radiation therapy for example) where the same dose given to the "whole body" would have fatal consequences. The repair of radiation damage to a localized area is well documented; unfortunately the damage is never completely repaired, and some residual damage persists within the irradiated tissues. The significance of this residual damage in terms of its potential for carcinogenesis is at present poorly understood.

To assess the potential risks of dental radiography, it is beneficial to compare the various known sources of human exposure to X-Radiation with regard to quantitative amounts. Such comparisons provide a useful point of departure when discussing the potential adverse effects of ionizing radiation on the dental patient, especially with regard to exposures of the head and neck outside the primary beam.

There are two main sources of whole body radiation: background radiation and radiation received from occupational exposures. Major sources of population exposure are listed in figure 6-1.

Sources of background radiation are cosmic rays derived from solar sources, external terrestrial radiation derived from the radioactive decay of materials composing the earth's surface, and internally deposited radioisotopes derived from the ingestion or inhalation of various radioactive substances. The dose of background radiation a person receives depends on many factors but in the United States the average annual dose is about 120 mrads, or 0.3 mrads per day. Other miscellaneous sources of whole body exposure to humans are very minor in overall contribution to whole body exposure compared to background, amounting to about 8 mrads.

Dentists, dental auxiliaries, radiologists, and X-Ray technologists are exposed daily as a result of their occupations to small amounts of radiation to the whole body. This is a chronic type of exposure and is measured by the use of film badges. Maximum permissible limits for radiation exposure to radiation workers have been discussed in the previous section.

Aside from background radiation, medical and dental diagnostic radiographic procedures contribute the next highest somatic and genetic doses to members of the population. Diagnostic radiography, however, seldom involves exposures to the entire body and is confined to well-localized areas of the body so that the potential risk depends significantly on the organs and tissues irradiated.

In order to assess the potential risks of dental radiography, it will be necessary to discuss the amount of radiation an individual might receive utilizing current dental radiographic procedures. Unfortunately, it is necessary to stipulate that the quantities mentioned will be average quantities and may not relate to doses delivered under the wide range of practices

CMRS = Complete mouth radiographic survey.

Textbook of Dental Radiology

TYPICAL VALUES IN MREMS

	Whole Body mrem/year	Gonads mrem/year
I. Natural Background		
Cosmic Rays	38-75	
Terestrial Gamma	20-215	
Total	58-215	

The *average* annual whole body and genetically significant dose for the U.S. population is between 102 and 120 mrem/year.

	Whole Body mrem/year	Gonads mrem/year
II. Medical and Dental Radiation		
Medical	72	20
radiopharmaceuticals	1	0.26
Dental	—	0.15
Total	73	20.4
III. Miscellaneous Sources		
Nuclear power plants	1.0	1.0
Nuclear Testing (fallout)	4.0	4.0
T.V. & Consumer products	2.6	2.6
Total	7.6	7.6
Total Exposure All Sources:	138.6-295.6	

Source: Effects on populations of exposure to low levels of ionizing radiation, National Academy of Sciences, Washington, D.C., 1972.

IV. Doses associated with Dental Radiographic Procedures

    Dose per film — 200 mrads
    Highest reported dose to any given region per CMRS — 1500 mrads (maxillary central incisor)
    Genetically significant dose — no lead apron — 0.5 mrads per CMRS
    Genetically significant dose — with lead apron — 0.01-0.03 mrads per CMRS
    Average occupational exposure for:
        Medical personnel — 200 mrem/year
        Dental personnel — 50 mrem/year
        M.P.D. occupational workers — 5 rem/year
        M.P.D. non-occupationally exposed individuals — 0.5 rem/year (1/10th of occupational)

    Note: M.P.D. specifically excludes background and medical exposures

Figure 6-1. Sources of population exposure to ionizing radiation.

currently found in private dental practices. However, *if* "D" speed film is used, along with time-temperature processing, long shielded open cylinders (cones), and proper collimation and filtration of the beam of radiation using 80-85 kVp, then

areas marked in blue are in the center of the beam.

1 rad = 1000 mrad

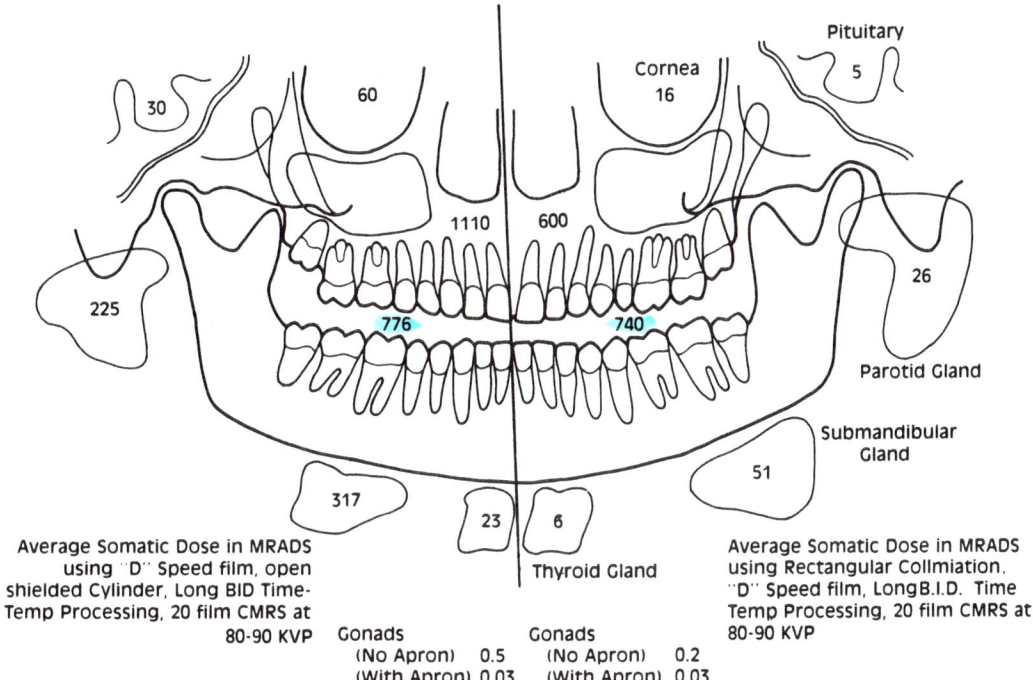

Figure 6-2. Comparison of radiation doses at various anatomic sites using an open shielded cylinder (left) and rectangular collimation. (From Smith, Q.W. et al.:*Radiological Tech*, Sept. 1983.)

the following doses may be used for making estimates of potential doses to patients from dental radiographic procedures. When lower kilovoltages are used in the vicinity of 60-70 kVp, patient doses would be approximately 30-50 percent higher than those described.

As a basis for risk estimation, consideration will be given to the estimated dose received by each of the critical organs or tissues previously discussed. They are the skin, eye, and hematopoietic, thyroid, and genetic tissues. It is important to remember that in order to produce a diagnostically acceptable radiograph under the conditions cited above, a certain amount of radiation must reach the dental film and the patient will receive a certain dose through the absorption of radiation by the tissues as the x-ray photons pass through on their way to strike the film and produce the latent image. Available literature indicates that patients will receive a dose of approximately 200 mrads for each radiograph taken. Averaged doses to various anatomic sites from various literature sources are depicted in Figure 6-2 for a complete mouth radiographic survey and Figure 6-3 for panoramic radiographic procedures.

see page 207

Risk Estimate for the Skin

During a twenty-one film complete mouth radiographic survey (CMRS), the tube head is repositioned about the patient's face in order to radiograph the various regions. Different portions of the head and neck will, therefore, receive differing amounts of radiation depending on

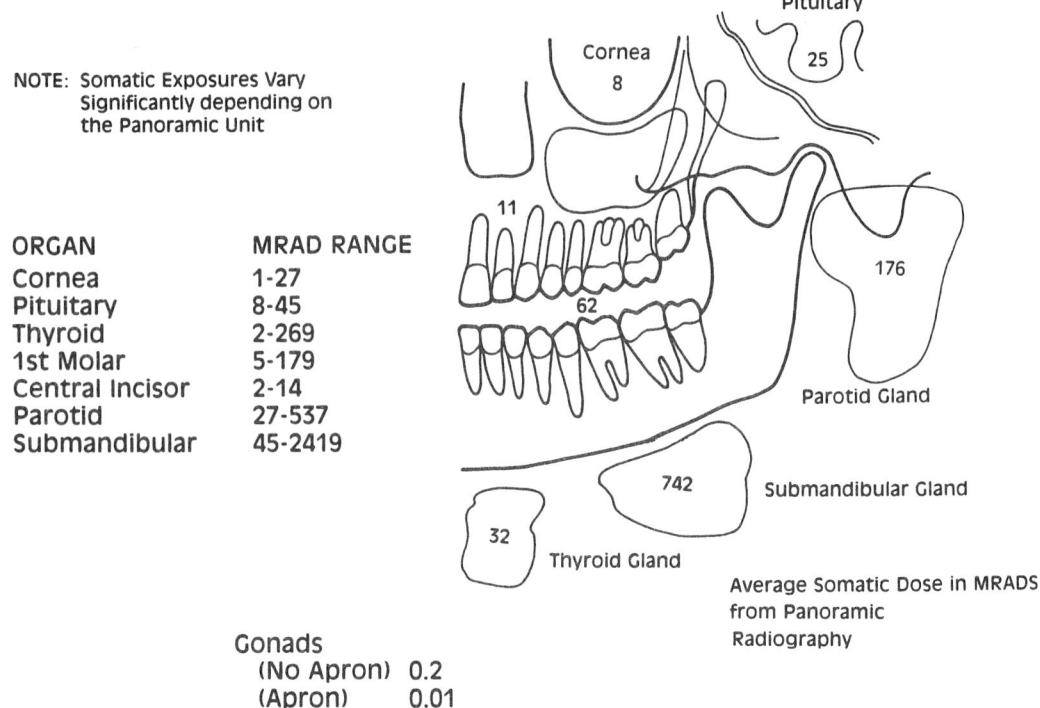

Figure 6-3. Averaged radiation dose to various anatomic sites from panoramic radiography. (From Smith, Q.W. et al.: *Radiological Tech*, in press.)

the number of films taken in any specific region. Available literature indicates that the highest somatic doses to the patient's face will probably be in the vicinity of 1000-1500 mrads. When rectangular beam collimating devices are used, the total dose may be reduced 25-45 percent. The risk of any potential harmful effects to the patient's face arising in terms of carcinoma induction would therefore be derivable from this relatively small dose. Available literature suggests that increased risks of skin cancer cannot be statistically demonstrated at dose levels below 25 rads (25000 mrads).

Risk Estimate for the Eye

Dental exposures to the lens and cornea of the eye are primarily from scattered radiation and are reported to be approximately 60 mrads when open shielded cones are used. Rectangular collimating instruments will reduce eye exposure to 16 mrad, while pointed plastic cones will increase this dose to approximately 300 mrads (5 times increase). The potential risk of dental X-Rays inducing cataracts in the lens of the eye must be related to the 60 mrads dose. Available literature indicates that it requires more than 200 rads (200,000 mrads) to induce clinically significant cataracts in the lens of the eye. As a consequence, the risk of dental procedures contributing significantly to the development of this problem is very unlikely.

Hematopoietic Tissue Dose Estimates

The region of the mandible and maxilla involved in dental radiography contains a very small percentage of the active bone marrow. The risk of leukemogenesis is directly associated with the amount of hematopoietic tissue irradiated and the dose. Bureau of Radiologic Health publications estimate the average bone marrow dose from periapical radiography to be approximately 1-3 mrads/film and 9-14 mrads/CMRS. Reports indicate an increased risk of leukemia induction following relatively low doses of whole body exposure, in the vicinity of 5 rads (5,000 mrads). A study by Linus as recently as 1980 found no significant increase in leukemia risk following bone marrow doses of 0-300 rads when administered in small doses over long periods of time.

Risk Estimates for the Thyroid Gland

Under most circumstances, the thyroid gland is not irradiated by the primary beam of radiation during dental radiography; the dose to the gland is reported to be approximately 23 mrads (open cone), 6 mrads with rectangular collimation, and approximately 60 mrads with the pointed plastic cone. The incidence of thyroid cancer has been reported to increase with doses in the vicinity of a few rads. Thyroid cancer is rarely fatal.

Risk Estimates for the Genetic Tissues

Genetic tissues receive irradiation from dental procedures as a result of scattered radiation from the face or pointed plastic cone. Approximately 1/10,000 of the dose received by the face will be scattered to the reproductive tissues (1/15,000 for females). In numerical terms, this is approximately 0.5 mrad for the open cone, 0.2 mrad for rectangular collimation, and 1.0 mrad for pointed plastic cones. Application of the lead apron reduces all values to approximately 0.01-0.03 mrad. It should be remembered that more than 98 percent of all genetic exposures are the result of medical, not dental, diagnostic exposures.

Risk Estimates for Pregnancy

Exposure to a fetus during gestation would be similar in magnitude to the genetic tissues. Current recommendations by the National Council on Radiation Protection Report Number 54 suggest that the production of congenital defects from doses below 10 rads is very small when compared to the normal risk of 4-6 percent and is negligible at 5 rads or less.

Summary

Available evidence indicates that all radiation, no matter how small the dose, has the potential for producing undesirable effects on both somatic and genetic tissues. Although repair processes occur within the cell, complete recovery from the effects of radiation does not occur and the residual damage persists and is cumulative. As a patient's dose increases, the risk of developing some adverse sequelae such as the induction of carcinoma, leukemia, cataract, or mutated reproductive tissues increases. The severity of the consequences can be minimized by utilizing every means to minimize patient exposure no matter how small, insignificant, or unimportant we may consider the modification. The next section describes those factors that contribute significantly to reducing patient and operator exposures.

Patient Radiation Protection

The following recommendations are

designed to minimize the somatic and genetic exposures to patients from dental diagnostic radiographic procedures. Many of the factors have been discussed elsewhere in the book and are included in this section as a means of integrating information on radiation protection. It should be noted that all suggestions will secondarily minimize the exposure of dental office personnel, and consequently, the results may be considered of potential double benefit to the patient and the dentist/auxiliary.

Recommendatins to Minimize Somatic Exposure

1. "E" Speed Film
   "E" speed film is presently the highest speed, most sensitive X-Ray film commercially available. Using this, or in the future other higher speed films, the practitioner may produce diagnostically acceptable radiographs with less exposure compared to available "D" speed film. "E" speed film will reduce patient exposure by about 40 percent compared to "D" speed film.
2. Correct Film Processing Procedures
   This recommendation must of necessity include a wide variety of subcategories because each factor will significantly improve the quality of the radiograph. If neglected, these same factors will severely degrade the quality of the radiograph.
   a. Darkroom free from light leaks
      White light should not be allowed to leak in around doors, plumbing, air conditioning ducts, windows, etc., because it will produce film fog.
   b. Adequate darkroom safelighting
      An appropriate safelight filter should be used in the darkroom to permit the operator to work in the dark without producing film fog during various stages in film processing.
   c. Time-temperature processing
      When radiographs are to be processed by hand (dip method) time-temperature processing is absolutely essential because it is the only way to assure maximum development of the radiographic image. When used with recommendation 1, this will assure that the patient receives the absolute minimum amount of radiation necessary to produce a diagnostically acceptable radiograph. It has been estimated that to shorten developing time by one minute it would be necessary to increase the patient's exposure by at least 30 percent, an extremely unwise reduction in processing time.
      i. This recommendation mandates the presence and use of a timer and thermometer in the darkroom.
      ii. Sight or visual development techniques are to be prohibited because it encourages overexposure and underdevelopment of the radiographic image.
      iii. Automatic film processors may be substituted for hand processing procedures, provided care is taken to keep solutions at optimal concentrations and wash water fresh.
   d. Processing solutions
      Processing solutions should be changed regularly, stirred thoroughly twice each day, kept covered to prevent oxidation when not in use, and not subjected to excessively high temperatures. Weekly quality control checks

should be performed to assure optimal processing and quality radiographs (daily for automatic processors).

e. Cleanliness

The darkroom should be immaculate and the counters devoid of wet or dried chemicals, which could adversely affect the quality of the films before or after processing.

3. Beam of Radiation

The beam of radiation should be restricted or collimated to no larger than 7 cm (2.75 inches) in diameter when measured at the patient's skin or 2.5 inches at the end of the cone. The area of skin irradiated at the recommended beam diameter is approximately 37.4 cm^2 (6 in^2).

a. Rectangular collimation. A rectangular field the size of the film is preferable to a circular field of radiation because a smaller area of the patient's face is irradiated with each exposure. For example, the area covered by the Rinn rectangular cone is 14.6 cm^2 (3.5 in^2) and the area of the precision instrument is 11.4 cm^2 (1.8 in^2). Thus, by utilizing rectangularly collimated beams a 60-70 percent reduction in the area of a patient's face may be achieved. When translated into terms of patient dose, a reduction of 45-95 percent, depending on anatomic site, may be achieved compared to circular fields.

4. Type of Cone to be Used on the Tube Head

a. Open end lead-lined cylinders or rectangles are the preferred method of visualizing the direction and location of the beam of radiation relative to the film plane and the patient's face. Long open end cones (12-16 inches in length) are preferred because they will reduce somatic exposure because of less divergence of the beam of radiation and consequently a smaller volume of the patient's face will be irradiated when compared with shorter (8 inch) cones. For example, a long open circular cone will irradiate 27 percent less volume than a short cone of similar diameter, and rectangular cones will irradiate approximately 80-85 percent less tissue than short circular cones.

b. Pointed plastic cones

Pointed plastic cones *are not recommended* because they increase scattered radiation to all areas of the patient's head, neck, and reproductive organs. In addition, a much greater volume of tissue is irradiated due to scattered radiation penumbra from the pointed cone; Weissman (1972) estimates that the total irradiation field for a cone of this type is 251 cm^2.

5. Aluminum Filtration

The purpose of the aluminum filter in the X-Ray tube head is to selectively absorb long wavelength, poorly penetrating X-Rays that are mainly absorbed by the soft tissues of the face and that increase the patient's somatic exposure. The filter significantly reduces somatic exposure, by some estimates as much as 57 percent.

By federal regulation, X-Ray units capable of operating at 70 kVp or higher must be filtered with a total equivalent of at least 2.5 mm of aluminum. X-Ray units not capable of producing 70 kVp must be filtered with 1.5 mm of aluminum.

6. Exposure timers

An accurate timer is essential to produce consistent quality diagnostic radiographs with minimal exposure to

the patient.
   a. Electronic timers
      Electronic timers are preferred and recommended because they accurately reproduce short exposure times required by the use of D and E speed film, time-temperature processing, and short (8 inch) cones.
   b. Mechanical (spring wound) timers
      Mechanical timers are not recommended because they cannot accurately and consistently reproduce short exposure times.
7. X-Ray Units
   X-Ray units whose kilovoltage is not capable of being adjusted to produce higher than 60 kVp X-Rays are not recommended. Low kVp X-Ray units will produce somatic exposures as much as 45 percent higher than an X-Ray unit operating at 80 kVp or higher!
8. Film Holding Devices
   The use of film holding devices for intraoral radiographic techniques is recommended to prevent unnecessary exposure to the patient's fingers. Secondarily, these devices produce more stable film placement in the mouth under a wide variety of clinical circumstances. Such devices are mandatory if rectangular collimation is used.
9. Thyroid Shields
   The use of thyroid shielding is suggested to reduce exposure to the thyroid gland. Recent studies indicate a 50 percent reduction in thyroid dose may be achieved when this type of shielding is used. The dose to the thyroid is reported to be approximately 20-50 mrads without the shield, 10-25 mrads with the shield.
10. Lead Apron
    The primary purpose of the lead apron is to reduce exposure to the reproductive organs from scattered radiation; however, a secondary benefit may be derived from the apron's ability to prevent scattered radiation from reaching sites of hematopoiesis in the chest and abdomen (Fig. 6-4).

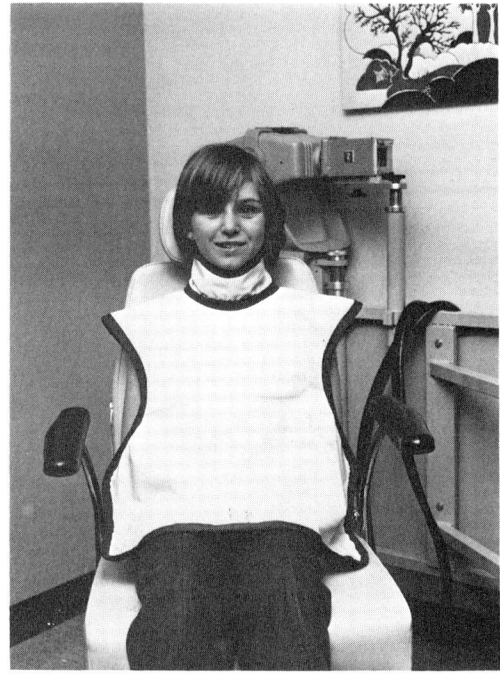

Figure 6-4. Example of a protective leaded lap apron and thyroid collar.

11. Discretionary Factors
    a. Radiographing patients on a "routine" annual or semiannual basis is not recommended. Radiographs should be taken only when there is a clinically justifiable need for diagnostic information that cannot be obtained by any other mechanism. Decisions to radiograph should therefore be based only on an individual basis.
    b. Postoperative radiographs should

be taken only when there is a clinical indication and not as verification for third-party payment plans.

c. Pregnant patients should not be radiographed unless there is a justifiable clinical need for diagnostic information that can not be achieved by any other means. When radiographs are necessary only the minimum number of films required to diagnose and treat the specific complaint should be taken.

Recommendations to Minimize Genetic Exposure

1. Lead Apron
   The lead apron is useful in minimizing the exposure of reproductive tissues to scattered radiation and is recommended for children and all adults with reproductive potential.
   Comment: With the lead apron in place, a twenty-one film survey will result in a dose of 0.01-0.03 mrad to the gonads of a male. When the lead apron is not used, the same survey will result in a genetic exposure of 1.0 mrad from a pointed plastic cone, 0.5 mrad from a long open shielded cone, and 0.2 mrad from a rectangularly collimated beam. The average daily exposure of an individual to background radiation is approximately 0.3-0.5 mrad per day.
2. Recommendations 1 through 5 above will significantly reduce the patients' somatic exposure; consequently, there will be less radiation scattered from the face to the reproductive tissues.

Operator Radiation Protection

The operator of dental X-Ray equipment may be potentially exposed to primary radiation from the useful beam, leakage radiation from the tube housing, and secondary or scattered radiation primarily from the patient's face. There are several procedures operators can utilize to minimize their occupational exposure in the dental office:

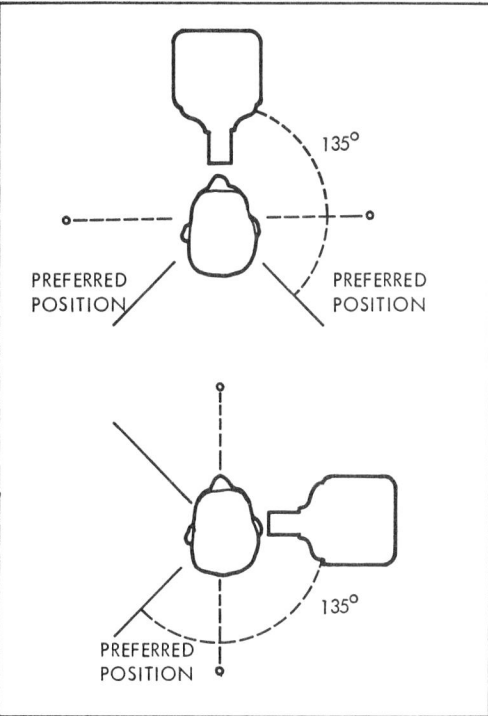

Figure 6-5. Positions of greatest safety for operator during X-Ray exposure to patient. The small circle represents the 90 degree position; the operator should stand in the area designated "preferred position," at least 6 feet away from the cone tip.

1. The most effective way of reducing operator exposure to primary radiation is to enforce strict application of the position and distance rule, i.e. stand at least 6 feet away from the patient at an angle between 90 and 135 degrees to the primary beam (Fig. 6-5).

a. If the operator cannot stand at least six feet from the patient during the exposure, he/she should stand behind an appropriate protective barrier or outside the operatory.
2. Forbid personnel to: (a) hold films in the patient's mouth, (b) hold or stabilize the tube head or cone during exposure, or (c) stand directly in line with the primary beam of radiation.
3. Monitor Office Personnel. Subscribing to one of the many film badge services provides an excellent tangible way for the practitioner to express concern for reducing and monitoring radiation exposure to office personnel. Quarterly reports (monthly or semiannually are also available) from a film badge service provide appropriate legal documentation that employees have or have not received radiation exposure during their employment in the office. These reports also serve as a direct way of monitoring the employees' willingness to abide by office safety rules regarding radiation exposure procedures. An additional advantage to monitoring office personnel is that a series of radiation reports indicating little or no exposure serves to allay any apprehensions the office staff may have about receiving potentially damaging exposure to X-Radiation.

It *is not* an acceptable personnel monitoring procedure to attach a coin or paper clip to a dental film for purposes of monitoring occupational exposure. Dental film and processing procedures in the dental office are not rigidly controlled nor sensitive enough to permit detection of operator exposures at moderate to low levels of occupational exposure encountered in typical dental situations.

Office Design

A properly designed dental office protects the X-Ray operator—along with patients and staff in adjacent operatories, reception area, and office areas—from exceeding the appropriate maximum permissible dose limits. Sources of radiation in the operatory consist of primary, secondary, and tube head leakage radiation—for radiation protection purposes. The walls of the dental operatory X-Ray cubicle may be designated either primary or secondary barriers. Primary barriers are those walls intended to absorb radiation from the primary beam; secondary barriers are intended to absorb only secondary and leakage radiation. In general, a primary barrier is any wall potentially in a direct line with the beam of the X-Ray unit. Typically three walls of the cubicle—behind the patient's head, and to the right and left—are primary barriers. Secondary barriers typically include the floor, ceiling, and on fixed position chairs the wall adjacent to the patient's feet.

Determination of appropriate radiation barrier thicknesses requires knowledge about five essential factors: (1) workload, (2) maximum kVp, (3) distance to the person to be protected, (4) radiation status of the person to be protected, and (5) occupancy factor of the areas adjacent to the X-Ray unit. Barrier requirements are determined separately for each X-Ray unit in the office.

Workload

The determination of X-Ray machine workload is an important measure of the total amount of radiation produced by the unit. It is determined by multiplying the milliamperage, exposure time, and the *average* number of films taken by the unit *per week*.

$$\text{workload} = \text{mA} \cdot \text{exposure time per film} \cdot \text{number of films per week} = \text{mAs}$$

The exposure time used for determining workload should be the exposure time used to produce a diagnostically acceptable periapical radiograph of the maxillary molar region. If a particular X-Ray unit is used for both periapical and extraoral types of radiographs, then two workloads must be determined, one for intraoral radiography and one for extraoral radiography; the sum of the two workloads would become the total workload of the X-Ray unit.

The total workload of a dental unit will vary from office to office because of such variables as cone length, kilovoltage, film speed, filtration, processing, and use of xeroradiography, all of which would influence the acceptable exposure time for a particular radiograph. The unit of measurement for workload is the milliampere-second (mAs).

Kilovoltage

The operating kilovoltage of the dental X-Ray unit is important because this determines the penetrating ability of the radiation. For office design purposes, the highest kilovoltage used in intraoral or extraoral radiographic techniques is the one used for this factor. The higher the kilovoltage the greater the penetrating ability of the beam and consequently the thicker the protective barrier required.

Distance

For barrier design purposes, the distance to the person to be protected is very important. Because X-Rays obey the inverse square law, the farther the person to be protected is from the source of radiation, the thinner the barrier will need to be.

Radiation Status

The radiation status of the person to be protected is an important consideration in barrier determinations because of differences in MPD allowed between occupationally and nonoccupationally exposed persons. In principle, the barrier serves to prevent the protected person from exceeding the MPD. Consequently, barriers designed to protect nonoccupationally exposed persons will be heavier than those intended to protect occupationally exposed persons. For the practitioner wishing to optimize radiation protection in the office, all potential radiation barriers may be designed to protect nonoccupationally exposed persons regardless of the person's actual radiation status.

Occupancy Factor

The occupancy factor is a measure of how frequently the area adjacent to the X-Ray cubicle is in use. Within the dental office all areas are considered to have an occupancy factor of 1—full utilization. Office areas adjacent to the actual dental office may vary in their use from 1 to 1/16. It should be obvious that protective barriers adjacent to relatively unoccupied areas would not have to be as thick as those adjacent to fully occupied areas.

Once the above five factors have been properly determined, appropriate tables in the National Council on Radiation Protection Handbook Number 35 may be consulted and the appropriate thickness of either primary or secondary barriers obtained. Handbook 35 provides barrier thicknesses in terms of their absorbing properties in millimeters of lead or inches of concrete. It is important to recognize that these tables do not mean that the protective barriers must be "lined" with the specified thickness of lead or concrete; the table only says that the barrier must absorb the same amount of radiation as the specified thickness of lead or concrete. In principle, marshmallows could be used for a radiation barrier as long as the marshmallow layer was thick enough to absorb the same amount of radiation as the specified amount of lead or concrete. The absorptive properties of various thicknesses of lead and some common office building materials are provided in Tables 6-V and 6-VI.

Table 6-V

MM Lead	%Absorption 90 kVp
0.1	66
0.2	83
0.3	90
0.4	93
0.5	95
0.7	97
1.0	99
1.5	99.8
2.0	99.9
2.5	99.99

Table 6-VI

Wall Section	%Absorption 90 kVp
1/8" veneer paneling (2 sheets on 2x4 studs) (total thickness 1/4 inch)	4
3/4" pine board (2 boards on 2x4 studs) (total pine thickness 1.5 inches)	20
1/2" dry wall/sheet rock (2 on 2x4 studs) (total dry wall 1 inch)	66
1/2" dry wall/sheet rock + 5 inches fiberglass insulation on 2x4 studs (total dry wall = 1 inch)	70
5/8" dry wall/sheet rock 4 thicknesses 2x4 studs (total 2.5 inches)	89
3-5/8" cinder block wall	98
3-5/8" ceramic tile brick	95
5-5/8" cinder block	98
5-3/4" ceramic tile brick	97
Brick and mortar wall	99
Mortar on metal lath	92

Panoramic dental X-ray units, in general, do not require special protective cubicles primarily because they utilize a very narrow beam of radiation that is always directed toward the film cassette, which is backed by lead. Manson-Hing and Greer (1977) report operator exposures of 0.1 mR per film at 1 meter; with the operator standing at 2 meters, this would decrease to 0.025 mR per film. For the average dental office with low work loads and numbers of films, no special shielding of the panoramic units is required. Shielding may be required for heavy use clinic operations where large numbers of patients are radiographed weekly.

Most dental offices have relatively low radiation workloads; as a result, adequate protection may be derived from use of several thicknesses of common construction materials such as "dry wall or sheet rock." For example, four thicknesses of 5/8 inch dry wall are roughly equivalent in absorbing capacity to 0.3 mm of lead. Wood paneling or wood products of any type do not make adequate radiation protection barriers by themselves; they should be veneered to lead or some other good radiation absorber. Table 6-VII provides a simple method to determine the barrier requirements of a dental office.

Table 6-VII

STEPS IN DETERMINING BARRIER REQUIREMENTS

---

1. Who is to be protected?
    a. occupationally exposed _____
    b. nonoccupationally exposed _____
2. How far are they from the source of radiation? _____ ft.
3. What is the maximum kVp of the dental X-Ray unit? _____ kVp
4. What is the weekly workload of the unit?
    a. How many films are exposed per week? _____ films/week
    b. What is the average exposure time? _____ sec.
    c. What is the X-Ray unit milliamperage? _____ mA

Calculate workload:
   1. Ave. exp. time per film · mA = mAs/film
   2. mAs/film · film/week = mAs/week or workload

5. Assume occupancy factor of 1

When all of the above are known, Appendix B, Tables 3 and 4, p. 30, 31 NCRP Handbook No. 35 may be used to calculate primary barrier thickness. For secondary barriers use Tables 5 and 6, p. 32, 33 of NCRP Handbook No. 35.

Table 6-VII continued

Page 30/ APPENDIX B/NCRP HANDBOOK No. 35

TABLE 3—*Lead primary protective barriers*

Workload (mAs/week)	Distance from Target to Area of Interest						
	ft	ft	ft	ft	ft	ft	ft
20,000	3.5	5	7	10	14	20	28
10,000		3.5	5	7	10	14	20
5,000			3.5	5	7	10	14
2,500				3.5	5	7	10
1,250					3.5	5	7
625						3.5	5
313							3.5

Thickness of Lead							
	mm	mm	mm	mm	mm	mm	mm

Full Occupancy

Occupationally exposed persons							
50 kVp	0.1	0.1	0.1	0.0	0.0	0.0	0.0
70 kVp	0.4	0.3	0.2	0.2	0.1	0.1	0.1
100 kVp	0.9	0.7	0.5	0.4	0.2	0.1	0.1
Non-occupationally exposed persons							
50 kVp	0.3	0.2	0.2	0.1	0.1	0.1	0.1
70 kVp	0.8	0.7	0.5	0.4	0.3	0.2	0.2
100 kVP	1.6	1.4	1.2	1.0	0.8	0.6	0.4

Partial Occupancy

Non-occupationally exposed persons							
50 kVp	0.2	0.1	0.1	0.1	0.1	0.1	0.0
70 kVp	0.5	0.4	0.3	0.2	0.2	0.1	0.1
100 kVp	1.2	1.0	0.8	0.6	0.4	0.3	0.2

Occasional Occupancy

Non-occupationally exposed persons							
50 kVp	0.1	0.1	0.1	0.1	0.0	0.0	0.0
70 kVp	0.3	0.2	0.2	0.1	0.1	0.1	0.0
100 kVp	0.8	0.6	0.4	0.3	0.2	0.1	0.0

Courtesy of National Council on Radiation Protection and Measurements, 1970.

Table 6-VII continued

Page 31/ APPENDIX B/NCRP HANDBOOK No. 35

TABLE 4—*Concrete primary protective barriers*
(Concrete density: 147 lbs/ft³)

Workload (mAs/week)	Distance from Target to Area of Interest						
	ft	ft	ft	ft	ft	ft	ft
20,000	3.5	5	7	10	14	20	28
10,000		3.5	5	7	10	14	20
5,000			3.5	5	7	10	14
2,500				3.5	5	7	10
1,250					3.5	5	7
625						3.5	5
313							3.5
	Thickness of Concrete						
	inches	inches	inches	inches	inches	inches	inches
Full Occupancy							
Occupationally exposed persons							
50 kVp	0.5	0.4	0.2	0.0	0.0	0.0	0.0
70 kVp	1.4	1.0	0.7	0.5	0.3	0.2	0.1
100 kVp	2.9	2.3	1.7	1.1	0.6	0.3	0.1
Non-occupationally exposed persons							
50 kVp	1.2	1.0	0.8	0.6	0.4	0.3	0.2
70 kVp	2.8	2.4	2.0	1.5	1.1	0.7	0.5
100 kVp	5.1	4.5	3.8	3.1	2.5	1.8	1.2
Partial Occupancy							
Non-occupationally exposed persons							
50 kVp	0.8	0.6	0.4	0.3	0.2	0.1	0.0
70 kVp	2.0	1.5	1.1	0.7	0.5	0.4	0.3
100 kVp	3.8	3.1	2.5	1.8	1.2	0.8	0.4
Occasional Occupancy							
Non-occupationally exposed persons							
50 kVp	0.4	0.3	0.2	0.1	0.0	0.0	0.0
70 kVp	1.1	0.7	0.5	0.4	0.2	0.1	0.0
100 kVp	2.5	1.8	1.2	0.8	0.4	0.1	0.0

Courtesy of National Council on Radiation Protection and Measurements, 1970.

Table 6-VII continued

Page 32/ APPENDIX B/NCRP HANDBOOK No. 35

TABLE 5—*Lead secondary protective barriers*

Workload (mAs/week)	Distance from Target to Area of Interest						
	ft	ft	ft	ft	ft	ft	ft
20,000	3.5	5	7	10	14	20	28
10,000		3.5	5	7	10	14	20
5,000			3.5	5	7	10	14
2,500				3.5	5	7	10
1,250					3.5	5	7
625						3.5	5
313							3.5
	Thickness of Lead						
	mm	mm	mm	mm	mm	mm	mm
Full Occupancy							
Occupationally exposed persons							
50 kVp	0.2	0.1	0.0	0.0	0.0	0.0	0.0
70 kVp	0.4	0.2	0.0	0.0	0.0	0.0	0.0
100 kVp	0.5	0.4	0.2	0.0	0.0	0.0	0.0
Non-occupationally exposed persons							
50 kVp	0.3	0.2	0.2	0.1	0.1	0.1	0.0
70 kVp	1.0	0.8	0.6	0.4	0.3	0.1	0.0
100 kVp	1.3	1.1	0.8	0.6	0.4	0.2	0.1
Partial Occupancy							
Non-occupationally exposed persons							
50 kVp	0.2	0.1	0.1	0.1	0.0	0.0	0.0
70 kVp	0.6	0.4	0.3	0.1	0.0	0.0	0.0
100 kVp	0.8	0.6	0.4	0.2	0.1	0.0	0.0
Occasional Occupancy							
Non-occupationally exposed persons							
50 kVp	0.1	0.1	0.0	0.0	0.0	0.0	0.0
70 kVp	0.3	0.1	0.0	0.0	0.0	0.0	0.0
100 kVp	0.4	0.2	0.1	0.0	0.0	0.0	0.0

Courtesy of National Council on Radiation Protection and Measurements, 1970.

Table 6-VII continued

Page 33/ APPENDIX B/NCRP HANDBOOK No. 35

TABLE 6—*Concrete secondary protective barriers*
(Concrete density: 147 lbs/ft³)

Workload (mAs/week)	Distance from Target to Area of Interest						
	ft	ft	ft	ft	ft	ft	ft
20,000	3.5	5	7	10	14	20	28
10,000		3.5	5	7	10	14	20
5,000			3.5	5	7	10	14
2,500				3.5	5	7	10
1,250					3.5	5	7
625						3.5	5
313							3.5

	Thickness of Concrete						
	inches	inches	inches	inches	inches	inches	inches

Full Occupancy

Occupationally exposed persons							
50 kVp	0.4	0.2	0.0	0.0	0.0	0.0	0.0
70 kVp	1.0	0.5	0.0	0.0	0.0	0.0	0.0
100 kVp	1.6	1.1	0.5	0.0	0.0	0.0	0.0
Non-occupationally exposed persons							
50 kVp	1.1	0.9	0.7	0.5	0.3	0.1	0.0
70 kVp	2.7	2.2	1.7	1.2	0.7	0.2	0.0
100 kVp	4.0	3.3	2.6	1.9	1.3	0.7	0.2

Partial Occupancy

Non-occupationally exposed persons							
50 kVp	0.7	0.5	0.3	0.1	0.0	0.0	0.0
70 kVp	1.7	1.2	0.7	0.2	0.0	0.0	0.0
100 kVp	2.6	1.9	1.3	0.7	0.2	0.0	0.0

Occasional Occupancy

Non-occupationally exposed persons							
50 kVp	0.2	0.1	0.0	0.0	0.0	0.0	0.0
70 kVp	0.7	0.2	0.0	0.0	0.0	0.0	0.0
100 kVp	1.3	0.7	0.2	0.0	0.0	0.0	0.0

Courtesy of National Council on Radiation Protection and Measurements, 1970.

Bibliography

Accident Facts. Chicago, National Safety Council, 1979.

Alcox, Ray W.; and Jameson, Wayne R.: Patient exposures from intraoral radiographic examinations; *J Am Dent Assoc, 88*:568, March 1974.

Altonen, M.; Heikkila, M.: and Mattila, K.: A comparative study of radiation doses received during examinations with the pantomograph, orthopantomograph, panorex, status x and conventional roentgen apparatus. *Proc Finn Dent Soc, 70*:67, 1974.

Antoku, S.; et al.: Doses to critical organs from dental radiography: *Oral Surg, 41*:251, 1976.

Beckmann, Peter: *The Non-Problem of Nuclear Wastes.* Boulder, CO, Galem Press, 1979.

Bonnell, J.A.; and Horte, G.: Occupational exposure to ionizing radiation, the risk in perspective. *Lancet*, pp 1032, May 13, 1978.

Cancer Statistics. *Ca Cancer J Clin.*, Jan, Feb. 1979.

Casarett, A.P.: *Radiation Biology.* Englewood Cliffs, NJ, P-H, 1968.

Christensen, Ralph C.: Shielding calculations below 100 kVp in concrete equivalent materials. *Health Phys, 36*:69, Jan 1979.

Christensen, Ralph C.; and Sayeg, Joseph A.: Attenuation characteristics of gypsum wallboard, *Health Phys, 33*:595, May 1979.

Danforth, R.A.; and Gibbs, S.J.: Diagnostic dental radiation. What's the risk? *California Dent Assoc J, 28*:1980.

Dertinger, H.; and Jung, H.: *Molecular Radiation Biology.* New York, Springer-Verlag, 1970.

Dunster, H.J.: Dose equivalent unit. *Health Phys, 36*:536, 1979.

Ennis, LeRoy M.; Berry, Harrison; and Phillips, James E.: *Dental Radiology*, 6th ed. Philadelphia, Lea & Febiger, 1967.

Glaze, Sharon A.; Schneiders, Nicholas J.; and Bushong, Stewart, C.: Use of gypsum wallboard for diagnostic X-Ray protective barriers. *Health Phys, 30*:587, May, 1979.

Gray, Joel E.: The radiation hazard in perspective. *J Am Dent Assoc, 100*:490, March, 1980.

Greer, David F.: Determination and analyses of absorbed doses resulting from various intraoral radiographic techniques. *Oral Surg, 34*:146, July 1972.

Gregg, Earl C.: Radiation risks with diagnostic X-Rays. *Radiology, 123*:447, 1977.

Hall, Eric J.: *Radiobiology for the Radiologist*, 2nd ed. Scranton, PA, Har-Kow, 1978.

Jerman, Albert C.; Kinsley, Earl L.; and Morris, Charles R.: Absorbed radiation from panoramic plus bitewing exposures vs full-mouth periapical plus bitewing exposures. *J Am Dent Assoc, 86*:420-423, Feb 1973.

Johns, Harold E.; and Cunningham, John R.: *The Physics of Radiology*, 3rd ed. Springfield, Charles C Thomas, 1969.

Kelsey, C.A.: Comparison of relative risk from radiation exposure and other common hazards. *Health Phys, 35*:428 Aug, 1978.

Lee, Wah: Comparative radiation doses in dental radiography. *Oral Surg, 37*:962, June, 1974.

Lindell, Bo: Radiation and man. *Health Phys, 31*:265, Sept, 1976.

Linus, Athena; et al.: Low dose radiation and leukemia. *N Engl J Med, 302*:1101, May 15, 1980.

MacDonald, John C.F.; Reid, John A.; and Berthoty, Dean: Drywall construction as a dental radiation barrier. *Oral Surg, 55*:319, March 1983.

Manson-Hing, L.R.; and Greer, D.F. Radiation exposure and distribution measurements for three panoramic machines. *Oral Surg, 44*:313, 1977.

Medwedeff, Fred M.; Knox, William H.; and Latimer, Paul: A new device to reduce patient irradiation and improve dental quality. *Oral Surg, 15*:1079, Sept 1962.

Medwedeff, Fred M.; and Knox, William H.: Radiation reduction for children. *J Tenn State Dent Assoc, 42*: Oct 1962.

National Academy of Sciences, Committee on Biological Effects of Ionizing Radiation: *The Effects on Populations of Exposure to Low Levels of Ionizing Radiation.* Washington, D.C., NAS, 1980.

National Council on Radiation Protection and Measurements: *Report No. 35, Dental X-Ray protection.* Washington, D.C., NCRP Publications, March 1970.

National Council on Radiation Protection and Measurements: *Report No. 39, Basic Radiation Protection Criteria.* Washington, D.C., NCRP Publications, Jan. 1971.

National Council on Radiation Protection and Measurements: *Report No. 54, Medical Radiation Exposure of Pregnant and Potentially Pregnant Women.* Washington, D.C., NCRP Publications, 1977.

Pizzarello, Donald J.: and Witcofski, Richard L.: *Medical Radiation Biology, 2nd ed.*, Philadelphia, Lea & Febiger, 1982.

Preece, J.W.: and Morris, C.R.: Efficient and effective use of X-Radiation in the dental office, part I patient protection. *GP Texas Acad*

Gen Dent Pub, 6(1): April 1980.

Preece, J.W.; and Morris, C.R.; Efficient and effective use of X-Radiation in the dental office, part II assessing dental radiation risks. *GP Texas Acad Gen Dent Pub,* 6(2): August 1980.

Preece, J.W.; and Morris, C.R.; Efficient and effective use of X-Radiation in the dental office, part III. *GP Texas Acad Gen Dent Pub,* 6(3): Dec 1980.

Proceedings of the Public Meeting to Address a Proposed Federal Radiation Research Agenda vol. 2. Bethesda, Science Projection Papers, Interagency Radiation Research Committee, National Institutes of Health, March, 1980.

Radiation hygiene and practice in dentistry: I. *J Am Dent Assoc,* 74:1032, April 1967.

Radiation hygiene and practice in dentistry: II. *J Am Dent Assoc,* 75:1197, Nov 1967.

Radiation hygiene and practice in dentistry: III. *J Am Dent Assoc,* 76:115, Jan 1968.

Radiation hygiene and practice in dentistry: IV. *J Am Dent Assoc,* 76:363, Feb 1968.

Radiation hygiene and practice in dentistry: V. *J Am Dent Assoc,* 76:602, March 1968.

Richards, Albert G.: Radiation protection via the pin hole camera. *Oral Surg,* 13:953, Aug 1960.

Shleien, B.; Phoom, D.; Tucker, T.; and Johnson, D.W.: *The mean active bone marrow dose to the adult population of the United States from diagnostic radiology.* FDA Publication 77-8013. Washington, D.C., U.S. DHEW, 1977.

Smith, Q.W.; Preece, J.W.; Hefley, D.C.; and Fasser, C.E.: Radiation exposure in the dental setting: an update, *Radiol Technol,* 55:546, Sept. 1983.

Surgeon General's Report on Smoking and Health. Washington, D.C., U.S. HEW, 1979.

Thunty, Kavas H.: and Weinberg, Roger: Sensitometric comparison of dental films of groups D and E. *Oral Surg,* 54:250, Aug, 1982.

Wall, B.F.; et al.: Doses for patients from pantomographic and conventional dental radiography. *BS Radiol,* 52:727, 1979.

Weissman, Donald D.; and Sobkowski, Frank J.: Comparative thermoluminescent dosimetry of intraoral periapical radiography. *Oral Surg,* 29:376, March 1970.

Weissman, Donald D.; and Feinstein, Richard D.: X-Ray beam profiles and oral radiography. *Oral Surg,* 31:546 April 1971.

Weissman, Donald D: Comparative absorbed doses in intraoral periapical radiography, *JSCDA,* 39:886, Nov 1971.

Weissman, D.D.: Comparative absorbed doses in periapical radiography II panorex. *Oral Surg,* 33:661, 1972.

Whitcher, B.L.; Gratt, B.M.; and Sickles, E.A.: Leaded shields for thyroid dose reduction in intraoral dental radiography. *Oral Surg,* 48:567, 1979.

Whitcher, Bruce L.; Gratt, Barton M.; and Sickles, Edward A.: A leaded apron for use in panoramic dental radiography. *Oral Surg,* 49:467, May 1980.

White, S.C.; and Rose, T.C.: Absorbed bone marrow dose in certain dental radiographic techniques. *J Am Dent Assoc,* 98:553, 1979.

Wuehrmann, Arthur H.; and Manson-Hing, Lincoln R.: *Dental Radiology,* 4th ed. Mosby, St. Louis, 1977.

Wycleaff, H.O.: The international system of units. *Radiology,* 128:833, 1978.

Zelac, R.E.: Panoramic dental X-Ray installation, structural shielding and operator protection requirements. *Health Phys,* 25:52, 1973.

Chapter 7

INTRAORAL RADIOGRAPHIC TECHNIQUES

INTRAORAL RADIOGRAPHS are made by placing the film packet inside the oral cavity and projecting the X-Ray beam at various angles from a position outside the mouth through the anatomical region of interest toward the film packet. There are three types of intraoral projections: (1) periapical, (2) bitewing, and (3) occlusal projections.

Periapical radiographs record images of the outlines, position, and mesiodistal extent of the teeth and surrounding tissues. It is the best available means whereby the apices of the teeth and their surrounding tissues can be shown. It is essential in a periapical radiograph to obtain the full length of the tooth and at least 2 mm of the periapical bone (Fig. 7-1).

Bite-wing radiographs record, on a single film, images of the outlines, position, and extent of the crowns and the coronal one-third of the interalveolar bone and roots of the maxillary and mandibular teeth (Fig. 7-2). They are valuable for revealing the presence of interproximal caries, recurrent caries, overhangs on restorations, periodontal conditions, calculus deposits, the chronic resorption of interalveolar bone, pulp stones, and the occlusal relationship of the teeth. Bite-wing radiographs are particularly valuable for the detection of incipient carious lesions that are difficult or impossible to find by other clinical methods.

Occlusal radiographs record images of the incisal edges and the occlusal sur-

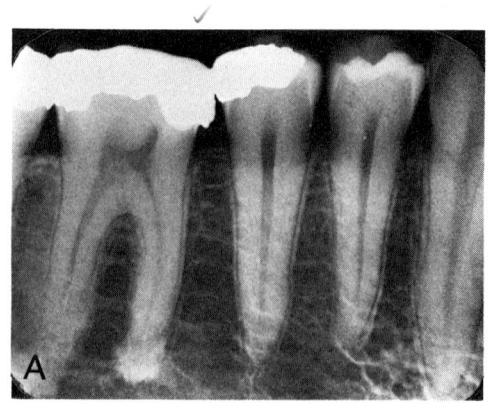
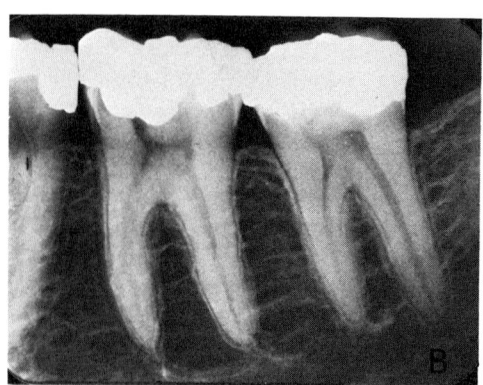

Figure 7-1. Periapical radiographs. **(A)** Topographical maxillary view. **(B)** Molar region.

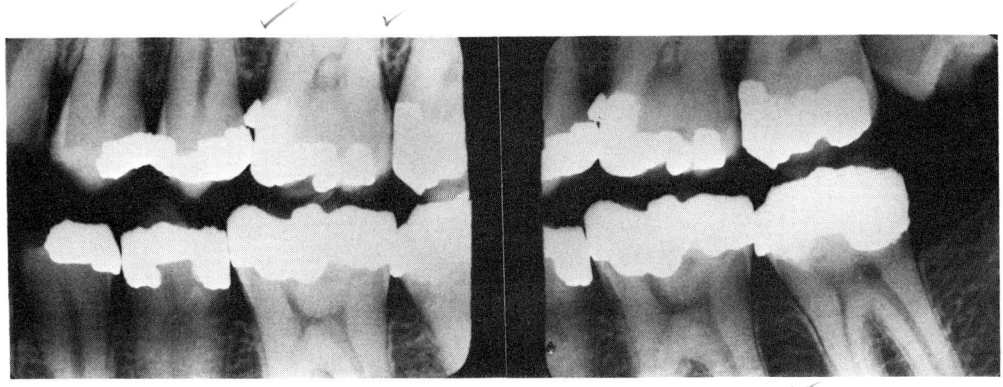

Figure 7-2. Bite-wing radiograph.

faces of the teeth, and a cross section of the distal arches. The maxillary occlusal radiograph (Fig. 7-3A) depicts images of the hard palate, bones, upper lip, and the base of the nose; the mandibular occlusal radiograph (Fig. 7-3B) records images of the tongue, floor of mouth, and lower lip. Occlusal radiographs are used to detect the presence and relative positions of impacted or embedded teeth, foreign borders, fractures, stones in the salivary ducts, and other gross conditions or lesions in the jaws.

A complete mouth survey is composed of several single periapical radiographs. A radiographic survey should completely cover all the teeth and the tooth-bearing alveolar bone of both arches. Some dentists take as many as twenty-two periapical radiographs per complete mouth survey while others take as few as ten radiographs. We recommend a minimum of fourteen and a maximum of seventeen periapical radiographs per complete radiographic survey, accompanied by two or four bite-wing radiographs. At the University of Texas Dental School at San Antonio, we use a complete radiographic survey composed of sixteen periapical and four bite-wing radiographs (Fig. 7-4). A complete radiographic survey composed of fourteen radiographs is usually sufficient to cover the totally edentulous arches (Fig. 7-5). However, it should be

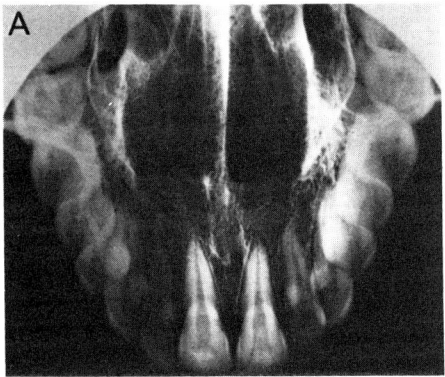
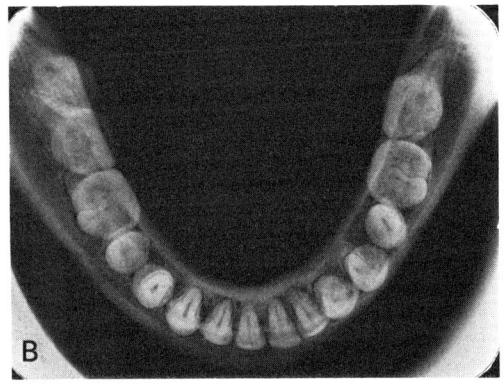

Figure 7-3. Two occlusal radiographs. (A) Topographical maxillary view. (B) Mandibular cross-sectional view.

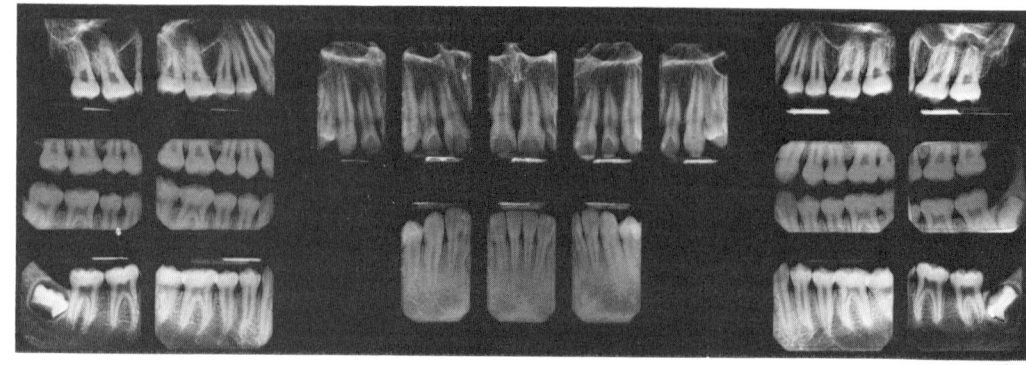

Figure 7-4. Complete mouth X-Ray survey and posterior bite-wings of dentulous mouth (20 films).

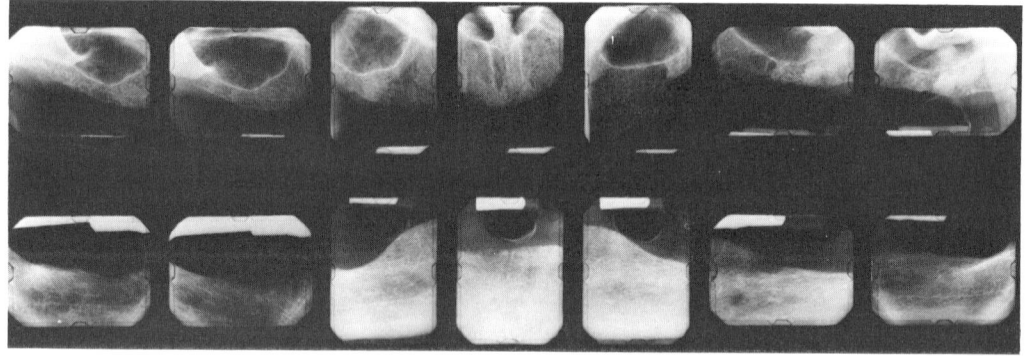

Figure 7-5. Complete mouth X-Ray survey of edentulous mouth (14 films).

kept in mind that the number of radiographs needed for a complete radiographic examination of a patient will depend on the technic used, the number of teeth present, the age of the patient, and the individual anatomical variations.

CRITERIA FOR ORDERING RADIOGRAPHS

The frequency of intraoral radiographic examinations is made on an individual basis and will vary with circumstances. This judgment is left to the dentist. Dental radiographs should only be taken after a dentist has examined the patient and has established by clinical indication the need for the radiographic examination. Radiographs must never be ordered routinely using a set time interval, such as regular patient recall visits, as the only criterion for ordering radiographic examinations. Automatic and routine use of radiographs without prior consideration of the patient's medical and dental history or clinical signs or symptoms is unjustified. Exposure to X-Rays should be kept to a minimum while obtaining the maximum amount of necessary diagnostic information. Thus, the dentist is responsible for deciding the need, for ensuring technical competence, and for developing within himself the ability to adequately interpret radiographs.

IMPORTANCE OF DENTAL RADIOGRAPHS

It is important for the dentist to realize that dental radiographs are essential to the diagnosis and treatment conditions that threaten a patient's oral and general health. There are many disease conditions of the teeth and jaws that may **not** be apparent in the clinical examination alone without radiographs. Such conditions as small carious lesions, periapical lesions, cysts, tumors, and bone destruction from periodontal disease may go unnoticed until more obvious signs and symptoms develop. By the time these disease processes become more apparent clinically, treatment would be more time-consuming, extensive, expensive, and in some cases, life-threatening, than if the disease process was detected earlier by the use of radiographs.

PERIAPICAL INTRAORAL RADIOGRAPHY

Basic Principles

There are certain basic principles that must be considered in the performance of **periapical intraoral radiographic techniques**. They include (1) the anatomy of the teeth and jaws, (2) patient head position, (3) X-Ray beam angulations, and (4) point of entry of X-Ray beam.

Anatomic Considerations

There are two anatomic considerations the operator must take into consideration prior to the placement of the film into the patient's mouth. They are —

1. location of the long axes of the teeth; and
2. location of the apices of the teeth.

Location of the Long Axes of the Teeth

Intraoral radiography depends upon the operator's knowledge of the approximate positions of the long axes of the teeth in the oral cavity. Practically all of the teeth in the maxillae are usually tilted outward (Fig. 7-6). The flatter the palatal

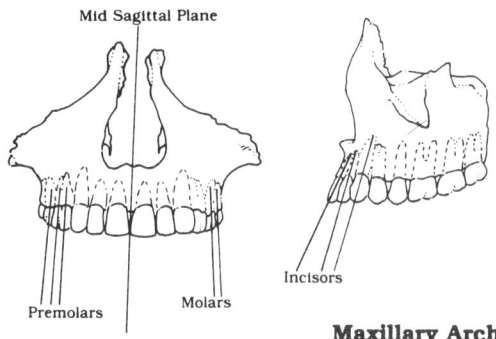

Figure 7-6. Drawing of long axes of teeth in the maxillary arch.

vault of the maxillae the greater the tendency for the teeth to tilt outwards.

In the mandible the six anterior teeth are usually tilted outward; on occasion, they sometimes are tilted backwards. The mandibular premolars, on the other hand, are usually positioned more nearly vertical, and the molars tilt inward slightly (Fig. 7-7). Also, the operator should be aware that crown or apparent axis of the tooth is different from the root or true axis of the tooth (Fig. 7-8). A line

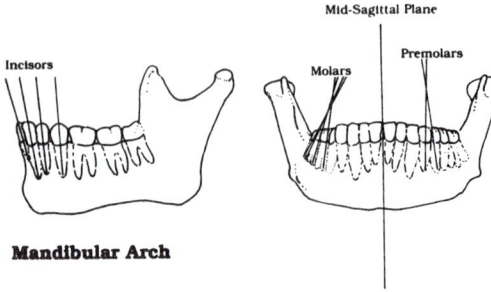

Mandibular Arch

Figure 7-7. Drawing of the long axes of teeth in the mandibular arch.

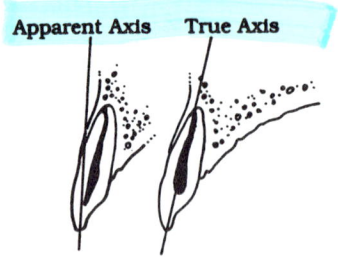

Figure 7-8. Drawing of apparent and true axis of tooth.

drawn through the vertical axis of the crown of the tooth and one drawn through the root forms an angle (crown-root angle) that generally varies from 5 to 20 degrees. Furthermore, the greater the tilt of the tooth, the greater the crown-root angle.

Location of Apices of Teeth

The apical region of the maxillary teeth are located on an imaginary line drawn from the tragus (earlobe) of the ear to the ala (wing) of the nose (Fig. 7-9). To localize each maxillary tooth apical region, a line is dropped from various landmarks on the face to the tragal-ala line (Fig. 7-10). The landmarks for each tooth are as follows:

Maxillary Second Molar: Drop a line to the tragal-ala line from a point 1 cm distal to the outer **canthus** of eye. (Canthus is the angle at the end of the fissure between eyelids.)

Maxillary First Molar: Drop a line to the tragal-ala line from the outer canthus of the eye.

Maxillary Second Premolars (region between apices): Drop a line to the tragal-ala line from the outer edge of the eye ball.

Maxillary Canine: The line is on the tragal-ala line 5 mm distal to ala of nose.

Maxillary Incisors: The landmark is the region just below the nasal cavity (*see* Fig. 7-6).

The location of tooth apices of the mandible is less complicated because it is easier to see the teeth. The apices of the mandibular teeth are 0.5 cm above the lower border of the mandible. Also, the same landmarks used for localizing the

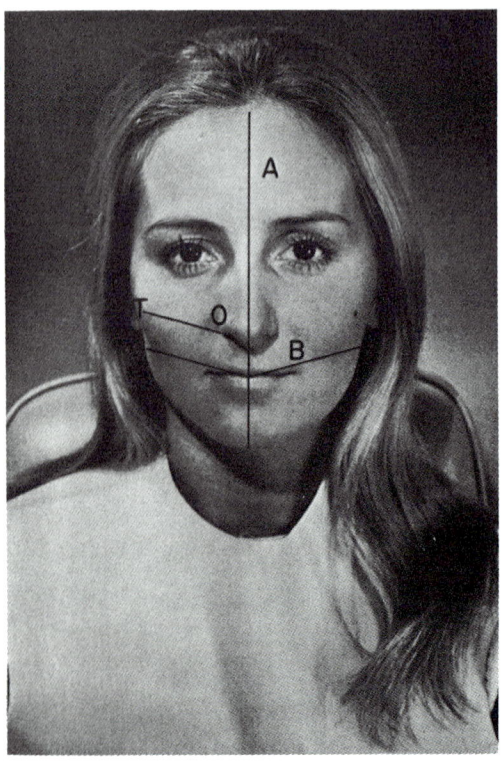

Figure 7-9. The head divided into four quarters by sagittal plane *A* and the occlusal plane *B*. The line *TO* is the tragal-ala line, which is parallel to the occlusal plane B.

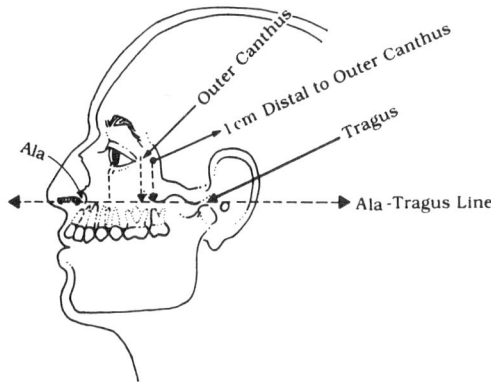

Figure 7-10. Drawing of apices of maxillary teeth.

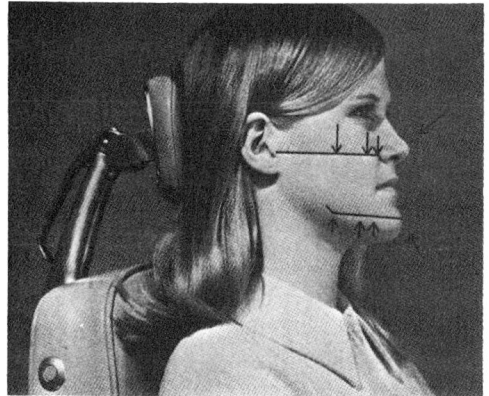

Figure 7-11. Localization of apical regions of teeth of both jaws. In the mandible the root apices can be established by estimating the points of entry from the lower border of the mandible. This is usually the width of the thumb (1/4 inch).

maxillary teeth may be used in the mandible (Fig. 7-11).

Head Position

In almost all of the intraoral periapical techniques, it is recommended that the patient be placed in an upright position, with the occlusal plane of the teeth to be radiographed parallel to the floor, and the sagittal plane of the head perpendicular to the floor. The **maxillary orientation line** is an imaginary line drawn from the tragus of the ear (cartilagenous projection located just before the ear hole or external auditory meatus) to the ala of the nose (wing of the nose). This line should be parallel to the floor when radiographing the maxillary teeth (*see* Fig. 7-9).

The **mandibular occlusal plane** changes when the mouth is opened. Therefore, tilt the patient's head slightly backwards so the occlusal plane of the mandible will be parallel to the floor when the mouth is opened. Make sure that the patient does not open too wide as this will contract the muscles of the floor of the mouth and make it difficult to place the film. If the patient tenses the muscles of the floor of the mouth, have him relax these muscles by swallowing.

The **sagittal plane** of the skull divides the skull vertically in the midline into right and left halves. The sagittal plane of the skull should be perpendicular to the floor prior to placing films into mouth for the bisecting-digital technic (*see* Fig. 7-9).

X-Ray Beam Angulation

The X-Ray tube head has two directional projections: **vertical** angulation and **horizontal** angulation. **Vertical** angulation is the movement of the tube head up and down in relation of the occlusal plane, which is parallel to the floor (Fig. 7-12). The changes in vertical angulation are measured in degrees and recorded on a dial located on the side of the X-Ray tube. A downward angulation of the cone is a positive or plus (+) angulation; an upward angulation of the cone is a negative or minus (−) angulation. **Horizontal** angulation is the movement of the X-Ray tube head around the patient's head in relation to the sagittal plane, when the patient is in an upright position (Fig. 7-13). Improper horizontal angulation will cause overlapping of the tooth images (Fig. 7-14).

Point of Entry

The point of entry of the X-Ray beam should be directed through the center of the region being radiographed. The objective is to completely cover the film with the beam of radiation. If this is **not** done, a "cone cut" or "partial image" will be seen in the resultant radiograph (Fig. 7-15).

Quality Evaluation Criteria for IntraOral Radiography

There are certain general characteristics of a quality dental radiograph that should be the objective of all persons taking intraoral radiographs. Some of these are listed below.

Adequate Image Contrast, Density, and Sharpness

These will permit—with standard illumination—differentiation between the various structures of the teeth, the periodontal ligament spacings, the lamina dura, the supporting bone, and normal anatomic landmarks.

Film Coverage

All crowns and roots, including apices, are fully depicted together with interproximal alveolar crests, contact areas, and surrounding bone regions.

Minimal Image Defects

Images of all teeth and other structures are shown in proper relative size and con-

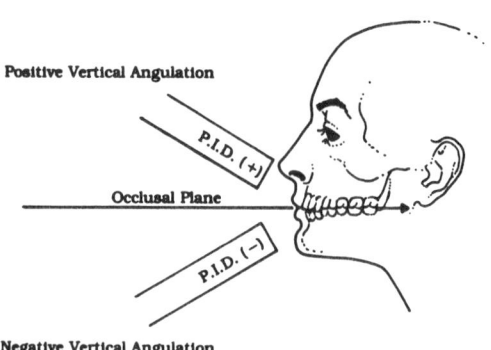

Figure 7-12. Vertical angulation.

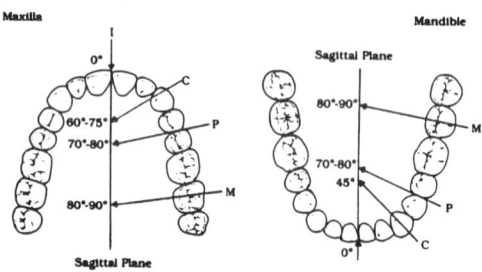

Figure 7-13. Horizontal angulation.

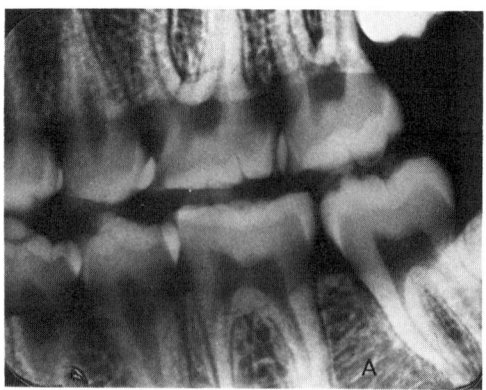
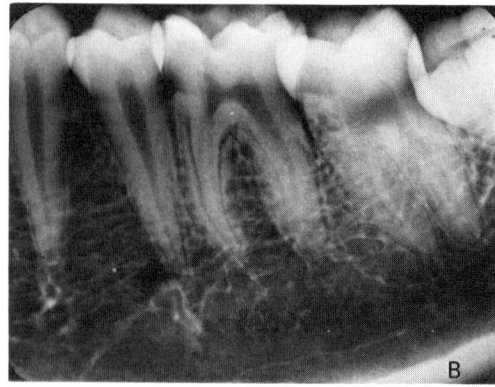

Figure 7-14. Overlapping. (A) Bite-wing. (B) Periapical radiograph.

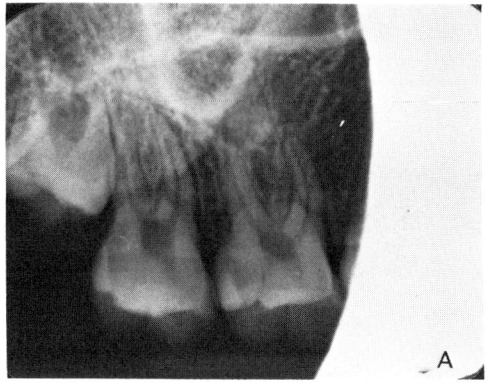
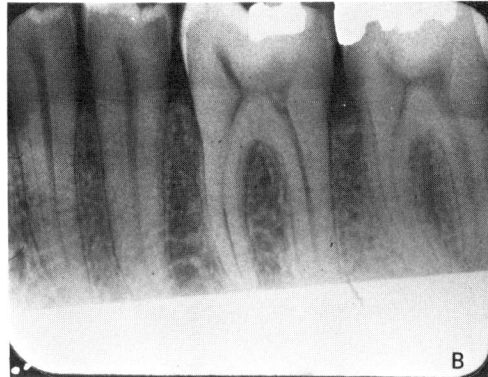

Figure 7-15. "Cone-cut" or partial image. **(A)** Round cone too far posteriorly. **(B)** Rectangular P.I.D. (too high).

tour with minimal distortion without overlapping images where anatomically possible, and without partial images (cone cuts).

Anatomical Accuracy

A radiograph is said to have anatomical accuracy when —

1. the facial and lingual cemento-enamel junctions of the anterior teeth are superimposed;
2. the facial and lingual cusps of posterior teeth (especially the molars) are superimposed;
3. the contacts of the teeth are opened in at least one of the projections of a given area;
4. the facial portion of the alveolar crest is superimposed over the lingual portion of the alveolar crest; and
5. there is no superimposition of the zygomatic bone over the roots of the maxillary molar teeth.

X-Ray Procedural Technique in Intraoral Radiography

There are sequential steps that an operator must accomplish in the exposure of an intraoral film.

1. Seat the patient in the dental chair, adjust the head rest; obtain a short history, wash hands, and conduct a brief clinical examination.
2. Have patient take out removable dental appliances and remove eyeglasses (not contacts).
3. Place patient in upright position; position head so occlusal plane of the jaw is parallel to the floor. Generally it is better to adjust the chair in the low position for the maxillary projections and high position for the mandibular projections.
4. Place lead apron and cervical shield (Fig. 7-16).
5. Set machine to proper exposure factors (kVp, mA, and exposure time) as designated on the exposure chart. Be sure the exposure chart is designed for film speed (D or E) and cone length (short or long) in use.
6. Position the film in mouth directly behind the teeth to be recorded on the radiograph. Place the film or film holder into position, and stabilize the film either by the patient's fingers or by having the patient bite firmly against the bite-block of the film

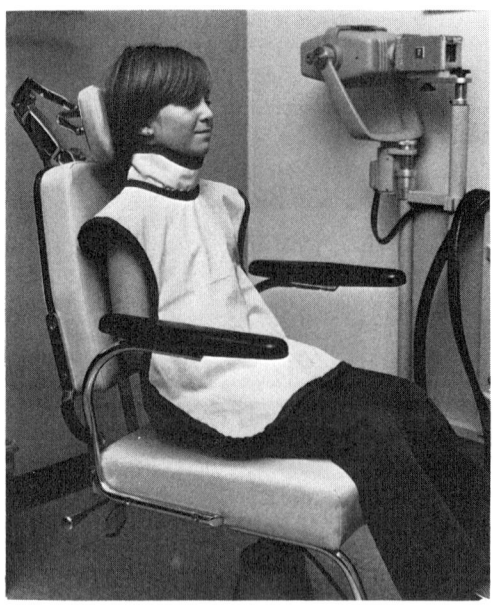

Figure 7-16. Leaded apron and thyrocervical shield.

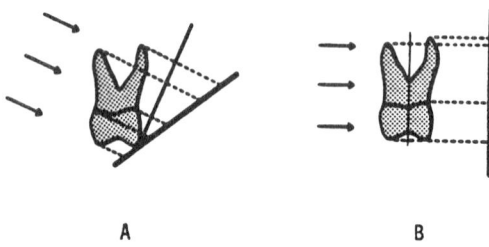

Figure 7-17. Diagram of bisecting and paralleling technics. **(A)** Bisecting principle. **(B)** Paralleling principle.

holder. In the paralleling technic, place the film parallel to the long axis of the teeth; in the bisecting angle technic, place the film against the teeth and dental arch to be included in the projection (Fig. 7-17).

7. Align the cone (circular or rectangular) for the desired vertical angulation of the X-Ray beam. In the paralleling technic, direct the X-Ray beam at right angles to the film surface; in the bisecting angle technic, direct the X-Ray beam at an imaginary line bisecting the angle formed by the intersection of the plane of the tooth and the film (Fig. 7-17).
8. Align the cone (circular or rectangular) for the desired horizontal angulation of the beam as determined by the film position and the anatomy of the teeth to be radiographed.
9. Check to determine whether the cone of radiation covers the film packet. The **point of entry** of the X-Ray beam on the surface of the face is determined by the film position and anatomical area of interest.
10. Proceed to an area outside the exposure of primary and secondary radiation (see Chapter 6 on Radiation Protection).
11. Quickly check the exposure conditions again (X-Ray panel, patient, film placement, cone position, and apron) and make necessary adjustments. Tell patient to remain motionless.
12. Push exposure button. Keep pressure on exposure button until audible or light signal ceases.
13. Remove film from patient's mouth and dry film with paper towel.
14. Keep exposed and unexposed films separate from each other to prevent double exposures.
15. If a complete mouth radiographic survey (CMX) is to be taken, a regular sequence should be followed. Some operators like to take the anterior projections first because they cause less discomfort to the patient. After finishing with an X-Ray procedure, move the X-Ray tube out of the way, and remove leaded apron and cervical shield from patient.
16. Process the film or films, and retake films as required.

Periapical Radiography

There are two intraoral periapical techniques that are employed in periapical radiography to minimize shape distortion of the radiographic image: the **paralleling** technic and the **bisecting angle** technic. The **paralleling** technic is prefered because it produces a more accurate and less distorted radiographic image than the **bisecting** angle technic. However, there are advantages and disadvantages to both techniques and there are anatomic variations from patient to patient or within the oral cavity of the same patient that present circumstances for modification of the projection technique used by the operator.

Paralleling or Right Angle Technic

The paralleling or right intraoral radiographic technic is based upon the paralleling principle. The paralleling principle in essence follows the five rules of accurate image formation (discussed in Chapter 4) to minimize the undesirable image characteristics of **unsharpness, magnification**, and **shape distortion** (Fig. 7-18).

Basically the **two** fundamental rules for the paralleling technic are these:

1. The film is placed in the mouth in a position that is parallel to the long axes of the teeth.
2. The central ray of the X-Ray beam is directed perpendicular or at right angles to both the long axes of the teeth and the plane of the film.

In order to achieve parallelism between the film and the long axes of the teeth, the object-film distance will have to be increased (especially in the maxillary arch). Of course, this goes against one of the five rules of accurate image formation, which states: "The film must be as

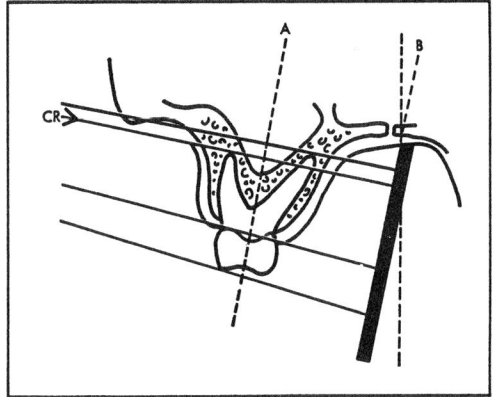

Figure 7-18. Diagram of paralleling technique. Diagram illustrating the relationship of the film and teeth in the paralleling (right angle) technique.

close to the object as possible." Therefore, to compensate for the undesirable image characteristics of geometric unsharpness and magnification caused by this procedure, the source-film distance is **increased**. This is probably why this technic has been referred to as the "long cone" technic in the past, but in reality this is a misnomer because the extension cone is not the basis of the technic; it is only a secondary feature of the technic. Source-film distances of 18 and 20 inches have been used in the past, but the source-film distance of **16 inches** seems to be the most practical distance to be used in most dental offices.

Film Holders

As you may suspect, the most common problem experienced in the past with the paralleling technic has been the proper retention and placement of the film packet in the mouth. The film must be placed as nearly parallel to the long axes of the teeth as possible, maintaining a flat plane at all times, and retaining the film in position until it is properly exposed. Various film holders have been designed to overcome

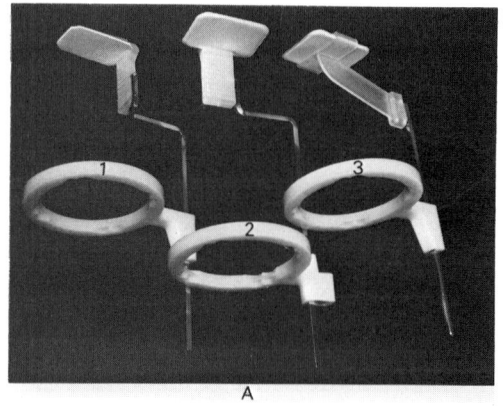

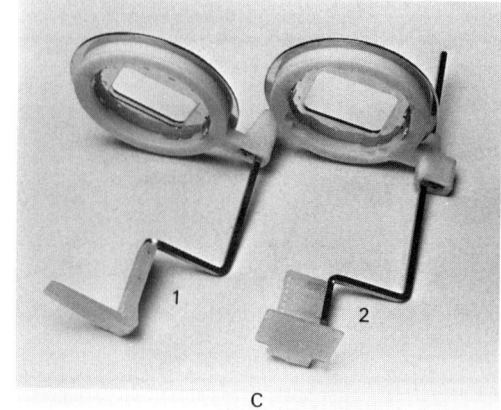

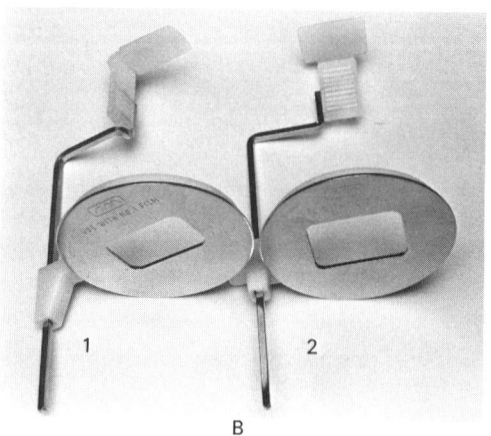

Figure 7-19. The Rinn XCP Instruments. (A) (#1) Anterior, (#2) posterior, (#3) bite-wing instruments assembled. (B) Stainless teel collimator attachment (#1) anterior instrument, (#2) posterior instrument. (C) Stainless steel collimator attachment (posterior view).

these problems associated with film retention and alignment:

1. the *XCP* instruments (Rinn) (Extension Cone Paralleling) (Fig. 7-19);
2. the *Precision* (Masel Corp.) rectangular collimating instruments, which restrict the beam size at the patient's face (Fig. 7-20);
3. the *Stabe* disposable film holder (Greene Corp) (Fig. 7-21);
4. the *VIP* film holder (UP-Rad Corp) (Fig. 7-22);
5. the *Snap-A-Ray* film holder (Ada Corp) and *EEZEE Grip* Film Holder (Rinn) (Fig. 7-23);
6. the *Fitzgerald* paralleling instruments, using hemostat and bite-blocks (Fig. 7-24); and
7. the *Uni-Bite* film holder (Rinn Corp) (Fig. 7-25).

The first two instruments (Rinn XCP and Masel Precision) have an added benefit in radiation reduction to patient by **rectangular collimation** (*see* Fig. 7-26). Of course, the Rinn XCP instruments must be used with a rectangular B.I.D. (Beam Indicating Device) for this to occur. However, a special stainless steel collimator may be purchased for the XCP alignment ring, which will provide rectangular collimation (Fig. 7-19 B, C). The Masel Precision instrument collimates the X-Ray beam at the skin surface (Fig. 7-20).

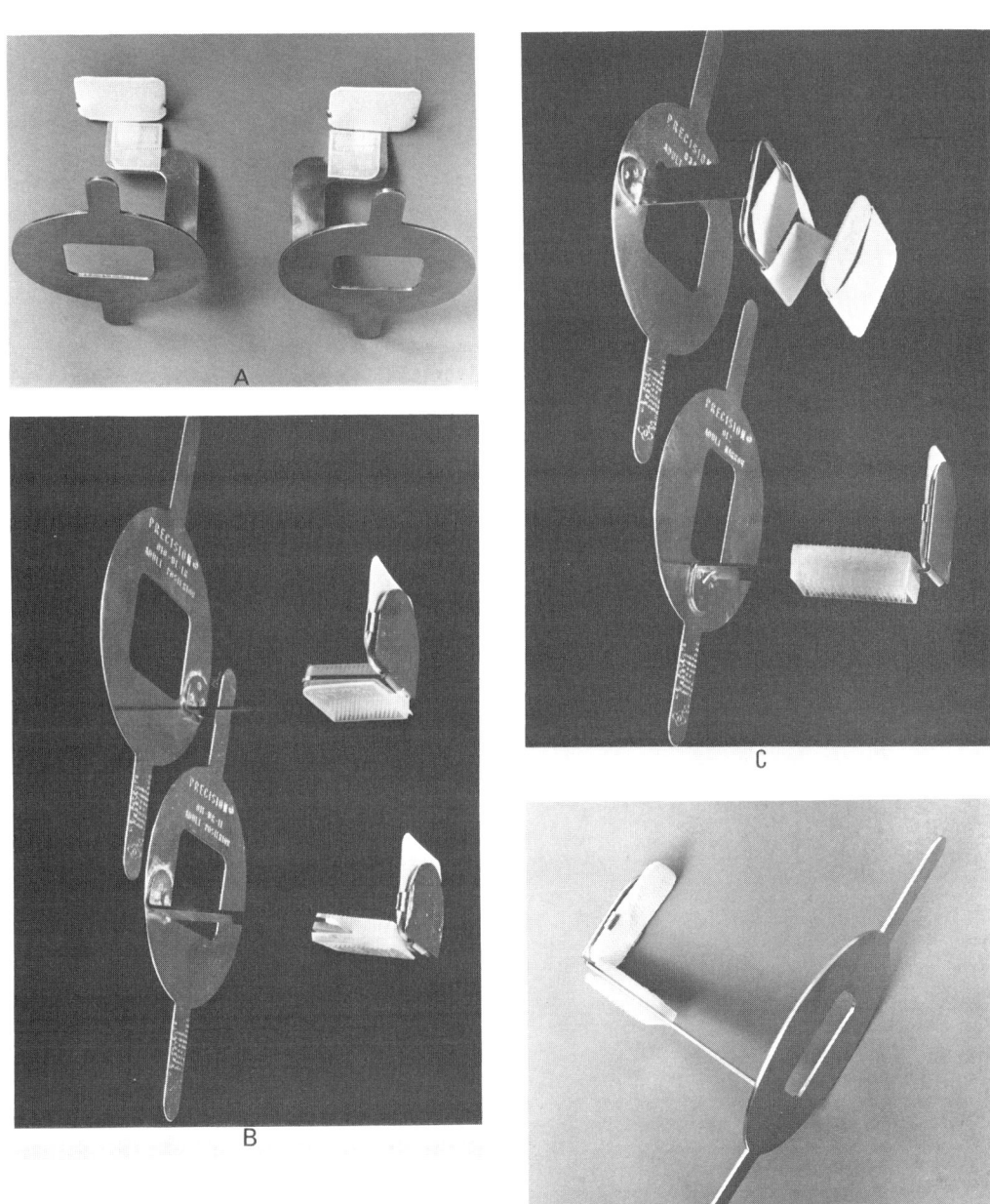

Figure 7-20. Precision film Holders (Masel). **(A)** Posterior instruments, front view. **(B)** Posterior instruments, back view. **(C)** (Top) bite-wing instrument; (bottom) anterior instrument. **(D)** Anterior instrument, oblique view. **(E)** Demonstrates the use of anterior precision instrument in maxillary anterior region. **(F)** Demonstrates the use of the posterior precision instrument in posterior maxillary region. **(G)** Demonstrates use of PBW precision instrument.

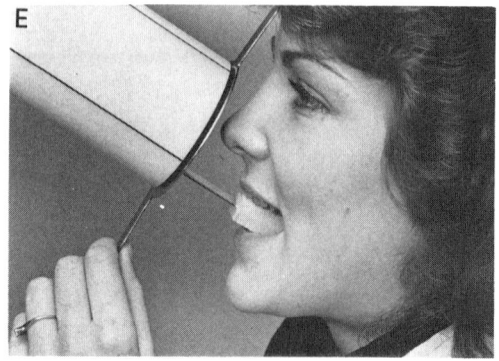
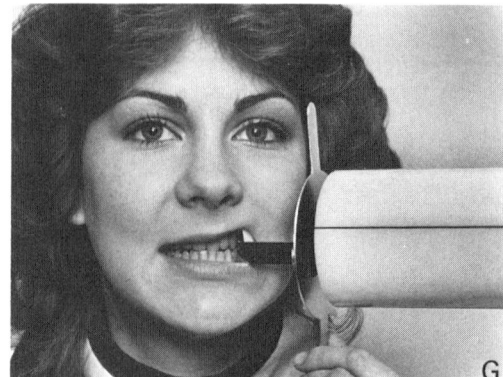
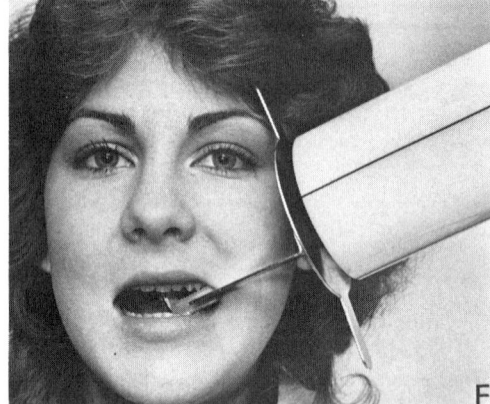

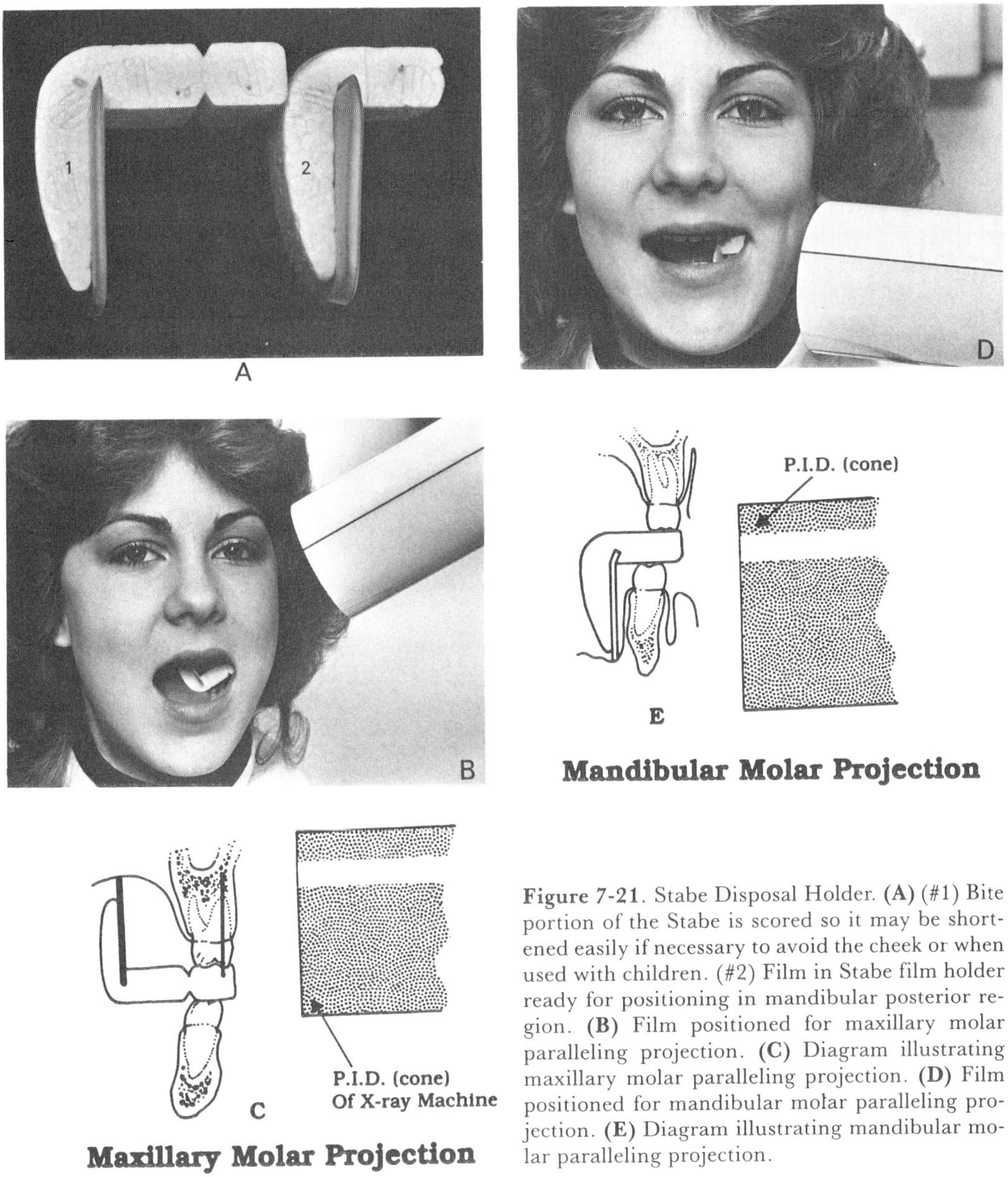

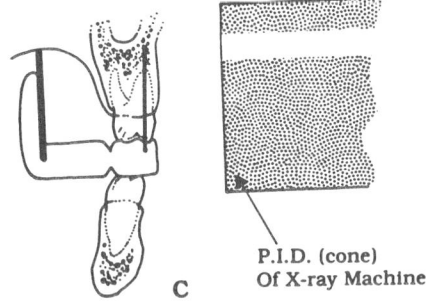

Mandibular Molar Projection

Maxillary Molar Projection

Figure 7-21. Stabe Disposal Holder. (**A**) (#1) Bite portion of the Stabe is scored so it may be shortened easily if necessary to avoid the cheek or when used with children. (#2) Film in Stabe film holder ready for positioning in mandibular posterior region. (**B**) Film positioned for maxillary molar paralleling projection. (**C**) Diagram illustrating maxillary molar paralleling projection. (**D**) Film positioned for mandibular molar paralleling projection. (**E**) Diagram illustrating mandibular molar paralleling projection.

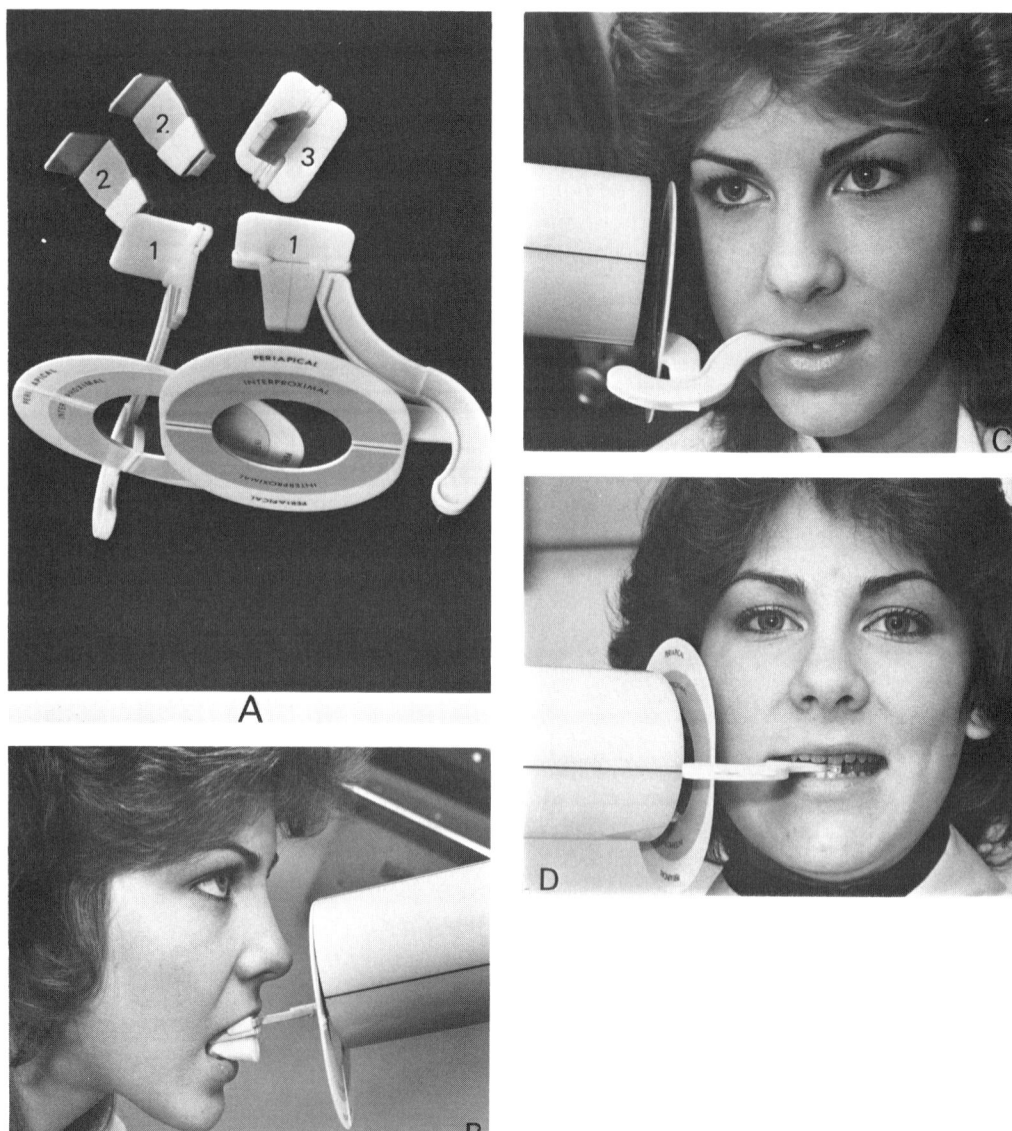

Figure 7-22. VIP (UpRad) Film Holders. **(A)** (#1) Posterior assembled instruments using the versatile (white) film holder, which has metal backing plates to prevent film bending. The versatile film holders are used in special cases, such as low palates, shallow mandibular sulci, children, edentulous, and bite wings. Films can be adjusted vertically to accommodate areas requiring less film coverage. (#2) All purpose (blue) film holder, which will accommodate all sizes of film positioned vertically or horizontally, making it possible to take all exposures with one film holder. NOTE built-in backing support to prevent film bending. Backing on right has been cut down to accommodate No. 1 film horizontally for child. Also, notice attached bite pads, which are used on the film holders for patient comfort and film stability. (#3) Versatile film holder assembled for No. 2 film horizontal bite-wing radiography. (Two other Versatile film holders are available for vertical bite-wing radiography using No. 1 and No. 2 film). **(B)** Maxillary anterior projection using VIP system. **(C)** Maxillary posterior projection using VIP system. **(D)** Posterior horizontal bite-wing projection using VIP system.

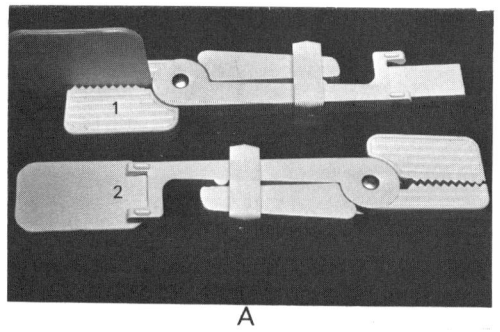
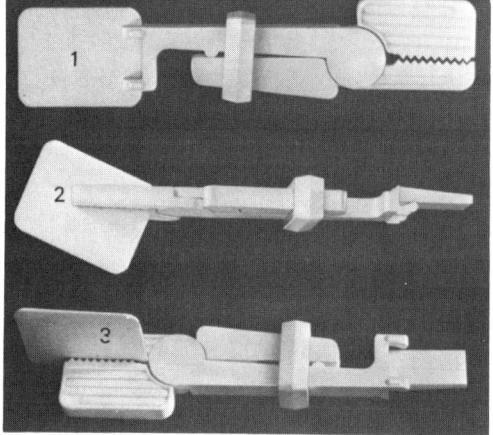
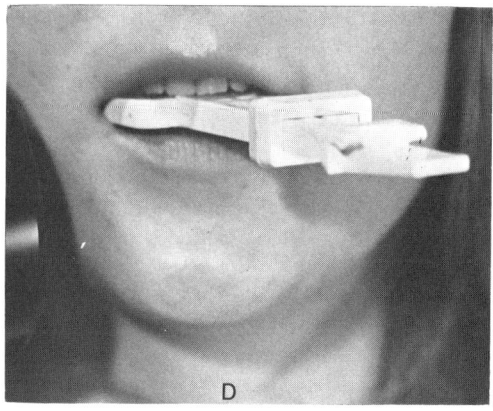
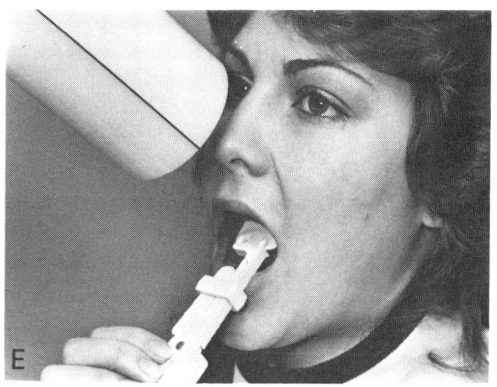
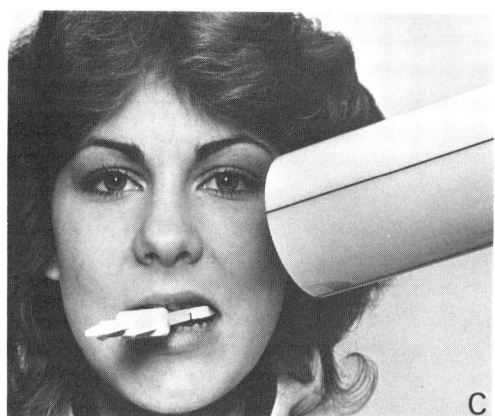

Figure 7-23. (A) Ada Snap-A-Ray (#1) Posterior projection (#2) Anterior projection (B) Rinn EEZEE Grip - (#1) anterior projection; (#2) mandibular third molar projection; (#3) posterior projection. (C) Maxillary posterior projection (Ada Snap-A-Ray). (D) Mandibular posterior projection, Rinn EEZEE Grip. (E) Maxillary anterior, Ada Snap-A-Ray.

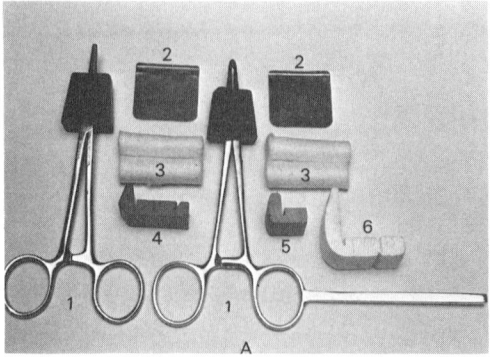
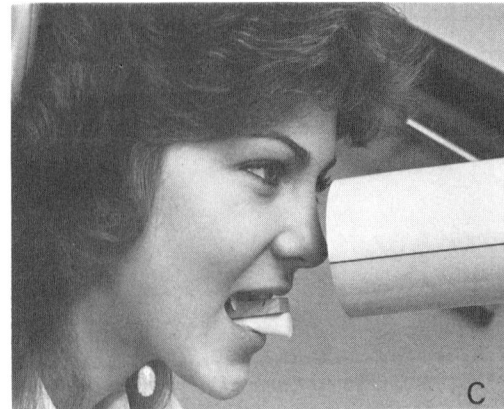
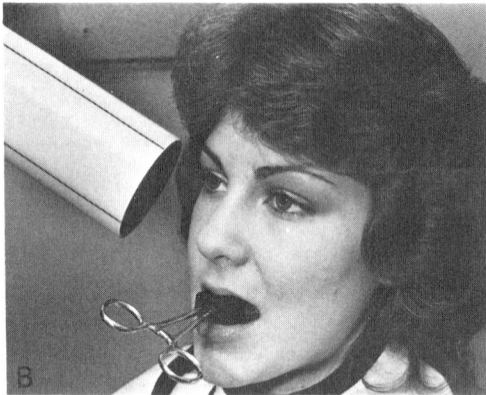

Figure 7-24. (A) Fitzgerald paralleling instruments: (#1) hemostats, (#2) metal backings, (#3) cotton rolls, (#4) anterior and (#5) posterior wooden bite blocks, and (#6) Stabe film holder. (B) Fitzgerald hemostat, posterior projection. (C) Fitzgerald wooden bite-block, anterior projection.

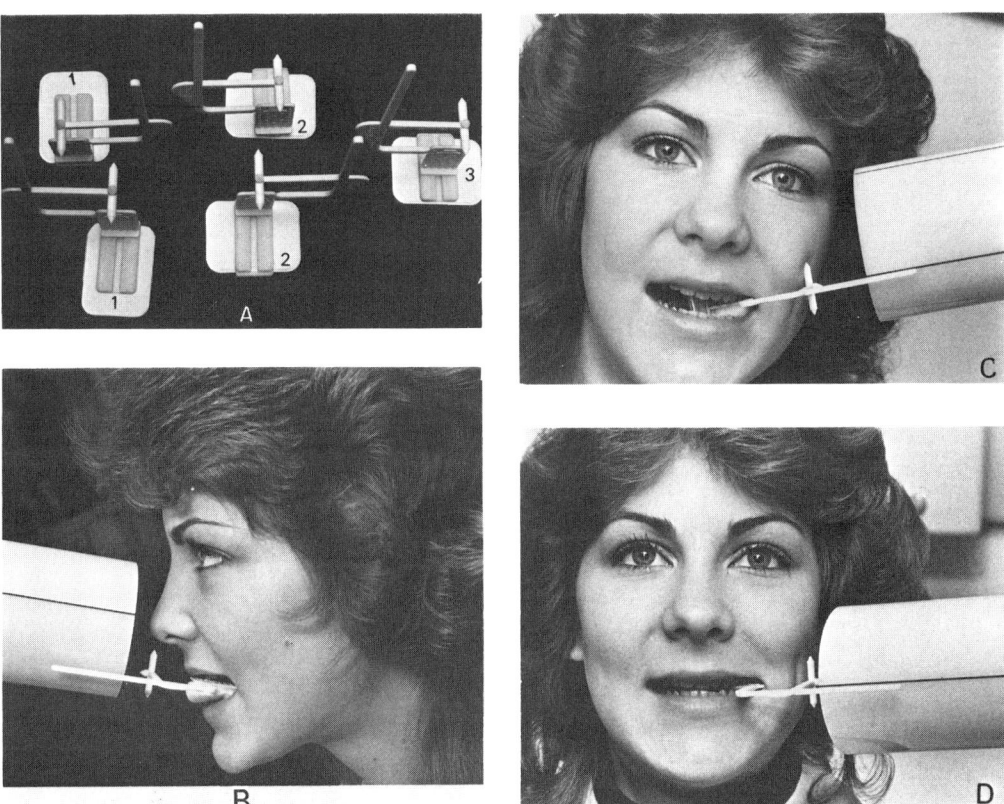

Figure 7-25. Rinn Unibite Film Holder. **(A)** Universal film holder, the sliding film carrier is adjustable to accommodate exposures of maxillary as well as mandibular teeth, posterior as well as anterior teeth, periapicals as well as bite-wings. (#1) anterior; (#2) posterior; (#3) bite-wing. **(B)** Maxillary anterior, Unibite projection. **(C)** Maxilary posterior, Unibite projection. **(D)** Bite-wing Unibite projection.

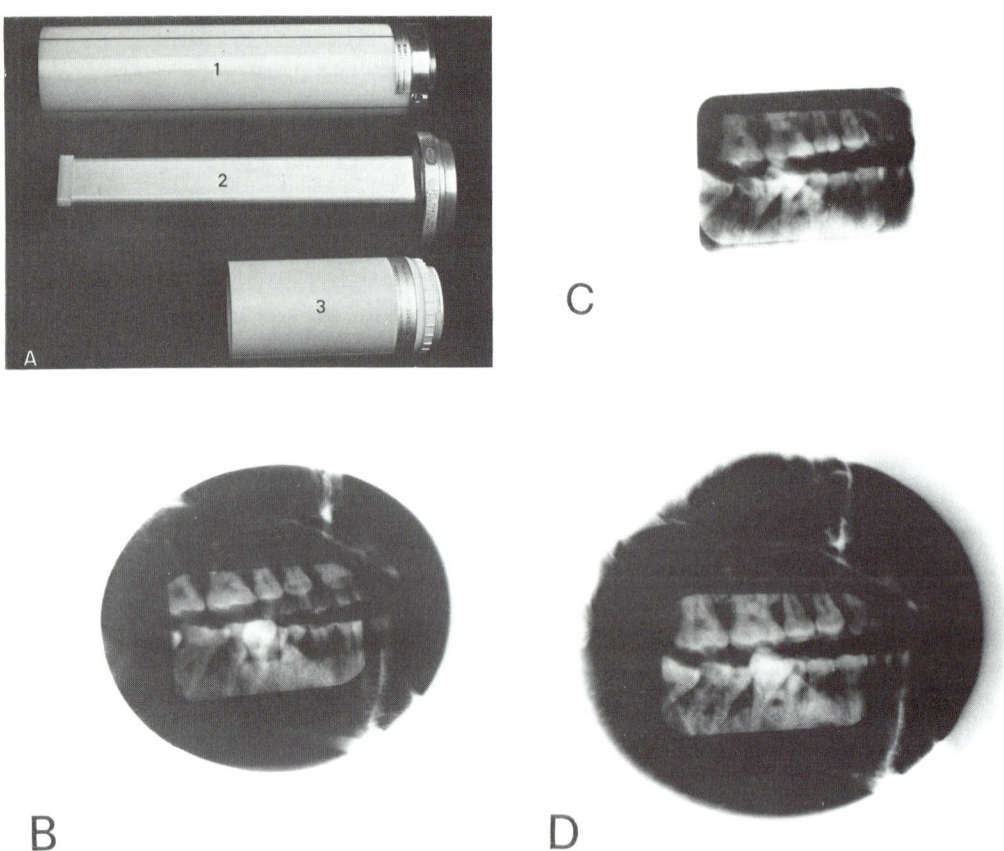

Figure 7-26. (**A**) Three types of cones or B.I.D.s. 1, long round cone; 2, long rectangular cone; 3, short round cone. (**B**) Exit radiation dose, long round cone. (**C**) Exit radiation dose, long rectangular B.I.C. or P.I.D. (**D**) Exit radiation dose, short round cone. Notice the exit dose is much smaller by using the long rectangular B.I.D.

Parallelling or Right Angle Technic Mount

A typical complete mouth radiographic survey using the paralleling technic consists of sixteen periapical projections and four bitewing projections (Fig. 7-27):

Six Rules to Follow in Paralleling Technic

The first three of the rules have to do with *placement of the film* in the patient's mouth, and the last three rules have to do with *positioning* the beam "cone" or P.I.D. or B.I.D. (Positioning or Beam Indicating Device).

Rule Number One: Place the film so that it covers the prescribed teeth to be examined for each region of the oral cavity. Each specific region of the CMX should inlcude the specific areas.

MAXILLARY MOLAR REGION: All crowns and roots of the maxillary third molar or tuberosity, second and first molar including the apices are fully depicted together with the interproximal alveolar crests, contact areas, and surrounding

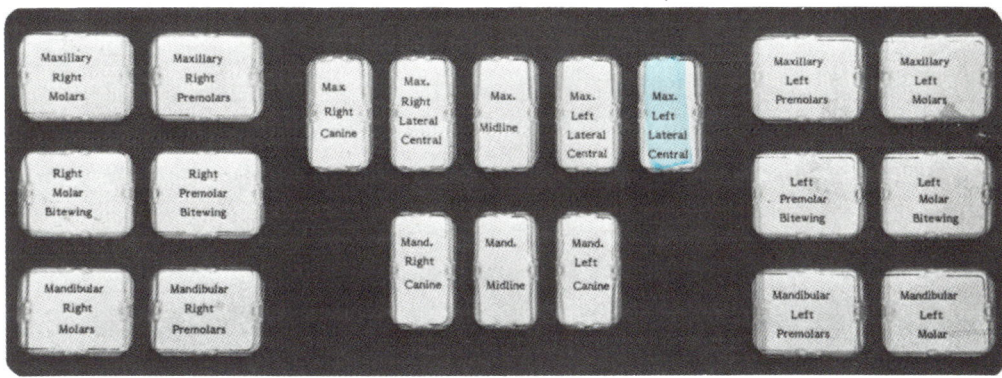

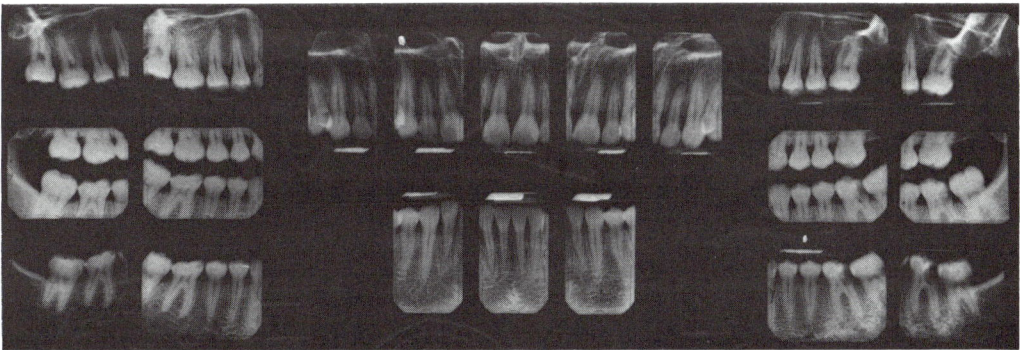

Figure 7-27. **(A)** Typical complete radiographic survey using the paralleling technique. (Note that the No. 1 narrow film is used in anterior.) **(B)** Typical CMX (8 posterior films, 8 anterior films, and 4 posterior bite-wings).

bone regions. There is no superimposition of the zygomatic bone over the roots (Fig. 7-28).

MAXILLARY PREMOLAR REGION: All crowns and roots of the maxillary premolars and first molars, including the apices, are fully depicted together with interproximal alveolar crests, contact areas, and surrounding bone. In the maxillary premolar projection, the **distal** surface of the canine must be seen (Fig. 7-29).

MAXILLARY CANINE REGION: All of the crown and root of the maxillary canine, including the apex, is fully depicted together with the interproximal alveolar crest between the maxillary canine and ther maxillary lateral incisor, the contact area, and surrounding bone region. The distal surface of the maxillary lateral inci-

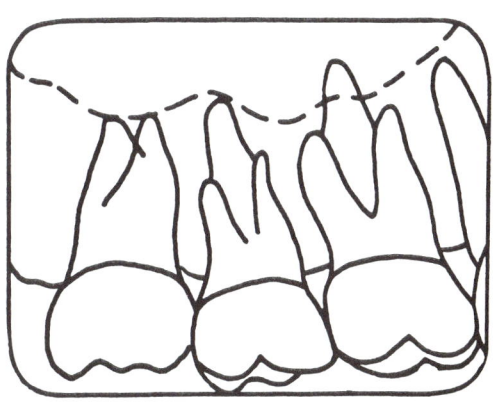

Figure 7-28. Maxillary molars.

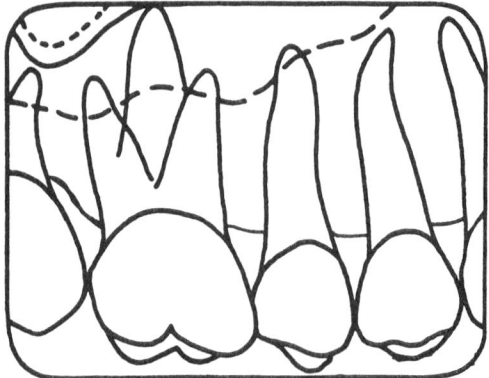

Figure 7-29. Maxillary premolars.

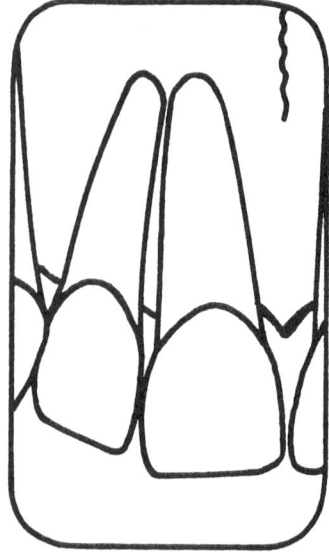

Figure 7-31. Maxillary central lateral incisors.

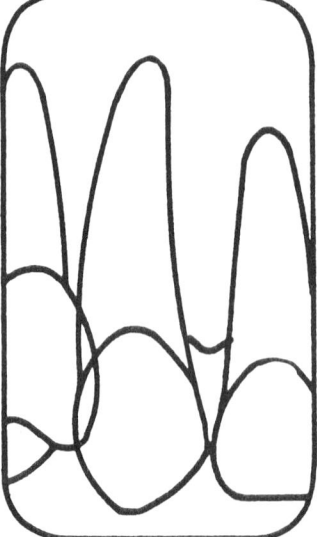

Figure 7-30. Maxillary canine.

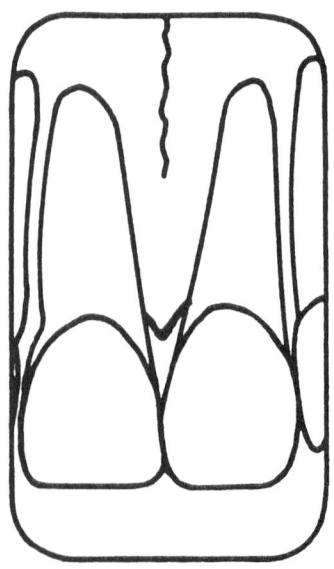

Figure 7-32. Maxillary midline area.

sor should be seen but it is not necessary for the distal surface of the maxillary canine to be seen. Usually the lingual cusp of the first premolar is **superimposed** over the distal surface of canine in this projection (Fig. 7-30).

MAXILLARY LATERAL INCISOR REGION: All of the crown and root of the maxillary lateral incisor, including the apex, is fully depicted together with the interproximal alveolar crests between the adjacent maxillary central incisor and maxillary canine, the contact areas, and the surrounding bone regions. The distal surface of the adjacent maxillary central incisor and the mesial surface of the maxillary canine should be seen on this projection (Fig. 7-31).

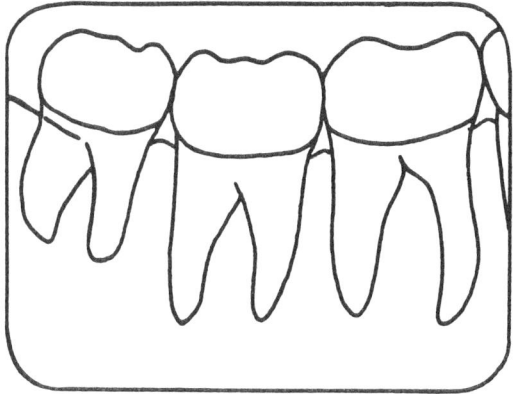

Figure 7-33. Mandibular molars.

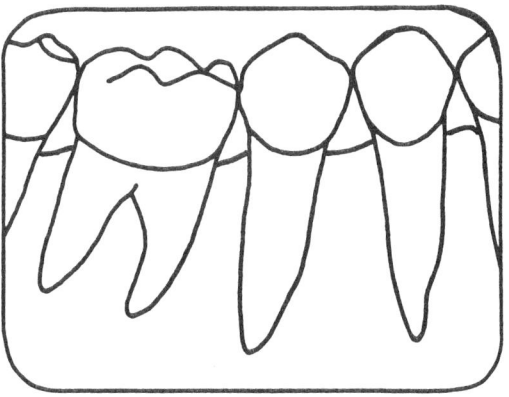

Figure 7-34. Mandibular premolars.

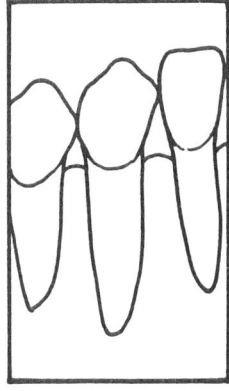

Figure 7-35. Mandibular canine region.

MAXILLARY MIDLINE REGION: All crowns and roots, including apices, of the maxillary central incisors are fully depicted together with interproximal alveolar crests, contact areas, and surrounding bone regions (Fig. 7-32).

MAXILLARY MOLAR REGION: All crowns and roots, including apices of all three mandibular molars, are fully depicted together with interproximal alveolar crests, contact areas, and surrounding bone regions (Fig. 7-33).

MANDIBULAR PREMOLAR REGION: All the crowns of the mandibular premolars, including the apices, are fully depicted together with interproximal alveolar crests, contact areas, and surrounding bone regions. The distal surface of the canine should be seen in this projection (Fig. 7-34).

MANDIBULAR CANINE REGION: All of the crown and the root of the mandibular canine, including the apex, is fully depicted together with the interproximal alveolar crests and contact area between the maxillary lateral incisor and mandibular canine, and surrounding bone region. The distal surface of the mandibular lateral incisor should be seen; however, it is not necessary for the distal surface of the mandibular canine to be seen (Fig. 7-35).

MANDIBULAR MIDLINE REGION: All crowns and roots, including apices of the central and lateral incisors, are fully depicted together with interproximal alveolar crests, contact areas, and surrounding bone regions. In most cases, it is not necessary to see the distal surfaces of the mandibular lateral incisors (Fig. 7-36).

PREMOLAR POSTERIOR BITE-WINGS: All crowns of the maxillary and mandibular premolars are fully depicted together with the interproximal crests and contact areas. The distal surfaces of the maxillary and mandibular canines are seen. The

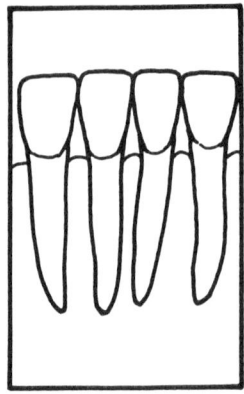

Figure 7-36. Mandibular midline region.

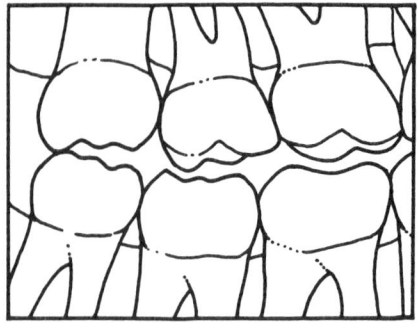

Figure 7-38. Molar bite-wing.

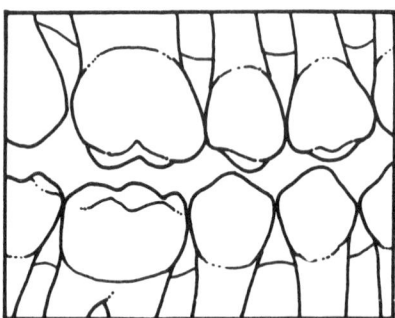

Figure 7-37. Premolar bite-wing.

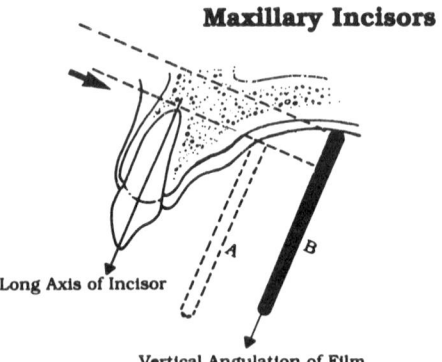

Figure 7-39. Maxillary incisor film vertical angulation: The angulation of tooth apices will not show in the radiograph when the film packet is placed in *A* position; with an increased object-film distance as shown in the *B* position, it is possible to demonstrate the apices of the teeth and structures beyond.

images are without overlapping where anatomically possible. (Fig. 7-37)

MOLAR POSTERIOR BITE-WING: All crowns of the maxillary and mandibular molars are fully depicted together with the interproximal crests and contact areas. It is preferable to see the distal surfaces of the maxillary and mandibular second premolar teeth. The images are without overlapping where anatomically possible (Fig. 7-38).

Rule Number Two: Position the vertical plane of the film parallel to the long axes of the teeth being radiographed. In the maxillary arch, because of the slight facial outward inclination of the long axes of the teeth, it is necessary to increase the tooth-film distance in order to achieve parallelism (Figs. 7-39 and 7-40). When the film is positioned parallel to the long axis of the posterior maxillary teeth (usually a vertical angle of 6-22 degrees from the mid-sagittal plane), the tissue edge of the film packet is beyond the median palatal suture line away from the teeth being radiographed. The film placement is altered when a low, flat palate is present. Fortunately, many low palatal

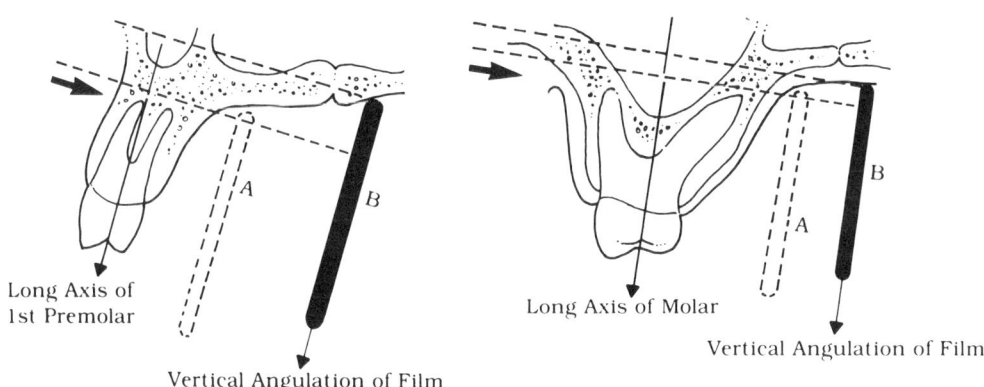

Figure 7-40. Maxillary premolar and molar film vertical angulation: increasing the object-film position from A to B, the film can be positioned vertically to approach parallelism between long axis of tooth and vertical plane of film and prevent the apices of the teeth from being cut-off.

vaults are also wider laterally, making it possible to obtain good results by shifting the film packet even farther across the mouth, away from the teeth being radiographed.

In the **mandibular posterior** region, the mandibular premolars are usually positioned nearly parallel to the midsagittal plane (positioned straight up and down) and the mandibular molars tilt slightly inward toward the midsagittal plane. Therefore, the film packet in the mandibular posterior region can be positioned close to the dental alveolar ridge and remain parallel vertically to the long axis of the teeth (Fig. 7-41).

In the mandibular incisor region, because of the outward vertical inclination of the teeth, the film is required to be placed well back in the mouth under the

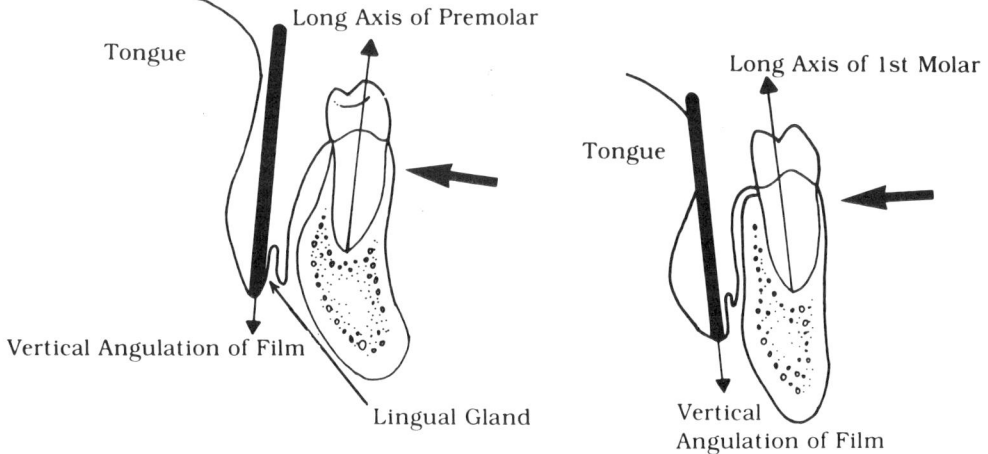

Figure 7-41. Vertical angulation of film in mandibular posterior region.

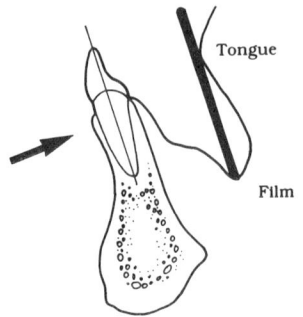

Mandibular Incisor

Figure 7-42. Vertical angulation of film in mandibular incisor region.

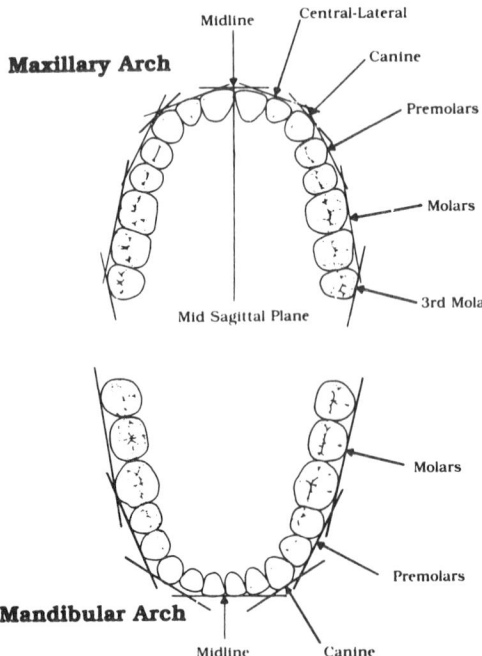

Figure 7-43. Maxillary and Mandibular mean tangents.

tongue to achieve parallelism of the vertical plane of the film packet with the long axes of the incisor teeth (Fig. 7-42).

Rule Number Three: Horizontal placement of film behind teeth to be radiographed. The correct horizontal position of the film in relation to the teeth is different in various regions of the oral cavity because the teeth form a curved arch and all the teeth will not have the same tangent. In this instance, the mean tangent plane is defined as the plane joining the most exterior points of the curved facial surfaces of teeth in a particular region of the oral cavity. It is easily seen that the mean tangent of the premolar teeth is not quite the same as that of the molars, and the tangent of the canine and the incisors is not the same as that of the premolars (Fig. 7-43). Naturally, the horizontal placement of the film packet, in most cases, must be parallel to the mean tangents. There are **two exceptions**—the maxillary molar and mandibular molar regions. In these regions, first place the film packet parallel to the mean tangent of the molars and then move the anterior edge of the film 15-20 degrees toward the other side of the arch. If this is not done, the embrasures between the molars will be opened in a majority of the projections taken (Fig. 7-44).

Rule Number Four: Vertical angulation of cone or P.I.D. Align the cone or P.I.D. surface parallel to the film packet or direct the X-Ray beam perpendicular to the plane of the long axis of the teeth and film packet. The proper vertical angulation of the cone will help minimize shape distortion of the resultant radiographic image produced on the radiograph (Fig. 7-45).

Rule Number Five: Horizontal angulation of X-Ray tube. Direct the X-Rays through the embrasures between the teeth. If this is not done correctly, the interproximal surface of the teeth will be overlapped (*see* Fig. 7-14).

After the films have been placed horizontally correctly (Fig. 7-44) the horizontal angulation of the films is easily determined by paralleling the outer surface of the cone or P.I.D. with the horizontal film plane or directing the X-Ray beam perpendicular to the film (Fig. 7-46).

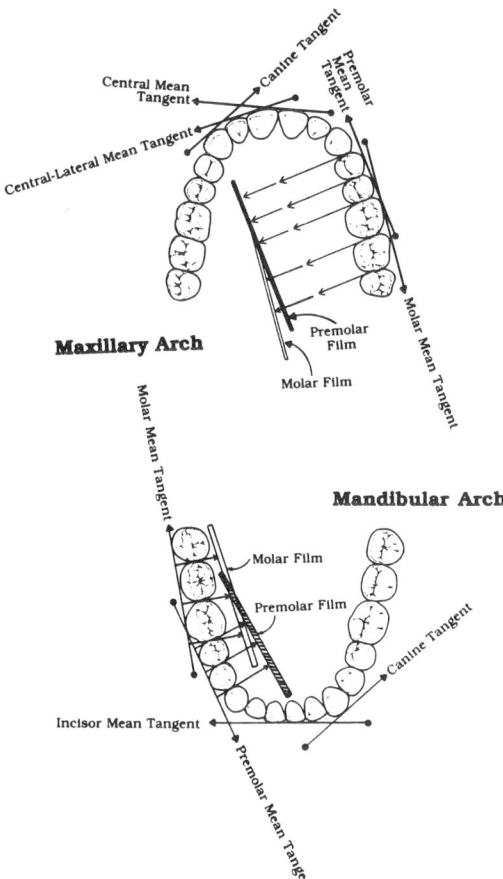

Figure 7-44. Proper horizontal placement of films in molar regions. Anterior edge of film placed 15-20° toward other side of arch.

Rule Number Six: Center the X-Ray beam on the film and be sure to cover the film packet completely with the X-Ray beam (Fig. 7-46). Failure to do this will cause "cone-cutting" or a partial image on the radiograph (*see* Fig. 7-15).

Procedure for Using Paralleling Technique Utilizing the Rinn XCP Instruments and Rectangular P.I.D. (B.I.D.)

The following is a procedure to be followed to take a complete radiographic series using the paralleling technique utilizing the Rinn XCP instruments. The

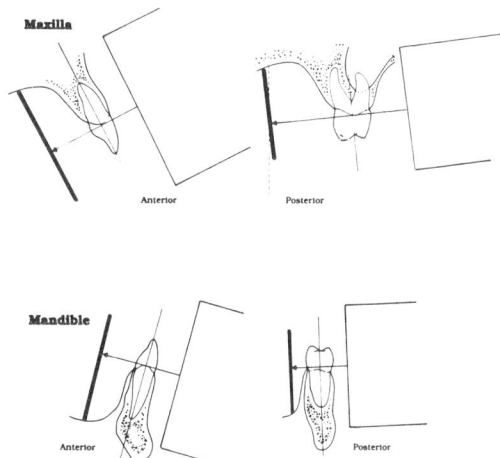

Figure 7-45. Proper vertical angulation of cone (P.I.D.)

same principles illustrated may be applied to the other film holders listed. A rectangular (P.I.D.) collimating device is used because it reduces the integral absorbed dose to patient by approximately one-half to two-thirds (Fig. 7-26).

A routine sequence of taking radiographs for a CMX (complete mouth survey of X-Rays) should be decided upon by the operator. This will save time and make sure that all the radiographs are taken without overlooking some of the projections. Some persons like to start in the upper right, proceed around to upper left, then down to the lower left, and end the procedure in the lower right quadrant. This is all right if the patient is cooperative; however, to start with the maxillary molar projection sometimes will cause the patient to gag prematurely, and subsequently cause the patient to lose confidence in the operator at the beginning of the procedure.

Rinn XCP Instruments (Extension Cone Paralleling) Film holding instruments such as the Rinn XCP instruments provide an external guide for positioning of the cone vertically and horizontally, as well as automatically establishing the

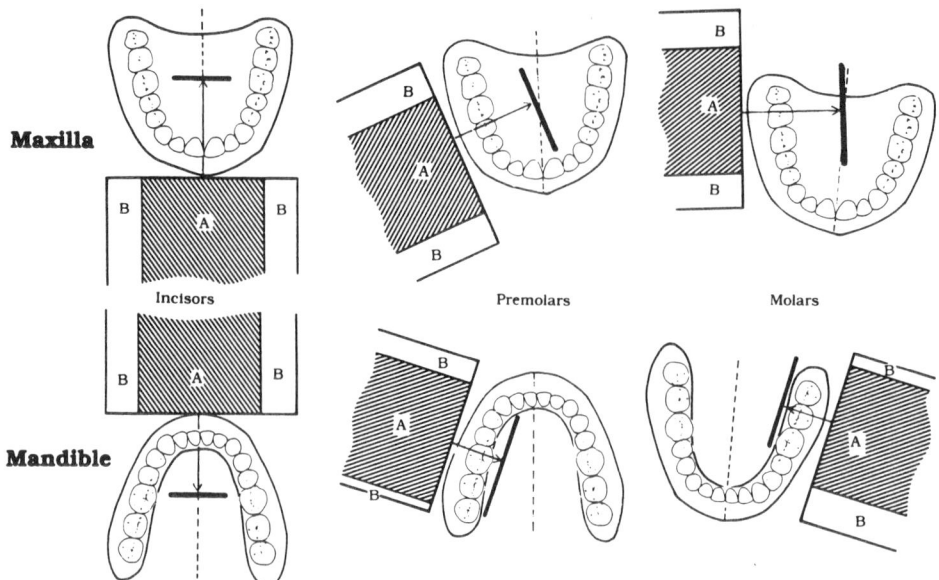

Figure 7-46. Proper horizontal angulation of P.I.D. and film coverage with X-Ray beam. A, size of smaller rectangular P.I.D. (cone); B, size of larger circular P.I.D. (cone).

point of entry of the X-Ray beam (*see* Fig. 7-19).

The Rinn XCP instruments were designed by Dr. William Updegrave, Professor Emeritus of the School of Dentistry, Temple University at Philadelphia. Each instrument consists of three parts:

1. *Anterior and posterior plastic bite-blocks*. These are designed to retain the film packet by means of tension created by a semiflexible plastic backing.
2. *Indicator rod*. These are made of stainless steel and are used to align the X-Ray cone with film. There is an anterior offset rod and a posterior right-angle rod designed to insert into the receptacle holes of their respective bite-blocks.
3. *Locator ring*. They are made for sliding on to the rods to establish alignment of the cone with the film. This also prevents "cone cutting."

The Rinn XCP locator ring or aiming device can accept either a round cone or a **rectangular-shaped** extension P.I.D. (Fig. 7-19). To aid in the alignment of the P.I.D. with the locator ring, the P.I.D. can be rotated on its own axis. This modification will simplify P.I.D. and film alignment.

The following is the recommended procedure using the Rinn XCP instruments for each region of the oral cavity.

Maxillary Central Incisor Region

1. Assemble anterior instrument and insert No. 1 film vertically in the anterior bite-block.
2. Center film with maxillary midline, and parallel to long axes of the central incisors. Entire length of block should be utilized to position film in region of the first molar (Fig. 7-47A, B).
3. With block resting on incisal edges of teeth to be radiographed, insert cotton roll between mandibular incisors and block, and instruct the patient to

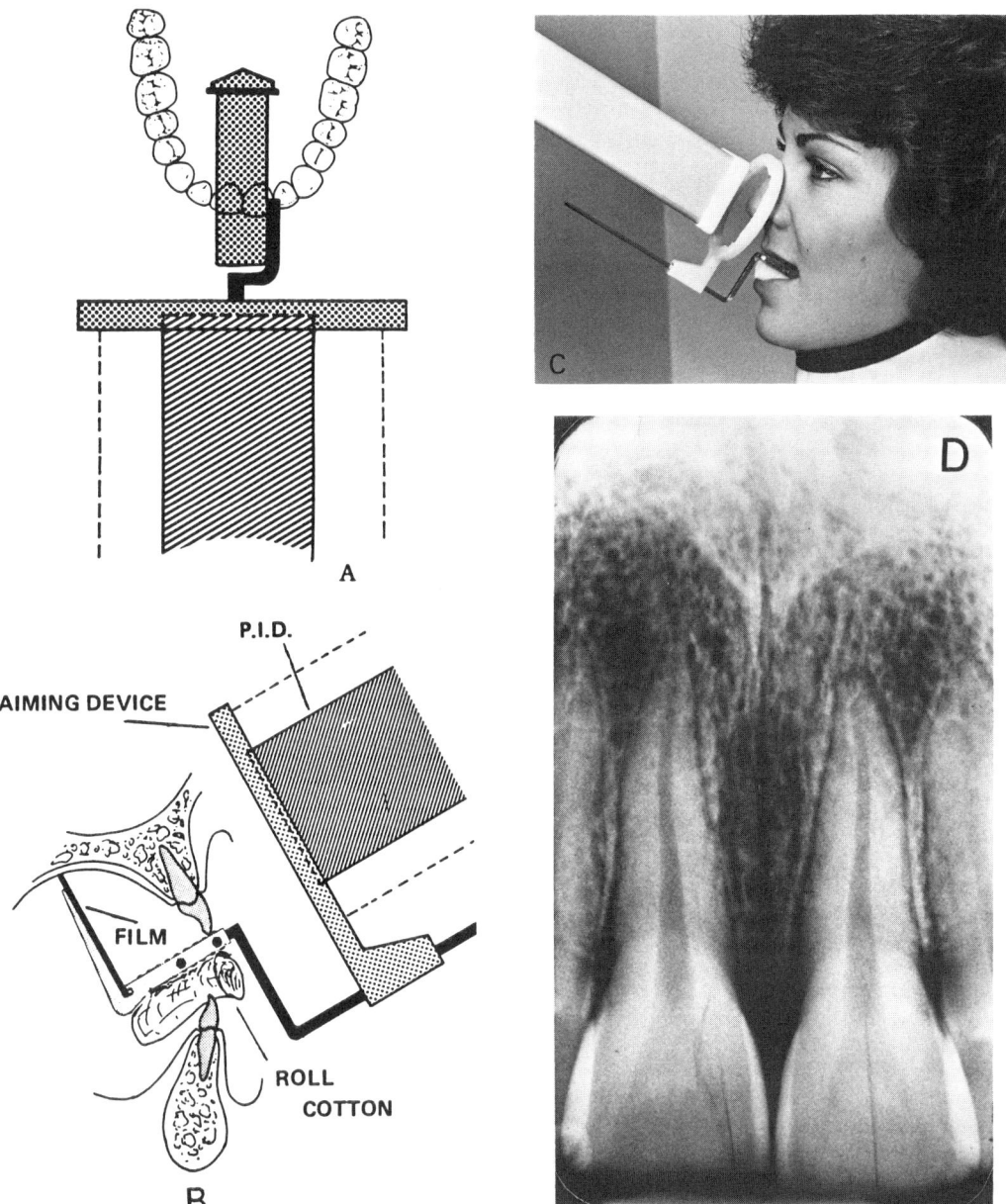

Figure 7-47. Maxillary midline region. **(A)** Horizontal film and P.I.D. placement. **(B)** Vertical film and P.I.D. placement. **(C)** Proper alignment of P.I.D. with Rinn XCP instrument. **(D)** Resultant radiograph.

close firmly to retain established position of film (Fig. 7-47B).
4. Slide the aiming device down the indicator rod to approximate skin surface, and turn P.I.D. vertically. Align P.I.D. with indicator rod and aiming device in both vertical and horizontal planes (Fig. 7-47C).
5. Make exposure (Fig. 7-47D).

Maxillary Lateral Region
1. Assemble anterior instrument and insert No. 1 film vertically in anterior bite-block.
2. Center lateral incisor on film and parallel with long axis of the lateral incisor. Entire length of block should be utilized to position film in region of the first molars.
3. With block resting on incisal edges of teeth to be radiographed, insert cotton roll between mandibular incisors and block, and instruct patient to close firmly to retain established position of film.
4. Slide the aiming device down the indicator rod to approximate skin surface.

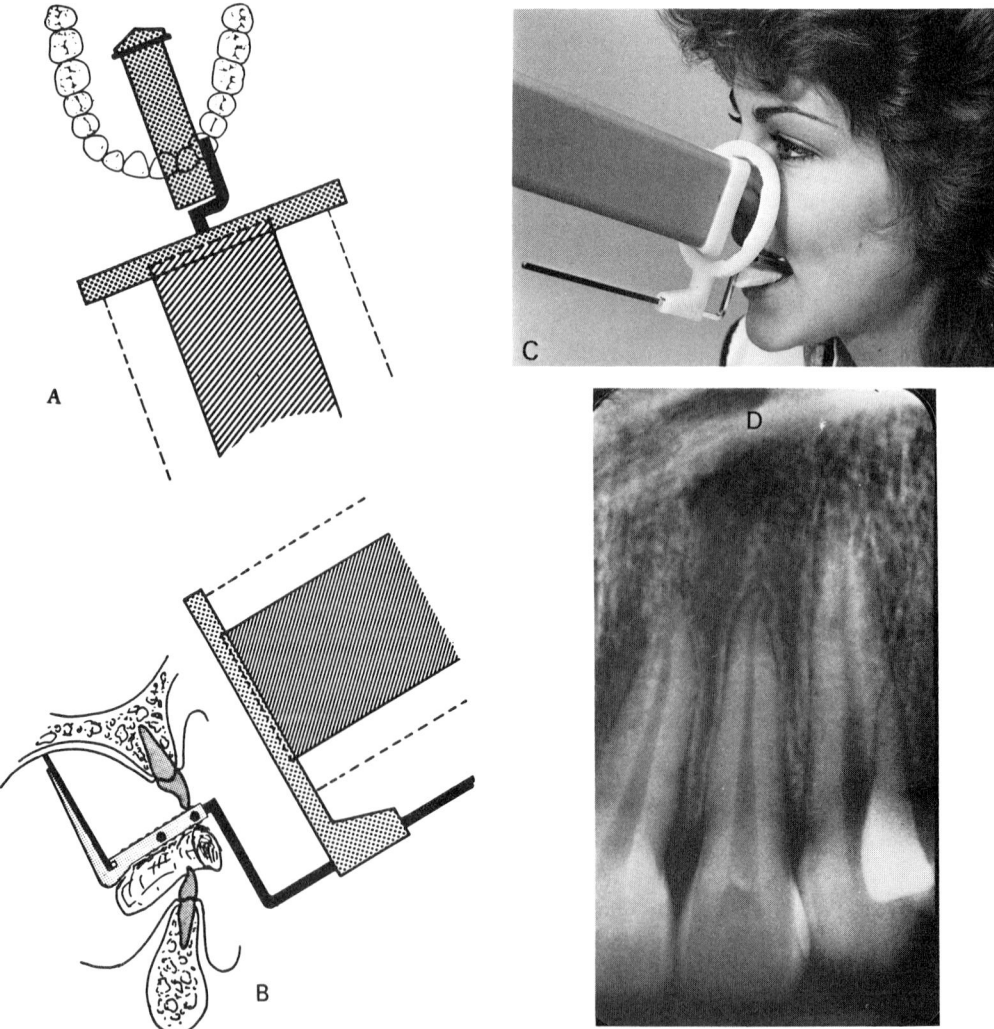

Figure 7-48. (**A**) Horizontal film and P.I.D. placement. (**B**) Vertical film and P.I.D. placement. (**C**) Alilgnment of P.I.D. with XCP instrument. (**D**) Resultant radiograph.

Turn P.I.D. vertically, and align it with indicator rod and aiming device in both vertical and horizontal planes (Fig. 7-48C).
5. Make exposure (Fig. 7-48D).

Maxillary Canine Region
1. Assemble anterior instrument and insert No. 1 film vertically in anterior bite-block.
2. Center canine on film and parallel with long axis of tooth (Fig. 7-49A,B).
3. With block resting on maxillary canine, insert cotton roll between mandibular teeth and block, and instruct patient to close firmly to retain established position of film.
4. Slide aiming device down indicator rod to approximate skin surface. Turn P.I.D. vertically, and align with indicator rod and aiming device in both vertical and horizontal planes (Fig. 7-49C).
5. Make exposure (Fig. 7-49D).

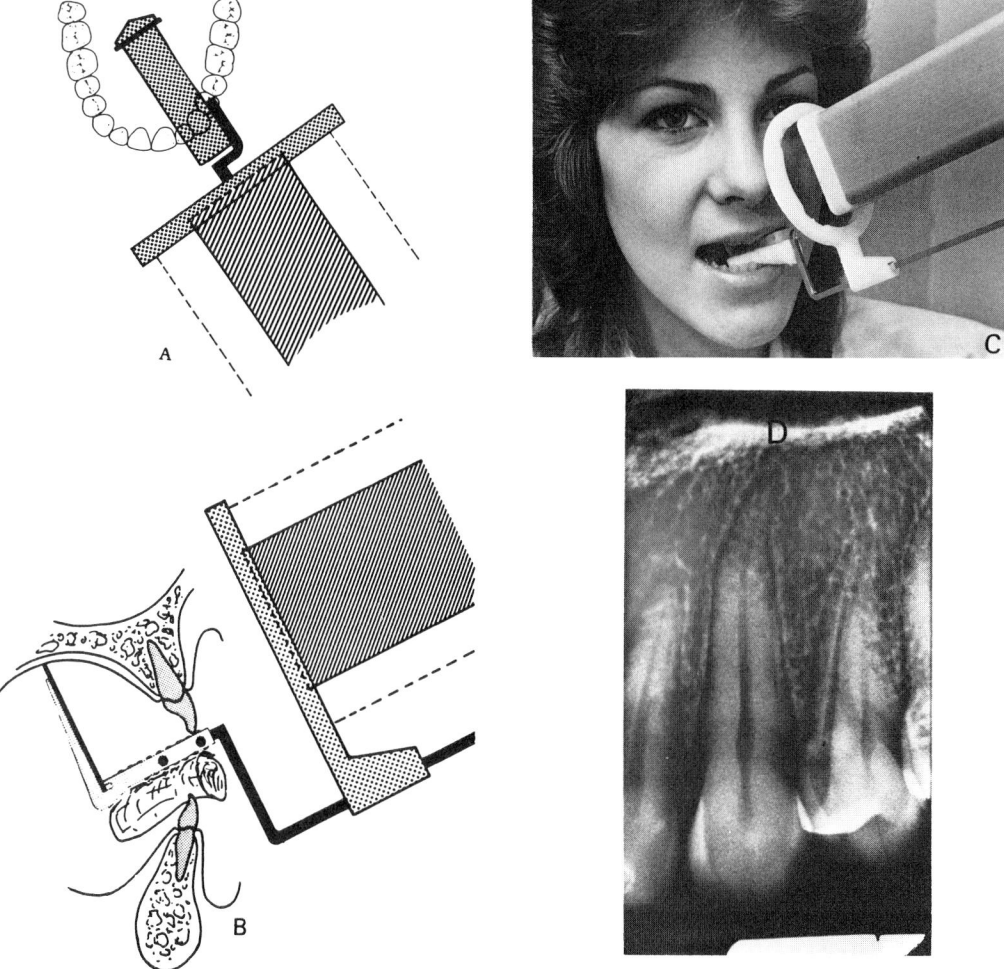

Figure 7-49. Maxillary canine region. **(A)** Horizontal film and P.I.D. placement. **(B)** Vertical film and P.I.D. placement. **(C)** Alignment of P.I.D. with XCP instrument. **(D)** Resultant radiograph.

Maxillary Premolar Region

1. Assemble posterior instrument and insert No. 2 film horizontally in posterior bite-block. Position film holder in mouth with second premolar centered on film (Fig. 7-50A).
2. Parallel film horizontally with mean tangent of the premolars and vertically with long axis of the premolars (Fig. 7-50A,B).
3. With bite-block held against the occlusal surfaces of the premolars and first molar, insert cotton roll between underside of block and mandibular teeth, and instruct patient to close firmly to retain established position of film.
4. Slide aiming device or locator ring down indicator rod to approximate the skin surface (usually takes two hands). Rotate P.I.D. in horizontal position, and align it with both the rod and aiming device in both horizontal and vertical planes (Fig. 7-50C).
5. Make exposure (Fig. 7-50D).

Maxillary Molar Region

1. Assemble posterior instrument, and insert No. 2 film horizontally in posterior bite-block. Position in mouth with anterior edge of film at middle of second premolar, and if need be move film posteriorly to cover the maxillary third molar or maxillary tuberosity if third molar is not visible clinically.
2. Position film at or past midpalatal su-

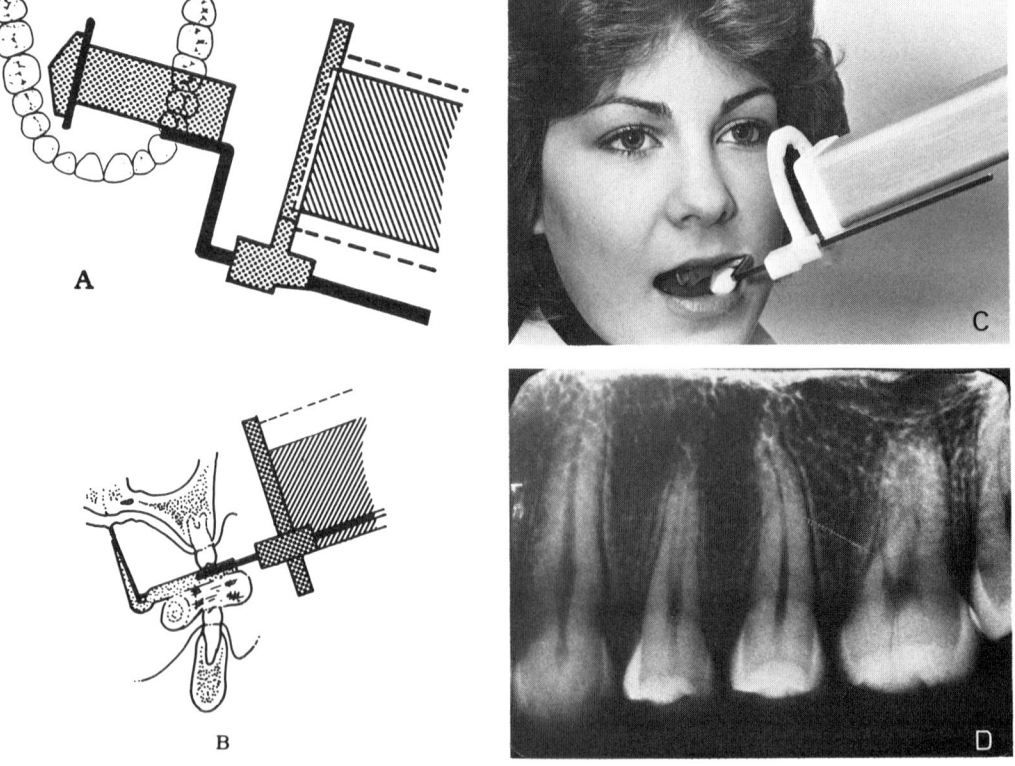

Figure 7-50. Maxillary premolar region. **(A)** Horizontal film and P.I.D. placement. **(B)** Vertical film and P.I.D. placement. **(C)** Alignment of P.I.D. with XCP instrument. **(D)** Resultant radiograph.

ture line and parallel to mean tangent of the molars. Then, move anterior edge of film 15-20 degrees toward other side of arch. (This will assure that you open the embrasure spaces between the molars.) The next step is to make sure the vertical plane of the film is parallel to the long axes of the molars (Fig. 7-51A,B).
3. Slide aiming or locator device down indicator rod (usually takes two hands) to approximate skin surface. Rotate P.I.D. to horizontal position, and align it with both the indicator rod and aiming device on horizontal and vertical planes (Fig. 7-51C).
4. Make exposure (Fig. 7-51D)

Mandibular Incisor Region

1. Assemble anterior instrument, and insert No. 1 film vertically in the anterior bite-block. Procedure is similar to maxillary anterior technic except for the inversion of holder in order to position the film lingual to the mandibular anterior teeth.
2. Center film with midline, parallel with long axes of the central incisors. Lingual placement of film packet to region of second premolars will accomplish this relationship (Fig. 7-52A).
3. With block resting on incisal edges of teeth to be radiographed, insert No. 2 cotton roll between top of block and

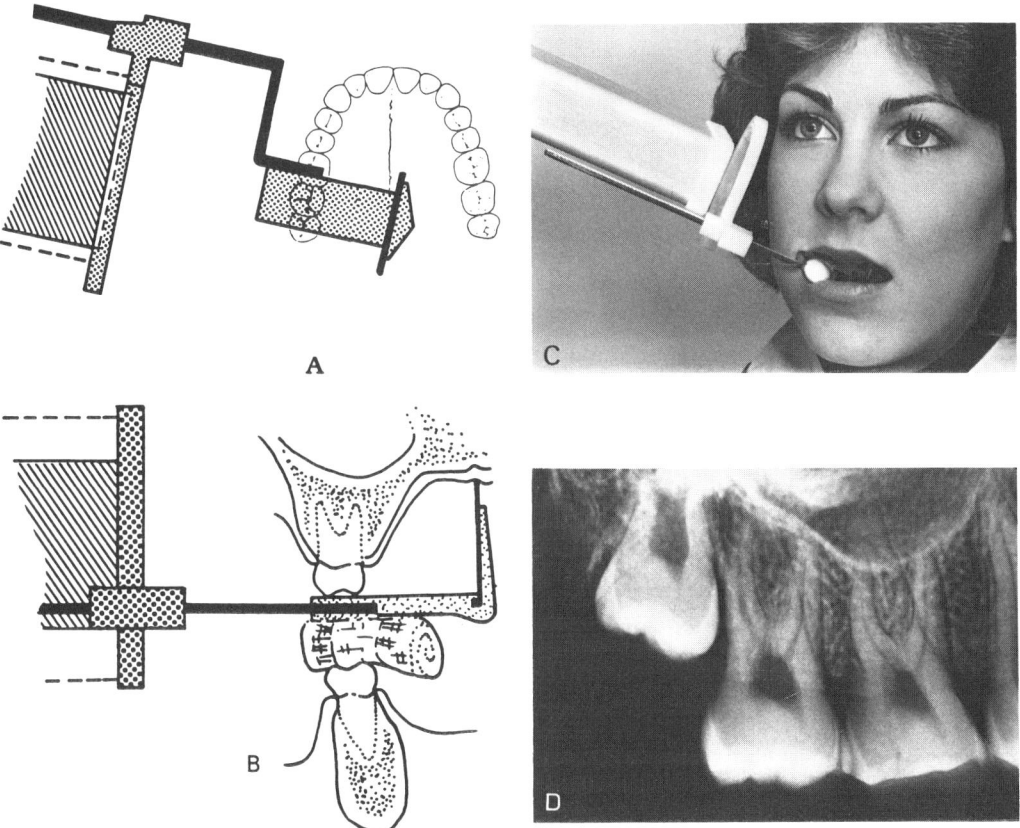

Figure 7-51. Maxillary molar region. **(A)** Horizontal film and P.I.D. placement. **(B)** Vertical film and P.I.D. placement. **(C)** Alignment of P.I.D. with XCP instrument. **(D)** Resultant radiograph.

maxillary incisors, and instruct patient to close firmly to retain established position of film (Fig. 7-52B). Place the film against the floor of the mouth, and rotate the film into position as patient bites on bite-block. Do not force this procedure. This procedure may be simplified by raising the chair and tilting the patient's head backwards.

4. Slide aiming device down indicator rod to approximate skin surface and

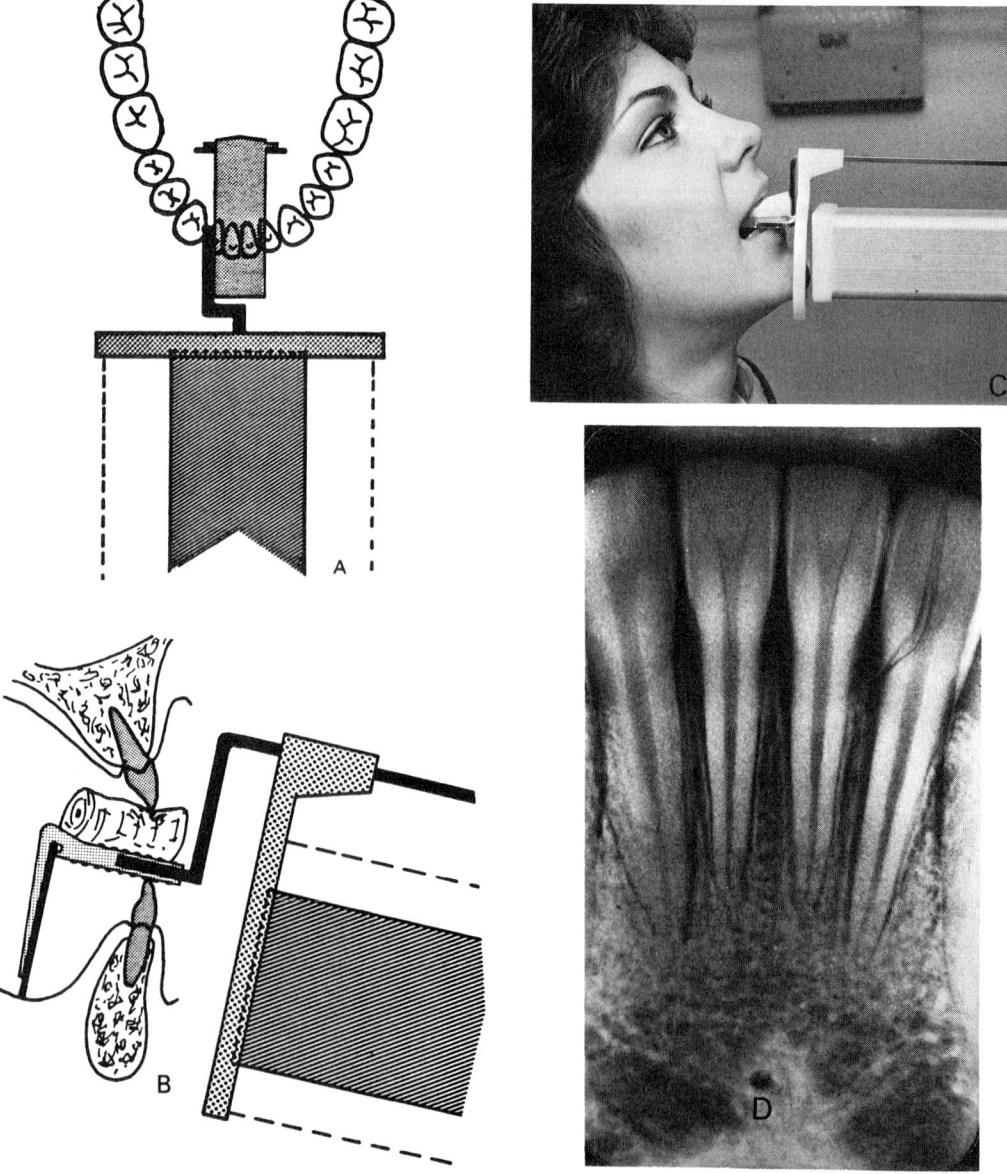

Figure 7-52. Mandibular incisor region. **(A)** Horizontal film and P.I.D. placement. **(B)** Vertical film and P.I.D. placement. **(C)** Alignment of P.I.D. with XCP instrument. **(D)** Resultant radiograph.

align the P.I.D. of the X-Ray unit with indicator rod and aiming device on vertical and horizontal planes (Fig. 7-52C). Rotate P.I.D. to vertical position.
5. Make exposure (Fig. 7-52D).

Mandibular Canine Region

1. Assemble anterior instrument and insert No. 1 film vertically in anterior bite-block.
2. Center canine on film, parallel with long axis of tooth (Fig. 7-53A,B).
3. With block resting on mandibular canine, insert cotton roll between block and maxillary teeth, and instruct patient to close firmly to maintain establshed position of film.

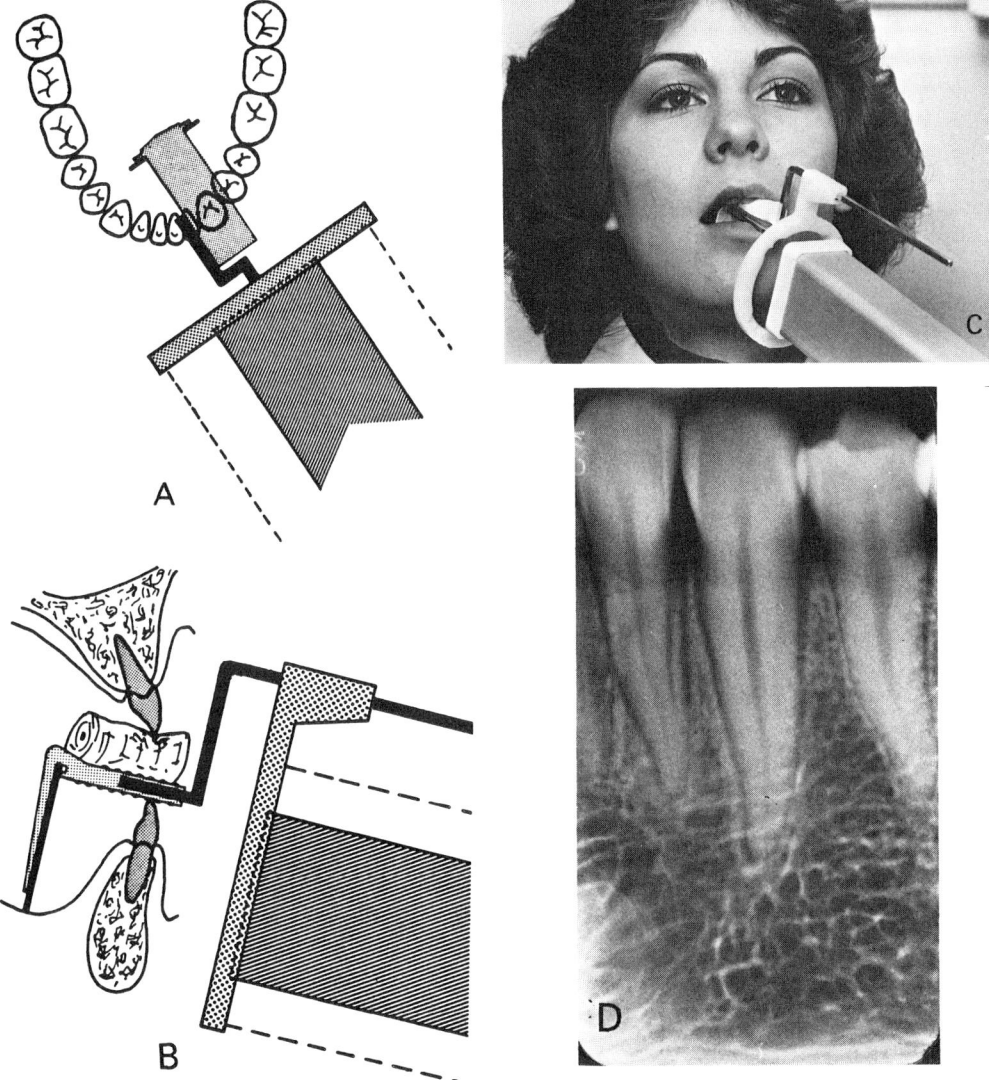

Figure 7-53. Mandibular canine region. (A) Horizontal film and P.I.D. placement. (B) Vertical film and P.I.D. placement. (C) Alignment of P.I.D. with XCP instrument. (D) Resultant radiograph.

4. Slide aiming device down indicator rod to approximate skin surface, and align the P.I.D. of the X-Ray unit with indicator rod and aiming device on vertical and horizontal planes. Make sure P.I.D. is rotated vertically (Fig. 7-53C).
5. Make exposure (Fig. 7-53D).

Mandibular Premolar Region
1. Assemble posterior instrument, and insert No. 2 film horizontally in posterior bite-block. Position in mouth with second premolar centered on film. Relief of the lower anterior corner of the film packet will facilitate positioning.
2. Parallel film horizontally to the mean tangent of the premolars and vertically to long axes of premolars (Fig. 7-54A,B).
3. With the bite-block held on the occlusal surfaces of the mandibular bicuspids, insert cotton roll between the block and maxillary teeth, and in-

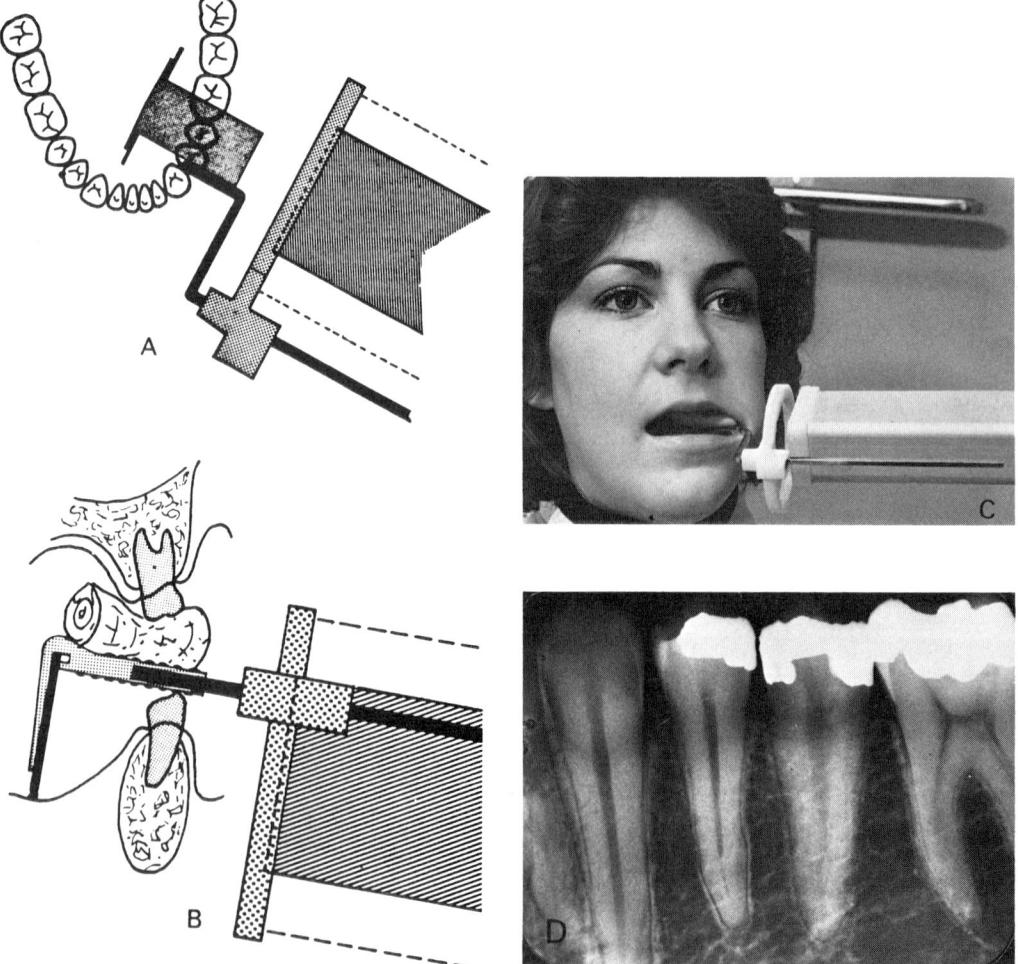

Figure 7-54. Mandibular premolar region. (A) Horizontal film and P.I.D. placement. (B) Vertical film and P.I.D. placement. (C) Alignment of P.I.D. with XCP instrument. (D) Resultant radiograph.

struct patient to close firmly to retain established position of film.
4. Slide aiming device down indicator rod to approximate skin surface. Rotate P.I.D. horizontally and align with both indicator rod and aiming device in both horizontal and vertical planes (Fig. 7-54C).
5. Make exposure (Fig. 7-54D).

Mandibular Molar Region

1. Assemble posterior instrument and insert No. 2 film horizontally in posterior bite-block. Position in mouth with anterior edge of film in vicinity of first molar-second premolar embrasure; however, the film must cover all of the third molar.
2. Parallel the film horizontally with the mean tangent of the molar and move anterior edge of film 15 to 20 degrees toward tongue. This is done to ensure that molar embrasures are open on the resultant radiograph (Fig. 7-55A). Parallel film vertically with long axes of molars. (The occlusal surfaces of molars are usually at right angles to their long axes so if the block is rested flat across the occlusal surfces the plane of the film automatically assumes a position parallel to the long axes of the teeth.) The film packet is

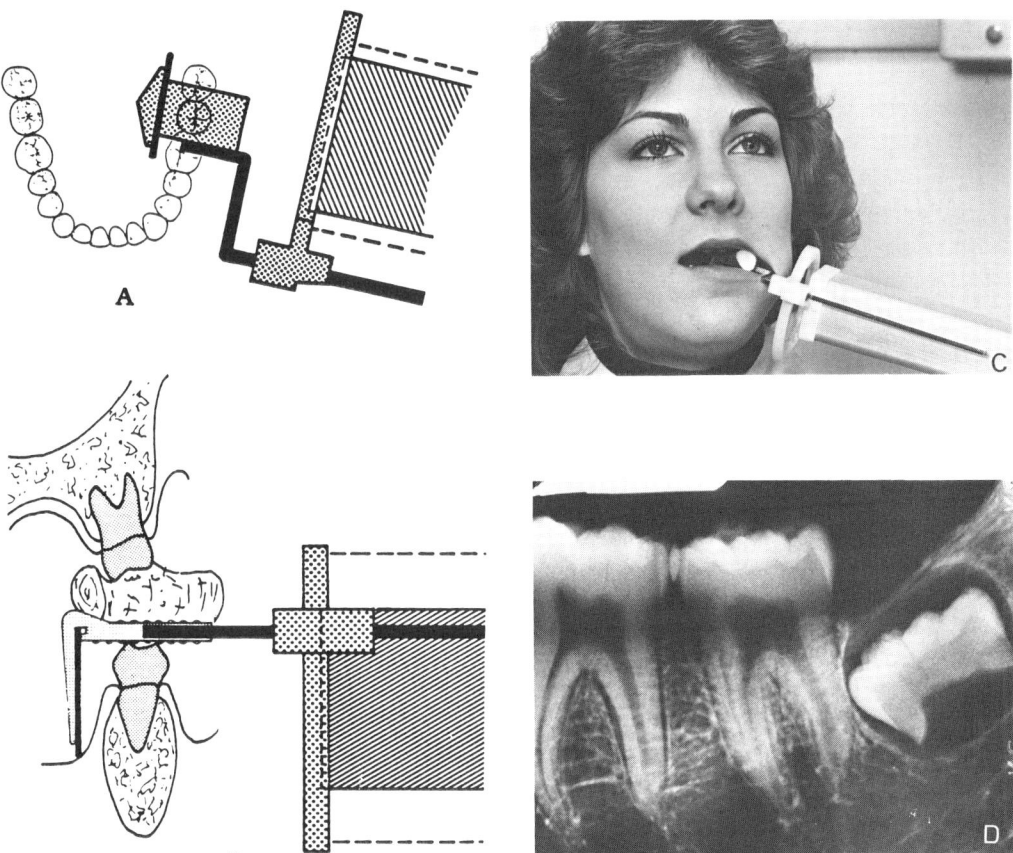

Figure 7-55. Mandibular molar region. (A) Horizontal film and P.I.D. placement. (B) Vertical film and P.I.D. alignment. (C) Alignment of P.I.D. and XCP instrument. (D) Resultant radiograph.

positioned in the sulcus between the teeth and tongue (Fig. 7-55B).
3. Place a cotton roll between the block and opposing maxillary teeth and instruct the patient to close firmly to retain established position of film.
4. Slide aiming device down indicator rod to approximate skin surface. Rotate P.I.D. to horizontal position and align with indicator rod and aiming device in both horizontal and vertical planes (Fig. 7-55C).
5. Make exposure 9Fig. 7-55D).

Modifications in Rinn XCP Technique to Accommodate Variations in Anatomical Conditions

Low and Shallow Palates. The angle between the film and the bite-block in the Rinn XCP instrument is 90 degrees. Therefore, when the film is positioned with the superior edge of the film placed in contact with the palate, and the bite-block against the occlusal surface, the film should be nearly parallel to the long axes of the teeth to be radiographed. However, this is usually not the case, because tilting of the bite-block is produced, which is directly influenced by the height of the palate.

Absolute parallelism between the film and long axes of the teeth is difficult to accomplish in patients with low maxillary palatal vaults. However, if the discrepancy of parallelism between the film and the long axis of the tooth does not exceed 20 degrees, the resultant radiograph is usually acceptable (Fig. 7-56).

In those unusual cases where the patient has a very low palate, it has been suggested that by using two cotton rolls (one on each side of the block), the film can be paralleled with the long axes of the teeth. This technic also reduces the area of periapical coverage and should only be used when the teeth have short roots. It is a technic that is **not** recommended by the authors (Fig. 7-57).

Another method to use in case of a very low maxillary palate is to increase the vertical angulation to 5-15 degrees greater than the instrument indicates. However, by doing this, it will increase the shape distortion of the anatomic structures in the region and a portion of the

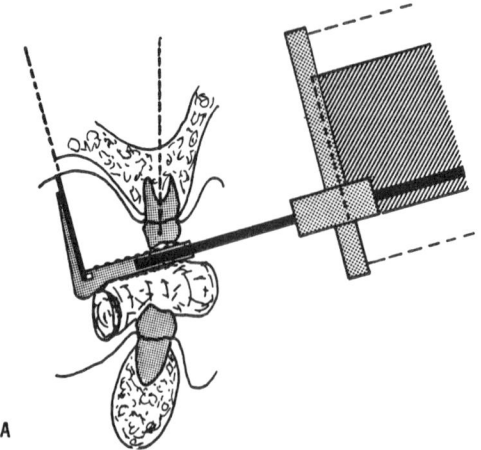
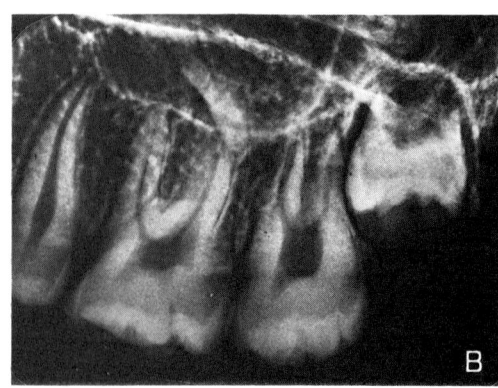

Figure 7-56. Maxillary low palates. **(A)** If the discrepancy does not exceed 20 degrees, the resultant radiograph is usually acceptable. **(B)** Radiograph taken of patient with low maxillary palate, but which did not exceed parallelism by 20 degrees.

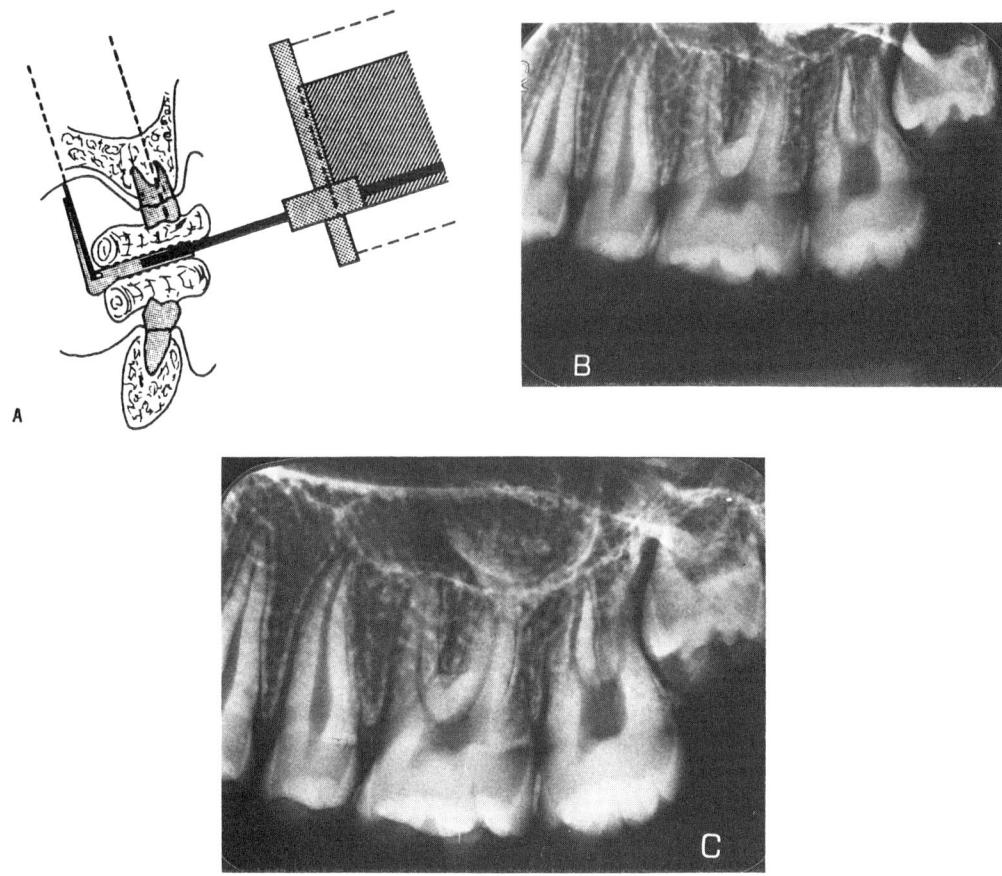

Figure 7-57. Two cotton roll technique for low maxillary palates. **(A)** One cotton roll is placed on each side of the bite-block, which allows film to be more nearly parallel to long axes of the teeth. **(B)** The periapical coverage is reduced using the two cotton roll technic as shown in this radiograph (which is usually not acceptable). **(C)** Same region of the same patient with low palate using conventional XCP technic and increasing the object-film distance. Although the zygomatic arch is superimposed over the apices of the first and second molars, there is greater periapical coverage. (In this case, the conventional method of increasing and the object-film distance is better than two cotton roll method).

cusps may be "cut off" (Fig. 7-58). This is a good method for compensating for shallow palates with extremely long roots.

Maxillary Toris. This is a form of **exostosis** (extra bone growth) at maxillary palatal sutural lines. It is seen in 20 percent of the general population and 60 percent of the American Indians/Eskimos. It is usually round, may be flat, spindle-shaped, nodular, or lobular in shape. It provides a problem in taking radiographs of the maxilary molars with the XCP paralleling technic. It is suggested that the film be placed on the far side of the torus prior to exposing the film. Do not try to place it on the torus itself (Fig. 7-59).

Distal Surface of Canine. It is important to cover the distal portion of the canine with the film when taking the maxillary and mandibular premolar periapical radiographs because the canine periapical film will not reveal the distal portion of the canine with the XCP paralleling technic. Sometimes this is difficult to do with

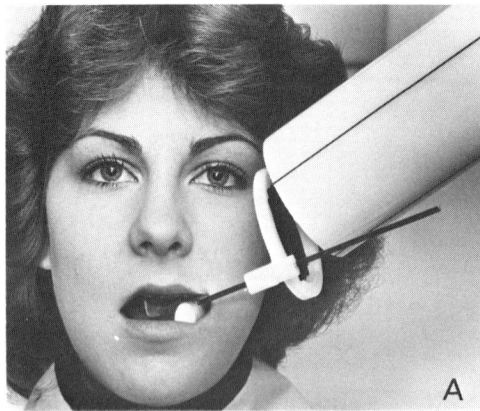
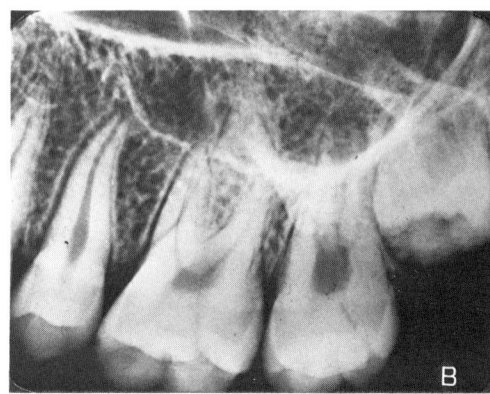

Figure 7-58. Increasing vertical angulation in patients with low palates to increase periapical coverage. (A) Front view of increasing vertical angulation to compensate for low palate. (B) Resultant radiograph by increasing vertical angulation by 10 degrees. Notice downward movement of zygoma, buccal cusps, and buccal roots by increasing the vertical angulation.

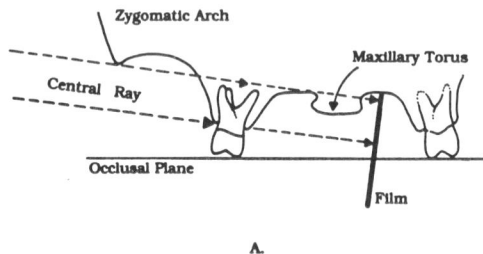

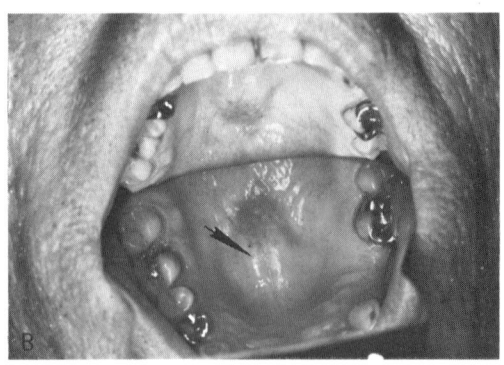

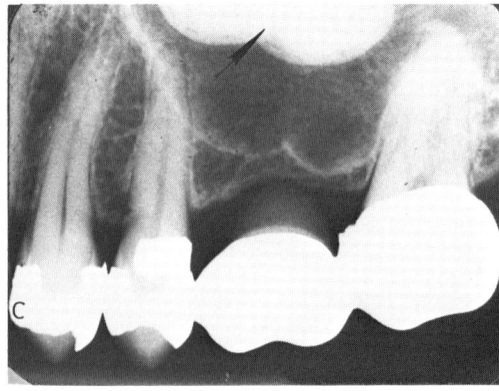

Figure 7-59. (A) Drawing of maxillary torus and placement of film. (B) Photograph of maxillary torus (arrow). (C) Radiograph of maxillary torus (arrow).

some patients who have anatomical limitations. One suggestion is to slightly **offset** the film in the bite-block slot toward the anterior region of the jaws. This procedure will aid the operator in positioning the film more anteriorly to cover the distal of the canine. Remember to slightly offset the P.I.D. anteriorly to cover the film to prevent a "cone-cut" (Figs. 7-60, 7-61). Controlled shaping (bending) of the apical corners wil prevent undue discomfort to the patient (especially if the film is of

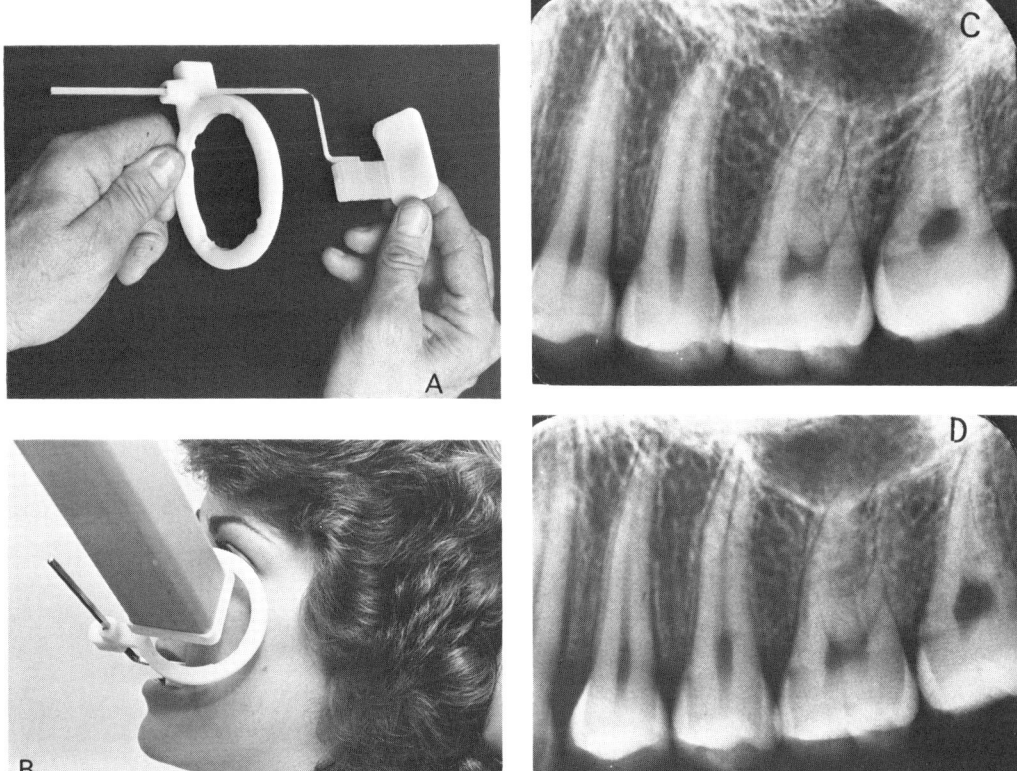

Figure 7-60. Procedure to cover distal surface of maxillary canine. **(A)** Offset film in bite-block (maxillary premolar projection). **(B)** Offset P.I.D. to compensate for anterior placement of film in bite-block (maxillary premolar projection). **(C)** Radiograph of maxillary premolar region with distal surface of canine missing. **(D)** Radiograph of maxillary premolar region with distal surface of canine showing.

the poly-soft type).

Maxillary Third Molar Region Off-set Method. There are some patients in which the XCP bite-block cannot be placed posteriorly far enough in the maxillary arch to cover the maxillary tuberosity or an impacted third molar because of anatomical limitations or gagging. One suggested method to solve these problems is to "off-set" the film posteriorly in the bite-block. In many cases, this will allow the operator to place the film posteriorly enough to cover the third molar region. This procedure will require the posterior placement of the P.I.D. to cover the film, or a "cone-cut" will result (Fig. 7-62).

The Maxillary Third Molar Distal Oblique Technic. The distal oblique projection is recommended for the maxillary unerupted or impacted third molars. The distal oblique projection should show the distal half of the first molar, the second molar, and all of the third molar regardless of its position in the tuberosity. The tuberosity, the distal wall and a portion of the floor of the maxilary sinus, the hamular process of the sphenoid bone, and the coronoid process of the ramus of the mandible may be in evidence also. Usually the contacts will be closed because of the distal projection of the X-Ray beam.

The Ada Snap-A-Ray, Rinn EEZEE

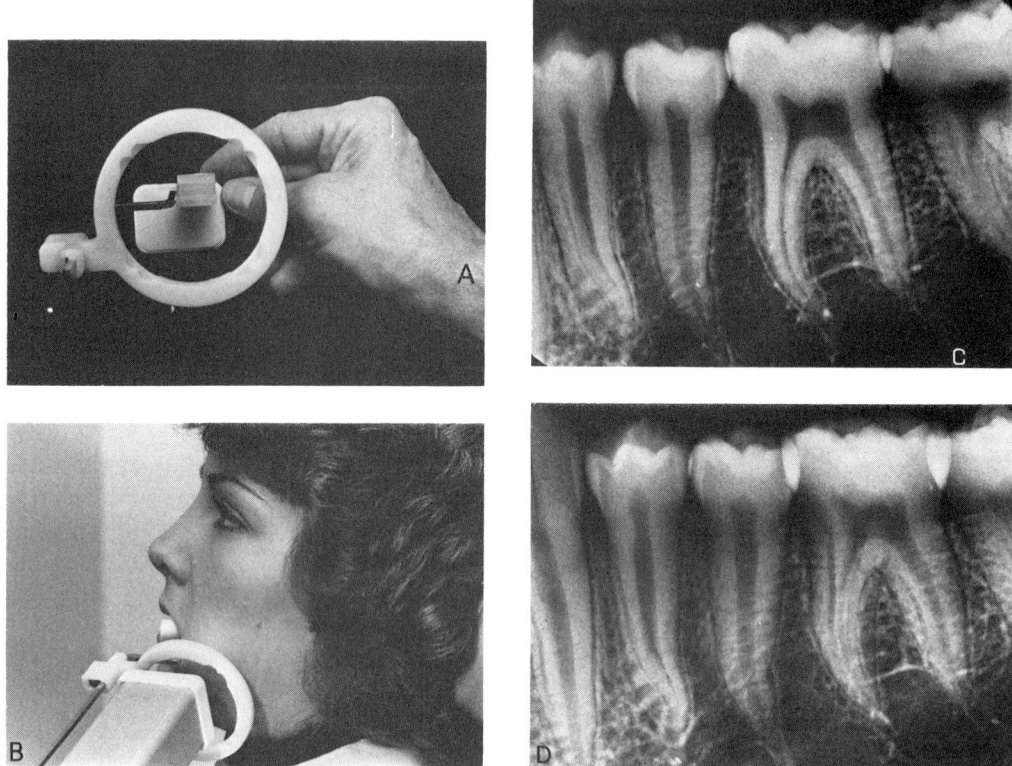

Figure 7-61. Procedure to cover distal surface of mandibular canine. **(A)** Offset film in bite-block. **(B)** Offset the P.I.D. **(C)** Radiograph of distal surface of the mandibular canine not revealed. **(D)** Radiograph of mandibular distal surface of the canine revealed.

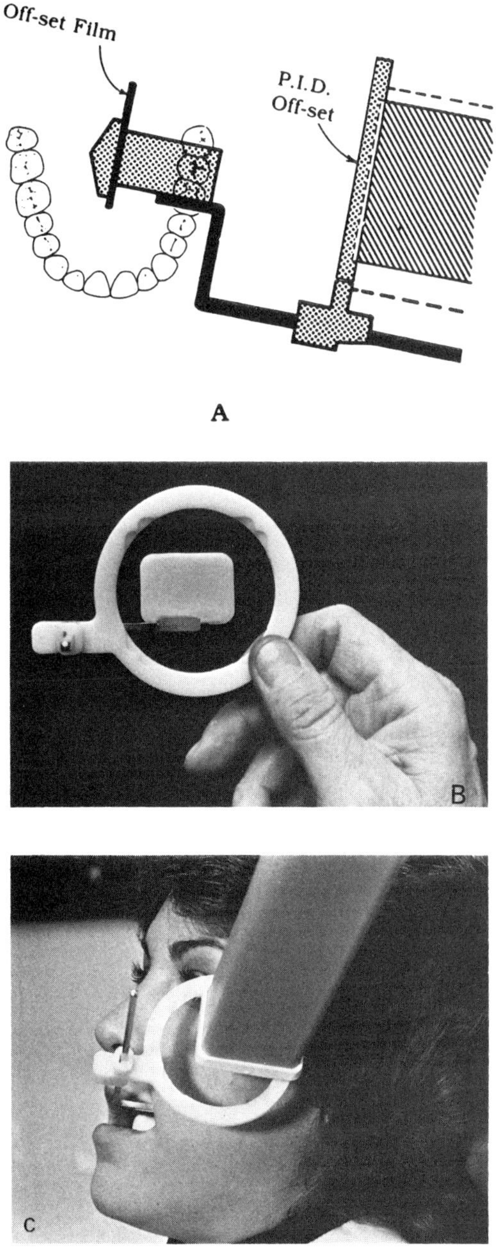

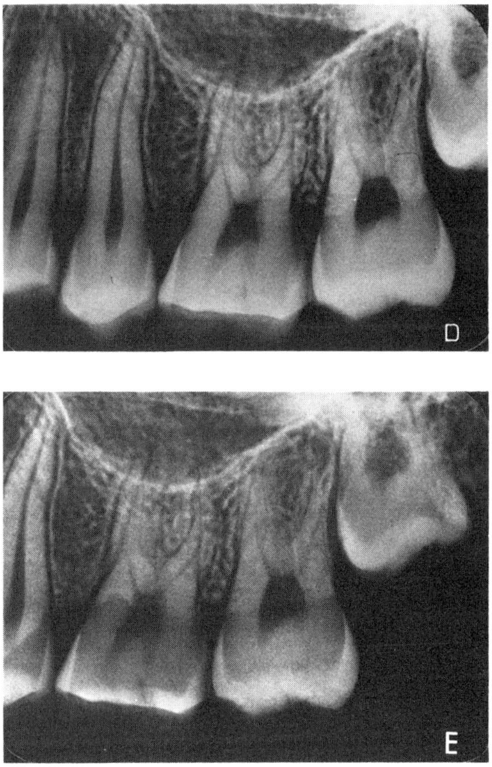

Intraoral Radiographic Techniques

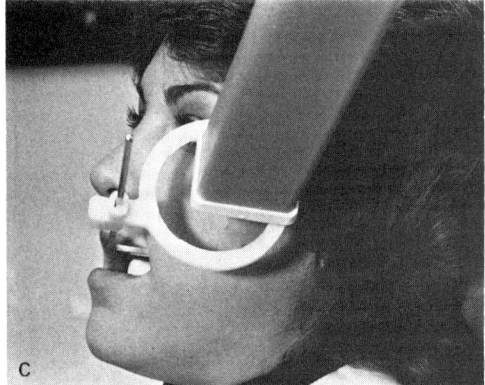

Figure 7-62. Procedure using XCP paralleling technic to extend film farther posteriorly in maxillary arch to cover third molar region. (A) Diagram of "offset" film technique in maxillary molar region. (B) Offset film farther posteriorly to cover third molar region; (C) Offset P.I.D. to cover film to prevent cone-cut; (D) Radiograph in which all of third molar **not** showing. (E) Radiograph revealing third molar after using offsetting film technic.

Grip, or the Fitzgerald hemostat film holders are the instruments of choice (Fig. 7-63); however, the Rinn XCP posterior instrument can be used.

Position the film holder so the plane of the film is parallel to the long axis of the third molar. If the third molar is erupted, its inclination is used as the guide in film positioning. Generally, the alignment of the long axis of the maxillary third molar is tipped more buccally than the second molar; therefore, it is necessary to also take a lateral projection to establish the true relationship of the second and third maxillary molars. If the third molar is not erupted, it is routine practice to incline the film packet to a greater degree in order that all of the maxillary tuberosity will be completely in evidence on the radiograph (Fig. 7-64B).

The tissue edge of the film packet should be beyond the midpalatal suture line forming an angle to it. The apex of the angle is formed by the mesial portion of the film packet (Fig. 7-64A). This is accomplished by placing the film as far posteriorly as you would for a lateral projection of the molar region; then, using the mesial corner of the film packet as a pivot, shift the distal portion of the film

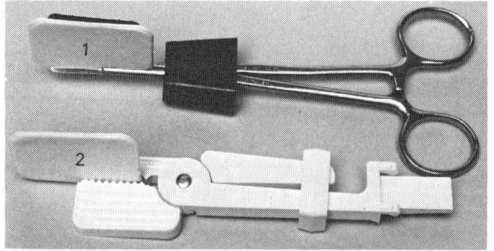

Figure 7-63. Fitzgerald hemostat (#1) and Ada Snap-A-Ray (#2) used for distal oblique projection of third molars.

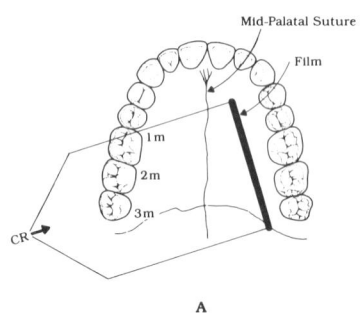

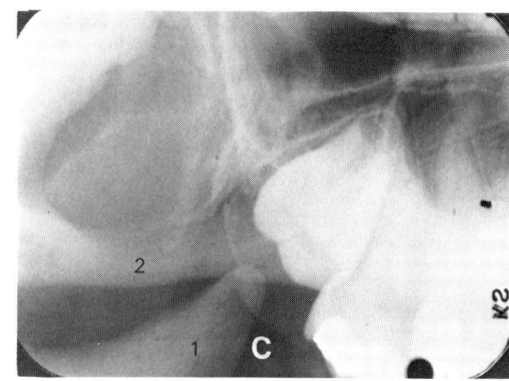

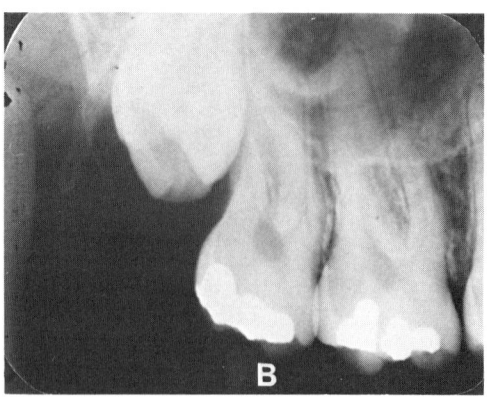

Figure 7-64. Maxillary molar distal oblique technic. (A) Horizontal film placement of distal oblique projection of maxillary third molar. (B) Conventional maxillary molar region radiograph. All of third molar **not** shown. (C) Distal oblique radiograph of same patient as (B). Note that all of third molar is revealed as well as (1) coronoid process and (2) zygomatic process.

laterally across the palate so that the distal portion of the film is positioned against the opposite maxillary tuberosity.

The correct vertical angulation of the P.I.D. is determined by the vertical inclination of the film. The operator can estimate this angulation after the patient has closed down on the bite-block. The range of the vertical angulation varies from a plus 20 degrees to a plus 36 degrees. A plus 30 degree vertical angulation usually is a good starting angle to use.

The long extension cone is directed downward and forward so the X-Ray beam is directed just under the notch of the inferior border of the zygomatic arch. The notch is about a finger's width anteriorly to the mandibular condyle.

The X-Ray beam is directed toward the apices of the third molar. Parallel the film with the open face of the extension cone to minimize distortion (Fig. 64C).

Mandibular Third Molar Region Offset Method. There will be times, because of anatomic limitations or gagging, that the film in the XCP holder cannot be placed posteriorly far enough to cover an impacted third molar. In these instances one suggested method to use is the "offset" film technic as recommended for the maxillary molar region. In this technic the film is positioned further posteriorly in the bite-block than usual, and the P.I.D. or cone is aligned posteriorly to the aiming device to compensate for the posterior positioning of the film (Fig. 7-65).

Mandibular Third Molar Distal-Oblique Technic. This projection will provide a view of the mandibular third molar and retromolar area of the mandible, but in most cases the first and second molars will be overlapped because of the distal oblique projection of the X-Ray beam. It is primarily designed for the detection and/or examination of impacted mandibular third molars and/or pathologic conditions in this area rather than examination of the first and second molars themselves.

The Ada Snap-A-Ray, Rinn EEZEE Grip or one of similar design is the film holder of choice, but the Rinn XCP instrument can be used. The film packet is placed well back in the lingual vestibule between the dental ridge and the tongue. It is important to remember that the lower edge of all mandibular films must be positioned away from the sensitive lingual gingiva covering the bones. This will prevent undue discomfort to the patient. If possible the mesial border of the film packet should be aligned with the lingual grooves on the crown of the first molar. In small mouths this will not be possible, but an effort should be made to place the film as far distally as practical. To improve the projection, the posterior margin of the film is rotated toward the midline, causing some displacement of the tongue.

The X-Ray beam is directed at right angles to the surface of the film, which is positioned parallel to the long axis of the third molar. Since the third molar usually has a greater lingual inclination than the first and second molars, the vertical angulation of the X-Ray beam is in most cases a positive or downward angulation. A vertical angulation of +17 degrees is used as a good starting angulation (Fig. 7-67).

Sensitive Mandibular Premolar Region. In the mandibular premolar projection, the lower border of the film packet is placed under the tongue and away from the sensitive lingual gingiva covering the bone. The anterior border of the film is moved far forward to cover the distal surface of the canine. The apical border of the film may be bent or shaped to the XCP plastic backing to prevent excessive irritation and pain sensations.

The XCP instrument should be positioned in the mandibular arch in the fol-

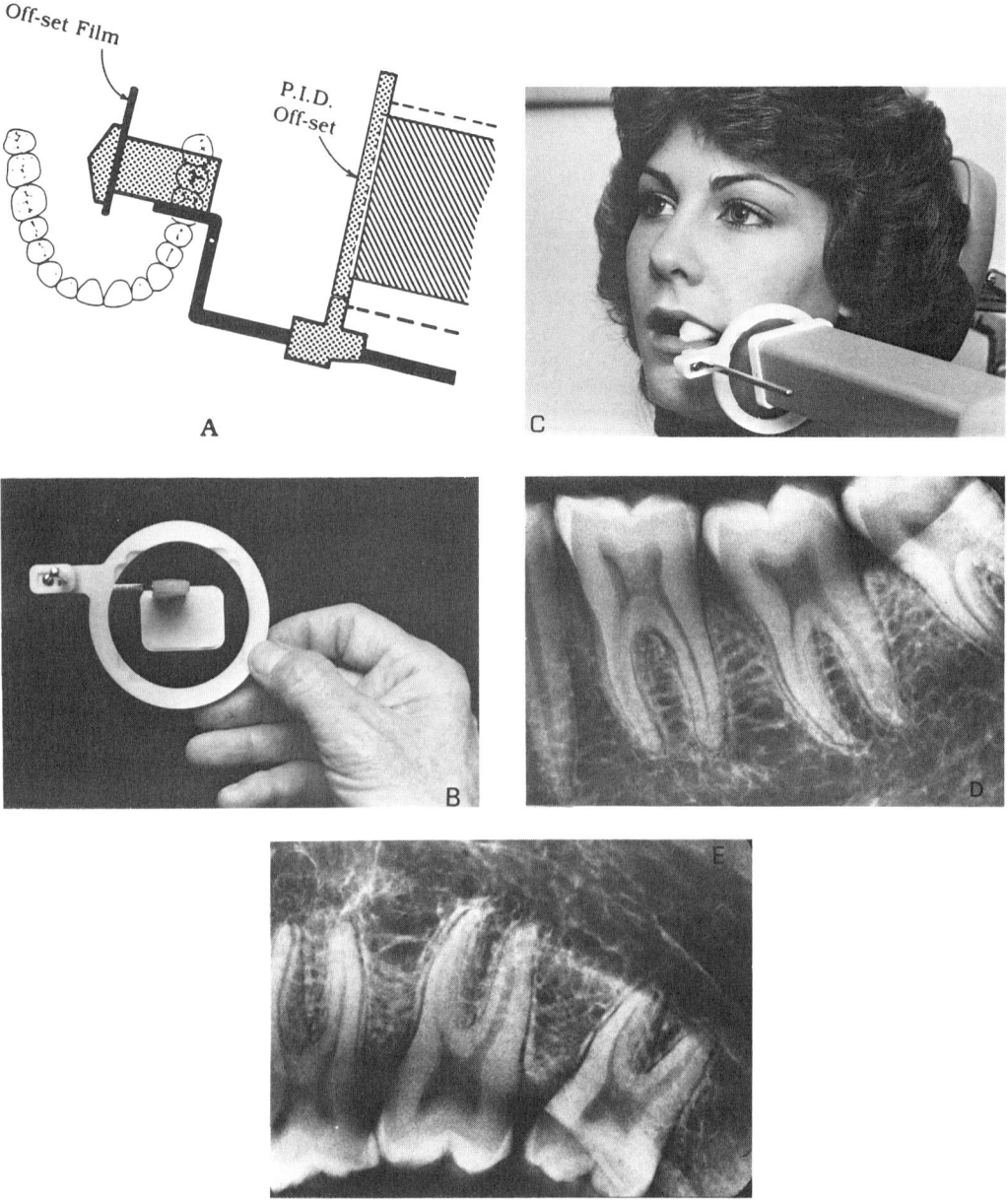

Figure 7-65. Procedure using XCP paralleling instruments to extend film farther posteriorly in mandibular arch to cover the mandibular third molar. (A) Diagram of "offset" film method in mandibular molar region. (B) Offset film farther posteriorly to cover third molar region and (C) offset P.I.D. posteriorly to prevent cone-cutting. (D) Conventional XCP paralleling radiograph in which tip of roots of third molar were not covered. (E) "Off-set" technic radiograph of same patient in which tips of roots of third molar were covered.

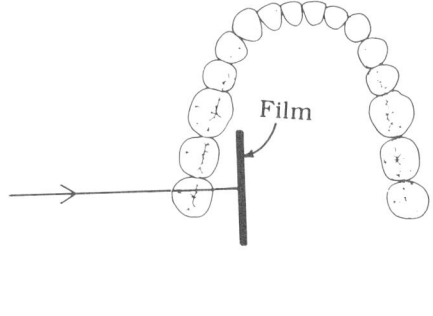

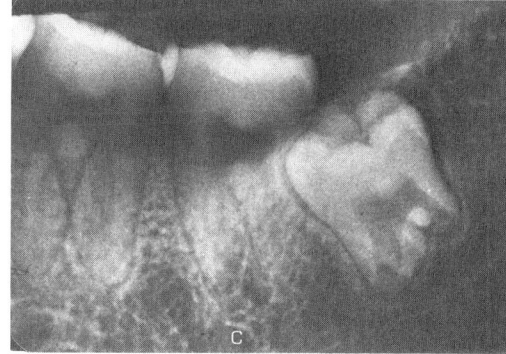

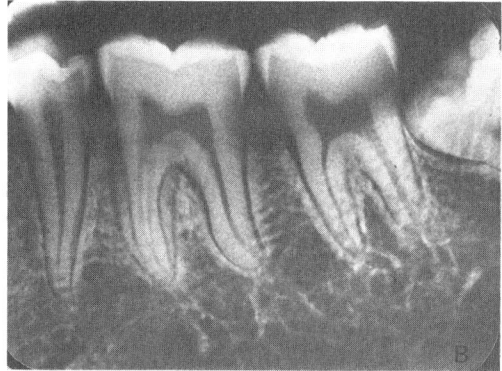

Figure 7-66. Distal oblique projection of mandibular third molar. (A) Distal oblique positioning of film to cover mandibular third molar. (B) Conventional XCP paralleling radiograph of mandibular third molar region. (C) Distal oblique projection of mandibular third molar (same patient as in B). The third molar is an evidence, but notice overlapping of first and second molar.

lowing manner. First, the XCP bite-block is brought in firm contact with teeth to be examined, and the film at this stage should exert very little pressure on the soft tissues (Fig. 7-68A). The film is brought to its terminal position by a tilting action of the instrument (using the bite-block as a fulcrum) as the patient is asked to close on the bite-block. The operator coordinates the movement of the film with the patient's jaw movements. As the patient closes, the muscles of the floor of the mouth relax, enabling the film to be brought to place without discomfort (Fig. 7-68B).

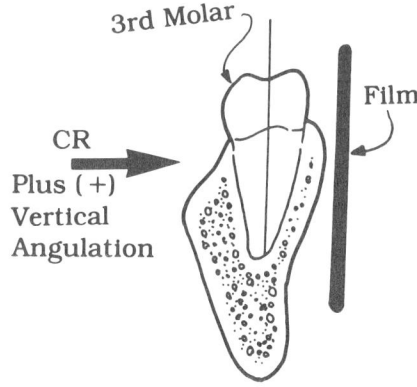

Figure 7-67. Lingual inclination of third molar requires a positive or downward vertical angulation of beam.

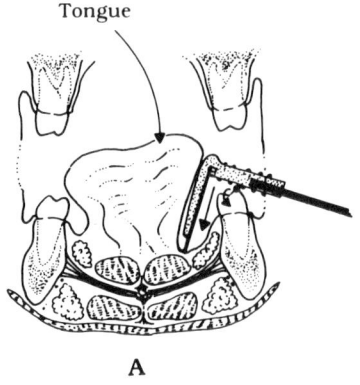

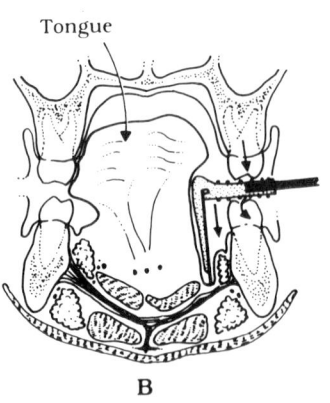

Figure 7-68. Positioning XCP paralleling instrument in posterior region. (**A**) Initial position. (**B**) Terminal position (sometimes a cotton roll between opposing teeth and biteblock may be used. (Adapted from Th. W. Jensen: Reliable low dose dental radiograph. *Dentomaxillofac Radiol,* *11*:57, 1982, Figs. 3 and 5.)

Inadequate Periapical Coverage in Mandibular Premolar Region. When there is an excessive mandibular occlusal curve, high muscle attachments, or long premolars, the conventional XCP paralleling technique may result in inadequate periapical coverage in the premolar region (Fig. 7-69A). One method to overcome this problem is to increase the vertical angle negatively (upward movement) 5-15 degrees greater than the instrument indicates (Fig. 7-69B,C). The Ada Snap-a-Ray may be substituted for the XCP in the mandibular premolar region with some success because the mandibular premolars are positioned more vertically in the alveolar bone with very little lingual inclination allowing for adequate paralleling of the film with the long axes of the teeth without increasing the object-film distance (Fig. 7-70).

Mandibular Tori. The mandibular torus is an extra growth of bone (exostosis) found primarily on the lingual alveolar surfaces of the mandibular premolar teeth. It is usually bilateral and one-third as freqent as the palatal type (torus palatinus) (Fig. 7-71A). The mandibular tori can cause a problem in the insertion of the film into premolar vestibule between the mandibular premolar teeth and tongue if the tori are large. It is important **not** to place the apical border of the film on top of the mandibular torus as it will be irritating and painful to the patient. Insert the film between the lingual gland and the tongue away from the torus, increasing the object-film distance (Fig. 7-71B,C).

Sensitive Mandibular Incisor Region. The mandibular incisor intraoral radiography using the XCP instrument can be very sensitive to a patient if the XCP film holder is not positioned correctly. The XCP bite-block should be brought in firm contact with the incisal edge of the mandibular incisor teeth. At this stage, the apical portion of the film packet should exert little or no pressure on the soft tissues of the floor of the mouth (Fig. 7-72A). Next, the film is brought into the final position by a tilting movement of the XCP instrument as the patient slowly closes her/his mouth. The film can be placed into position without sensitivity by coordination of the movement of the film with the patient's jaw movement. The muscles of the floor of the mouth relax as the mouth

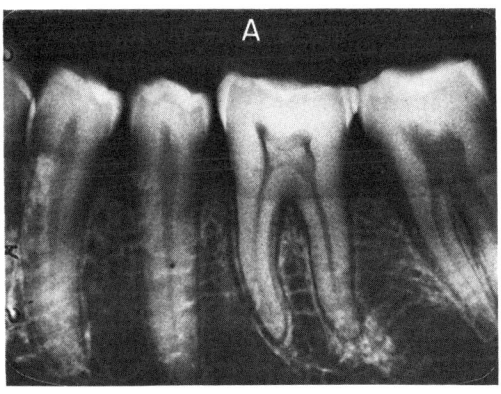
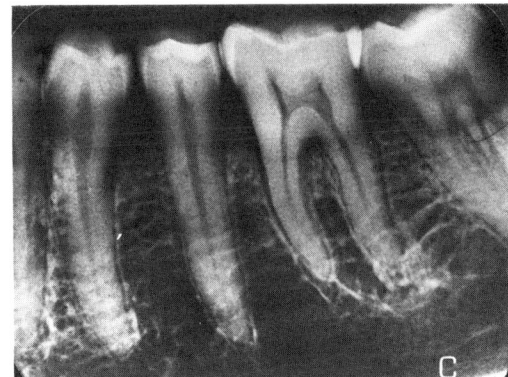
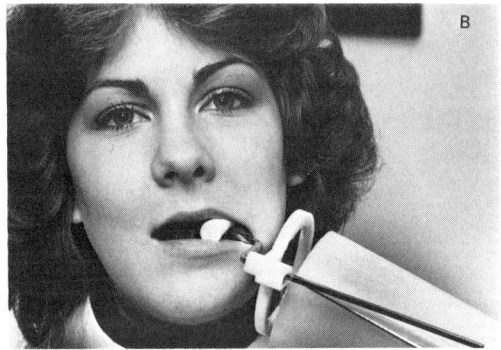

Figure 7-69. Inadequate periapical coverage in mandibular premolar region. (A) Inadequate coverage. (B) Increasing negative angulation. (C) Resultant radiograph of B.

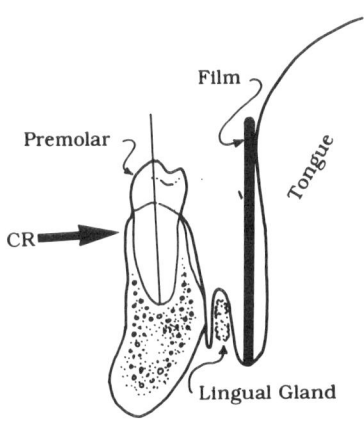

Figure 7-70. Mandibular premolars are more vertically positioned in arch than mandibular molars, allowing for greater convenience in paralleling film with long axes of premolars.

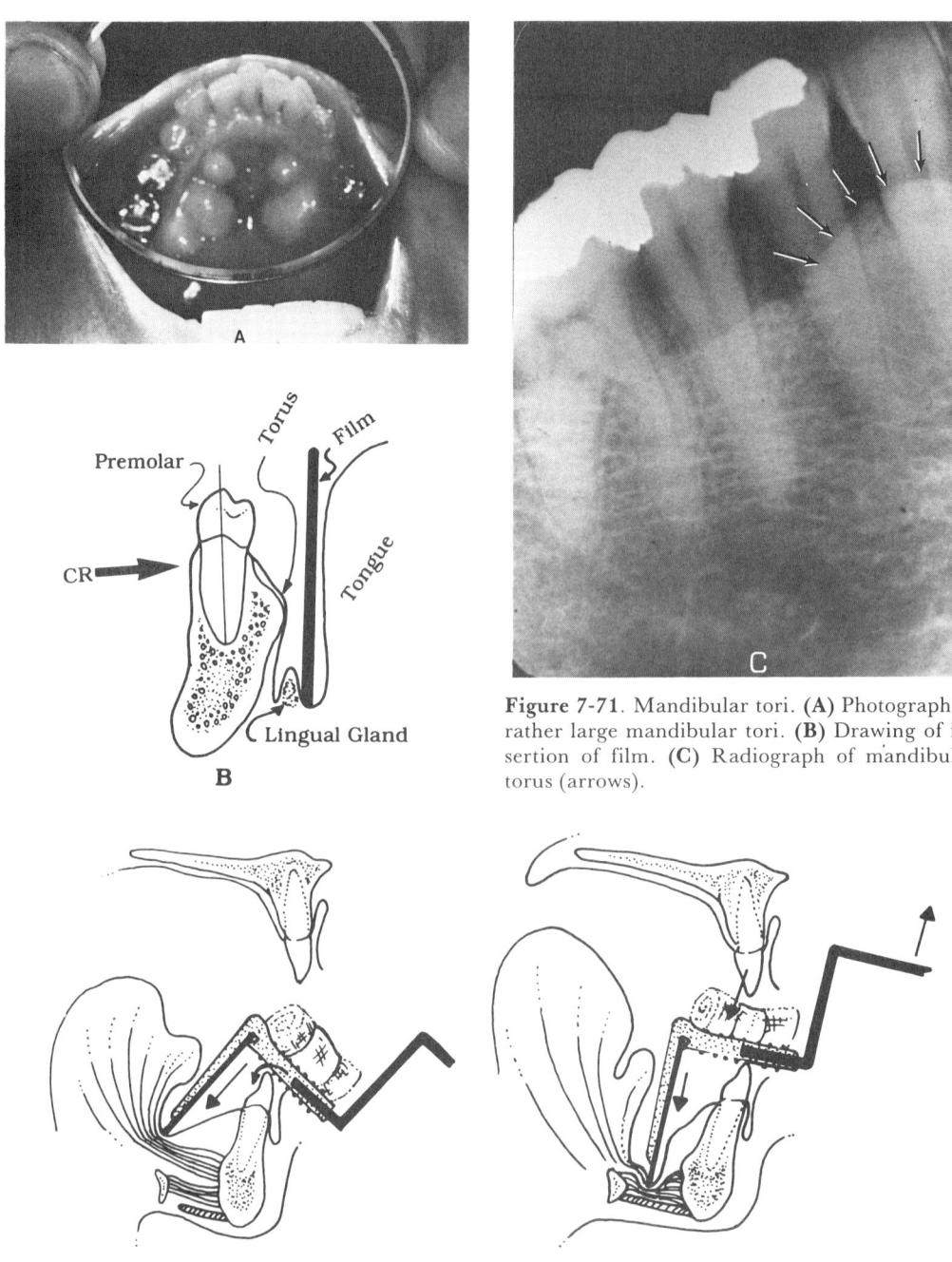

Figure 7-71. Mandibular tori. (A) Photograph of rather large mandibular tori. (B) Drawing of insertion of film. (C) Radiograph of mandibular torus (arrows).

Figure 7-72. Positioning anterior XCP instrument in mandibular incisor region. (A) Starting position. (B) terminal position.

closes and provides adequate room for the film packet (Fig. 7-72B).

Bisecting Angle Technic

The bisecting principle is based upon the geometric principle that states that two triangles are equal if they have two equal angles and a common side. It is called the "rule of isometry." (Isometry is defined as equality of measurement.) (See Fig. 7-73.)

In 1904, Dr. Weston Price, a Cleveland, Ohio dentist, first applied the **rule of isometry** to intraoral radiographic projection technic. When this rule is applied to dental radiography, it is used to determine the **correct vertical angulation** of the tube and cone. (Vertical angulation is the up and the down movement of the tube and cone.)

When the bisecting principle of isometry is applied to an intraoral radiographic technic the rule is: "The central ray is directed through the median plane of the tooth, perpendicular to a line bisecting the angle formed by the plane of the long axis of the tooth and the plane of the film" (Fig. 7-74).

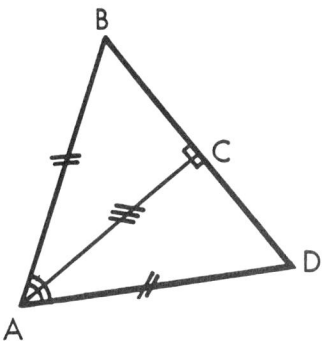

Figure 7-73. The Rule of Isometry: Angle (A) is bisected by line AC. Line AC is perpendicular to line BD. Angle DAC is equal to Angle CAB, and Angle ACD is equal to ACB. If two triangles have two equal angles and a common side, then it can be said that the two triangles are equal. Therefore, triangle DAC is equal to triangle CAB. (Courtesy of Dr. Leroy M. Ennis)

This rule applies admirably to plane surfaces that have only length and width, but it has certain shortcomings when applied to structures such as the teeth that also have depth. Nevertheless, this procedure has served the profession well and does have certain advantages.

If the bisecting angle rule is neglected in the slightest manner, the resulting radiographic image will be distorted. Elongation of the length of the actual image of the tooth will result if the X-Ray beam is directed perpendicular through the plane of the long axis of the tooth rather than through the bisecting line.

Foreshortening or shortening of the radiogrpahic image will occur when the X-Ray beam is directed perpendicular to the plane of the film rather than the bisecting line (Fig. 7-75).

The bisecting technic is for the most part practiced with the short cone (8 inches SFD). If the short cone is used, it should have an open, flat face.

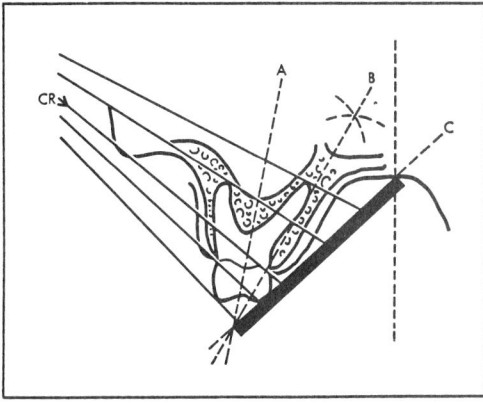

Figure 7-74. The rule of isometry applied to the intraoral radiographic technic commonly called the bisection-of-the-angle technic. Line A = long axis of the tooth; Line C = long axis of the film; Line B = the bisecting line; CR (path of the central ray) directed perpendicular to Line B.

The long or extension cone may also be used with the bisecting technic. Source-film distances of 20 and 18 inches have been used in the past, but the 16 inch source-film distance seems to be the most practical distance to use in most dental offices. The advantage of the extended source-film distance is that it minimizes geometric unsharpness and magnification of the radiographic image (Fig. 7-76).

Procedures

In order to determine the correct alignment of the central beam, the film, and the teeth, using the bisecting technic, the following procedures must be considered:

1. head position;
2. film placement;
3. vertical angulation of the tube;
4. horizontal angulation of the tube; and
5. the point of entry of the central beam.

Head Position. When using the bisecting technics with the digital (finger) method of holding the films in the mouth, the head position is quite important. The rule for head position is as follows: The occlusal plane of the teeth to be radiographed should be parallel to the floor; and the sagittal plane of the head should be perpendicular to the floor.

The **maxillary orientation line** is an imaginary line drawn between the tragus of the ear (cartilagenous projection located just before the ear hole or external auditory meatus) and the ala of the nose (wing of the nose). This line should be parallel to the floor when radiographing the maxillary teeth (Fig. 7-9). The **mandibular occlusal plane** changes when the mouth is open. Therefore, tilt the patient's head slightly backwards so the occlusal plane of the mandible will be parallel to the floor when the mouth is opened. Make sure that the patient does not open too wide as this will contract the muscles of the floor of the mouth and make it difficult to place the film. If the patient tenses the muscles of the floor of the mouth, have him/her relax these mus-

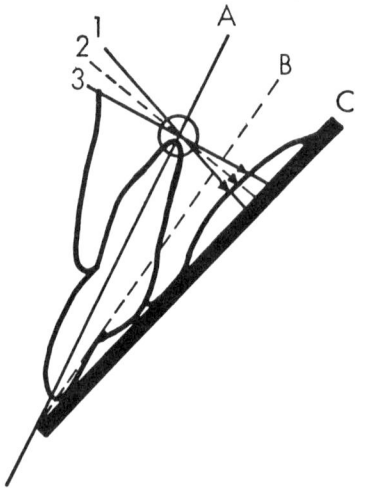

Figure 7-75. In the bisecting angle technic, if the central ray is directed as photon (1) perpendicular to the film, the radiographic image will be *foreshortened*; if the CR is directed as photon (3) perpendicular to the tooth, the radiographic image will be elongated. (Courtesy of Dr. LeRoy M. Ennis.)

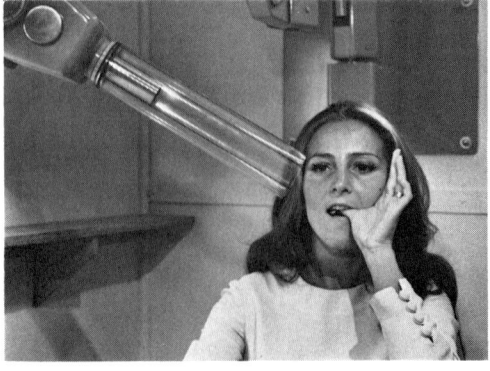

Figure 7-76. The long cone can be used with the bisecting technic.

cles by swallowing.

The **sagittal plane** of the skull divides the skull vertically in the midline into right and left halves. The sagittal plane of the skull should be perpendicular to the floor prior to placing films into the mouth for the bisecting-digital technic (*see* Fig. 7-9).

Film Placement. The rule for film placement in the bisecting-digital technic is this: The center of the film is positioned behind the center of the region to be radiographed.

The most popular complete periapical examination (often called the full-mouth survey) using the bisecting technic is the fourteen-film survey (Fig. 7-77). The films are of the No. 2 (1.2) or standard periapical film size. The following areas are covered:

> One film in each of the 4 molar areas = 4 films
> One film in each of the 4 premolar areas = 4 films
> One film in each of the 4 canine areas = 4 films
> One film in each of the 2 midline incisor areas = 2 films
> TOTAL: 14 films

The No. one (1.1) (0.9 by 1.6 inch) narrow film size is much more desirable than the No. two (1.2) (1.2 by 1.6 inch) regular size for use in the anterior portion of the mouth. It may require one or two more projections; however, it prevents distortion from film bending, and it is much easier to place.

In positioning the films in the mouth for the molar and premolar projections, place the long axes of the film packets horizontally to the long axes of the teeth. The canine and incisor projections require the placement of long axes of the film packets vertically to the long axes of the teeth (Fig. 7-77).

When using the bisecting technic, the film packets may be held in the mouth by the patient's fingers (digital method) or by means of film holders. The digital method has been popular for many years, but it is the most undesirable. It places the patient's hand in the primary beam of radiation.

The film is held in the mouth by the patient's thumb for the maxillary projections and by the patient's forefinger for the mandibular projections. In radiographing the right side of the mouth the

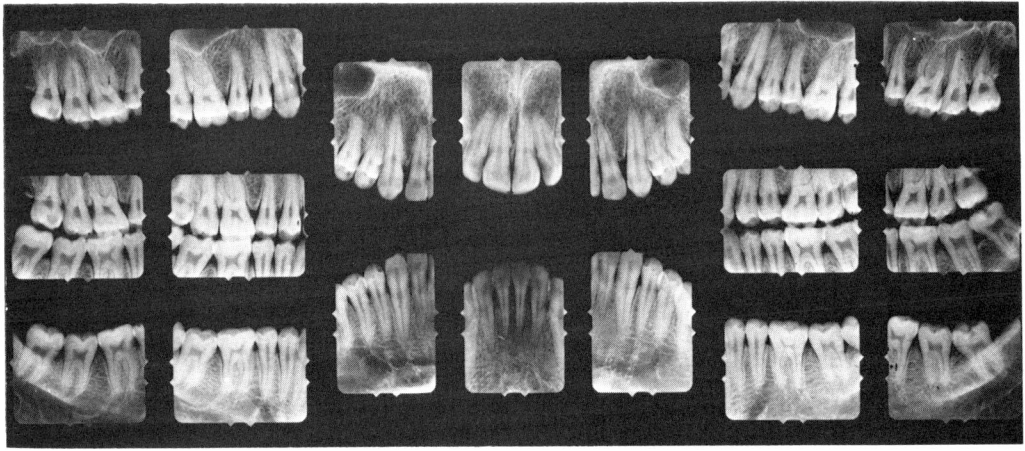

Figure 7-77. Typical complete radiographic survey taken by bisecting angle technic utilizing a short cone (8-inch SFD). (Note that No. 2 regular film is used throughout the survey).

patient's left hand is used, and vice versa. It is always a good suggestion to have the patient wash his/her hands before this technic is used because he/she will be placing his/her fingers into his/her mouth.

Always make sure that approximately 1/8 inch of the film appears below or above the occlusal plane of the teeth. If this is overlooked, partial images of crowns of the teeth will be seen on the finished radiograph.

Many times the film for the maxillary premolar teeth is intentionally bent sharply across the upper anterior corner, which is placed in the region of the lingual surface of the opposite lateral incisor. The premolar projection must reveal the distal surface of the canine because this surface is usually not seen on the canine projection (Fig. 7-78).

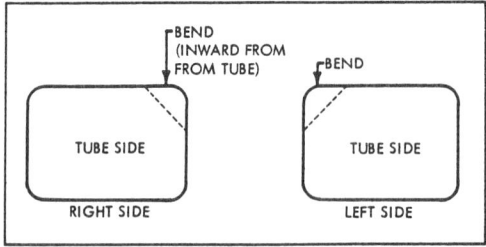

Figure 7-78. In the digital bisecting technic, bend the film in the upper mesial corner for the maxillary premolar as shown here.

In taking he maxillary canine projections with No. 2 (1.2) regular film, it may be necessary to bend the film in the upper anterior corner in order for the film to fit lingually to the opposite premolar region. The patient holds the film with his/her thumb on the bend to make sure that the film is not placed too far back in the mouth, which will result in missing the lateral incisor in this projection (Fig. 7-79).

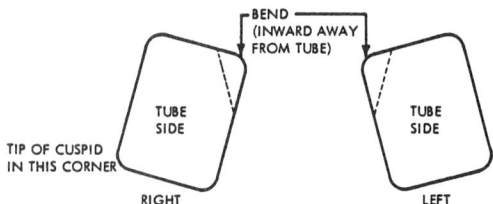

Figure 7-79. In the digital bisecting technic, bend the film in the upper mesial corner for the maxillary canine projection as shown here.

Two cotton rolls may be placed between the film and the teeth in the anterior projections to prevent distortion from film bending.

Vertical Angulation of the Tube or cone. The rule for vertical angulation in the bisecting technic is this: Direct the central beam through the center of the field under examination, perpendicular to the line bisecting the angle formed by the planes of the long axes of the tooth and the plane of the film.

Due to variations in the arrangement, inclination, and angulation of the teeth in the jaws, the angle formed by the plane of the film and the long axes of the teeth for any given area of the mouth varies from one patient to another.

In the normal maxillary arch, the roots of the teeth are inclined palatally from the vertical with the premolars having the most perpendicular roots. The maxillary incisors have the greatest inclination, and the maxillary first molars rarely tilt more than 15 degrees from the vertical. Also, the palatal depth is much higher in the posterior region of the maxilla than the incisor region, which has an effect on the angle formed by the film and the long axes of the teeth. Therefore, the vertical angulations in the maxilla are governed by the inclinations of th teeth from vertical and the palatal depth.

In the mandible, the inclinations of the

teeth are not as pronounced from the vertical as in the maxillary arch. The roots of the anterior teeth slant inwards, the premolars are fairly vertical, and the roots of the molars slant outward slightly. The muscle attachments in the floor of the mouth modify the mandibular vertical angles more than the inclinations of the teeth.

The muscle attachments in the floor of the mouth are deep in the molar region, less deep in the premolar region, and high in the incisor region. The angle formed by the long axes of the teeth and the film is much greater in the regions where the muscle attachments are high. Consequently, the vertical angulations of the tube will be greater in areas where the muscle attachments are high in the mandible. As you can see, it is very difficult to devise routine vertical angulations that will be accurate for any given region for every patient.

To aid the operator, certain ranges of vertical angulatins have been devised into which the majority of the patients fall. These ranges are used only as a guide by the operator; the exact angle to be used for each region for each patient must be determined after the film has been placed in the mouth. The ranges of prescribed vertical angulations for both the long and the short cone bisection of the angle technics are listed in figures 7-80 and 7-81. The long cone vertical angulations are generally less than those listed for the short cone.

Horizontal Angulation. The rule for horizontal angulation is this: As the tube moves around the arch, the X-Ray beam is directed perpendicular to the mean tangents of the facial surfaces of the teeth under examination. The flat face of the cone should be placed parallel to the horizontal plane of the film.

If there is an error in the horizontal angulation, overlapping of the radio-

FILM	MAXILLARY RANGE	MAXILLARY STARTING ANGLE	MANDIBULAR RANGE	MANDIBULAR STARTING ANGLE
Molar	+25° to 30°	+30°	0°	0°
Bicuspid	+35° to 40°	+40°	-5° to -10°	-10°
Cuspid	+45° to 50°	+50°	-15° to -30°	-15°
Incisor	+55° to 65°	+55°	-15° to -30°	-20°
P. Bitewing		+10°		

Figure 7-80. Ranges of vertical angulation for short cone bisecting technic.

FILM	MAXILLA	MANDIBLE
Molar	+25°	+5° (Fixed Angle)
Bicuspid	+35°	-5°
Cuspid	+45°	-10°
Incisors	+45°	-15°
P. Bitewing	+10°	

Figure 7-81. Starting angles (adults) long cone (16 inch SFD), bisection of the angle technic. The +5 degree vertical angulatin is a fixed angle, meaning that practically every mandibular molar shot is taken at +5 degrees above the horizontal.

graphic images will result. The mean tangents of the facial surfaces of the teeth will vary from one region to another.

As you move around the dental arches, the mean tangents of the facial surfaces of the teeth will not be the same. The mean tangents will generally be the same for the following groups of teeth: molars, premolars, canines, and incisors. Therefore, the horizontal angulation must be adjusted for each of these regional exposures. Since the dental arches vary so much as to size and shape from one person to another, no predetermined set of angles can be used. The correct horizontal angulation is easily visualized in the mandibular regions. It is most difficult to visualize the correct horizontal angulations for the maxillary regions. Therefore, it is helpful for the operator to

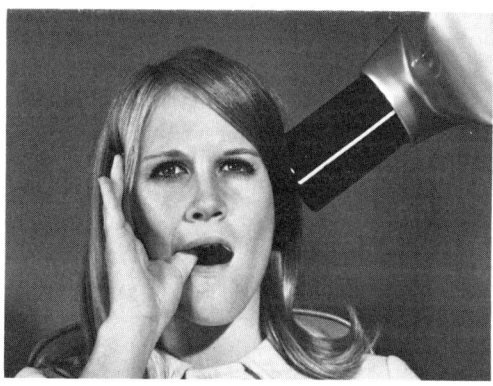

Figure 7-82. Maxillary molar projection. (Digital bisecting short cone technic.)

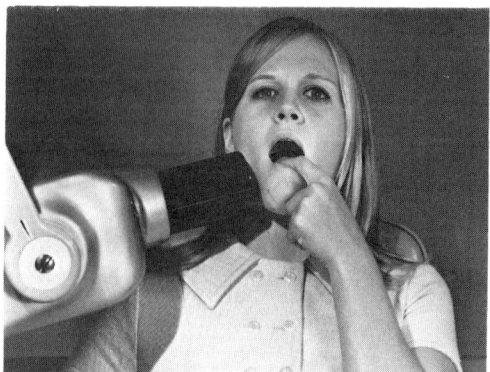

Figure 7-85. Mandibular premolar projection. (Digital bisecting short cone technic.)

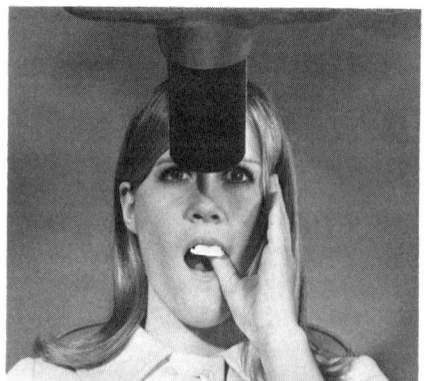

Figure 7-83. Maxillary midline projection. (Digital bisecting short cone technic.) Notice the use of two cotton rolls between film and teeth.

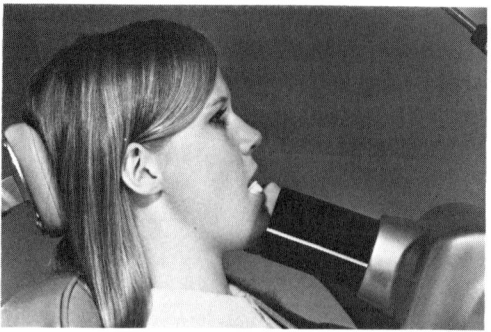

Figure 7-84. Mandibular midline projection. (Digital bisecting short cone technic.)

learn the average horizontal angulations in the maxillary arch (*see* Fig. 7-13).

Point of Entry. The rule for the point of entry in the bisecting technic is this: The X-Ray beam is directed through the center of the area to be radiographed.

The objective here is to completely cover the film with the cone of radiation. If this is not done, a "cone-cut" or partial image will be seen in the finished radiograph.

Bisecting Angle Digital Retention Technic

The bisecting-angle technic using the digital (finger) retention method is illustrated in Figures 7-82 to 7-85. In placing films into the floor of the mouth, care must be taken not to injure these sensitive tissues. Never force films into place; glide them gently and firmly into place. Then guide the patient's index finger to the proper position to hold the film.

It may be necessary to crease the lower anterior border of the premolar film prior to placement. This is the most sensitive area in the floor of the mouth. The situation is complicated even more if a mandibular torus (bony projection) is present.

Use of Film Holders with Bisecting Angle Technic

Film holders have been devised to use with bisecting angle technic. Two such film holders are (1) the Rinn BAI film hodlers and the (2) Greene Stabe disposable periapical X-Ray film holder.

The Bisecting Angle Technic Using the Rinn BAI Instruments

The Rinn BAI instruments are designed to aid in the determinatin of horizontal and vertical angulations, minimize distortion from film bending, and prevent "cone-cutting." A set of Rinn BAI (Bisecting Angle Instruments) instruments consists of anterior and posterior periapical bite-blocks, indicator rods, and aiming devices (Fig. 7-86).

By use of the Rinn BAI instruments, vertical and horizontal P.I.D. angulations need not be memorized and head positioning is not critical. Moreover, correct film placement and retention is accomplished with lesss strain on the patient. A long or short P.I.D. (cone) can be used with the bisecting technic. If a short cone is all that is available for use, the bisecting angle technic is recommended over the paralleling technic.

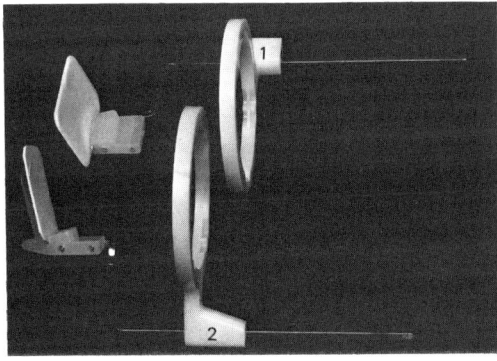

Figure 7-86. (#1) Posterior and (#2) Anterior BAI (bisecting angle) instruments.

Maxillary and Mandibular Anterior Region. Insert No. 2 (1.2) or No. 1 (1.1) film vertically in anterior bite-block, center with midline or canine, and position against lingual surface of crown of teeth as anatomy permits. Instruct patient to protrude mandible and close firmly to retain film in place. A cotton roll may be inserted between opposing teeth and block to increase stability. Slide aiming device on rod to approximate skin surface and align P.I.D. (cone) of X-Ray unit with rod and aiming device on vertical and horizontal planes (Figs. 7-87 and 7-88).

Maxillary and Mandibular Posterior Region. With No. 2 (1.2) size film placed horizontally in the posterior Rinn BAI bite-block, insert into mouth, positioning block on occlusal surface of first molar tooth for molar projection and second premolar for premolar projection and as close to the lingual surfaces of the teeth as the anatomy permits. Relief of the anterior upper or lower corner of the film packet for the premolar projections (maxillary or mandibular) will facilitate positioning. Instruct the patient to close firmly on block to retain film in place. A cotton roll may be inserted between opposing teeth and block to insure stability. Slide aiming device on rod to approximate skin surface and align the P.I.D. of the X-Ray unit with rod and aiming device on vertical and horizontal planes (Fig. 7-89 and 7-90).

Bisecting Angle Technique Using Stabe Film Holder

The Stabe film holder (Greene Products, New York) is made of an expanded rigid polystyrene plastic material. It is soft, allowing the patient's teeth to penetrate the bite-block portion of the film holder, locking it into position (Fig. 7-21).

The Stabe film holder can be used in the bisecting angle technic by placing the film as shown in Figure 7-91. The remov-

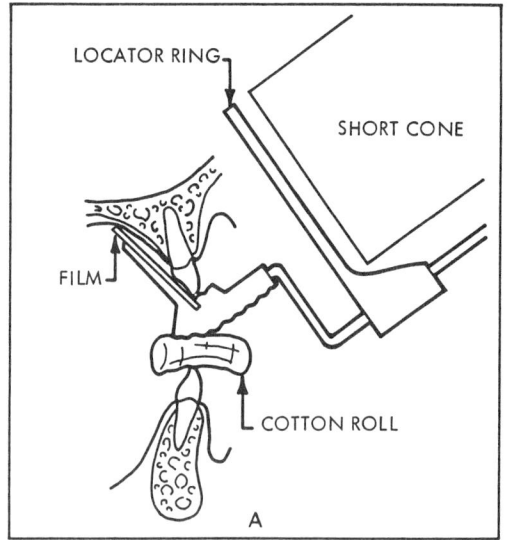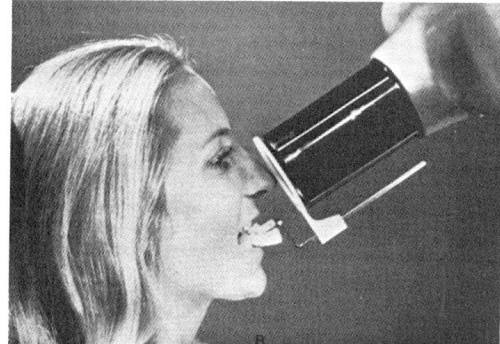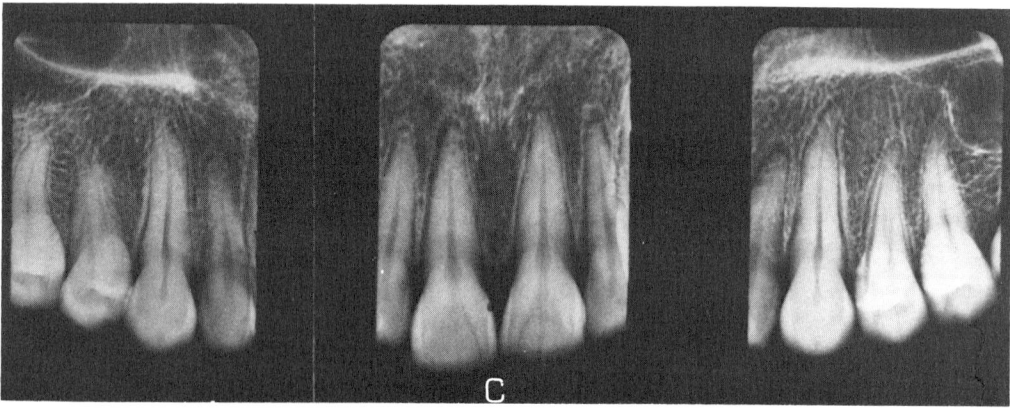

Figure 7-87. Maxillary anterior projections using Rinn Bisecting Angle anterior instrument. (**A**) Diagram showing the correct positioning of Rinn bisecting film holder and cone for maxillary incisor region. (**B**) Maxillary anterior region. (Rinn Bisecting Instrument used with round cone.) Note use of cotton roll on opposing teeth to stabilize the film holder. (**C**) Radiographs of maxillary anterior teeth taken with Rinn BAI anterior instrument.

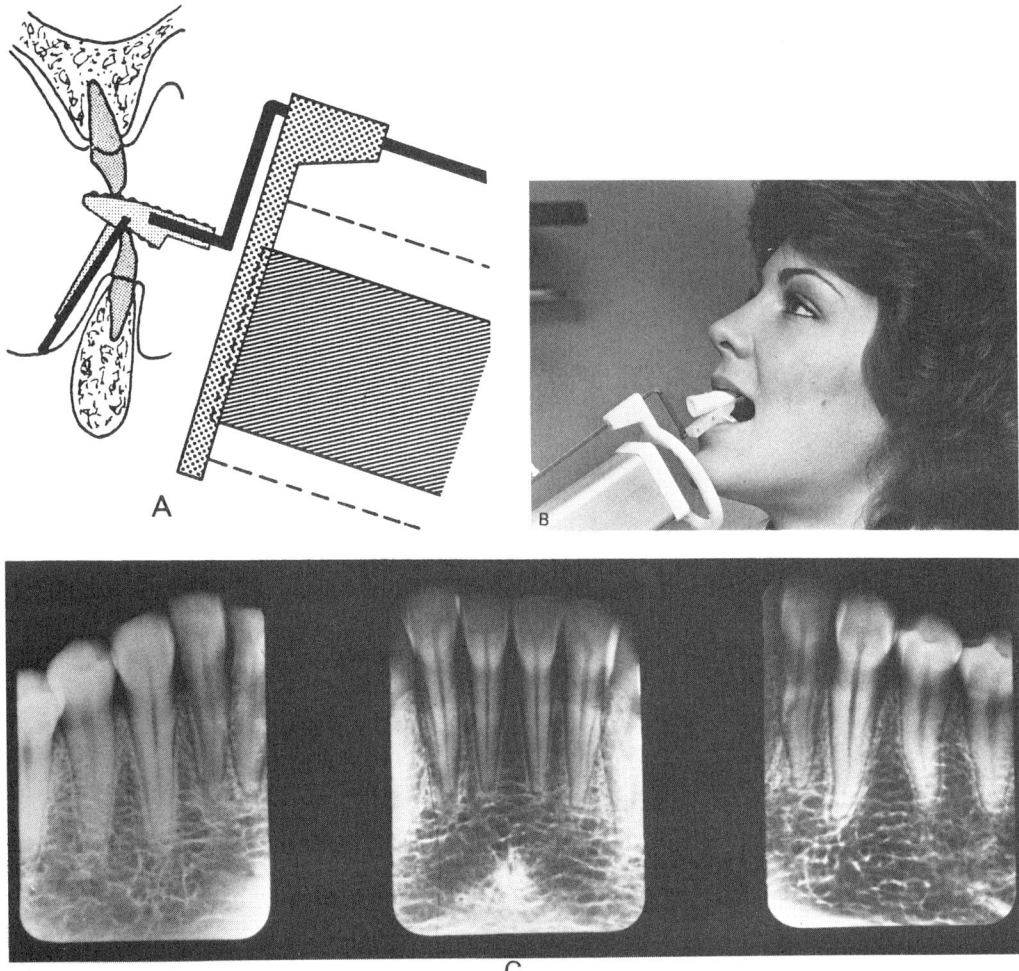

Figure 7-88. Mandibular anterior proejctions using Rinn Bisecting Angle anterior instrument. **(A)** Diagram showing the correct positioning of Rinn Bisecting Film Holder and cone (P.I.D.) in mandibular anterior region. **(B)** Mandibular anterior region. (Rinn Bisecting Instrument used with rectangular P.I.D.) **(C)** Mandibular anterior radiographs taken with Rinn (BAI) bisecting angle instruments.

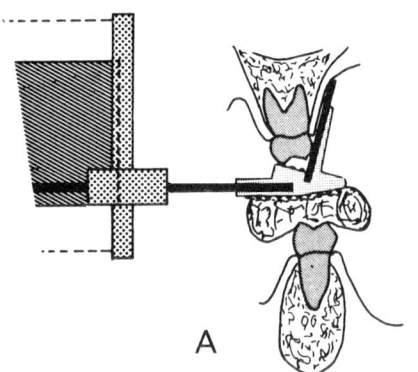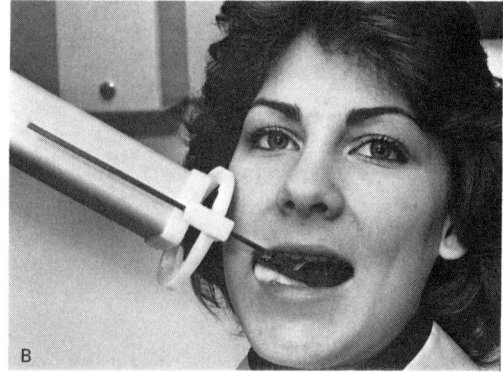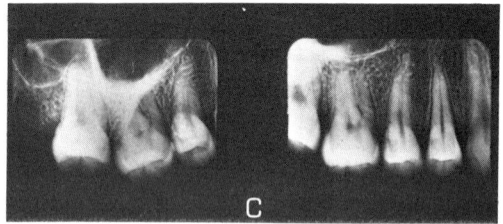

Figure 7-89. Maxillary posterior region using Rinn bisecting angle posterior instrument. (A) Diagram showing the correct positioning of Rinn bisecting film holder and PID for maxillary molar region. (B) Maxillary premolar region (Rinn bisecting instrument). (C) Radiographs of maxillary molar and premolar region using Rinn bisecting posterior instrument.

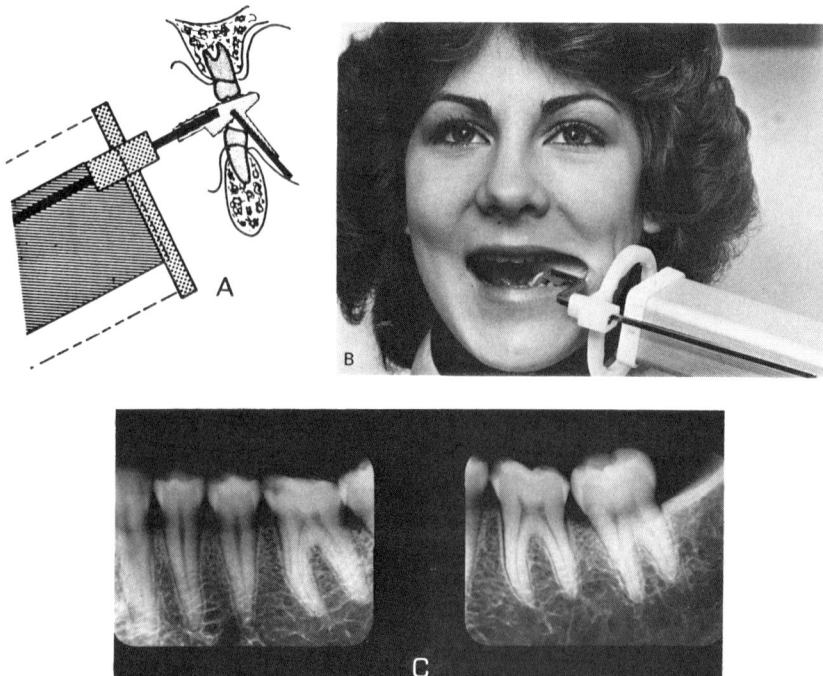

Figure 7-90. Mandibular posterior region using Rinn Bisecting Posterior Instrument. (A) Diagram showing correct positioning of Rinn Bisecting Film Holder and cone for mandibular Premolar region. (B) Mandibular premolar region (Rinn bisecting instrument). (C) Radiographs of mandibular premolar and molar regions (BAI technic).

able end of the Stabe is removed for placement of all periapical packets with this technique. With film in the Stabe film holder, place the film as close to the teeth as possible without bending the film. Have patient close gently on the bite portion of the film holder. Direct the X-Ray beam perpendicular to the plane, bisecting the angle formed by the plane of the film and the long axes of the teeth (Fig. 7-91). Position the cone (P.I.D.) horizontally so the flat portion of the X-Ray P.I.D. is parallel to the facial surfaces of the teeth. The vertical angulation of the cone will change depending on anatomic region being radiographed. Remember that the use of the bisecting angle method requires careful positioning of the patient's head. The sagittal plane must be perpendicular to the floor, and the occlusal plane of arch being radiographed must be parallel to the floor.

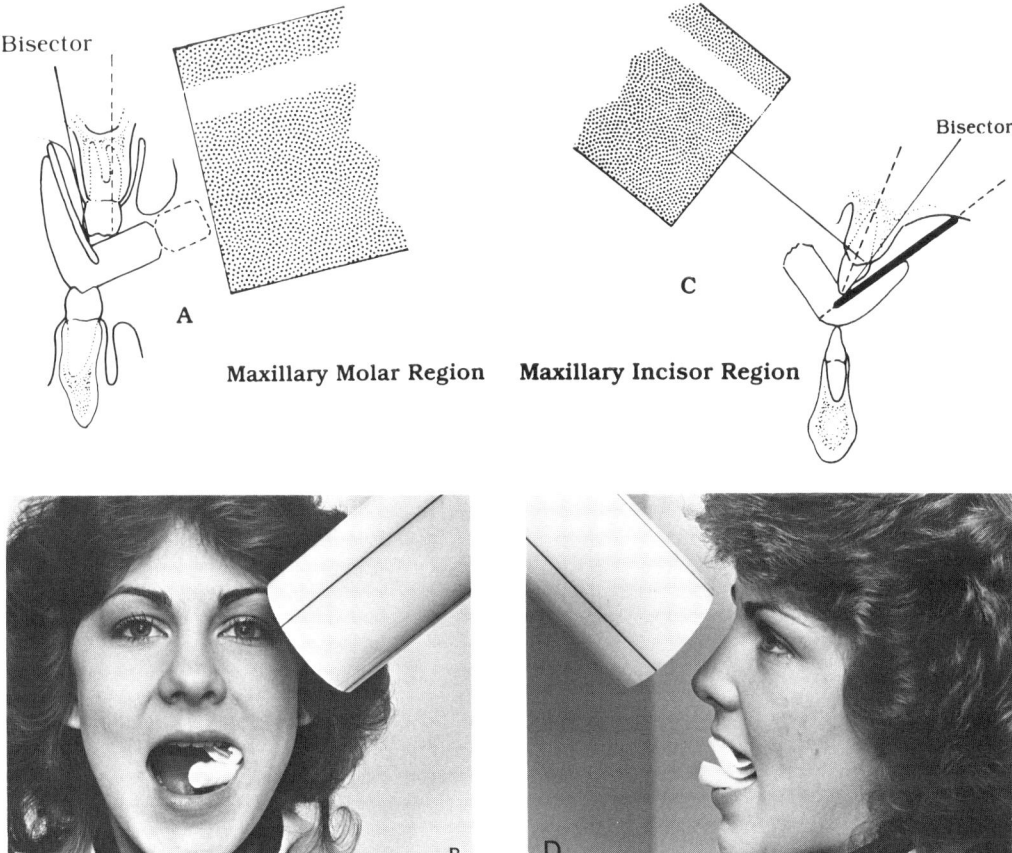

Figure 7-91. Bisecting angle technique using the Stabe film holder. **(A)** Maxillary molar Stabe bisecting technic. **(B)** Stabe bisecting angle technic in maxillary molar region. **(C)** Maxillary incisor Stabe bisecting technic. **(D)** Stabe bisecting angle technic in maxillary central incisor region.

POSTERIOR BITE-WING FILM TECHNIC

In 1926, Dr. Howard Raper of Indiana University and Albuquerque, N.M., proposed the bite-wing technic for detecting interproximal caries. The posterior bite-wing film reveals the crowns and adjacent tissue of the teeth of both jaws on one film.

Bite-Wing Tab Technic

A bite-wing film has a wing or tab attached to the pebbled side of the film.

When the tab is placed on the occlusal surfaces of the mandibular posterior teeth, and the patient closes on the tab, the film will be held in a lingual position to the maxillary and mandibular crowns.

There are two sizes of adult bite-wing films:

1. **Adult or No. 3 (2.3) Bite-Wing Film** is designed to record the crowns of all the posterior teeth, both maxillary and mandibular. This type of bite-wing film is **not** recommended because there is a slight amount of distortion in the film from conforming to a curved arch, and many times this film does not reveal all of the interproximal surfaces of all the posterior teeth.
2. **No. 2 (2.2) or Standard Size Bite-Wing Film**, one of which is not long enough to record all posterior crowns in an adult mouth; thus, in the adult, one No. 2 bite-wing film should be used in the molar region, and one No. 2 bite-wing film should be used in the premolar region.

Head Position

Regardless of the type of cone you may be using, the sagittal plane should be perpendicular to the floor, and the tragal-ala line should be parallel to the floor.

Film Placement and Retention

Step 1: Place the bite-wing tab or wing on the occlusal surface of the mandibular molars or premolars with the lower edge of the film packet placed in the vestibule between the tongue and the teeth. The anterior edge of the premolar bite-wing film should extend to the mesial surface of the mandibular canine, and the anterior edge of the molar bite-wing film should be placed at the midline of the mandibular second premolar.

To avoid overlapping of the contact points, the film should be positioned perpendicular to invisible lines drawn through the embrasures of the teeth. To do this, in the molar bitewing projection, the anterior border of the film packet should be a greater distance from the lingual surfaces of the teeth than the posterior border.

If the person has a shallow vault, the film should be placed even a greater distance away from the lingual surfaces of the teeth. This will enable the person to close down on the bite-wing tab with less difficulty.

Step 2: fold down half of the bite-wing tab over the buccal surface of the teeth. This should be done before the tab is placed on occlusal surfaces of the teeth. With the index finger of one hand, press against the lower lingual border of the film to keep it upright. Use the index finger of the other hand to press the tab against the buccal surface of the mandibular teeth.

Step 3: Now remove the finger that is pressing against the back of the film, and instruct the patient to close slowly against the bite-wing tab in a normal bite. The patient will not close against your index finger because it is pressing against the buccal surfaces of the lower teeth. After the patient has closed against the bite-wing tab, remove your finger from the tab.

Vertical Angulations

Short Cone (8 inch SFD): +10 degree vertical angulation.

Long Cone (16 inch SFD): +8 degrees for molar region and +6 degrees for premolar region.

If the palate is shallow, the upper border of the film will be forced lingually by the palate on closure. The vertical angle may have to be increased in this case to prevent shape distortion of the maxillary crowns.

Usually the maxillary premolars and molars tilt bucally (sometimes as much as 15 degrees from the vertical) while the mandibular premolars and molars slant very little from the vertical. Therefore, in order to compensate for this descrepancy, and to prevent distortion of the crowns, a compromise vertical angulation is used for the bite-wing projections (Fig. 7-92).

Horizontal Angulation

Direct the central beam through the interproximal embrasures of the crowns of the teeth under examination. The flat face of the cone should be horizontally parallel to the film packet.

Point of Entry

Direct the central beam through the occlusal plane of the teeth toward the center of the film packet. In order to prevent "cone-cutting," gently pull back the corner of the lips, and observe whether the anterior periphery of the cone is covering the anterior border of the film. In the molar projection, attach the tab flush with the anterior margin of the film. This will serve as a landmark for the anterior border of the film, when the patient's teeth are closed together. In the premolar projection, the anterior margin of the film can be readily seen.

In order to prevent cone cutting, use the teeth as landmarks in the following manner:

Molar No. 2 Bite-Wing Film: Align the anterior margin of the cone with the interproximal space between the maxillary first premolar and the maxillary canine. Direct the central ray through the occlusal plane of maxillary and mandibular teeth (Fig. 7-93A).

Premolar No. 2 Bite-Wing Film: Align the anterior margin of the cone with the interproximal space between the maxillary lateral and central. Direct the central ray through the occlusal plane of the maxillary and mandibuar teeth (Fig. 7-93B).

Bite-Wing Technic Using Film Holder

There are several bite-wing instruments that can be used instead of the bite-

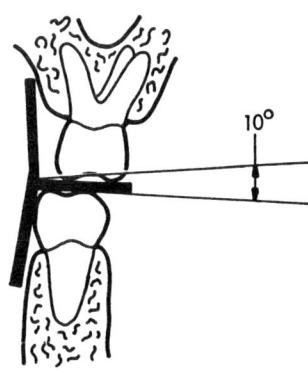

Figure 7-92. Short cone vertical angulation for posterior bite-wing radiograph.

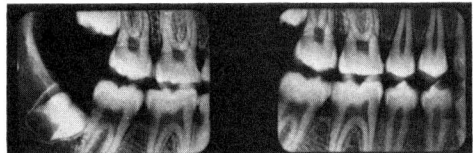

Figure 7-93. Molar and premolar bite-wing radiograph using bite-wing tab.

268   Textbook of Dental Radiology

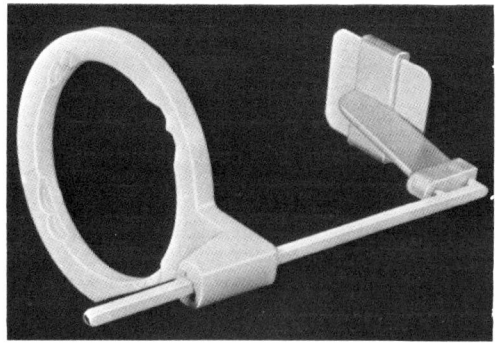

Figure 7-94. Rinn bite-wing film holder assembled with film in place.

wing tab. They are the Rinn Bite-wing instrument (Fig. 7-94), the Precision (Masel) Bite-wing instrument (*see* Fig. 7-20), VIP (Up-Rad) bite-wing instrument (*see* Fig. 7-22), and the Rinn Unibite film holder (*see* Fig. 7-25).

Rinn Bite-Wing Instrument Technic

The interproximal examination is considered the least difficult of the intraoral technics, yet the results of incorrect alignment of the film, teeth, and X-Ray beam are frequently seen on the finished radio-

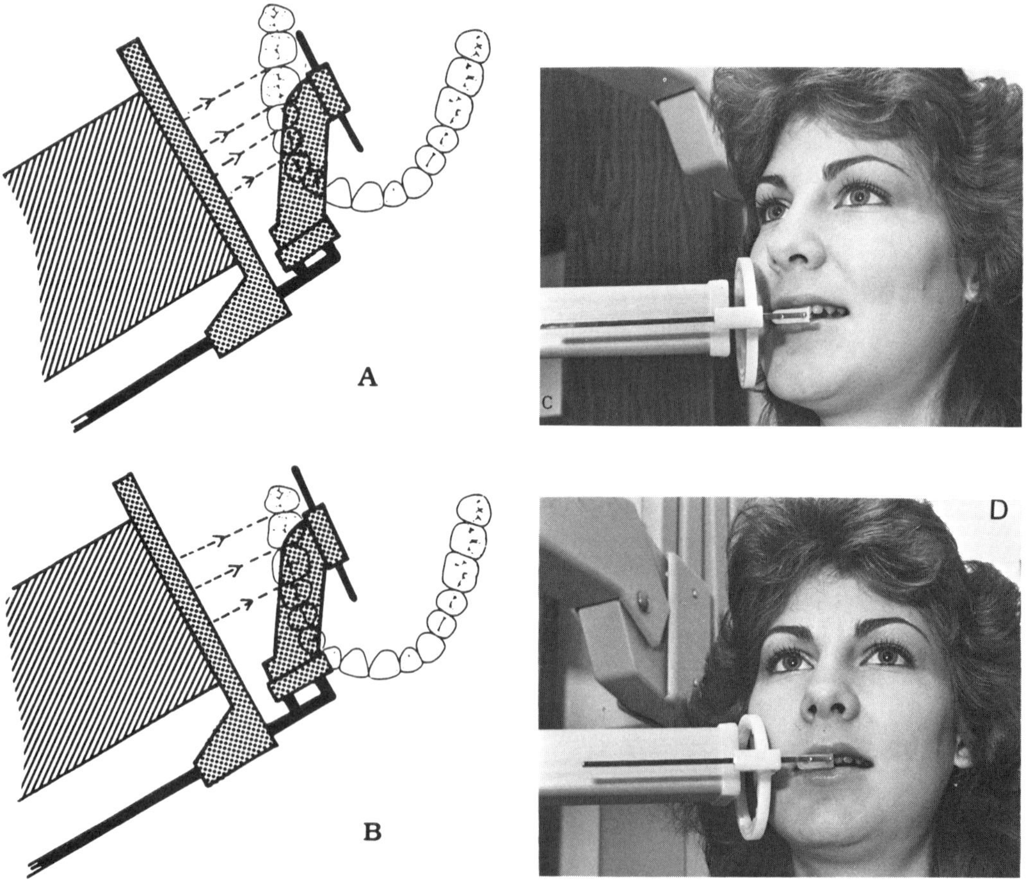

Figure 7-95. The correct positioning of film holder and film for premolar and molar bite-wing projections using the Rinn bite-wing instrument. (A) Premolar bite-wing positioning. (B) Molar bite-wing positioning. (C) Premolar bite-wing projection. (D) Molar bite-wing projection. (E) Premolar and molar bite-wing radiographs.

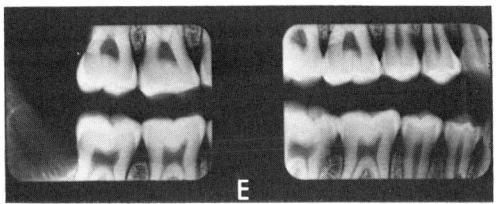

graph. These errors are manifested as "cone-cutting", closed interproximal areas, overlapping of crowns of teeth, and occlusal surfaces recorded diagonally on the film. Bite-wing instruments such as the Rinn Bite-wing instrument were designed to reduce these errors to a minimum.

Assemble the Rinn Bite-wing instrument as shown in Figure 7-94. The film is inserted into position with imprinted side (lead side) facing *away* from the aiming device. Two bite-wing projections are taken, one for the premolar area and one for the molar area. With the biting portion resting on the occlusal surfaces of the mandibular teeth, position the film for each projection as shown in Figure 7-95A,B. Instruct the patient to close firmly to retain the film in position. Slide the aiming device on the rod to approximate skin surface and align the P.I.D. of the X-Ray unit with rod and aiming device on vertical and horizontal planes (Fig. 7-95C,D,E).

OCCLUSAL RADIOGRAPHY
(INTRAORAL OCCLUSAL RADIOGRAPHY)

The occlusal film is much larger than the regular periapical film. It is 3 by 2.25 inches in size, and its film emulsion speed is the same as the speed of periapical films (D group or E group speed film). The film is placed between the occlusal surfaces of the teeth and held in place by the patient's teeth. If the patient has no teeth the film is held in place by the patient's finger (thumbs for maxillary projection and forefinger for mandibular projection). In general, the occlusal radiograph is used to visualize large areas of the maxilla and mandible that cannot be seen on the smaller periapical film.

The occlusal radiograph is indicated in the follwoing cases:

1. in location of fractures of maxilla and mandible;
2. in location of impacted teeth (especially canines and third molars), supernumerary teeth, retained roots, foreign bodies, and calculi in salivary ducts;
3. in cases where patients cannot open mouth wide enough to take regular intraoral dental radiographs;
4. in determining the extent of such pathoses as cysts, osteomyelitis, and bone tumors;
5. in observing the condition of the maxilla following surgery for closure of cleft palates.

Three occlusal intraoral radiographic technics will be described. Of course, there are several other modifications of these three basic occlusal technics that can be used by the operator depending on the clinical situation.

Maxillary Topographical Projection

Purpose. To observe a much larger area of the maxilla than can be observed with intraoral periapical radiographs.

Head Position. Line from tragus of ear to ala of nose is horizontal and is parallel to the floor. The midsagittal plane is per-

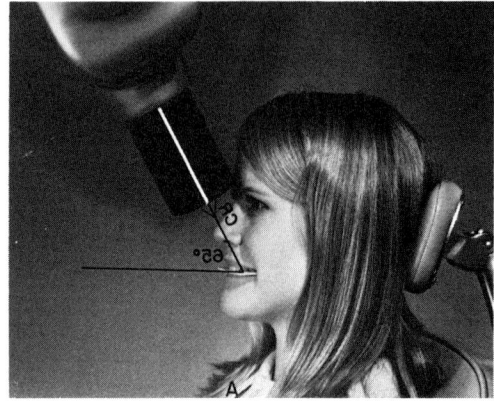
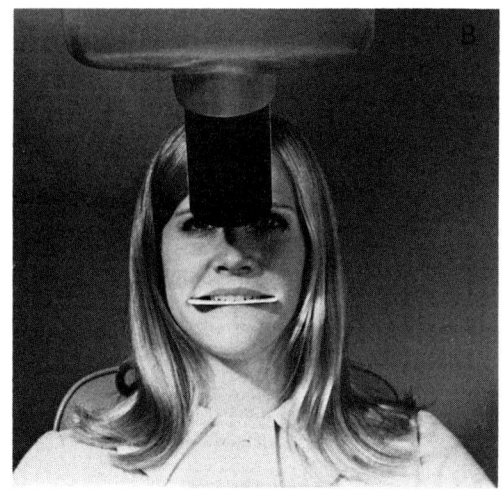
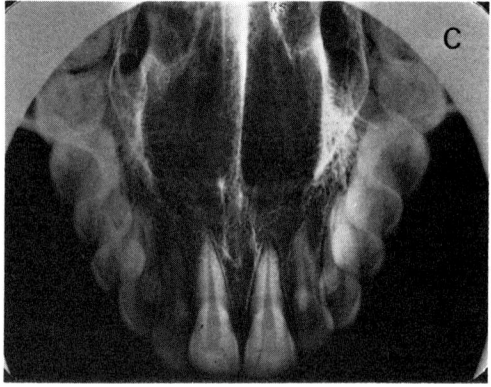

Figure 7-96. Maxillary topographical occlusal radiograph. (A) Side View. (B) Front view. (C) Radiograph of maxilary topograhpical-occlusal projection.

pendicular to the floor.

Film Retention and Placement

Film is placed in the mouth with the longer axis of the film running laterally from side to side, with the pebbled side against the maxillary teeth and inserted posteriorly as the inner vestibule will permit. Patient bites down gently to hold in position. If edentulous, have patient use thumbs to hold film against edentuluous ridges (Fig. 7-96).

Projection of the Central Ray

The principle involved is the same as that used in the bisecting angle technic in intraoral radiography. The central ray of the beam of radiation is directed through, or at the level of, the apex of the maxillary incisor teeth so that it is perpendicular to the bisector of the angle formed by the film and the long axes maxillary incisor teeth.

Direct the **central ray** at a vertical angle of approximately +65 degrees, through a point in the midsagittal plane between the top of the nose and the nasal bridge, to the center of the packet (Fig. 7-96).

Approximate Exposure Factors

Radiographic Factors

Film: Kodak Occlusal Film (D or E speed film)

Source-Film Distance: 9 inches (short

cone) (If you use long cone, use your bite-wing premolar exposure settings.)

Exposure	Adult Impulses	(D speed film) Seconds
65 kV, 10 mA	30	1/2
90 kV, 10 mA	9	3/20

If 15 mA is used, reduce exposure time by one-third. Reduce exposure by 40 percent if E speed film is used, and 25 percent in edentulous patients.

Mandibular Cross-Sectional Projection

Purpose: The projection shows the relationship of an object to the teeth in horizontal plane and thus provides the information that, when coupled with that obtained from the intraoral periapical survey, accurately localizes the position of an object within the mandible. It is also very important in the diagnosis of sialoliths in the submandibular gland duct (Wharton's) and of calcifications within the gland itself (Fig. 7-97).

Head Position. Head is tipped backwards until occlusal plane of maxillary teeth is vertical and at right angles to median plane.

Film Retention and Placement

An occlusal packet is inserted with the pebbled side adjacent to the mandibular occlusal surfaces; short center axis is coincident with midsagittal plane; posterior edge of packet is against anterior aspect of rami. Patient slowly closes on packet with gentle end-to-end bite. Edentulous patients should hold film against ridge with their forefinger.

Projection of the Central Ray (CR)

The central ray enters beneath the chin, approximately one inch posterior to the mental symphysis at the midline. The central ray is directed perpendicular to the occlusal film (*see* Fig. 7-97).

Radiographic Factors

Film: Kodak Occlusal (D or E Speed Film)

Source-Film Distance: 10 inches (short cone) (If you use long cone, use your premolar bite-wing exposure settings.)

Exposure	Adult Impulses	(D speed film) Seconds
65 kV, 10 mA	30	1/2
90 kV, 10 mA	9	3/20

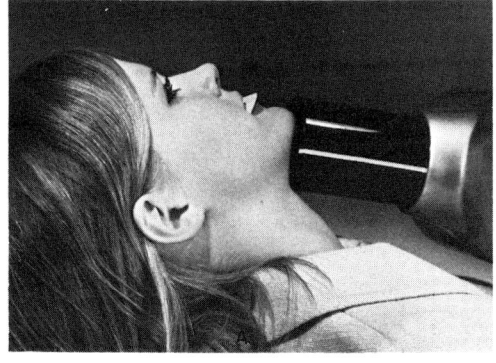 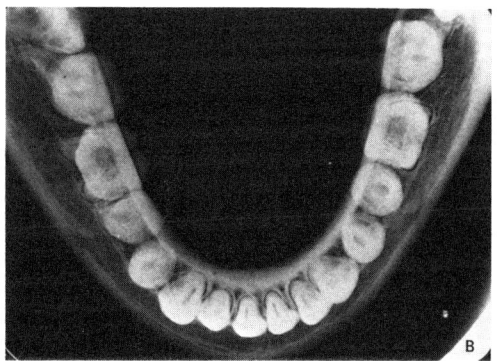

Figure 7-97. Mandibular cross-sectional occlusal radiograph. **(A)** Cone and film placement. **(B)** Resultant radiograph of mandibular cross-sectional occlusal projection.

If 15 mA is used reduce exposure time by one-third. Reduce exposure by 40 percent if E speed film is used, and 25 percent in edentulous patients.

Mandibular Symphysis Projection

Purpose: To get an enlarged view of the mandibular incisor region (Fig. 7-98B).

Head Position: Tilt chair backwards until occlusal plane of the maxillary teeth forms an angle of 55 degrees to the horizontal plane. The midsagittal plane should be perpendicular to the floor(Fig. 7-98A).

Film Placement and Retention

An occlusal packet is inserted with the pebbled side adjacent to the mandibular occlusal surfaces. Long center axis is coincident with midsagittal plane. Patient slowly closes down on packet with gentle end-to-end bite.

Projection of the Central Ray

Use a – 20 degree **vertical angulation** of the cone and direct the central ray parallel to the sagittal plane through the symphysis to the approximate center of the packet. The film packet and the central ray should form an approximate angle of 55 degrees (Fig. 7-98A).

Radiographic Factors

Film: Kodak Occlusal Film (Speed D or E)

Source-Film Distance: 10 inches (short cone) (If you use long cone, use your premolar bite-wing exposure settings.)

Exposure	Adult Impulses	(D speed film) Seconds
65 kV, 10 mA	30	1/2
90 kV, 10 mA	9	3/20

If 15 mA is used reduce exposure time by one-third. Reduce exposure by 40 percent if E speed film is used, and 25 percent in edentulous patients.

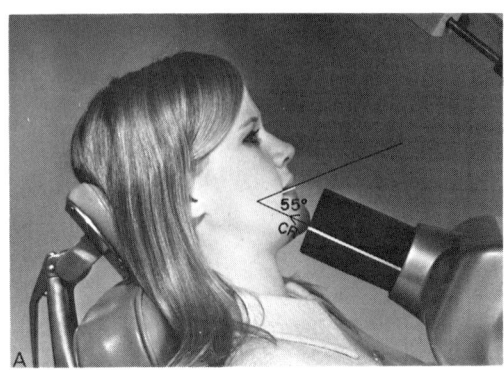
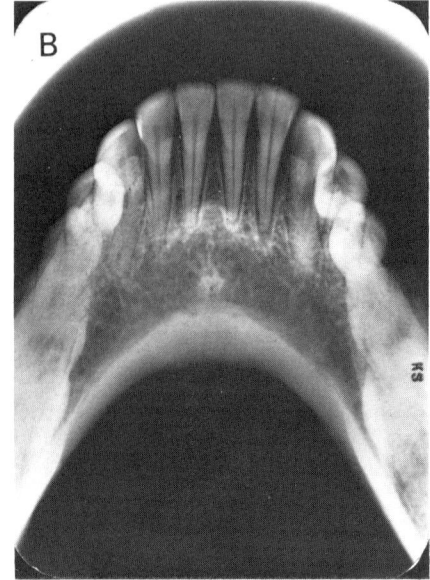

Figure 7-98. Mandibular symphysis occlusal radiograph. **(A)** Cone and film placement. **(B)** Resultant radiograph of mandibular symphysis.

EXTRAORAL OCCLUSAL RADIOGRAPHY

Occlusal films can also be used outside the oral cavity. This procedure, in most cases, should be avoided because it requires a much higher exposure time to produce an image with occlusal films than with extraoral cassettes utilizing intensifying screens. There are times, however, when extraoral occlusal radiography is useful. Some of these projections follow.

Reverse Symphysis Occlusal Radiograph

This is made by placing occlusal film under the chin and projecting the X-Ray beam perpendicular to a line bisecting the angle formed by the plane of the film and the long axis of the teeth. (Fig. 7-99). The radiograph is useful in patients who cannot open their mouths for some reason because of trismus or previous intermaxillary fixation of the jaws.

Lateral Jaw Radiograph of Children

Since the jaws of a child are quite small, an occlusal radiograph many times will suffice as a film large enough for a lateral jaw projection (Fig. 7-100). The technic for the lateral jaw projection is described in Chapter 14.

Actually, lateral jaw radiographs of children should be taken with a five by seven inch screen cassette and screen film because this technic greatly reduces the X-Ray exposure to the child as compared to the occlusal extraoral film technic.

Anterior Profile or "Tangential" Projection

Purpose: To aid in the buccolingual localization of maxillary canine impactions to maxillary incisors (Figs. 7-101B and 7-102).

Head Position: Line from tragus of ear to ala of nose is horizontal.

Film Placement and Retention

Patient holds the pebbled side of the film against the cheek parallel to the midsagittal plane and centered over the region of interest (usually the canine area). The long axis of the film should coincide with the midsagittal plane (Fig. 7-101A).

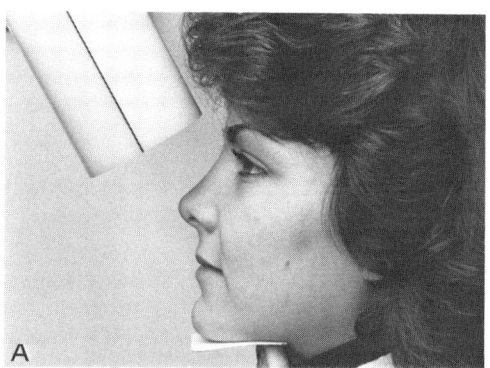
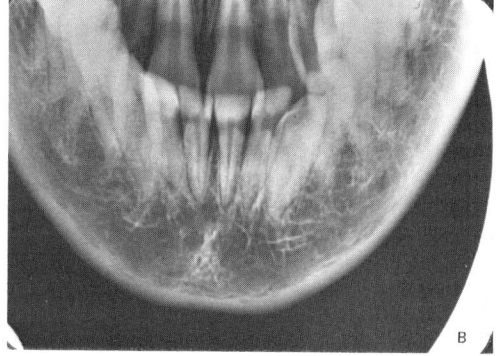

Figure 7-99. Reverse symphysis occlusal radiography. (A) Photo of patient with film under chin. (B) Radiograph of reverse symphysis occlusal radiograph.

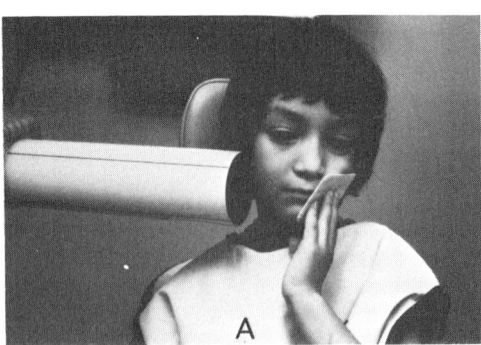 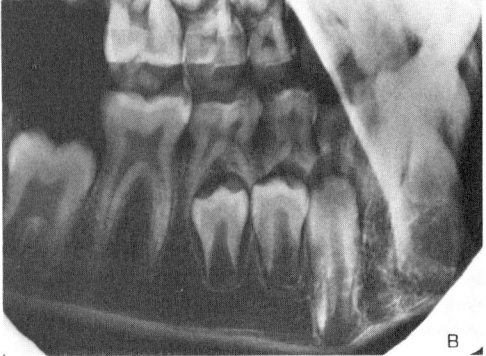

Figure 7-100. Lateral jaw technic in child using an occlusal film. **(A)** Photo of child holding occlusal film for lateral jaw technic. **(B)** Lateral jaw radiograph of child using occlusal film.

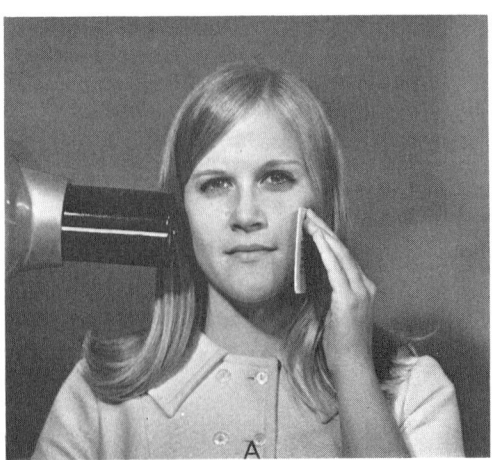 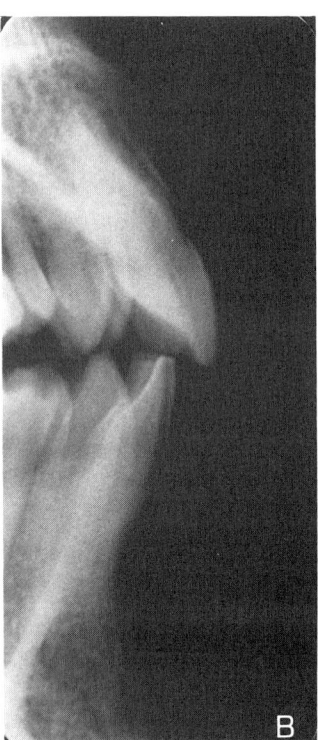

Figure 7-101. Anterior profile or "tangential" projection. **(A)** Position of head, cone, and film. **(B)** Radiograph.

Projection of the Central Ray (CR)

The central ray is directed from the other side of the face through the apices of the teeth of the maxillary or mandibular anterior region perpendicular in both the horizontal and vertical planes to the center of the film. (Fig. 7-101).

Radiographic Factors

Film: Kodak Occlusal Film (D or E speed) (A No. 2 regular periapical film may be used.)

Source-Film Distance: 13 inches (short cone)

Exposure Factors	Adult(D speed film)
65 kV, 10 mA	1/2-3/4 seconds

Reduce exposure by 40 percent if use E speed film.

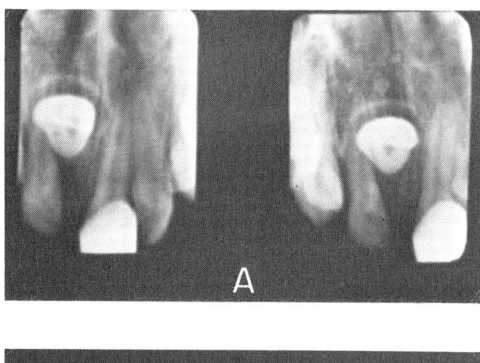
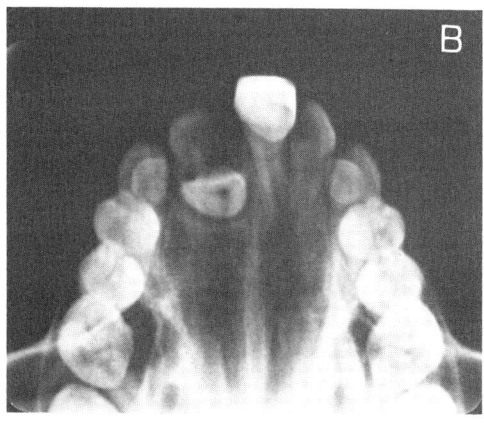
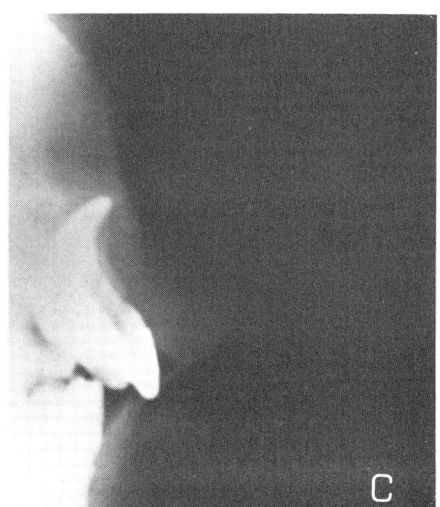

Figure 7-102. **(A)** Periapical radiographs. **(B)** Maxillary occlusal radiographs. **(C)** Anterior profile or "Tangential" projections (localizing malposed tooth).

MANAGEMENT OF RADIOGRAPHIC PATIENTS

In order to reduce radiographic retakes, the operator must know how to manage each patient individually. There are certain patient variations that should be considered before beginning any radiographic procedures. Some of these have been discussed earlier in this chapter.

Anatomical Variations

1. maxillary and mandibular tori;
2. maxillary palatal vault shape, size, and depth;
3. height of muscle attachments in floor of mouth;
4. size of the tongue and whether patient has "tongue thrust" habit;
5. height of the patient (a tall person will oftentimes have longer rooted teeth; the crowns of the teeth may give some indication);
6. edentulous patient will require less exposure time to avoid high density films;
7. people with ruddy, red complexions have more blood in these tissues and may require more exposure time to avoid low density films;
8. larger patients and patients with "fat cheeks" (obese individuals) will require more exposure time to avoid low density films;
9. small patients and thin patients will usually require less exposure time to maintain the desired density.

Age of Patient

The recommended exposures are based on requirements for adults twenty to fifty years of age, average build, and with teeth present. For patients under twelve years of age, the exposure time may have to be decreased to maintain the desired film density. For patients over fifty years of age, the exposure time may have to be increased to maintain the desired film density—the pulps of these teeth have reduced in size considerably. However, many elderly individuals have a condition called osteoporosis of the bone. In this condition, the cortex of the bone becomes thin and the trabeculae of the cancellous bone becomes reduced in number. Naturally, the exposure time should be reduced in a patient with this condition.

Apprehensive Patient

Usually, apprehensive patients are highly nervous individuals who have hypersensitive mouths. They usually have a low pain threshold. The dentist's first contact with these individuals should be a pleasant one, and extreme care should be used in the placement of the films in the mouths of these patients.

It is imperative to employ a rapid and accurate radiographic technic.

Gagging Patient

Gagging is the involuntary effort to vomit. It is caused by the gag reflex and is very annoying in intraoral radiography. Some patients have an extremely low threshold for the gag reflex.

The receptors for the gag reflex are located in the soft palate, the lateral posterior one-third of the tongue, and the region of the retromylohyoid space. The ninth or the glossopharyngeal cranial nerve governs the sensibility of these areas and also controls the reflex movement of swallowing, gagging, and vomiting (Fig. 7-103).

The mechanism of the gagging reflex is set off by initial irritation to the soft palate or the posterior third of the tongue, and it is subsequently conveyed by afferent nerves to the gag center in the medulla oblongata. There is an outflow from this nerve center by way of efferent nerve fibers to the muscles involved in gagging. The gag reflex proceeds by a series of reactions:

1. First, there is the cessation of respiration.
2. This is followed by the contraction of

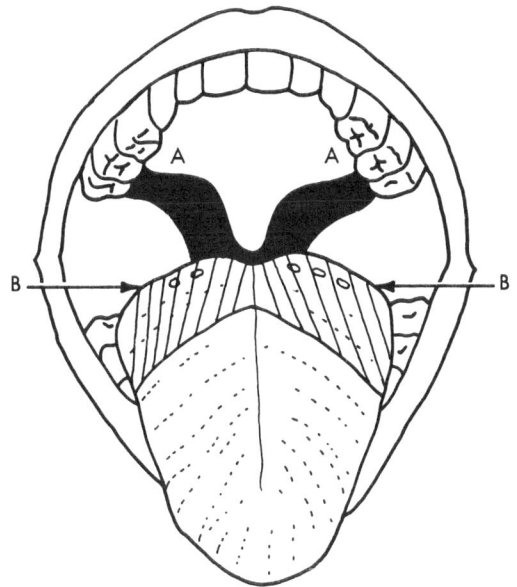

Figure 7-103. Areas of the oral pharynx and the posterior one-third of the tongue where the receptors for the gag reflex are located. These areas are innervated by the ninth or glossopharyngeal nerve—see areas (A) and (B).

the thoracicoabdominal and oropharyngeal muscles. (Sometimes food is regurgitated into the larynx, the oropharynx, and the mouth.)

The two stimuli that commonly initiate the gag reflex are (1) the psychic stimuli and (2) the tactile stimuli.

In order to eliminate or diminish the gag reflex, we must diminish or eliminate these stimuli from the patient. How is this accomplished?

Reducing the Psychic Stimuli

People with accentuated gag reflexes are usually highly nervous and highstrung individuals with very hypersensitive oral tissues. The following methods will aid in the management of these individuals:

1. The first contact with these patients should be a pleasant one, and every effort should be made to give the person confidence in the dentist's ability to perform the service about to be rendered. Discuss the problem in a kindly and sympathetic manner, and try to gain the patient's confidence.

2. Do the anterior regions of the oral cavity first and the most sensitive maxillary molar regions last. Perhaps by then the patient's fears from psychic stimuli will be forgotten, and these sensitive areas in the oral cavity may be radiographed without incident.

3. Try to divert the patient's attention from the unpleasant prospect of gagging to some other interest or preoccupation:

   a. Tell the patient to think of something else.
   b. Have him/her bite hard on the bite-block; the pain may divert his/her attention.
   c. Instruct the patient in breathing exercises. These will keep his/her mind off the dental procedures, and besides, if the patient is breathing, he/she cannot gag. Remember that the first reaction in the gag reflex is the cessation of breathing. An excellent method is to tell the patient to breathe "rapid and shallow." The breathing should be audible to the operator. This should be demonstrated to the patient.

Reducing the Tactile Stimuli

Some people have accentuated gag reflexes because of hypersensitive pharyngeal areas. Patients suffering from chronic sinus trouble (the well-known postnasal drip) are the worst gaggers. An accumulation of mucus and saliva into the nasal or oropharynx may initiate the gag reflex with these people.

Methods to alleviate the tactile stimuli follow.

1. The film should be placed positively

and firmly in the mouth and retained in position without movement. Carry the film into the mouth parallel with the plane of teeth axes, until in proper position, then rotate the film to touch the palate. Film holders such as the Ada Snap-A-Ray are very useful in the positive placement and retention of the film.

2. The exposure of the film should be done as quickly as possible by using a rapid radiographic technic. The timer is preset; the cone is placed for the approximate horizontal and vertical angulations; the film is placed into the mouth and then exposed as quickly as possible. Most people can stand the uncomfortable feeling for a few seconds. For example, for projections in the maxillary molar region:

    a. Preset the timer.
    b. Place film in Ada Snap-A-Ray holder.
    c. Place patient's head in correct position (midsagittal plane perpendicular to the floor and tragal-ala line parallel to the floor).
    d. Adjust the vertical angulation of the cone to +30 degrees and place center of cone over the point of entry (apices of maxillary second molar). Adjust the horizontal angulation by paralleling the face of the flat-ended cone to the buccal surface of the maxillary molar crowns.
    e. Place film quickly and firmly into position to cover maxillary molar region. Have patient close firmly on bite-block.
    f. Expose film quickly.

3. If these procedures do not work, use the following methods:

    a. Give the patient a drink of ice water, which is supposed to dull the sensory nerve endings.
    b. Place ordinary table salt on the tip of the tongue.
    c. Use a topical anesthetic, which may be of the viscous or spray type. When using the spray type topical anesthetic, spray the anesthetic on the palate and the posterior third of the tongue and have the patient EXHALE WHILE DOING THIS. Wait a minute for the anesthesia to take effect. Benzocaine is the active ingredient of this topical anesthetic. The anesthesia lasts for approximately twenty minutes. Use caution in the use of the spray topical anesthetic: (1) do not give it to any individuals who are allergic to benzocaine or have a tendency toward bronchial complications; (2) if the topical spray is inhaled it could cause an aspiration pneumonitis, an inflammation of the air passages of the lungs which could be quite serious. The topical anesthetic procedure is used infrequently, however.

Extreme Cases with Accentuated Gag Reflexes

There are some patients with accentuated gag reflexes. It is usually impossible to take an intraoral periapical radiograph on these individuals. This happens infrequently, but when it occurs, use one of the following technics:

    a. right and left lateral jaw radiographs.
    b. maxillary topographical occlusal radiograph.
    c. mandibular incisor occlusal radiograph.
    d. attempt bite-wing films using a smaller sized film (size No. 1 or No. 0 films).
    e. panoramic radiograph.

Bibliography

Appleman, R.M.: The extended tube technique in intraoral Roentgenology. *AJR,* 62(6):881-889, December, 1949.

Bachman, L.H.: Pedodontic radiography. *Dent Radiogr Photogr,* 44:51-56, 1971.

Barr, J.H.; and Gron, P.: Palate contour as a limiting factor in intraoral X-Ray technique. *Oral Surg,* 12:459-472, 1959.

Bean, L.R.: Comparison of bisecting angle and paralleling methods of intraoral radiology. *J Dent Educt,* 33:441-445, 1969.

Carr, J.D.; et al.: *Manual for Dental Radiology.* Indiana University, School of Dentistry, 1960.

Dempster, W.T.; Adams, W.J.; and Duddles, R.A.: Arrangement in the jaws of the roots of the teeth. *J Am Dent Assoc,* 67:779, December, 1963.

Dresen, O.M.: Control of the gagging patient. *Texas Dent J,* 65:332-333, 1947.

Ennis, L.M.; Berry, H.; and Phillips, J.E.: *Dental Roentgenology,* 6th ed. Philadelphia, Lea & Febiger, 1967.

Ennis, L.M.: The bisecting technique versus paralleling. *Dent Clin North Am,* 779-781, November, 1969.

Ennis, L.M.; and Berry, H.: Necessity for routine roentgenographic examination of the edentulous patient. *Oral Surg,* 7:3-19, 1949.

Fitzgerald, G.M.: Dental roentgenography. I. An investigation in adumbration, or the factors that control geometric unsharpness. *J Am Dent Assoc,* 34:1-20, 1947.

Fitzgerald, G.M.: Dental roentgenography, II. Vertical angulation, film placement and increased object-film distance. *J Am Dent Assoc,* 34:160-170, 1947.

Fitzgerald, G.M.: Dental roentgenography. III. *J Am Dent Assoc,* 38(3):293-303, March, 1949.

Fitzgerald, G.M.: Dental roentgenography. IV. *J Am Dent Assoc,* 41(1):19-28, July, 1950.

Fitzgerald, G.M.: Roentgenographic rebuttal. *Oral Surg,* October, 1960.

Gilbert, R.R.; and Hanan, L.: Duplication and quality control for intra-oral roentgenographic use in clinical periodontics. *Oral Surg,* 26:31, July, 1968.

Kaletsky, T.: A simple way to produce consistently accurate intraoral roentgenograms and a modification of the technic of dental roentgenography. *J Am Dent Assoc,* 26:390, March, 1939.

Landa, J.S.: *Practical Full Denture Prosthesis.* Brooklyn, N.Y., Dental Items of Interest Publishing Co., 1947, pp. 268-279.

LeMaster, C.A.: A modification of technic for radiographing upper molars. *J Natl Dent Assoc,* 8:328, 1921.

Lozier, M.: Etiology and control of gagging reflex in the practice of intraoral roentgenography. *Oral Surg,* 2:766-769, 1949.

Manson-Hing, L.R.: On the evaluation of radiographic technique. *Oral Surg,* 27:631-634, 1969.

McCall, J.; and Wald, S.: *Clinical Dental Roentgenology,* 4th ed. Philadelphia, Saunders, 1957.

McCormack, D.W.: Mechanical aids for obtaining accuracy in dental roentgenology. *J Am Dent Assoc,* 40:144-153, 1950.

McCormack, F.W.: A plea for a standardized technique for oral radiography, with an illustrated classification of findings and their verified interpretation. *Br Dent J,* 2:467-510, 1920.

McCormack, D.: Dental roentgenology: A technical procedure for furthering the advancement toward anatomical accuracy. *J Calif State Dent Assoc,* 89:May-June, 1937.

Medwedeff, F.M.; Knox, W.H.; and Latimer, P.: A new device to reduce patient irradiation and improve dental film quality. *Oral Surg,* 15:1079-1088, September, 1962.

Medwedeff, F.M.; and Ellan, P.D.: A precision technic to minimize radiation. *Dent Surv,* 43:45, October, 1967.

Moss, A.A.: The confident dentist can eliminate gagging by making hypnotic suggestion. *Dent Surv,* 26:198-199, 1950.

Mourshed, F.: Clinical evaluation of two bitewing instruments. *Oral Surg,* 34:972-977, 1972.

Pature, B.: Roentgenographic evaluation of alveolar bone changes in periodontal disease. *Dent Clin North Am,* March 1960.

Peterson, S.: *Clinical Dental Hygiene.* St. Louis, Mosby, 1959.

Price, W.A.: The technique necessary for making good dental skiagraphs. *Dental Items of Interest,* 26:161-171, 1904.

Raper, H.R.: Uses of bitewing radiographs. *Dent Surv,* 30:763, June, 1954.

Raper, H.: Advantages and disadvantages of three radiodontic technics. *Dent Surv,* 1404, November, 1955.

Raper, H.: Critical analysis of three radiodontic technics — introduction. *Dent Surv,* 731, June, 1955.

Raper, H.: Criticism of mathematical angulation technic. *Dent Surv,* 986, August, 1955.

Raper, H.: Mathematical angulation technic.

Dent Surv, 863, July, 1955.

Richards, A.: The control of gagging in dental radiography. *Dent Radiogr Photogr*, (2):1950.

Richards, A.: New concepts in dental X-Ray machines. *J Am Dent Assoc, 73*:69076, 1966.

Scandrett, F.R.; Tebo, H.G.; Miler, J.T.; et al.: Radiographic examination of the edentulous patient. Review of the literature and preliminary report comparing three methods. *Oral Surg, 35*:266-274, 1973.

Scandrett, F.R.; Tebo, H.G.; Quigley, M.B.; et al.: Radiographic examination of the edentulous patient. Differences in number and location of root fragments. *Oral Surg, 35*:872-875, 1973.

Shawkat, A.H.; Nolting, F.W.; Phillips, J.D.; et al.: Evaluation of the utilization of the supine position in intraoral radiology. *Oral Surg, 43*:963-970, 1977.

Shawkat, A.H.; and Phillips, J.E.: Bisecting and paralleling technics for improved periapical examination. *Pa Dent J, 36*:129-133, 1969.

Silha, R.E.: The versatile occlusal dental X-Ray film. III. A new pedodontic survey. *Dent Radiogr Photogr, 39*:40-43, 1966.

Silha, R.E.: Paralleling long cone technic. *Dent Radiogr Photogr, 41*:3-19, 1968.

Silha, R.E.: Special radiographic surveys. *Dent Radiogr Photogr, 45*:23-33, 1972.

Silha, R.E.: Paralleling technic with a disposable film holder. *Dent Radiogr Photogr, 48*:27-35, 1975.

Silha, R.: Roentgenographic service gor gagging patient. *Oral Surg*, 64, January, 1962.

Spear, L.B.; and Hannah, R.: Practical and improved periapical technic. *Dent Radiogr Photogr, 26*:212-25, 1953.

Stafne, E.C.: *Oral Roentgenographic Diagnosis*, 3rd ed. Philadelphia, Saunders, 1969.

Stephens, D.W.: Physiological and psychological approach to the problem of gagging. *Dent Surv, 25*:1795-1797, 1949.

Updegrave, W.J.: Radiographic examination. *Current Therapy in Dentistry*, Vol. II. St. Louis, Mosby, 1966.

Updegrave, W.J.: *Dental radiography with the Rinn bisecting angle instruments*. Elgin, Illinois, Rinn Corp. 1967.

Updegrave, W.J.: Paralleling extension cone technique in intraoral dental radiography. *Oral Surg, 4*:1250-1261, October, 1951.

Updegrave, W.J.: High and low kilovoltage. *Dent Radiogr Photogr*, (4):33-71, 1960.

Updegrave, W.J.: Higher fidelity in intraoral roentgenography. *J Am Dent Assoc, 62*:1-22, January, 1961.

Updegrave, W.J.: Simplifying and improving intra-oral roentgenography. *Oral Surg, 12*:704-716, 1959.

Updegrave, W.J.: *New horizons in periapical radiography*. Elgin, Ill, Rinn Corp, 1966.

Updegrave, W.J.: Simplified and standardized bisecting angle technic for dental radiography. *J Am Dent Assoc, 75*:1361-1368, 1967.

Updegrave, W.J.: Right-angle dental radiography. *Dent Clin North Am, 12*:571-579, 1968.

Updegrave, W.J.: A plea for a standard intraoral radiography with reduced tissue irradiation. *J Am Dent Assoc, 85*:861-869, 1972.

Updegrave, W.J.: The versatile No. 1 X-Ray film. *Dent Radiogr Photogr, 48*:60-62, 1975.

van Aken, J.: Optimum conditions for intraoral roentgenograms. *Oral Surg, 27*:475-491, 1969.

Venokur, P.C.; Einbender, S.; and Myers, B.S.: Modified X-Ray technique for dentistry with patients in the supine position. *Oral Surg, 32*:148-150, 1974.

Voorhees, R.S., Jr.: Occlusal radiography. *Dent Radiogr Photogr, 3*:3-6, 1930.

Waggener, D.T.; and Ireland, R.L.: Intraoral roentgenography for children. *J Am Dent Assoc, 47*:133-139, 1953.

Walton, R.E.: Endodontic radiographic technics. *Dent Radiogr Photogr, 46*:51-59, 1973.

Weissman, D.D.; and Longhurst, G.E.: Clinical evaluation of a rectangular field collimating device for periapical radiography. *J Am Dent Assoc, 82*:580-582, 1971.

Weissman, D.D.; and Sobkowski, F.J.: Comparative thermoluminescent dosimetry of intraoral periapical radiography. *Oral Surg, 29:376-386, 1970.*

Winkler, K.G.: *Influence of rectangular collimation and intraoral shielding on radiation dose in dental radiography. J Am Dent Assoc, 77*:95-101, 1968.

Wuehrmann, A.H.: The long cone technic. *Practical Dental Monographs*. Chicago, Year BK Med, 1977.

Wuehrmann, A.H.: Evaluation criteria for intraoral radiographic film quality. *J Am Dent Assoc, 89*:345-352, 1974.

Wuehrmann, A.H.; and Curby, W.A.: Radiopacity of oral structures as a basis for selecting optimum kilovoltage for intraoral roentgenograms. *J Am Dent Assoc*, 1952.

Wuehrmann, A.H.; and Manson-Hing, L.R.:*Dental Radiology*, 4th ed. St. Louis, Mosby, 1977.

Chapter 8

FILM PROCESSING AND DUPLICATION

EVEN if the finest x-ray equipment is used and the most exacting radiographic technic is employed, the radiograph produced may be of inferior quality if the processing of the exposed x-ray film is carelessly executed.

Processing the film completes what the exposure started. It produces a visible, lasting image of the latent image created by the x-rays. When the x-rays strike the light-sensitive silver salts (AgBrI) in the film emulsion, the energy is stored in the form of a latent image. The latent image becomes visible after the film is immersed in certain chemical solutions that change the exposed silver halide salts into particles of metallic silver. The term for the several operations that collectively produce the visible, permanent images is **processing**.

Processing, automated or manual, consists of developing, fixing, washing, and drying operations and they are all carried out in a darkroom, unless, of course, an automatic processor with a **daylight loader** is used.

Darkroom or Processing Room

The darkroom or processing room should be clean, efficient, and well equipped. Spots, streaks, fog, and other artifacts on the processed radiograph can be traced to poor darkroom conditions.

It is very important that the darkroom be designed to make film processing an efficient, precise, and standardized procedure. Since the processing operations are carried out in near-total darkness, every piece of equipment must be in its specific place. Figure 8-1 illustrates a well-designed darkroom. For efficiency's sake, the room should be large enough to avoid crowded conditions and the equipment should be arranged so as to expedite the flow of work. The size of an x-ray darkroom for a dental office can be as small as three by three feet for an individual dentist; however, for a group practice, installation of a four by six foot darkroom would be more adequate and convenient.

Processing rooms cannot be used as storage rooms or for any other procedure in the dental office that will contaminate the films with dust or fumes. The darkroom must provide adequate bench space and facilities for proper developing, fixing, washing, and drying of the films.

If development and drying are done in the same room, it is recommended that some means of ventilation be provided to supply the room with fresh air as well as exhausting the heated air from the dryer. A room temperature of 70°F is recommended. If humidity is a problem, especially in parts of the country where the

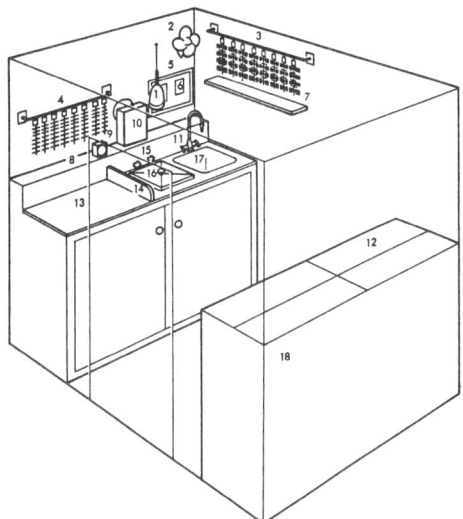

Figure 8-1. (1) Darkroom lamp, (2) Electric fan, (3) Rack for drying films, (4) Storage rack for intraoral hangers, (5) Bulletin board, (6) Exposure and processing chart for dental x-ray films, (7) Drip pan, (8) Shelf, (9) Timer, (10) Utility safelight lamp, (11) Gooseneck faucet, (12) Area for automatic processor, (13) Loading tank, (14) Splashboard, (15) Hot and cold water valves, (16) 8 × 10 dental processing tank, (17) Utility sink, (18) Supply cabinet for chemicals, cassettes, and other accessories. (Courtesy of Eastman Kodak Company.)

climate is hot and humid, air conditioning is a necessity. When the temperature of the processing room exceeds 90°F, the x-ray films may become sensitized by heat alone.

There are certain minimum requirements that every darkroom should have:

1. lighttight room;
2. processing tanks;
3. hot and cold running water;
4. accurate thermometer and interval timer;
5. both white light and safelight illumination;
6. means of viewing wet radiographs;
7. adequate storage space for chemical solutions, film hangers, and cassettes;
8. film drying rack or film dryer;
9. provision for automatic processing; and
10. lighttight drawer for storage and protection of unexposed extraoral film (includes panoramic film).

Lighttight Processing Room

The first requisite of a processing room is the exclusion of all external light. Dental film emulsions are extremely sensitive to visible light, and any light leaking around a door or window will fog and spoil the films. Possible sources of white light leaks are doors, windows, keyholes, ventilators, joints in walls, partitions, and unsafe or damaged safelights. It is advantageous to have a lock on the darkroom door in order to eliminate the possibility of someone opening the door unexpectedly.

Light leaks in the darkroom may be tested in the following manner: Place unexposed films half covered with the black protective paper in various locations in the room where films are normally loaded and unloaded. Leave for three minutes in the dark and process in the usual manner. Any visible degree of fog in that portion of the film not covered by the black paper is indicative of light leaks.

Fluorescent lights should **not** be used as overhead lights in the darkroom because there is often a short afterglow that may fog the first few films opened after the light has been turned off. For the same reasoning, fluorescent illuminators in the darkroom are also contraindicated.

Processing Tanks

There are two methods used in processing x-ray film: automatic and manual processing. Most automatic processors utilize a roller transport system to move the film through the developer, fixer,

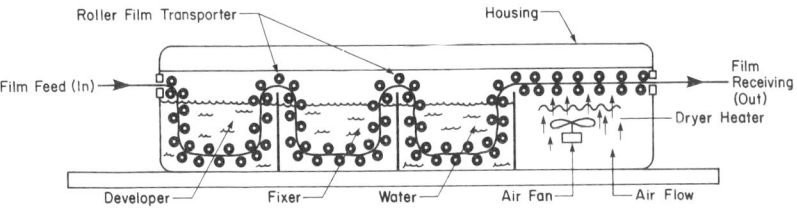

Figure 8-2. Diagram of automatic film processor (From Kasle, M.; and Langlais, R.: *Basic Principles of Oral Radiology,* Vol. 4, Exercises in Dental Radiology. Philadelphia, W B Saunders, 1981).

wash, and dry cycles (Fig. 8-2).

Manual processing is the simplest and probably the most efficient method to develop, rinse, fix, and wash dental films under accurate control. The processing tank is the most important piece of equipment in manual processing. There are many sizes and types of tanks available commercially. The most practical processing tank for a dental office consists of a master tank and two removable insert tanks with a one gallon capacity. The master tank holds the running water for rinsing and washing, and the insert tanks are for the developer and fixer (Fig. 8-3).

Processing tanks are made of polyethylene, fiberglass, or stainless steel (AISI type 316 stainless steel with 2-3% molybdenum). Do not use tanks or other containers that have been soldered, because the reaction of the solution with the solder metals causes chemical fog on the film.

Cleaning Processing Tanks

The action between the mineral salts in the water and carbonate in the developing solutions produces a deposit on the inside walls of the developing tanks. A commercially prepared stainless steel tank cleaner can be used to remove these deposits. After using the tank cleaner, rinse the tank with fresh water and wipe out the tank with a clean cloth. Do not use abra-

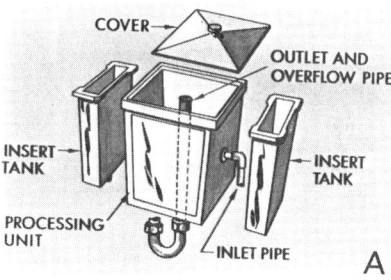

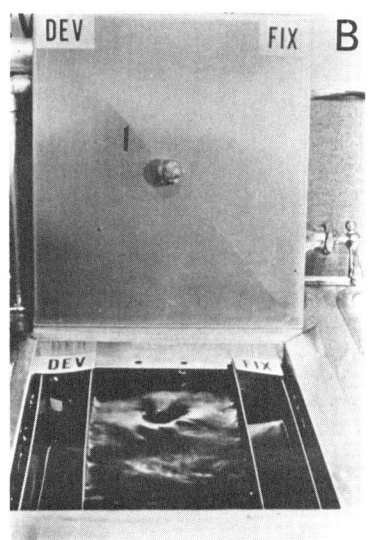

Figure 8-3. Typical dental processing tank. **(A)** Master tank and two insert tanks. Drainage is through an overflow pipe that empties into waste line. The master tank may be emptied for cleaning. **(B)** Master tank filled with running water and left tank filled with developing solution and right tank with fixing solution. (Courtesy of National Audiovisual Center, Washington, D. C.)

sives such as "kitchen cleansers" in the tanks. These abrasives react unfavorably with the developing solution.

Running Hot and Cold Water

X-ray processing solutions are most effective when used with a comparatively narrow range of temperatures. Below 60°F, some of the chemicals are definitely sluggish in action, which may cause underdevelopment and inadequate fixation. Above 75°F, they work too rapidly and may produce fogging of the film. A temperature of 70°F is recommended for three reasons:

1. The optimum quality of the radiograph is attained at this temperature. The contrast and density of the film are most satisfactory and fog is kept to an acceptable low level.
2. The processing time is practical.
3. With modern solution-tempering devices, a temperature of 70°F is usually conveniently maintained. The temperature of the water in the master tank is controlled by a thermostatic or manual mixing value in the water supply (Fig. 8-4). This is the reason hot and cold running water is essential. The temperature of the water in the master tank in turn controls the temperature of the processing solutions in the insert tanks.

Thermometers and Interval Timer

Proper control of the processing time is dependent upon the temperature of the solutions, and a good thermometer is an indispensable processing room accessory. There are two types: (1) a tank thermometer that is plainly marked with both Centigrade and Fahrenheit scales, and has a steel clip on the back formed into a hook to hang the thermometer in the tank, (2) the floating, stirring rod type of thermo-

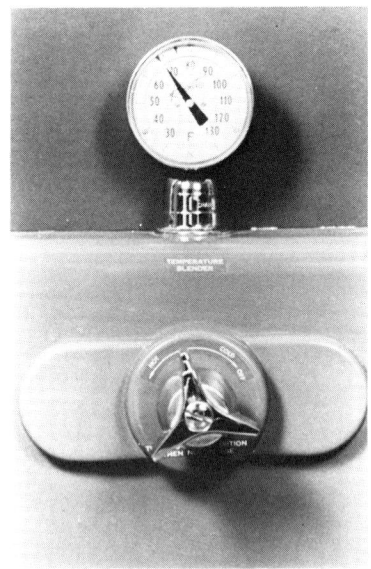

Figure 8-4. Typical mixing value to blend incoming hot and cold water to correct temperature. The water is piped into the bottom of the master tank. (Courtesy of National Audiovisual Center, Washington, D. C.)

meter that is all glass and can also be used for stirring small quantities of processing solutions. An *interval timer* is also important to control time of development and fixation.

Correct Illumination

The processing room must be provided with both white and safelight illumination. White light is desirable when such work as cleaning the tanks and preparing the solutions is done. An illuminator (viewbox) is desirable for reading wet radiographs. This saves time in carrying wet radiographs from darkroom to the dental operatory and reduces the trail of chemical or water spots on the floor. The safelight, with the proper filter, should be placed over the loading bench, no closer than four feet.

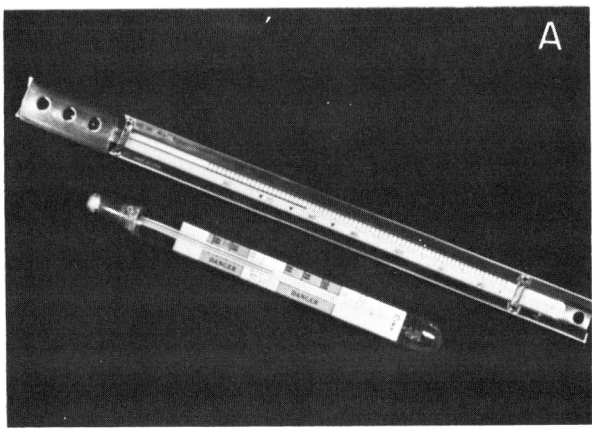

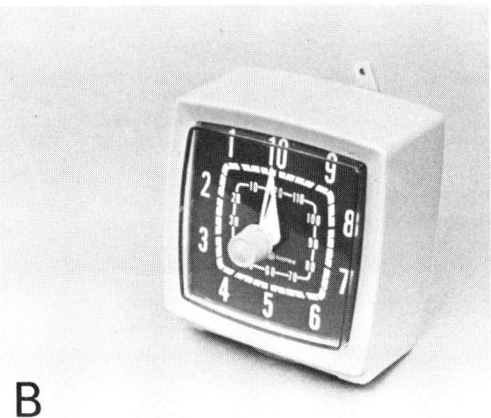

Figure 8-5. Thermometers and Interval Timers. (A) Upper: Floating thermometer. Lower: Tank thermometer. (B) Interval timer.

Safelighting

The function of a safelight is to provide enough illumination in the darkroom so essential processing activities may be accomplished with a minimum amount of errors, but without fogging the film.

Safelight filters are designed to transmit light outside the normal color-sensitivity ranges of film emulsions handled in their light. X-ray emulsions are primarily sensitive to blue and green light, and they are less sensitive to light in the opposite region of the spectrum—yellow and red light. Therefore, safelights are safest when made with amber or red filters. However, most films have some sensitivity to all colors of light transmitted by filters recommended for use with them. Therefore, it is necessary to keep safelight illumination (wattage to bulb) and film handling times under the safelights at a safe, practical minimum. Most dental films have an emulsion characteristic that enables them to be used in more light than with extraoral (panoramic) screen films. Dental films may be used under the Kodak Morlite (ML-2) light-orange filter. This filter transmits a light orange light that is closer to green than red in the light spectrum, permitting a higher level of illumination than a red filter. As a result, darkroom efficiency is increased, and the likelihood of errors is reduced.

The Kodak Morlite (M-2) light-orange filter cannot be used with panoramic or extraoral screen films because it transmits light in the color-sensitivity range of these screen film emulsions.

The Kodak Safelight filter GBX (red) is a new, universal safelight filter that can be used in darkrooms where both intraoral and extraoral films are used. The GBX filter permits higher levels of illumination than the older Wratten 6B (Brown) filter, but lower levels of illumination than this ML-2 (light orange) filter.

Although the GBX filter was designed primarily for darkrooms with automatic processors, it may be used successfully in manual processing darkrooms, provided the films are not handled under safelight conditions for over 2.5 minutes.

Safe illumination in the darkroom is also dependent on the **wattage** of the bulb and the **distance** the safelight is from the workbench (Fig. 8.6).

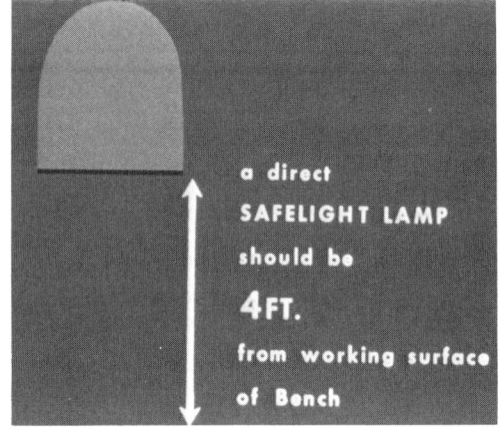

Figure 8-6. Correct distance for safelight over the working bench is 4 feet.

Direct light safelights require a standard 15 watt bulb for most intraoral, panoramic, and extraoral films, while a 25 watt bulb may be used for indirect (reflected from ceiling) light (Fig. 8-7). Kodak SB (single coated, blue sensitive) film requires a 7.5 watt bulb.

The direct safelight should be placed at a minimum of four feet from the workbench. Never shorten this distance unless compensation is made by using a bulb of

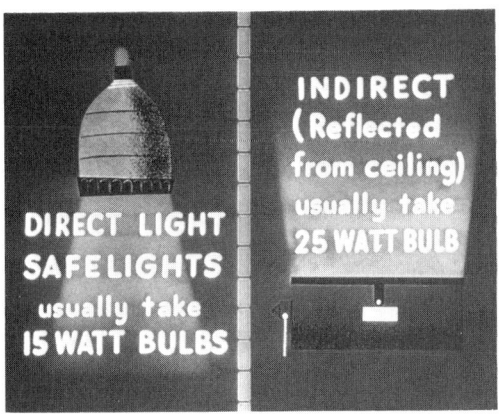

Figure 8-7. Wattage of safelight bulb (15 watt bulb for direct safelight and 25 watt for indirect safelight).

face of the bench beneath the safelight lamp. Place a small coin on each film. Expose one film each to the safelight illumination for the following exposure times: 1, 1.5, 2, 2.5, 3, and 3.5 minutes. Develop the films in the usual manner. After the films have been cleared in the fixing bath, examine each film before an illuminator. If the outline of the coin on the film exposed to the safelight illumination for one minute can be seen, the safelight is **not** safe (Fig. 8-9). Next,

lower wattage. Remember, the inverse square law applies to light illumination: The intensity of light varies inversely as the square of the distance (Fig. 8-8).

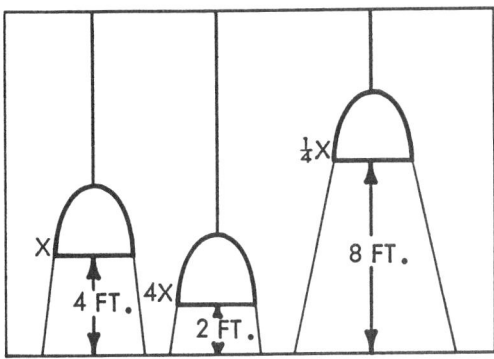

Figure 8-8. Inverse Square Law in Safelight Illumination. If we have X intensity at 4 feet, we have $4X$ the intensity at 2 feet and $\frac{1}{4}X$ intensity at 8 feet.

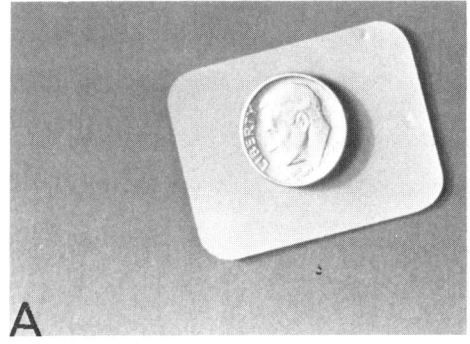

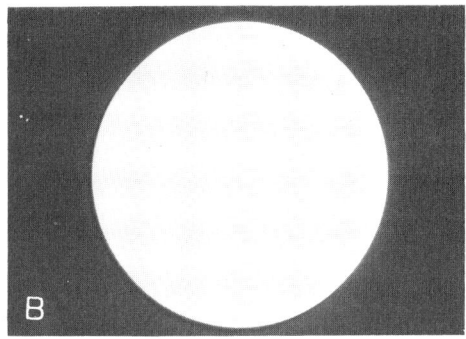

Figure 8-9. Safelight Test. (A) Coin placed on film. (B) Illustration of an unsafe safelight at particular time film was exposed to the film.

Safelight Check

A simple method of checking the safety of illumination of the safelight follows: Remove six dental x-ray films from their packets and lay them on the working sur-

determine, in which film fogging can first be seen—this will indicate the time that is safe for film to be exposed to the safelight.

If the safelight is not safe, the following

things must be done to correct the problem:

1. Replace the bulb with one of lower wattage.
2. Raise the safelight lamp higher from the working surface.
3. Check the filter—the filter may be transmitting light within the color-sensitivity range of the film being used, or the filter may be damaged or broken.

Manual Film Processing

Processing Hangers

Processing hangers for manual processing are available in several sizes to accommodate intraoral and extraoral films (Fig. 8-10A). The intraoral film hangers are made of stainless steel with white cellulose identification tabs (Fig. 8-10B).

Occasionally, pieces of gelatin from the film emulsion adhere to the clips on the hangers. This prevents the clips from getting a good grip on the film with the result that the film may loosen during processing and fall into the tank. A solution of sodium hypochlorite, or Clorox®, will remove gelatin particles from hanger clips. Also, film hangers that have not been washed after use will retain the chemicals of the processing solution on them, and crystallize when they dry. This will cause streaks on the film.

Film hangers should not be placed too close to each other during development, fixing, and drying procedures. If two films stick to each other, artifacts on the film will result.

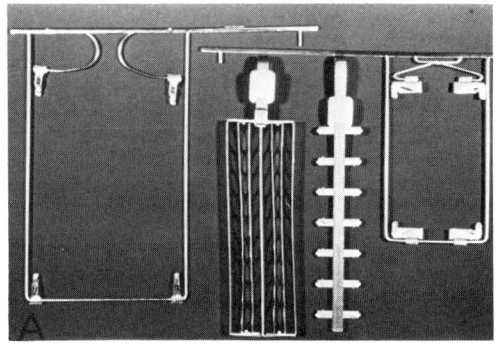

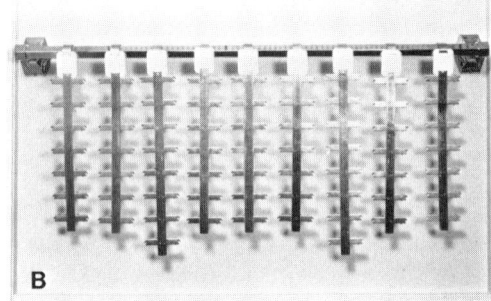

Figure 8-10. Processing hangers for intraoral and extraoral films. (**A**) Assortment of processing hangers. (**B**) Intraoral film hangers with white cellulose identification tabs.

Film Processing

Film processing refers to the entire procedure of (1) conversion of the latent image to a visable image (Fig. 8-11) and (2) the preservation of the visible image. This primarily involves development, rinsing, fixing, washing, and drying. The sequence of steps in manual processing is outlined in Table 8-I.

Table 8-I

SEQUENCE OF STEPS IN MANUAL PROCESSING

STEP	PURPOSE	APPROX. TIME
Wetting	Alkaline developing solution softens and opens up gelatin so developing agents can act on silver halide crystals	15 sec
Development	Production of visible image from latent image; exposed silver halide crystals are reduced to metallic silver, forming radiographic image	5 min
Rinsing	Termination of development and removal of excess chemicals from emulsion	30 sec
Fixation	Removal of unexposed silver halide crystals from emulsion; hardening of gelatin	10 min
Washing	Removal of excess chemicals (if fixing agent [ammonium thiosulfate] is left in emulsion, it will eventually change deposited black silver to brown silver sulfide)	30 min
Drying	Removal of water and preparation of radiograph for viewing	30 min

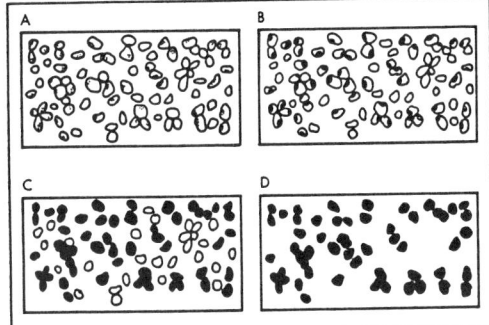

Figure 8-11. Diagram of processing action in x-ray film emulsions: (**A**) Schematic distribution of silver bromide crystals. The gray areas indicate latent image produced by exposure—the silver bromide crystals that have been exposed to x-radiation. (**B**) Partial development begins to produce metallic silver (black) in exposed grains. (**C**) Development completed. The greater the action of the rays on the film, the greater will be the amount of metallic silver left. (**D**) Unexposed silver bromide crystals have been removed by fixing. The fixing solution dissolves the excess silver salts and fixes the metallic silver upon the film by stopping the action of the developer. (Courtesy of Eastman Kodak Co.)

Development

The basic action of development is the reduction (addition of electrons) of the silver in the AgBr or AgI crystal into black metallic silver as follows:

Ag^+ (ion in x-ray-exposed AgBr crystal) + electron (from developing agents) = Ag (metallic)

The silver in an AgBr or AgI crystal that is not exposed (i.e. does not contain the latent image) can be reduced by the developing agents but does so at a much slower rate. Therefore, **time** is a significant factor in the developing process (Fig. 8-12).

Other important factors in the development process include the temperature and concentration of the developer. Manufacturers of radiographic film and developing chemicals have carefully established the optimum conditions of time, temperature, and concentration of chemicals for proper development. By following the manufacturer's directions, the devel-

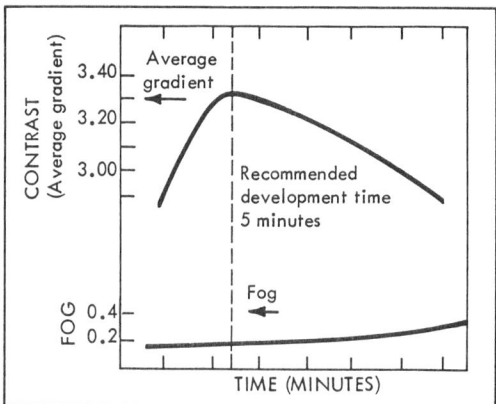

Figure 8-12. This graph illustrates that overdevelopment of the film will cause chemical fog on the film.

opment action will stop when the difference between the exposed (developed) crystals and the unexposed (undeveloped) crystals is the greatest.

The developer or reducing solution used in manual processing is a mixture of hydroquinone and Metol® (Elon). This mixture has a faster development rate than the sum of the development rate of each agent alone. As the developing agents reduce the silver ions to metallic silver, they become inactivated by the process of oxidation. Along with this chemical reaction is a liberation of hydrogen ions. Sodium carbonate is added to developer to serve as a buffer to control the hydrogen ions liberated during the development reaction. A combination of hydroquinone and Phenidone® (rather than Metol) is used in automatic processing because the speed of this combination is of value in the rapid processing of film.

In addition to developing agents, the developer contains (1) an alkali (Na_2CO_3) to maintain the pH in a range of 10 to 11.5; (2) a preservative (sodium sulfite) to decrease the rate of oxidation of developing agents, especially hydroquinone; and (3) restrainers (potassium bromide) to prevent the development of unexposed silver halide crystals, which would cause fogging of the radiographic image (Table 8-II).

Table 8-II

TYPICAL DEVELOPER COMPOSITION

MANUAL X-RAY DEVELOPER (normally used at 68°-78°F)

General Function	Chemical	Special Function	
Reducing Agents	Metol	Quickly builds up gray tones in the image.	The developing agents convert the exposed silver halide crystals into black metallic silver.
	Hydroquinone	Slowly builds up black tones and contrast in the image.	
Activator	Sodium Carbonate	Swells and softens the emulsion so that the reducing agents may work more effectively. Provides required alkalinity for reducing agents.	
Restrainer	Potassium Bromide	Restrains the reducing agents from developing unexposed silver halide to produce fog.	
Preservative	Sodium Sulfite	Prevents rapid oxidation of the developing agents.	
Solvent	Water	Liquid for dissolving chemicals.	

(Table 8-II *continued*)

AUTOMATIC X-RAY DEVELOPER (normally used at 80°-84°F—4½-7 minute cycle
90°-94°F—90 second cycle)

General Function	Chemical	Special Function	
Reducing Agents	Phenidone	Quickly builds up gray tones in the image.	The developing agents convert the exposed silver bromide crystals into black metallic silver.
	Hydroquinone	Slowly builds up black tones and contrast in the image.	
Activator	Sodium Carbonate	Swells and softens the emulsion so that the reducing agents may work more effectively. Provides required alkalinity for reducing agents.	
Hardener	Glutaraldehyde	Controls emulsion swelling to allow better transportation of films through the processor.	
Restrainer	Potassium Bromide	Restrains the reducing agents from developing unexposed silver halide which produces fog.	
Preservative	Sodium Sulfite	Prevents rapid oxidation of the developing agents.	
Solvent	Water	Liquid for dissolving chemicals.	

The developer is affected by rate of oxidation (by use and aeration), number of films processed, contaminants, and accumulation of by-products of development reactions including oxygen, hydrogen ions (causing reduced alkalinity of solution), and bromine ions. All of these factors weaken, or exhaust, the developer. Unless measures are taken to compensate for this exhaustion, underdevelopment will result, adversely affecting the contrast of the films. Also, some of the developer is removed from the developing tank with each film, which lowers the level of the developer.

Replenishment System

It used to be emphasized that the replenisher solution should not merely be original-strength developer. The older replenishers were free of bromide because this ion accumulates in the developer, and they contained higher concentrations of hydroquinone, Metol or Phenidone, and alkali because these ingredients are disproportionately exhausted with continued use of the developer. However, the newer developing solutions such as the Kodak GBX (Green-Blue X-ray) Developer/Replenisher can be used interchangeably as a developer or a replenisher and the need for a separate replenisher solution is unnecessary. This is accomplished by increasing the replenishment rate by 20 percent. It is recommended that six ounces of developer be added each morning to a one gallon tank of the developer solution whether the tank has been used or not. If the tank level is at its maximum, remove six ounces of the old GBX developer and add six ounces of a new solution of the GBX developer. The replenisher performs the double function of maintaining both the liquid level in the developing tank and the activity level of the developer. After adding the replenisher, the developer must be stirred thoroughly.

With the replenishment method, the films should be removed from the developer quickly, not allowing the excess solution to drain back into the tank. Replenisher solution should be stirred vigorously after each addition.

Replenishment should not be continued indefinitely. The developer should be discarded after three months because of the accumulation of gelatin, sludge, and impurities.

Rinsing

After development, the film should be rinsed in clean, circulating water for thirty seconds. This will remove most of the adhering chemicals. Without thorough rinsing after development, the acidity of the fixer is rapidly reduced because the alkali of the developer will gradually neutralize the acid in the fixer. The fixer then will not act evenly on the emulsion, and the radiograph will be streaked and stained.

Fixation

During fixation, the unexposed silver salts are dissolved out of the emulsion and the gelatin is hardened to prevent damage from future handling. A common fixer, which forms stable complexes with silver ions, is thiosulfate in the form of a sodium or ammonium salt. The fixer is called the clearing agent because it clears up the milky appearance of the film. It changes the unexposed and undeveloped silver halide crystals in the emulsion (milky appearance) to soluble silver salts, which are readily removed by washing the film in water. The fixer or clearing agent (hyposulfite or sodium thiosulfate— $Na_2S_2O_3$) is called hypo, a name given by photographers years ago.

A typical reaction of the hypo with a silver bromide crystal is as follows:

silver bromide + sodium thiosulfate (hypo) = silver thiosulfate complex + sodium bromide

The time required for the fixing agent to dissolve the undeveloped silver halide on the film (clear up the original milky opacity) is called the clearing time. As the clearing action subsides, the hardening action begins, resulting in the shrinking and hardening of the gelatin emulsion containing the silver image, which is untouched by the fixing agent. Do not turn the white light on in the darkroom until the film is entirely clear (can see through clear areas) or it will become fogged (darker density) by the light exposing the unexposed silver halide crystals.

The hardener is usually a chromium or aluminum compound. The fixing solution also contains an acid, a stablizer, and a buffer (to maintain the acid pH level).

Fixing time depends on the age and number of films processed. A freshly mixed fixer should clear a screen film in less than one or two minutes. It takes an equal amount of time to harden the film. Thus, the total fixing time is approximately twice the clearing time.

Fixing time can be kept at a minimum by replenishing the fixer (periodically adding fresh fixer after an equal volume of old fixer is removed). Replenishment also prolongs the life and maintains the activity level of the fixer.

The level of the fixing solution generally remains constant, since films and film hangers carry about the same amount of liquid into the fixer tank as they carry out of it when removed. Therefore, it is important to remove an equal amount of the exhausted solution before adding the replenisher.

When the original clearing time has increased by a factor of three, the fixer is exhausted and should be replaced.

Fixing, like developing, must be properly timed. Too short a fixing time can result in inadequate hardening, slower dry-

Table 8-III

TYPICAL FIXER COMPOSITION

MANUAL X-RAY FIXER (temperature same as developer)
AUTOMATIC X-RAY FIXER (fix and wash 5° below developer temperature)

General Function	Chemical	Special Function
Fixing Agent	Ammonium Thiosulfate	Clears away the unexposed silver halide crystals.
Acidifier	Acetic or Sulfuric Acid	Stops development by neutralizing developer. Provides required acidity.
Hardener	Aluminum Cloride or Sulfide	Shrinks and hardens the emulsion.
Preservative	Sodium Sulfite	Maintains chemical balance of the fixer chemicals.
Solvent	Water	Liquid for dissolving chemicals.

ing, and the possible loss of permanence of the image. Prolonged fixing may cause the hypo to be bound to the emulsion so that it cannot be removed in washing, thereby causing an eventual brown discoloration on the radiograph. Also, if the film is left in the fixing solution, for instance, for an hour or more, it will cause bleaching of the image, resulting in a loss in density (Table 8-III).

Washing

The object of washing is to remove residual processing chemicals and silver salts from the radiograph. If these chemicals are not removed, the radiograph will discolor, impairing its value as a permanent record.

Radiographs that have turned brown with age are a result of improper washing. The retained hypo in the emulsion reacts with the silver image to produce a brown silver sulfide in much the same way as silverware tarnishes when exposed to the hydrogen sulfide of cooking gas. The general reaction is:

    hypo + silver = silver sulfide (brown)
                    + sodium sulfide

The washing procedure requires clear water running at a rate of approximately eight tank volumes per hour. Hangers should be well spaced and completely immersed in the tank so that chemicals can be removed from the tops of the hangers. The time required in the wash tank depends on water temperature, rate of flow, and type of fixer. Washing is usually complete in twenty to thirty minutes.

Drying

In most offices, films are dried by merely hanging a rack in the darkroom above a drip tray designed to catch the run-off excess water. Other offices use an ordinary fan to dry the film. However, the fan should not blow directly on the films.

Cabinet dryers are available that are equipped with a fan and heating elements, temperature not to exceed 120°F (49°C). Usually this type of dryer should be vented to the outside to prevent moisture condensation in the darkroom. Moderately warm air is preferred to hot air.

It should be remembered that wet films are subject to damage from scratching and abrasion if not handled properly. If there is dust in the air, dirt will become easily embedded within the emulsion. Do not remove wet radiographs from their

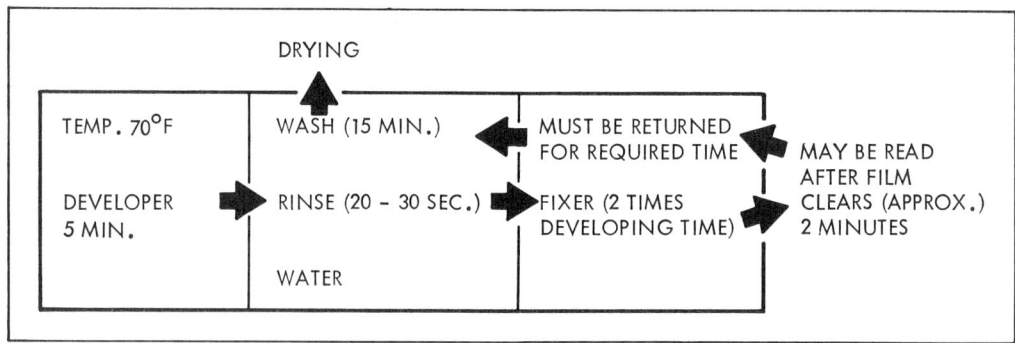

Figure 8-13. Basic steps in processing x-ray film manually.

hangers until they are completely dry.

Films can be rapidly dried by two methods:

Wetting agents will decrease the drying time and prevent drying marks. It works by reducing the surface tension of water on the film so the water will drain more rapidly from the film after washing. There are a number of wetting agents on the market such as Kodak's Photo-Flo® and General Electric's Supermix Wetner®. The wetting agents are actually detergents. A small amount of the wetting agent is placed in the final rinse water. After thirty seconds in the final rinse, the radiograph is placed in the dryer. This will decrease the normal drying time of the film.

Alcohol: This method is used when a dry film is needed in an emergency situation. Use a 70% concentration by volume of any good grade denatured alcohol. Thoroughly drain the films after the final wash and immerse the films in a tray of alcohol with the temperature under 70°F for two minutes. Rock the tray to make sure the films do not stick to the bottom of the tray and so both sides of the films are thoroughly bathed. Remove and place films in a second tray of alcohol. This will remove the last remnants of the water. After draining the films, hang the films up for drying. The alcohol will evaporate quickly leaving a dry film.

Manual Processing Procedure

In most darkrooms the developer will be in the left-hand tank as you face the tank, the water bath in the center, and the fixer in the right-hand tank. In strange darkrooms, the developing solutions can be identified by its slippery feeling, the fixer by its vinegary odor when fresh.

Processing involves chemical reactions that, like all chemical reactions, are critical and require careful attention to details.

The steps employed in tank processing x-ray films are summarized in the following paragraphs (Fig. 8-13).

1. *Stir solutions:* Stir developer and fixer solutions to equalize their temperature. (Use separate paddle for each to avoid possible contamination.) There is a tendency for the temperature at the bottom of the tank to be less than the upper areas.

2. *Check the solution level* of the developer—if it is low, the correct level should be maintained by adding replenisher. Keep a bottle of replenisher solution on hand for this purpose. Do not add water to devel-

oper to maintain proper level. This practice will dilute the developer and slow down the developing action on the films.

3. *Check temperature* of the solutions and adjust, if possible, to 70°F before development. Never place ice in the solutions to cool them down—this will dilute the solution. One way to cool the solutions in warm weather would be to place ice cubes in a rubber glove and then place in solutions. Be sure to stir the solutions, though, in order to equalize the temperatures in the solutions after cooling.

4. *Exclude all white light* in the processing room and turn on safelights. (Use only safelights with GBX filters for screen film. This includes the panoramic films.)

5. *Remove exposed film* from its packet and clip into processing hangers (Fig. 8-14).

6. *Set the interval timer* so it will ring at the end of the desired time of development. Consult the manufacturer's table, which is based on the temperature of the developer. When employing regular x-ray developer, the time of development is five minutes at 70°F. If rapid x-ray developer is used, the development time is three minutes at 70°F.

7. *Immerse the film* smoothly into the developer solution and start the timer. Agitate film hanger by raising and lowering it several times to break up residual air bubbles and permit the solution to bathe both surfaces of the film. Agitating the film will also drive away the accumulated bromide ions that form near the surface of the film and prevent the developing agents from getting to the film emulsion. Do not crowd film in the developing tank—films may rub together and

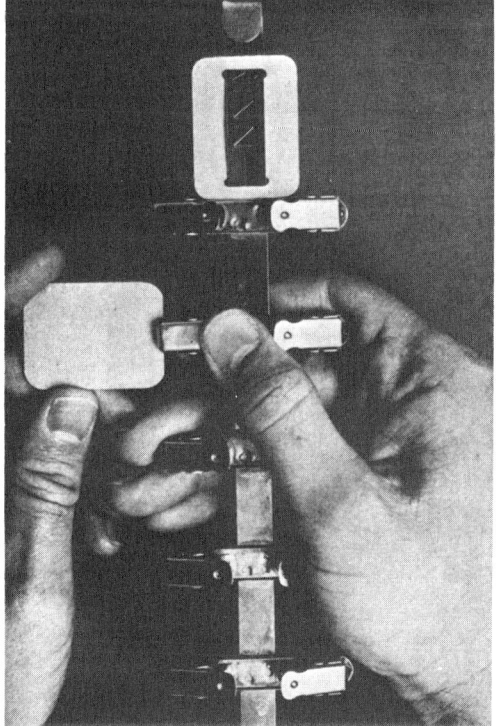

Figure 8-14. After the name of the patient has been placed on the hanger tab, the film is removed from the film packet and placed in the clip of the film hanger. Avoid finger marks, scratches, and film bending.

become stuck. Allow at least one inch of space between films.

8. *Remove hanger* from developer when bell rings, indicating the termination of the development period. Do not remove films from the developer tank too rapidly because excess solution is carried away from the tank. Allow five seconds for the excess solution to drain back into the developing tank.

9. *Immerse the film* in the circulating rinse water and agitate. This will take approximately fifteen to twenty seconds. A **stop bath**, such as Kodak Indicator Stop Bath, can be used in place of a water rinse. A stop bath retards development faster and more

uniformly than water rinse.
10. After rinsing, *place the film in the fixer solution* and agitate until fixer has thoroughly bathed both film surfaces. **Do not expose to white light until the film has cleared.** The time required for the fixer to dissolve the undeveloped silver halide in the film (the original milky opacity of film disappears) is the clearing time. An equal amount of time is required for the silver salt to diffuse out of the emulsion and for the gelatin to be hardened. Thus, the total fixing time for a film usually is approximately twice the clearing time. It takes approximately one to two minutes to clear a film in the fixer. It is possible to view the radiograph in white light at this point, but additional fixing is needed to preserve the image and to harden the emulsion properly. If the films are viewed wet, they must be returned to the fixer and allowed to remain for the recommended time. Too short a fixing time can cause inadequate hardening, slower drying, and possible loss of permanence in the image. If left too long in fixing bath, for instance, for an hour or more, the image may lose radiographic density. The fixer should always be discarded when fixing requires too long a time. Use of an exhausted fixer can result in inadequate hardening with abnormal swelling and slow drying as well as stained or otherwise damaged films. (NOTE: Be sure to recover silver before discarding used fixer solution.)
11. Upon completion of fixation, *remove film to the washing compartment.* Let it remain until it is completely washed in circulating water. Allow adequate time for thorough washing (15-20 minutes). Proper washing time for x-ray films depends principally upon the frequency with which the water is changed. The rate of flow of the water should be adjusted so that the water in the tank changes completely approximately ten times each hour. To determine the rate at which the water changes in the wash tank, measure the time it takes to fill the tank once. If this is six minutes, the tank volume will be replaced ten times in an hour. Under these conditions, films should be washed at least twenty minutes, the time being computed from the moment the last of the group of films is placed in the wash tank. A temperature of approximately 70°F is recommended. Also, prolonged washing tends to make the emulsion soft, especially if left in the wash overnight.
12. *Remove film from final wash* — allow films to drain for two or three seconds after being lifted from the wash water.
13. *Hang up films to dry*, or place in a dryer that supplies circulating, clean dry air.
14. *Remove the dry radiographs* from the hanger by **opening** the clips. Do not pull film from clips since clips may be broken or portions of film remain to clog them later when another film is to be processed.
15. *Place films* into special film mounts.

X-Ray Checker

The analysis of film quality can be done rather simply by use of an "x-ray checker" as devised by Wainwright and Villanyi in 1960 (Fig. 8-15). The three parts of the "x-ray checker" are as follows:
1. *Lead* (total absorber) $1/32$ inches thick, $9/16$ by $1 1/4$ inches in size) — clear area used to analyze fog;
2. *Aluminum* (specific absorber) (4 mm

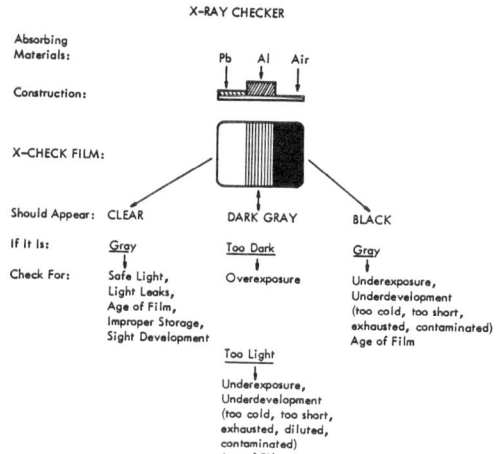

Figure 8-15. The x-ray checker (Courtesy of William W. Wainwright.)

thick, $9/16$ by $1\,1/4$ inches in size) — gray area used to analyze density changes;

3. *Acetate* (air absorber) ($1/32$ inch thick, $1\,1/4$ by $1\,3/4$ inches in size) — black area to analyze developing technic.

In order to obtain a standard radiograph using the Wainwright X-Ray Checker, place the "x-ray checker" over a No. 2 regular film and position the x-ray P.I.D. one inch from the film. Expose the film for the same amount of time normally used for the lower molar region. Process the film with the regular processing technique. If a good standard film cannot be obtained with the technique used, take the "x-ray checker" to another dental office known for producing good films and have them expose and process a film. This will provide a standard film to compare with radiographs taken from time to time. Proper use of the "x-ray checker" will aid in "trouble-shooting" for problems associated with the processing (Table 8-IV) and exposure techniques used.

Automatic Film Processing

Manual film processing is gradually being replaced by automatic processing. There are many reasons for this. First, automatic processors shorten the processing time from 50-60 minutes to 1.5 to 5 minutes. Second, the automatic processing cycle produces constant end-results. Of course, this is dependent on proper maintenance of the equipment. Automatic processors require less floor space than manual processors and have daylight-loading capabilities. Also, film hangers and film dryers, used in manual processing, are not required in automatic processing. Still another decided advantage is that automatic processing eliminates wet reading of films, which drips solution all over the office. Furthermore, a dry film is more useful diagnostically than a wet film.

The basic mechanism of automatic processors is usually a series of rollers that transport the films through the various sections — developer, fixer, washer, and dryer (Fig. 8-16). These rollers are driven by a series of gears, chains, and pulleys; any change in their speed, size, or tension alters the rotating speed of the rollers, which in turn affects the processing time in each section. Spacing of the rollers must be carefully adjusted to prevent jamming and slipping of the film during transport.

In addition to assuring continued movement, the rollers have other functions. They provide a massaging action, which contributes to the uniform processing of the films in the developing and fixing sections. Also, there are special squeegee rollers that remove processing solutions from the film surfaces, which reduces the amount of solution carry-over from one tank to the next. This prolongs

Table 8-IV

MANUAL FILM PROCESSING TROUBLE CHART

Condition	Cause
1. **Low Density and contrast**	a. **Underdevelopment** 　1) time too short 　2) temperature too low 　3) combination of both 　4) inaccurate thermometer b. **Exhausted developer** c. **Diluted developer** d. **Incorrectly mixed developer**
2. **Fog** (generalized darkening of film)	a. **Exposure to light leaks** in darkroom b. **Unsafe safelight** (too high bulb wattage, incorrect filter, crack in filter, too short safelight-to-workbench distance) c. **Exposure of films to white light** before films are cleared by fixer d. **Exposure of films to unwanted x-radiation** (store films safe distance from x-ray source or in lead-lined boxes) e. **Chemical fog**: 　1) overdevelopment (time) 　2) development at high temperatures 　3) oxidized, exhausted developer (may stain emulsion brown) 　4) repeated inspection of films during development 　5) contaminated, corroded tanks
3. **Stain**	a. **Yellow or brown**: exhausted developer, oxidized developer; insufficient rinsing; exhausted fixer (hypo later reacts with silver to produce silver sulfide); prolonged fixing b. **Variegated (different colors in streaks or spots)**: careless rinsing, causing fixer to act unevenly on emulsion; exhausted developer or fixer; contaminated developer or rinse water c. **Green**: insufficient washing d. **Grayish white scum**: incomplete rinsing (excess developer carried into fixer precipitates hardening agent, resulting in white sludge in solution and white scum on film; can be prevented by proper rinsing)
4. **Marks or defects**	a. **Crinkle marks**: curved black or white lines caused by film bending or rough handling of film b. **Static marks**: lightning or treelike marks on film caused by static electricity produced by friction between film and intensifying screen or when removing fresh film from box; usually occurs during periods of low humidity c. **Water marks**: caused by water droplets on film d. **Screen marks**: white spots on film caused by dust particles, small foreign objects, defects in screen e. **Streaking (uneven density)**: 　1) failure to rinse films prior to fixation 　2) failure to stir processing solutions thoroughly after replenishment 　3) failure to agitate films in developer and fixer 　4) unclean film hangers

*Streaking from improper rinsing is due to the fact that one or two minutes may elapse before the alkali in the developer carried over by the film is neutralized by the acid in the fixer bath. During this time, development of the film will continue, causing streaks on the film.

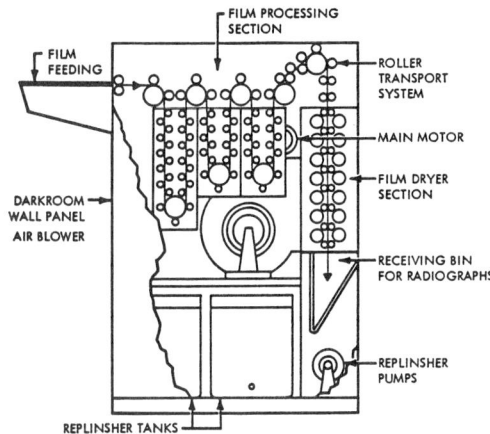

Figure 8-16. Section through a Kodak X-OMAT automatic processor model. (Courtesy of Eastman Kodak Co.)

the life of the fixer and increases the effectiveness of the washing procedure. The squeegee rollers in the wash section remove most of the water from the film emulsion prior to transport of the film to the drying section, allowing the film to dry uniformly and rapidly. In the drying section, the film is quickly dried by jets of heated air before the film drops into the discharge receptacle.

Since the total processing time is reduced in automatic processing, the chemical concentration and temperature of the solutions must be increased. Phenidone is substituted for Metol (Elon) as a developing agent because, when combined with hydroquinone, it provides the rapid chemical reaction necessary for automatic processing (Table 8-2). In the ninety-second automatic processors, the temperature is kept at 90-94°F in the developer, fixer, and wash sections and 135°F in the dryer section. The longer-cycle automatic units process at temperatures of approximately 83°F for a 4.5 minute cycle.

To prevent the emulsion from softening and sticking to the rollers, a special hardening chemical, glutaraldehyde, is added to the developer. Sulfate compounds are also added to the developer to minimize the swelling of the emulsion so that the films can be transported by the rollers uniformly.

With automatic processors, a rigid schedule of replenishment is necessary to maintain the proper concentrations of the solutions and to neutralize the unwanted by-products of each reaction. To maintain the alkalinity of the developer, the acidity of the fixer, and the chemical strength of both solutions, a replenisher must be added at a constant rate for each film processed.

If continued satisfactory results are expected, automatic processors must be cleaned routinely and preventative maintenance procedures followed. Experience has shown that the greatest cause of automatic processor breakdown is failure to keep the rollers clean. A schedule should be established for cleaning the rollers and replenishment and changing of solutions. A proposed schedule is listed below.

1. Replenish solutions and check levels and temperature daily. Temperature of developer should be 81-83°F for longer-cycle automatic processors (80°F for 5.5 minute cycle, and 83° for 4 minute cycle). It is best to drain water section each night. Always run a cleaning film through each morning before use.
2. Clean roller racks with warm running water weekly. Soak and wash roller sections thoroughly for 10-15 minutes only. If you have an ultrasonic radiographic tabletop cleaning unit (Health-Sonics Corp.), the roller racks can be cleaned in five minutes. Remember to run at least two panoramic cleaning films through processor before use (exposed films will do).

3. Change solutions every two to four weeks, depending on rate of use of processor. Be sure to use rapid-processing developer and fixer solutions specially made for automatic processors. Do not use processing solutions or films designed for manual processing.
4. Monthly cleaning
    a. Clean developer section with special developer cleaner. (Failure to do so will cause foggy or streaked films.)
    b. Clean fixer section with warm water only. This will prevent crystals from forming on fixer rollers.
    c. Clean washing section with household bleach/water solution. This will prevent scum forming in the water and leaving spots and artifacts on films.
    d. Rinse all racks thoroughly with water after removing from cleaning solutions.
    e. Visually check dryer; dust as needed.

Preventive maintenance procedures are important and a few of them are listed for your convenience.

1. Check each day to see if transport sections are aligned properly. The films will fall through to the bottom of the tanks if the transport sections are not aligned properly.
2. Lubricate moving parts monthly. Gears, sprockets, idlers, bearings, drive mechanisms, and ring points must be lubricated on a regular basis. Failure to do so will cause excessive wear of moving parts and will eventually slow down the speed of the rollers and, in turn, affect film quality. Do not allow any oil to get on rollers.
3. Replenish the solutions on a regular basis according to the rate of films processed. After four panoramic films, add approximately 6 ounces. Failure to do so will result in low levels of exhausted developer and fixer. This will cause smudgy, low-density films.
4. Check the temperature of the processing solutions regularly. Changes in temperature of the developer will cause changes in density of the processed film. (It only takes a change in temperature of a few degrees to affect the density. It is important to be sure that the thermostat on the processor is accurate.)
5. Keep the cover open slightly when the processor is not in use. After each day's operation, leave cover slightly open so the chemical fumes can escape. Failure to do so could lead to fogging (blackening) of films.

The following is a quick test to check an automatic processor. First, process an unexposed film. It should be clear, clean, and dry. If it is not, check (1) solutions (exhausted developer will create and increase film fog); (2) safelight; (3) darkroom light leaks; and (4) rollers (they may need to be cleaned). If the film is not dry, check dryer temperature and fixer. Second, process a film that has been exposed to light. It should be black and dry. If it is not, check solutions and dryer temperature.

Here are a few important recommendations for feeding the film into the processor.

1. Feed the films slowly and carefully. Enter the panoramic films into the processor in a straight line with the roller system. Failure to do so could cause a jam-up in the processor.
2. If film is bent, insert the unbent side of the film into machine first.
3. Do not feed damp or wet films into machine, as it will contaminate rollers

and cause streaking of subsequent films.
4. Do not feed films too quickly in succession. They may stick to each other and jam the machine.

Several brands of automatic processors are available (Table 8-V). Since they are competitive in performance and price, the decision of which brand to buy usually rests on the availability of competent repair service. See Figure 8-17 for photographs of some of the major commercially available dental automatic processors. Table 8-VI lists problems commonly encountered with automatic film processing.

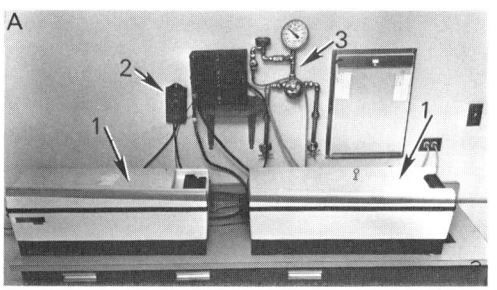

(A) The Xonics (Xonics Medical Systems) automatic processor with replenishment systems. (1) Xonics automatic processor (P-6). Processing time is $4^{1}/_{2}$ minutes to dry. Does not require hard plumbing, but utilizes flexible plastic tubing for wash drain and wash water supply. (2) Replenishment system uses a diaphragm-type pump. Replenisher solutions located in cabinets below processors. Activation of system is related to film usage. (3) Mixing valve plumbing system to control water temperature.

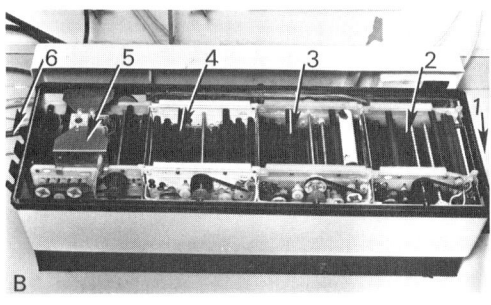

(B) Xonics processors are gear driven via a belt from main drive motor to drive shaft. The individual rack rollers are belt driven. A roller transport system is used to carry film. Daylight loaders are available for all size dental films. (1) Film inserted at this end. (2) Development rack. (3) Fixer rack. (4) Wash rack. (5) Dryer. (6) Film exit.

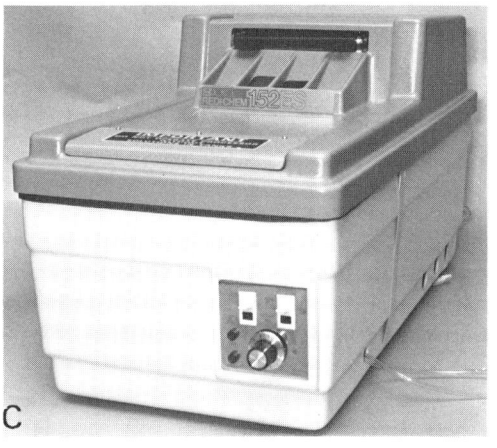

(C) Xonics REDI-CHEM 152ES automatic processor (1981 model).

Figure 8-17. Commercially available dental automatic film processors.

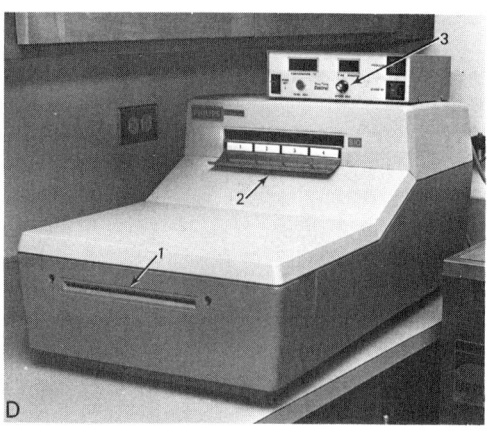

(D) Philips 810 automatic processor (Philips Dental Systems). May be installed with external plumbing into water and drain hook-ups or with an optional water recirculator, eliminating the need for external plumbing. Processing time and temperature can be varied from 50 seconds to 6 minutes (20-35°C [68-95°F]). An archival-quality film is provided in 4½ minutes at 28°C (83°F). (1) Film is inserted here. (2) Film exits here. (3) Time/temperature control system.

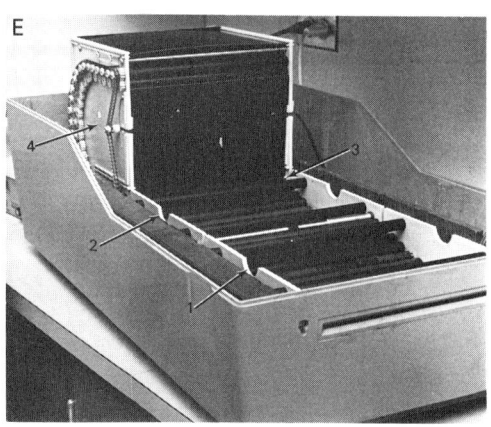

(E) Philips 810 employs a bicycle and ladder-type drive system with stainless steel chains and gears. The film transport system uses plastic and rubberized rollers. Two daylight loaders are available, one for the larger panoramic and 8 × 10 films and one for intraoral films only. (1) Developer transport module. (2) Fixer transport module. (3) Washer module underneath dryer module (4) which employs a patented spray-wash. (4) Dryer module.

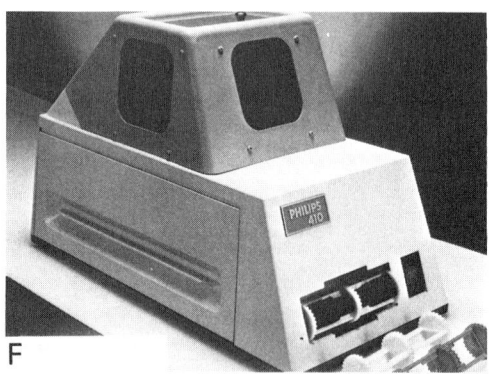

(F) New Philips 410 automatic processor for intraoral x-ray film only (1981 model). Provides wet reading in 3½ minutes and dry film in 6½ minutes.

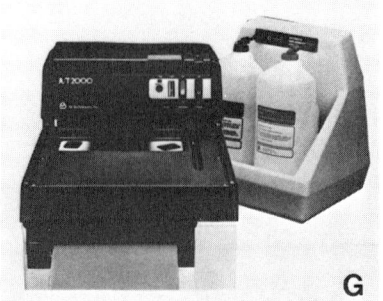

(G) A/T2000 (Air Techniques, Inc.) automatic processor requires water and waste hook-ups. Processing time preset at the factory from 5 minutes, dry to dry. This time can be changed to 2½ minutes by changing the pulleys on the main motor drive and the amid drive shaft. An automatic replenisher system is available as show here. It maintains the proper chemistry level and strength automatically. (Courtesy of Air Techniques, Inc., Hicksville, NY.)

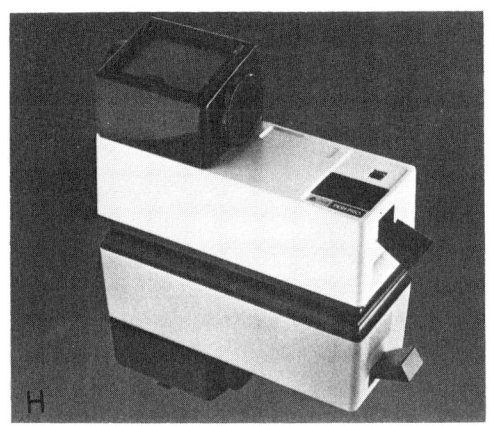

(H) Peri-Pro II (Air Techniques, Inc.) automatic processor used for intraoral film only (1983 model). Optional daylight loader is shown on top. (Courtesy of Air Techniques, Inc., Hicksville, NY.)

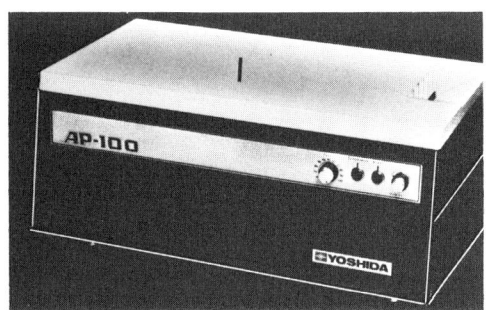

(I) Yoshida/Kaycor AP100 automatic film processor (Yoshida Dental Mfg. Co., Ltd., Tokyo, Japan) handles intraoral, panoramic, and cephalometric films. Adjustable speed from 90 seconds to 5.75 minutes. Optional daylight loader and replenisher system available. (Courtesy of Kaycor International Ltd., Evanston, IL.)

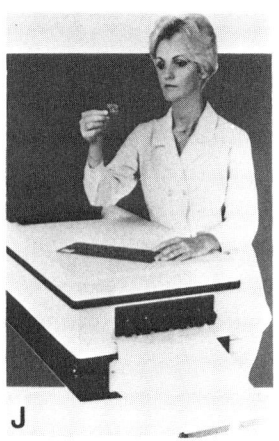

(J) Hope Processor (P-10) handles intraoral panoramic and 8 × 10 inch size films. Optional replenisher system and daylight loader available.

Table 8-V

RAPID DENTAL FILM PROCESSING DEVICES
CURRENT PRODUCTION MODELS
(September 1982)

Manufacturer	Model	Film Sizes	Cycle Time	Cycle Control	Solution Temp (°F)	Temp. Control	Drying Mechanism	Recommended Chemistry	Recommended Changing Sol.	Replen. System
Air Techniques	Peri-Pro	Intraoral only (no occl.)	7 min	No	Room: 70°-82°	No	Yes	Peri-Pro	2 weeks or 300-350 films	Manual
Air Techniques	Peri-Pro II	Intraoral only (no occl.)	6.25 min.	No	Not stated	No (heater bar)	Yes	Peri-Pro	2 weeks or 300-350 films	Manual
Air Techniques	A/T 2000	Intraoral, pano's, ceph's	5 min., Option: 2.0 min.-90 sec.	Yes	80°	Yes	Yes	Co. Brand	3 weeks to 3 months	Option – extra cost
Philips	810	Intraoral, Extraoral-8" W	4.5 min.	Yes	83°	Yes	Yes	Most R.P. chemicals	Weekly	Option – extra cost
Philips	410	Intraoral only (no occl.)	6.5 min. (wet in 3.5 min.)	No	80°	No	Yes	Most R.P. chemicals	Weekly	Manual
Hope Industries	P-6	Intraoral + pano's 6" W	4.0 min.	No	80°	Yes	Yes	Hope A&B	Monthly	Yes-Push Button
Hope Industries	P-10	Intraoral, Extraoral-10" W	4.0 min.	No	80°	Yes	Yes	Hope A&B	2-4 weeks	Yes-Push Button
Xonics (Redi-Chem)	152-ES	Intraoral + pano's 6" W	4.5 min.	No	Variable	Yes	Yes	Xonics A&B (Redi-Chem)	2-4 weeks	Option – extra cost
Siemens	Procomat	All intraoral	6 min. (wet)	No	65°-74°	Yes	No	Most R.P. chemicals	2 weeks	Manual
Siemens	Pantomatic	Intraoral, Extraoral-8" W	4.5 min.	No	86°	Yes	Yes	Most R.P. chemicals	2 weeks	Automatic
Yoshida (Kaycor)	AP100	Intraoral, Extraoral	Min.-90 sec.	Yes	86°	UNK.	Yes	Not spec.	UNK.	Automatic

(Two newer processor models are the Fisher DP-1 (8" dental processor) and the Philips 810XL with a built-in light-activated replenisher.)

Table 8-VI

AUTOMATIC FILM PROCESSING TROUBLE CHART

Condition	Cause
1. Low-density films	a. Solution temperature too low b. Exhausted developer (underreplenishment) c. Improper agitation or massaging action of rollers d. Processing too fast
2. High-density films	a. Solutions overheated b. Light leaks in processor cover c. Too much replenisher
3. Wet or tacky films	a. Dryer and developer temperatures too low b. Dryer thermostatic control or heater inoperative c. Dryer air circulation inadequate (high humidity in dryer section) d. Wrong chemistry and/or film e. Processing too fast
4. Film discoloration (brown)	a. Contamination of fixer in developer
5. Film discoloration (greenish yellow)	a. Fixer solution exhausted (underreplenishment) b. Processing too fast c. Wrong type of film for processor
6. Fogged films (unwanted density)	a. Incorrect or defective safelight filter or bulb b. Light leaks in darkroom c. Developer temperature too high d. Improper storage of films
7. Streaking (uneven density)	a. Underreplenishment b. Rollers and crossovers encrusted with chemical deposits c. Dirty wash water d. Film not hardened properly by chemicals
8. Surface marks	a. Foreign materials or irregularities on surface of rollers b. Rough handling of film prior to processing
9. Shiny films	a. Excessive hardening b. Wash water not turned on
10. Films chalky or dirty	a. No wash water or dirty wash water b. Precipitate in fixer
11. Jams or failure of film to transport	a. Chemicals contaminated or diluted b. Chemical temperature too high c. Films excessively soft and not adequately hardened; when enough gelatin lubricates the rollers, films will jam up with one another d. Dirty rollers e. Racks not seated properly f. Dirty wash water g. Incorrect dryer temperature h. Hesitation in drive assembly, causing film to pause in transit i. Film not tracking through processor in straight course (improper feeding of films)

Identification

Identification of Films and Identification of Right and Left Side of Patient

Since nearly all films used in dentistry are double coated emulsion films, for identification purposes intraoral films have a raised, embossed dot. The raised, or convex, side of the dot is always placed toward the beam of radiation and, therefore, identifies the side of the film toward the teeth. Knowing this, the right and left side of the patient can easily be identified.

Extraoral films do not have the embossed dot for identification purposes. Therefore, these films must be identified at the time of exposure by placing a lead letter "R" or "L" on the tube side of the cassette (Fig. 8-18). The panoramic film also has to be identified as to the right or left side of the patient. This can be done by placing a lead "R" and "L" on the cassette holder, the cassette itself, or the head holder device of a panoramic unit (Fig. 8-19).

Identification of Patient

The patient's name and relevant information can be identified on extraoral films in several ways. One method is to use commercial leaded tape, which is placed on the cassette with the desired information typed or written on the tape. When the film is exposed, the information will be photographically imprinted on the film (Fig. 8-20). Another method is to use a commercial imprinter, which records the pertinent information on the panoramic radiograph by means of a semitransparent card placed between the film and the imprinter light. Care must be taken not to imprint the information on an area of the film that will block out

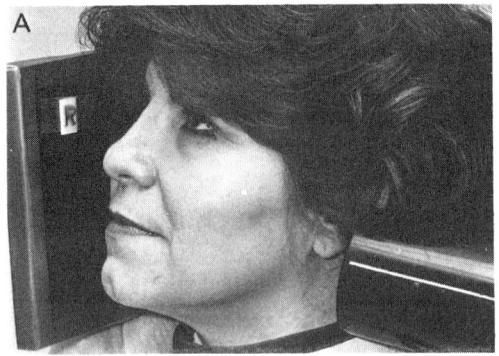
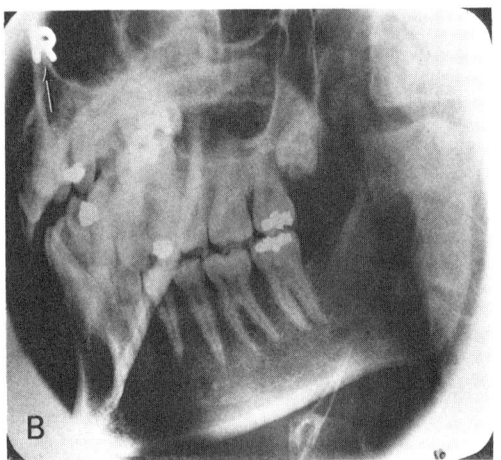
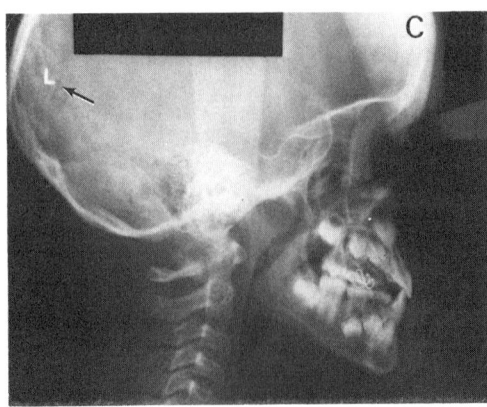

Figure 8-18. Identification of extraoral film. **(A)** Letter "R" placed on cassette prior to exposure. **(B)** Letter "R" on radiograph identifies right side of patient in this lateral jaw radiograph. **(C)** Letter "L" on this cephalometric radiograph identifies left side of patient.

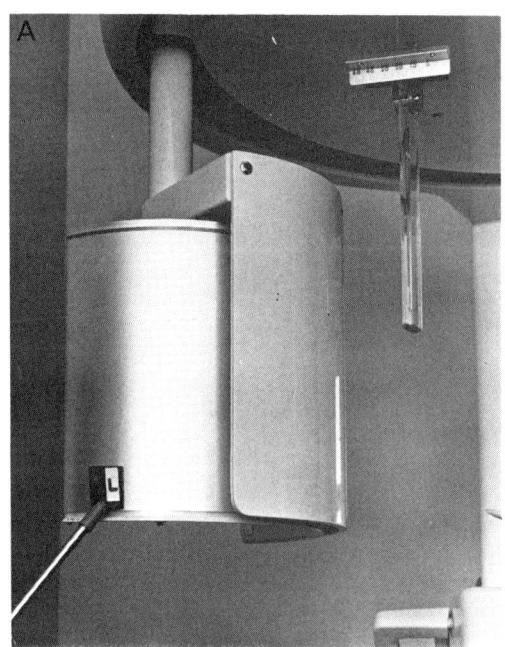

Figure 8-19. Identification of panoramic radiographs. **(A)** Placing lead "L" on the plastic cassette holder of the Ritter/Sybron Panoral panoramic unit. **(B)** G.E. Panelipse radiograph identified with "R" and "L" lead markers on the plastic head positioner guides. **(C)** Panorex I radiograph identified by placing lead markers "LEFT" on cassette holder.

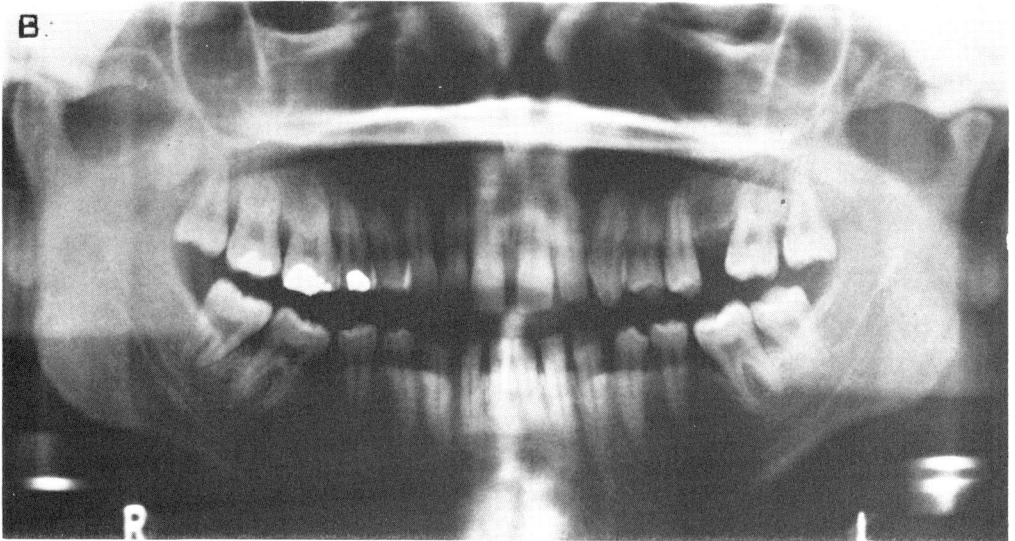

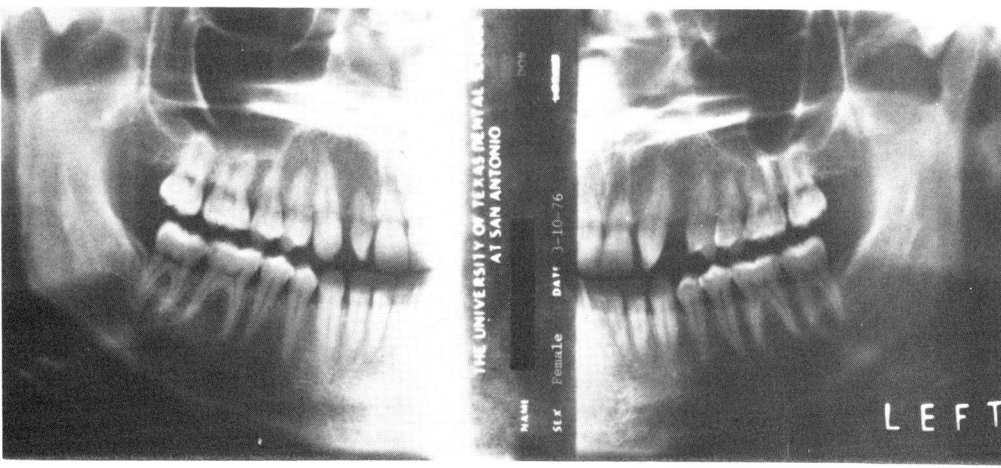

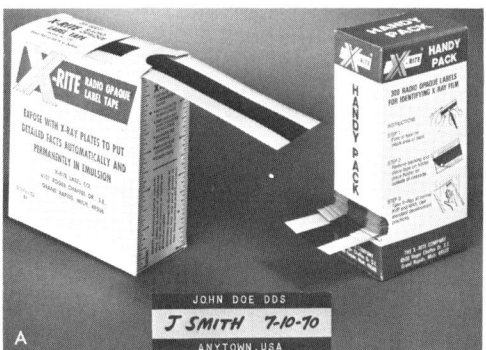

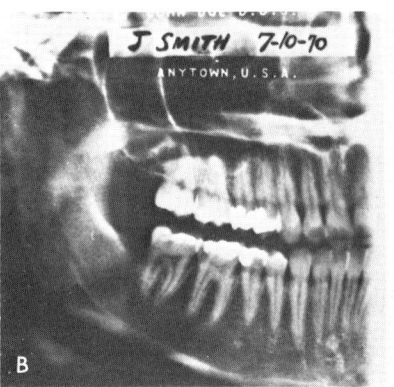
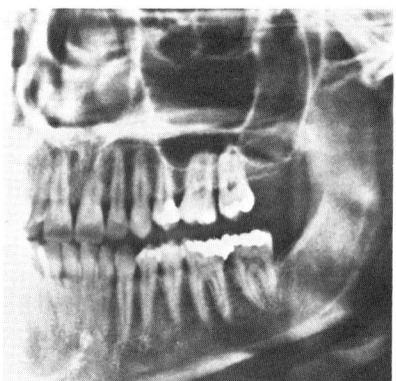

Figure 8-20. Identification of patient using a leaded tape on cassette. (A) Use of leaded-type labels to identify x-ray film provides positive legal identification at time of exposure. Print or type on black area of tape. Remove backing and place tape on a special holder. Place holder on cassette and take radiograph in normal manner. (B) A Panorex radiograph taken with radiopaque identification label. (Courtesy of X-Rite Label Co., Grand Rapids, MI.)

diagnostic information (Fig. 8-21).

Mounting Dental Radiographs

The following are reasons dental radiographs should be mounted:

1. There is less chance for an error in interpretation because each film is mounted in normal anatomic relation to each other.
2. It prevents finger marks, scratches, and abrasions because radiographs are not handled as much.
3. Repeated study and comparison of single radiographs with each other is time-consuming. It results in inefficiency and confusion.
4. Mounts exclude illumination around the individual radiographs. This is an aid in interpretation as it prevents glare.
5. Radiographs in mounts are easy to file. Therefore, they are instantly available for study during an operative procedure and consultation.
6. It has a psychological effect on patients. The impression that mounted radiographs have upon the patient is in itself sufficient reason for mounting them. It cannot be expected that a handful of small radiographs that are shuffled in and out of an envelope will be valued very highly.

Radiograph Mounting Problems

Mounting intraoral radiographs is a relatively simple procedure, when the in-

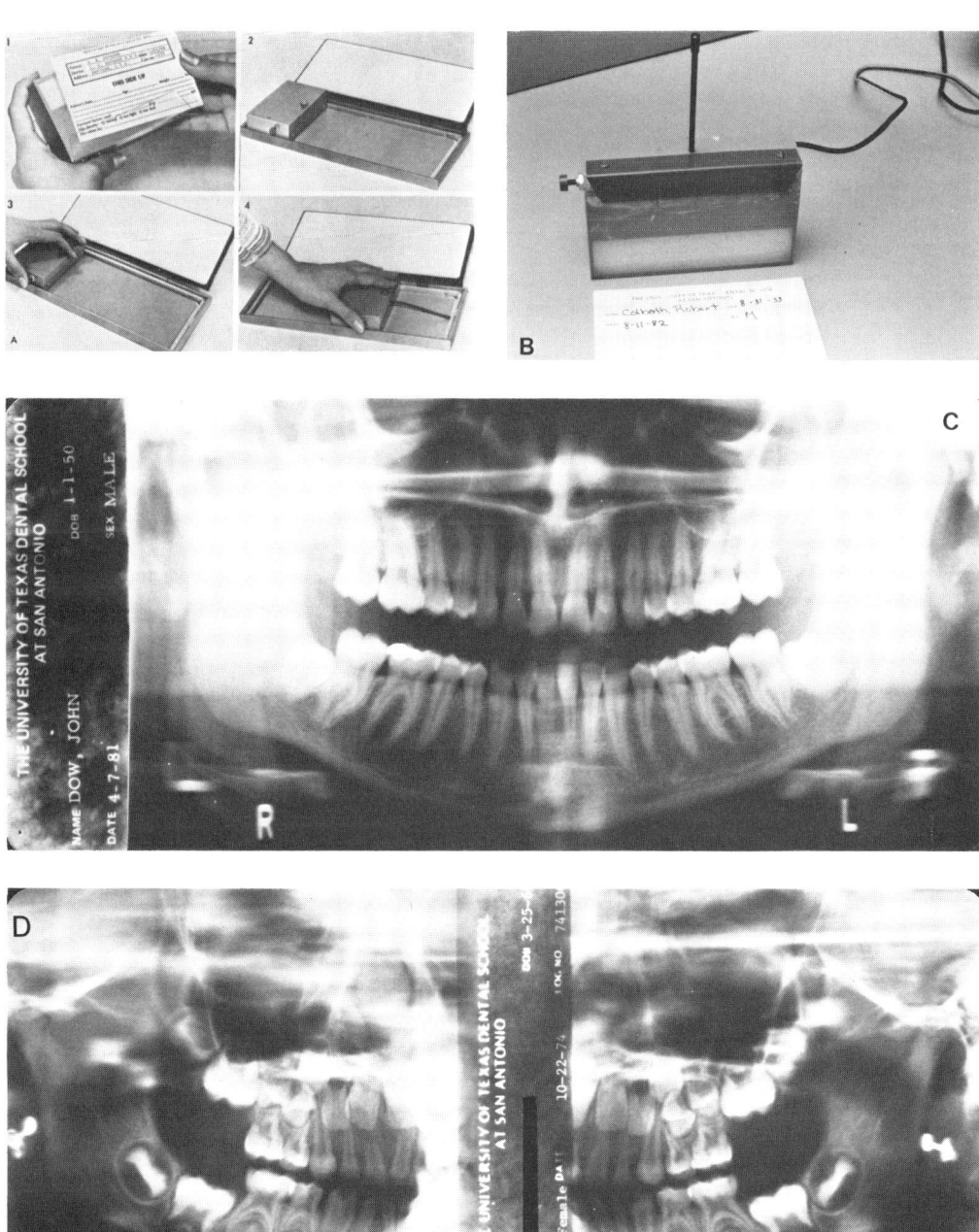

Figure 8-21. (A) S.S. White R.D.F. printer. (A) Patient information types on card, and card placed over illumination window. (2) Illuminator placed on exposed film under safelight conditions. (3) Illuminator exposing film for imprinting side of radiograph. (4) Imprinter exposing white band area in middle of Panorex radiograph. (Courtesy of S.S. White Dental Products Division, Pennwalt Corp., Philadelphia, PA). (B) S.S. White light card imprinter. (C) Card imprinter used on side of a Panelipse radiograph. The area where patient information is to be imprinted must be blocked out with lead on outside of the cassette. (D) Card imprinter used in middle, clear area of Panorex I (S.S. White/Pennwalt) radiograph. (E) Card imprinter used to identify cephalometric radiograph. (Area to be imprinted must be blocked out with lead at time of exposure.)

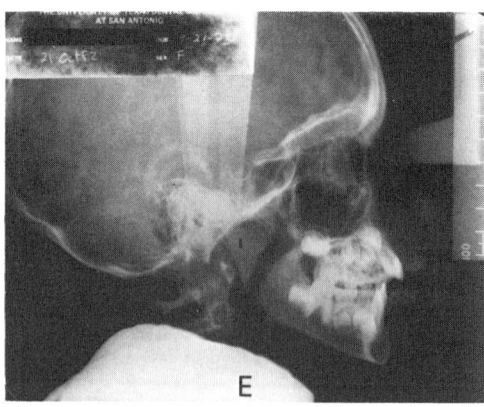

E

dividual responsible has some knowledge of the normal radiographic anatomical landmarks for each region of the mouth and can recognize tooth morphology. Each anatomical region of the jaws has identifying anatomic landmarks (Fig. 8-22).

Anatomic Landmarks

Maxillary Molar Area:
 a. posterior wall of the maxillary tuberosity
 b. hamular process
 c. coronoid process of mandible
 d. maxillary sinus
 e. zygomatic process

Maxillary Premolar Area
 a. maxillary sinus

Maxillary Incisor Area
 a. incisive foramen
 b. cartilage of nose
 c. nasal septum
 d. nasal fossae

Mandibular Molar Area
 a. external oblique line
 b. mylohyoid ridge
 c. mandibular canal

Mandibular Premolar Area
 a. mylohyoid ridge
 b. mental foramen

Mandibular Incisor Area
 a. mental ridges
 b. lingual foramen
 c. genial tubercles

Prior to preparation to mount radiographs, it is important to know from what aspect the radiographs will be viewed. The radiographs can be mounted for viewing two ways:

1. The radiographs may be mounted with the depressed or concave sides of the embossed dots toward the viewer. The viewer, then, is observing the radiographs from the lingual aspect, with the tube side of the film toward the back of the mount, as if inside the patient's mouth looking out. The reasons given for mounting the films this way are twofold: (a) objects nearing the film during exposure record sharper images than those farther from it; thus, the true relation of the objects is best seen by viewing from the lingual aspects since the lingual aspect of the teeth are closer to the film; (b) it is easier to visualize the effect of angulation by viewing from an opposite direction to that which the x-rays travel.

2. In the second method of mounting, the radiographs are mounted with all of the raised or convex sides of the embossed dots toward the viewer. The viewer, then, is observing the radiographs from the facial aspect with the tube side of the film toward the viewer. This is as though the viewer is looking directly at the patient. The films are mounted in this way at The University of Texas Dental School at San Antonio because it is easier to view the radiographs in the same direction that the rays were projected. Another advantage is that the films are mounted in the same relationship as the teeth are

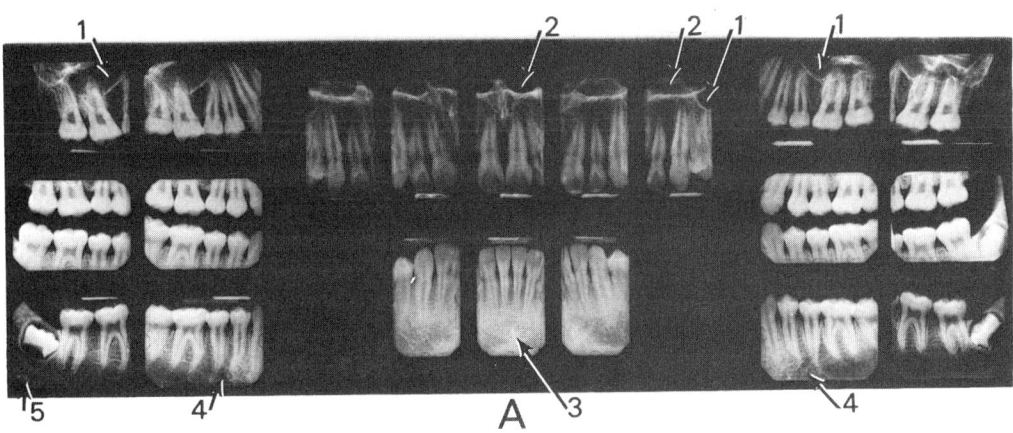

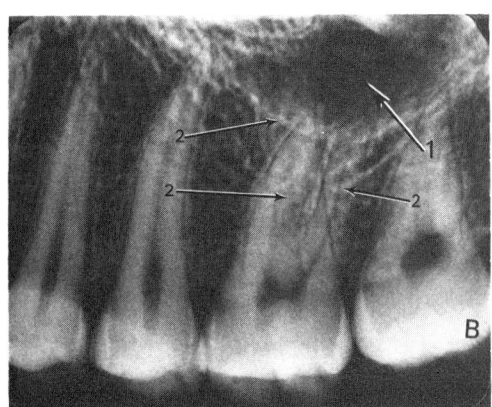

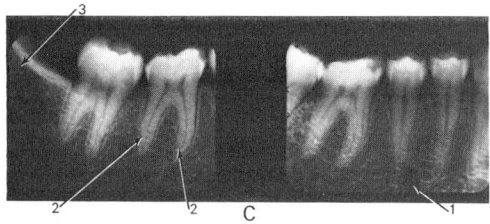

Figure 8-22. Normal anatomical landmarks. (**A**) Complete radiographic survey: **1**, maxillary sinus; **2**, nasal cavities; **3**, genial tubercle; **4**, mental foramen; **5**, mandibular canal. (**B**) Maxillary premolar region: **1**, maxillary sinus; **2**, three-rooted maxillary molar. (**C**) Mandibular premolar-molar region: **1**, mental foramen; **2**, two-rooted mandibular molars; **3**, ramus of mandible.

dry, care must be taken to avoid fingerprinting the radiographs; consequently, radiographs should be handled *only* by their edges with *clean, dry* fingers or with mounting gloves.

Once the radiographs are removed from the automatic processor or from the film drying cabinet, the following sequence is suggested for mounting the radiographs into an appropriate film mount. The mounting procedure described is the one where the radiographs are mounted as though the viewer is looking directly at the patient.

Step 1. Arrange all radiographs of the complete mouth radiographic survey (**CMX**) on a flat view box with the *embossed dot* or bump *upward.*

Step 2. Arrange the radiographs on the viewbox in order of anatomic site, e.g. select out and arrange in groups all maxillary radiographs according to posterior or anterior regions.

recorded on the examination chart. This makes for less chance for error.

However, it depends upon previous training and preference as to which method of mounting radiographs is used. The mount can be turned over if the way mounted is not desired.

Once the processed radiographs are

Step 3. Take all maxillary posterior radiographs and arrange them with the crowns of the teeth toward the bottom of the viewbox. With all embossed dots up and the crowns of the teeth oriented downward, it will be necessary only to identify mesial or distal anatomic landmarks of teeth in order to distinguish right from left. Posterior radiographs with the more mesial structures are mounted in the premolar position; those with more distal landmarks are mounted in the molar positions. (Fig. 8-22 A, B).

Step 4. Identify the five maxillary anterior radiographs and rotate the incisal portion of each film down toward the bottom of the viewbox (Fig. 8-23).

Step 5. Identify the maxillary central incisor radiograph and mount it in the center of the anterior section of the mount; next identify the R and L lateral and canine radiographs and mount them with mesial anatomic structures always directed toward the middle of the mount.

Step 6. Identify the four posterior

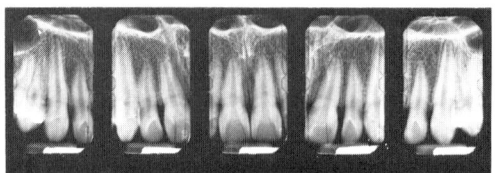

Figure 8-23. Identification of the five maxillary anterior teeth.

mandibular radiographs. Rotate these radiographs around until the coronal portion of the film is directed toward the top of the viewbox. Identify mesial and distal structures and arrange in appropriate areas of the mount (Fig. 8-22C).

Step 7. Rotate the three mandibular anterior radiographs until their incisal edges are directed toward the top of the viewbox; identify the central incisor region and mount it in the center window of the mount. Next mount the canine projections. (Fig. 8-24).

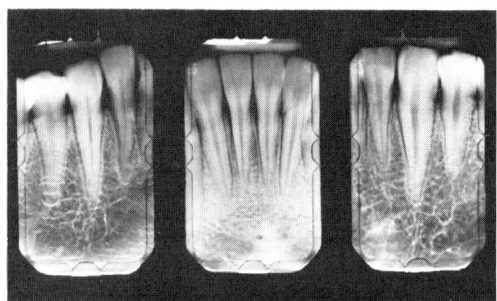

Figure 8-24. Three mandibular anterior radiographs.

Step 8. The remaining four films are interproximal radiographs. Orient these radiographs with the curve of spee (occlusal plane between maxillary and mandibular teeth) directed upward toward the distal. If the occlusal plane is flat, attempt to identify characteristics of the respective crowns; frequently, the bifurcation of the mandibular molar is distinguishable and may serve as a valuable aid in distinguishing mandibular from maxillary teeth.

Once the appropriate arch is identified the film can be properly oriented. The direction of the most mesial structures is used to identify right from left and premolar from molar regions (Fig. 8-22A).

Interpretation

Radiologic interpretation is the translation of the variations from normal density into terms of diagnostic significance. This implies two things: that the dentist knows normal radiologic anatomy and that an accurate clinical examination of the patient has been made.

Radiologic interpretation is a difficult

process to learn, mainly because the dentist is examining two-dimensional images of three-dimensional structures. The radiograph lacks depth; therefore, all of the anatomic structures are superimposed on each other.

Because disease is a continuous process, the radiograph reveals only an instantaneous glimpse of this process. For example, in caries the radiograph reveals a radiolucent area on a tooth, which represents decalcification of the tooth, not the carious process. Only the destruction of the tooth from the carious process is seen. An abnormal radiolucency in the bone may be the result of an inflammatory, noninflammatory, cellular, or mechanical process.

The diagnostician must train himself to evaluate the underlying process contributing to the abnormal variation in density on the radiograph so that he may become more accurate in his interpretative abilities.

Quality

The radiograph must have diagnostic quality, i.e. it must have proper contrast and density, maximum definition and detail, minimum distortion, and an adequate number of views of the area in question.

Conditions of Viewing

Manson-Hing (1962) listed several factors that help to improve the dentist's visual acuity in radiologic interpretation (*see* Fig. 8-26). Some of these factors are the following:

1. The view box or illuminator must have opal glass to diffuse the light and a variable intensity rheostat or other means of varying the light intensity to compensate for density variations in the radiograph. Radiographs of low density can be viewed better if the illumination is reduced; conversely, the illumination should be increased when the films are of high density.
2. All glare spots arising from direct light or reflections of light should be avoided. This can be done by reducing the overhead lights in the room and masking the complete radiographic survey with opaque material to allow the light of the illuminator to show only through the radiographs. This prevents glare and permits better visualization of the mounted radiographs.
3. A magnifying lens is particularly helpful in the evaluation of small changes in density on the radiograph.
4. Concentration is important in radiologic interpretation. The radiographs should be viewed in quiet surroundings without interruption. Inattention will cause the observer to become, for all intents and purposes, blind.
5. Fatigue has a detrimental effect on visual acuity. The dentist should not try to interpret a whole group of films after a busy day of work.
6. The radiographs should be studied carefully before a decision is reached. Once an individual makes a choice by visual observation, it is difficult for him to consider other possibilities (Renshaw, 1964).

Viewing Procedure

The following is a suggested sequential viewing procedure (*see* Fig. 8-22A):

1. Start in the upper left, move horizontally to the upper right, move down to the lower right and across again to the lower left.

2. Use a series of circuits in which you examine for a specific area on the radiograph for each circuit.
    a. Examine for unerupted, missing, and impacted teeth.
    b. Examine all the crowns of the teeth for caries, size and shape of pulps, and interproximal contacts.
    c. Examine the interseptal bone areas for evidence of periodontal destruction and local irritating factors. These include cratering of the interseptal crestal bone, overhanging restorations, and calculus.
    d. Examine all of the roots and the periapical bone areas for condition of lamina dura, periodontal membrane space, and size and shape of pulpal canals and roots.
    e. Examine all regions not previously examined, such as the sinuses and the remaining bone of the jaws.
    f. Read the complete survey from a distance. Subtle density changes in the cancellous bone may sometimes be discovered by this procedure.

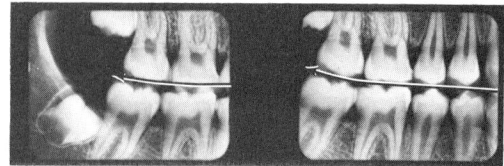

Figure 8-25. Posterior bite-wing illustrating that "Curve of Spee" curves upwards from an anterior to posterior direction.

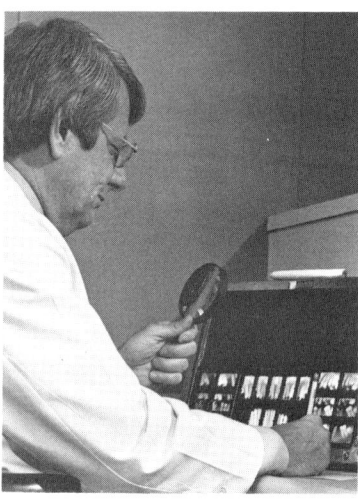

Figure 8-26. Proper use of the view box in radiographic interpretation. Note that the complete radiographic survey has been masked and that a magnifying glass is being used.

Copying or Duplicating Radiographs

Since the discovery of x-rays, people have been trying to reproduce radiographs. A single radiograph series may seem sufficient at the time taken; however, it may become necessary to refer or transfer a patient while keeping the original radiographs. Also, as third party payments increasingly become a part of every practice, it becomes necessary to find a simple and inexpensive way to copy original radiographs. The advantages of copying radiographs are —

1. to refer patients for consultation and treatment;
2. to transfer a patient moving to another area;
3. to eliminate retakes, which reduces unnecessary radiation to the patient;
4. to comply to peer review committee requests;
5. to place many small radiographs on one sheet of film (8 × 10 inch size film);
6. to use as teaching aids.

Films can be duplicated by the use of a special duplicating film called direct-reversal films, which have been solarized by a chemical treatment of the emulsion. The exact processes are trade secrets.

Years ago, solarization was done by exposing a film to direct light for a prolonged period of time.

Solarization of a film is exposing the film (chemically or by light) beyond that which produces maximum density until a decrease in density occurs. Solarization of the individual grains of the film emulsion means that the increased exposure has actually destroyed the developable state of that which had been induced by the earlier part of the exposure (Fig. 8-27). The explanation of solarization is up for debate, but current evidence favors the rebromination hypothesis. It states in essence that during overexposure of the emulsion, bromine builds up in the spaces between the emulsion grains, and eventually reacts with the metallic silver at the latent-image centers on the surface of the grain. This coats the latent-image center with a layer of silver bromine and prevents the action of the developing agent on the grain.

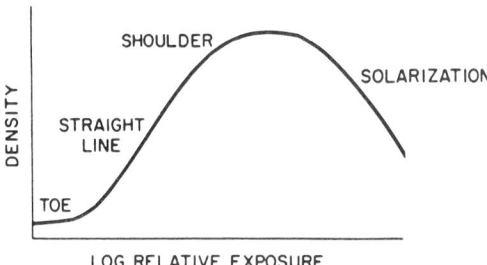

Figure 8-27. Characteristic curve extended into the region of solarization where increased log relative exposure produces decreased density. (From Fig. 22-1, pg. 302, Christenson, Curry & Dowdy, *An Introduction to the Physics of Diagnostic Radiology*, 2nd edition. Philadelphia, Lea & Febiger, 1978.)

The important thing to remember about solarized film is that more light exposure produces **less** density, which is just opposite of standard radiographic film exposures.

Halation

Radiographic duplicating film has a solarized emulsion side (purple side) on a blue-tinted polyester film base, and an antihalation coating (shiny side) on the opposite side. Halation is light reflected back from air after it has passed through the duplicating film. Halation light spreads out beyond the boundaries of the image and causes unsharp edges. Halation can be prevented by coating the back side of the film base with a layer of gelatin that contains a dye, which absorbs the reflected light to which the emulsion is sensitive, thus the name: antihalation side of the duplicating film.

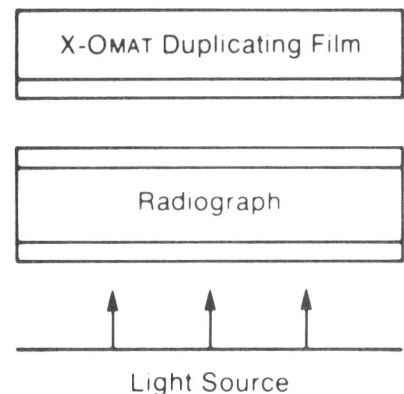

Figure 8-28. Technic of duplicating film.

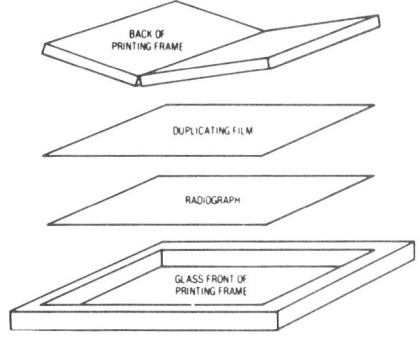

Figure 8-29. Assembly of components for exposure in a printing frame.

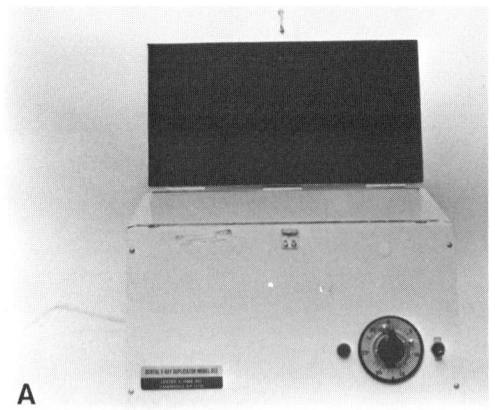

(A) Lid open.

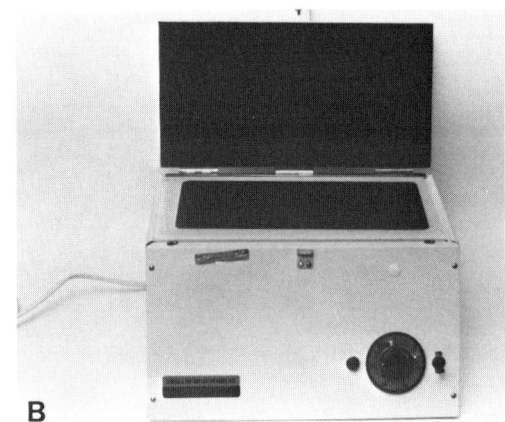

(B) Placement of Panoramic film on illuminator surface.

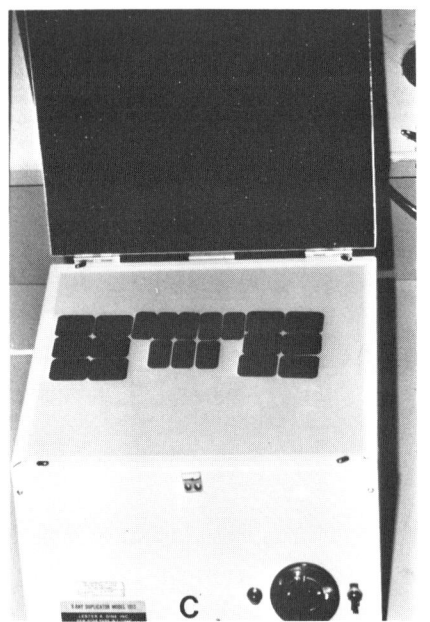

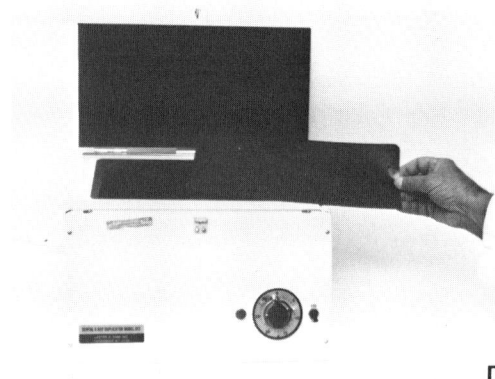

(D) Placement of duplicating film — solarized side down on film.

(C) Full mount survey.

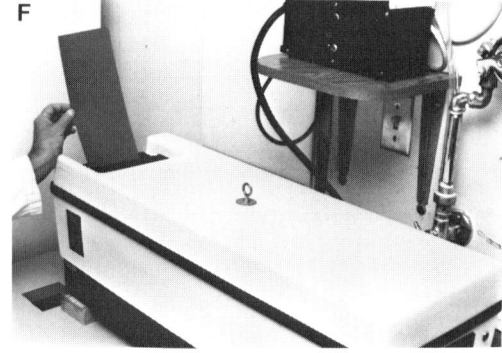

(F) Film developed as usual.

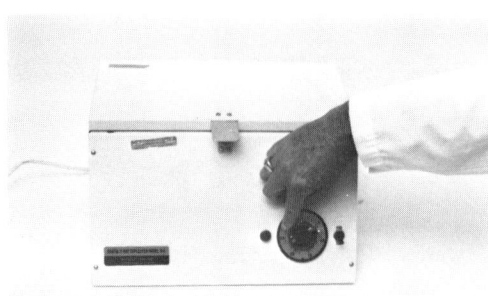

(E) Time set and exposure made.

Figure 8-30. Duplication procedure using Lester Dine duplicator.

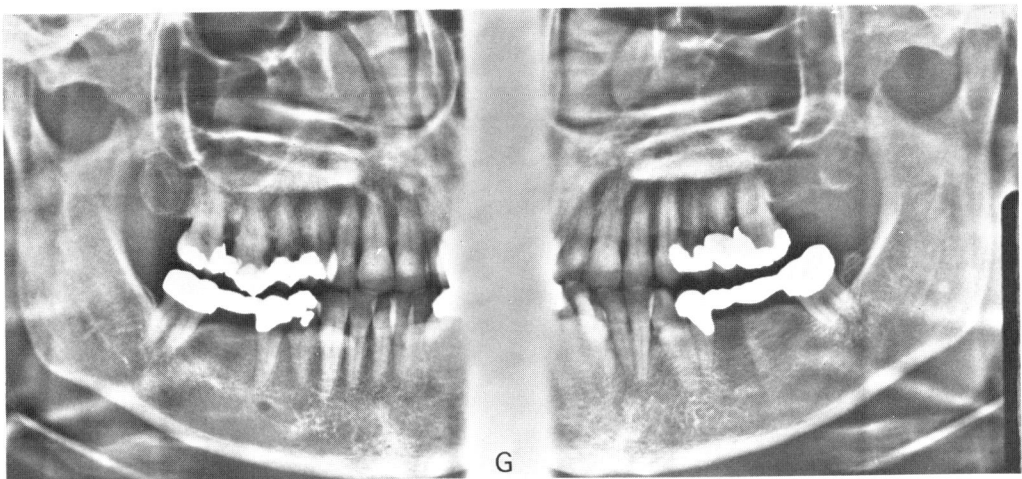

(G) Duplicated Panoramic film.

Duplication Procedure

The basis for the duplicating technic is to expose a special duplicating film by a light that has passed through the original film. The duplicating film is designed to be exposed with an ultraviolet light source, such as BLB ultraviolet fluorescent lamp (Fig. 8-28).

A typical radiograph illuminator having two F15T8BLB fluorescent lamps may be used as an exposure source. The radiograph to be duplicated must be held in close contact with the emulsion side of the single-coated duplicating film during exposure to prevent blurring. This may be accomplished by use of a photographic printing frame (Fig. 8-29) or one of the commercially available contact printers (Fig. 8-30) such as those manufactured by Rin Corp., Lester A. Dine, Inc., Ada Products, and Star X-Ray Company. Kodak X-OMAT duplicating film is available in seven sizes, fifty sheets per package (Fig. 8-31). The common sizes used in dentistry are the 5 × 12 inch, 8 × 10 inch, and 10 × 12 inch sizes. The 10 × 12 inch size divides into two panoramic film sizes (5 × 12 inch). Because duplicating film is a direct positive or reversal film, increasing exposure reduces the density produced on a duplicating film. Therefore, a duplicate that is too low in density can be corrected by decreasing the exposure. If the density of the copy is too high, the exposure should be increased to lower the density.

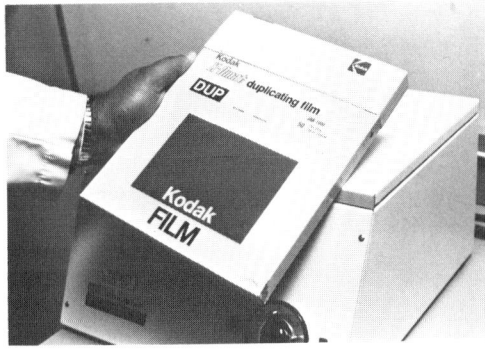

Figure 8-31. Kodak X-OMAT duplicating film.

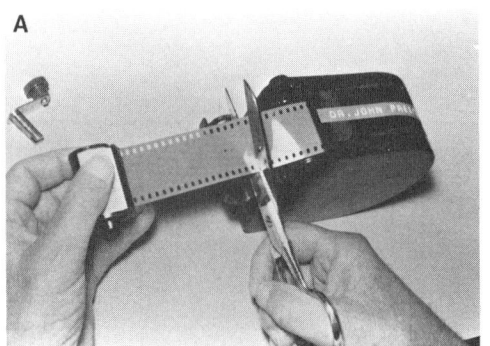
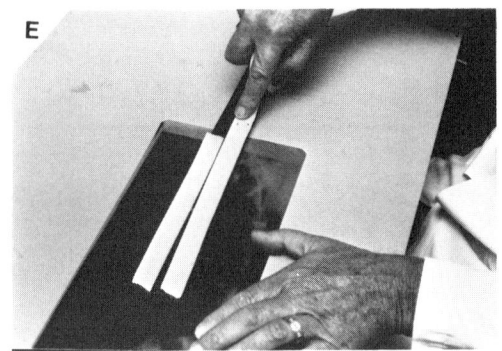
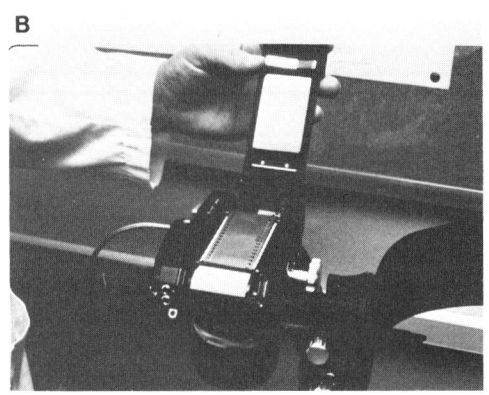
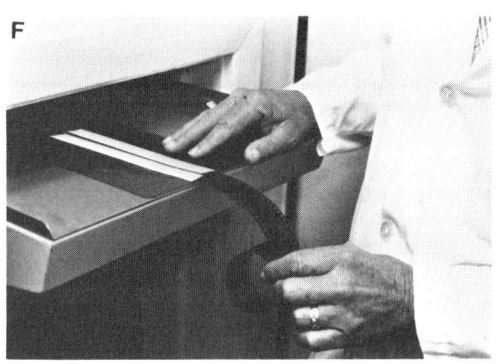
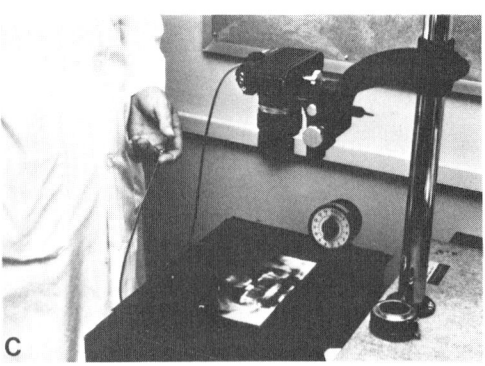
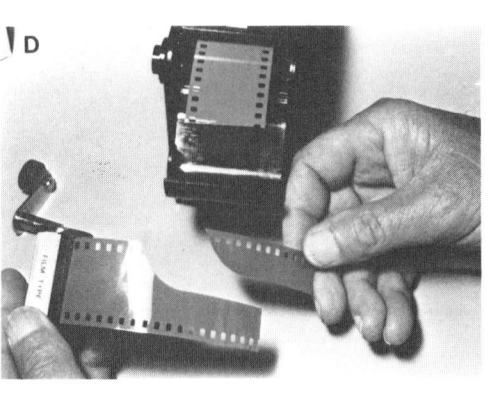

Figure 8-32. Procedure for producing slides from radiographs using direct-reversal 35 mm roll-type film. **(A)** Kodak S0185 (RPC) rapid processing copy film can be purchased in 36 exposure magazines or obtained in 150 foot rolls. First, the film when purchased in a 150 foot roll is loaded from daylight loader into a 35 mm film cassette. **(B)** Load film into 35 mm camera. **(C)** Using a standard viewbox for a light source, exposure time averages approximately 30 seconds for a panoramic film with the lens aperture set at F/3.5 (wide open). If the original radiograph has light density, use 20 seconds to darken film, and 40 seconds to lighten the density of a dark original radiograph. **(D)** After completing film exposures, unload the camera. **(E)** Tape the exposed film under darkroom conditions (GBX filter) to a film leader (panoramic filter). **(F)** Feed film into automatic processor with duplicating film emulsion side down. (This is a Kodak X-OMATIC processor—90 seconds dry-to-dry.) **(G)** Cut the processed film roll to place in slide mounts. **(H)** Mounting film. **(I)** Completed film mount ready for projection.

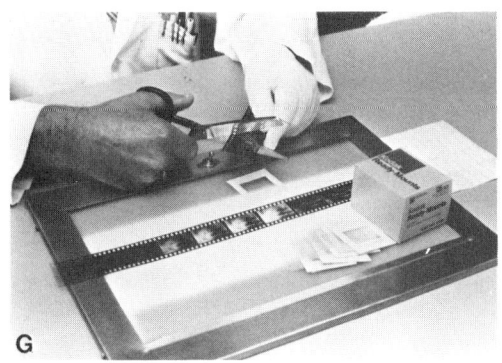
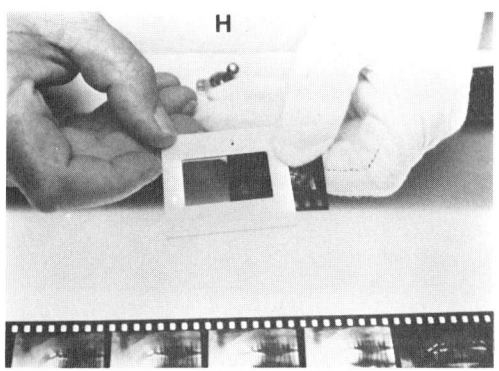
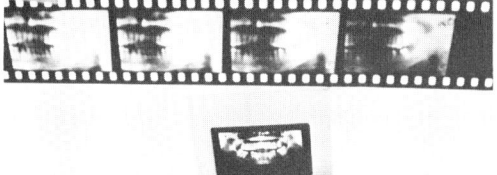
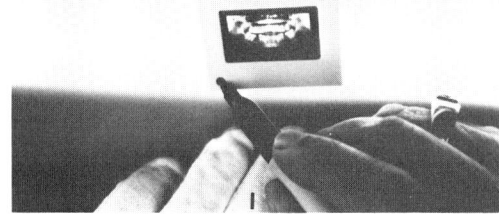

Rapid Processing Copy Film SO-185RPC and DuPont Cronex DP35. Both of these films can be processed in automatic processors. The exposed film must be taped to a film leader 5 × 12 inch (panoramic size) or larger. The leader and film (emulsion side up) are then fed into the automatic processor. After processing the film, it is easily cut and mounted as slides. Using these copy films it is possible to produce a slide ready for projection in about ten minutes (Fig. 8-32).

Slides

At this time Eastman Kodak and DuPont have available direct-reversal (solarized emulsion) 35 mm films that are designed to permit production of 2 × 2 inch slides of good quality from radiographs with a minimum of time and effort: Kodak

Bibliography

Allen, M.J.; and Silha, R.E.: New copiers for dental radiography duplicating film. *Dent Radiogr Photogr, 49*:14, 1976.

A Look at X-ray Film Processing. Milwaukee, General Electric Company, X-ray Department.

Beck, J.O.: *Syllabus of Oral Radiology.* University of Minnesota School of Dentistry, 1970.

Bloom, W.L.; Hollenbach; and Morgan, J.A.: *Medical Radiographic Technic*, 3rd ed. Springfield, Charles C Thomas, 1969.

Bushong, S.C.: *Radiologic Science for Technologists.* St. Louis, Mosby, 1975.

Cahoon, J.B.: *Formulating X-ray Technics.* Durham, N.C., Duke University Press, 1953.

Carr, J.D.; and Norman, R.D.: Effective use of the darkroom. *Dent Clin North Am*, 363-370, July 1961.

Christensen, E.E.; Curry, T.S.; and Dowdey, J.E.: *An Introduction to the Physics of Diagnostic Radiography.* Philadelphia, Lea & Febiger, 1978, pp. 110-151.

Clark, H.A.: Radiographical duplication of radiographs. *Br Dent J, 102*:229, 1957.

Copying Radiographs. Kodak Publ. No. M3-24, Rochester, NY, Eastman Kodak Company, 1973.

Darkroom Techniques for Better Radiographs Processed Manually or Automatically. El DuPont DeNemours & Co., Inc.

Dillon, C.: Reproduction and duplication of radiographs. *Dent Digest, 64*:16, 1958.

Erales, F.A.; and Manson-Hing, L.R.: A study of the quality of duplicated radiographs. *Oral Surg, 47*:98, 1979.

Ennis, L.; Berry, H.; and Phillips, J.E.: *Dental Roentgenology*, 6th ed. Philadelphia, Lea & Febiger, 1967, pp. 307-320.

Esworthy, S.; and Fox, J.: Duplicating dental radiographs. *Dent Assistant, 37*:26, 1968.

Fertman, A.: Direct positive duplication of x-ray film. *J Pract Orthod, 3*:200, 1969.

Fuchs, A.W.: *Principles of Radiographic Exposure and Processing,* 2nd ed. Springfield, Charles C Thomas, 1979.

Gibson, H.L.: Direct duplicates of dental radiographs. *Dent Radiogr Photogr, 38*:60, 1965.

Hartley, J.B.: Film viewing 1966. *Rontgenblatter, 20*:96, 1967.

Herz, R.M.: *The Photographic Action of Ionizing Radiations.* New York, Wiley-Interscience, 1969, pp. 396-399.

Hurtgen, T.P.: Safelighting in the dental darkroom. *Dent Radiogr Photogr, 52*(4):9, 1979.

Jacobi, C.A.: *X-ray Technology,* 2nd ed. St. Louis, Mosby, 1960, p. 65.

Kasle, M.J.; and Langlais, R.P.: *Exercises in Dental Radiology,* Vol. 4, Basic Principles of Oral Radiography. Philadelphia, Saunders, 1980.

Kodak Safelighting Filter Type GBX: New For The Radiographic Darkroom. (Code M3-143). Rochester, N.Y., Eastman Kodak Company.

Lane, E.J.; Proto, A.V.; and Phillips, T.W.: Mach bands and dentistry perception. *Radiology, 121*:9, 1976.

Lawrence, D.J.: Kodak X-Omatic and Lanex screens and Kodak films for medical radiography. *Med Radiogr Photogr, 53*(1):2, 1977.

Lynch, P.A.; Automatic view box. *Am J Roentgenol, 106*:218, 1969.

Manson-Hing, L.R.: *Panoramic Dental Radiography.* Springfield, Charles C Thomas, 1976, pp. 157-164.

Manson-Hing, L.R.: Vision and oral roentgenology. *Oral Surg, 15*:173, 1962.

Manual Processing of Extraoral Kodak Dental X-Ray Films. Rochester, NY, Eastman Kodak Co., 1977.

Mattsson, O.: Aspects of the interpretation of contrast and detail in radiographs. *Acta Radiologica, 38*:477, 1952.

McCall, J.; and Wald, S.: *Clinical Dental Roentgenology,* 4th ed. Philadelphia, Saunders, 1957, pp. 113-128.

Milder, J.J.: One step roentgenogram duplication method. *J Am Dent Assoc, 58*:93, 1959.

Pappas, C.G.: Duplicating film in dentistry. *Dent Clin North Am,* 613-623, 1968.

Peterson, S.: *Clinical Dental Hygiene.* St. Louis, Mosby, 1959, pp. 240-252.

Radiology Specialist. Washington, D.C. U S Government Printing Office, Department of the Air Force, pp. 8-15.

Recovering Silver from Photographic Materials. Kodak Publication No. J-10. Rochester, NY, Eastman Kodak Co., 1980.

Reid, J.A.: and Ruprecht, A.: Duplication of radiographs: Simple methods to be used in dental offices. *J Can Dent Assoc,* (6): 278-281, 1977.

Reiter, E.N.: Simple radiographic reproduction. *Tx Dent J., 94*:21, 1976.

Renshaw, S.: *Psychological Optics,* Vols. 1-3. Duncan, OK: Optometric Extension Prognosis, 1964.

Richards, A.G.: Duplication of radiographs. *J Mich Dent Assoc, 57*:337, 1975.

Riebel, F.A.: Use of the eyes in x-ray diagnosis. *Radiology, 70:*252, 1958.

Roberts, E.P.; Davidson, J.B.; and Lambeck, C.E.: Composite film prints from dental radiographs. *Dent Radiogr Photogr, 26:*26, 1953.

Rohler, R.: Psysiological problems in viewing radiographs. *Rontgenblatter, 20:*79, 1967.

Rouff, L.N.: Copying x-rays, *NY State Dent J, 41:*484, 1975.

Seidberg, B.H.; Andres, E.; Alibrandi, B.V.; Carter, W.; and Goldstone, R.: How to duplicate radiographs. *Dent Surv, 51:*24, 1975.

Selman, J.: *The Fundamentals of X-Ray and Radium Physics,* 6th ed. Springfield, Charles C Thomas, 1978.

Sensitometric Properties of X-Ray Films. Rochester, NY, Eastman Kodak Co., 1974.

Silver Recovery with the KODAK Chemical Recovery Cartridge, Type P. Kodak Publication No. J-9. Rochester, NY, Eastman Kodak Co., 1979.

Simpson, C.O.: The advantages of mounting dental radiographs. *Dent Radiogr Photogr,* (1). 1937.

Sivasriyanond, C.; and Manson-Hing, L.R.: Microdensitometric and visual evaluation of the resolution of dental films. *Oral Surg, 45*:811, 1973.

Skucas, J.; and Gorski, J.: Applications of modern intensifying screens in diagnostic radiology. *Med Radiogr Photogr, 56*(2):25, 1980.

Stafne, E.: *Oral Roentgenographic Diagnosis,* 3rd ed. Philadelphia, Saunders, 1969, pp. 380-386.

Sweet, A.P.: Processing technic. *Oral Surg,* May, 1950.

Sweet, A.P.: Safelights reconsidered. *Dent Radiogr Photogr,* (2), 1962.

Sweet, A.P.: X-ray processing solutions. *Dent Radiogr Photogr,* (2):27, 1955.

The Fundamentals of Radiography. Rochester, NY, Eastman Kodak, 1980, pp. 93-106.

Thunthy, K.H.; Fortier, A.P.; and Knapp, W.B.:

Automatic film processing in the dental office. *Quintesence Int.* (9):75, 1977.

Tuddenham, W.J.: The visual physiology of roentgen diagnosis. A. Basic concepts. *AJR, 78:*116, July 1957.

Wainwright, W.W.; and Villanyi, A.A.: The simplest radiographic analyzer: The x-ray checker. *J So Calif Dent Assoc, 28*(4):122, 1960.

Wuehrmann, A.H.; and Manson-Hing, L.R.: *Dental Radiology.* St. Louis, Mosby, 1977, pp. 30-33, 183-201.

X-rays in Dentistry. Rochester, NY, Eastman Kodak Co., 1962, pp. 66-80.

Chapter 9

ANALYSIS OF ERRORS AND ARTIFACTS

FILMS lacking in diagnostic quality should be avoided for the following reasons:

1. Retakes expose the patient to unnecessary radiation.
2. Retakes waste the time of the dentist and his auxiliaries.
3. Retakes waste film, which is costly.
4. Faulty radiographs interfere with accurate interpretation.

The four major causes of unsatisfactory radiograps are faulty projection of the beam, incorrect technique, exposure problems, and improper processing.

The following is a table of common errors and their corrections. Hopefully, this list will help those who take radiographs to identify and eliminate the causes of their errors.

Study the list and the illustrations. Note that separate lists are provided for intraoral and panoramic techniques, as well as for manual and automatic processing.

INTRAORAL PROJECTION OR TECHNIQUE ERRORS

Error	*Cause*	*Correction*
1. *Apical ends of teeth "cut off"* (Fig. 9-1, 9-2).	Film placed too close to teeth in maxillary arch in paralleling technic.	Move film away from the teeth.
	Too flat a vertical angulation, which causes elongation.	Increase vertical angulation (especially shallow vaults).
2. *Overlapping of teeth* (Fig. 9-3).	Plane of film not parallel to lingual surface of teeth.	Place film horizontally, parallel to lingual surface of teeth, and direct the central ray of the x-ray beam perpendicular to the facial surfaces of the teeth.
	Incorrect horizontal angulation of cone.	

Analysis of Errors and Artifacts 323

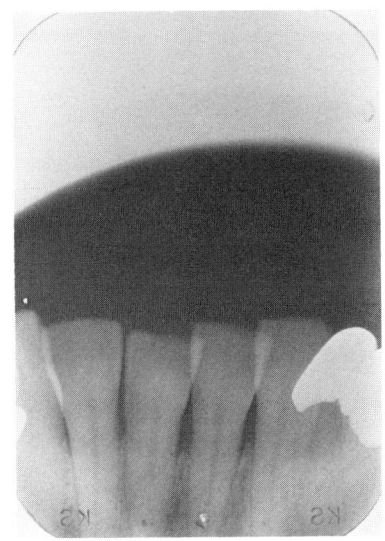

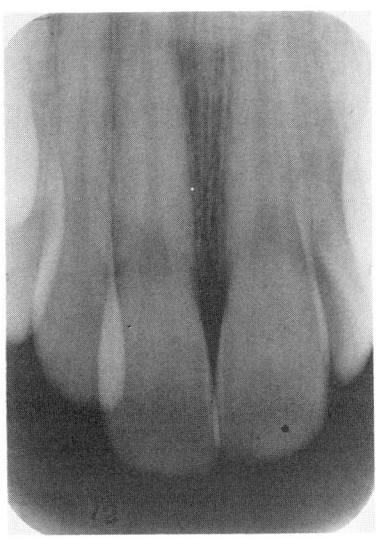

Figure 9-2. Improper beam alignment: elongation causes apices to be projected off film.

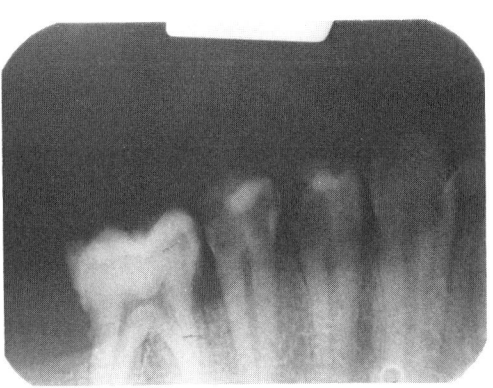

Figure 9-1. Incorrect film placement and retention. **(A)** Film not placed into floor of mouth. Note the cone cut. **(B)** Inadequate periapical coverage.

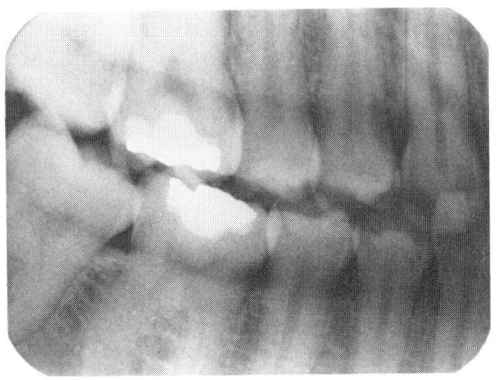

Figure 9-3. Incorrect horizontal angulation of the beam: overlapping of contacts.

3. *All of specific region not showing* (Fig. 9-4).	Faulty film placement.	Center the film over teeth to be radiographed.
4. *Crowns of teeth not showing* (Fig. 9-5).	Not enough film showing below or above the crowns of the teeth.	Increase amount of film showing below and above the crown of the teeth (Approximately 1/8 inch

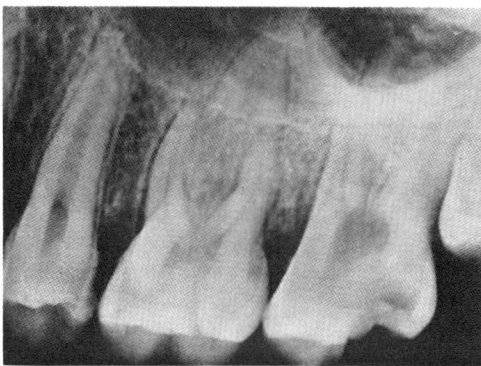

Figure 9-4. Incorrect film placement: maxillary third molar cut off.

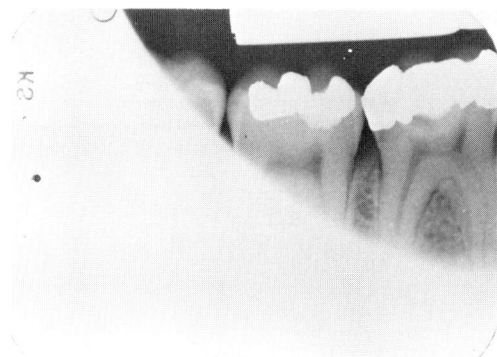

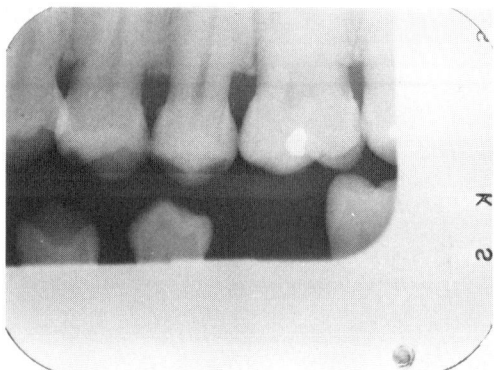

Figure 9-6. Improper beam alignment: **(A)** Cone cut, round cone. **(B)** Cone cut, rectangular cone.

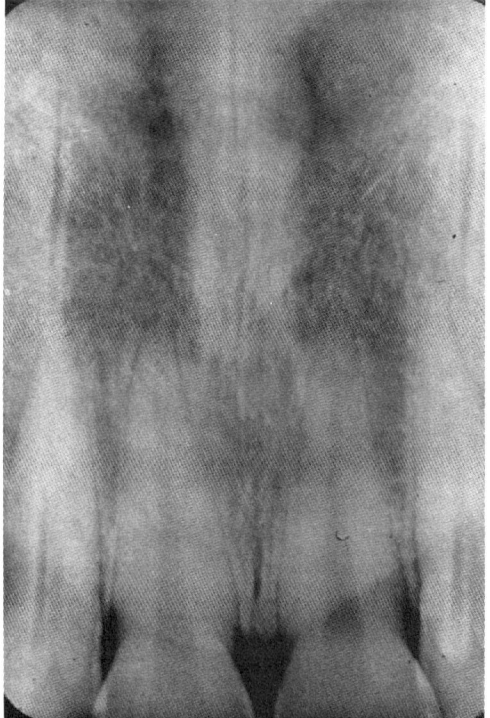

Figure 9-5. Incorrect film placement: Crowns of maxillary incisors cut off.

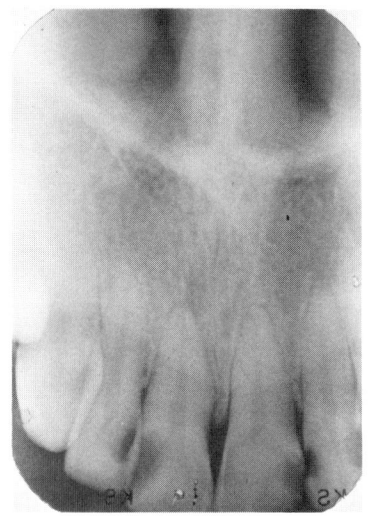

Figure 9-7. Improper beam alignment: Foreshortening due to excessive vertical angulation.

		showing).
	Vertical angulation too steep.	Decrease vertical angulation.
5. *Partial image "cone cut"* Fig. 9-6).	Cone of radiation not covering area of interest.	Make sure vertical and horizontal position of cone covers film.
6. *Shape Distortion* a. Foreshortening (Fig. 9-7).	*Bisecting Technic:* Vertical angulation of cone too acute.	Reduce vertical angulation.
	Paralleling Technic: Film not paralleling with long axes of teeth.	Place film parallel to long axes of teeth — it is difficult in shallow palatal vault case.
	Paralleling Technic: Long cone is not positioned correctly.	Position long cone so CR strikes film at right angle.
b. Elongation (Fig. 9-8).	*Bisecting Technic:* Vertical angulation of cone is too flat.	Increase vertical angulation of cone.
	Paralleling Technic: Film not positioned parallel to long axes of teeth.	Place film parallel with long axes of teeth.
	Paralleling Technic: Long cone not positioned correctly.	Position long cone so CR strikes film at right angle.
d. Dimensional Distortion (Fig. 9-10).	Inherent error in bisecting angle technic, produces elongation of palatal roots and foreshortening of buccal roots of molars in same view.	Use long cone paralleling technic. Place film parallel to long axes of molars.
c. Image Distorted (Fig. 9-9).	Film is bent as patient bites on film holder or biteblock or as patient holds film in mouth.	Use a film backing.

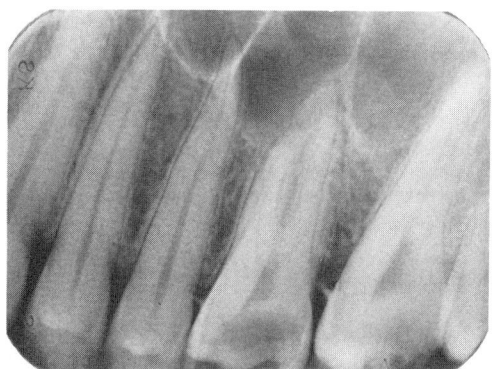

Figure 9-8. Improper beam alignment: Elongation due to inadequate vertical angulation.

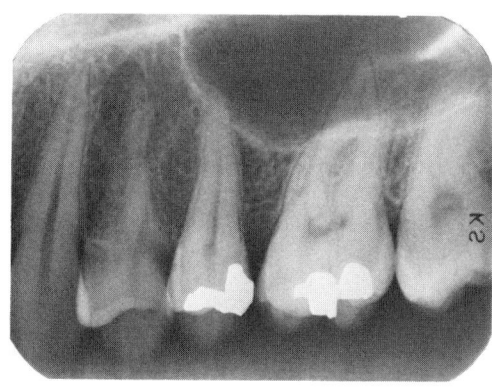

Figure 9-11. Improper beam alignment: Fuzzing-out of roots due to improper horizontal angulation of the beam for anterior one-third of the film.

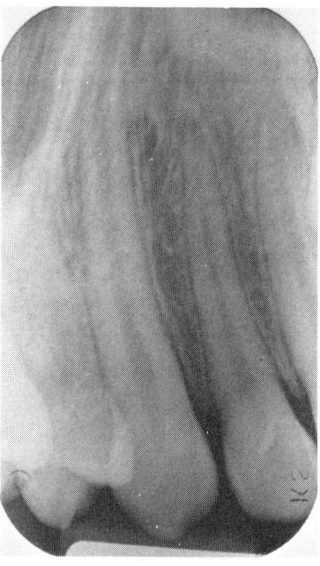

Figure 9-9. Improper film placement and retention: "Fuzzing-out" of the image due to distortion from finger pressure.

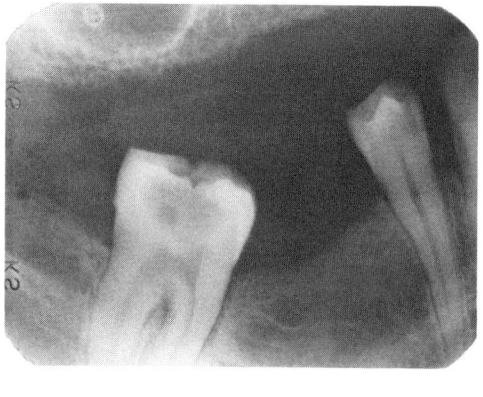

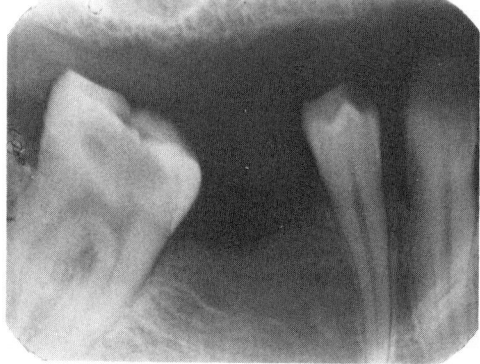

Figure 9-12. Magnification: **(A)** Poorly exposed radiograph; **(B)** Second poorly exposed radiograph of same area with magnification.

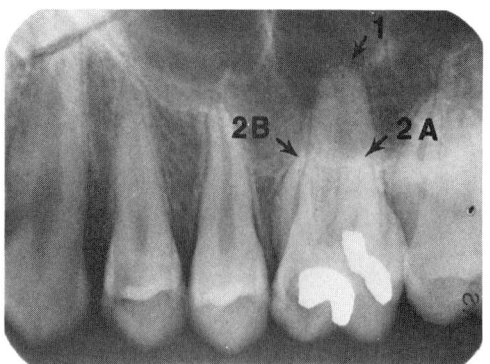

Figure 9-10. Dimensional distortion. (1) Elongated palatal root. (2A) Foreshortened distal buccal root. (2B) Foreshortened mesial buccal root.

e. Fuzzing-out of roots (Fig. 9-11).	Seen in maxillary bicuspid region due to improper horizontal angulation of beam.	Use correct horizontal angulation.
	Film not parallel to teeth in anteroposterior direction.	Proper film placement.
7. *Magnification* (Fig. 9-12).	Inadequate control of geometric factors.	Use machine with small focal spot.
	Usually seen with short cone and excessive object film distance.	Use of long a cone as possible. Use as short an object film distance as possible.
8. *Herring-bone effect or tire track.* (Fig. 9-13).	Printed back side of film placed toward cone of radiation (film reversed).	Placed pebbled or front side of film toward cone of radiation.
9. *Black dot in apical area* (Fig. 9-14).	Manufacturers identifying mark on film placed toward apical area of teeth.	Place black dot on film toward the occlusal or incisal surfaces of teeth.
10. *Artifacts on Radiograph* a. Writing lines on radiograph (Fig. 9-15).	Writing on film packet with ball point pen or lead pencil before exposure.	Use a crayon-type pencil or plastic marker pen to mark on film packet.
b. Black marks on radiograph (Fig. 9-16).	Moisture contamination (failure to blot film packet).	Blot film packet immediately after removal from patient's mouth.
c. Black lines on radiograph (Fig. 9-17).	Bending of film to reduce patient discomfort.	Avoid unnecessary film bending.
d. "Phalangioma" (Patient's finger in image) (Fig. 9-18).	In holding film, patient's finger placed between film and teeth.	Insure that patient holds film on back side only.
11. *Double images on radiographs* (Fig. 9-19).	Film exposed twice to radiation.	Place exposed film in receptacle.

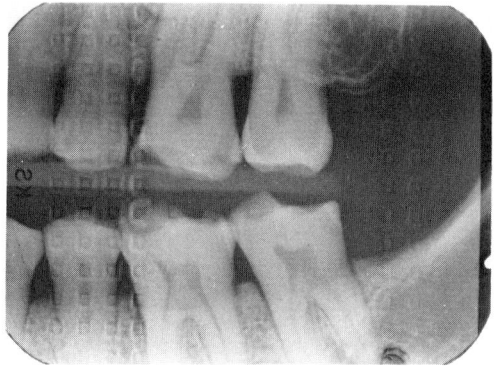

Figure 9-13. Improper film placement: "Tiretracks"; film placed back to front.

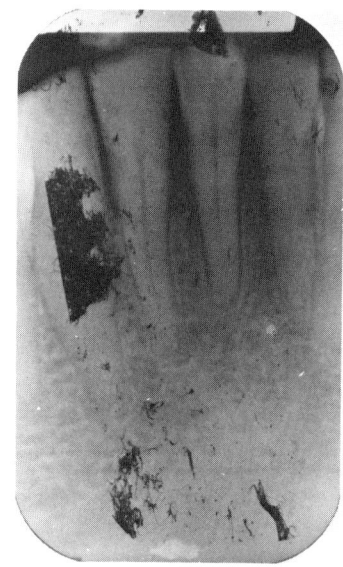

Figure 9-16. Moisure contamination.

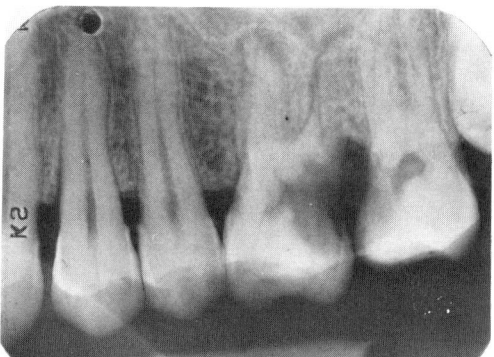

Figure 9-14. Improper film placement: Black dot on apex; locating dot should be placed toward the occlusal.

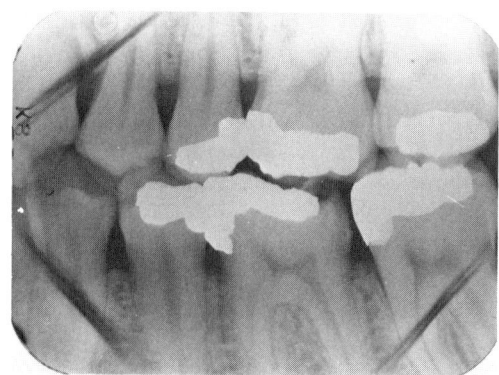

Figure 9-17. Film bending.

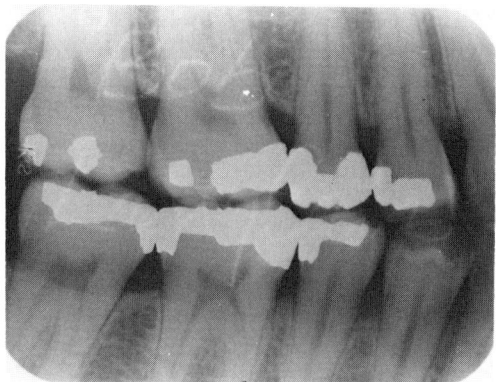

Figure 9-15. Writing on film: Due to writing on film packet before exposure of the film.

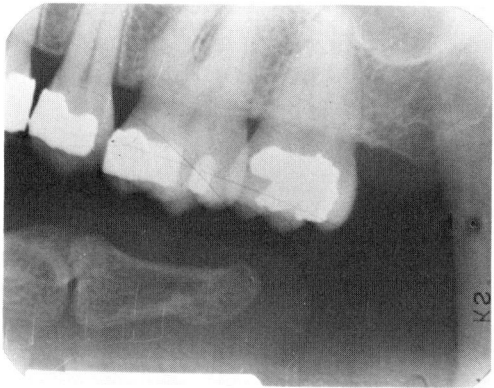

Figure 9-18. "Phalangioma": The patient's finger was placed between the film and the beam of radiation.

Analysis of Errors and Artifacts 329

12. *No image on radiograph* (Blank image).	Failure to fully depress exposure button. Failure to turn machine on.	Fully depress exposure button, wait for machine to turn on and off before letting go. Listen for audible exposure signal.
13. *Blurred image on radiograph* (Fig. 9-20).	Movement of film, patient, or tube during exposure.	Instruct patient properly; immobilize patient and tube. Repeat radiograph if you notice patient moving during exposure.
14. *Radiopaque artifacts on radiograph* (figs. 9-21, 9-22, 9-23).	Leaving dental appliance in mouth and/or glasses on person.	Instruct patient to remove dental appliances and glasses before exposure.
	Zirconium prophy paste in gingival sulcus.	Take radiograph prior to prophy or on another visit. More thorough rinsing of prophy paste.

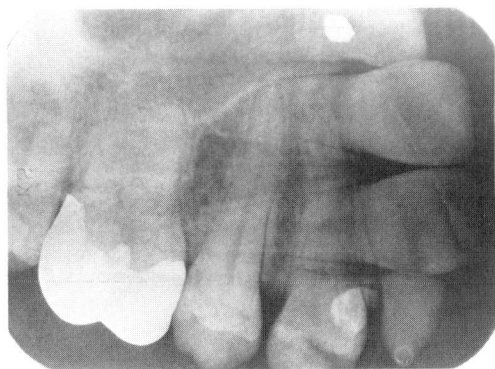

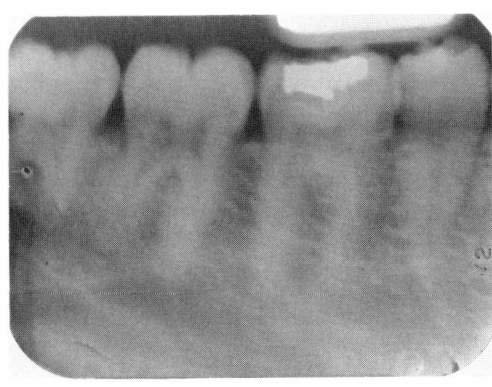

Figure 9-20. Movement: of film, patient, or tube head.

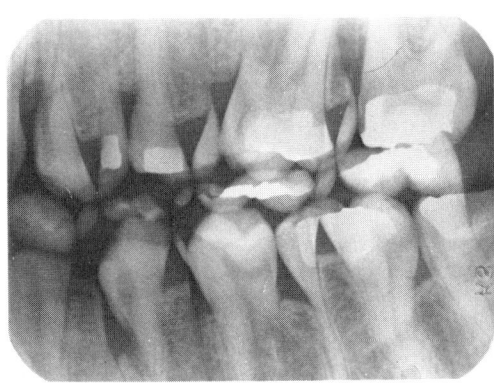

Figure 9-19. Double exposure: **(A)** Images taken at right angles to each other; **(B)** Images taken parallel to each other.

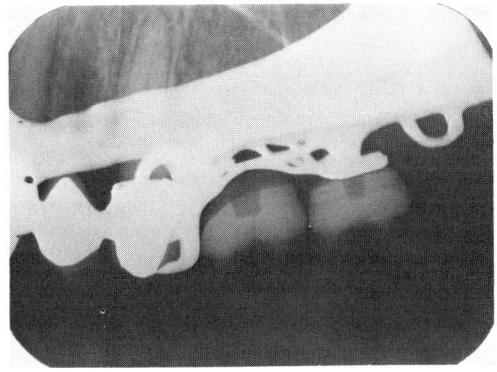

Figure 9-21. Removable appliance left in.

330 Textbook of Dental Radiology

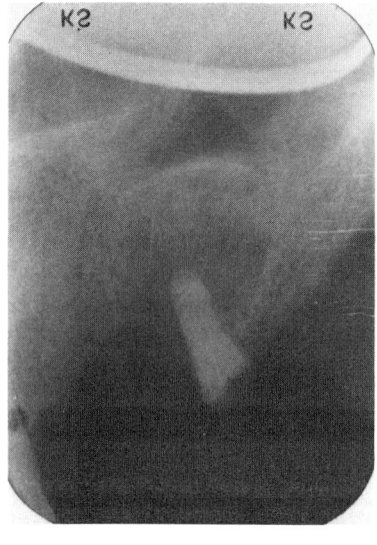

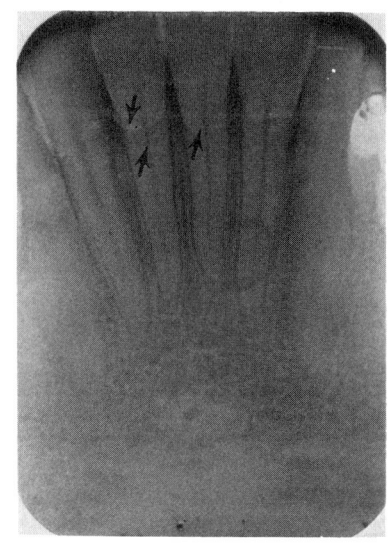

Figure 9-23. Zirconium prophy paste.

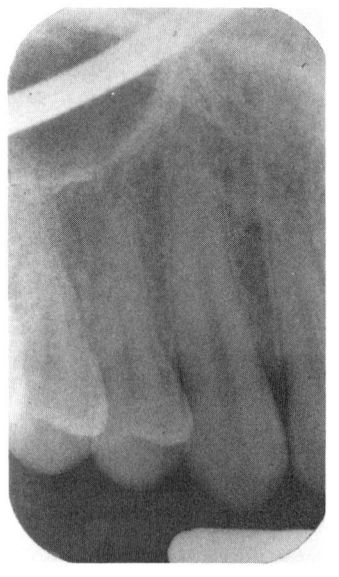

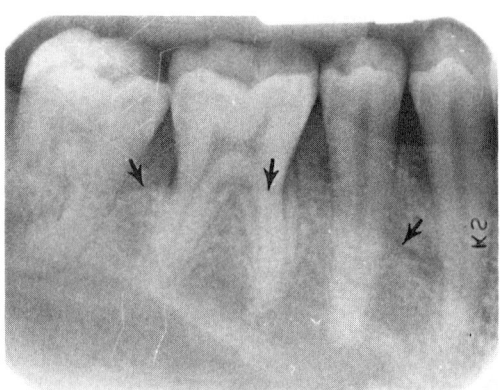

Figure 9-24. Improper film placement: Tongue image.

Figure 9-22. Eyeglasses left on: (A) Eyeglasses made of glass (radiopaque); (B) Eyeglasses made of acrylic (lenses not seen).

15.	*Tongue image* (Fig. 9-24).	Placing film on top of tongue.	Place film beneath tongue.
16.	*Cervical burnout* (Fig. 9-25).	Not a true error. Due to bell-shaped roots, allowing more radiation to penetrate and expose film.	Alter horizontal angle. Reduce kilovoltage. Reduce mAs if possible.

INTRAORAL EXPOSURE AND MANUAL PROCESSING ERRORS

Error	*Cause*	*Correction*
1. *Low Density or Light Films* (Fig. 9-26).	*Underexposure* a. Too short exposure.	Hold button for complete exposure. Set exposure time correctly and/or check calibration of exposure time.
	b. Source-film distance too great.	Check source-film distance.
	c. Too low kVp.	Increase kVp by approximately 5 kVp.
	d. Too low mA.	Increase mA or exposure time (mAs is one factor).
	e. Film packet placed backward in mouth.	See herring-bone effect error.
	f. Drop in line voltage. (1) Elevators, furnaces, blowers, etc. on same circuit as x-ray unit.	Use separate circuit for x-ray units.
	(2) Insufficient amount of power.	Increase size of power line and/or transformers.
2. (Fig. 9-27).	*Underdevelopment* a. Improper development	
	(1) Time too short.	Set darkroom timer correctly (check accuracy).
	(2) Low developer temperature.	Raise temperature to 70°F.
	(3) Inaccurate thermometer.	Replace thermometer.
	b. Exhausted and/or contaminated developer.	Replace developer.

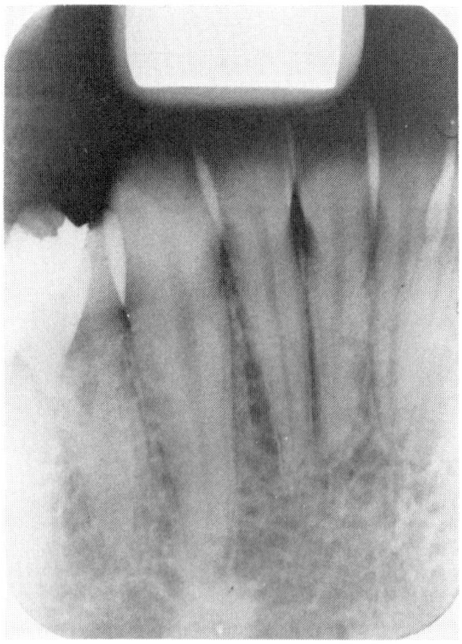

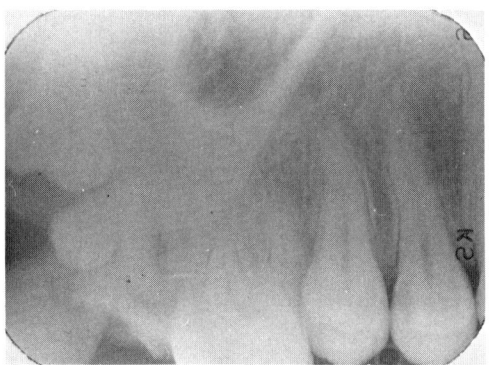

Figure 9-25. Improper film placement: Cervical burn-out.

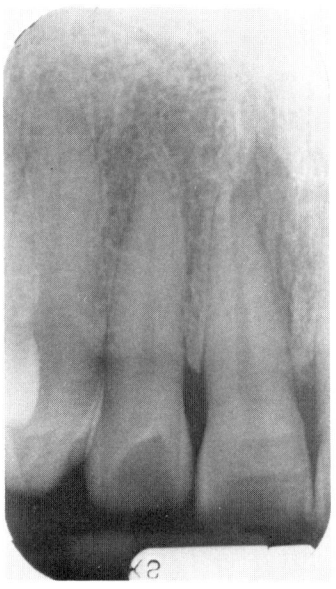

Figure 9-26. Underexposed radiograph.

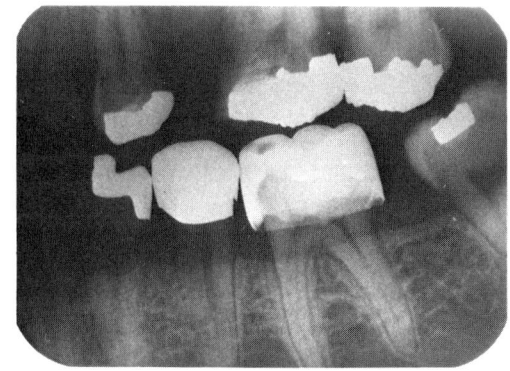

Figure 9-28. Overexposed radiograph.

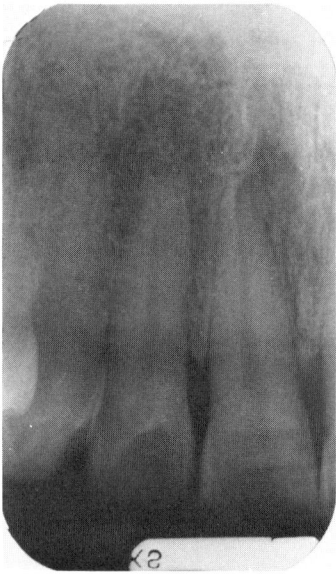

Figure 9-29. Overdevelopment (simulated photographically).

Figure 9-27. Underdevelopment (simulated photographically).

Analysis of Errors and Artifacts 333

    c. Diluted developer

(1) Water added to raise level of developer.	Add replenisher or replace developer.
(2) Insufficient developer solution added to water.	Add more developer solution.

3. *High Density or Dark Films* (Fig. 9-28).

    Overexposure

a. Exposure time too long.	Set timer correctly and/or reduce exposure time.
b. kVp too high for exposure time.	Reduce kVp.
c. Source-film distance too short for exposure time.	Measure source-film distance and adjust exposure time accordingly.
d. Timer inaccurate.	Check timer with spinning top and adjust exposure time accordingly.
e. mA too high for exposure time.	Reduce mA or exposure time.

4. (Fig. 9-29).

    Overdevelopment

a. Developing time too long.	Use time-temperature method with darkroom timer.
b. Developer temperature too high.	Lower developer temperature to 70° F.
c. Combination of a. & b.	
d. Inaccurate thermometer.	Replace thermometer.
e. Overstrength developer.	Check tank capacity and mixing directions (*see* Chapter 8 under processing tanks).

5. *High Contrast* (Fig. 9-30).

a. Insufficient penetration.	Increase kilovoltage.

	b. Overdevelopment.	See correction above (underdevelopment).
	c. Use of film and/or intensifying screens of too high contrast.	Use lower contrast films or slower speed screens.
	d. Too long exposure.	Timer inaccurately set, or timer out of calibration.
6. *Low Contrast* (Fig. 9-31).	a. Excessive penetration.	Decrease kilovoltage.
	b. Underdevelopment.	See correction above (underdevelopment).
	c. Use of film having insufficient contrast and/or cassettes with too slow intensifying screens.	Use of higher speed screens.
	d. Scattered radiation.	Check diaphragm size and use suitable cone.
		Develop by time-temperature method.
7. *Fog* (Fig. 9-32).	*Light*	
	a. Light leaks in darkroom.	Check doors and walls for leaks.
	Improper safelight.	Reduce wattage of bulb.
	Improper filter in safelight.	Check type of filter and examine for cracks in filter (Wratten 6B type for screen film).
	b. Turning overhead (white) light on too soon.	Fix films 1-2 minutes before turning on the white light.
	c. Prolonged exposure of films to safelight.	Reduce exposure time of films to safelight.
8. (Fig. 9-33).	*Radiation*	
	a. Insufficient protection.	Store unexposed film in lead receptacles.

Analysis of Errors and Artifacts

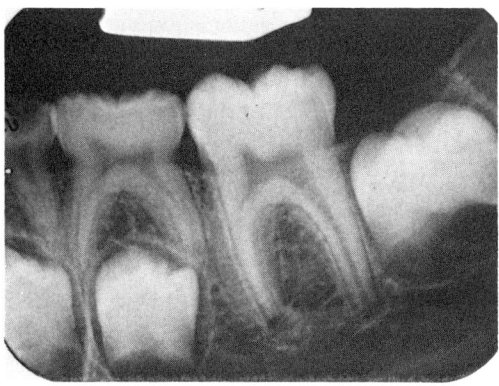

Figure 9-30. High contrast.

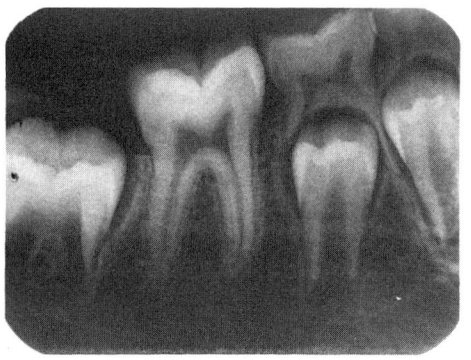

Figure 9-31. Low contrast.

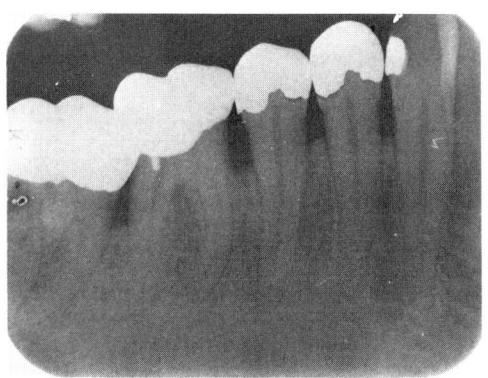

Figure 9-32. Low contrast.

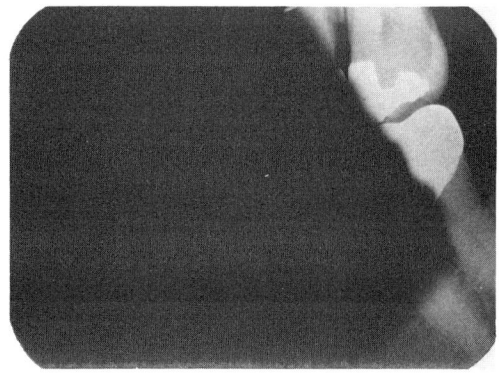

Figure 9-33. Light contamination: Exposure of film to light after taking radiograph, before processing.

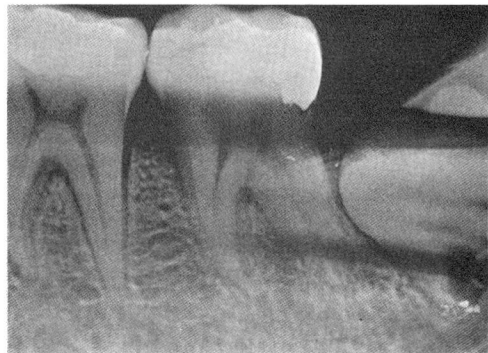

Figure 9-34. Developer contamination: Hanger clips contaiminated with developer.

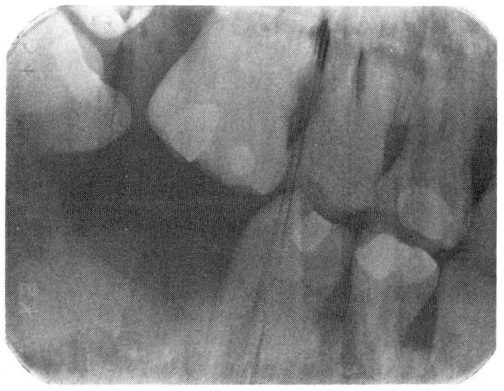

Figure 9-35. Inadequate fixing.

336 Textbook of Dental Radiology

9. *Chemical*

   a. Developer temperatures too high. — Reduce temperature of developer to manufacturer's optimum temperature (70°F).

   b. Overstrength developer. — Check tank capacity and mixing directions.

   c. Prolonged development.

   d. Contaminated developer. — Clean developer tank periodically.

10. *Deterioration of Film*

    a. Temperature of storage area too high. — Store film in a cool place (70° F) or use refrigerator for storage of film.

    b. Humidity of storage area too high. — Store films in dry place (50% relative humidity. Use refrigerator.)

    c. Strong fumes (ammonia, paint). — Keep films away from fumes.

    d. Outdated film. — Limit supply and use older films first.

11. *Streaks on film.*

    a. Failure to agitate film during development. — When first immersed in developer, agitate films.

    b. Undue amount of inspection of film during development. When films are held in front of safelight during development, the developer solution runs across the films producing uneven reduction of emulsion. — Use time-temperature method of development. This reduces the need to inspect film during development.

Analysis of Errors and Artifacts 337

	c. Chemical deposits on hanger clips (Fig. 9-34).	Keep hanger clips clean.
	d. Excessive drying temperature.	Reduce air flow over films.
	e. Insufficient fixing (Fig. 9-35).	Usually the fixing time is twice the developer time.
	f. Dirty or contaminated wash water.	Wash films in fresh running water.
	g. Premature exposure of film to white light before fixing process is complete.	It usually requires approximately 2 minutes to clear film in fixing solution.
12. *Air Bubbles* (Fig. 9-36).	Air bubbles trapped on film surfaces preventing uniform reduction of emulsion.	Agitate films upon immersion into developer.
13. *White spots and lines on film.*	a. Grit or dust present on films or upon screens.	Keep darkroom clean to prevent dust and dirt particles from settling on films. Periodically clean screens with commercial screen cleaner.
	b. Emulsion tears from rough handling of films in processing tank (Fig. 9-37).	Do not rub films up against sides of tanks or on other film hangers.
	c. Fixer artifact (Fig. 9-38).	Avoid splashing fixer on film before developing.
14. *Black spots on film.*	a. Grit or dust in contact with undeveloped film.	Prevent fine particles of developer coming in contact with film (dry chemicals).
	b. Film splashed with developer before being placed in developer tank (Fig. 9-39).	Careful handling of solutions and clean work area.

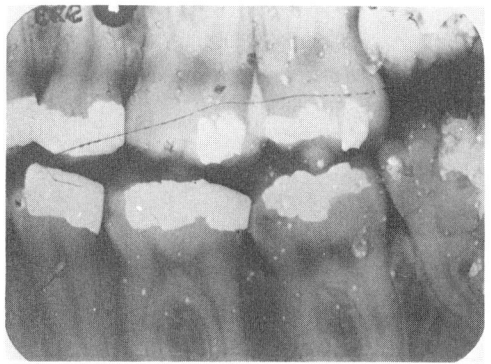

Figure 9-36. Air bubbles.

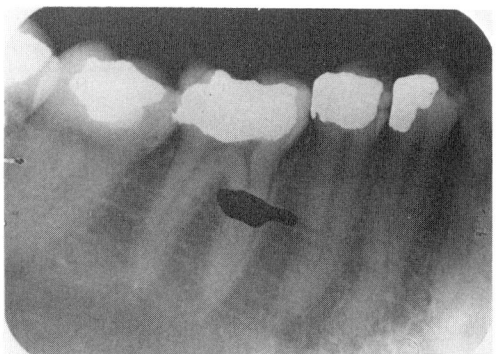

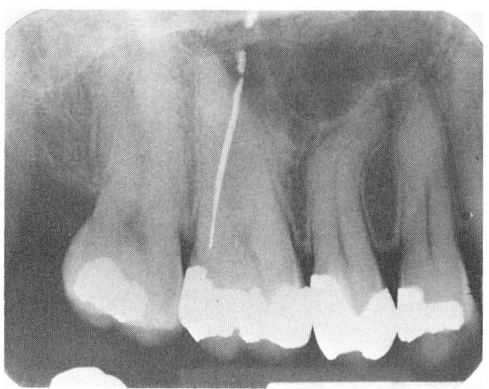

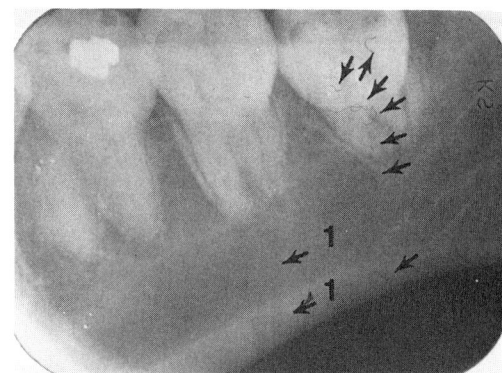

Figure 9-37. Torn emulsion. Scratch

Figure 9-39. Developer artifact: **(A)** Black developer stain; **(B)** 1. Developer stain mimics fistulous tract; 2. Other arrows: static electricity.

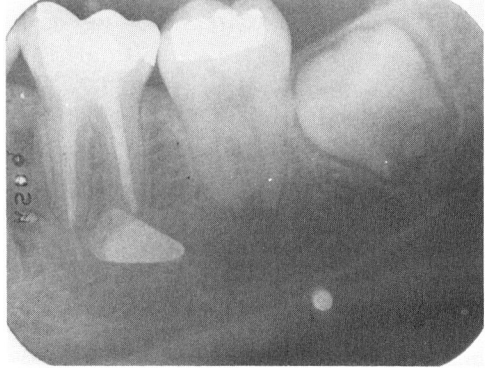

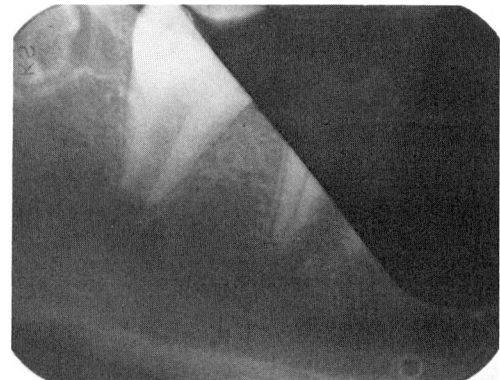

Figure 9-38. Fixer artifact.

Figure 9-40. Films stuck together.

Analysis of Errors and Artifacts

	c. Films touching during fixing (Fig. 9-40).	Films should not touch in processing tanks.
15. *Artifacts from processing.*		
a. Black cresents (Fig. 9-41).	Rough handling of film.	Handle film by edges only.
b. Smudge marks or fingerprints on film.	Fingerprints or finger abrasions.	Have fingers dry when handling film (processing and mounting).
Black (Fig. 9-42A).	Contamination with fluoride containing prophy paste.	Wash hands before processing.
Grey-black (Fig. 42-B).	Contamination with developer.	Clean area to avoid contamination of hands.
White (Fig. 9-42C).	Contamination with fixer.	Handle film by edges.
c. Black lines (Fig. 9-43).	Static electricity. Too rapid removal of film from packet in air with dry humidity.	Slow removal of film from packet. Humidify darkroom.
16. *Stains on film*		
a. Yellow or brown	Exhausted developer.	Replace developer solution.
	Oxidized developer. Prolonged developer.	Keep developer covered. Use correct development time.
	Insufficient rinsing.	Rinse films 15-20 seconds in fresh running water.
	Exhausted fixer solution.	Replace fixer solution frequently.
b. Dichromic (showing two colors).	Old or exhausted developer.	Replace developer solution.
	Nearly exhausted fixer.	Replace fixer solution.
	Developer containing small amounts of scum or fixer.	Remove scum and/or replace fixer solution.

	Film partially fixed in weak fixer, exposed to light, and washed.	Replace fixer solution: follow recommended processing cycle.
	Prolonged intermediate rinse in contaminated rinse water.	Use fresh, running water and recommended cycle.
17. *Deposits on film*	Contaminated solutions (oil, impurities).	Mix new solution.
	Chemical deposits on hangers.	Clean clips and hanger tops.
	Grit from dirty water.	Use fresh, running water.
	Metallic deposits (oxidized products from developer).	Replace developer solution.
	Fixer contains excessive amounts of silver.	Replace fixer solution.
	White deposits: use of fixer that has milky appearance; this is caused by excessive amounts of precipitated aluminum sulfite.	Follow manufacturer's recommendations for mixing fixer solution. Use premixed liquid solution.
	Excessive amounts of developer carried into fixer on film emulsion.	Rinse properly and allow developer solution to drip into water a few seconds before placing film in fixer.
18. *Brittleness of finished radiographs.*	Excessive drying temperature.	Reduce dryer temperature.
	Excessive drying time; incoming air too humid and cold air velocity too low.	If use dryer, reduce drying time and adjust incoming air. Use a wetting agent prior to placing films in dryer.
	Excessive fixer acidity.	Replace fixer solution.

Analysis of Errors and Artifacts

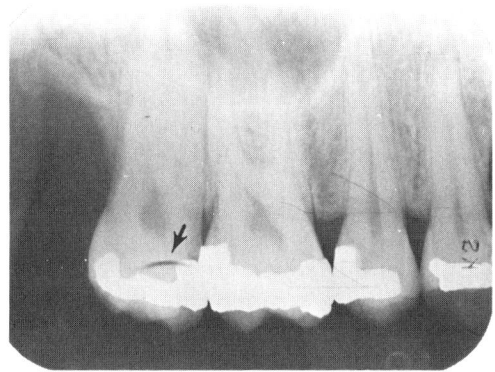

Figure 9-41. Fingernail artifact.

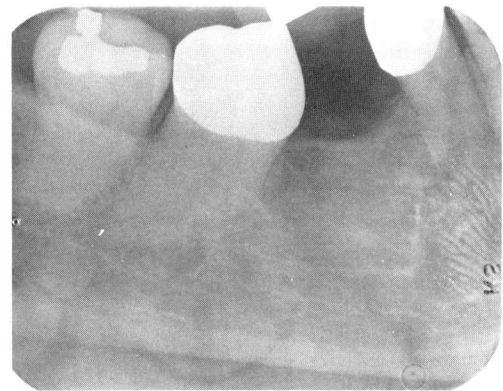

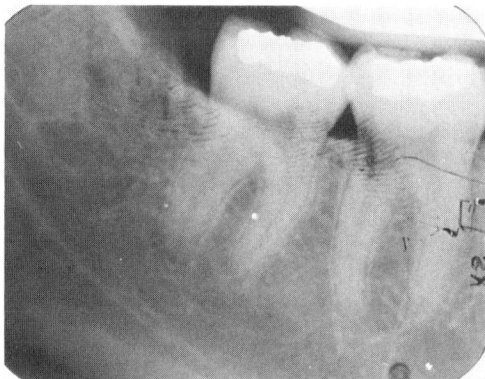

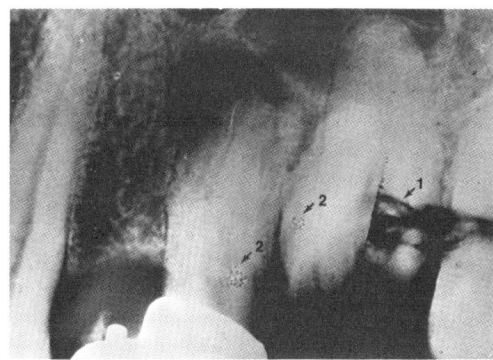

Figure 9-43. Static electricity: (1) Linear form; may appear as thin, lintlike lines or as lighteninglike streaks. (2) Punctuate form; may appear as a group of little black dots; as a larger black dot; or a black dot with one or many straight lines radiating from it.

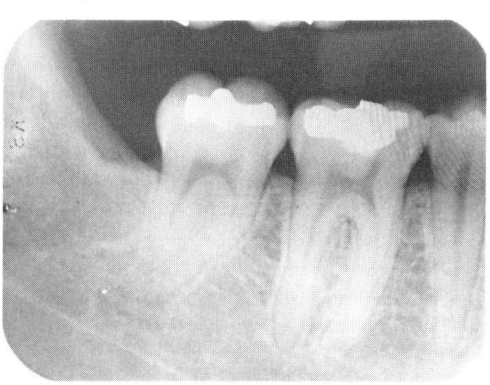

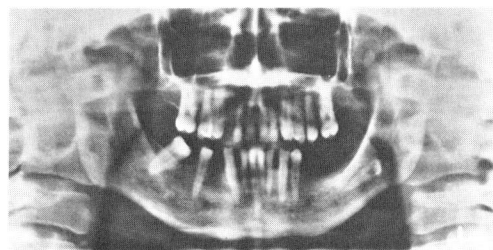

Figure 9-42. Fingerprints: (A) Fluoride contamination (Stannous); (B) Developer contamination; (C) Fixer contamination.

Figure 9-44. Patient positioning error: Patient too far forward.

19. *Faded image on finished radiograph.*	Exhausted fixer.	Replace fixer solution.
	Inadequate fixing.	Fix films three times the clearing time.
	Insufficient final wash.	Wash film in fresh, running water for a minimum of 15-20 minutes.

PANORAMIC PATIENT POSITIONING ERRORS

Error and Cause	*Identifying Features*	*Correction*
1. Patient too far forward (Fig. 9-44).	Narrow blurred anterior teeth. Superimposition of spine on ramus. Bicuspid overlap bilaterally.	Use incisal bite guide. Line up incisal edge of teeth with notch. In edentulous, bite about 5 mm behind notch.
2. Patient too far back (Fig. 9-45).	Wide, blurred anterior teeth.	Use incisal bite guide. Line up incisal edge of teeth with notch.
3. Chin tipped too low (Fig. 9-46).	Excessive curving of occlusal plane. Loss of image of roots of lower anterior teeth. Narrowing of intercondylar distance and loss of head of condyles at top of film.	Tip chin down, but ala-tragus line should not exceed -5 to -7 degrees downwards. Use chin rest.
4. Chin raised too high (Fig. 9-47).	Flattening or reverse curvature of occlusal plane. Loss of image of roots of upper anterior teeth. Lengthening of intercondylar distance and loss of head of condyles at edges of film. Hard palate shadow superimposed on apices of maxillary teeth.	Tip chin down -5 to -7 degrees. Use chin rest.

Analysis of Errors and Artifacts 343

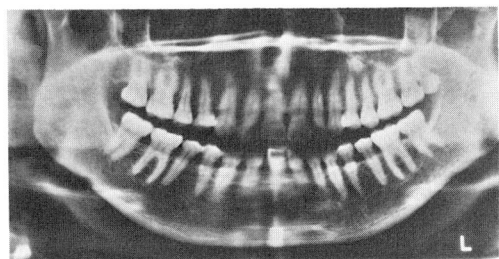

Figure 9-45. Patient positioning error: Patient too far back.

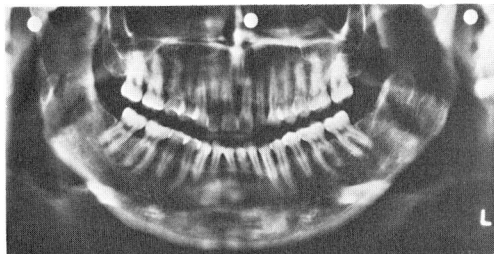

Figure 9-46. Patient positioning error: Chin tipped too low.

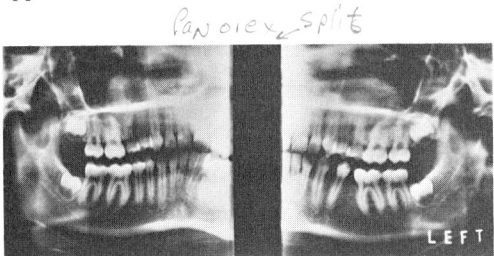

Figure 9-47. Patient positioning error: Chin raised too high.

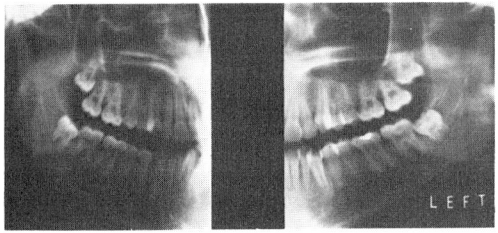

Figure 9-48. Patient positioning error: Head twisted.

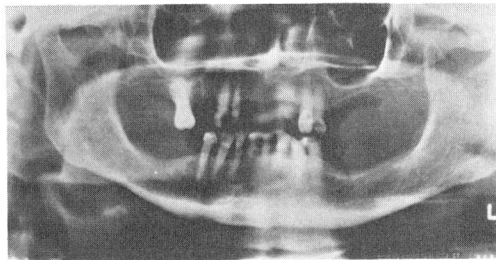

Figure 9-49. Patient positioning error: Head tilted.

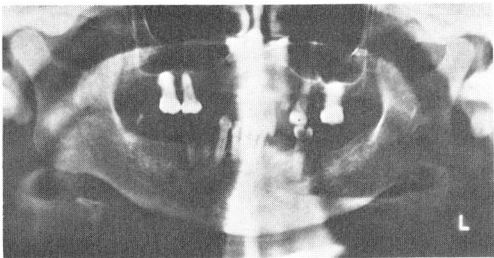

Figure 9-50. Patient positioning error: Slumped position.

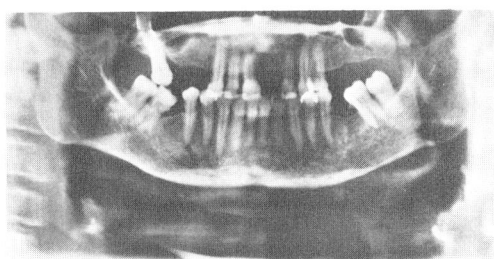

Figure 9-51. Patient positioning error: Chin not on chin rest (machine too low).

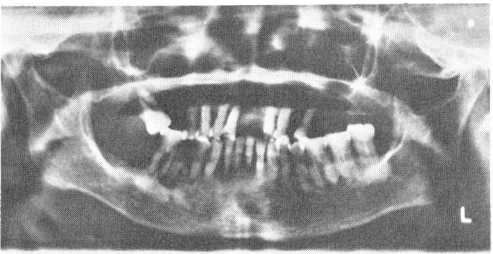

Figure 9-52. Patient positioning error: Bite guide not used. In this case a sufficient number of cotton rolls should have been placed in the maxillary midline area to cause a separation of the posterior teeth when the lower incisors are placed in the notch of the bite guide.

5. Head twisted (Fig. 9-48).	Unequal right-left magnification. Particularly teeth and ramus. Severe overlap of contact points and blurring.	Line up patient's midline with middle of incisal bite guide.
6. Head tilted (Fig. 9-49).	Mandible appears tilted on film. Unequal distance between mandible and chin rest at a given point on right and left sides.	Position chin firmly on both sides of chin rest.
7. Slumped position (Fig. 9-50).	Ghost image of cervical spine superimposed on anterior region.	Stand-up machines — have patient step forward or place feet on markers. All machines — be certain patient is sitting or standing erect.
8. Chin not on chin rest (Fig. 9-51).	Sinus not visible on film; top of condyle cut off; excessive distance between inferior border of mandible and lower edge of film.	Position chin on chin rest.
9. Bite guide not used (Fig. 9-52).	Incisal and occlusal surfaces of upper and lower teeth overlapped.	Use bite guide. Compensate for missing anterior teeth with cotton rolls.
10. Machine too high (chin rest too low) (fig. 9-53).	Inferior border of mandible cut off at lower edge of film.	Adjust machine to correct vertical height. Chin rest in position for special technique. With 6 inch cassette and 5 inch film, tap film down to bottom edge of cassette.
11. Tongue not on palate (Fig. 9-54).	Relative radiolucency obscuring apices of maxillary teeth (Palatolglossal air space).	Place tongue firmly against palate.

Analysis of Errors and Artifacts

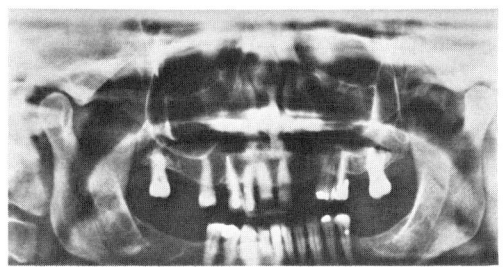

Figure 9-53. Patient positioning error: Machine too high (chin rest too low).

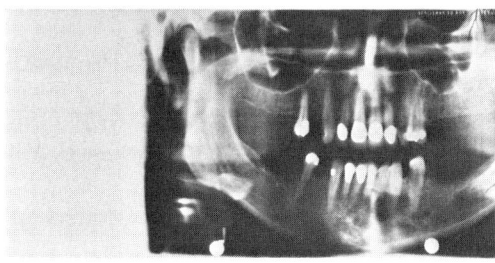

Figure 9-57. Operator error: Not starting at home base.

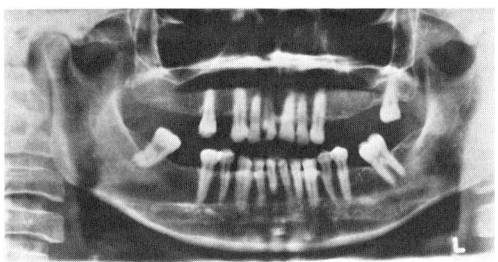

Figure 9-54. Patient positioning error: Tongue not on palate; lips open.

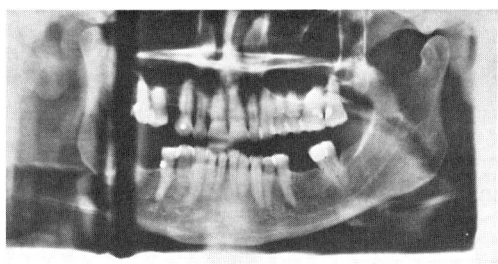

Figure 9-58. Operator error: cassette resistance

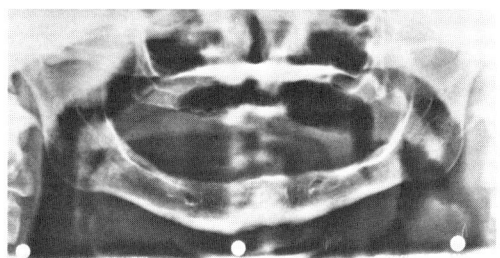

Figure 9-55. Patient positioning error: Patient movement.

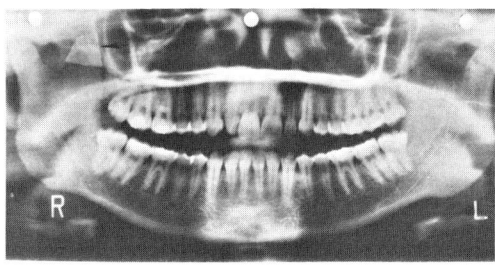

Figure 9-59. Operator error: Paper or lint in screen.

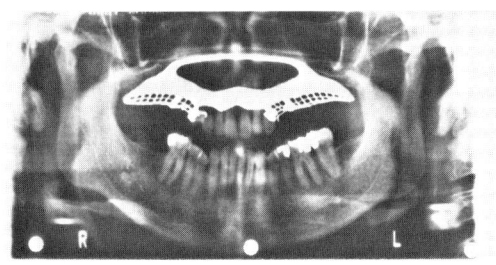

Figure 9-56. Patient positioning error: Prostheses left in.

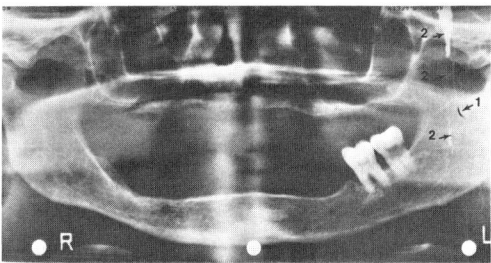

Figure 9-60. Operator error: Fingernail artifact; film crimping. (1) fingernail artifact or film crimping; (2) cracked screen.

346   Textbook of Dental Radiology

12. Lips open (Fig. 9-54).	Relative radiolucency on coronal portion of of upper and lower teeth.	Close lips
13. Patient movement (Fig. 9-55).	Wavy outline of cortex of inferior border of mandible. Blurring of image above wavy cortical outline.	Ask patient to hold still. Explain function of machine to avoid startling patient. Be certain patient is relatively comfortable.
14. Prostheses (Fig. 9-56).	Evidence of prostheses in film. Acrylic denture teeth and bases do not show.	Remove all complete and partial dentures and eyeglasses.

COMMON PANORAMIC OPERATOR ERRORS

Error and Cause	*Identifying Features*	*Correction*
1. Not starting at home base (Fig. 9-57).	A portion of film is blank; a portion of anatomy is lost at edge of film.	Align machine and/or cassette with starting point.
2. Cassette resistance: (Fig. 9-58).	One or several dark vertical bands on film. These represent areas of overexposure as the cassette is stopped, but radiation continues to be emitted until the end of the cycle.	Be certain to remove thickly padded items of clothing. In stocky patients with a short neck, the cassette may need to be raised slightly above the ideal position.
3. Paper or lint in screen (Fig. 9-59).	Radiopacity of unusual shape and location. Foreign object prevents complete exposure of film by fluorescent screen.	With envelope-type soft cassettes, periodic inspection and cleaning of screens.
4. Fingernail artifact (Fig. 9-60).	Cresenct shaped radiolucency.	Avoid using fingernails to remove film from cassette.
5. Film crimping (Fig. 9-60).	Cresent shaped radiolucency.	Avoid forcefully pushing film into the cassette; or bending the leading edge upon removal of film from cassette.

Analysis of Errors and Artifacts

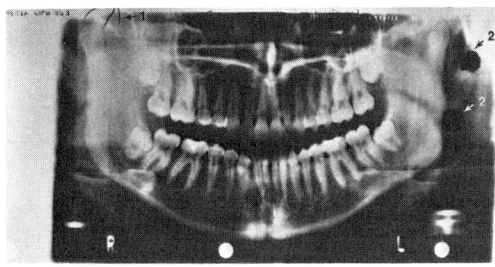

Figure 9-61. Operator error: Static electricity (1) linear form; (2) punctate form.

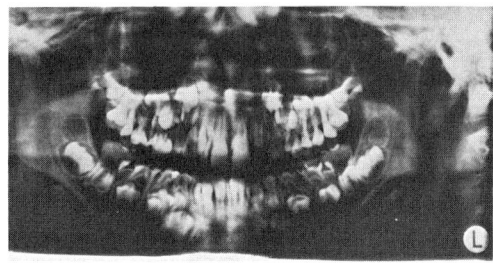

Figure 9-63. Operator error: Double exposure.

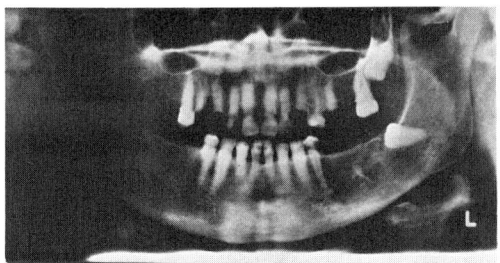

Figure 9-62. White-light exposure.

6. Static electricity (Fig. 9-61).	Lightninglike radiolucency; Dotlike radiolucencies.	Dry air in darkroom can be humidified with a humidifier or large bowl of water. Avoid rapid pulling-out of film from envelope-type cassettes.
7. White-light exposure (Fig. 9-62).	A portion of the film appears overexposed.	Avoid smoking near film. Check other sources of light leaks in darkroom, i.e. unsafe safelight, etc.; check integrity of cassette.
8. Double exposure (Fig. 9-63).	Two images on same film.	Always place exposed films in the same location and where they may not be mistaken for unexposed films.
9. Underexposed	Film too light.	Increase kV and/or mA depending upon machine. Place film in between screens, not to one side only.

10. Overexposed.	Film too dark.	Decrease kV and/or mA depending upon machine.
11. No name.	Patient's name or identification number not on film.	Use film imprintor, special labeling tape, or special pen.

OPERATOR'S TROUBLESHOOTING GUIDE FOR AUTOMATIC PROCESSORS*

Section I — Film Density Problems

Error	*Cause*	*Correction*
1. *Decrease of film density (overall light films).*	a. Developer temperature low.	Increase heat in the developer. NOTE: Check the temperature of the developer solution with a thermometer of known accuracy.
	b. Developer reaching exhaustion.	Drain and thoroughly clean tank; install new developer solution.
	c. Developer contamination — the most likely reason for contaminated developer is fixer solution splashed or dripped into the developer.	Drain and thoroughly clean tank and rack; install new developer solution.
	d. No agitation in developer tank.	Be sure the agitator paddle drive belt is in the proper position in the pulleys.
2. *Increase in film density (overall dark films).*	a. Developer temperature too high.	Water turned off. Check temperature of incoming water supply and adjust from 75° to 78° F. Decrease the heat in the developer solution. NOTE: Check the temperature of the developer solution with a thermometer of known accuracy.

*From Profexray's Automatic Dental Film Processor's Manual.

3. *Fogged film.*

a. Developer solution contaminated with fixer.

Drain and thoroughly clean tank and rack; install new developer solution.

b. Processor light leaks.

Be sure processor cover is secured firmly in place.

c. Light leaks in other areas.

Check light tightness of darkroom.

d. Improper safelight.

Use 7½ watt frosted bulb in safelight with proper filter, mounted no closer than 4 feet from working area.

e. Heat fog.

Make sure film storage area is not excessively hot.

f. Excessively high developer temperature.

Readjust developer thermostat and water to proper temperature.

Section II — Film Drying Problems

1. *Films are not dry.*

a. Depleted fixer.
b. Insufficient water flow (film not properly washed).

Install new fixer solution. Check incoming water lines and valves.
NOTE: The incoming water flow must be a minimum of ½ gallon-per-minute — or a maximum of 1 gallon-per-minute.

c. Dryer temperature setting too low.

Increase dryer temperature.

d. Chemical imbalance (either developer or fixer).

Replace with new solution.

e. Improper type of film for time cycle of processor.

Check with dealer for information regarding proper type of film. (It is not recommended for film with acetate film base or any other film not designed for automatic processing.)

Section III — Abnormal Film Surface Marks

1. *Peeling of film emulsion.*

   a. Developer temperature too high. — Reduce developer temperature to proper level.

   b. Improper fixer strength or depleted fixer. — Replace fixer solution.

   c. Heavy developer deposits on developer rack rollers above solution level. — Be sure to follow the recommended housekeeping and cleaning procedures.

   d. Improper film. — Check with dealer for information regarding proper type of film.

2. *Pressure marks.*

   a. Foreign material or rough spot on roller. — Clean rollers and/or remove rough area on roller.

   b. Rough handling or excessive hand pressure on film before processing. — Film emulsions are extremely sensitive, particularly after exposure and before processing. Good habits in gentle handling of film must be practiced.

3. *Cloudy or smudge appearance or film surface (greenish or yellowish)*

   a. Depleted fixer.
   b. Improper type of film for time cycle of processor.

   — Replace fixer solution. Check with dealer.

4. *White cloudy appearance over film surface.*

   a. No water in wash tank. — Check incoming controls and lines. Be sure drain plug in wash tank is inserted in drain outlet.

5. *Scratches on film surface.*	a. Foreign material on roller(s).	Clean rollers.
	b. Improper handling of film before processing.	Proper, gentle handling of film must be practiced.
	c. Damaged or defective film.	Hand develop film(s) of the same batch or box. This may pick up defects that could be characteristic of the particular box or batch of film.
	d. Stalled or sticking roller.	Inspect racks, gears, and gear mesh. correct as required.
6. *Drying pattern on film surface.*	a. Dryer too hot.	Reduce dryer temperature.
	b. Characteristic of film.	Process film of same box through another processor and chemicals to determine consistency of pattern.

References

A Look At X-ray Film Processing. Milwaukee, X-ray Department, General Electric Co.

A Textbook of Selective X-ray Technique. Rochester, New York, Ritter, pp. 136-138.

Bloom, William L.; Hollenbach, John L.; and Morgan, James A.: *Medical Radiographic Technic,* 3rd ed. Springfield, Charles C Thomas, 1969, pp. 127-128.

Darkroom Technique for Better Radiographs. Wilmington, Delaware, Photo Products Department, E. I. du pont de Nemours and Co.

Du Pont Guide for Dental X-ray Darkrooms. Wilmington, Delaware, Photo Products Department, E. I. du Pont de Nemours and Co.

Fuchs, Arthur W.: *Principles of Radiographic Exposures and Processing,* 2nd ed. Springfield, Charles C Thomas, 1958, pp. 199-258.

McCall, John; and Wald, Samuel: *Clinical Dental roentgenology,* 4th ed. Philadelphia, W. B. Saunders, 1957, pp. 124-126.

Peterson, Shailer: *Clinical Dental Hygiene.* St. Louis, Mosby, 1959, pp. 239-247.

Radiodontic Pitfalls. Rocheser, N.Y., Eastman Kodak Co., X-ray Division.

Chapter 10

QUALITY ASSURANCE

W. Doss McDavid and Emily E. Taylor

What Is Quality Assurance?

QUALITY assurance, as applied to diagnostic radiology, refers to those steps that are taken to make sure that a radiological facility will produce consistently high quality radiographs at minimum cost and minimum patient exposure. In Chapters 4 and 9, the common causes of unsatisfactory radiographs have been discussed. Many of these, such as improper angulation and film positioning, result primarily from human error. Others, such as exposure and processing problems, may result from equipment failure. Since even the most skilled operator will be unable to produce radiographs of consistently high quality if the various factors such as kilovoltage, tube current, and exposure time are not accurate and repeatable or if variations in processing chemistry have taken place, these types of problems are, in a way, primary. The term **quality assurance** has come into general use to describe the administrative and technical efforts that are made toward identifying and correcting equipment problems before they have become so severe as to affect the diagnostic quality of the radiographs being produced.

Quality assurance may be divided into two major categories: (1) quality control, and (2) quality administration (Fig. 10-1). Quality control summarizes the techniques used for the routine physical testing of the X-Ray system. Quality administration refers, on the other hand, to the management aspect. It includes those steps taken to make sure that testing techniques are properly performed and that the results of such tests are used effectively to maintain a consistently high level of image quality.

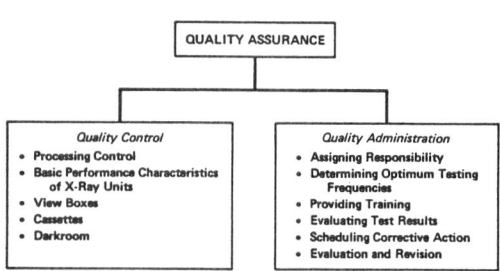

Figure 10-1. Components of a quality assurance program.

Establishing a Quality Assurance Program

A diagnostic radiology quality assurance program involves periodic testing of the various components that make up a system for diagnostic X-Ray imaging. This includes the entire chain of components from the X-Ray generator to the viewing room. The use of the Wainwright X-Ray Checker, as described in Chapter 8, is one very simple form of quality control. If used routinely, this simple method can help identify a number of problems. Unfortunately, it has the disadvantage of not being able to distinguish between problems that originate in the darkroom and problems that are connected with the radiographic equipment. There are a number of other testing methods that may be used to provide more specific information about problems. In the next few pages we will examine some of these tests and the equipment used to perform them. The specific tests employed in a particular facility and the frequency of testing is a highly individual matter and will depend on the resources and workload of a particular institution or office. This has been recognized by the Bureau of Radiological Health (1979) in formulating its recommendations for quality assurance programs:

> The parameters to be monitored in a facility should be determined on the basis of the expected benefits and costs. Such factors as the size and resources of the facility, the type of examinations conducted, and the quality assurance programs that have occurred in that or similar facilities should be taken into account in establishing the monitoring system. The monitoring frequency should also be based upon need and can be different for different parameters.

Similarly, the personnel utilized to carry out the testing procedures can be adapted to the special requirements of a given facility. For example, since the monitoring of processing procedures should be a daily matter, these processing tests can be accomplished by in-house personnel. Tests of parameters such as kVP and focal spot size can be carried out at much longer time intervals by qualified outside personnel such as consultants or industrial representatives. A list of qualified experts capable of performing X-Ray equipment tests at a moderate cost is generally available from state agencies overseeing the use of ionizing radiation. Here it should be emphasized that the choice of outside personnel for this task is usually one of convenience and economics. It is not based on the technical complexity of the testing procedures since these require only a minimum of training to be performed effectively. An alternative possibility, which can be quite effective in performing tests other than the daily monitoring or processing, is the sharing of the essential test instruments between a group of private practitioners and rotating the quality control "kit" between offices.

Although the details will vary from one facility or office to the next, there are five key components of the X-Ray system that should be monitored: (1) film processing, (2) basic performance characteristics of the X-Ray unit, (3) cassettes, (4) view boxes, and (5) the darkroom. We will consider each of these in the following sections.

Film Processing

By instituting effective processing control measures, incipient changes in film processing may be noted early in order that corrective actions may be taken. Many of the variables affecting processing (temperature regulation, chemistry, replenishment, etc.) change so slowly that it is only by daily monitoring that they can be detected before the radiographs have begun to deteriorate in diagnostic quality.

Processing quality control can be carried out at a number of levels of sophistication. A simple and inexpensive method is the use of a "reference film" produced under "ideal" conditions. A "good quality" periapical or bite-wing radiograph should be attached to a viewbox where the dentist or his auxilliaries can easily compare it to recently processed radiographs. Changes in film density between test films and the reference film can be identified, as can changes in overall film quality. A reference film for each specific type of radiograph (e.g. panoramic, cephalometric, etc.) should be maintained. Processing solutions should be changed when there is visual evidence of reduced quality of the test film.

A more sophisticated and effective method of quality control of processing is the use of control strips exposed using a sensitometer. A sensitometer is simply a device that exposes an X-Ray film to a highly reproducible step pattern of light intensity (Figs. 10-2 and 10-3). When films are exposed by a sensitometer and developed in a consistent manner, they will appear identical. A film from a box reserved for this purpose should be exposed the first thing in the morning using a sensitometer and developed imme-

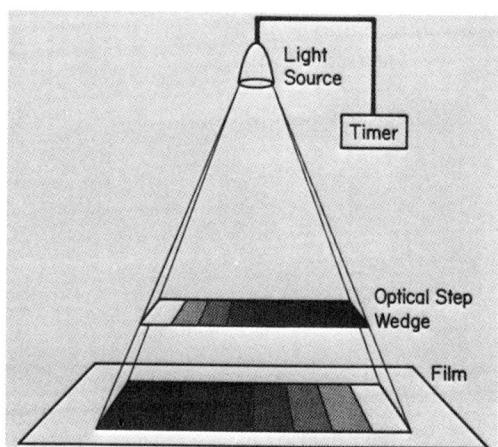

Figure 10-3. Schematic diagram of a sensitometer.

diately (Fig. 10-4). The film is then compared visually with a reference film or, better yet, the optical density of the exposed areas of the film is read with a densitometer (Fig. 10-5). A densitometer is a device for measuring optical density as defined in Chapter 3 and consists of a

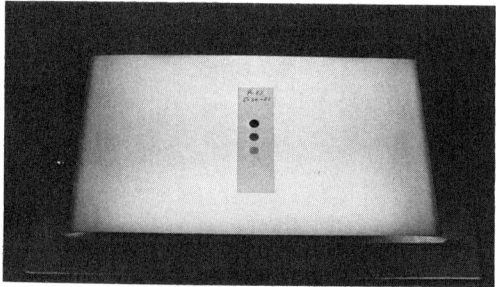

Figure 10-4. A test film exposed using a sensitometer.

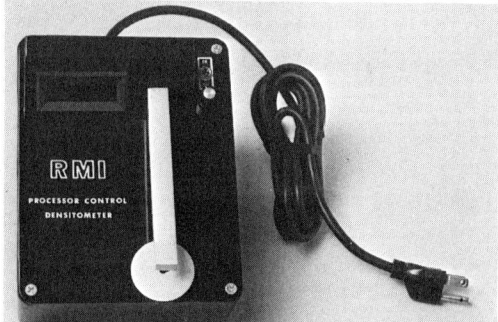

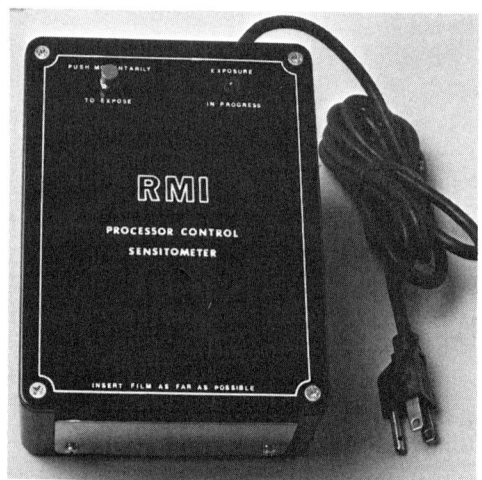

Figure 10-2. A sensitometer for quality control of processing.

Figure 10-5. A densitometer for quality control of processing.

light source and a photocell that measures the transmitted light.

If the sophisticated method is used, it is generally recommended that a record be kept of the density of a particular sensitometer step (speed index), the difference between adjacent steps (contrast index), and the fog level (Fig. 10-6). A log should also be kept of the temperature of the developer. Measurements outside of tolerance limits indicate problems that must be corrected. In general, the developer temperature must be within ±1°F of the manufacturer's recommended value, density variations must not exceed ±0.1, and the fog level must not exceed 0.3. In addition to the early morning test, it may also prove worthwhile to process additional strips at other times during the day to detect any significant changes that may have occurred.

Basic Performance Characteristics of X-Ray Units

The following tests should be routinely performed (at least once yearly) in order to assure that the X-Ray equipment is functioning properly. This should be followed by corrective action and reexamination of those units that failed to meet the required standards. A log should be maintained on each X-Ray unit showing the date and results of quality assurance testing, as well as the date and nature of corrective measures taken. At more frequent intervals, comparison of a test film, exposed and developed under standard conditions, against a reference film will indicate machine problems, providing processing quality control is being performed on a daily basis.

Measurement of Output and Half-Value Layer

The radiation output of an X-Ray system may vary as a result of a failure of

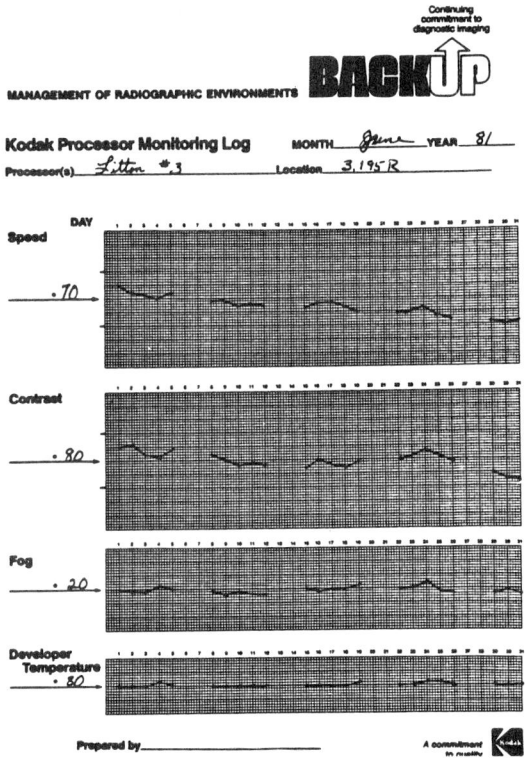

Figure 10-6. A processor monitoring log. Deterioration of processing chemistry results in a gradual decrease in recorded optical density.

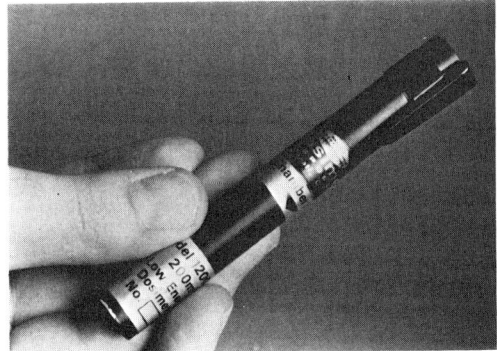

Figure 10-7. A pocket dosimeter for measuring radiation output.

electronic components, removal of a required filter, or drift from the manufacturer's X-Ray calibration values, as well as from other causes. Radiation output can be checked quickly and easily using a low-energy pocket dosimeter (Fig. 10-7). This type of dosimeter is a cylindrical device containing a simple optical system permitting the user to view the internally mounted quartz fiber that serves as a radiation indicator (Fig. 10-8). When the dosimeter is charged (the charger is purchased separately), the quartz fiber is electrostatically repelled away from the U-shaped frame on which it is mounted, since they both receive a positive charge (Fig. 10-9). As a result, the hairline image moves to the "zero" position as indicated on a scale consisting of a glass disk with calibrated graduations, typically from 0 to 200 mR. When X-Rays enter the sensi-

THE DOSIMETER

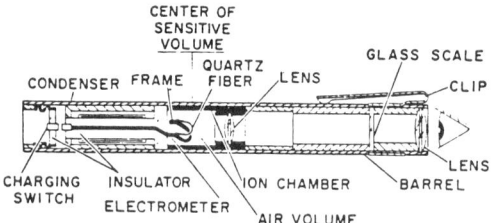

Figure 10-8. Schematic diagram of a pocket dosimeter.

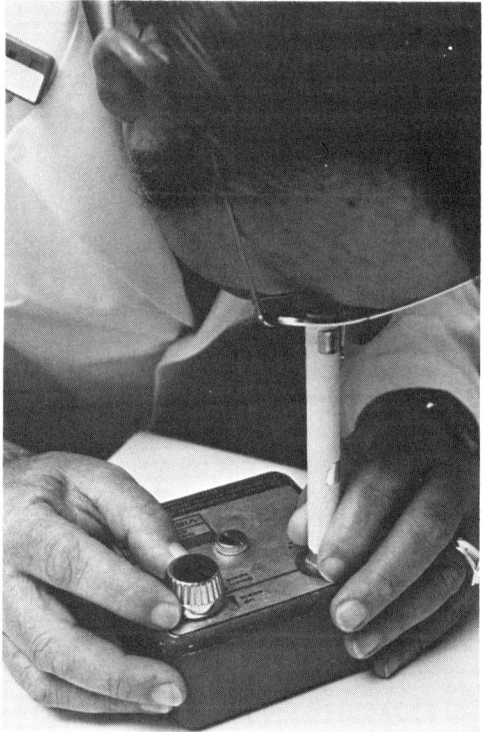

Figure 10-9. A pocket dosimeter being charged before use.

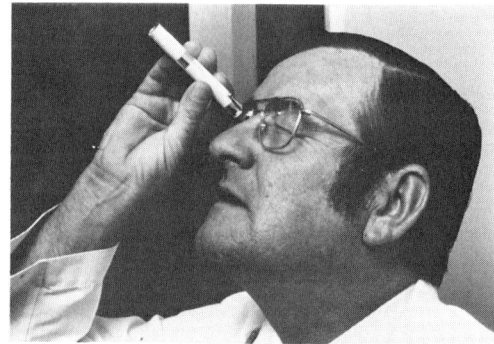

Figure 10-10. A pocket dosimeter being read after exposure.

tive volume of the detector, positive and negative ions are produced in the air surrounding the frame and the fiber. The negative ions (electrons) migrate to the positively charged central frame/fiber and the positive ions to the negatively charged wall of the chamber, discharging the chamber to some extent. As a result, the fiber moves toward its frame and, therefore, away from the zero position as viewed on the scale (Fig. 10-10).

Radiation output should be checked periodically, being careful to use a fixed and reproducible geometry. Always make the measurement in exactly the same way.

Table 10-I

Mean milliroentgens per milliampere-second at 12 inches by kilovolt peak and filtration categories for dental X-Ray units

Total filtration (millimeters of Al equivalent)	\multicolumn{9}{c}{Kilovolt peak}								
	50	55	60	65	70	75	80	85	90
0.5	91.11	96.03	101.44	107.59	114.73	123.10	132.94	144.49	158.00
1.0	58.38	63.32	68.54	74.27	80.75	88.24	96.98	107.20	119.15
1.5	36.61	41.64	46.72	52.09	57.99	64.66	72.35	81.30	91.75
2.0	23.26	28.45	33.45	38.52	43.89	49.81	56.52	64.25	73.27
2.5	15.79	21.19	26.19	31.01	35.92	41.14	46.93	53.52	61.16
3.0	11.65	17.33	22.37	27.02	31.52	36.12	41.04	46.55	52.88
3.5	8.30	14.32	19.47	24.01	28.17	32.19	36.32	40.80	45.88
4.0	3.19	9.61	14.94	19.43	23.30	26.82	30.21	33.73	37.62
4.5	-----	.67	6.24	10.73	14.39	17.46	20.18	22.80	25.56

Under normal circumstances, there should not be a variation of more than ±15 percent in the measured value. In making output measurements with a pocket dosimeter, it is a good idea to make three or four measurements and average the results. The values listed in Table 10-I provide an indication of the levels of radiation that will be measured for dental X-Ray units.

Determination of the half-value layer can be carried out easily using a pocket dosimeter. The half-value layer is the thickness of aluminum required to reduce the exposure of the X-Ray beam to one-half of its initial value. The half-value layer is a useful index of filtration of the X-Ray beam (Table 10-II). It is measured by inserting a series of aluminum filters into the beam and plotting the diminishing exposure measurements as a function of the thickness of aluminum intercepting the beam (Fig. 10-II).

Table 10-II

Half-value layers as a function of filtration and tube potential for diagnositc units

Total filter (mm Al)	Half-value layers (mm Al)				
	45 kVp	50 kVp	70 kVp	90 kVp	100 kVp
0.5	0.5	0.6	0.8	0.9	1.0
1.0	0.9	0.9	1.2	1.5	1.6
1.5	1.2	1.2	1.6	1.9	2.1
2.0		1.5	1.9	2.3	2.5
2.5		1.7	2.2	2.6	2.8

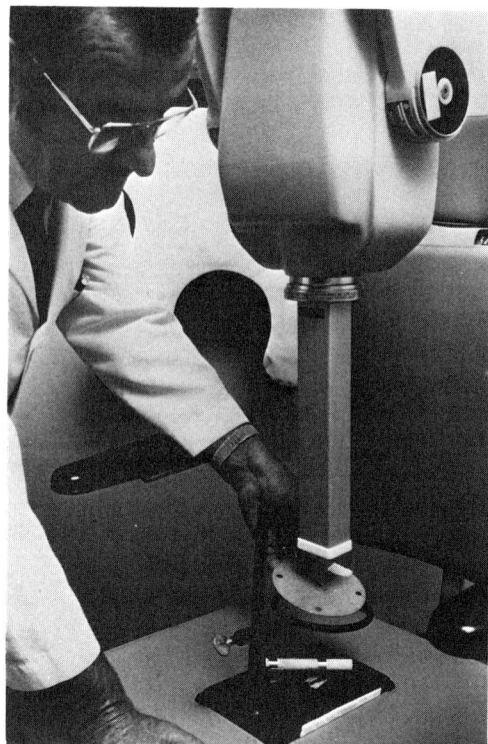

Figure 10-11. Procedure for measuring the half-value layer of an x-ray beam.

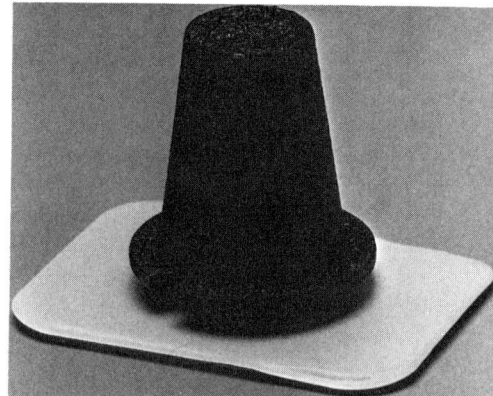

Figure 10-12. A spinning top for measuring exposure time.

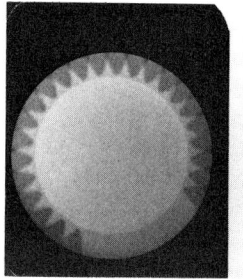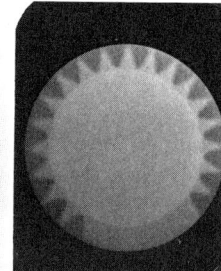

Figure 10-13. Images exposed using a spinning top. The film on the left was exposed using twenty-four impulses, while the film on the right was exposed using nineteen impulses.

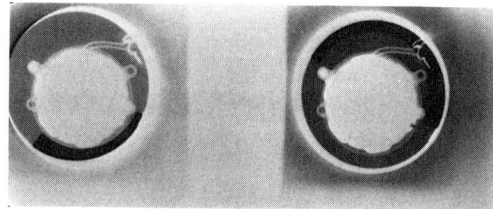

Figure 10-14. A radiograph of a mechanical spinning top exposed using a constant potential dental X-Ray unit.

Determination of Exposure Time

The accuracy and precision of the timer on diagnostic X-Ray equipment is important since exposure time directly influences the mAs and therefore the quantity of radiation produced. Unsatisfactory timer reproducibility may lead to erratic radiographic results, which may be erroneously attributed to other causes. A well-known and simple method for testing exposure time involves the use of a spinning top consisting of a metal disk containing a single hole or slit (Fig. 10-12). If the top is radiographed while it is spinning, the resulting radiograph will show a distinct black spot for each pulse of the X-Ray unit. The spacing of the black spots will depend on the waveform and rectification of the X-Ray tube. A single phase X-Ray generator with full wave rectification will give rise to a black spot for every

1/120 second pulse of the X-Ray unit, while a self-rectified dental unit will produce a black spot each 1/60 second. The number of spots can then be used to determine the "on" time of the X-Ray generator, which can then be compared to the value set on the timer (Fig. 10-13). Timers for constant potential X-Ray units are measured using a motor-driven top that rotates at a known speed. The resulting radiograph shows a continuously exposed arc (Fig. 10-14). The angle subtended by this arc is proportional to the exposure time. For example, if the top is rotating at 1 revolution (360 degrees) per second, then an exposure time of 0.25 second will result in an angle of 90 degrees. If the angle is measured using a protractor, the exposure time can be calculated using the expression:

$$\text{measured exposure time (sec)} = \frac{\text{measured angle}}{360 \cdot \text{rev./sec}}$$

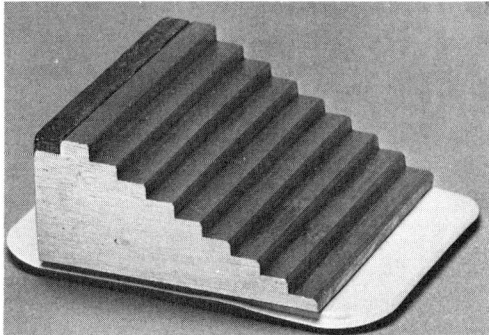

Figure 10-15. An aluminum stepwedge for checking mAs reciprocity.

The following criteria are recommended by the American Association of Physicists in Medicine (AAPM) (1978) for the evaluation of timers:

Timer Range	Acceptable Range
0-1/4 sec	± 1 pulse
1/4-1/2 sec	± 2 pulses
longer than 1/2 sec	± 5% of set time

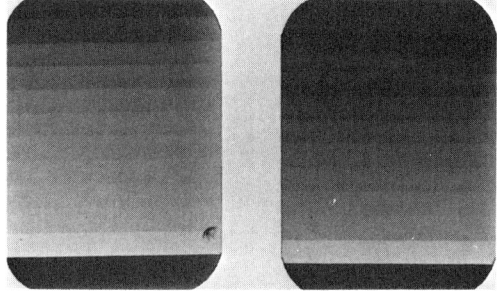

Figure 10-16. Radiographs exposed to check mAs reciprocity. The radiograph on the left was exposed using 10 mA and 15 impulses while the one on the right was exposed using 15 mA and 10 impulses. The test results indicate that at least one of the mA settings is out of calibration.

Evaluation of mA Calibration

The other factor involved in setting the desired mAs is tube current or milliamperage (mA). Variation in this factor will have the same effect on the final radiograph as variation in exposure time. If the preceding exposure time test has been performed so that one accurately knows the "on" time of the X-Ray unit at the various timer settings, it is possible to detect variations in tube current. To do this, an appropriate step wedge (Fig. 10-15) is radiographed using different mA settings but with the timer set in such a way as to give the same mAs. If the mA is set properly, the radiograph images of the step wedge should be identical. If this is not the case, one or both of the mA settings may be out of calibration (Fig. 10-16). Tube current cannot be checked in this way for dental units that have a single, fixed value of milliamperage. In units of this type, variations in tube current may be seen in altered exposure values as measured using a pocket dosimeter as described previously. If the timer settings and kVp are satisfactory, such alterations may indicate that the tube current is out of calibration.

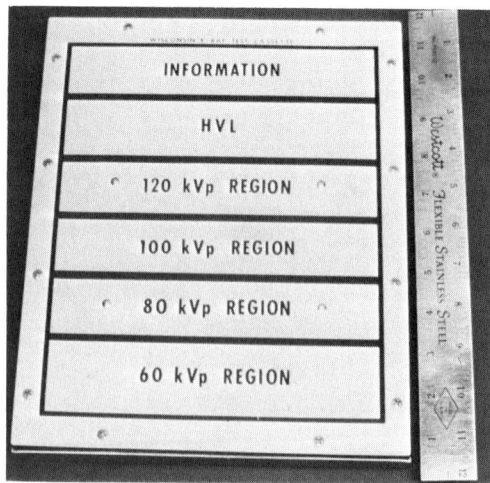

Figure 10-17. A Wisconsin Test Cassette for determining kVp.

TEST CASSETTE DESIGN

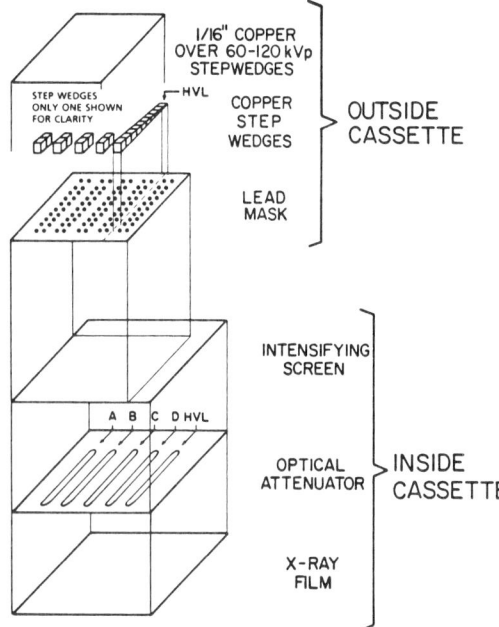

Figure 10-18. Schematic diagram showing the design of the Wisconsin Test Cassette.

Determination of Operating Peak Kilovoltage (kVp)

The X-Ray tube kVp is a very critical

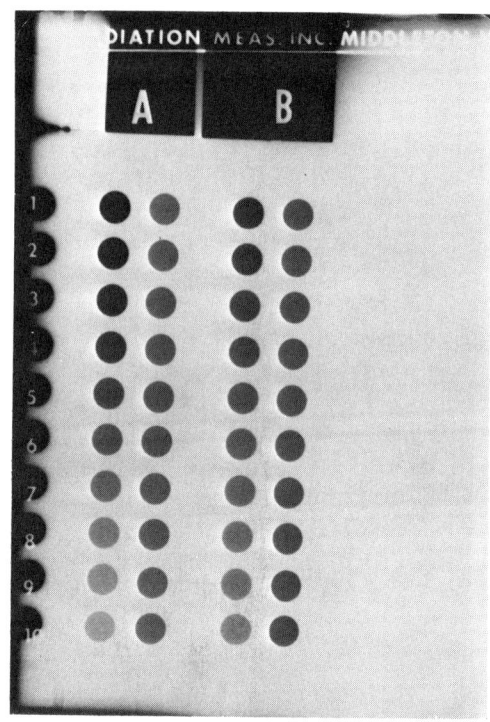

Figure 10-19. A film exposed using the Wisconsin Test Cassette.

factor, since a small error in its value will have a more dramatic effect on the final X-Ray image than a comparable variation of any of the other factors (such as mA or exposure time). A convenient method for measuring kVp involves the use of a modified form of the test cassette described by Ardran and Crooks (Fig. 10-17). Test cassettes of this type are commercially available from a number of suppliers.

The components of a kVp test cassette are shown in Figure 10-18. The X-Ray beam first passes through a copper filter, which reduces the fraction of low energy photons present in the beam. The beam then passes through two rows of holes in a lead mask and impinges on an intensifying screen. The light from the intensifying screen then exposes the test film. A copper step wedge is placed in front of one row of holes while an optical filter, which reduces the light emitted by the screen by a factor of 3 before it strikes the test film, is placed behind the screen of the other row. A comparison of optical densities corresponding to the consecutive pairs of holes (Fig. 10-19) allows one to determine the copper third-value layer of the beam (the thickness of copper that reduces the intensity of the beam by a factor of 3). This quantity, which increases as a near-linear function of kVp, can then be used to estimate the peak kilovoltage with a high degree of accuracy. A calibration chart is provided by the manufacturer for each cassette (Fig. 10-20). For example, the nearest match in optical densities of the test radiograph shown in Figure 10-19 occurs at step 6. Referring to Figure 10-20, it will be noted that a match at step 6 corresponds to a peak kilovoltage slightly greater than 60 kV.

Verification of Focal Spot Size

An alteration in focal spot size from its accustomed value can indicate the deterioration of the X-Ray tube. Focal spot size can be checked with relative ease by using a test object containing a number of bar patterns (Fig. 10-21). The American Asssociation of Physicists in Medicine paper on quality assurance (1978) recommends the use of a set of slots in a metal mask ranging from 0.6 to 3.35 line pairs/mm or more. Perpendicular sets of bars at

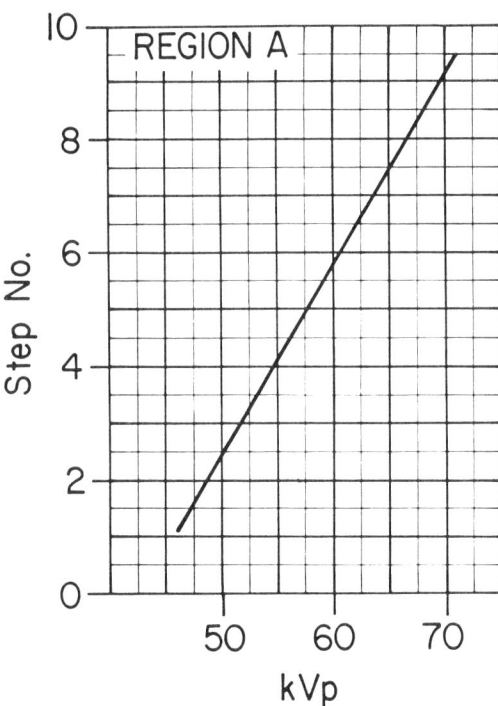

Figure 10-20. Calibration chart for a Wisconsin Test Cassette. The step where the densities match is plotted versus kVp.

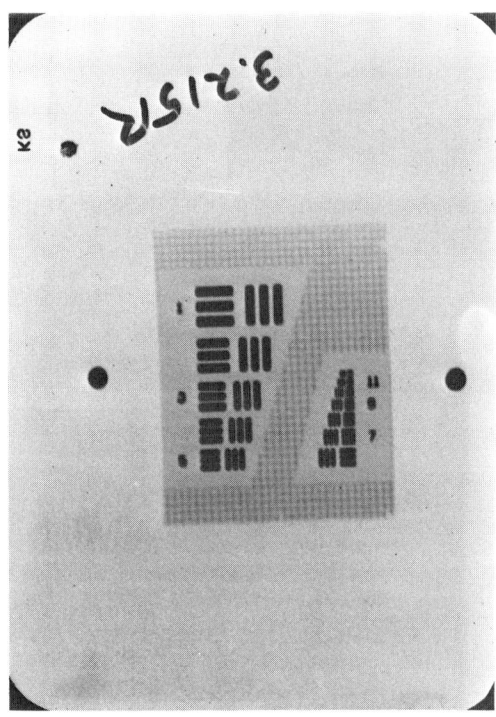

Figure 10-21. Test film exposed using the test pattern for measuring focal spot size.

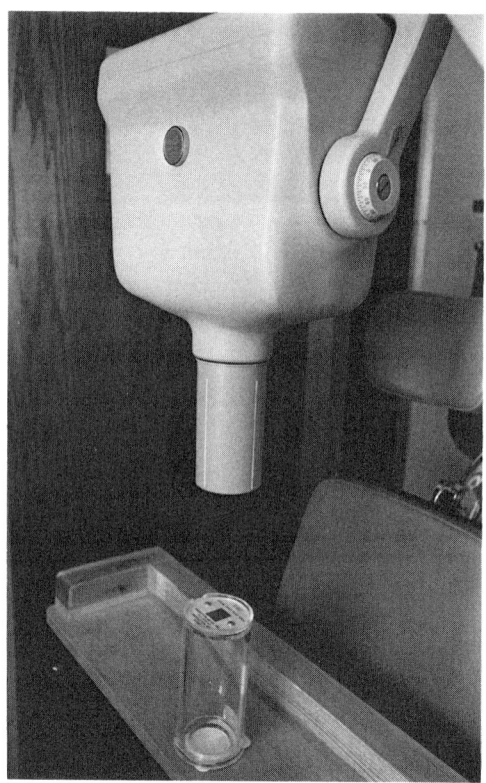

Figure 10-22. Test arrangement for measuring focal spot size.

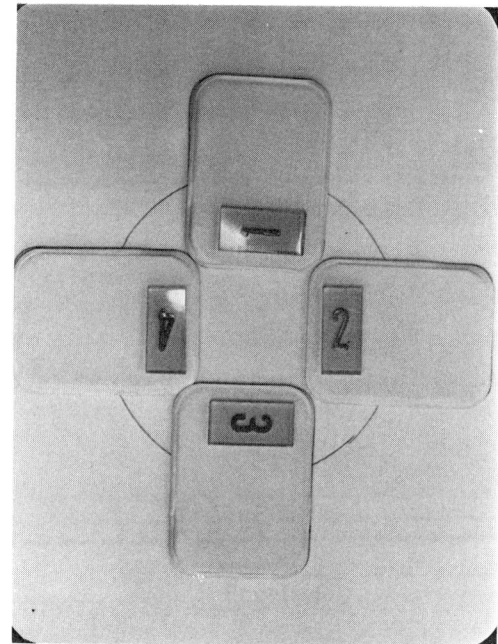

Figure 10-23. Arrangements of films for testing beam alignment.

Table 10-III

Determination of focal spot size from resoluting pattern

	Group (lp/mm)	Nominal Focal Spot Size (mm)	
1.	0.6	2.0	(or smaller)
2.	0.7	2.0	"
3.	0.85	2.0	"
4.	1.0	2.0	"
5.	1.15	1.8	"
6.	1.4	1.5	"
7.	1.7	1.3	"
8.	2.0	1.0	"
9.	2.5	0.8	"
10.	2.8	0.6	"
11.	3.35	0.5	"

each spacing are used to measure resolution (fine detail) parallel and perpendicular to the anode-cathode axis of the X-Ray tube. The bar pattern is radiographed using nonscreen film at a target-to-object distance of 18 inches and object-to-film distance of 6 inches (Fig. 10-22). Resolution (ability to separate images of small objects placed close together) can then be related to focal spot size using Table 10-III. Test devices conforming to these specifications are available from a number of suppliers.

Verification of Beam Alignment

It is important that the X-Ray field be approximately congruent (same shape and size) with the directing cone and that the useful beam be restricted to a diameter of 2.75 inches when measured at the end of the cone (*see* Chapter 6). This can be verified by radiographing four No. 2 dental films placed on a piece of paper in the form of a cross (Fig. 10-23). The position indicating device and the location of

Quality Assurance

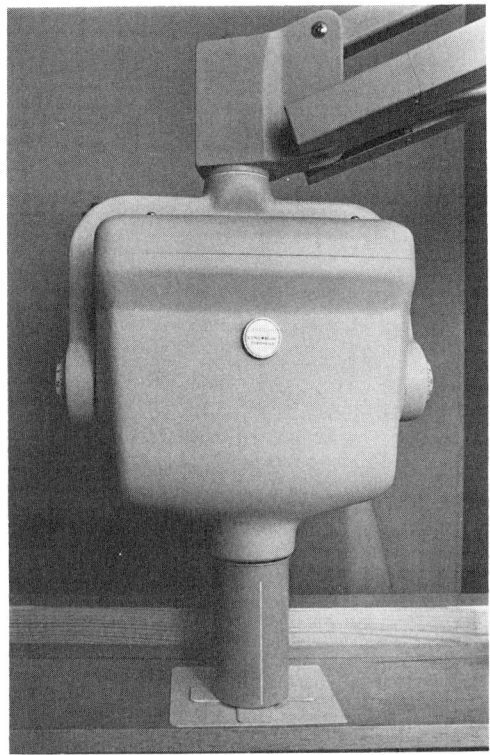

Figure 10-24. Arrangement of equipment and film for testing beam alignment.

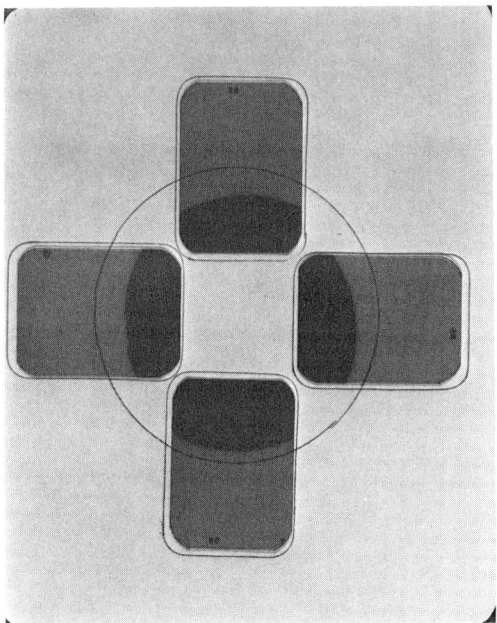

Figure 10-25. The location of the X-Ray field within the position indicating device.

Figure 10-26. Test radiograph showing light leaks in a defective cassette.

each film should be traced on the paper and the films should be identified with numbers so each can be returned to its proper place after exposure. The tube is positioned to cover approximately half of each film packet, touching the packets (Fig. 10-24). The films are exposed using one-half of the maxillary anterior exposure, processed, and returned to the paper in proper order (Fig. 10-25). If the exposed area is greater than 2.75 inches in diameter, the lead collimator opening is too large and should be replaced. If the exposed area is obviously out of alignment with the circumference of the cone, the collimator or the X-Ray focal spot may be malpositioned and the problem should be brought to the attention of service personnel.

Cassettes

Warped cassettes, fatigue of foam or felt compression material, worn closures, dirt, light leaks, etc., frequently produce unsharp or fogged radiographs to the

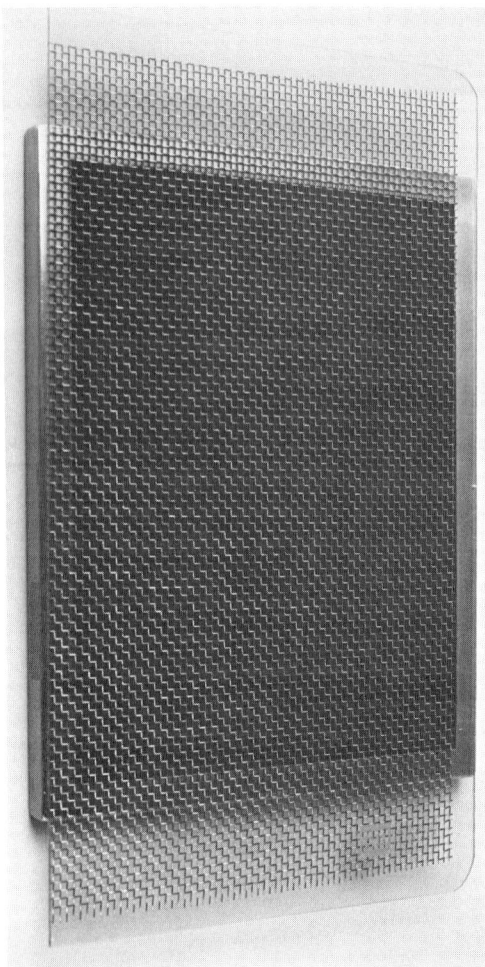

Figure 10-27. Wire mesh used for checking screen-film contact.

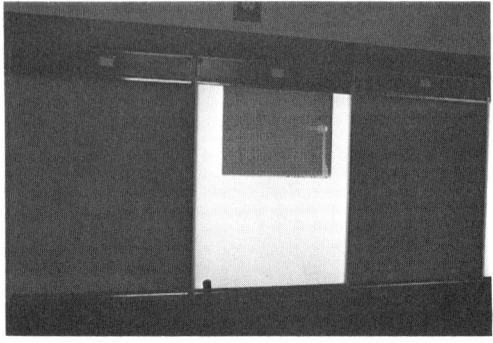

Figure 10-28. Radiograph of wire mesh for checking screen-film contact.

point where the cassettes or screens should be replaced (Fig. 10-26). Screens should be periodically inspected for worn areas, stained areas, or yellowing due to age. At this time, screens should be cleaned and treated with antistatic solution (commercially available). Before acceptance of new cassettes, and periodically thereafter, film/screen contact should be tested using a piece of 1/4 inch galvanized wire mesh (Fig. 10-27) exposed for a background density of about 1.0 (*see* Chapter 3 for explanation of density). Mesh test films (Fig. 10-28) are viewed from a distance of 6-8 feet and inspected for dark areas containing blurred images of the wire mesh. Cassettes showing poor contact involving large area should be designated for replacement.

View Boxes

The conditions under which a dentist views radiographs may influence diagnostic accuracy and stamina. Viewing conditions include the brightness of the illuminators as well as the ambient room light level. Testing should be accomplished by surveying the brightness and color of all illuminators in a given area by visual means and, when necessary, using a photographic light meter to compare relative illuminator brightness in different viewing areas. Illuminator opal glass fronts should be cleaned regularly and illuminator fluorescent tubes showing blackening at the ends should be replaced.

Darkroom

In addition to processing procedures and chemistry, the effective operation of a darkroom depends on correct safelighting procedures and adequate lighttightness of the room. For this reason, the darkroom should be periodically checked for lighttightness and proper safelighting. Safelights should be "safe" for the films that are to be processed (intraoral or extraoral). A 15 watt bulb at 48 inches from working area (where film is unwrapped) is considered optimal. The safelight should be visually inspected for cracks in the filter, proper bulb size, and white light leaks. To insure that the safelighting is safe, a dental film should be unwrapped and placed on the working surface with a radiopaque object (coin, number, etc.) on top. After five minutes (maximum time to unwrap a CMX) the film should be processed in the normal manner and examined. If an image is visible, the light is not safe and should be replaced or repaired. It is also important to pay attention to the spectral characteristics of the safelight as discussed in Chapter 8.

General Condition of the Facility

In addition to these specific items, the general condition of the facility should be checked. The following list, extracted from the AAPM Quality Assurance protocol (1978) contains some of the most important of the common sense items that should be checked:

Mechanical integrity. A general observation of the diagnostic system should be made. Key items to look for are the presence of loose or absent hardware that may have been improperly installed or worked loose due to use. The functioning of meters, dials, pilot lights, and other indicators should be checked.

Mechanical stability. To obtain a diagnostic quality radiograph, it is important to minimize relative patient motion. Of key importance from the equipment side is the stability of the X-Ray tube hanger.

Electrical safety. The electrical safety of the system should be checked. Key areas include power cords, the wires to the exposure hand switch, cables to the tube head, and the proper grounding of all components.

Record Keeping

In carrying out a quality assurance program, it is necessary to do a certain amount of record keeping. A daily log of retakes is a useful way to identify problem areas that need attention. Important information that should be recorded includes date, operator, reason for retake, and corrective action. Using this log, repeated errors can be identified and systems corrected or technicians given added instruction (i.e. technician instructed on improving film placement when projecting a mandibular premolar radiograph).

An individual room log should be maintained for each X-Ray unit. This room log should be conveniently located so that it is available to all personnel involved (dentists, auxilliaries, equipment service personnel, etc.). The room log should contain the following information:

1. Equipment data
   a. Identification of major components
      (1) Manufacturer
      (2) Model number
      (3) Serial number
      (4) Date installed
   b. Technical specifications (such as pulsating or constant potential, focal spot size, mA and kVp settings, etc.)
   c. Tube heat loading charts
   d. Equipment operating instructions
2. An outline of the quality assurance program
3. A log of quality assurance tests
   a. Specific test performed
   b. Date performed
   c. Test results
   d. Individual performing test
4. A log of all service work
   a. Malfunction
   b. Service performed
   c. Date of service
   d. Individual performing service

Benefits of Quality Assurance

The need for quality assurance in dental radiology is illustrated by the results of

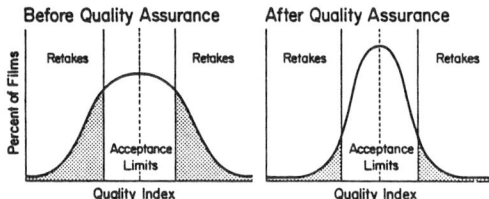

Figure 10-29. Diagram illustrating the benefits of a quality assurance program.

a study of preauthorization dental radiographs submitted to Pennsylvania Blue Shield (Biedeman et al., 1976). This study showed that more than 50 percent of the films submitted were inadequate for determining the efficacy of the proposed treatment. A more detailed follow-up study showed that 20 percent of the radiographs were unsatisfactory for reasons most likely related to poor equipment performance. Since the primary objective of quality assurance is to reduce this kind of problem, it is apparent that the institution of effective quality assurance programs should be an important factor in improving the performance of dental radiology facilities. The effect of quality assurance may be illustrated using a conceptual model described by Goldman (1977). Goldman suggested that if values of a hypothetical "index" of quality were plotted as a function of their frequency of occurrence, the result would be a bell-shaped curve (Fig. 10-29), which ideally would have its peak at some "optimum" value. At either extreme there are limits of acceptability. Beyond these limits, films are rejected and must be repeated. The effect of quality assurance is to reduce the variability in radiographic quality and therefore to narrow the width of the bell-shaped curve. As a result, the distribution will fall more completely within the acceptance band. The number of retakes is decreased and the average deviation from optimal quality of the accepted radiographs will decrease.

The implementation of quality assurance programs should lead to improved diagnostic performance as well as a substantial savings in cost since every retake is an additional expense and wastes valuable time. Such programs have been shown to lower the level of radiation to which the patient is exposed by decreasing the number of retakes and by preventing overexposure of the patient in an attempt to compensate for processing deficiencies. With these benefits in mind, the Food and Drug Administration's Bureau of Radiological Health has recommended quality assurance programs for all diagnostic radiology facilities (1979).

Bibliography

American Association of Physicists in Medicine: *Basic Quality Control in Diagnostic Radiology*, AAPM Report No. 3. AAPM, 1978.

Beideman, R.W.; Johnson, O.N.; and Alcox, R.W.: A study to develop a rating system and evaluate dental radiographs submitted to a third party carrier. *J Am Dent Assoc,* 93:1010-1013, 1976.

Bureau of Radiological Health: *Diagnostic Radiology Quality Assurance Catalog,* HEW Publ FDA 77-8028. Rockville, MD, US Dept HEW, July 1977.

Bureau of Radiological Health: *Radiological Health Handbook.* Washington, DC, US Government Printing Office, 1970, p. 158.

Bureau of Radiological Health: Quality assurance programs for diagnostic radiology facilities, final recommendations. *Federal Register,* 44:71728-78740, 1979.

Burkhart, R.L.: A proposed recommendation for quality assurance programs in diagnostic radiology facilities. In Society of Photo-Optical Instrumentation Engineers: *Optical Instrumentation in Medicine VI.* Bellingham WA, Photo-Optical, 1977, pp. 266-170.

Goldman, L.W.: Effects of film processing variability on patient dose and image quality. In *Second Image Receptor Conference: Radiographic Film Processing* (Proceedings of a conference held in Washington, D.C., March 31-April 2, 1977). Washington, DC, US Government Printing Office, 1977, pp. 55-63.

Gould, R.G.; and Gratt, B.M.: A radiographic quality control system for the dental office. *Dentomaxillofac Radiol,* 11:123-127, 1982.

National Council on Radiation Protection and Measurements: *Dental X-Ray Protection,* NCRP Report No. 35, Washington, DC. NCRP Publications, 1970, p. 35.

Chapter 11

PRINCIPLES OF INTERPRETATION OF PATHOLOGIC CONDITIONS

VIEWING THE RADIOGRAPH

IN order to obtain the greatest amount of information from radiographs, the following principles should be observed when viewing them:

1. Interpret only from properly exposed and processed radiographs.
2. Use multiple views, when these are required to fully demonstrate all of the radiographic features.
3. View the radiographs in a quiet area with subdued lighting.
4. The viewbox should provide a uniform degree of light. A variable intensity light should be available for viewing darker radiographs.
5. All extraneous light should be blocked out from around the edges of the film on the viewbox.
6. Use a good magnifying glass.
7. Restrict the size of the viewing field.
8. Obtain supplemental studies when the standard views fail to illustrate completely the structure being studied. Some supplemental studies include arthrography, tomography, sialography, barium swallow, xeroradiography, nuclear scans, C.A.T. scans, and N.M.R. images.

Radiographic interpretation is a subjective skill. For example, in respect to caries, one might expect the interpretation of this condition to be relatively straightforward. In a study conducted by the authors, several sets of bite-wing radiographs were displayed for interpretation by faculty teaching operative dentistry, general practice, oral diagnosis, and radiology. Their radiographic findings were reported on a standardized form. After studying the data it was found that there was very little agreement among the approximately thirty participating faculty as to the size of the carious lesions, their depth into dentin, and their proximity to the pulp. Indeed, for several surfaces, some faculty could identify no carious lesions, while the same surfaces were reported to have deep caries involvement approaching the pulp by other faculty. In spite of the previous statement, the one conclusion that could be drawn from this study is that the greatest area of agreement was regarding the presence or absence of disease, while the greatest disagreement occurred over the degree of disease present.

The primary objective of radiographic interpretation is to identify the presence or absence of disease, based upon a previous physical examination of the patient. Radiographs are best studied when appropriate viewing conditions are provided. Once an abnormality has been identified on the radiograph, further information as to the nature and degree of disease will depend to a great deal upon the experience and skill of the person interpreting the radiograph. The authors have included the following concepts in order to further enhance the dentist's skill in radiographic interpretation of bony conditions as they affect the jaws.

IDENTIFICATION OF THE BASIC RADIOGRAPHIC PATTERN

In another publication, the authors have described and illustrated all the conditions about to be named. Their classification of the basic radiographic patterns is based upon the classic presentation of a disease in its mature form. The classification is limited primarily to diseases as they present in the jaws; note the conditions that may be suspected in association with each pattern.

Radiolucent Lesions

Periocoronal Radiolucencies

do not tend to contain radiopaque flecks
Normal follicular space (Fig. 11-23)
Osteitis associated with pericoronitis
Dentigerous cyst (Fig. 11-23)
Ameloblastic fibroma

may contain radiopaque flecks
Ameloblastic fibroodontoma
Adenomatoid odontogenic tumor
Calcifying epithelial odontogenic tumor
Keratinizing and calcifying odontogenic cyst

Radiolucencies with Distinct Borders

Variations in trabecular patterns and marrow spaces
Early stage tooth crypts
Postextraction socket (Fig. 11-2)
Focal osteoporotic bone marrow defect of the jaws
Fibrous healing defect (Fig. 11-4)
Developmental lingual mandibular salivary gland depression (Fig. 11-14).
Primordial cyst
Lateral periodontal cyst
Incisive canal cyst
Median palatal cyst
Globulomaxillary cyst
Median mandibular cyst
Residual cyst
Traumatic cyst (Figs. 11-2, 11-30)
Neuroma, neurofibroma, neurilemoma

Multilocular Radiolucencies

Odontogenic keratocyst
Ameloblastoma (Figs. 11-3, 11-13)
Central giant cell granuloma (Figs. 11-29, 11-30)
Cherubism
Odontogenic myxoma
Aneurismal bone cyst
Central hemangioma and vascular lesions

Radiolucencies with Indistinct or Ragged Borders

Osteomyelitis (Fig. 11-15)
Osteoradionecrosis
Primary intraalveolar carcinoma
Metastatic disease (Fig. 11-5)
Histiocytosis-X group
Multiple myeloma

Lymphosarcoma
Fibrosarcoma
Burkitt's lymphoma
Histiocytic lymphoma
Ewing's sarcoma

Radiopaque Lesions

Periapical Radiopacities

Idiopathic osteosclerosis
Condensing osteitis
Hypercementosis (Fig. 11-27)
Periapical cemental dysplasia (Fig. 11-28)
Benign cementoblastoma (Fig. 11-26)
Benign osteoblastoma
Central cemento-ossifying fibroma (Fig. 11-9)

Separate Single or Multiple Radiopacities

Radiopacities associated with the jaws
Exostosis
Enostosis
Osteosclerosis
Osteoma
Chondrosarcoma
Osteosarcoma
Foreign bodies
Root fragments
Odontoma (Fig. 11-24)
Ameloblastic odontoma
Garrés osteomyelitis (Fig 11-11)

Radiopacities outside the jaws
Rhinoliths, antroliths, sialoliths
Soft tissue calcifications
Eagle's syndrome (Fig. 11-10)

Generalized or Diffuse Radiopacities Involving One or More Quadrants

Chronic diffuse sclerosing osteomyelitis
Fibrous dysplasia
Osteopetrosis
Paget's disease of bone
Hyperparathyroidism (Fig. 11-20)
Dominant craniometaphyseal dysplasia

Van Buchem's disease

Once the basic radiographic pattern has been identified or classified, a variety or other changes may be seen in association with this basic pattern. For example, is there a well-corticated peripheral outline? Are there dimensional changes, such as expansion? Is the outer cortex affected? What is the involvement of erupted or unerupted teeth? In the remainder of this chapter, these questions will be outlined and discussed with respect to an overview of radiographic interpretation.

Nature of the Peripheral Outline

CORTICATED: Smooth
               Irregular
                 scalloped
                 (wavy)
                 multilocular
NONCORTICATED: Punched-out
               Indistinct

When the peripheral outline is corticated, a slow, benign process may be suspected, although one notable exception to this is the chondrosarcoma. Some examples of conditions with well-corticated outlines are most types of cysts (Fig. 11-1)

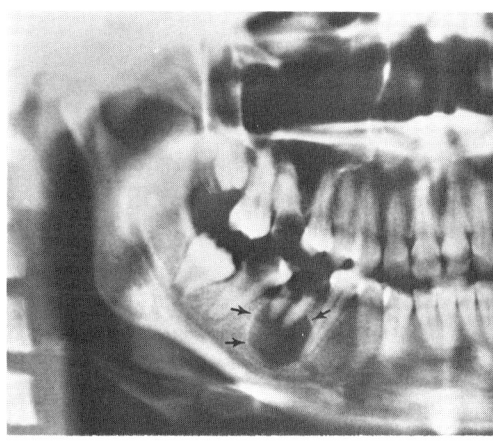

Figure 11-1. Smooth Corticated Outline: This is an example of a periapical cyst.

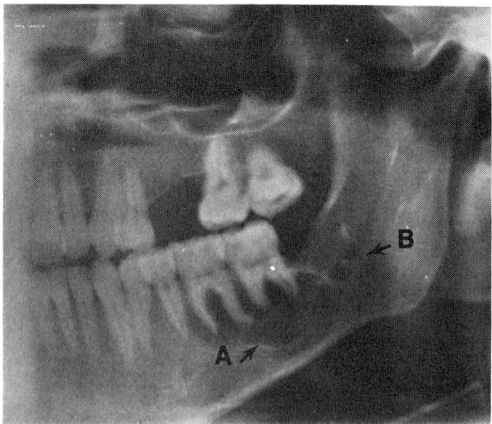

Figure 11-2. Irregular Corticated Outline: The irregularity of the cortical outline is provided by the superior portion of this traumatic cyst (arrowA), and by the adjacent lamina dura outlining a recent extraction socket (arrow B). (Courtesy of Dr. Guss Pappas, Columbus, Ohio).

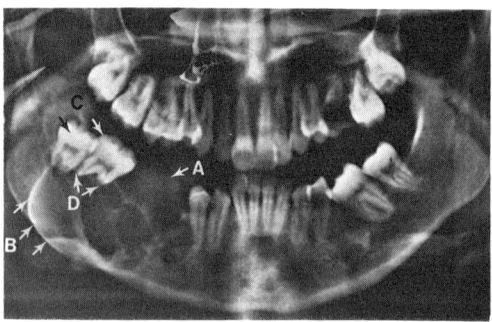

Figure 11-3. Multilocular Corticated Outline:This ameloblastoma also demonstrates the following features: **(A)** perforation with herniation of soft tissue material; **(B)** expansion; **(C)** tooth displacement; **(D)** root resoprtion. (Courtesy of Dr. Gus Pappas, Columbus, Ohio.)

and some benign central neoplasms. When the corticated outline is scalloped or wavy, an odontogenic keratocyst or a traumatic cyst (Fig. 11-2) may be suspected, while a variety of lesions will produce a multilocular outline (Fig. 11-3).

When a radiolucent lesion is described as punched-out, it remains well defined but without a distinct peripheral cortical outline. Several classic punched-out radiolucencies include fibrous healing defect (Fig. 11-4), salivary gland depressions, particularly the anterior

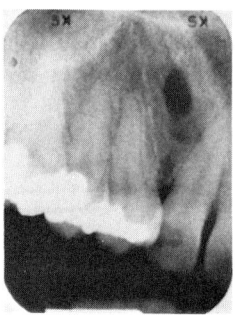

Figure 11-4. Punched-out Noncorticated Outline: This fibrous healing defect occurred as a sequel to the surgical extraction of the impacted cuspid.

type, eosinophilic granuloma, and multiple myeloma. When the peripheral outline is indistinct or ragged, osteomyelitis or osteoradionecrosis may be suspected. However, an indistinct peripheral border to any lesion is a hallmark of malignancy (Fig. 11-5) and a high level of suspicion

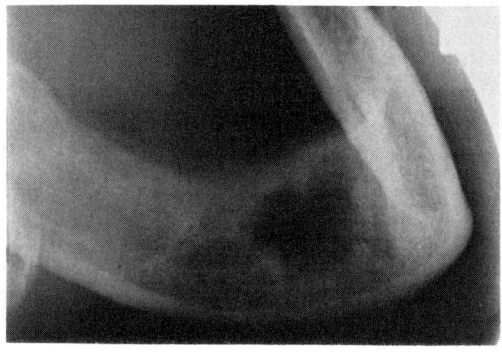

Figure 11-5. Indistinct Noncorticated Outline: This lesion was a metastatic adenocarcinoma of the breast in a fifty-two-year-old female. Nonpainful, rubbery, matted submandibular nodes were present. The breast had been removed three months prior to the discovery of this lesion.

should be maintained until such a possibility has been confirmed or ruled out by further diagnostic studies such as biopsy.

Dimensional Changes

DECREASES IN SIZE: Overall
                     Focal
INCREASES IN SIZE: Expansion
                     Other
                       causes
                         overall
                         focal

A dimensional change implies an increase or decrease in size of a portion or of the whole of the structure being studied. Overall decreases in size may be seen in hypoplsia, which is developmental in natue (Fig. 11-6) or is due to some acquired defect such as seen in radiation stunting or alveolar resorption following extraction of all of the teeth (Fig. 11-7).

A focal decrease in size of the condyle may occur as a result of a variety of joint diseases, while other examples of focal decreases in size include alveolar resorption

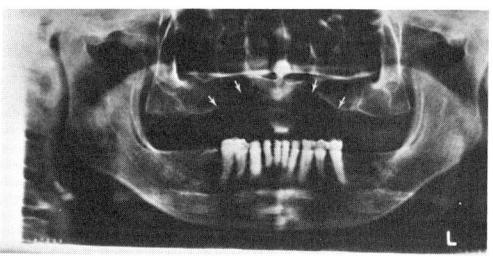

Figure 11-7. Focal Decrease in Size: In this case there is a focal resorption of the anterior maxillary alveolar ridge due to the excessive trauma produced by the remaining mandibular natural teeth. Note that there is no corresponding resorption of the maxillary posterior ridge since the mandibular poserior teeth were never replaced.

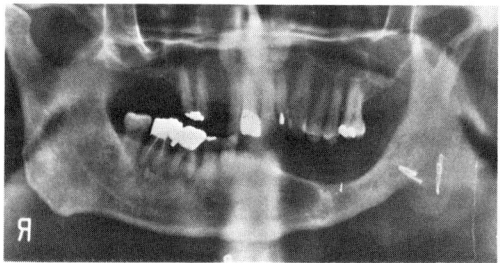

Figure 11-6. Overall Decrease in Size: This is a case of hemiatrophy in which cosmetic soft tissue implants have been placed to improve facial symmetry.

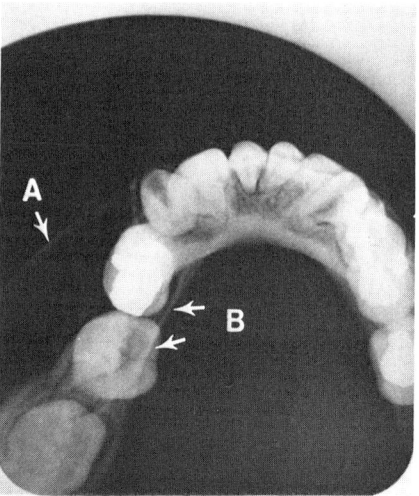

Figure 11-8. Expansion: This was due to a dentigerous cyst associated with the unerupted second bicuspid in this twelve-year-old female. In this case there is a marked expansion and thinning of the buccal cortical plate (arrow A), and a slight expansion of the lingual cortical plate (arrow B). (Courtesy of Dr. Dale A. Miles, Dalhousie University, Halifax, N.S.)

due to tooth extraction; resorption of the coronoid process, condyle, or ramus due to scleroderma; and resorption of the ramus due to fibrosis following radiation therapy.

Expansion is a term used to characterize a localized bulging-out of the cortex, rather than actual cortical growth. Expansion occurs usually as a result of a resorption and remodeling process in which the bone is attempting to contain a lesion.

Expansion tends to be a benign feature, but it is not present in all benign conditions. Expansion is a feature of more active or locally destructive benign processes (Fig. 11-8). Most of the multilocular lesions are also expansile and most cysts may eventually cause expansion. Expansion is a highly characteristic feature of the central cemento-ossifying fibroma, particularly of the inferior border of the mandible in the standard view (Fig. 11-9).

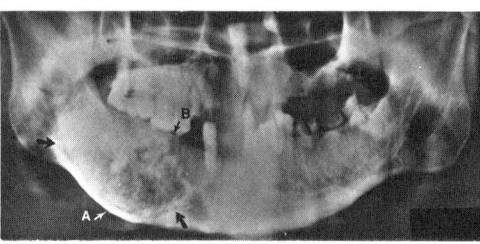

Figure 11-9. Expansion: Note that this central ossifying fibroma is a radiopaque lesion. In a comparison of the right and left sides, the viewer will note expansion of the interior cortex of the mandible (arrow A), and expansion of the crestal portion of the alveolar ridge (arrow B). (Courtesy of Dr. Gus Pappas, Columbus Ohio.)

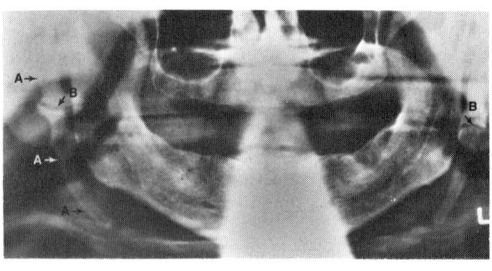

Figure 11-10. Generalized Increase in Size: This fifty-six-year-old male patient has symptomatic elongated styloid processes (Arrows A). This condition is known as Eagle's syndrome. This presentation has been classified as type-2 or pseudoarticulated (Arrows B). (Courtesy of Dr. Dale A. Miles, Dalhousie University, Halifax, N.S.)

Bones may also demonstrate a generalized increase in size in association with conditions such as Paget disease, acromegaly, dominant craniometaphyseal dysplasia, hypertrophy, van Buchem's disease, and Eagle's syndrome (Fig. 11-10). Localized increases in size may occur at the angle of the mandible in association with masseter hypertrophy or at the mandibular condyle as a result of a hypertrophic response to inflammation.

Alterations of the Outer Cortex

CORTICAL ENLARGEMENT: Periosteal reactions
Cortical proliferation

CORITCAL LOSS: Perforation
Cupped-out areas
Cortical destruction

The outer cortex of the jaws consists of dense compact bone. When viewed in the standard radiograph, it not only provides the radiopaque outline of the peripheral margins of the bone but also the "trabecular pattern." The loose spongy bone between the cortical plates does not contribute to the radiographic image. For example, if a radiolucency is noted in the mandible, then destruction of the inner or outer cortical plate has occurred. If there is an alteration of the trabecular pattern, then the change has occurred within the cortical bone.

Cortical enlargement may occur in association with subperiosteal deposition of new bone. This new bone tends to be deposited in layers and may occur as a result of inflammation as in Garré's osteomyelitis (Fig. 11-11) or as a result of proliferation in a malignant process such as osteosarcoma, chondrosarcoma, and

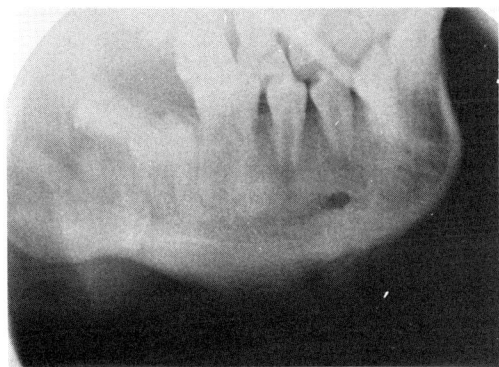

Figure 11-11. Periosteal Reaction: Note the laminations of superiosteal new bone in this case of Garré's osteomyelitis. Clinically, the facial swelling is "bony-hard" to palpation, and there is a loss of depth to the mucobuccal fold. (Courtesy of Dr. Chris Nortjé, University of Stellenbosch, Tygerberg, South Africa.)

Ewing's sarcoma. Localized proliferations of the cortex may be seen in exostoses, tori (Fig. 11-12), osteomas, and enostoses, while generalized cortical proliferation is seen in osteopetrosis and, classically, in van Buchem's disease.

Cortical loss may occur as a result of perforation by a lesion. Perforation of the cortex may be especially seen in association with expansion and is one of the characteristics of the larger odontogenic keratocysts and ameloblastomas (Fig. 11-13). Perforation without expansion may occur as a result of inflammation such as in a fistulous tract; however, perforation without expansion is an ominous sign characteristic of many malignant processes all associated with this feature.

Cupped-out areas are localized defects and may have a variety of interpretations depending upon the location. Cupped-out depressions at the crest of the alveolar ridge are an ominous finding and a high level of suspicion should be maintained until malignancy can be ruled out. Probably the most common cause of a cupped-

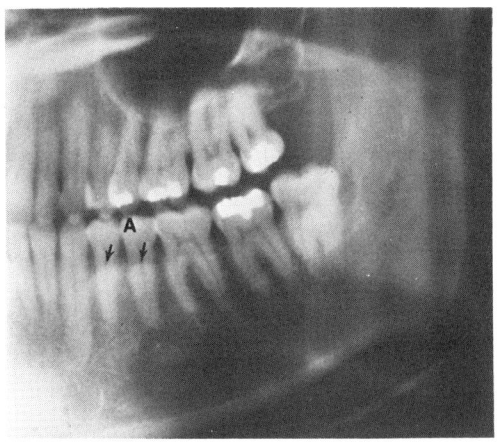

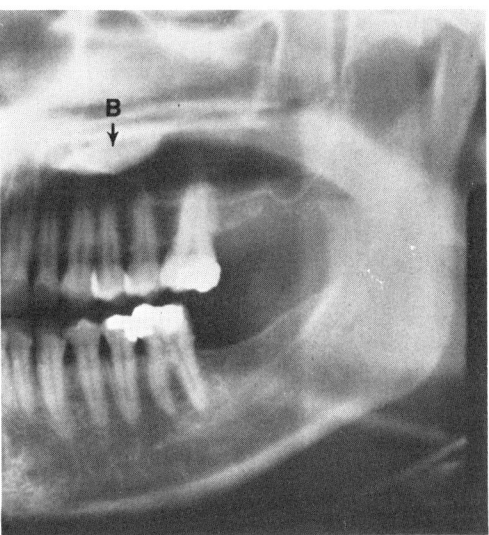

Figure 11-12. Localized Cortical Proliferation: (A) Mandibular torus (arrows A). (B) Palatal torus (arrow B).

out area at the crest of the ridge is localized periodontal disease following removal or loss of the tooth. However, exactly the same pattern is seen in locally invasive gingival carcinoma and in eosinophilic granuloma. A fibrous healing defect in an edentulous area may occur as a cupped-out lesion at the crest of the ridge due to alveolar resorption. A cupped-out depression at the inferior bor-

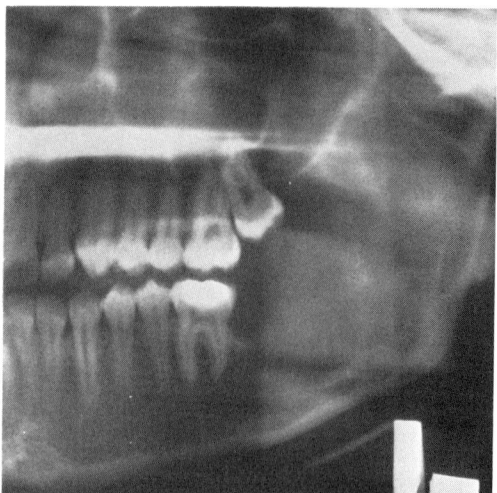

Figure 11-13. Cortical Perforation: This was an ameloblastoma.

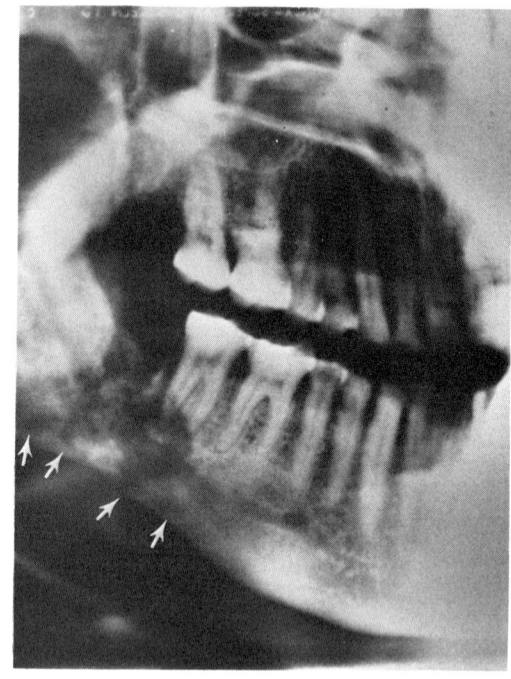

Figure 11-15. Cortical Destruction: Note the "moth eaten" appearance of this radiolucent lesion resulting from chronic osteomyelitis.

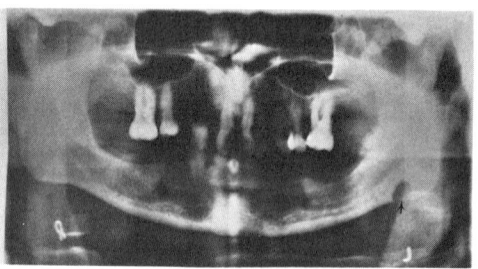

Figure 11-14. Cupped-out Cortical Depression: This was a developmental lingual mandibular salivary gland depression (Arrow).

der of the mandible may be seen in association with larger developmental lingual salivary gland depressions (Fig. 11-14) and similar lesions at the posterior border of the ramus may be seen in association with scleroderma and postirradiation fibrosis. Cortical destruction is an early feature of fibrous dysplasia.

Greater areas of cortical destruction may be seen in association with osteomyelitis (Fig. 11-15) and osteoradionecrosis. However, other conditions such as osteogenic sarcoma, epidermoid carcinoma, and other malignant processes may be associated with cortical destruction.

Involvement of the Supporting Structures of the Teeth

PERIODONTAL
MEMBRANE SPACE: Loss of
                   Enlargement
LAMINA DURA: Loss of
                   Enlargement
ALVEOLAR BONE: Loss of
                   Enlargement

Involvement of the supporting structures of the teeth is an important area of consideration in radiographic interpretation, since a variety of conditions characteristically cause changes in these structures. A loss of the periodontal membrane space is characteristic of ankylosis

Principles of Interpretation of Pathologic Conditions 375

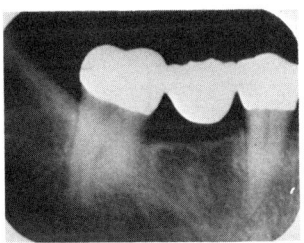

Figure 11-16. Loss of Periodontal Membrane Space: In this example the cause is ankylosis of the second molar.

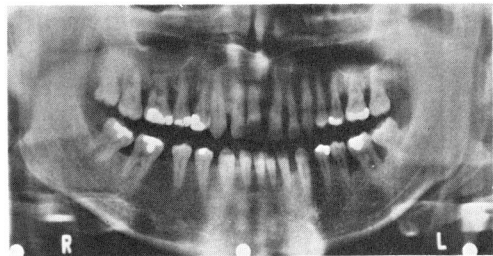

Figure 11-19. Generalized Loss of the Lamina Dura: This is a case of periodontitis. Note the degree of horizontal bone loss and the distal drift of the mandibular right premolars.

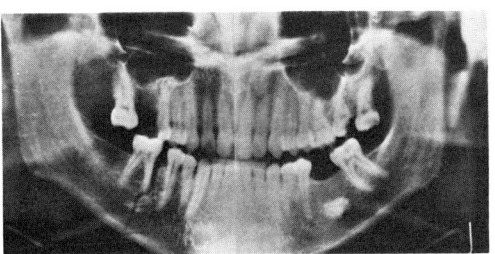

Figure 11-17. Localized Periodontal Space Enlargement: This was due to a compound fracture of the mandible.

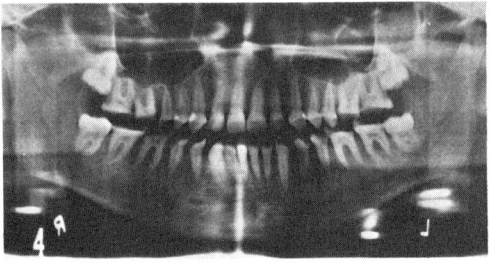

Figure 11-20. Generalized Loss of the Lamina Dura: This is a case of secondary hyperparathyroidism due to renal failure in this fifteen-year-old female. Note the accompanying "ground-glass" pattern of the alveolar bone. The unusual shape of the crown is due to severe erosion caused by chronic vomiting. All four third molars were unerupted and were therefore unaffected.

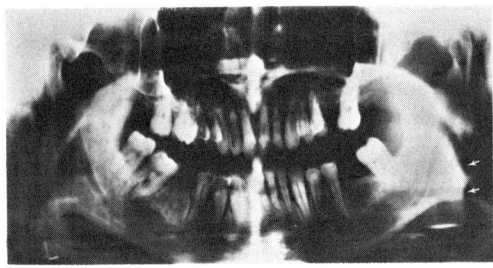

Figure 11-18. Generalized Periodontal Space Enlargement: This is a case of scleroderma. Note also the cupped-out areas at the posterior border of the ramus. These resorptive areas are also consistent with this deasease. (Courtesy of Dr. Robert Craig, Audie Murphy Veterans Hospital, San Antonia, Texas.)

and occurs particularly in embedded and submerged teeth (Fig. 11-16). However, a localized loss of the periodontal membrane space may also be due to a proliferative process such as chondrosarcoma or osteosarcoma. In the absence of periodontal or occlusal abnormalities, localized periodontal membrane space enlargement, particularly down one side of the tooth, may be an ominous sign of early malignancy, especially metastatic disease. On periapical films this may be an important sign of alveolar fracture (Fig. 11-17). Generalized enlargement of the periodontal membrane space has been classically described in association with some cases of scleroderma (Fig. 11-18).

A generalized or localized loss of the lamina dura is usually seen in association with periodontal disease, particularly periodontitis (Fig. 11-19). In the absence of

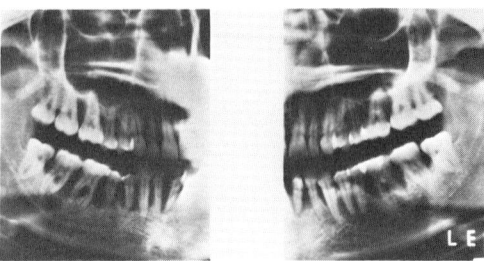

Figure 11-21. Generalized Loss of Alveolar Bone: This was due to advanced periodontitis.

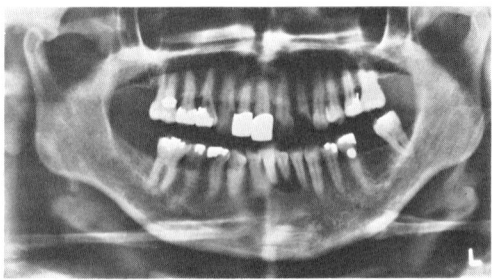

Figure 11-22. Localized Loss of Alveolar Bone: Floating tooth in this case was due to severe localized pulpal and periondontal disease.

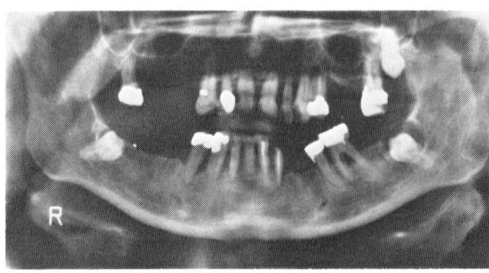

Figure 11-23. Pericoronal Lesion: The most common pericoronal radiolucent lesion is the dentigerous cyst. These may be associated with the crowns of erupting, unerupted, and impacted teeth. In this case compare the dentigerous cyst on the patient's left side to the normal follicular space on the other side.

periodontal disease, loss of the lamina dura may also be seen in association with

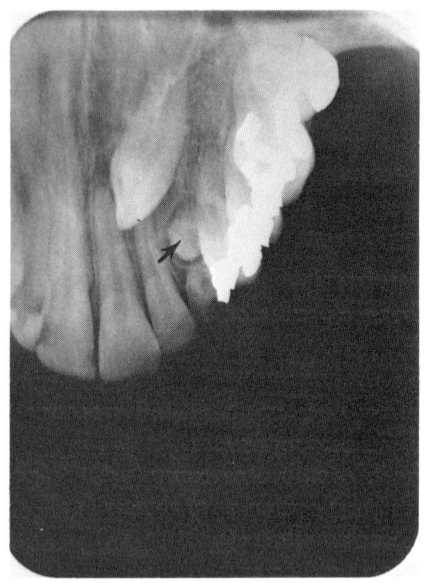

Figure 11-24. Association with an Impacted Tooth: This odontoma (arrow) is both associated with and probably the cause of the canine impaction.

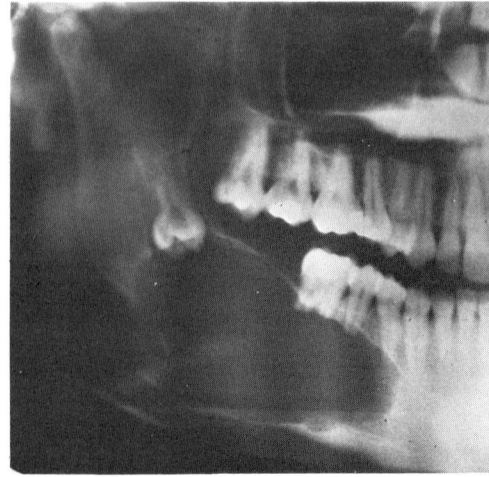

Figure 11-25. Resorption of Tooth Apices: Note the tooth resorption that has occurred in association with this ameloblastoma. Note also the bony expansion and displacement of the third molar. This mural ameloblastoma arose in the wall of a dentigerous cyst.

fibrous dysplasia, hyperparathyroidism, Paget disease, and dominant craniometaphyseal dysplasia (Fig. 11-20). All of these conditions may also be associated with a "ground glass" trabecular pattern at some stage of the disase. Enlargement of the lamina dura may occur locally due to occlusal trauma; in osteopetrosis, enlargement of the lamina dura is generalized.

Loss of alveolar bone is most frequently seen in association with periodontal disease (Fig. 11-21). A focal loss of alveolar bone may produce a "floating tooth" and may be caused by advanced localized periodontal disease; however, "floating teeth" are also seen in gingival carcinoma and eosinophilic granuloma (Fig. 11-22). A generalized loss of alveolar bone may be a sign of advanced periodontitis, juvenile periodontitis, Papillon-Lefevre syndrome, Chediac Higashi disease, agranolocytosis, cyclic neutropenia, and uncontrolled diabetes. A localized enlargement of the interdental crestal alveolar bone is an ominous sign and may be the only manifestation of early osteogenic sarcoma. It may also be seen in association with a peripheral cemento-ossifying fibroma.

Association with Teeth

CROWN:	Pericoronal
	Impacted
APEX:	Resorption
	Deposition
	Relationship to lesion
OVERALL:	Displacement
	Straddling
	Floating

The nature of the association of a lesion with one or more teeth may be helpful in interpreting the radiograph. For example, as we saw in our classification of lesions, a variety of conditions such as the dentigerous cyst or adenomatoid odontogenic tumor are associated with the crown of a tooth (Fig. 11-23). A variety of conditions may be associated with impacted teeth. For example, the ameloblastic fibroma is almost always associated with an impacted tooth. The Pindborg tumor is sometimes associated with an impacted tooth, and when this occurs it will be a tooth that is rarely impacted, such as the mandibular first or second molar. On the other hand, odontomas may be associated with unerupted teeth that are often impacted such as third molars and cuspids (Fig. 11-24). A variety of other conditions may also be associated with impacted teeth including dentigerous, Gorlin, and odontogenic keratocysts. Unerupted or impacted teeth are also seen in association with Gardner's syndrome, cleidocranial dysplasia, and osteopetrosis.

Resorption of the apex of one or several teeth in association with a lesion is a sign of a benign process (Fig. 11-25). Generally speaking, malignant disorders are too rapidly destructive and tend to move rapidly in the path of least resistance, thus precluding tooth resorption. A notable exception to this rule is the chondrosarcoma, which may have a well-corticated outline, be expansile, and cause root resorption.

Deposition of material upon the apex of a tooth is usually also an indication of a benign process. The classic example of this feature is the benign cementoblastoma, which in its mature classic presentation is radiographically pathognomonic (Fig. 11-26). In contrast to this, in periapical cemental dysplacia (cementoma) the deposition of radiopaque material is near and around the apex but not on the root of affected teeth. Hypercementosis does not usually obliterate the dentinal outline within the cemental mass (Fig. 11-27) while the benign cementoblastoma is characterized by the loss of the root outline. Benign osteoblastoma, periapical ce-

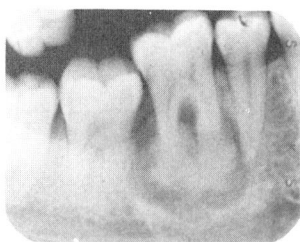

Figure 11-26. Deposition of Material on the Apex: This is a classic case of a benign cementoblastoma in the intermediate stage of development. The features are vital tooth, most frequently the mandibular first molar; the radiopaque cemental mass obliterates the dentinal outline of the root and root apex; this is surrounded by a radiolucent band; the outer periphery may be well demarcated by a sclerotic area of reactive bone.

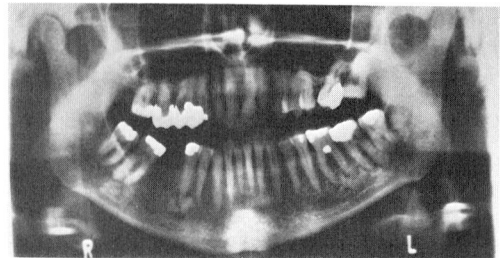

Figure 11-28. Deposition of Material Around or Near the Root Apex: This is a case of multiple cementomas (periapical cemental dysplasia) in a middle-aged black female. Note that the radiopaque cemental masses do not tend to interfere with visualization of the root apices. In dentate individuals, mature cementomas tend to be "croissant" or "half-moon" shaped, while removal of the teeth allows the cemental masses to grow apically and laterally to produce smaller roundish "tennisball" shapes or larger "globular" masses.

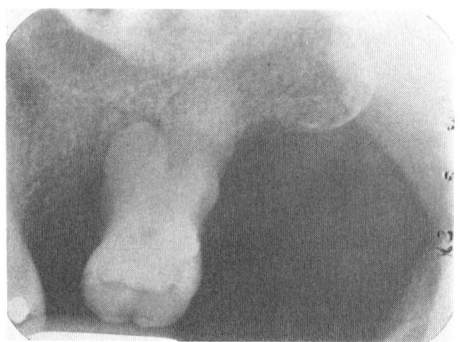

Figure 11-27. Deposition of Material on the Root: Hypercementosis. The cause here may be extrusion and/or advanced periodontal disease.

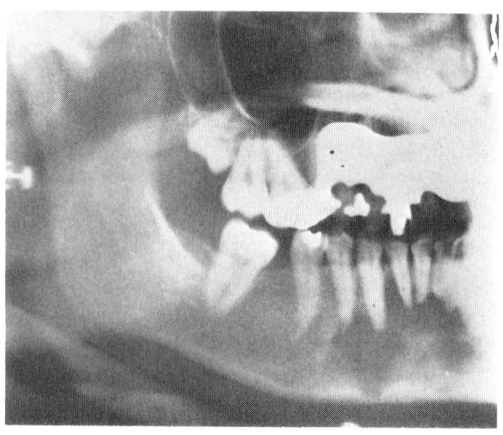

Figure 11-29. Relationship of Apices to the Lesion: In the case of this central giant cell granuloma, the apices are protruding into the radiolucent lesion. This is seen more frequently in neoplasms as opposed to cysts, although this finding is not always consistent.

mental dysplasia (Fig. 11-28), and central cemento-ossifying fibroma do not tend to alter the appearance of the apical portion of involved roots.

The relationship of the apex to a radiolucent lesion is notable. If the apex of one or more teeth appears to be protruding into a lesion, this may be a sign of neoplasia as opposed to cyst formation. If the apices do not project into a radiolucency which closely approximates them, then the lesion may consist of a cyst (Fig. 11-29).

If a lesion appears to be displacing erupted or unerupted teeth, this may be interpreted as a sign of a benign process. Classically, the central cemento-ossifying fibroma may cause displacement of adjacent erupted and unerupted teeth. Displacement is also seen in association with

Principles of Interpretation of Pathologic Conditions 379

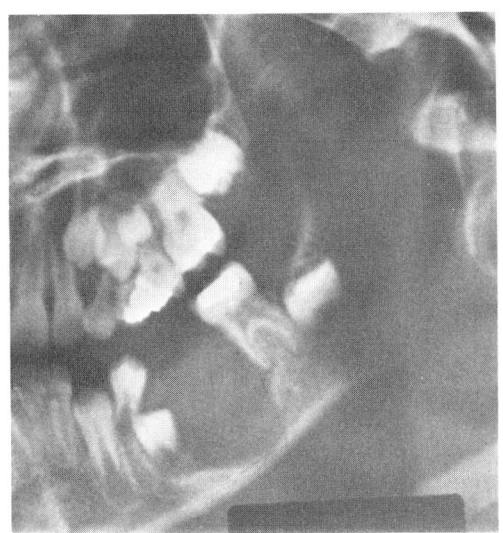

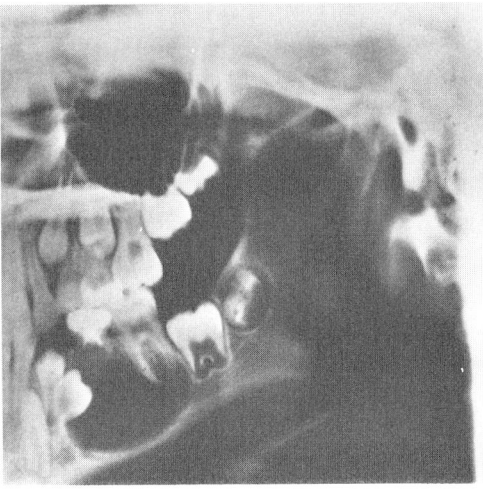

Figure 11-30. Tooth Displacement. Compare these almost identical lesions: **(A)** Central Giant Cell Granuloma; **(B)** Dentigerous cyst.

ameloblastoma, odontogenic myxoma, odontogenic keratocysts, and in the brown tumors of renal osteodystrophy in children. A variety of other conditions may cause tooth displacement (Fig. 11-30).

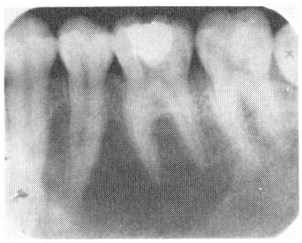

Figure 11-31. Tooth Straddling: This traumatic cyst illustrates this finding. By this we mean that the superior portion of the lesion creeps up between teeth and roots with a wavy or undulating border and does not tend to affect the lamina dura or displace the vital teeth.

There is one lesion that characteristically "straddles" teeth and consists of the traumatic cyst. Classically, the superior portion projects up between teeth without destruction of the lamina dura or displacement of adjacent teeth (Fig. 11-31).

Teeth may also be seen to be "floating" and, as was previously pointed out, should be considered an ominous finding until proven otherwise.

As was stated in the beginning of this chapter, radiographic interpretation is a highly subjective skill. Most changes are nonspecific. There are, however, a variety of findings that influence the significance of the radiographic findings. Some of these are pathognomonic and therefore suggest a specific diagnosis; others are indications of a benign process; and some findings are suggestive of malignancy. This chapter should serve as an introduction to interpretation of diseases of the jaws and should provide a nidus upon which a framework can be built in which all diseases can be studied, particularly in respect to the interpretation of changes they may produce on radiographs.

Chapter 12

NORMAL RADIOGRAPHIC ANATOMY

The Teeth and Supporting Structures

Enamel

ENAMEL is the most radiopaque natural material seen in radiographs and covers the coronal portion of the tooth. When a radiograph has been correctly exposed and processed, there is a difference in density between the enamel and underlying dentin. When enamel has been penetrated by caries, the affected area becomes more radiolucent or darker in the radiograph. **Carious enamel** is less dense, therefore more photons of X-Ray energy are allowed to pass through and expose the film. If more photons are allowed to expose the film, the area appears more radiolucent.

Once the crown has fully developed, no further enamel can be elaborated as a part of the tooth's defense or reparative mechanisms.

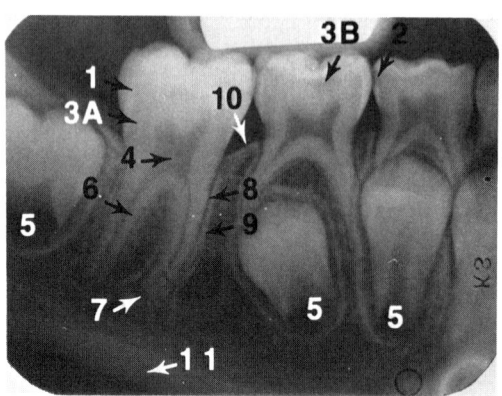

Figure 12-1. Normal Anatomy: (1) Enamel; (2) Carious enamel; (3A) Dentin; (3B) Carious dentin; (4) Pulp chamber; (5) Dental Papilla; (6) Root canal space; (7) Apex (incompletely formed); (8) Periodontal membrane space; (9) Lamina dura; (10) Crestal bone (alveolar crest); (11) Inferior cortex of mandible.

Cementum

Cementum covers the root portion of the tooth. Under normal circumstances, cementum is the same density as dentin and, therefore, cannot be distinguished from this material. When cementum is present in excessive amounts such as in hypercementosis, it can sometimes be distinguished from dentin.

Dentin

Dentin may be seen immediately beneath the enamel in the coronal portion of the tooth and it also makes up most of the root structure. In a correctly exposed and processed radiograph, dentin appears less dense or lighter than the underlying pulp, but darker than the overlying enamel. **Carious dentin** is more radiolucent than the surrounding normal dentin. Unlike enamel, new dentin may be laid down after the tooth has fully developed.

Secondary or **reparative dentin** is formed as part of the aging process, beneath deep restorations, or within portions of the pulp threatened by advancing caries. In such instances, the pulp horns become blunted in appearance and eventually disappear as they are no longer seen. Secondary or reparative dentin is also responsible for narrowing of the root canal space. As the process continues, the roof of the pulp chamber may become very close to the floor, and the entire pulp chamber may disappear completely. Radiographically, reparative or secondary dentin is indistinguishable from normal dentin except by its location.

Sclerotic dentin is produced by another defense mechanism whereby the existing dentin becomes more mineralized. This dentin is thus more radiopaque than the surrounding dentin and often resembles an arrowhead in its configuration, with the tip of the arrow pointing at the pulp and the base adjacent to the injurious process. This mechanism is usually stimulated by a low grade chronic pulpal irritation such as redecay beneath the leaky margin of a restoration.

Pulp

The pulp is contained within the pulp chamber and root canal portions of the tooth. The pulp tissue is not visible radiographically. The spaces that contain the pulp are the most radiolucent portions of the tooth. In younger individuals, the pulp spaces tend to be large and they decrease in size with advancing age. The **dental papilla** is that portion of the pulp seen at the widened apex of developing teeth.

Pulp stones are sometimes seen as radiopacities within the pulp space. They may be single or multiple and may occupy

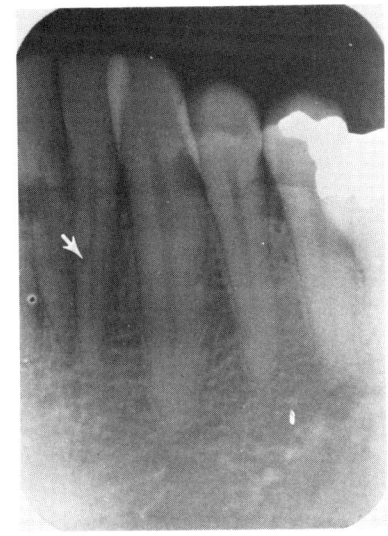

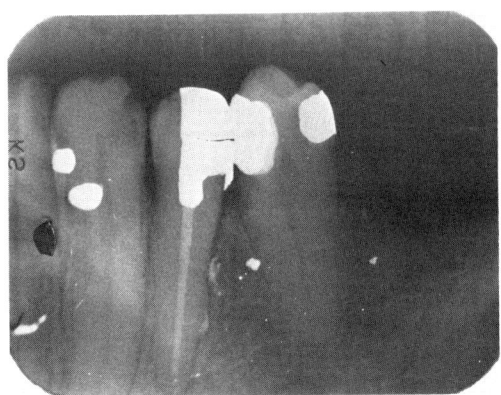

Figure 12-2. (A) Lateral Canals. (B) Lateral canals filled with root canal sealer.

much of the pulp space. Histologically, they may consist of dystrophic calcification or dentin. In either case, they are variations of normal and are of no known significance, although pulp stones are a feature of dentin dysplasia types 1 and 2.

The root canal space is usually seen as single and is centered within the root. In actual fact, many root canal spaces bifurcate to form two or more separate canals within the same root. In normal instances the root canal space is gently tapered toward the apex; when there is bifurcation, an abrupt change in the size of the root canal space will be seen. **Lateral canals** are lateral divisions of the root canal space and often communicate with the external aspect of the root. These should not be mistaken for root fractures. The **apex** of the tooth is the terminal portion of the root, while the **apical foramen** is the terminal portion of the root canal space, through which the vital elements of the tooth pass.

Periodontal Membrane Space

The periodontal membrane is not visible radiographically, but it is contained within the periodontal membrane space that is normally visible. It is seen as a distinct radiolucent line just outside the root portion of the tooth. The periodontal membrane space is wider in younger individuals and narrows with advancing age. It may become widened due to tooth mobility or due to the presence of disease such as scleroderma and early malignant disorders such as osteogenic sarcoma, chondrosarcoma, fibrosarcoma, and metastatic disease. It may completely disappear in conditions such as ankylosis.

Alveolar Process

This structure is made up of the inner and outer cortical plates, the cancellous or spongy alveolar bone, and the lamina dura. The **lamina dura** is a thin layer of compact or cortical bone seen as a distinct radiopaque line immediately surrounding the periodontal membrane space. The integrity of this structure is important in evaluating early abscess formation, periodontal disease, and other disorders in which the lamina dura is lost such as hyperparathyroidism, renal osteodystrophy, Paget disease, and fibrous dysplasia. The lamina dura becomes thickened in os-

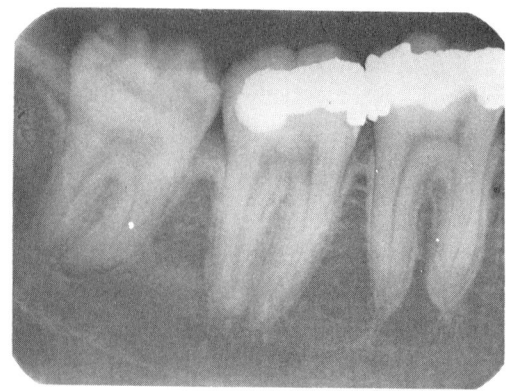

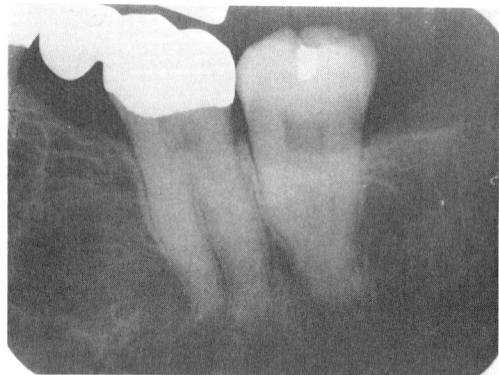

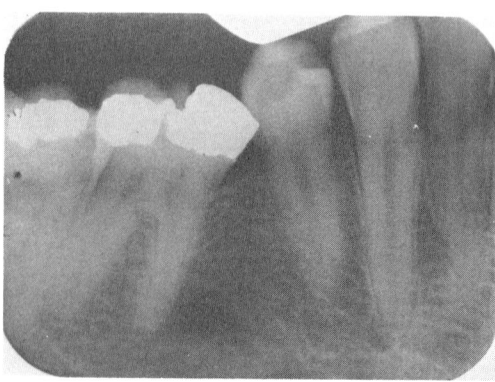

Figure 12-3. Trabecular Patterns. **A** Loose pattern. **B** Moderate pattern. **C** Dense pattern.

teopetrosis.

The **cortical plates** at the alveolar crest should be intact. A loss of alveolar cortical bone may be seen in periodontal disease, while a proliferation of osseous material in this region may be an indication of neoplasms such as peripheral ossifying fibroma or osteogenic sarcoma. The inner and outer cortical plates consist of a layer of compact bone covering the outer aspect of the jaws. These are evaluated when looking for fractures and for other conditions such as the submandibular and lateral fossae, lingual salivary gland depressions, and a variety of destructive processes. Additionally, various processes may stimulate subperiosteal reactions, which produce localized areas of cortical enlargement. Classic examples include Garré's osteomyelitis, osteogenic sarcoma, and Ewing's sarcoma (Fig. 12-3).

The **trabecular pattern** seen in intraoral radiographs is mainly a feature of the inner and outer cortical plates, rather than the loose cancellous or spongy bone contained within. The trabecular pattern is referred to as loose, moderate, or dense and these variations are of no significance. A further alteration consists of a stepladder pattern (Fig. 4A, 4B), and it is usually a variation of normal. This occurs most frequently between the roots of mandibular first molars and between the mandibular central incisors, in which case it is sometimes erroneously referred to as a vestigeal symphysis by some authors. A stepladder trabecular pattern is also reported to occur in association with thalassemia and sickle cell anemia. Other pathologic variations in the trabecular pattern have been variously described as ground glass, salt and pepper, orange peel (peau d'orange), and granular, as well as others including tubular, sun ray, honeycomb, and hair-on-end patterns.

Nutrient Canals

Nutrient canals may be seen in cross

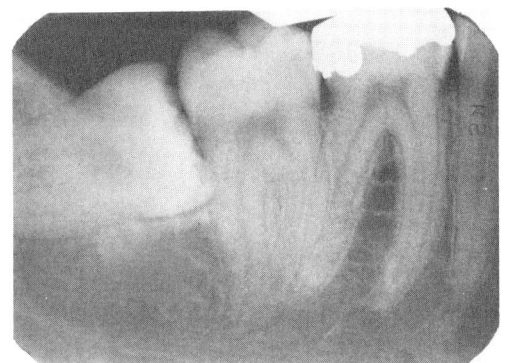

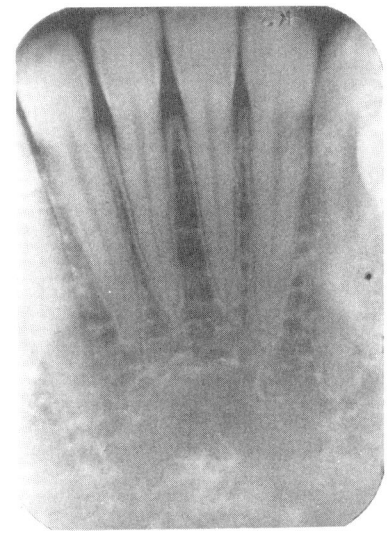

Figure 12-4. Step Ladder Trabecular Patterns. **(A)** First molar region. **(B)** Mandibular anterior midline region.

section, where they appear as **foraminae**. In the mandibular anterior area, the presence of multiple nutrient canals may be a variation of normal; however, they may be an indication of an increased susceptibility to or the presence of periodontal disease. In the area of the **maxillary sinus**, the canal of the posterior superior alveolar vessels and nerve may be seen. Within the **alveolar bone**, many nutrient canals may be seen leading to the apices of the teeth.

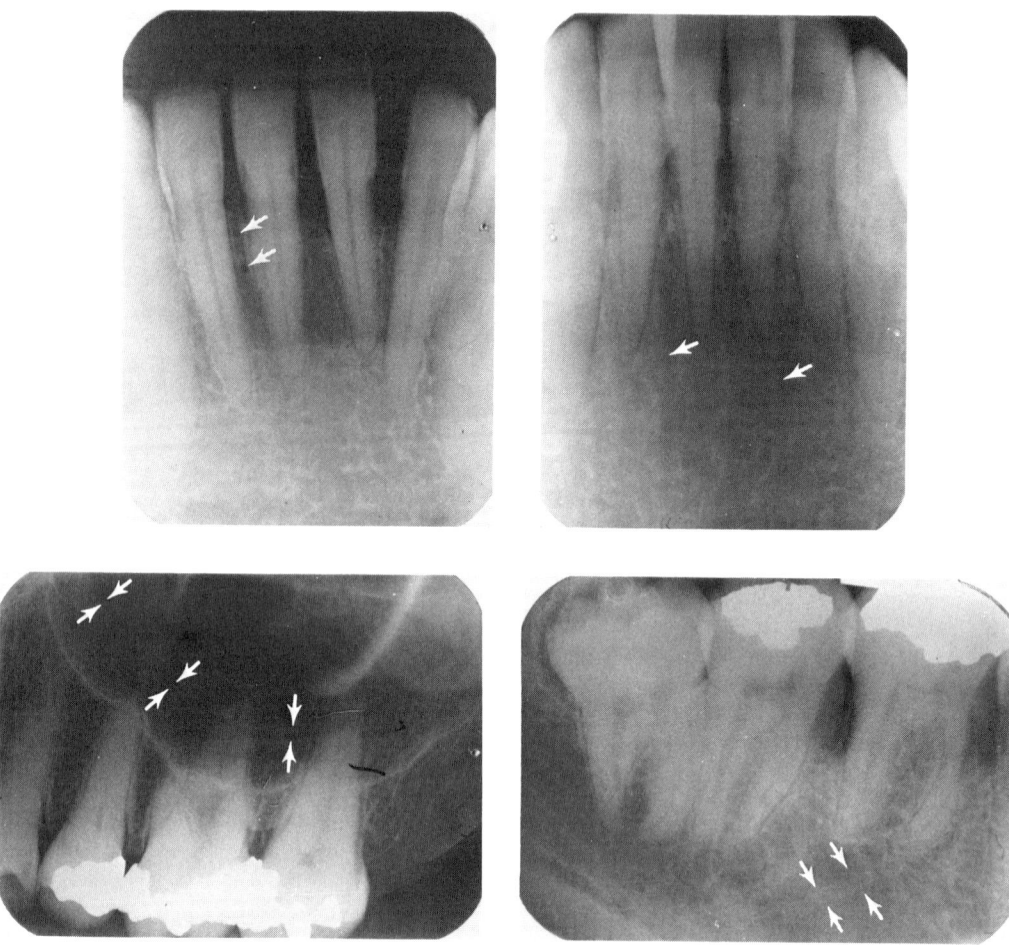

Figure 12-5. Nutrient Canals. **(A)** Foraminae of nutrient canals. **(B)** Mandibular anterior region. **(C)** Posterior superior alveolar canal. **(D)** At apex of a tooth.

The Midline Area

The **median maxillary suture** lies between the two processes of the maxilla in the midline of the palate. It consists of a thin radiolucent line, bounded by the thin outer cortical plate of the maxillary processes on either side. Sometimes there is a funnel-shaped widening at the anterior aspect, known as the **anterior median maxillary cleft**. This common finding is not classified as a true cleft palate. It may, however, be associated with a diastema between the maxillary central incisors and probably represents a variation of normal. The median maxillary suture is more apparent in younger individuals and may disappear with age.

The **incisive** or **nasopalatine foramen** is the oral terminal of the incisive canal. This foramen is located on the palatal aspect of the maxilla beneath the incisive papilla. In some individuals it may not be apparent, while in others it may be symmetrically round, oval, or heart-

The Maxilla

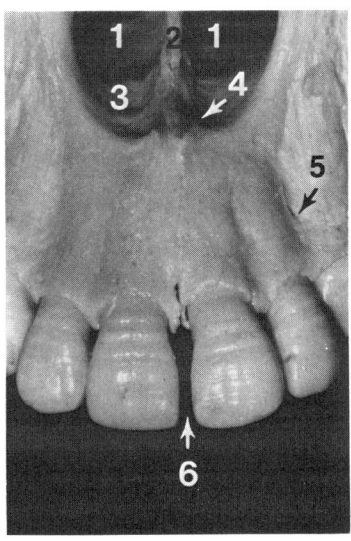
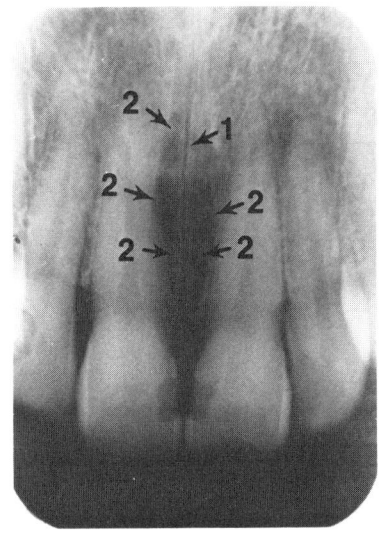

Figure 12-6. (A) Buccal view: (1) Nasal fossa; (2) Nasal septum; (3) Floor of nasal fossa; (4) Superior foramen of incisive canal; (5) Lateral fossa; (6) Diastema.

(C) (1) Median maxillary suture; (2) Incisive foramen.

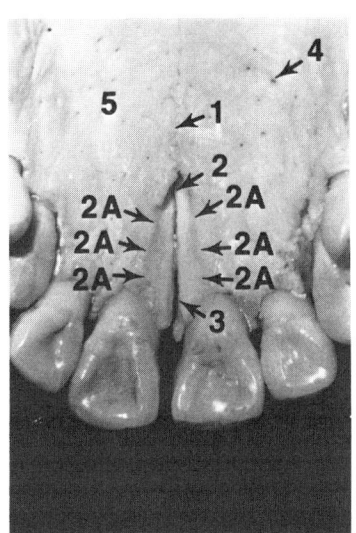
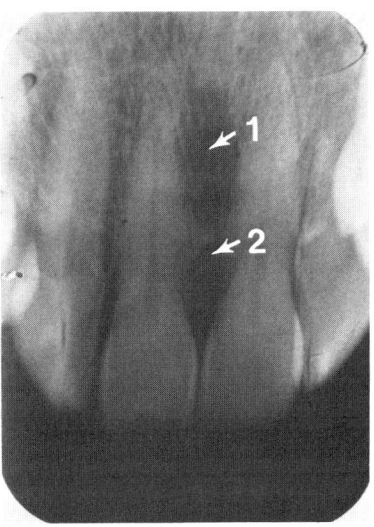

(B) Palatal view: (1) Median maxillary suture; (2) Incisive canal (most inferior aspect); (2A) Incisive foramen (resembles a fossa); (3) Anterior median maxillary cleft; (4) Foramen of a nutrient canal; (5) Hard palate.

(D) (1) Incisive foramen; (2) Foramen of nutrient canal.

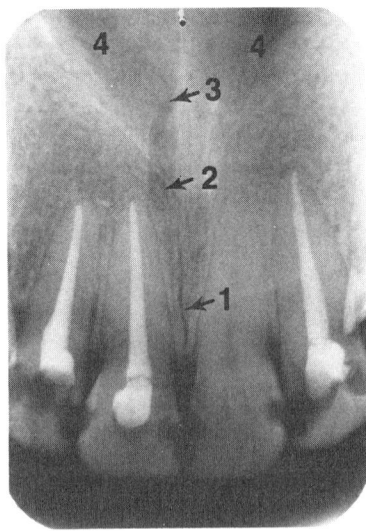

(E) (1) Median maxillary suture; (2) Incisive canal; (3) Superior foramen of incisive canal; (4) Nasal fossa.

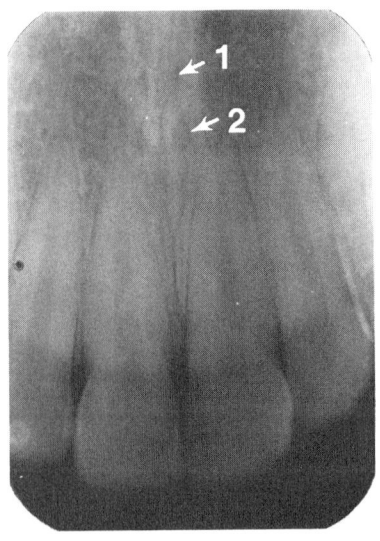

(G) (1) Foramen of Scarpa; (2) Foramen of Stensen.

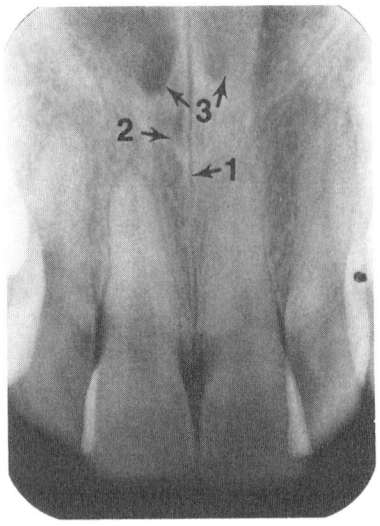

(F) (1) Median maxillary suture; (2) Incisive canal; (3) Superior foramen of incisive canal.

shaped and may be small or large. It rarely has a cortical outline. This normal structure should be distinguished from an incisive canal cyst, which it may greatly resemble. Features of the incisive canal cyst include an increase in size, displacement, or resorption of one or both central incisor roots, a loss of symmetry such as unilateral enlargement, and cortication of its outline. The incisive canal or nasopalatine duct runs within the anterior palate and terminates in the floor of the nose. There is one canal on each side of the midline and in some individuals each canal further subdivides into the **canals of stenson and scarpa**. The canals of stenson tend to be larger and more lateral, while the canals of scarpa tend to be smaller and more towards the midline. The **superior foramen of the incisive canal** may be found in the floor of the nasal fossa on either side of the midline. The superior foramen of the incisive canal may be superimposed on the apex of a central incisor and mistaken for periapical pathology.

Normal Radiographic Anatomy

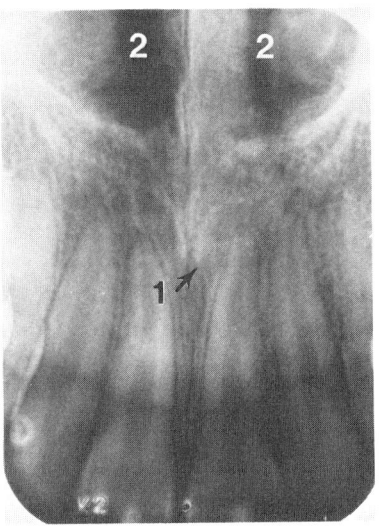

Figure 12-7. Maxillary Midline Region: (1) Anterior nasal spine; (2) Nasal fossa.

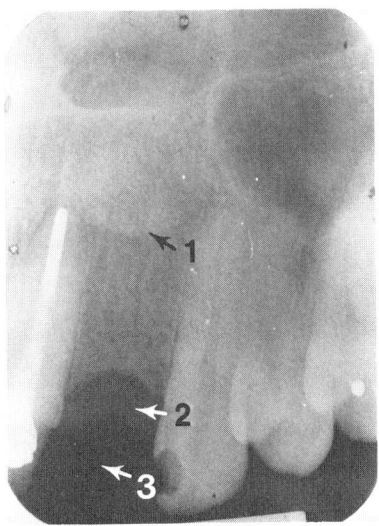

Figure 12-9. Maxillary Lateral Region: (1) Soft tissue outline of ala of nose; (2) Gingiva; (3) Upper lip.

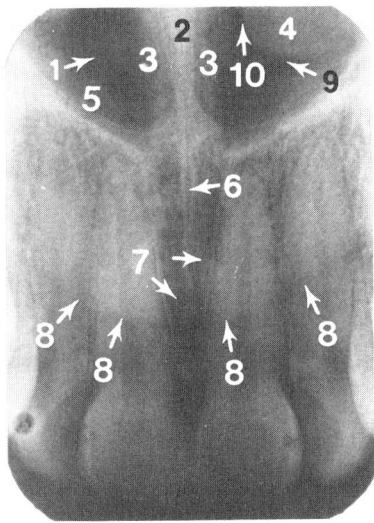

Figure 12-8. Maxillary Midline Region: (1) Nasal fossa; (2) Nasal septum; (3) Soft tissue lining nasal septum; (4) Inferior turbinate; (5) Soft tissue of floor of nose; (6) Median maxillary suture; (7) Incisive foramen; (8) Soft tissue outline of nose; (9) Inferior meatus; (10) Common meatus.

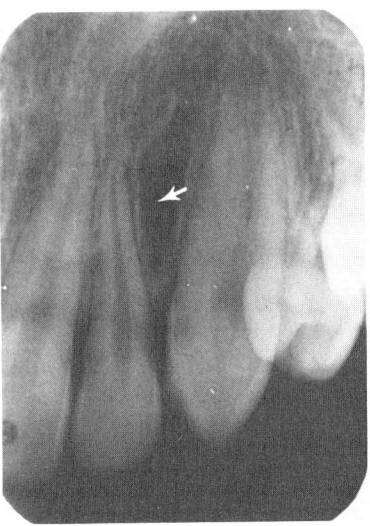

Figure 12-10. Maxillary Lateral Region: Lateral fossa

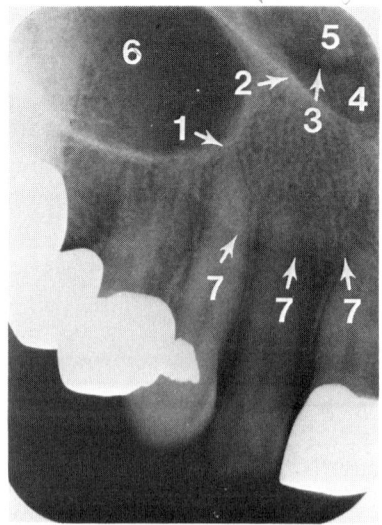

Figure 12-11. Maxillary Cuspid Region: Inverted "Y": (1) Anterior wall of maxillary sinus; (2) Floor of the nose; (3) Inferior meatus; (4) Soft tissue lining of floor of nose; (5) Inferior turbinate; (6) Maxillary sinus; (7) Soft tissue outline of ala of nose.

The **anterior nasal spine** is a V-shaped radiopacity in the midline at the level of or just above the apices of the central incisors. When there is a history of trauma, this structure is sometimes fractured; it may be better visualized with a right angle or Miller projection.

In some cases, particularly when excessive vertical angulation is used, the **nasal fossae** may be seen. These are divided by the **nasal septum** in the midline and often the **inferior turbinate** and **inferior meatus** of each fossa may be seen. In the midline area the following additional soft tissue outlines may be seen: **tip of the nose, columella, ala, gingiva**, and **upper lip**. In some instances the nares or nasal openings produce a relative radiolucency in the region.

The Maxillary Lateral-Canine Area

The **lateral fossa** represents a thinning of the cortical bone between the lateral incisor and cuspid teeth. This produces a relatively more radiolucent area, which

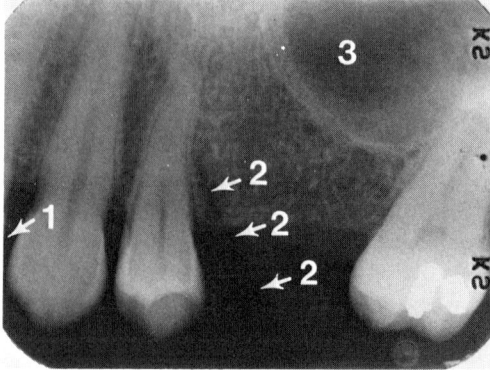

Figure 12-12. Maxillary cuspid region: (1) Maxillary primate space; (2) Nasoalveolar fold; (3) Maxillary sinus.

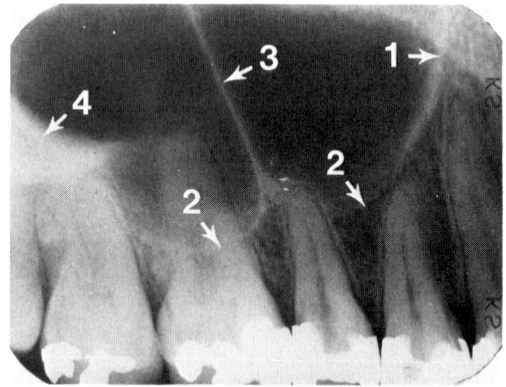

Figure 12-13. Maxillary Posterior Region: Maxillary Sinus. (1) Anterior wall of maxillary sinus; (2) Floor of maxillary sinus; (3) Bony septum; (4) Malar.

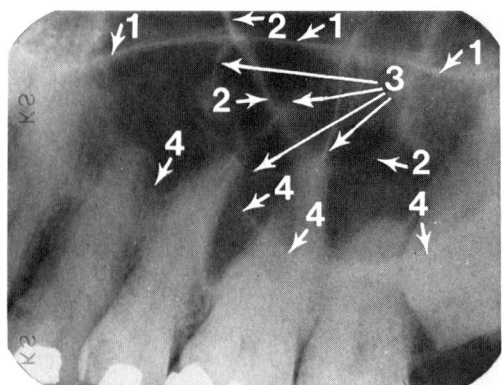

Figure 12-14. Maxillary Posterior Region: Maxillary Sinus. (1) Floor of the nose (hard palate); (2) Malar (3) Bony septae; (4) Floor of the sinus.

should not be mistaken for abnormalities such as a globulomaxillary cyst, periapical cyst, or lateral periodontal cyst. The **inverted Y** is an important anatomical landmark. It is especially useful in locating the cuspid area in edentulous surveys. It is formed by the cortical lining of the anterior wall of the maxillary sinus and the floor of the nasal fossa. A **diastema** is a space between any two teeth. In the maxilla, a specific diastema known as the primate space may be seen between the lateral incisor and cuspids of many normal individuals. The soft tissue outline of the **nasolabial fold** is another useful landmark in locating the canine area in edentulous patients. It may also produce a relative radiolucency as it angles across the roots of the maxillary cuspid or first bicuspid, thus mimicking a root fracture.

The Maxillary Sinus Area

In periapical films of the posterior teeth, **the cortical outlines of the anterior wall, floor and posterior wall** of the maxillary sinus may be seen. A lack of continuity of the floor of the sinus is seen in the antrooral fistula, and in other pathologic conditions. The maxillary sinus or maxillary antrum is an air-filled cavity that communicates with the nasal fossa via the maxillary osteum, an open-

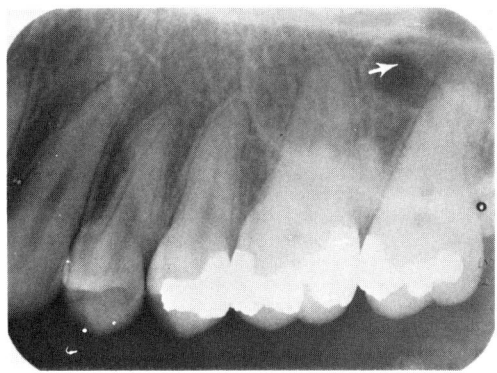

Figure 12-15. Maxillary Posterior Region: Maxillary Sinus. Sinus recess

ing that is not visible in periapical radiographs.

The maxillary sinus is sometimes divided into multiple smaller compartments by **bony septae**, which appear as thin radiopaque lines within the sinus cavity. The sinus may also be further compartmentalized by the presence of one or more **sinus recesses**. These are out-pocketings of the wall of the sinus and appear as well-circumscribed circular or ovoid radiolucencies within the maxillary sinus. When superimposed upon the apices of maxillary posterior teeth, sinus recesses may mimic periapical pathology. **Pneumatization** of the maxillary sinus occurs when the sinus space appears to be

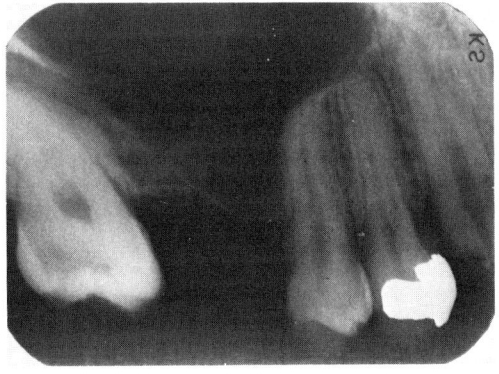
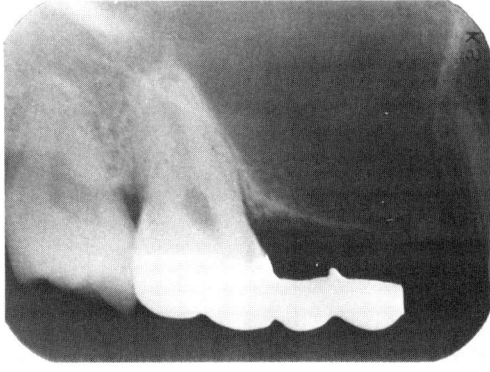

Figure 12-16. Maxillary Sinus: Pneumatization. **(A)** Clear sinus; **(B)** Cloudy sinus.

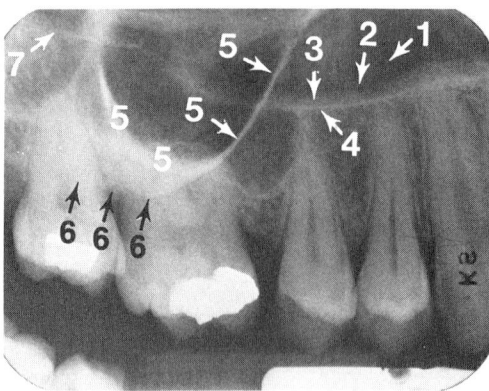

Figure 12-17. Maxillary Posterior Region: Maxillary Sinus. (1) Soft tissue shadow of inferior turbinate; (2) Inferior meatus; (3) Soft tissue lining of floor of nose; (4) Floor of nose; (5) Malar bone; (6) Inferior border of zygomatic arch; (7) Posterior border of hard palate.

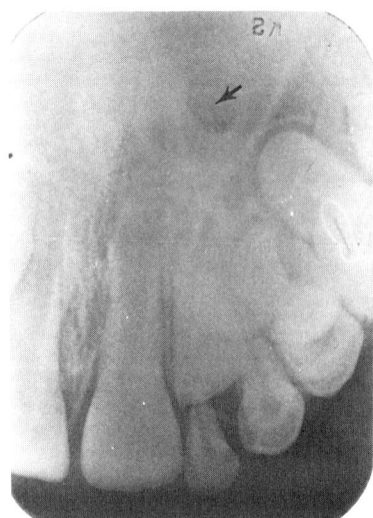

Figure 12-18. Maxillary Posterior Region: Lacrymal duct.

larger than normal. When the teeth are present, the cortical outline of the floor of the sinus appears to dip down between the roots of the adjacent teeth, while in edentulous cases, the floor of the sinus lies just below the crest of the ridge. Pneumatization may be associated with chronic sinus infections or allergy, but is of no significance when the sinus appears clear or radiolucent. A cloudy sinus is a significant finding and may occur in sinusitis due to filling with fluid or as a result of tumorification. A cloudy sinus appears more grey or opaque; when this is seen on periapical films it should be further investigated by taking panoramic views or a sinus series, which consists of the Waters, Caldwell, and lateral extraoral views.

The floor of **the nasal fossa** may be seen as a radiopaque line traversing the sinus in a horizontal anterior-posterior direction. This should not be mistaken for a septum or further compartmentalization of the sinus.

In younger individuals, the vault tends to be shallow and more excessive vertical angulations are necessary when taking some periapical films. In such instances the **lacrymal duct** may be seen in cross section in the area of the inverted "Y," above the lateral wall or floor of the nasal cavity. This should not be mistaken for periapical pathology or for an uncalcified supernumerary tooth bud.

The **zygomatic arch** and its component parts is another prominent structure that may be superimposed on the maxillary sinus. It is seen particularly when excessive vertical angulation is used. The U-shaped malar bone is usually in the area of the apex of the first or second maxillary molars and may obliterate these structures when excessive vertical angulation is used. The **inferior border of the zygomatic arch** extends posteriorly, an important landmark when trying to orient edentulous views. In some instances, the **zygomaticotemporal suture** may be seen marking the division between the maxillary and temporal portions of the zygomatic arch. This suture line should not be mistaken for a fracture of the zygomatic arch. In edentulous cases, the soft tissue

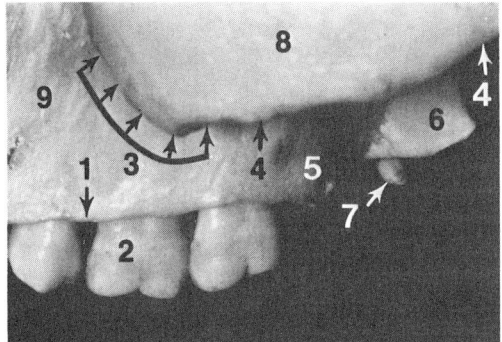

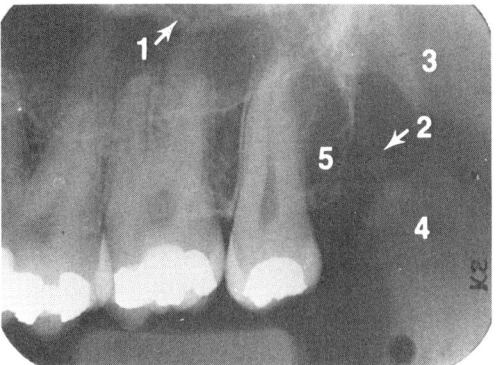

Figure 12-20. (1) Inferior border of zygomatic arch; (2) Hamular process of medial pterygoid plate; (3) Lateral pterygoid plate; (4) Coronoid process of mandible; (5) Maxillary tuberosity.

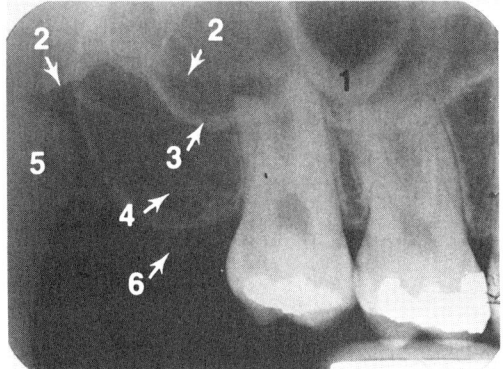

Figure 12-19. (A) Lateral view of gross appearance of region: (1) Crest of alveolar bone; (2) Maxillary first molar; (3) Malar process of zygomatic arch; (4) Inferior border of zygomatic arch; (5) Maxillary tuberosity; (6) Lateral pterygoid plate; (7) Hamular process of medial pterygoid plate; (8) Zygomatic arch; (9) Lateral wall of maxillary sinus. (B) (1) Malar process; (2) Inferior border of zygomatic arch; (3) Floor of maxillary sinus; (4) Maxillary tuberosity; (5) Coronoid process of mandible; (6) Soft tissue of maxillary tuberosity.

outline of the crest of the ridge is often seen.

Posterior Maxillary Area

The **maxillary tuberosity** is the terminal enlargement of the posterior portion of the maxilla. The size of the tuberosity appears relatively larger when the third molars are absent. However, in some cases further idiopathic enlargement of the maxillary tuberosity occurs and is of no significance unless there is impairment of function by impingement upon the coronoid process of the mandible upon opening, or when there is interference with the insertion of a denture.

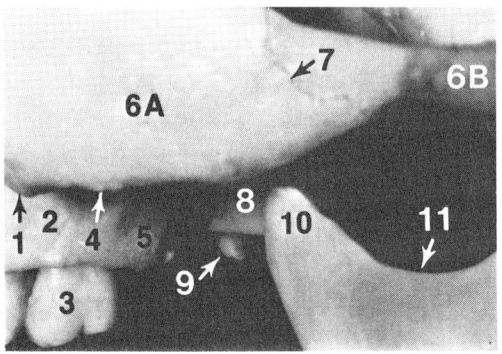

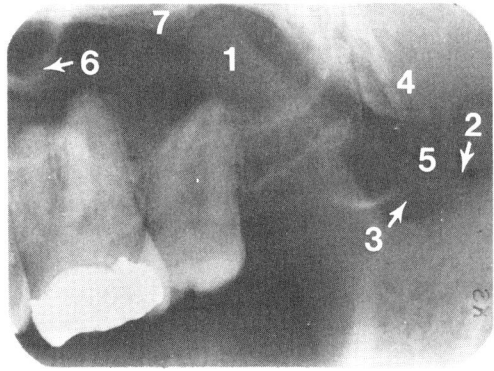

Figure 12-21. Maxillary Posterior Region: Lateral view of gross appearance of region. (A) (1) Inferior tip of malar process; (2) Maxilla; (3) Maxillary second molar; (4) Inferior border of zygomatic arch; (5) Maxillary tuberosity; (6A) Zygomatic arch; maxillary portion; (6B) Zygomatic arch; temporal portion; (7) Zygomaticotemporal suture; (8) Lateral pterygoid plate; (9) Hamular process; (10) Coronoid process; (11) Sigmoid notch. (B) (1) Coronoid process; (2) Sigmoid notch; (3) Medial sigmoid depression; (4) Lateral pterygoid plate; (5) Hamular process; (6) Malar process; (7) Zygomatic arch.

When the teeth have been extracted, periapical films in this region should always include all of the tuberosity area due to the possibility of the presence of residual or other pathology such as an odontoma or primordial cyst.

In some instances the inferior aspect of the **lateral pterygoid plate** and the **hamular process** of the medial pterygoid plate of the sphenoid bone may be seen. Occasionally, the hamular process may be elongated and may cause mild discomfort in the lateral aspect of the soft palate just distal to the maxillary tuberosity. In unusual cases, the **coronoid process, sigmoid notch**, and **medial sigmoid depression** of the mandible may be seen. The **soft tissue outline of the tuberosity** may be seen in some instances.

The Mandible

The Midline Area

In the midline the symphysis of the mandible is open at birth, and closes within the first six months of infancy. The **vestigeal symphysis** is a misnomer and represents a relatively more radiolucent trabecular pattern in the mandibular midline. This is rarely seen in edentulous cases.

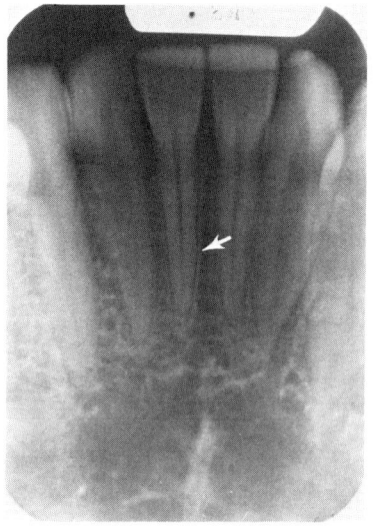

Figure 12-22. Mandibular Midline Region: Midline mandibular marrow space.

The **genial tubercles** are located in the midline on the lingual aspect of the mandible. They are four in number, the upper pair marking the site of attachment of the ligament of the genioglossus muscle and the lower pair marking the geniohyoid ligament. Radiographically, the genial tubercles produce a donut-shaped radiopacity usually well below the apices of the mandibular central incisors.

The **lingual foramen** lies between the upper and lower pairs of genial tubercles and is the radiolucent center of the donut-like genial tubercles. This foramen transmits a small lingual artery, which is a branch of the incisive artery and should not be confused with the larger lingual artery, which is a branch of the external carotid and supplies the tongue and sub-

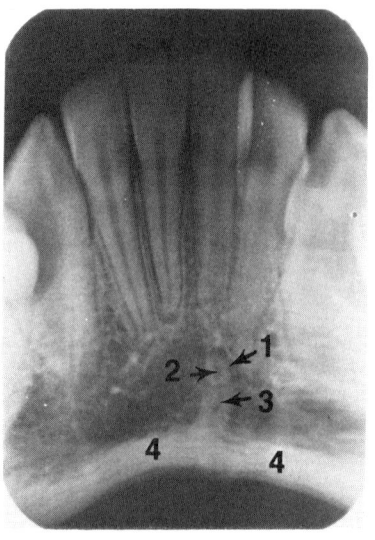

Figure 12-23. Mandibular Midline Region: (1) Genial tubercles; (2) Lingual foramen; (3) Lingual canal; (4) Inferior cortex of mandible.

Normal Radiographic Anatomy

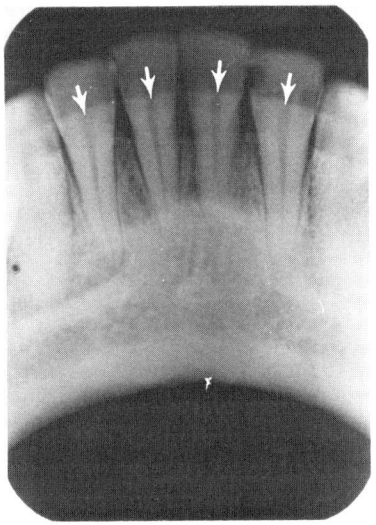

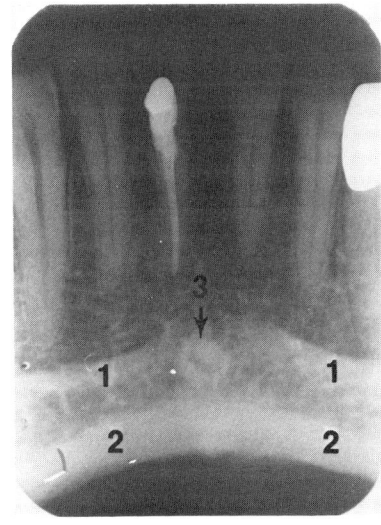

Figure 12-25. Mandibular Midline Region: (1) Mental ridge; (2) Cortical plate of inferior border of mandible; (3) Genial tubercles.

more radiopaque, due to the superimposed soft tissue shadow. In some instances, the outline of the **gingiva** may be seen, as well as the **dorsum of the tongue** when the film is inadvertently placed on top of the tongue, rather than beneath it.

The **mental ridges** are two prominent radiopaque lines above the inferior border of the mandible. These sometimes meet in the midline to form an inverted V shape.

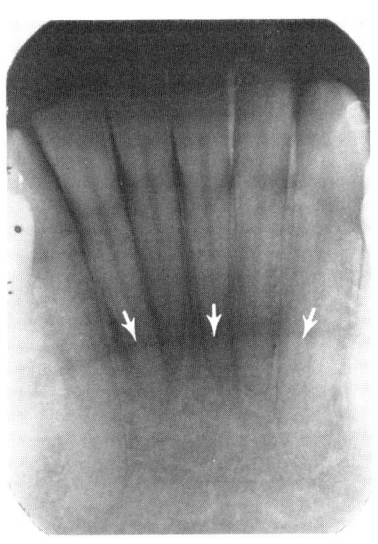

Figure 12-24. Mandibular Midline Region: Soft Tissue Outlines: **(A)** Lower lip. **(B)** Tongue.

lingual glands. The **lingual canal** is seen in rare instances and transmits the small lingual artery.

Transversing the mandibular midline, the following soft tissue outlines may be seen: The superior border of the **lower lip** usually causes the cervical and root portions of the mandibular incisors to appear

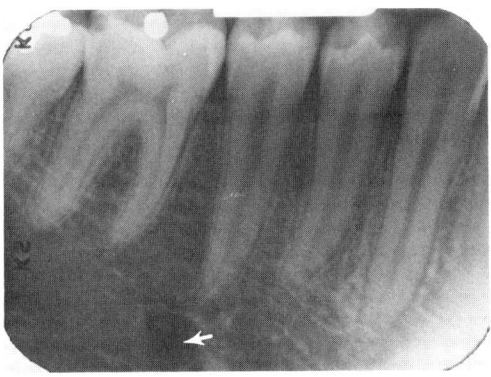

Figure 12-26. Mandibular Posterior Region: Mental foramen.

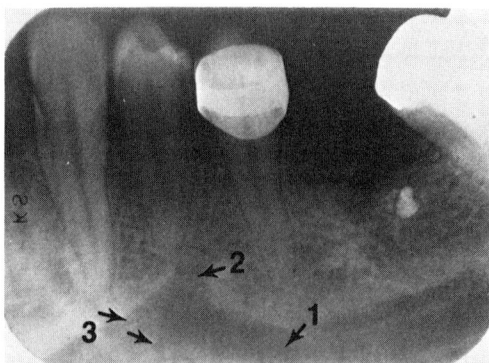

Figure 12-27. (1) Mandibular (inferior alveolar) canal; (2) Mental branch (contains mental nerve); (3) Incisal branches (note the bifurcation of the anterior or incisal branch; contains incisal nerve).

They correspond to a prominent ridge of cortical bone on the labial aspect of the anterior portion of the mandible. The mental ridges are seen when excessive vertical angulation is used. The **digastric fossae** are depressions on the lingual aspect of the mandible and may, in some instances, produce a relatively more radiolucent pattern in this area. These are lateral to the genial tubercles and beneath the apices of the lateral incisor and cuspid teeth. The digastric fossae mark the points of attachment of the anterior bellies of the right and left digastric muscles. When prominent, the digastric fossae should not be mistaken for anterior lingual mandibular salivary gland depressions.

The Mandibular Posterior Area

The **mental foramen** is on the buccal aspect of the body of the mandible in the bicuspid region. It is usually seen as a well-defined radiolucency and may be located anywhere between the distal of the canine and the anterior aspect of the mesial root of the first molar. It is usually in close proximity to the apex of the first or, more commonly, the second bicuspid and may mimic periapical pathology of pulpal origin. In edentulous cases the mental foramen may sometimes be located at the crest of the ridge and may be the source of pain when irritated by the overlying denture base or flange.

The **mandibular canal** is an important structure because it transmits the inferior alveolar vessels and nerve. It is important to note the relationship of the canal to teeth that are to be removed or to pathologic lesions that are to be excised. Occasionally, the canal may be perforated or displaced by pathologic conditions. In other instances the cortical outline of the canal is seen to be expanded or enlarged by conditions such as neuromas or hemangiomas arising within the canal. There may be bifurcation of the canal in the molar-ramus region, which is best seen on panoramic films. In the region of the mental foramen, where the inferior alveolar nerve bifurcates into its terminal branches, the **incisive and mental nerves**, further divisions of the canal are sometimes seen. The mandibular canal begins at the **mandibular foramen** midway up the medial aspect of the ramus, a landmark sometimes on panoramic films.

The **external oblique ridge** lies on the buccal aspect of the mandible and serves as the point of attachment of the most lateral fibers of the ligament of the buccinator muscle. It consists of a radiopaque line of varying thickness traversing the molar region and rarely extends more anteriorly than the second molar. In edentulous cases, the external oblique ridge may be continuous with and indistinguishable from the alveolar crest of the mandible.

The **mylohyoid ridge** is sometimes referred to as the **internal oblique ridge** and is located on the lingual aspect of the mandible. It serves as the point of attach-

Normal Radiographic Anatomy

ment of the mylohyoid muscle and extends from the molar region anteriorly to the biscupid area. Radiographically, it is a radiopaque line, often below the apices of the molar teeth. The mylohyoid ridge extends posteriorly to form the anterior lingual surface of the ramus, while the external oblique ridge forms the anterior buccal aspect of the ramus. Radiographically, these two lines sometimes join together posteriorly to form the apex of a triangle. The area between these two bony crests is called the **retromolar triangle**. The inner aspects of this triangle are referred to as the **buccinator crest** and provide attachment for the medial fibers of the buccinator muscle. The **submandibular fossa** is a relatively more radiolucent area beneath the mylohyoid ridge. It is a depression on the lingual aspect of the mandible to accommodate the submandibular gland.

The **inferior cortical plate** of the mandible is sometimes seen when excessive vertical angulation is used. In rare instances, the **gonial angle** of the mandible may be seen. This region is often relatively more radiolucent with large trabe-

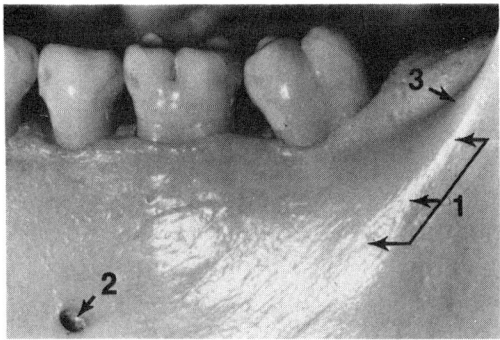
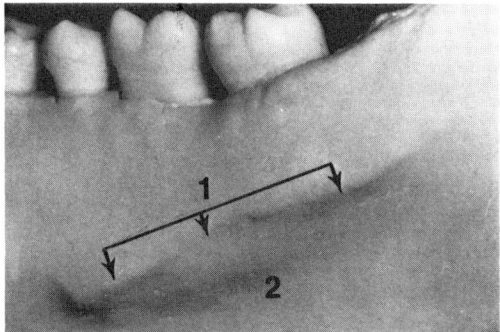
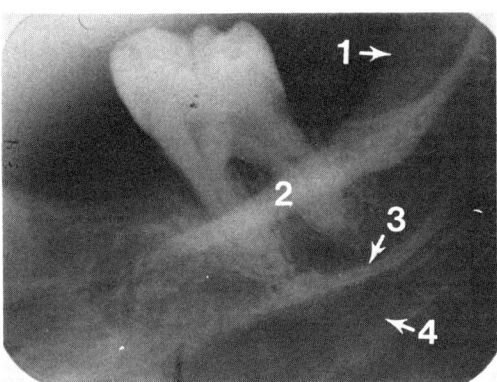

Figure 12-28. Mandibular Posterior Region: Gross appearance. **(A)** Lateral view: (1) External oblique ridge; (2) Mental foramen; (3) Buccinator crest. **(B)** Lingual view: (1) Internal oblique ridge (mylohyoid ridge); (2) Submaxillary fossa (submandibular fossa). **(C)** (1) Buccinator crest; (2) External oblique ridge; (3) Internal oblique ridge; (4) Mandibular canal.

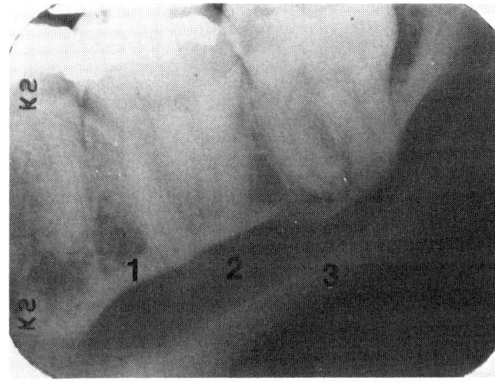

Figure 12-29. (1) Internal oblique ridge; (2) Submaxillary fossa; (3) Inferior cartex of mandible.

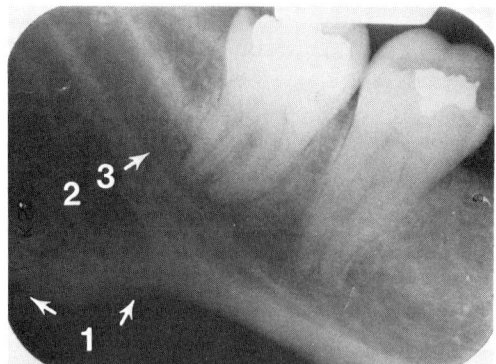

Figure 12-30. Mandibular Posterior Region: (1) Gonial angle; (2) Loose trabecular pattern of gonial angle; (3) Floor of mandibular canal.

cular spaces that should not be mistaken for pathology.

Distal mandibular pseudohyperostosis refers to a bony protuberance of the alveolar bone distal to the last tooth in the arch. This bony bump is seen in two situations: First, it represents the height of the remaining alveolar crest distal to which there is a depression due to a loss of alveolar height as a sequel of tooth extraction. Second, when a tooth has been lost mesial to the tooth in question, the remaining tooth tips mesially forming a mesial pseudopocket and on the tension side, a distal pseudohyperostosis develops.

The soft tissue **outline of the dorsum of the tongue** is sometimes seen in the posterior region when the film has been inadvertently placed on top of the tongue instead of beneath it.

Normal Anatomic Variations That Mimic Pathology

Bulbous roots may on occasion mimic hypercementosis. Note that normal amounts of cementum cannot be distinguished from dentin; when excessive quantities of cementum are present it can sometimes be distinguished from dentin and a dentinal outline of the root is seen within the enlarged area.

Uncalcified tooth crypts should not be mistaken for primordial cysts, residual cysts, or other radiolucent pathologic conditions.

The **dental papilla** at the apex of incompletely formed roots should not be mistaken for periapical pathology, particularly when obvious caries is present. Note that the cortical outline beyond the dental papilla is intact in the healthy tooth.

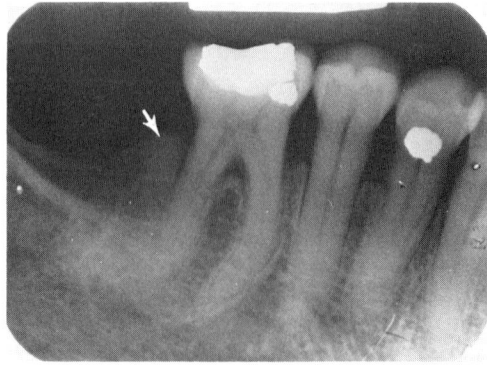
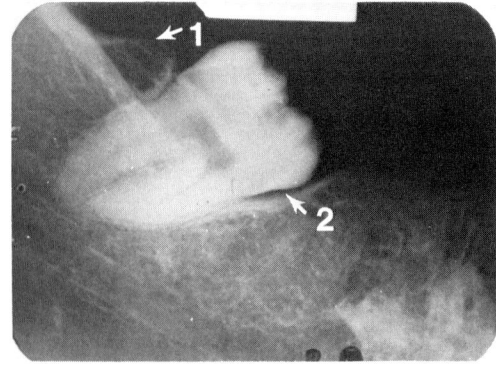

Figure 12-31. Mandibular Posterior Region: Distal Mandibular Pseudohyperostosis. **(A)** Type 1: Residual crestal bone. **(B)** Type 2: Excess crestal bone on tension side of tipped molar: (1) Distal mandibular pseudohyperostosis; (2) Mesial pseudopocket.

Lateral canals may, on occasion, mimic root fracture or fractures of the overlying cortical plate. In the second instance, the fracture line sometimes continues beyond the root area of the tooth, a helpful distinction when differentiating fractures of the alveolar plate from root fractures.

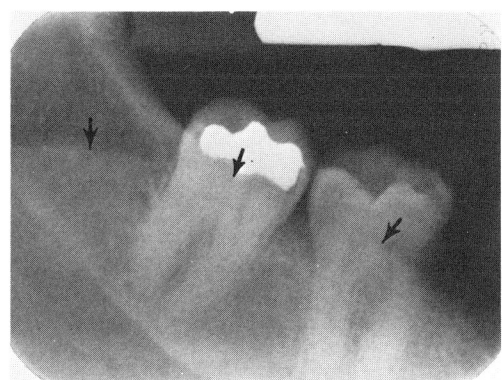

Figure 12-32. Mandibular Posterior Region: Tongue.

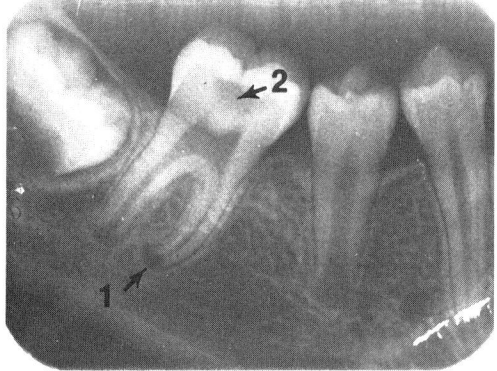

Figure 12-35. Variations Mimicking Pathology: (1) Dental papilla of incompletely formed apex (mimics periapical abcess); (2) Carious dentin.

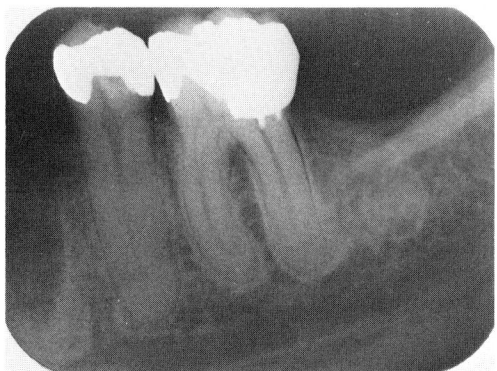

Figure 12-33. Variations Mimicking Pathology: Bulbous roots (mimic hypercementosis).

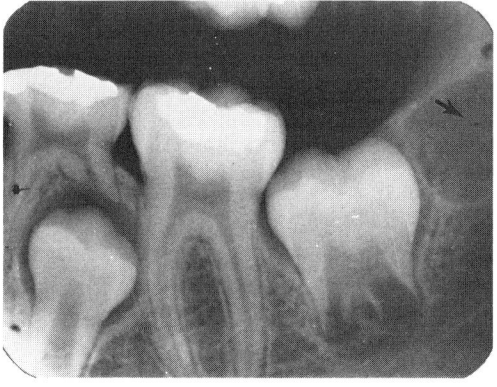

Figure 12-34. Variations Mimicking Pathology: Uncalcified tooth crypt (mimics primordial cyst).

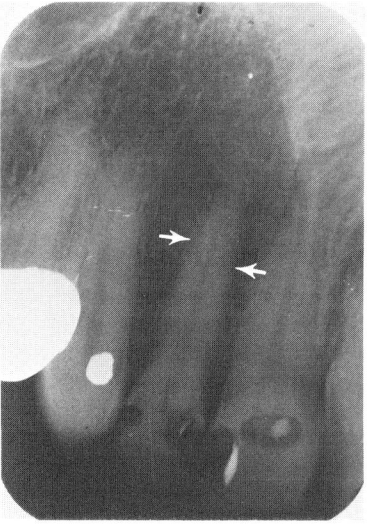

Figure 12-36. Variations Mimicking Pathology: Lateral canals (mimic root fracture).

A **double periodontal membrane space** may represent the outline of a second root in a tooth that usually has only one root. An important sign of this is the abrupt change in size of the root canal space. A double periodontal membrane space may also be seen in bell-shaped roots or in roots with a figure eight config-

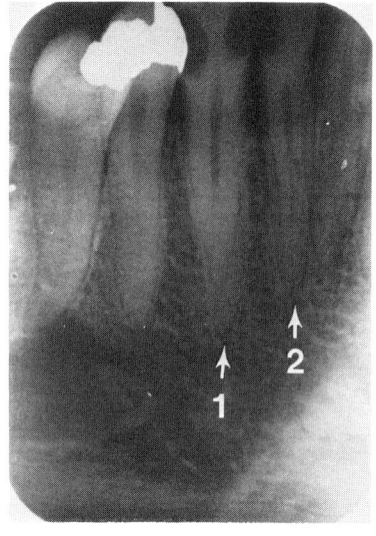

Figure 12-37. Variations Mimicking Pathology: Double periodontal membrane space. (1) Double roots (mimics root fracture); (2) Hourglass-shaped roots (mimics horizontal root fracture).

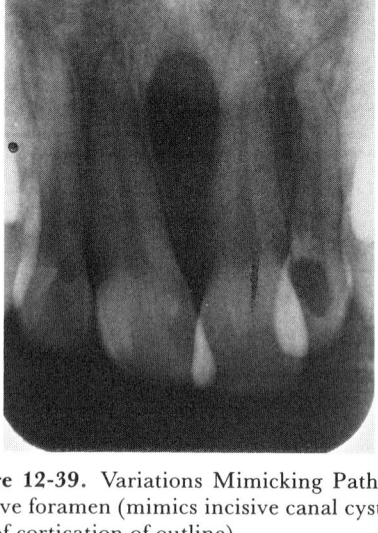

Figure 12-39. Variations Mimicking Pathology: Incisive foramen (mimics incisive canal cyst; note lack of cortication of outline).

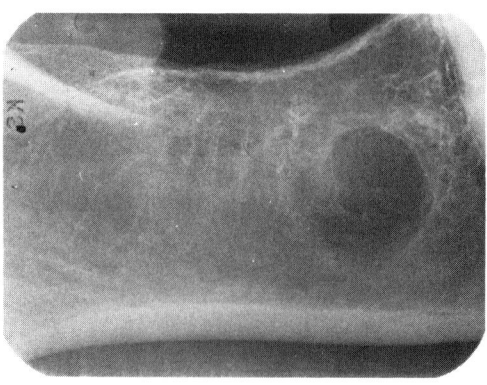

Figure 12-38. Variations Mimicking Pathology: Focally altered trabecular pattern (mimics residual cyst; focal osteoporotic bone marrow defect; others).

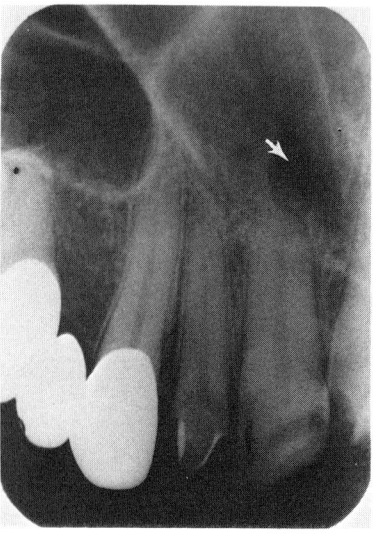

Figure 12-40. Variations Mimicking Pathology: Superior foramen of incisive canal (mimics periapical cyst, granuloma, or abcess).

Normal Radiographic Anatomy

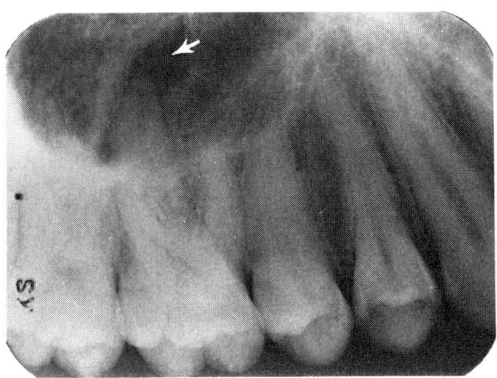

Figure 12-41. Variation Mimicking Pathology: Sinus recess (mimics periapical cyst, granuloma, abcess, and early cementoma).

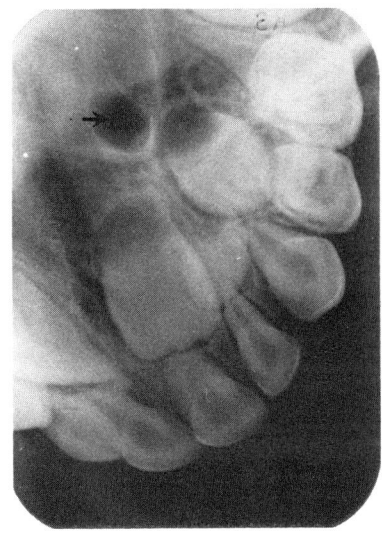

Figure 12-42. Variations Mimicking Pathology: Lacrymal duct (mimics uncalcified tooth crypt of supernumerary tooth).

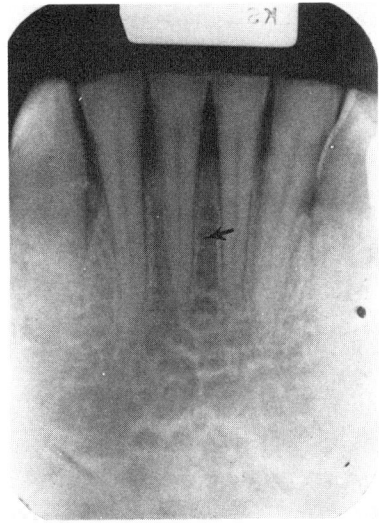

Figure 12-43. Variations Mimicking Pathology: Step-ladder trabecular pattern (mimics changes seen in thalassemina; sickle cell anemia).

uration, whereby the buccal and lingual aspects are not of the same width. In this instance, the variation may resemble a horizontal root fracture.

Alterations in trabecular pattern are rarely specific and may mimic a wide variety of pathological problems.

A well-defined **incisive foramen** may be mistaken for an incisive canal cyst or a radiolucency of pulpal origin.

When the **superior foramen of the incisive canal** is superimposed upon the apex of a central incisor, it may mimic periapical pathology. This is most often seen in periapical views of the lateral incisor, in which the central incisor is also seen and in which excessive vertical angulation was used. If the central incisor is healthy, the apical portion of the lamina dura may be seen to be intact.

Sinus recesses may be superimposed upon the apex of any maxillary posterior tooth whose roots appear to project into the antrum. The healthy tooth should have an intact periapical lamina dura.

The **lacrymal duct** is often seen in the cuspid-biscupid region of young children, within the nasal boundaries of the inverted "Y." It should not be mistaken for an uncalcified tooth crypt of a supernumerary tooth. In the midline anterior area

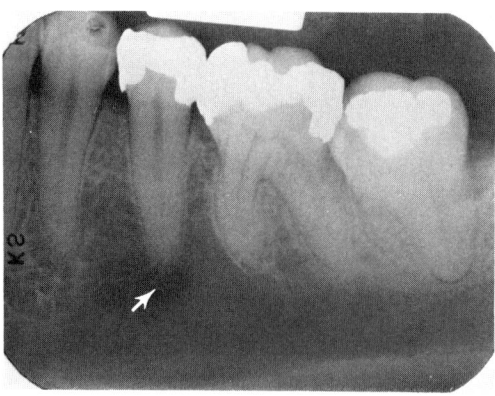

Figure 12-44. Variations Mimicking Pathology: Mental foramen (mimics periapical abcess, cyst, granuloma, or early cementoma).

of patients with teeth, a more radiolucent trabecular pattern may be seen. This is a variation of normal and should not be referred to as a **vestigeal symphysis**.

The **mental foramen** may be superimposed upon the apex of a tooth, particularly the mandibular second bicuspid, mimicking periapical pathology of pulpal origin.

Normal Edentulous Anatomy

The most difficult aspect of the edentulous survey is to orient the films for mounting purposes. The convexity of the dot is the first most important step. Make sure that *all* films are being viewed with the dot either convex or concave, depending upon the preferred method.

The **maxillary midline area** can be identified by the nasal structures, the incisive foramen, or by the soft tissue outlines of the nose. The **maxillary cuspid region** can be identified by the inverted "Y" or by the nasolabial fold.

The **maxillary posterior area** can be identified as right or left by remembering that the inferior border of the zygomatic arch extends posteriorly away from the malar process. Additionally, the malar process marks the previous position of the first or second molars. Other posterior

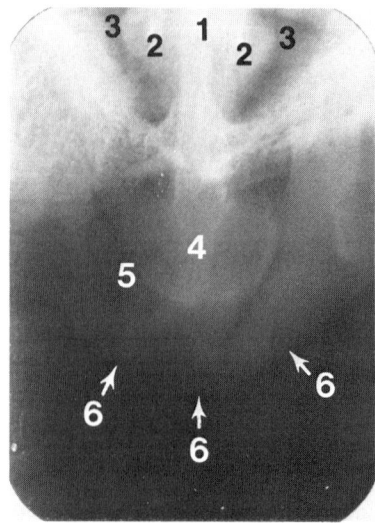
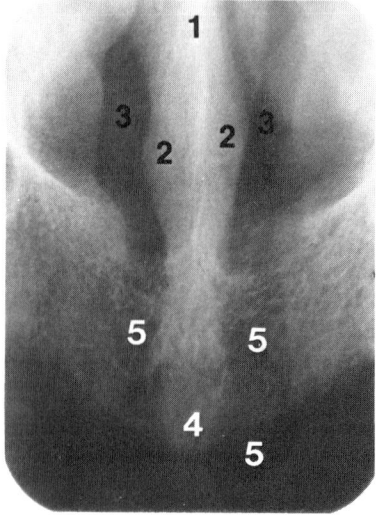

Figure 12-45. Edentulous — Maxillary Midline Region: **(A)** (1) Nasal septum; (2) Soft tissue lining of nasal septum; (3) Nasal fossa; (4) Columella of nose; (5) Nare (nasal orifice); (6) Tip of nose. **(B)** (1) Nasal septum; (2) Soft tissue lining of nasal septum; (3) Nasal fossa; (4) Columella of nose; (5) Nares.

landmarks such as the tip of the coronoid process, lateral pterygoid plate, or hamular process can sometimes be identified.

The **mandibular midline area** is indicated by the presence of the genial tubercles or mental ridge.

In trying to separate the bicuspid and molar regions in the **mandibular posterior area**, the mental foramen corresponds to the bicuspid region. Additionally, just as the curve of spee slopes upwards towards the posterior when the mandibular teeth are present, so too do the external oblique and internal oblique ridges, as well as the mandibular or inferior alveolar canal, thus indicating which side of the film is towards the posterior.

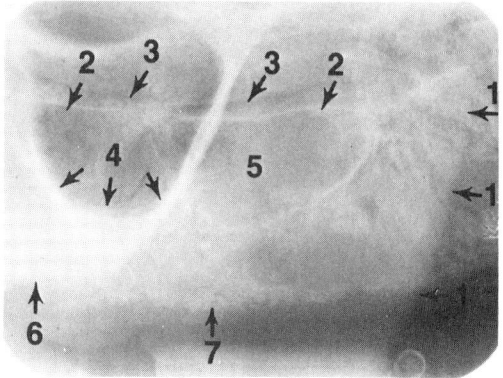

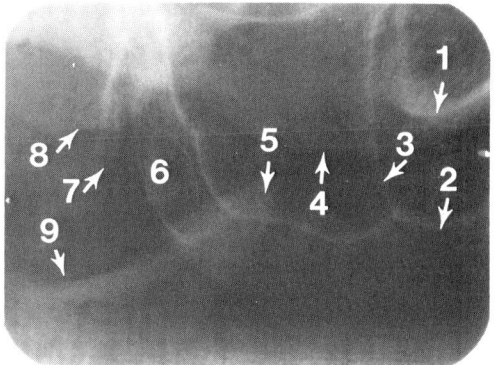

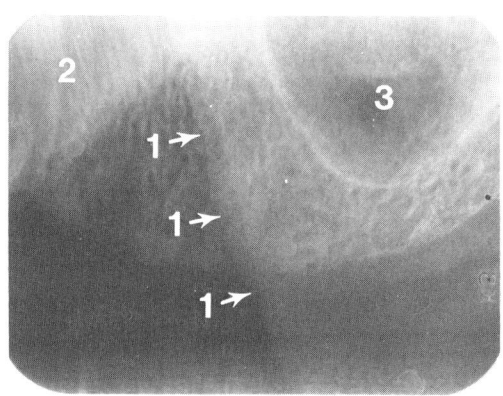

Figure 12-46. Edentulous—Maxillary Cuspid Region: (1) Nasolabial fold; (2) Film bending artifact; (3) Maxillary sinus.

Figure 12-47. Edentulous — Maxillary Posterior Region: **(A)** (1) Nasolabial fold; (2) Floor of nasal cavity; (3) Inferior meatus; (4) Malar process; (5) Maxillary sinus; (6) Inferior border of zygomatic arch; (7) Crest of alveolar ridge. **(B)** (1) Malar process; (2) Floor of maxillary sinus; (3) Bony septum; (4) Inferior border of zygomatic arch; (5) Tip of coronoid process; (6) Maxillary tuberosity; (7) Hamular process; (8) Lateral pterygoid plate; (9) Medial sigmoid depression.

NORMAL PANORAMIC ANATOMY

Introduction

Since the risk to the patient from one panoramic film is approximately equivalent to a set of four bite-wings, the use of this technique may represent a substantial savings in terms of radiation dose to the patient over the conventional full mouth survey. With the increased popularity of this technique, many clinicians have now

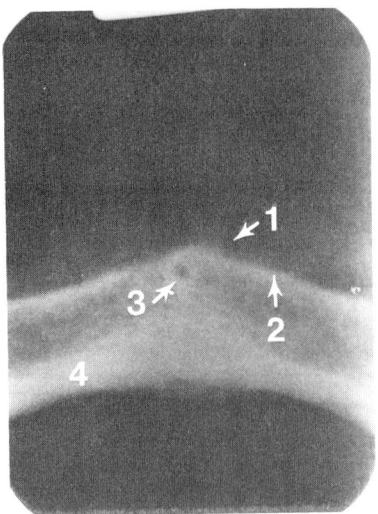

Figure 12-48. Mandibular Midline Region: (1) Nutrient canal; (2) Mental ridge; (3) Genial tubercle.

replaced the intraoral full mouth survey with a set of bite-wing films, a panoramic film, and selected periapical views as needed. We therefore feel compelled to include panoramic anatomy in this edition of the text.

When interpreting panoramic films, it is important to remember the following principles. Only correctly exposed and processed films should be used. The panoramic image is unique; therefore, anatomic relationships are different from those seen in conventional radiographs. The panoramic view also includes ghost images and other shadows peculiar to the technique. Additionally, the panoramic view provides an image of areas beyond the immediate tooth bearing region, to include much greater apical coverage and views of the whole ramus, temporomandibular joint, maxillary sinus, nasal cavity, and stylomandibular complex. Thus, the structures seen within these radiographs should be identified and recognized as the foundation upon which a meaningful interpretation of the panoramic image can be made.

Study the structures in the diagram in Figures 12-50 and 12-51, and then proceed with the text and illustrations of the various anatomic structures.

A Conceptual Approach to Normal Panoramic Anatomy

One way of learning normal panoramic anatomy is through a conceptual approach. Since the panoramic technique projects structures in a unique manner, simple osteology is an inade-

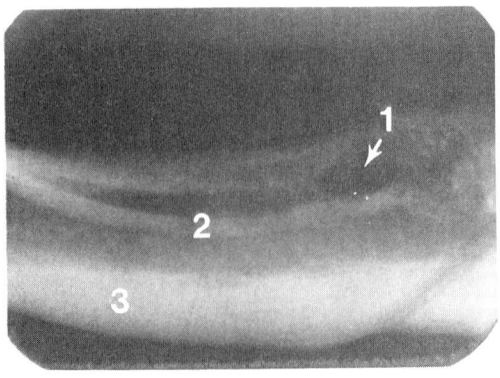 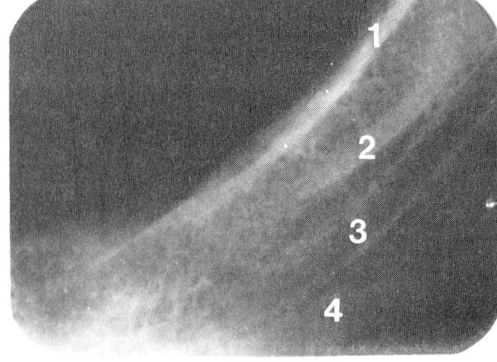

Figure 12-49. Mandibular Posterior Region: **(A)** (1) Mental foramen; (2) Internal oblique ridge; (3) Inferior cortex. **(B)** (1) External oblique ridge; (2) Internal obliqlue ridge; (3) Mandibular canal; (4) Inferior cortex.

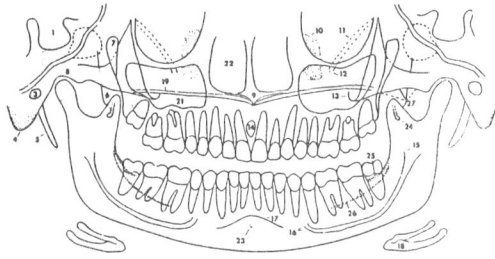

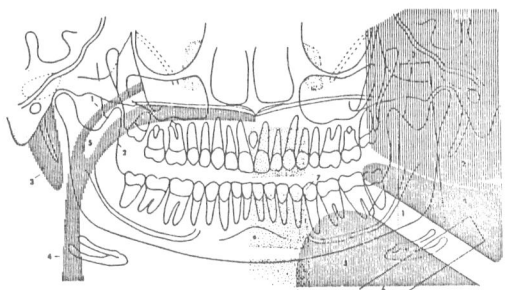

Figure 12-50. Normal Panoramic Anatomy: (1) Sella Turcica; (2) Sphenoid sinus; (3) External auditory meatus; (4) Mastoid air cells; (5) Stylohyoid ligament; (6) Lateral pterygoid plate; (7) Ptergomaxillary fissure; (8) Articular emminence; (9) Anterior nasal spine; (10) Ethmoid sinus; (11) Infraorbital canal; (12) Infraorbital foramen; (13) Malar process; (14) Incisive foramen; (15) Mandibular foramen; (16) Mandibular canal and mental foramen; (17) Mental ridge; (18) Hyoid bone; (19) Palate; (20) Infratemporal crest of temporal bone; (21) Maxillary sinus; (22) Nasal fossa; (23) Genial tubercles; (24) Hamular process; (25) External oblique line; (26) Internal oblique line; (27) Zygomatic arch. (Courtesy of Dr. John Preece, Department of Dental Diagnostic Science, UTHSC Dental School, San Antonio, Texas.)

Figure 12-51. Soft Tissue Shadows and Other Characteristic Features of the Panoramic Image: Soft Tissue Shadows: (1) Nasopharyngeal air space; (2) Palato-glossal air space; (3) Shadow of ear; (4) Glosso-pharyngeal air space; (5) Soft palate. Note: All artifact areas and shadows are bilateral. OTHER FEATURES: (1) Chin rest (opposite side); (2) Opposite mandible; (3) Pancentric (head positioner); (4) Soft tissue space below mandible and chin rest (opposite side); (5) Area of greater density (radiolucency) due to absence of superimposed structures; (6) Chin rest (same side); (7) Cervical vertebra and intervertebral space. (Courtesy of Dr. John Preece, Department of Dental Diagnostic Science, UTHSC Dental School, San Antonio, Texas.)

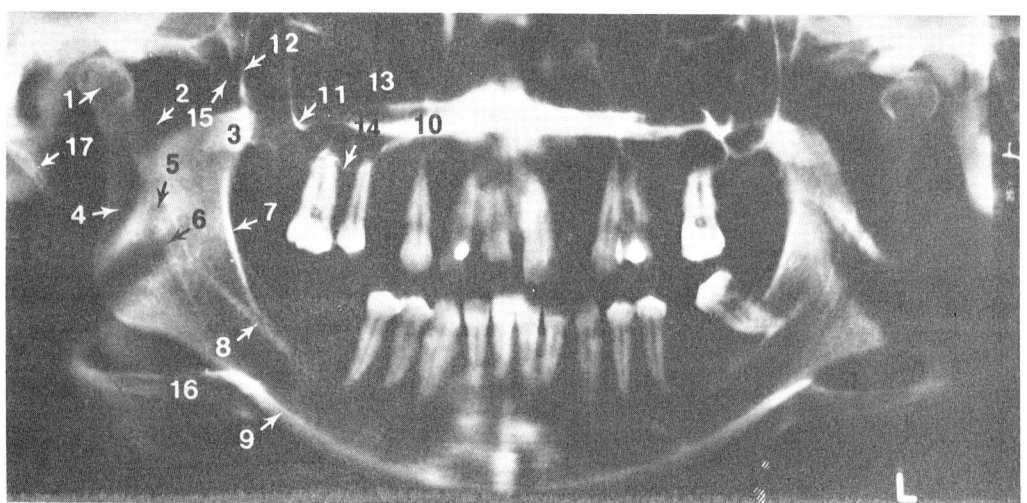

Figure 12-52. Concept 1: Structures are Flattened and Spread Out: Desirable Effects: (1) Head of condyle; (2) Sigmoid notch; (3) Coronoid process; (4) Ramus of mandible; (5) Mandibular foramen; (6) Mandibular (inferior alveolar) canal; (7) External oblique ridge; (8) Internal oblique (mylohyoid) ridge; (9) Inferior cortex of body of mandible; (10) Hard palate (floor of the nose); (11) Malar process; (12) Posterior wall of maxillary sinus; (13) Maxillary sinus; (14) Floor of maxillary sinus; (15) Inferior border of zygomatic arch; (16) Hyoid bone; (17) Styloid process.

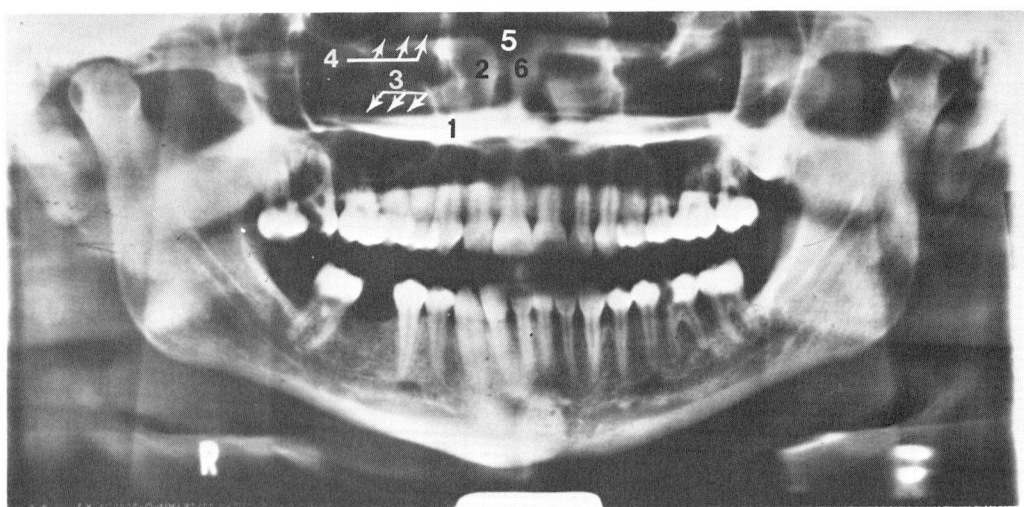

Figure 12-53. Concept 1: Structures are Flattened and Spread Out: Undesirable Effects: (1) Hard palate (floor of the nose); (2) Inferior turbinate; (3) Inferior meatus; (4) Middle meatus; (5) Common meatus; (6) Nasal septum.

quate basis for complete understanding of the panoramic image. Rather, osteology is a beginning point that, when combined with an understanding of certain panoramic principles, results in the following concepts. We have found these to be extremely useful in learning to interpret the normal panoramic image, through understanding rather than rote memorization.

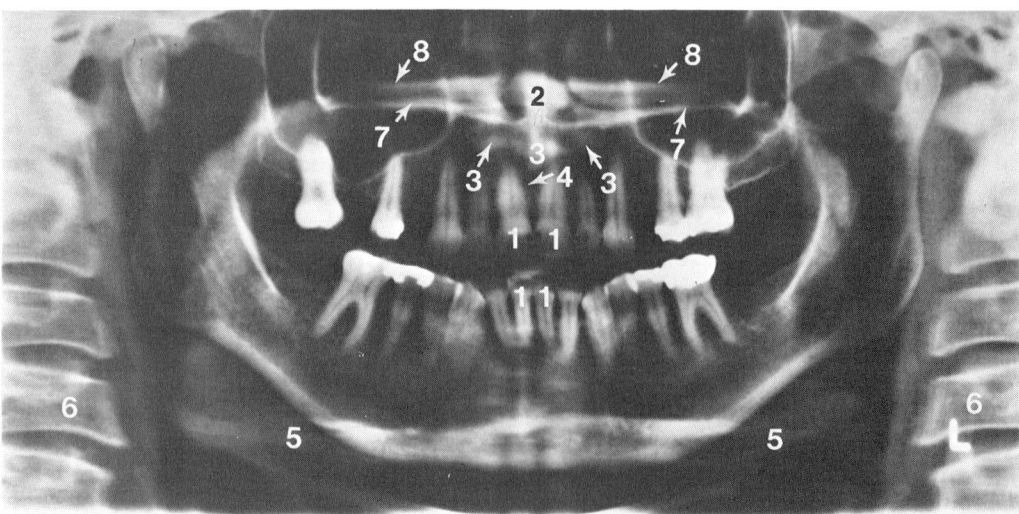

Figure 12-54. Midline Structures May be Projected in Two Ways: *Midline Single Images*: (1) Right and left central incisors; (2) Nasal septum; (3) Soft tissue outline of the nose; (4) Incisive foramen. *Bilateral Double Images*: (5) Hyoid bone; (6) Cervical spine; (7) Actual image of palates; (8) Ghost image of contralateral palates.

Concept 1: Structures Are Flattened and Spread Out

In some instances this feature of the panoramic image is **desirable**. For example, the mandible, mandibular canal, and zygomatic arches are all visualized within the same plane as the film and without any superimposition of the hard tissues of the right and left sides. This is also undesirable when the nasal turbinates and meati lie within the focal trough. In this instance, thick radiopaque bands bounded by thin radiolucent lines representing the inferior and middle turbinates and meati are spread across the maxillary sinus space. These may obliterate pathological changes and malignant tumors. The thin radiolucent lines representing the meati should not be misinterpreted as vascular canals or fracture lines.

Concept 2: Midline Structures May Be Projected in Two Ways

Some midline structures are projected **in the midline** as single images. Some of these include the central incisors, incisive foramen, anterior nasal spine, nasal septum, and soft tissue outline of the nose. These structures tend to be located towards the more anterior limits of the radiograph and lie between the center of rotation of the beam and the film only once during one exposure cycle.

Other midline structures are projected **bilaterally** as double images. Thus, the same structure is seen twice in the image. Some of these include the hyoid bone and epiglottis, cervical spine, hard palate, and palatal tori when present. If the cervical spine is superimposed upon the styloid process or mandibular ramus, an error in technique has occurred. In this double image concept, the midline structure falls within the focal trough twice. It is projected onto the image when the right side is being radiographed and once again as the machine rotates around the contralateral side. In each instance the contralateral twin image of the midline structure will appear in the correct panoramic relationship to other structures. Double images are produced because the object lies between the center of rotation and the

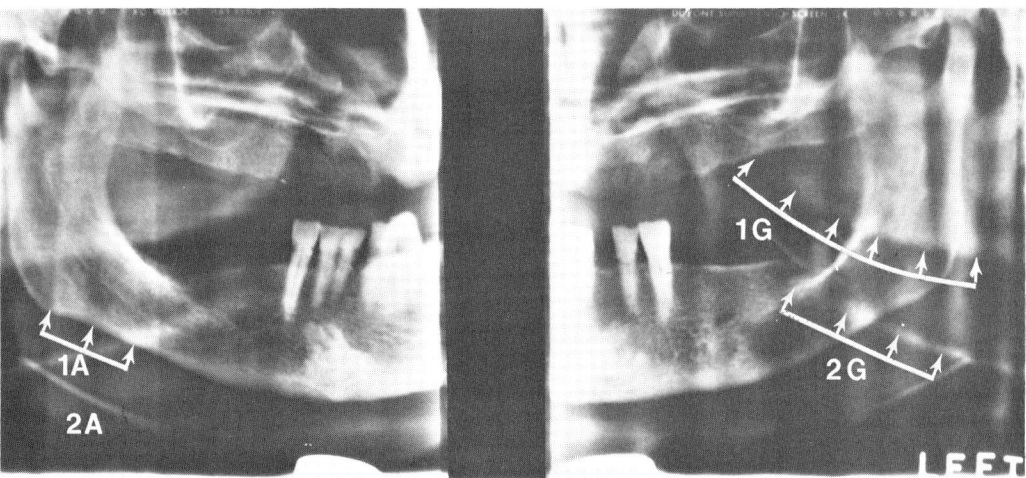

Figure 12-55. Concept 3: Ghost Images are Formed: (1A) Actual image of right inferior border of mandible; (1G) Ghost image of right inferior border of mandible; (2A) Actual image of chin rest; (2G) Ghost image of chin rest.

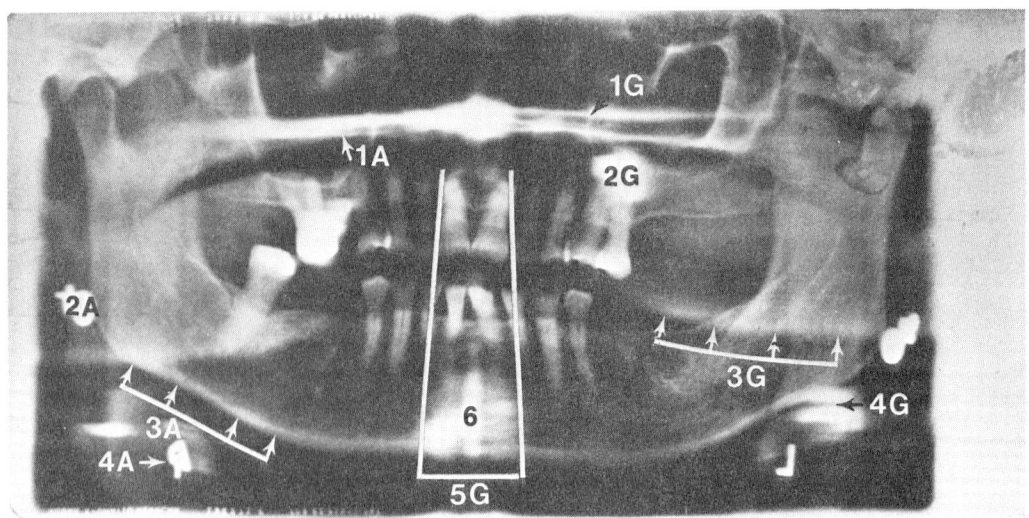

Figure 12-56. Concept 3: Ghost Images: (1A) Actual image of right palate; (1G) Ghost image of right palate; (2A) Actual image of right earring; (2G) Ghost image of right earring; (3A) Actual image of right inferior border of mandible; (3G) Ghost image of right inferior border of mandible; (4A) Actual image of right marker; (4G) Ghost image of right marker; (5G) Ghost image of cervical spine (increased opacity in outlined area); (6) Actual image of incisal guide post (not part of ghost image of cervical spine; occurs when profile index not set on profile index mark of G.E. panelipse).

film twice during one exposure cycle.

Concept 3: Ghost Images Are Formed

Some objects are imaged twice in the panoramic radiograph, in a manner that is different from the previous concept in which double imaging of some midline structures occurs. Ghosting occurs when objects are intercepted twice by the X-Ray beam: once when the object is be-

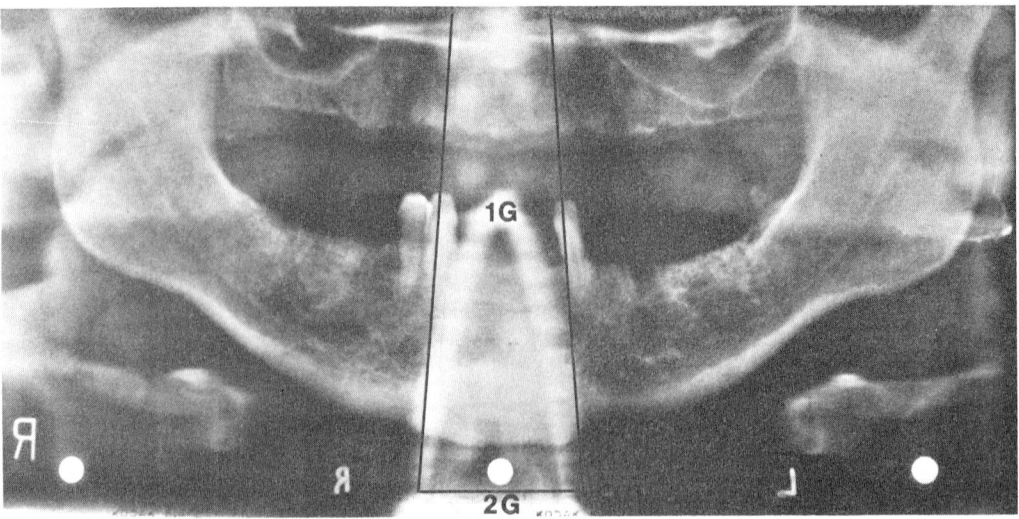

Figure 12-57. Ghost Images: (1G) Ghost image of napkin chain (actual image not seen); (2G) Ghost image of cervical spine (increased band of opacity in midline; actual image not seen).

tween the rotation center and the film, thus producing an actual image, and again when the same object lies between the X-Ray source and the rotation center, thus producing a ghost image. Some structures that are ghosted include the hyoid bone, cervical spine, inferior border of mandible, posterior border of the ramus, the hard palate, and the meati and turbinates. Other objects that may ghost are the chin rest and right and left markers of some machines, as well as earrings, napkin chains, neck chains, and protective aprons.

Ghost images have the following characteristics: The ghost image of a lateral structure is always seen in a location diametrically opposite to the true anatomic position; its outline is more blurred; it is magnified; it is above or superior to the actual image; and the ghost is spread out in exactly the same manner as the actual image. In the latter instance, when an anatomically bilateral structure such as the angle of the mandible is ghosted, the ghosted object resembles a mirror image of the actual image of the contralateral side. For example, the ghosted image of the right angle of the mandible is seen to be partially superimposed upon the left angle of the mandible and resembles a mirror image of the left angle of the mandible. Portions of the object that are narrow in the horizontal dimension will be poorly depicted in the ghost image.

Note the vertical (narrow) portion of the letter L in the ghost image in Figure 12-56 and compare it to the horizontal (wide) portion. The ghosted image is above the actual image because the X-Rays are directed from below and the angle of incidence is greater for objects closer to the X-Ray source. As a result, such objects are projected in a more superior location on the film.

In the machine with the split image mode, there is no ghosting of the cervical

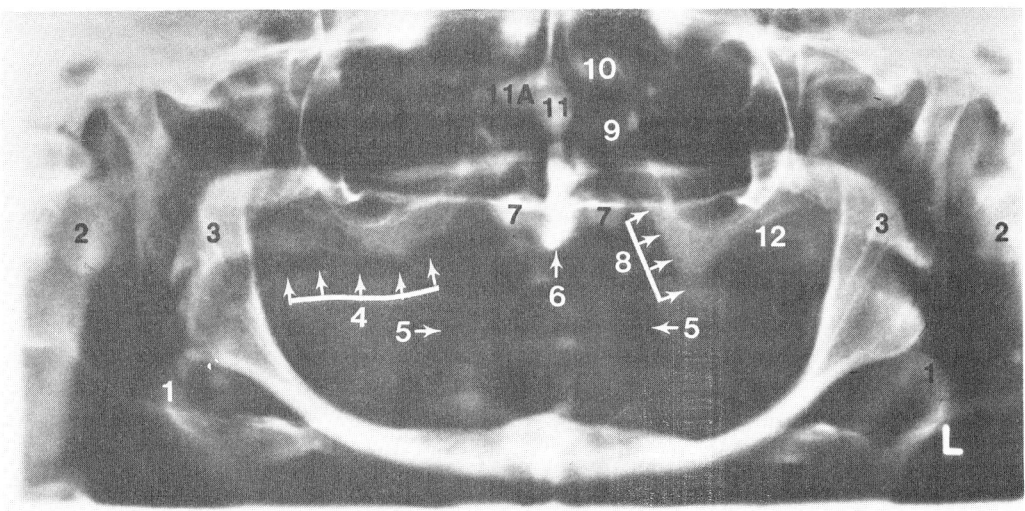

Figure 12-58. Concept 4: Soft tissue Outlines: (1) Epiglottis; (2) Ear lobe; (3) Soft palate; (4) Dorsum of tongue; (5) Upper and lower lips; (6) Tip of nose; (7) Ala of nose; (8) Nasolabial fold; (9) Inferior turbinate; (10) Middle turbinate; (11) Soft tissue of nasal septum (note spreading-out effect on right side); (12) Gingiva at crest of maxillary left ridge.

spine as the machine is designed so that no radiation is emitted when the cervical spine falls within the path of the beam. Ghosting of some structures cannot be avoided, since it results as a part of the design of the machine, particularly the location and path of the center or centers of rotation of the beam. When the cervical spine is ghosted as a vertical radiopacity approximately 2-4 cm wide in the anterior midline, it represents a technique error; when the hyoid bone is ghosted as a horizontal radiopaque line approximately 2 cm wide either below or within the body of the mandible, it represents a technique error.

Earrings should always be removed as the ghost image may be superimposed upon the maxilla or maxillary sinus; neck chains are ghosted in the midline mandibular area; and an improperly positioned shoulder covering of the protective apron may be ghosted onto either side of the midline mandibular region. Earring, neck chain, and apron ghosts represent errors in technique. In some cases, only the ghost image of an object is recorded on the film; examples include ghosts of the cervical spine and earrings.

Concept 4: Soft Tissue Outlines Are Imaged

In the panoramic technic, many soft tissue outlines are imaged. Some of these include the epiglottis, the ear and earlobes, soft palate, dorsum of the tongue, lips, nose, nasolabial fold, and the soft tissue of the nasal turbinates and septum. Additionally, the gingiva particularly at the crest of the ridge in edentulous areas and as the operculum of erupting teeth are also seen. In some instances, visualization of the dorsal aspect of the tongue, soft palate, lips, and nasal turbinates represent errors in technic.

Concept 5: Air Spaces Are Seen

Some of the air spaces that may be seen include those of the naso, oro, and

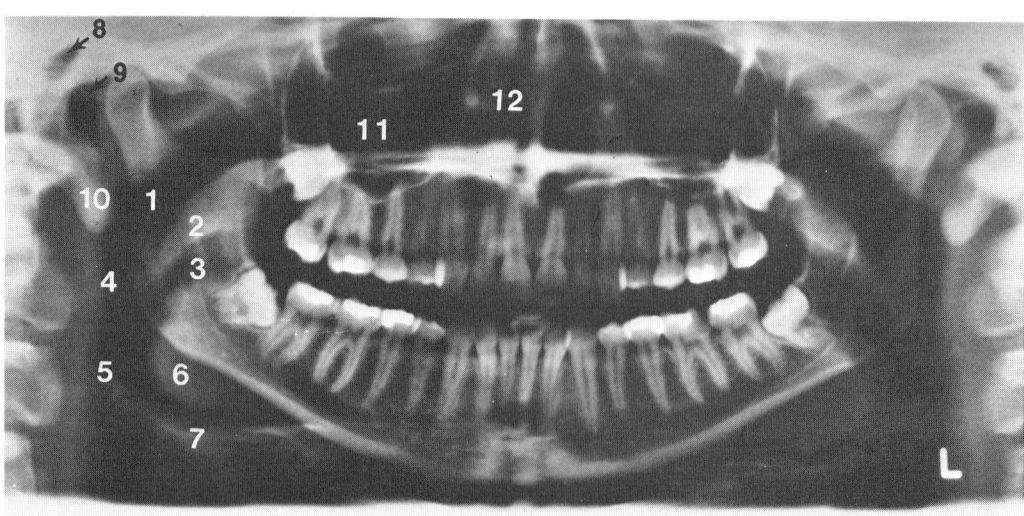

Figure 12-59. Concept 5: Air Spaces: (1) Nasopharyngeal air space; (2) Soft palate; (3) Palato-glossal air space; (4) Oropharynx; (5) Hypopharynx; (6) Base of tongue; (7) Hyoid bone; (8) External auditory meatus; (9) External opening of the ear; (10) Ear lobe; (11) Maxillary sinus; (12) Nasal fossa.

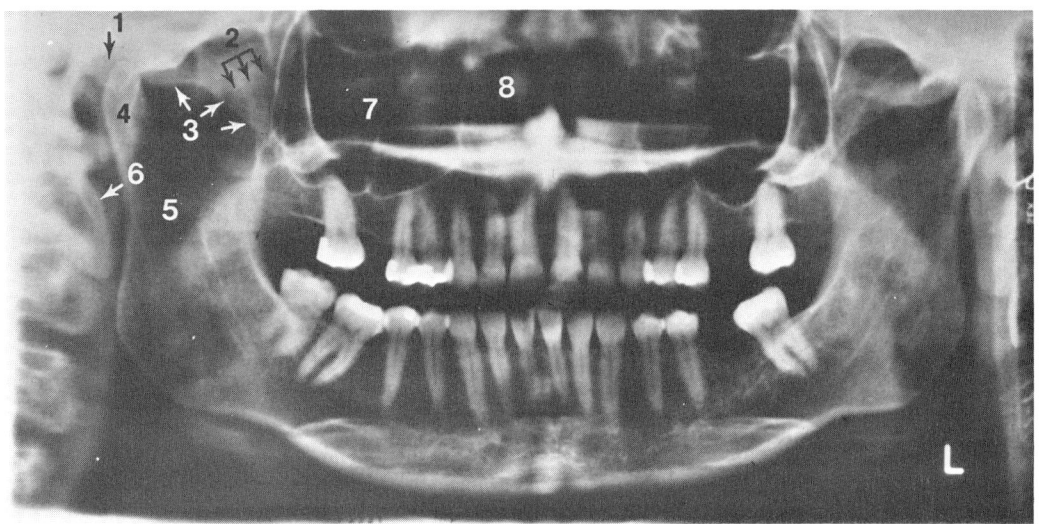

Figure 12-60. Concept 6: Adjacent Areas: (1) Temporomandibular joint; (2) Coronoid process; (3) Zygomatic arch; (4) Condyle; (5) Ramus; (6) Styloid process; (7) Maxillary sinus; (8) Nasal fossa.

hypopharynx, the external auditory canal and mastoid air cells, and the maxillary and ethmoid sinuses. If an air space is seen above the dorsum of the tongue, a technic error has been made. If the air space of the maxillary sinus is obliterated by the soft tissue outlines of the nasal turbinates, a technic error may have been made.

Concept 6: Areas Adjacent to the Tooth-Bearing Portions of the Jaws Are Visualized

A unique advantage of the panoramic image is that all of the teeth as well as many of the structures adjacent to them are seen in the one radiograph. Modern practitioners are no longer satisfied with the limits of periapical intraoral radiography. The teeth or their progenitor tissues may give rise to pathologic processes that primarily affect areas well beyond the periapical region. Additionally, other pathologic processes of nonodontogenic origin well away from the tooth-bearing areas are of interest. Some of these include the temporomandibular joint, coronoid process and upper ramus, the styloid process and calcified stylohyoid or stylomandibular ligaments, the peripheral borders of the body and ramus of the mandible, the maxillary sinus and nasal fossae, the zygomatic arches, and various calcifications such as calcified lymph nodes, sialoliths, tonsillitis, and calcifications of the walls of major vessels such as the common carotid and internal carotid arteries.

Concept 7: Relative Radiolucencies and Radiopacities Are Seen

As we have seen in the previous concepts, a great variety of structures are seen in the panoramic image. Although the hard tissues are flattened and spread out, usually without any superimposition of other hard structures, there is, however, superimposition of soft tissue outlines, ghost images, air spaces, and prostheses. Depending upon the machine used, parts of the apparatus itself such as

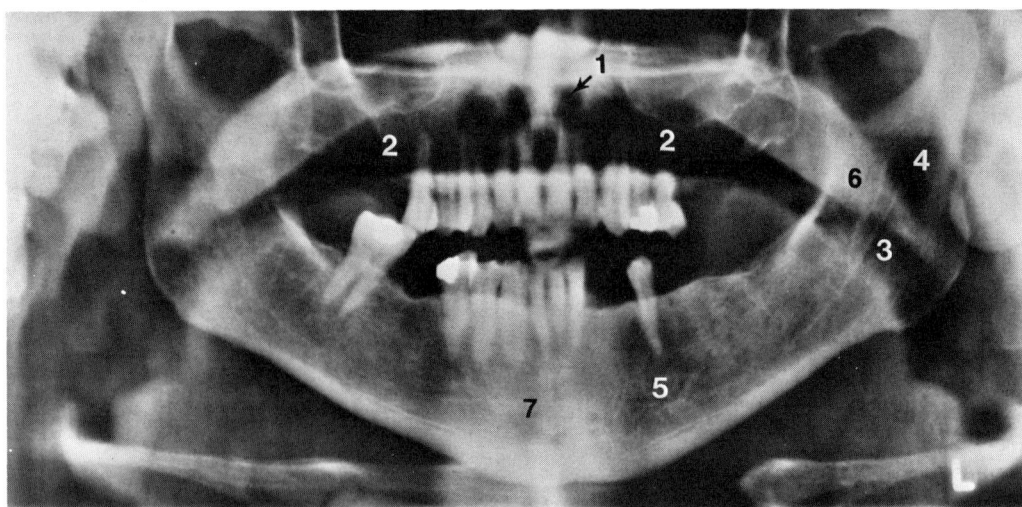

Figure 12-61. Concept 7: Relative Radiolucencies and Radiopacities: (1) Due to the orifice or nares of the nose (mimics periapical radiolucencies); (2) Palatoglossal airspace due to not having tongue against palate during exposure (obliterates apices of all maxillary teeth); (3) Palatoglossal airspace in ramus area; (4) Nasopharyngeal airspace in ramus area; (5) Relative radiolucency in biscuspid area due to diminished soft tissue thickness of the tongue and adjacent ghost image of spine; (6) Relative opacity due to soft palate in ramus area; (7) Relative opacity due to ghost image of cervical spine.

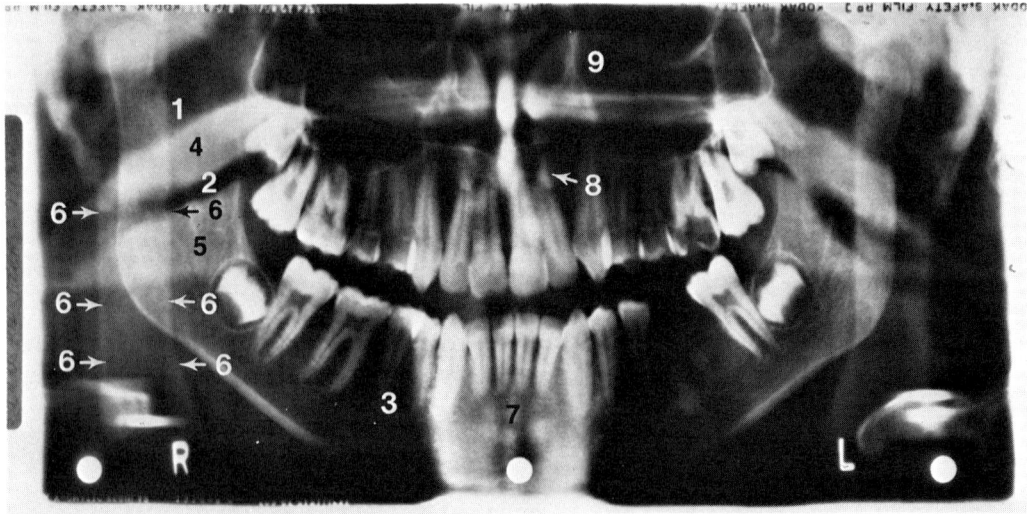

Figure 12-62. Concept 7: Relative Radiolucencies and Radiopacities: *Radiolucencies*: (1) Nasopharyngeal airspace on upper ramus; (2) Palatoglossal airspace on ramus; (3) Mandibular bicuspid burnout due to overexposure contrasted with the attenuation produced in the ghost imaging of the spine. *Radiopacities*: (4) Soft palate on upper ramus; (5) Body of the tongue on ramus; (6) Vertical head positioner; (7) Ghost of cervical spine; (8) Ala of nose (mimics periapical radiopacity); (9) Spreading out of inferior turbinate, occluding portions of the maxillary sinus.

the chin rest, vertical head positioner, or the vertical rod of the incisal bite guide may also be superimposed. These produce a number of relative radiolucencies or radiopacities within the teeth, jaws, and sinuses. These relative density changes may in some instances mimic pathology or even obliterate actual pathology. As outlined in the previous concepts, some of these can be minimized or eliminated by the use of correct technique. Relative density changes are seen in the mandibular bicuspid region, particularly when there is ghosting of the cervical spine; in the mandibular third molar region, particularly when there is ghosting of the contralateral mandible and chin rest; in the mandibular ramus when the pharyngeal air spaces are prominent; in the apical region of all of the maxillary teeth, particularly where the palatoglossal airspace is present because the tongue was not held tight against the hard palate; in the maxillary canine region when the nasolabial fold is prominent; and in the maxillary sinus when the nasal conchi are spread out. There are a great many other differences in density in the structures seen in the panoramic image. This concept deals with the main relative density changes that should be recognized and separated from pathologic change.

Chapter 13

DEVELOPMENTAL AND ACQUIRED ANOMALIES OF TEETH AND JAWS

Alterations in Tooth Morphology

Macrodontia and Microdontia

MACRODONTIA means teeth that are larger than normal. The condition may affect all of the teeth as may be seen in the pituitary giant or it may involve one or several teeth. The term macrodontia should not be applied to teeth that are enlarged due to magnification, gemination, or fusion. Relative macrodontia occurs when the teeth appear to be overly large due to micrognathia, where the jaws are too small to accommodate the teeth.

Microdontia means teeth that are smaller than normal. This condition is much more common than macrodontia. Microdontia may affect all of the teeth as may be seen in the pituitary dwarf. Relative microdontia occurs when the teeth appear to be too small to fill all of the space provided by the jaws. Microdontia of one or several teeth is more common than the generalized form. The most commonly affected teeth are the maxillary permanent lateral incisors, sometimes known as peg laterals, and the third molars. Peg laterals are usually cone shaped

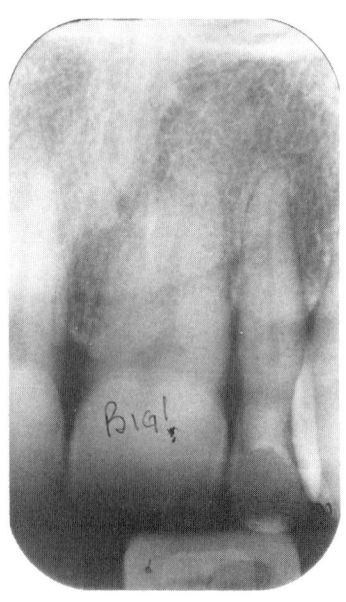

Figure 13-1. Macrodontia of the maxillary left central incisor.

and the condition is often bilateral and familial in occurrence. Cone-shaped microdontic teeth and many missing teeth are also seen in hereditary anhydrotic ectodermal dysplasia, chondroectodermal dysplasia, and incontinentia pigmenti. Often supernumerary teeth are microdontic. Microdontia may also be seen in teeth that received therapeutic doses of radiation (radiation therapy) during development.

Gemination (Schizodonitism)

Gemination consists of an aborted attempt by a single tooth bud to divide. It most frequently affects anterior teeth, particularly in the primary dentition. In gemination, the total number of teeth in the arch is normal. Radiographically, the crown is usually enlarged, and the incisal edge may be notched. The pulp chamber is often Y-shaped with two coronal portions and a single root canal space.

Fusion (Synodontism)

Fusion occurs as a result of the union of two adjacent tooth buds, by dentin

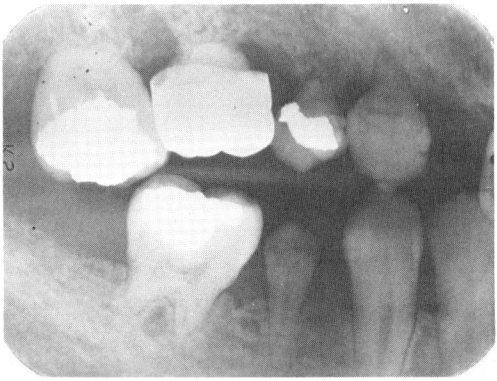

Figure 13-3. Microdontia, due to retarded development as a result of radiation therapy to the maxillary sinus at the age of twenty months. (Courtesy of Dr. Ivan Stangel, Montreal, Canada; and W.B. Saunders Co., Philadelphia, PA.)

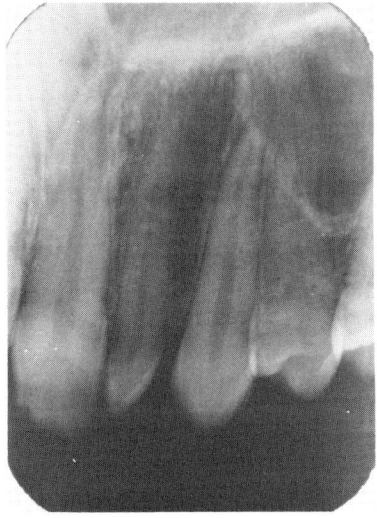

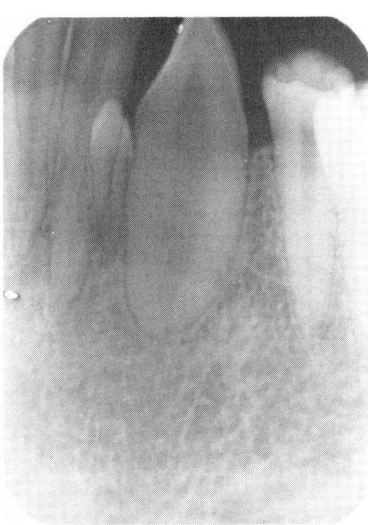

Figure 13-2. Microdontia. **(A)** Involving the lateral incisor, known as "peg laterals." **(B)** Involving a supernumerary mandibular cuspid.

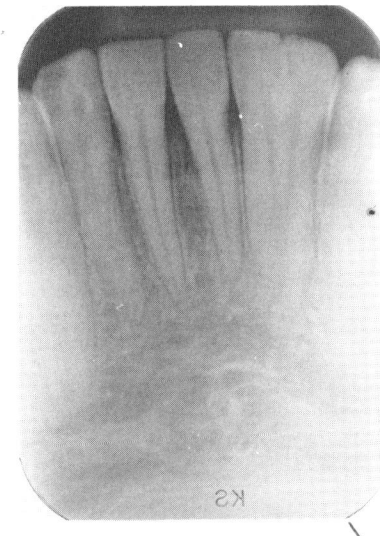

Figure 13-4. Gemination.

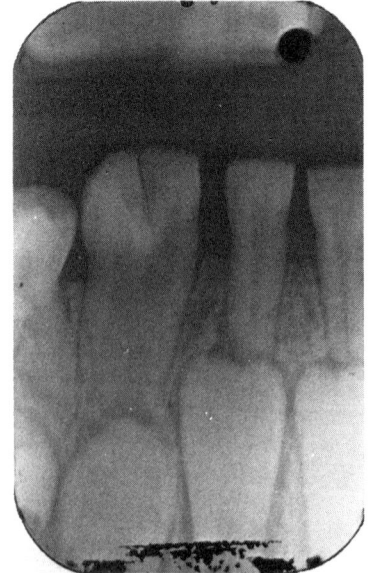

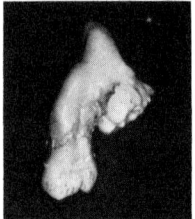

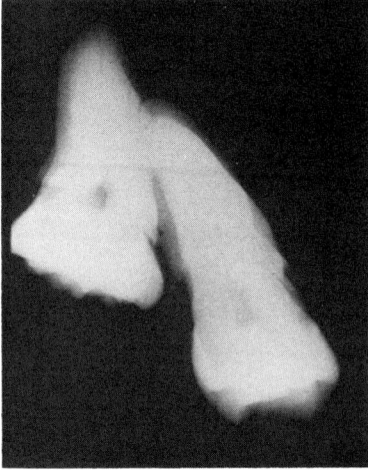

Figure 13-6. Concresence. (A) Gross specimen. (B) Radiograph of the same specimen.

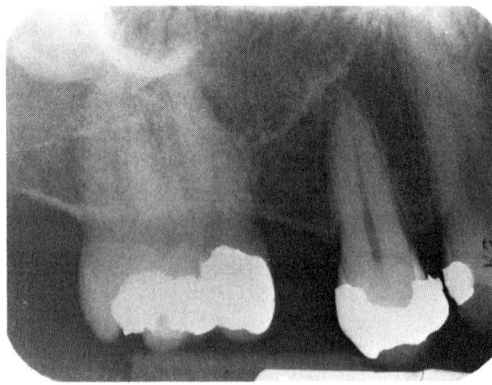

Figure 13-5. Fusion. (A) Between the primary lateral incisor and cuspid. (B) Between two permanent posterior teeth.

and/or enamel. If fusion occurs between two normal teeth, a reduced number of teeth will be present in the arch. If the union is between a normal tooth and a supernumerary tooth, the distinction between fusion and gemination may be impossible. Fusion occurs mainly in the anterior region, particularly in the primary dentition. The most reliable radiographic sign of this condition is seen when two separate root canal spaces and pulp chambers are seen.

Concresence

Concresence occurs when there is a union between the roots of two or more teeth by cementum only. In true concresence the union occurs during root development and/or eruption. In acquired concresence, the cemental union occurs after the completion of root formation, often as a result of hypercementosis.

Dilaceration

Dilaceration is a bent tooth. The root is most frequently involved, and it usually develops as a result of mechanical trauma during root formation and/or eruption. Some common causes include mechanical blockage of the path of eruption by the presence of neoplasms, cysts, supernumerary teeth, or orthodontic treatment. Dilaceration may occur at any location along the root.

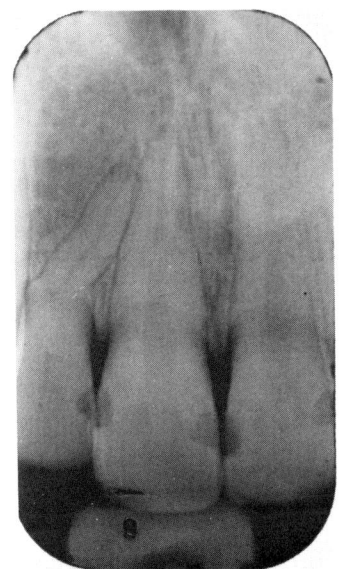

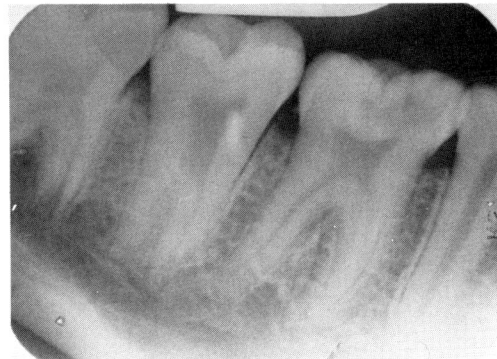

Figure 13-9. Taurodontism — mandibular second molar.

Taurodontism

Taurodontism refers to teeth that have an abnormally large pulp chamber and shortened roots. The condition often affects molar teeth and clinically the teeth appear normal. The pulp chamber appears rectangular in shape and lacks the usual constriction at the cervix. The roots are usually very short, although the overall length of the tooth is invariably normal.

Supernumerary Roots

Extra or supernumerary roots may occur on any tooth, but they are more frequently seen in mandibular permanent bicuspids and canines. Radiographic signs of supernumerary roots include a double periodontal membrane space on one side of the root; the periodontal membrane space crossing a root; an abrupt diminution in size of the root canal space with branching producing an inverted-Y shape of the apical portion of the root canal space.

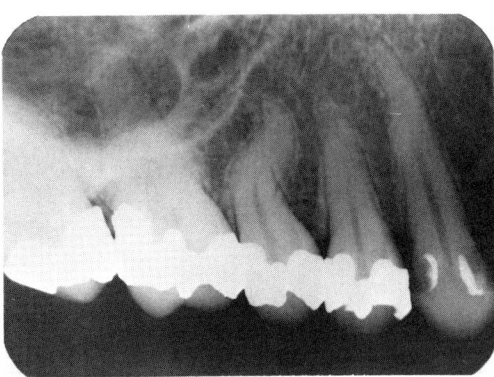

Figure 13-7. Dilaceration. (A) In a maxillary lateral incisor (B) In a maxillary second bicuspid.

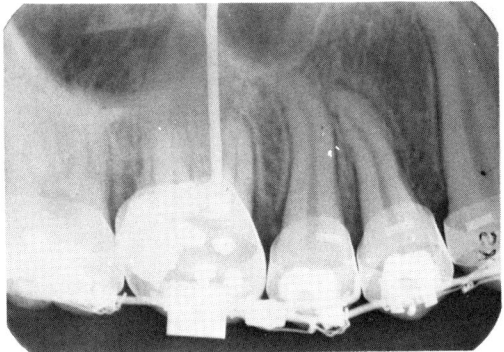

Figure 13-8. Dilaceration. This may have developed in association with the orthodontic treatment.

Enamel Pearls (Enameloma)

Enamel pearls consist of small round or ovoid radiopacities seen in the cervical portion of teeth, often molars. They are usually well defined and show the same degree of radiopacity as enamel. They may be superimposed upon the pulp

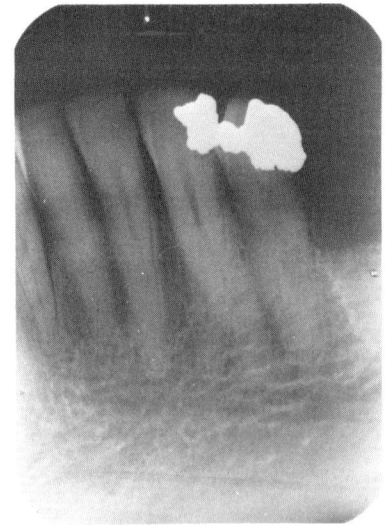

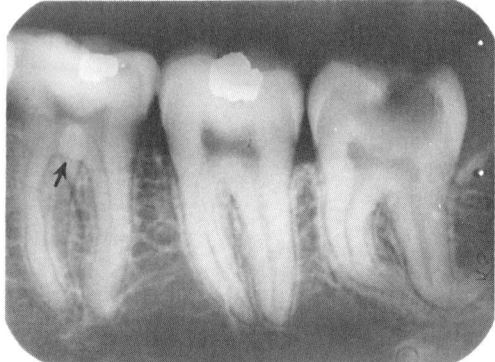

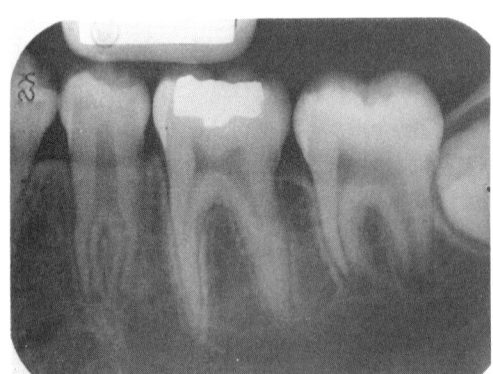

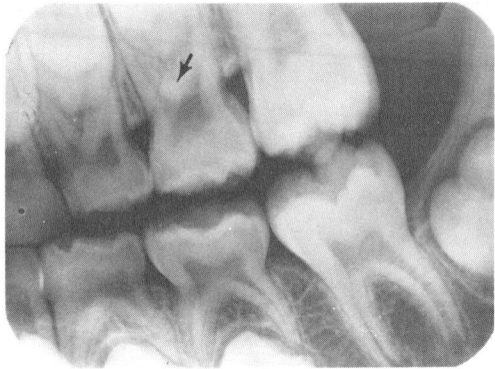

Figure 13-11. Enamel pearl. **(A)** On a permanent tooth. **(B)** On a primary tooth.

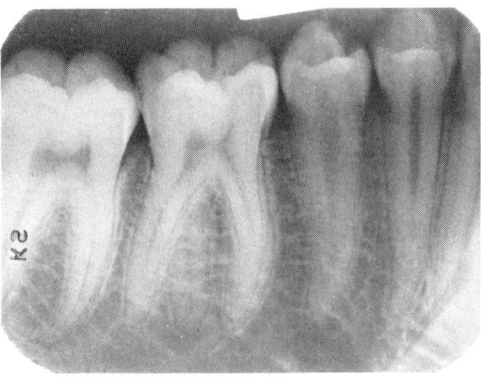

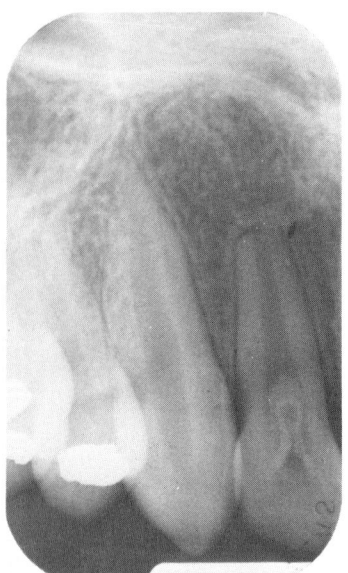

Figure 13-10. Supernumerary roots. **(A)** Note that the cuspid shows the periodontal membrane crossing the roots and inverted "Y" shape of the root canal space. The lateral incisor may also have a supernumerary root. **(B)** Developing supernumerary root. **(C)** In a mandibular first molar.

Figure 13-12. Dens in Dente.

chamber of affected teeth and may be mistaken for pulpal calcifications. Since the enamel pearl is on the outside of the tooth, it will move away from the pulp chamber when off angle views are taken, while pulp stones always remain within the confines of the pulp chamber or root canal space when supplemental views are taken.

Dens Invaginatus (Dens in Dente)

Dens invaginatus is a variation that arises as a result of an invagination or infolding of the tooth's surface prior to calcification. This condtion most frequently affects the coronal portion of permanent lateral incisors, may occur bilaterally, and is seen in 1-5 percent of the population. The invagination produces a deep lingual pit and the underlying pulp is more susceptible to exposure by caries or mechanically in the preparation of the tooth. Radiographically, a characteristic tear drop or hour glass shaped radiopaque line may be seen, with or without a thin layer of dentin beneath. There is often evidence of carious penetration of the base of the invaginated enamel and varying degrees of periapical disease of pulpal origin at the apex of the tooth.

Alterations in the Numbers of Teeth

Anodontia and Hypodontia (Oligodontia)

Anodontia means that all of the teeth are missing. In true anodontia, all of the teeth fail to develop, and this is an extremely rare occurrence. Acquired anodontia is very common and results from the extraction of all of the teeth.

Hypodontia means that one or several, but not all, teeth are missing. The most common congenitally missing permanent teeth are the third molars. Others include the premolars and maxillary lateral incisors. When the second premolars are missing, a submerged, ankylosed primary molar is sometimes present. As soon as the diagnosis of congenitally missing lateral and or central incisors is made, the child should be referred to an opthalmologist to test for Reiger's syndrome in which congenital glaucoma is a prominent feature. Early diagnosis and treatment may

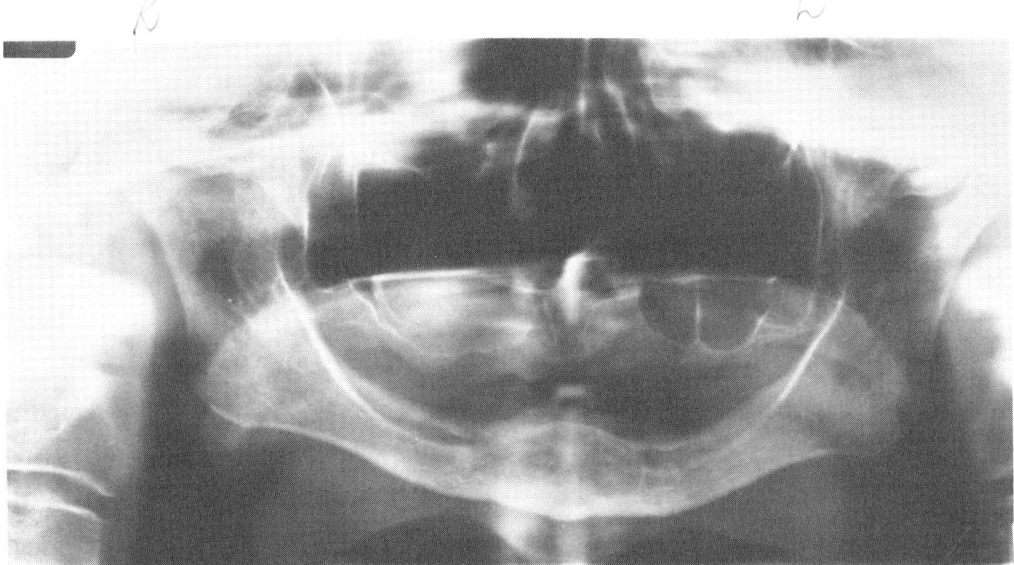

Figure 13-13. Acquired anodontia. The radiopacity in the right maxillary sinus was an extrinsic cyst of odontogenic origin.

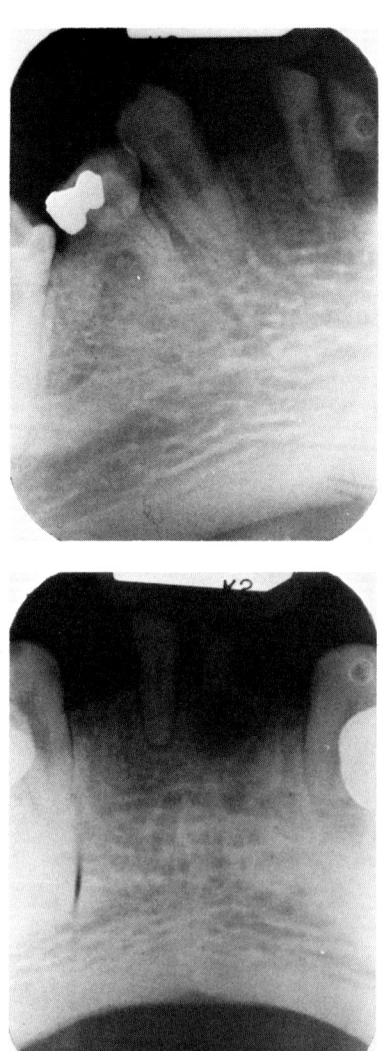

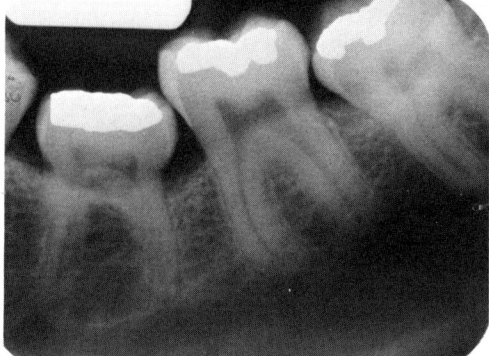

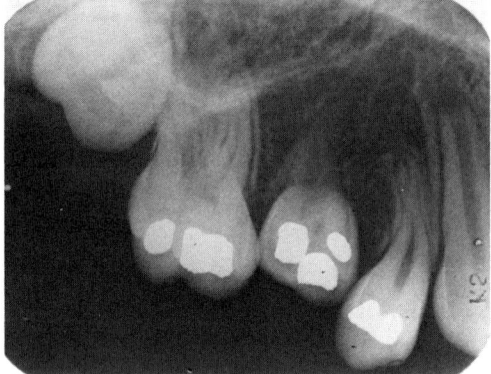

Figure 13-15. Hypondontia: **(A)** Of the mandibular second bicuspid producing a submerged and partly ankylosed primary molar. **(B)** Of the maxillary second bicuspid. Note the dilaceration of the adjacent first bicuspid.

Figure 13-14. **(A & B).** Hypodontia of multiple permanent teeth.

prevent blindness, which usually develops before the age of ten years. Other conditions associated with hypodontia are hereditary anhydrotic ectodermal dysplasia, chondroectodermal dysplasia, and incontinentia pigmenti.

Hyperdontia (Supernumerary Teeth)

Hyperdontia refers to one or more extra teeth. Hyperdontia affects males more frequently than females and occurs in as much as 3.5 percent of some population samples. Approximately 90 percent of all supernumerary teeth occur in the maxilla, particularly in the midline. The most common extra tooth is the maxillary mesiodens. Others include upper fourth molars and mandibular premolars. Upper fourth molars may resemble other maxillary molars or they may be small and conical in shape. These microdontic fourth molars are referred to as distomolars when they are distal to the third molar in location, or as paramolars when they are seen buccal or palatal to the maxillary molars.

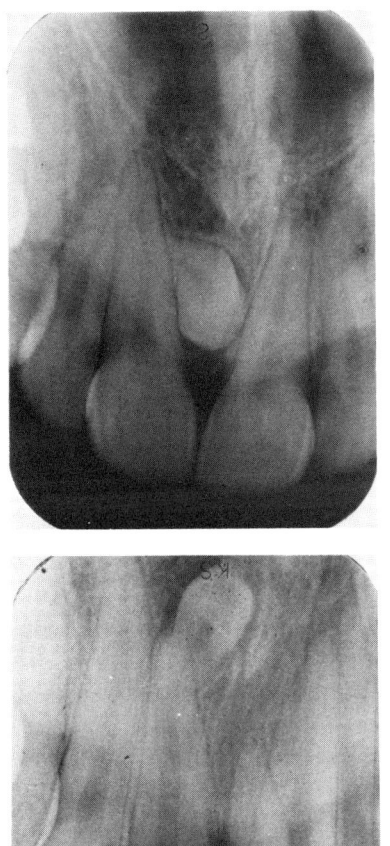

Figure 13-16. Hyperdontia. (A) Mesiodens. (B) Bilateral or double mesiodens formation.

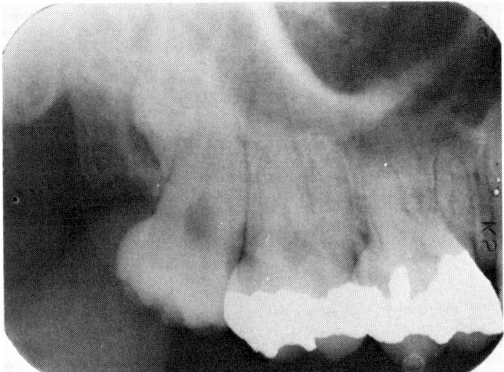

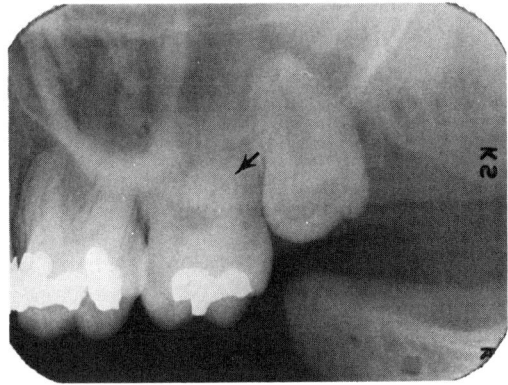

Figure 13-17. Hyperdontia. (A) Distomolar. (B) Paramolar. — Bu or Li location of extra molar

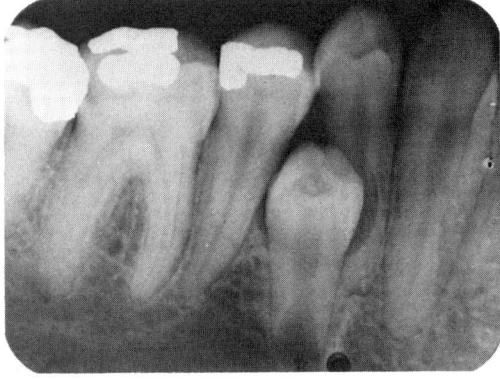

Figure 13-18. Hyperdontia — mandibular bicuspid.

Other conditions characterized by the presence of hyperdontia are cleidocranial dysplasia and Gardner's syndrome. In cleidocranial dysplasia there may also be delayed eruption of the permanent teeth, and the patient may be able to bring his/her shoulders together due to deficient or absent clavicles. In Gardner's syndrome, there may also be delayed eruption of some permanent teeth due to the presence of osteomas in the jaws and malignant intestinal polyposis may develop by the age of thirty years. Thus, the examination of siblings and genetic counseling may be beneficial for those who are affected by this hereditary condition.

Alterations of Tooth Structure

Enamel Hypoplasia

Enamel hypoplasia is an incomplete or defective formation of the organic enamel matrix of the teeth. This causes defects on the surface of the enamel that may range from a white spot to a more severe and generalized mottling, pitting, and grooving. Some specific forms of enamel hypoplasia due to various other causes in- and mulberry molars associated with congenital syphilis; mottled enamel due to fluorosis; Turner's hypoplasia due to trauma or local inflammation such as an abscessed primary molar; and enamel hypoplasia due to various other causes including nutritional deficiencies and high fevers. In many cases, the condition remains unexplained and is referred to as idiopathic.

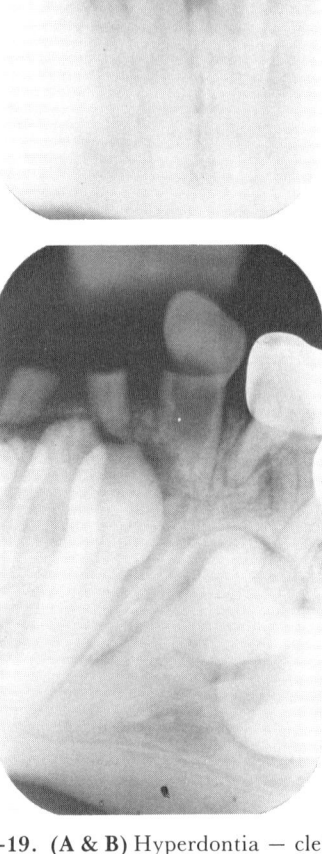

Figure 13-19. (A & B) Hyperdontia — cleidocranial dysplasia. (B) Note the toothbrush abrasion and internal resorption on the primary cuspid of this adult patient.

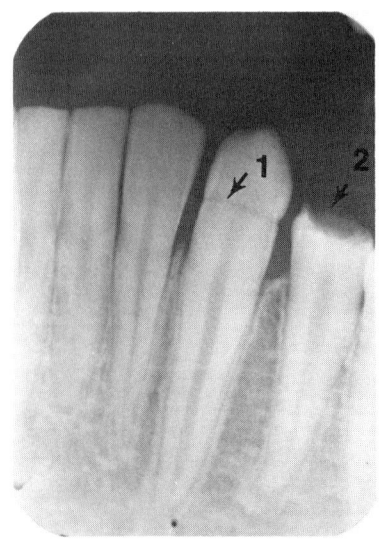

Figure 13-20. Enamel hypoplasia. (1) Linear or grooved type. (2) Turner type.

Amelogenesis Imperfecta

Amelogenesis imperfecta is a hereditary hypoplasia of the enamel that is transmitted as an autosomal dominant trait. There are two types of amelogenesis imperfecta: the hypoplastic type is characterized by the presence of a thin layer of normal enamel about the crowns of all of the teeth; the hypomineralized type consists of a normal amount of enamel that is poorly mineralized. In the latter type, the enamel may be pitted or chalky and tends to fracture. There is usually a greater resistance to caries than in normal teeth.

Dentinogenesis Imperfecta

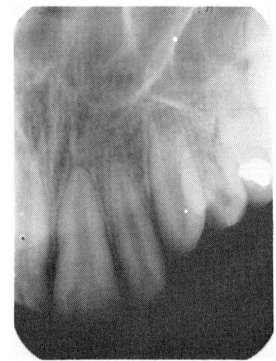

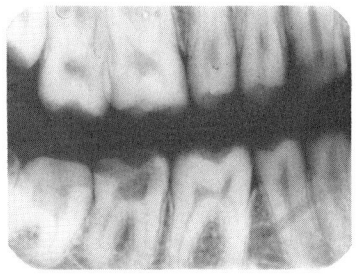

Figure 13-21. Amelogenesis imperfecta.

Dentinogenesis imperfecta is a hereditary disorder of dentin that is transmitted as an autosomal dominant trait. The dentin as well as the dentinoenamel junction are affected. Thus the teeth have a yellowish grey opalescent sheen and the enamel has a tendency to chip away. The condition may be associated with osteogenesis imperfecta, in which case there will be a history of susceptibility to fracture of the long bones, possible deformities due to multiple fractures, and blue sclera or "white of the eyes." The radiographic features of dentinogenesis imperfecta include enamel fractures, root fracture, bulbous crowns, shorter tapered roots, early obliteration of the root canal space, and normal susceptibility to caries. Dentinogenesis imperfecta is a generalized condition affecting all of the teeth including the primary and permanent denitions.

Acquired Defects of Teeth

Attrition

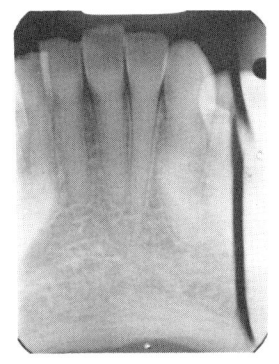

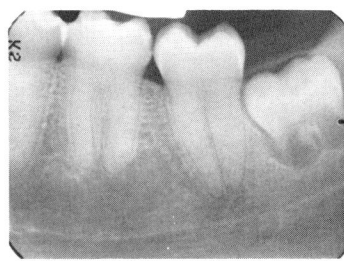

Figure 13-22. Dentinogenesis imperfecta.

Attrition is the physiologic wearing away of tooth structure as a result of normal function. Attrition that is confined to a single tooth or groups of teeth and that is caused by an abnormal function or position of the teeth is referred to as severe or pathologic attrition. Attrition most commonly affects the incisal or occlusal surfaces. It is also seen on the interproximal surfaces at the contact points. Pathologic attrition may be seen on the labial aspect of the maxillary central incisors in some patients with an Angle Class 3 malocclusion; it also on the labial surfaces of the mandibular incisors in some Angle Class 2 Division 2 malocclusions.

Radiographically, attrition is characterized by a flattening of the involved surfaces causing the teeth to appear worn down.

Abrasion

Abrasion is the pathologic wearing

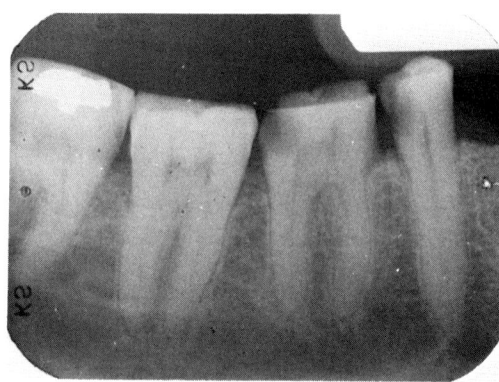

Figure 13-24. Attrition — posterior teeth

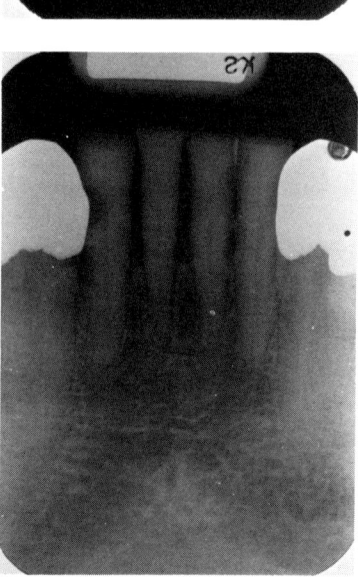

Figure 13-23. Attrition — anterior teeth. (A) Maxillary incisors (B) Mandibular incisors.

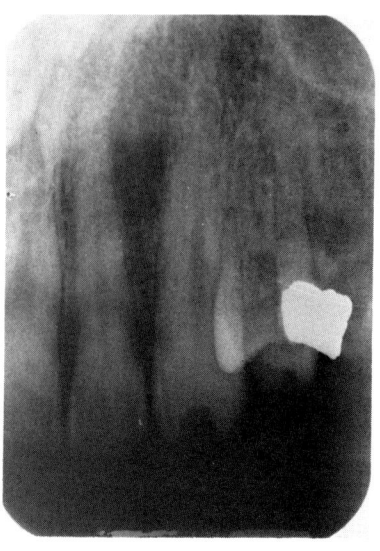

Figure 13-25. Occupational abrasion: bobby pin abrasion

Developmental and Acquired Anomalies of Teeth and Jaws 423

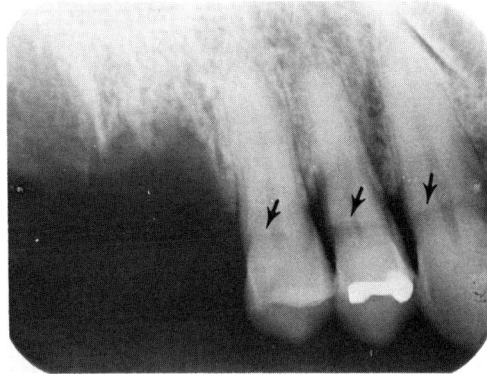

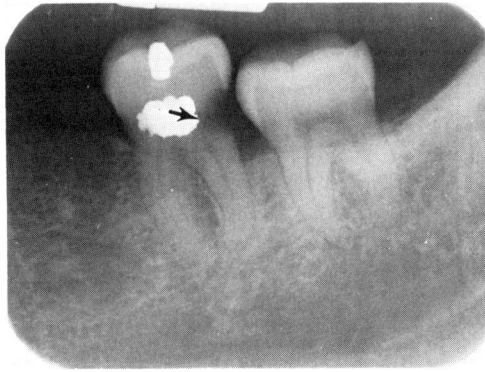

Figure 13-26. Habitual abrasion: **(A)** toothbrush abrasion; **(B)** toothpick abrasion.

away of tooth structure by a mechanical process or by the abrasive action of substances other than food. Some types of abrasion follow. Occupational abrasion is seen in seamstresses and tailors who hold needles and pins between their anterior teeth, hairdressers who use their teeth to open hairpins or bobby pins, shoemakers and carpenters who hold nails between their teeth, and others including glassblowers, musicians, sandblasters and farmers (dust).

Habitual abrasion is seen in pipe smokers, from opening hairpins, and from toothbrush and toothpick misuse. Clasp abrasion is caused by poorly designed removable partial denture clasps. Ritual abrasions are mostly seen in third world rural population groups.

Radiographically, the appearance varies greatly with the cause. Hairpins, nails, needles, and the like produce notched areas on the incisal edges. Pipe smoking, glass blowing, and the like produce an uneven wear pattern conforming to the shape of the object being held. Sandblasters and farmers may show an inordinate

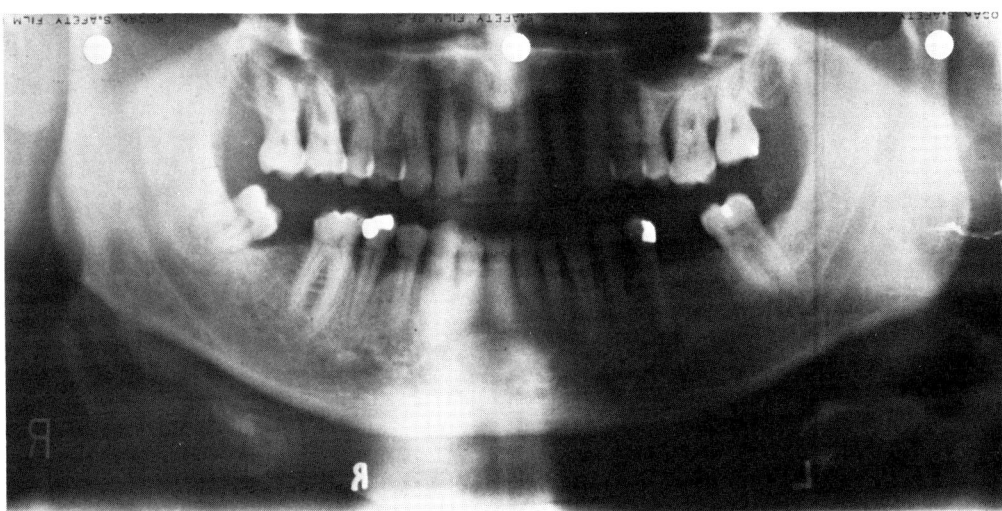

Figure 13-27. Toothbrush abrasion as seen on a panoramic radiograph. Note the prominent radiolucent lines at the cervical area of most of the mandibular teeth.

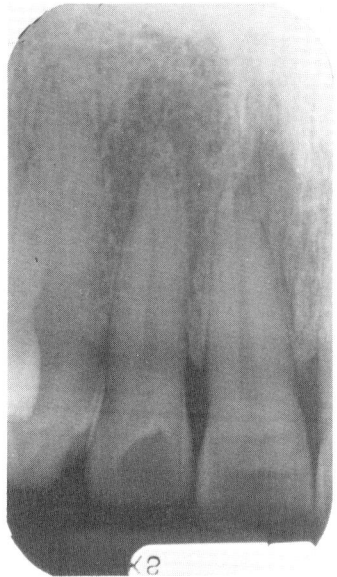

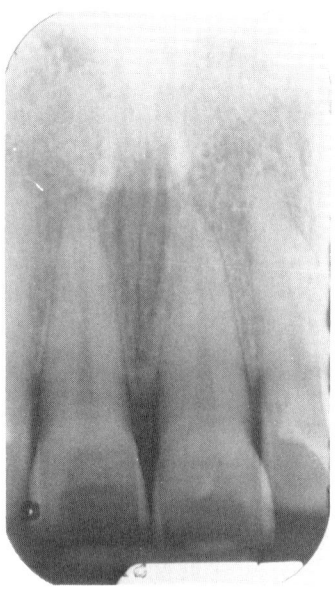

Figure 13-28. (A & B) Erosion. Note that erosion does not usually show prominent changes radiographically. The crown may be slightly less opaque. The horizontal radiolucent lines are seen in lemon sucking. The underlying dentin is more susceptible to toothbrush abrasion due to the erosion of the enamel.

degree of wear for their chronologic age due to the constant presence of grit in the mouth. In toothpick abrasion, the abnormal wear usually occurs beneath the contact points. Toothbrush abrasion produces a characteristic pattern in which there is a well-demarcated horizontal radiolucent line crossing the cervical area and is sometimes V-shaped in certain radiographic views.

Erosion

Erosion is the loss of tooth substance by a chemical process. Clinically, the teeth appear smooth and glistening and the underlying yellowish dentin may be exposed and sensitive, particularly to temperature changes. There may be a history of difficulty in retaining restorations. Known causes include chronic vomiting as in bulemia; chronic regurgitation as in hyatal hernia; excessive intake of acidic carbonated soft drinks; habitual lemon sucking; acidic medications such as dilute hypochloric acid and some iron preparations; and occupations in industries using acid. The radiographic findings are essentially nonspecific in most instances, although the crowns of the teeth may appear slightly more radiolucent than normal.

Retained Root Fragments

Retained root tips are usually well-demarcated by a periodontal membrane space and contain a root canal space within them. This helps to distinguish this condition from sclerotic bone in which these features are absent. Retained root fragments may appear to be floating entirely within soft tissue; may be partially embedded in alveolar bone; or may be completely surrounded by bone. They may also be seen within the maxillary sinus. A peculiar developmental pattern of retained root tips may be seen in association with second premolars in which the root tips of the primary teeth are retained, sometimes in all four quadrants in the same individual.

Foreign Bodies

When foreign bodies are metallic in nature they are easy to detect. The most common of these is probably amalgam fragments that fall into the socket of a tooth during extraction, or minute shavings that are implanted into the gingiva during the preparation of teeth with large amalgam restorations. Others include implants, bullet and shrapnel fragments, pellets from various types of firearms and air guns, and broken dental instruments or burrs. Occasionally, foreign bodies cannot be seen radiographically; some of

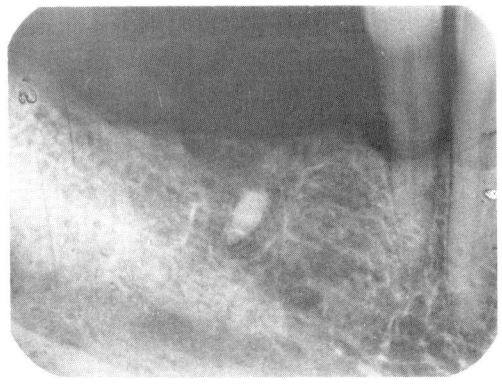

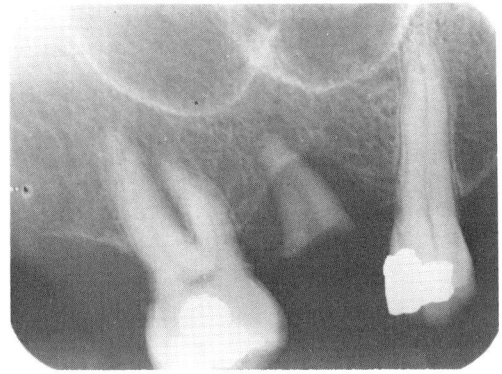

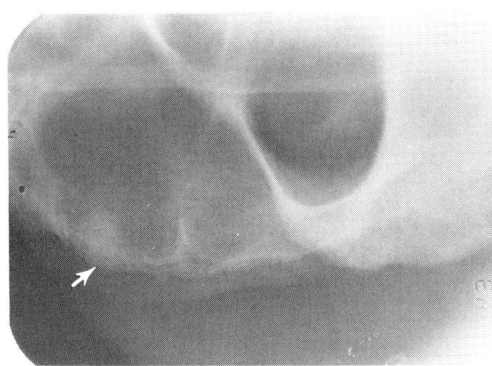

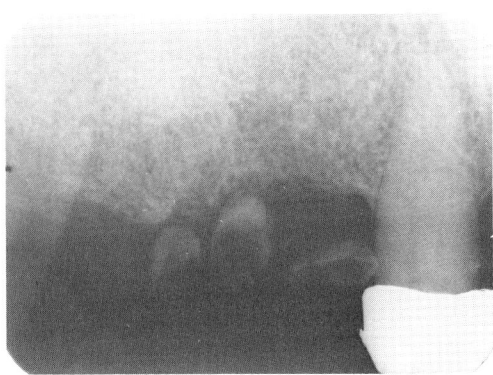

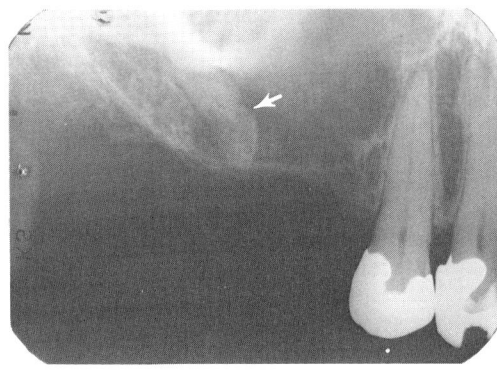

Figure 13-29. Retained root tips. **(A)** Entirely embedded in bone. **(B)** Partially embedded in bone. **(C)** "Floating" entirely within soft tissue.

Figure 13-30. Retained root tips. **(A)** Approximating the maxillary sinus. **(B)** Within the maxillary sinus.

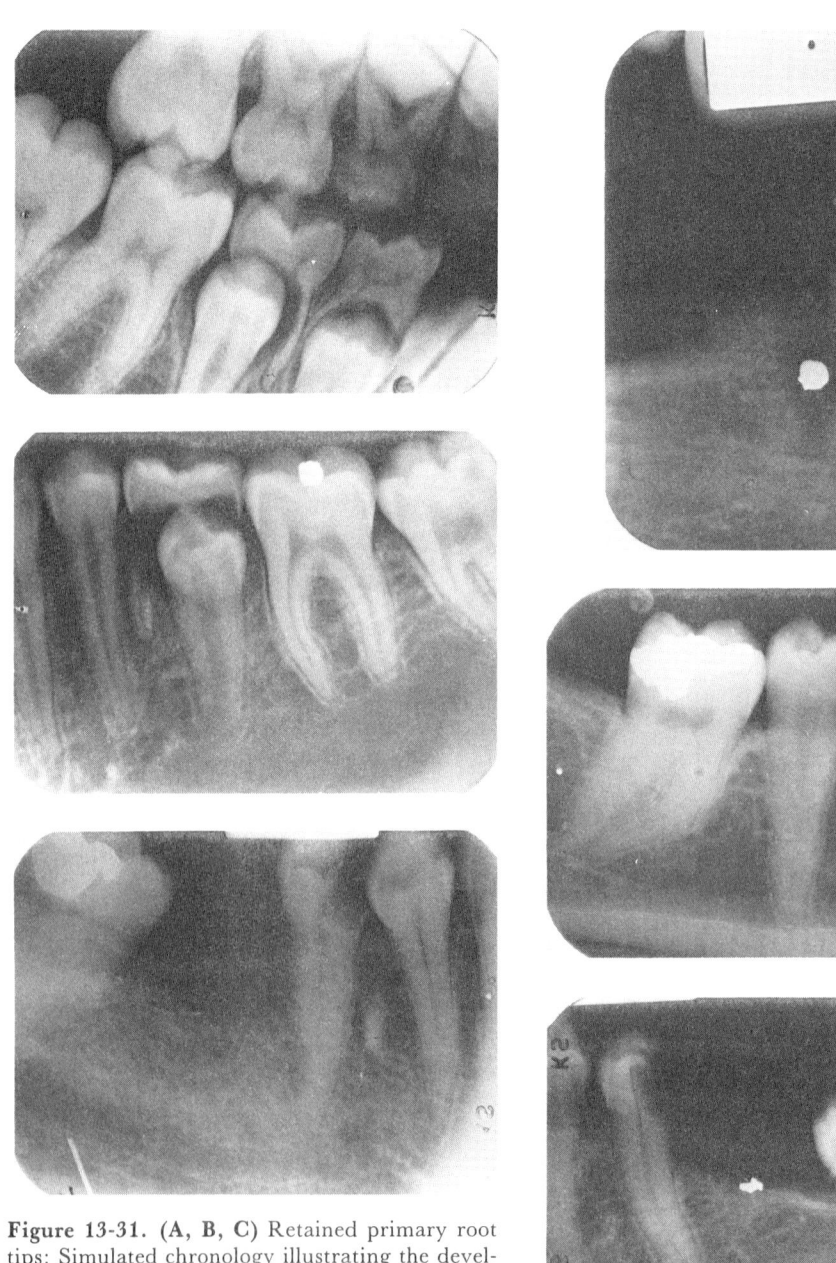

Figure 13-31. (A, B, C) Retained primary root tips: Simulated chronology illustrating the development of this condition, using three different patients.

Figure 13-32. (A, B, C) Foreign body — amalgam. Simulated chronology illustrating the development of an amalgam tattoo using three different patients. (A) Fragment falls into extraction socket. (B) Fragment within area of healed socket. (C) Fragment at crest of ridge due to bone loss.

Developmental and Acquired Anomalies of Teeth and Jaws

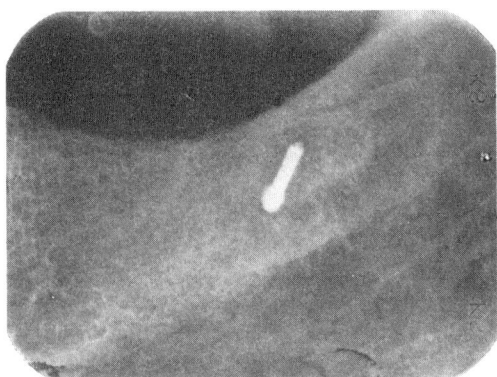

Figure 13-33. Foreign body — broken dental instrument.

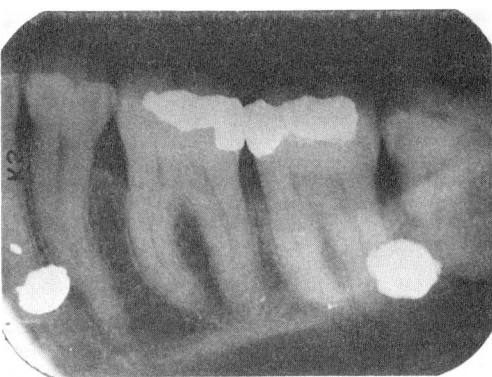

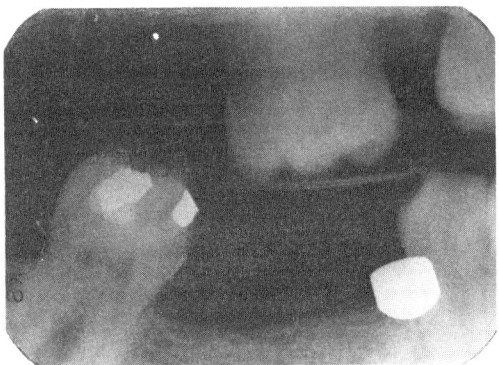

Figure 13-34. Soft tissue foreign bodies. **(A)** Several shotgun pellets contained entirely within soft tissue overlying the mandible. **(B)** Air gun pellet contained within the cheek for thirty-five years, prior to removal.

these include histoacryl bonding material, carberundum implants, acrylic, and unleaded glass.

Alterations in the Eruption of Teeth

Drift and Migration

Drift refers to the movement of an erupted tooth when either mesial or distal contact is lost. Distal drift is the most common and is frequently seen in mandibular second bicuspids.

Migration refers to an abnormal movement of an unerupted tooth. It may occur in a mesial or distal direction and is seen more frequently in the mandible. Migrated teeth usually remain embedded within the jaw.

Translocation (Transposition) and Ectopic Eruption

Translocation or transposition occurs when a tooth erupts into the normal position of another or where there is an interchange of position between two teeth. Since the translocated teeth occupy normal positions within the arch, crowding is often absent, and the curvature of the

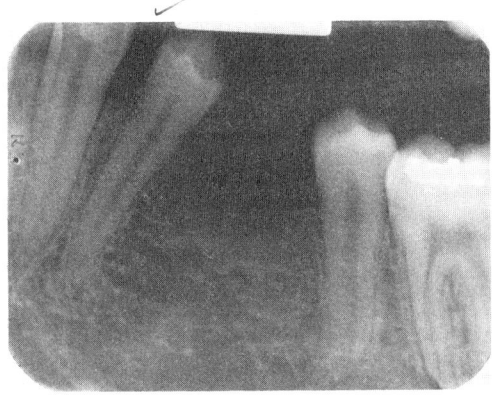

Figure 13-35. Distal drift — mandibular second bicuspid.

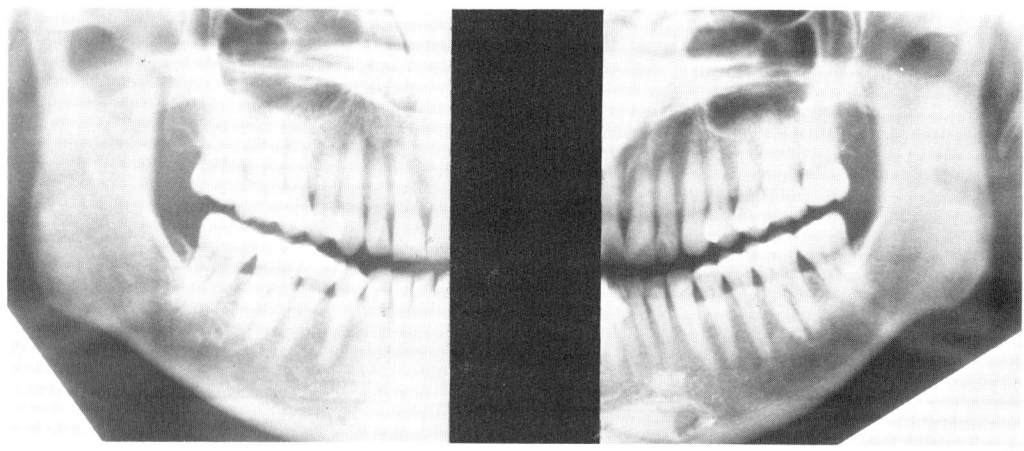

Figure 13-36. Migration — mandibular right cuspid.

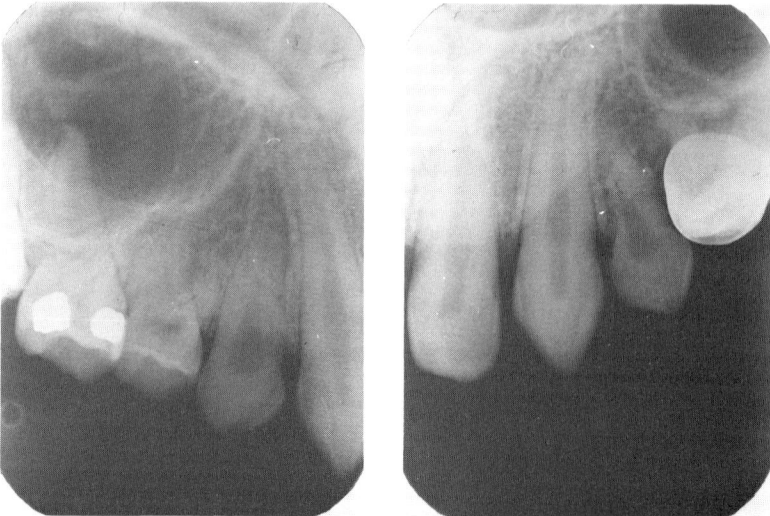

Figure 13-37. (A & B) Bilateral transposition of the permanent canines due to congenitally missing lateral incisors. Rule out the presence of Reiger's syndrome. Note the retained primary cuspids and primary molars.

arch remains normal.

Ectopic eruption refers to the eruption of a tooth into an abnormal position in the arch. In this instance there may be crowding and the wayward tooth may be located in a buccal or lingual position, producing a disruption of the even curvature of the arch.

Alterations of the Jaws

Mandibular Tori

Mandibular tori are bony protuberances that occur on the lingual aspect of the mandible in the cuspid-premolar region. They occur in approximately 25 percent of adults and affect males and females equally. Radiographically, they are seen as single or multiple well-defined radiopacities, usually superimposed on the roots of the canines or premolars. They are often round or ovoid in shape. Although usually well demarcated, they lack a radiolucent peripheral outline separating them from the surrounding structures. They are most often bilateral.

Maxillary Torus

Maxillary tori are a type of exostosis or bony outgrowth that occurs in the midline of the palate in approximately 40 percent of all adults. They are seen more frequently in females and may be lobulated. They may be seen as well-defined radiopaque structures in the apical area of the maxillary anterior views and within the maxillary sinus of maxillary posterior views. On occasion, they may contain laminations representing successive layers of new bone deposition.

Cleft Palate

Cleft palate may also be associated with clefting of the lip, soft palate, and uvula. They may be unilateral or bilateral. Often the cleft is seen in the maxillary lateral incisor region. Sometimes a

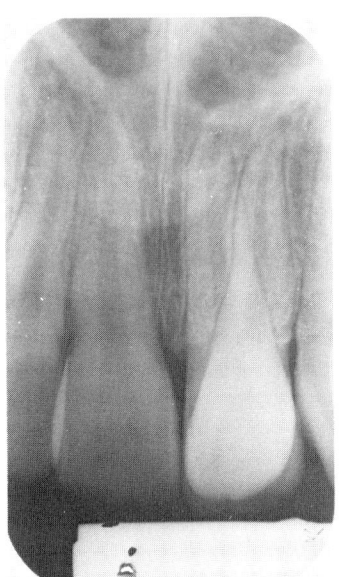

Figure 13-38. Ectopic eruption of the maxillary lateral incisor.

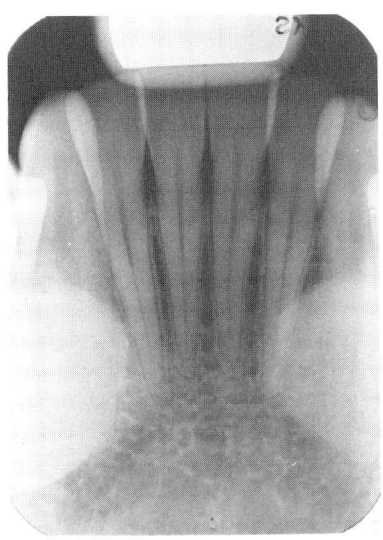
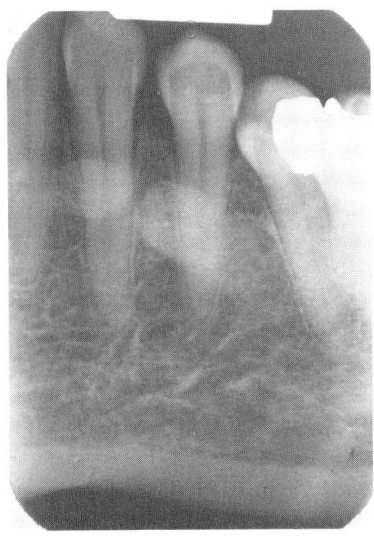

Figure 13-39. Mandibular tori. **(A)** Bilateral. **(B)** Bi-lobed.

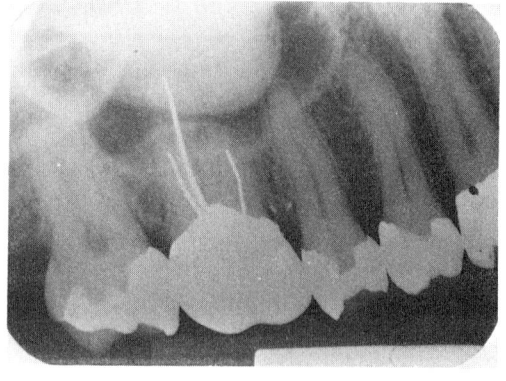

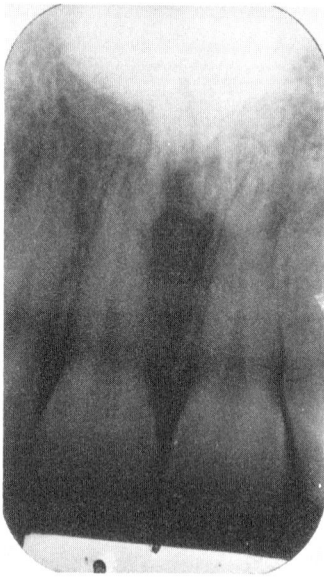

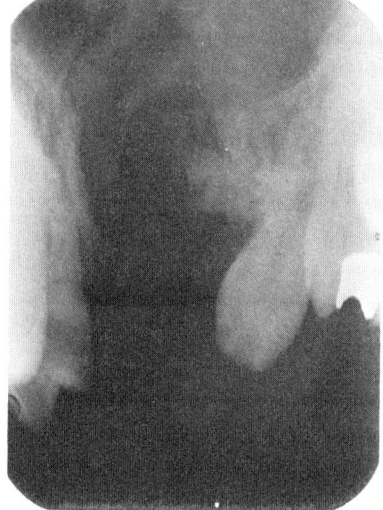

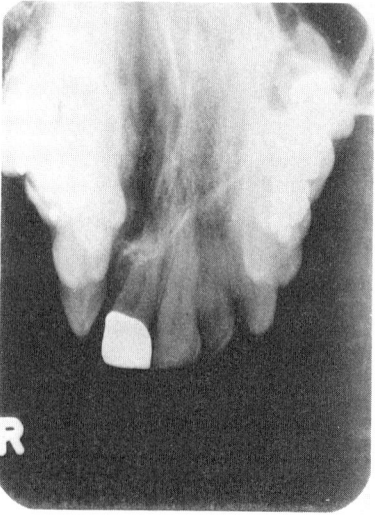

Figure 13-40. Maxillary torus. **(A)** As an opacity appearing within the maxillary sinus. Note the suggestion of a lamination at the outer perifore. **(B)** As an opacity in the periapical region of the maxillary midline area.

Figure 13-41. Unilateral cleft palate. **(A)** As seen in a periapical view. **(B)** As seen in an occlusal view in another patient.

microdontic lateral incisor may be present adjacent to the defect. Repaired clefts are often still present radiographically.

Anterior Median Maxillary Cleft

This condition occurs between the central incisors and probably represents a variation of normal. It is unrelated to other forms of cleft palate, but may be associated with a midline maxillary diastema. In some instances the condition may resemble an enlarged or funnel-shaped median maxillary suture line.

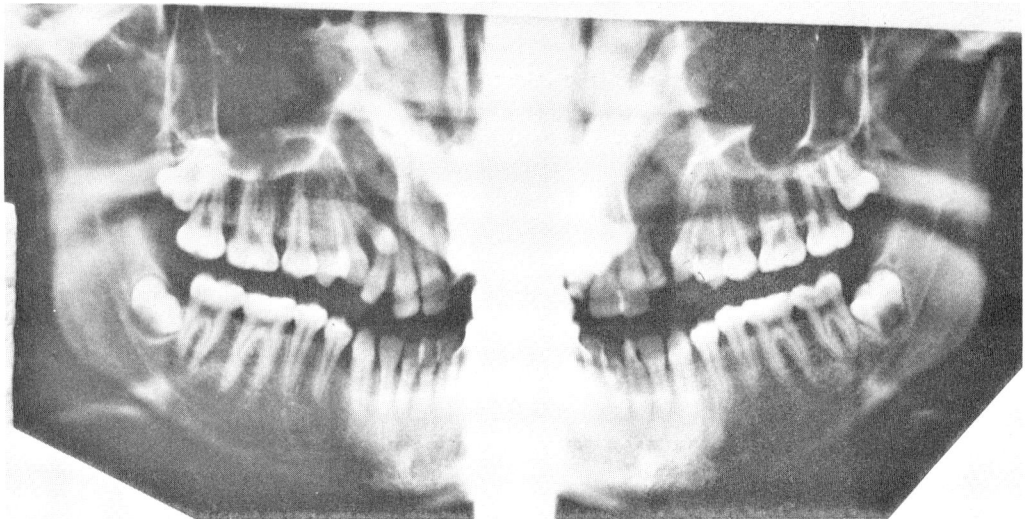

Figure 13-42. Bilateral cleft palate.

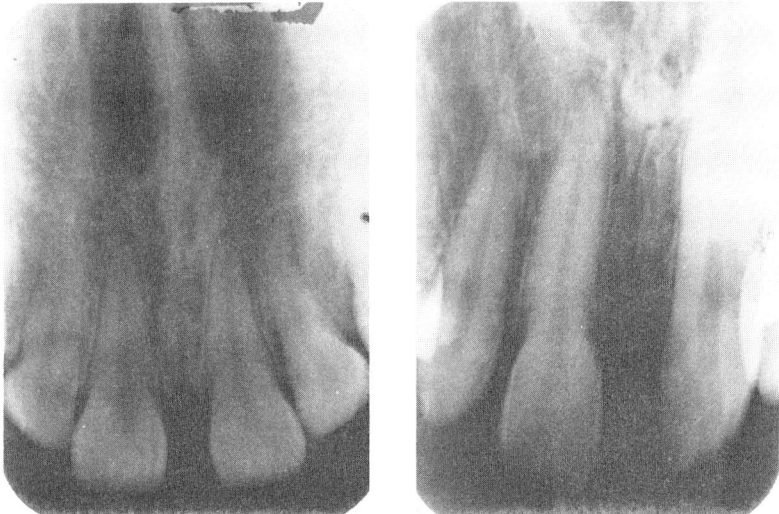

Figure 13-43. Anterior median maxillary cleft. (A) Minimal manifestation; note the diastema. (B) Moderate cleft; note the diastema.

Chapter 14

RADIOLOGIC INTERPRETATION OF DENTAL DISEASE

THE dental radiograph provides the dentist with essential information that cannot be received from any other source. However, the radiograph does have its limitations and the changes registered on the radiograph must be carefully interpreted with full consideration of the clinical data before a diagnosis can be made. One should not attempt a diagnosis from the radiograph only. It is only an aid in the diagnosis of the patient's dental disease.

The radiographic examination is useful to detect, to confirm, to classify, to define, and to localize a suspected disease.

It is helpful in establishing an early diagnosis, in finding the origin of symptoms, the etiology of disease, and the extent of the tissue involvement. Without radiographs it is often impossible to identify dental disease and plan appropriate treatment. Ths could result in (1) irreversible damage to teeth, alveolar bone, and other oral tissues, (2) compromised treatment, (3) increased risk of failure , and (4) more costly dental care.

A great percentage of the radiologic interpretation done in the dental office is devoted to acquiring information regarding dental caries, periapical disease, and periodontal disease.

Since studies conducted to determine the causes of tooth extraction (Brekhus, 1929; Allen, 1944) have reached similar conclusions — that caries, periapical dsease, and periodontal disease accounted for approximately 93 percent of the tooth loss — it is imperative that the dentist become competent in the radiologic interpretation of these dental diseases.

DENTAL CARIES

Dental caries is a pathological process of localized destruction of teeth by microorganisms. While many carious lesions are easily accessible for examination by explorer and mirror methods, a great percentage of them cannot be found by routine procedures. The intraoral radiograph (the bite-wing radiograph and the periapical radiograph taken by the paralleling technique) is indispensable in the detection of carious lesions, especially interproximal carious lesions. The bitewing film is the radiograph of choice for evaluating caries; however, it is important in many cases to use the periapical film of the same region for comparison. The periapical radiograph will produce a slightly different view of the same area, which will aid in the detection of caries.

The radiograph will reflect only the evidence of tooth destruction by the carious process, such as areas of demineralization and cavitation. The results of the action of the carious process reveals itself as radiolucent dark areas on the enamel, dentin, and cementum of the tooth.

The radiographic appearance of caries will be discussed according to the location of caries on the tooth: (1) interproximal surface, (2) occlusal surface, (3) facial/lingual surfaces, (4) pulpal, (5) root (cemental) surface, (6) recurrent or secondary (immediate vicinity of preexisting restoration), and (7) arrested caries (occlusal and interproximal surfaces).

Caries Location

Interproximal Carious Lesion

The interproximal carious lesion is the most easily recognized on the radiograph. It is also the most difficult to detect by use of clinical methods only. In a recent investigation by Hanson (1980), four times as many posterior interproximal carious lesions were found when posterior bitewings were used as compared to the number of lesions found by clinical observations alone.

The interproximal carious lesion is probably the most easily detected on the radiograph because there is lesser volume of normal tooth structure through which the x-rays must penetrate to reach the carious lesion on the interproximal surface than on any other tooth surface location. Interproximal caries usually begins just below the contact point and appears clinically as a chalky white spot that becomes slightly roughened due to early demineralization (Fig. 14-1). It is important to remember that the interproximal carious lesion begins on a small area located between the free gingival margin and the contact point of the tooth. The vertical

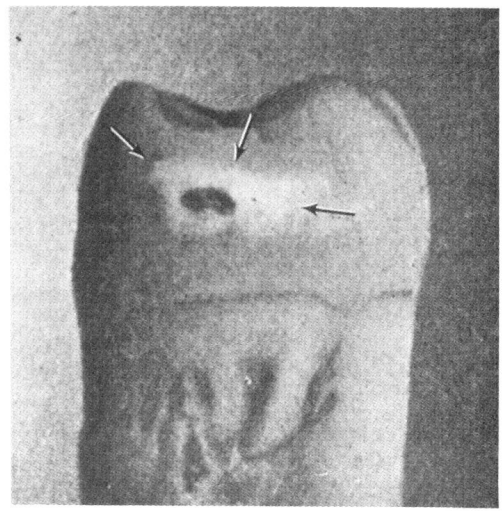

Figure 14-1. Early Carious Lesion. Notice the white chalky appearance with a stained cavitation area on interproximal surface between the contact point and cemento-enamel junction of this extracted tooth. (From Fig 164, page 346, Black, A. D.: Pathology of hard tissues of the teeth. *Oral Diagnosis,* 7th ed. Chicago, Medico-Dental Publ., 1936.)

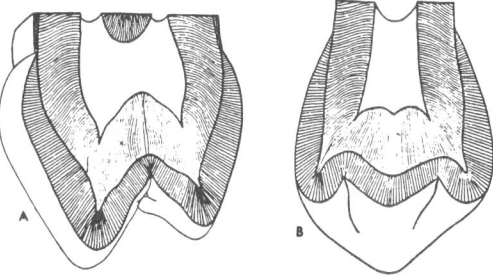

Figure 14-2. Arrangement of the enamel rods and dentinal tubules on a premolar sectioned buccolingually **(A)** and mesiodistally **(B)**. (From Noyes F: *Dental Histology and Empryology.* Philadelphia, Lea & Febiger, 1943.)

measurement of this lesion is most dependent on the recession of the free margin of the gingiva in this region. It may vary from one to several millimeters.

As the carious lesion grows, it forms a classical V-shaped appearance with the base of the triangle at the surface of the tooth with usually a rounded apex pointed toward the dentino-enamel junction. No reason can be given for this V-shaped configuration except that the carious process

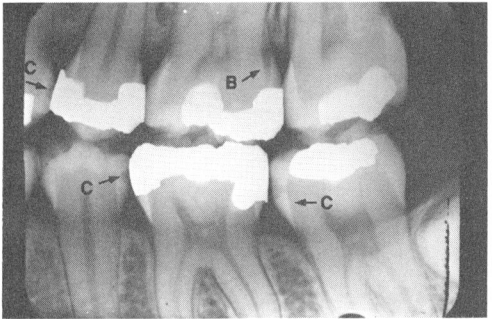

Figure 14-3. Note classical V-shaped caries (**C**) on mesial surface of mandibular second molar, and rounded triangular shaped caries (**C**) on distal surface of mandibular second premolar. The caries (**C**) on the distal surface of the maxillary first premolar has a broad base with a "scooped-out" appearance. The radiolucency on the distal surface of maxillary first molar is cervical burnout (**B**).

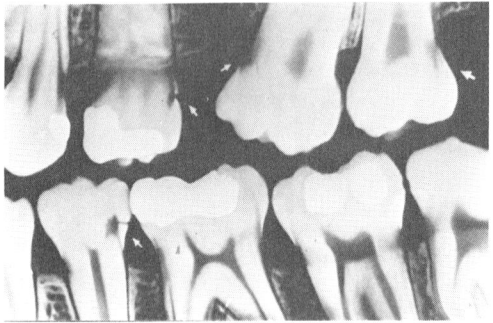

Figure 14-4. Bite-wing radiograph. Note "line-shaped" enamel caries with dentinal spread at DE junction of distal surfaces of maxillary and mandibular second premolar. Also, notice "cervical burnout" radiolucencies of mesial surface of maxillary second molar and distal surface of maxillary third molar.

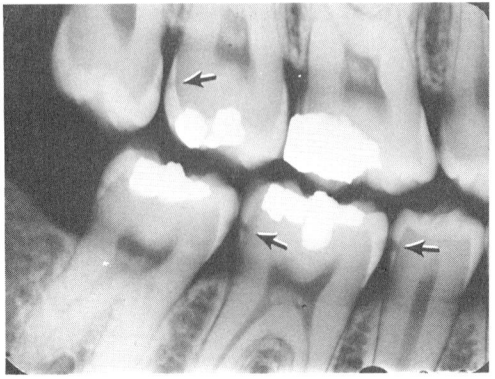

Figure 14-5. Acute caries. Note the small entrance of carious lesions on distal surfaces of lower first molar, second molar, and second premolar.

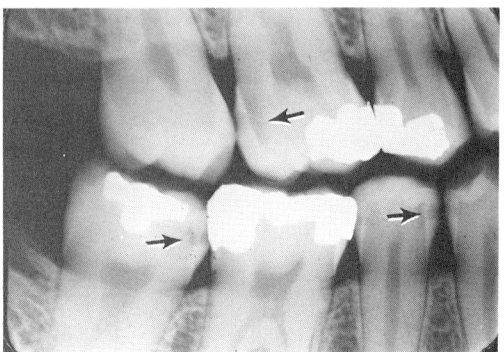

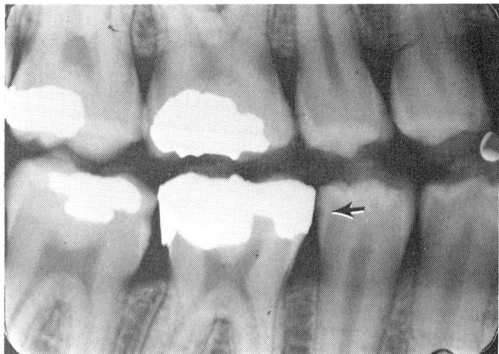

Figure 14-6. Chronic caries. (**A**) Note the large entrance of caries lesion at distal surface of upper first molar and mesial surface of lower second molar. (**B**) Note the large openings of chronic caries on mesial of lower second molar and distal of second premolar.

tends to follow the course of the enamel rods, which are usually aligned at right angles to the dentino-enamel junction (Fig. 14-2). Since the proximal surfaces are usually convex, the enamel rods tend to converge at the dentino-enamel junction, which in turn, produces the classical triangular V-shaped radiographic radiolucent appearance of interproximal caries (Fig. 14-3). However, there are exceptions to this rule, as many various shapes and sizes of proximal enamel carious lesions may be seen radiographically (thick line-shaped, W-shaped, flame-shaped, half-moon shaped, etc) (Fig. 14-4).

The shape of the lesion also has some bearing on the rapidity of the carious process. In most cases of acute caries, which are commonly seen in young adults between the ages of fifteen and twenty-five, there is rapid penetration through the enamel, and the initial entrance of the carious process remains small (Fig. 14-5). In chronic caries, however, which is commonly seen in adults, there is a slower progression of the lesion, and it has a larger entrance at the surface of the enamel (Fig. 14-6). After the carious lesion reaches the dentino-enamel junction, it usually first spreads laterally along the dentino-enamel junction, and proceeds toward the pulp with a tendency to follow the dentinal tubules toward the pulp. This forms another radiolucent triangle with its base at the dentino-enamel junction (Fig. 14-7).

Classification of Interproximal Dental Caries

There is need in private practice and teaching clinics for a caries scoring code to classify interproximal carious lesions according to their depth of penetration into a tooth. Not all early or incipient interproximal carious lesions detected radiographically should be restored. The determination whether the carious lesion

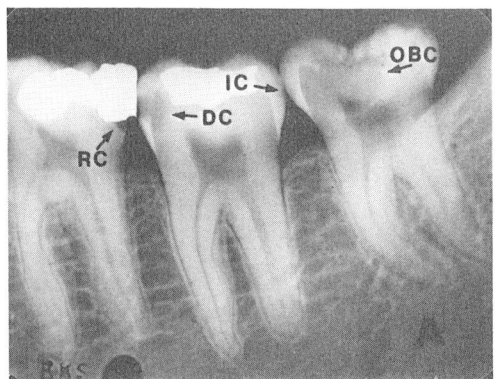

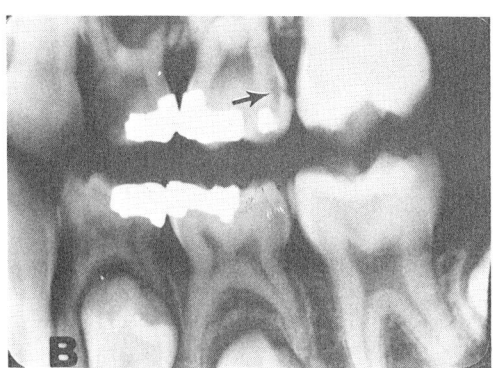

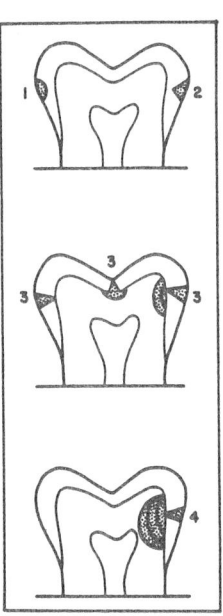

Classification of Radiographic Caries

C-1. Enamel Caries *less* than 1/2 way through enamel (sometimes called incipient caries) Do not record these lesions if doubtful of their existence.

C-2. Enamel caries penetrating at least 1/2 way through enamel, but *NOT* involving dentino-enamel junction.

C-3. Caries of enamel and dentine definitely at or through the dentino-enamel junction extending less than 1/2 way to pulp cavity.

C-4. Caries of enamel and dentine penetrating more than 1/2 way dentine toward pulp cavity.

Record the lesser score if there is doubt concerning depth of lesion.

Since occlusal caries is first seen radiographically when the caries penetrates the dentine, a score of C-3 or C-4 is given for occlusal caries.

Enamel caries of C-1 and C-2 cannot be scored if overlapping of interproximal surfaces occurs.

Figure 14-7. Dentinal caries (A) Note arrow at (DC). Notice spreading of caries at DE junction. (RC) is recurrent or secondary caries. (IC) is incipient caries. (OBC) is occlusal-buccal caries superimposed over pulp giving appearance of pulpal exposure. (B) Notice dentinal spreading at DE junction of distal surface of upper second primary molar.

Figure 14-8. A radiographic caries scoring code as recommended by Haugejorden and Slack in 1975. (From Haugejorden, O.; and Slack, G. L.: Progression of approximal caries in relation to radiogrpahic scoring codes. *Acta Odontologica Scandinavica, 33*:183-238, 1975.)

should be restored depends upon the results of the complete clinical examination and upon several other factors. In many cases the dentist may want to institute preventive caries measures rather than restorative procedures. If this is the case, it is important for the dentist to record in the patient's chart as objectively as possible the radiographic findings related to interproximal caries penetration. An example of a caries penetration scoring code is shown in Figure 14-8.

Each of the four classes of interproximal caries penetration is illustrated in Figure 14-9.

Occlusal, Facial, Lingual, and Pulpal Caries

Carious lesions of the occlusal, facial, and lingual surfaces of teeth are more readily found with the explorer; however the radiograph is an effective supplemental procedure because it alerts the dentist to areas of the mouth that may have been overlooked.

On the **occlusal surfaces** of teeth in the area of pits and fissures, the enamel rods diverge away from each other as they near the dentino-enamel junction. At this location, the carious lesion takes the appearance of a triangle with its base at the

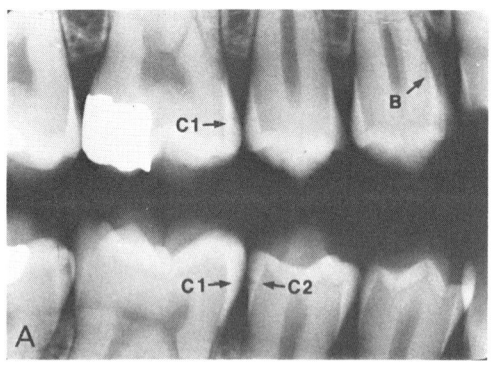
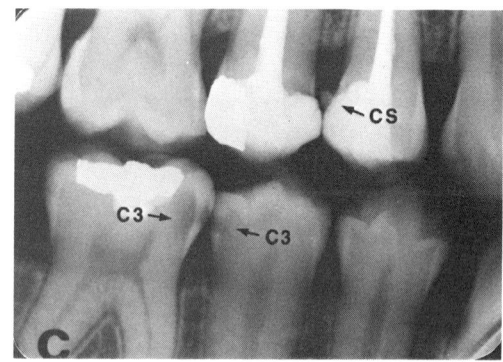
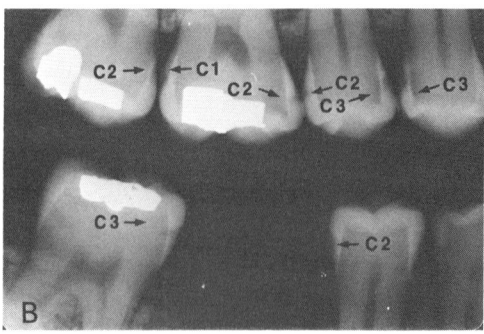
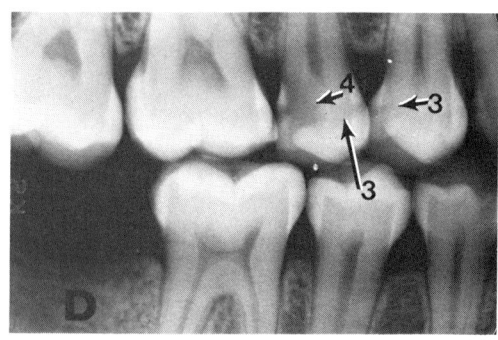

Figure 14-9. (A) Class I (Incipient) caries: (C-1) upper first molar, (B) cervical burnout, upper first premolar, (C-2) lower second premolar, (C-1) mesial, lower first molar. (B) Class II caries: (C-2) mesial upper second molar, mesial upper first molar, distal upper second premolar. Class III (C3) caries: mesial upper second premolar, distal upper first premolar, distal lower first premolar, mesial lower second molar. Class I (C-1) (incipient) distal upper first molar. (C) Class III caries (C-3): distal of lower second premolar and mesial of lower first molar. (CS) calculus spur. (D) Class IV caries: distal of upper second premolar; Class III caries, mesial of upper second premolar, distal, upper second premolar; Class II distal of upper canine.

Radiologic Interpretation of Dental Disease

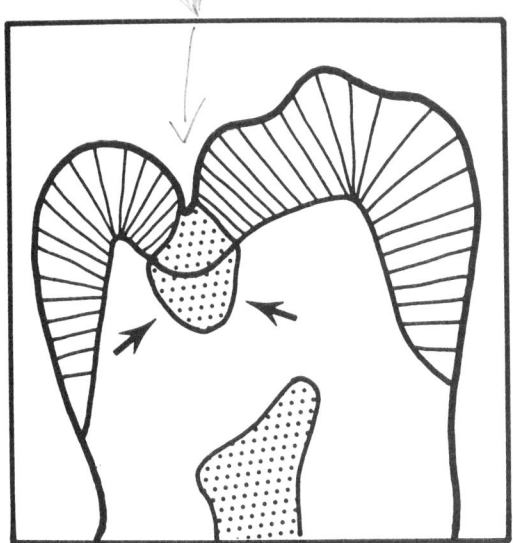

Occlusal Caries

Figure 14-10. Diagram showing the features of occlusal caries in posterior teeth.

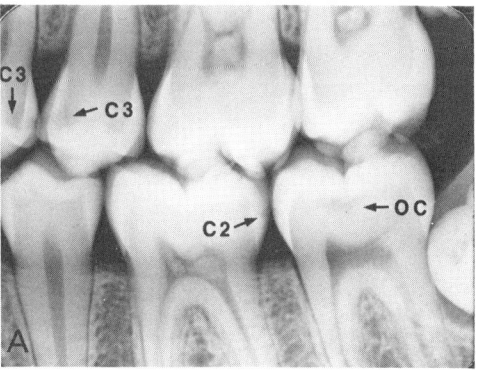

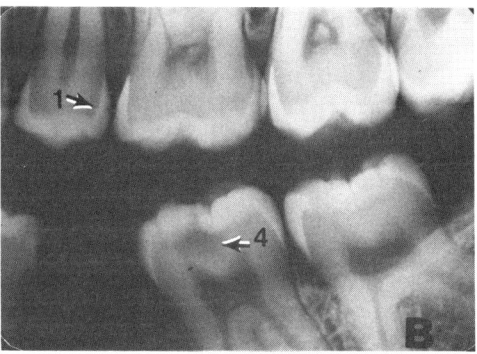

Figure 14-11. Occlusal caries. **(A)** Note radiolucent area under enamel cap (OC) of lower second-molar. There is class II caries on distal surface of lower first molar and Class II caries on distal surface of upper first premolar and mesial surface of upper second premolar. **(B)** Note occlusal caries in mandibular first molar. There is Class I caries on distal surface of upper second premolar.

dentino-enamel junction; this is the reverse of the appearance of smooth surface interproximal caries (Fig. 14-10). In most instances, enamel caries in fissures cannot be seen on the radiograph because of the thick layer of enamel that is superimposed over the occlusal surface of the teeth. Occlusal caries is in evidence on the radiograph only when the carious process has reached the dentino-enamel junction and spreads laterally in all directions. Evidence of occlusal caries is revealed when a dark radiolucent line can be seen under the enamel cap of the occlusal surface of the tooth (Fig. 14-11).

On the **facial and lingual surface** of the teeth, the enamel rods are essentially parallel to each other; therefore, the radiologic appearance of caries on these surfaces, in most instances, is a radiolucent dot or hole. The radiolucency will be more defined if the carious lesion is on the lingual surface because the film is in closer approximation to this surface (Fig. 14-12).

Cervical caries on the facial and lingual surfaces in most cases spreads in a circumferential fashion, leaving a curved semilunar radiolucency on the radiograph (Fig. 14-13).

It must be emphasized that the radiograph can only alert the dentist to the possibility of a carious **pulpal** involvement in a tooth; the actual verification of pulpal involvement must be done by carefully excavating the caries from the tooth (Fig.

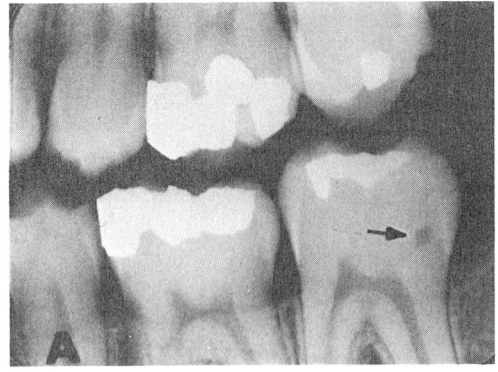

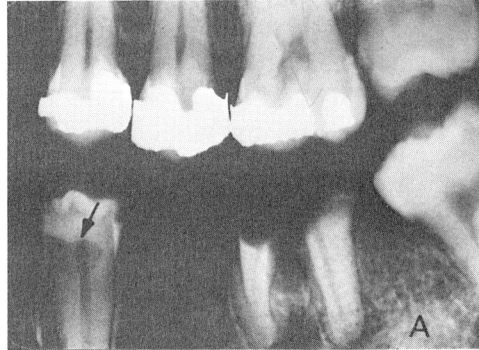

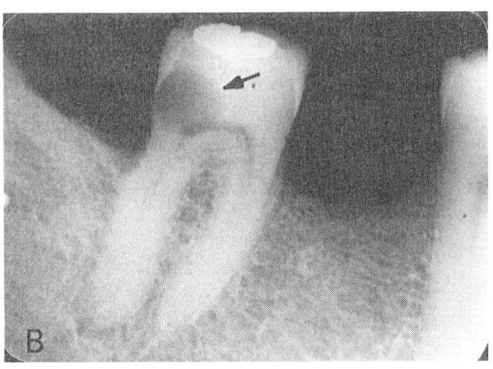

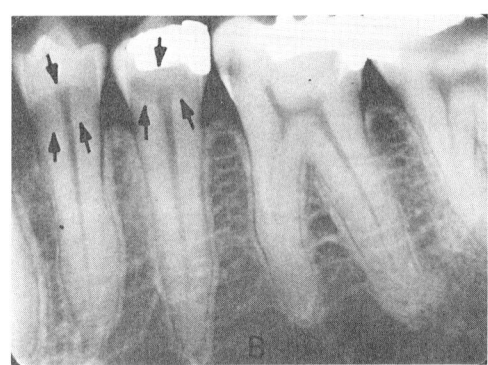

Figure 14-12. (A) Facial/Lingual Caries: Note the dark dot on facial/lingual surface of lower second molar. (Actually, it was a carious pit on the lingual surface of the tooth.) (B) Notice the round black circle on the facial/lingual surface of lower secnd molar (caries was on lingual surface).

Figure 14-13. Facial/Lingual Caries. (A) Note caries on facial/lingual surface of lower first premolar (caries was on facial surface of this tooth). (B) Note facial/lingual caries on first and second premolars (caries was on facial surfaces of teeth). There is Class III caries on mesial surface of first molar, sclerotic dentin under distal portion of DO restoration in first molar, and Class IV caries under restoration in second molar.

14-14).

Root (Cemental) Caries

These carious lesions affect the roots of teeth, involve the cementum, usually occur at interproximal spaces of teeth, and have a predilection for persons past middle age. This is why this type of caries is sometimes called "senile" caries.

It usually occurs in the elderly for two reasons: (1) advanced gingival recession exposing the cementum to the oral cavity, and (2) food packing areas caused by the loss of contact with adjacent teeth.

The enamel for various reasons in the elderly becomes almost caries immune, while the cementum does not enjoy this immunity. The cementum is formed in concentric layers and microorganisms tend to spread laterally between these various layers. The cemental carious process is similar to dentinal caries in that following decalcification, **proleotysis** of the remaining organic matrix occurs.

The loss of contact between teeth and

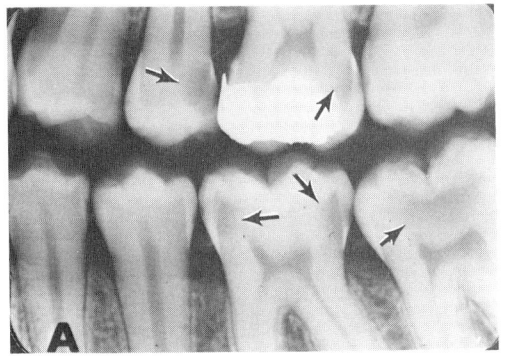

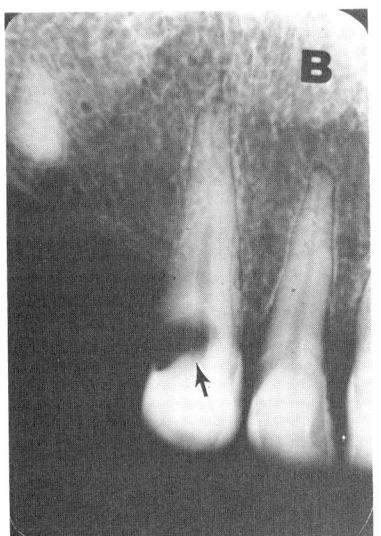

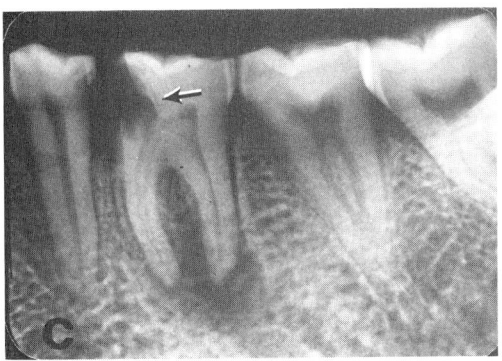

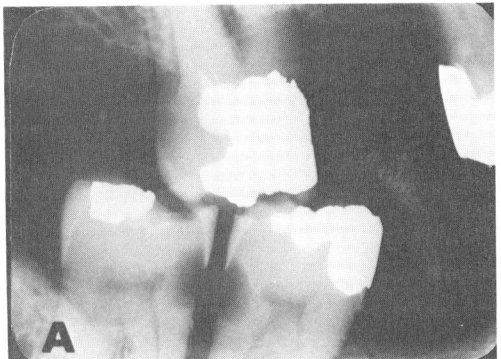

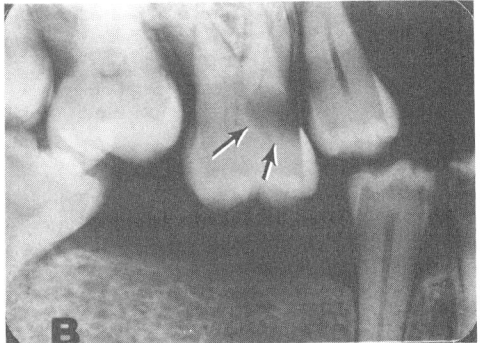

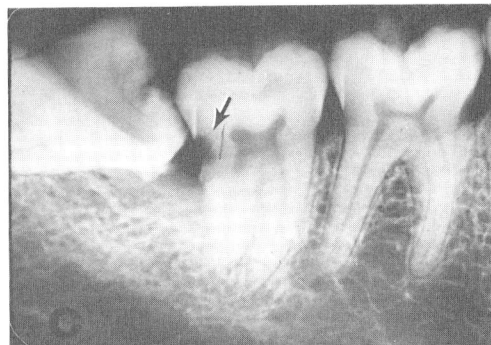

Figure 14-14. (A) Note large carious Class IV lesions with possible pulpal involvement in upper second premolar, upper first molar, lower first molar, and lower second molar. Also, notice calculus spurs on mesial of lower first and second molars and mesial of upper first molar. (B) Notice facial/lingual carious lesion on maxillary canine, which is superimposed over the pulp, which gives impression carious lesions have penetrated pulp. (C) Large carious lesion in first molar, which in all probability has reached the pulp because of the obvious apical pathology.

Figure 14-15. Root (cemental) caries. (A) Root or cemental caries with characteristic cupped-out appearance as seen on distal surface of lower first molar and mesial surface of lower second molar. Note the loose contact between the lower first and second molars and plunger cusp of upper second molar, which most likely forces food between lower molars. (B) Root (cemental) caries of mesial surfaces of the upper first molar. Food impaction was made possible between the upper first molar and the second premolar by the loss of contact between these two teeth when the upper first molar erupted into the space of the extracted lower first molar. (C) Radiograph of cemental caries with notched-out appearance as seen on distal surface of lower second molar. Impacted third molar should have been extracted earlier because it provided a food packing area distal to second molar (From Langland, O.E., Radiologic examination. In James W. Clark, (Ed.): *Clinical Dentistry,* Vol. 1, Philadelphia, Harper & Row, 1981, Fig 4-56, page 31.)

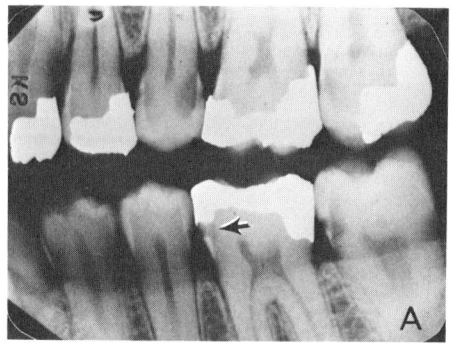

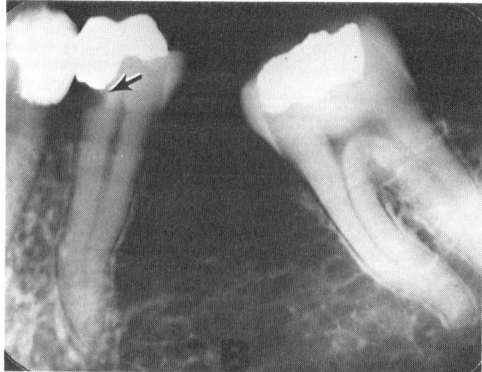

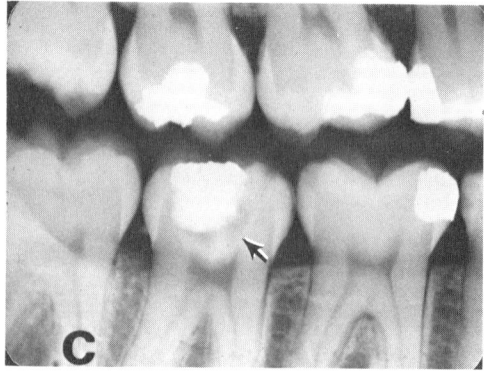

Figure 14-16. Recurrent (secondary) caries. **(A)** Note recurrent (secondary) caries on mesial surface of lower first molar and mesial surface upper first molar. There is Class III caries on mesial of upper second premolar, mesial upper second molar, and mesial of lower second molar. Also, Class IV caries on distal of upper second premolar. There is cervical burnout on distal lower second molar. **(B)** Large recurrent (secondary) caries on mesial of second premolar. Note cement (temporary) restoration in second premolar. **(C)** Notice radiolucent area under occlusal restoration in lower second molar. This is most likely recurrent (secondary) caries, which was not removed at the time of the cavity preparation. However, the radiopaque band under the radiolucency is most likely sclerotic dentin, which is a defensive response of the pulp to repel the carious process.

the resulting food packing areas in the elderly is usually made possible by severe attrition, large interproximal chronic carious lesions, or supraeruption of teeth.

The caries of the root (cementum) of teeth is usually described as saucer-shaped. It has a fairly rapid penetration and pulpal involvement is frequent. The caries is often leatherly and of brownish color.

Root (cemental) caries is usually revealed on the radiograph as an ill-defined radiolucent "cupped-out" or "saucer-shaped" area located in the interproximal region just below the cemento-enamel junction (Fig. 14-15A, B). If the clinical opening is small, the appearance of the carious lesion on the radiograph will have a more "notched" appearance than "saucer-shaped" appearance (Fig. 14-15C). Cemental caries does not involve the enamel except by extension laterally crownward along the dentino-enamel junction to undermine the cervical enamel. The unsupported cervical enamel usually fractures, resulting in a cavitation.

Sometimes root (cemental) caries is misinterpreted as "cervical burnout." Cemental caries is a more defined, darker radiolucent area than "cervical burnout," and is usually seen in an elderly person with loose contacts between adjacent teeth. However, a clinical exploration of the area will differentiate quite readily "cervical burnout" from root (cemental) caries.

Recurrent (Secondary) Caries

Recurrent or secondary caries originates in the immediate vicinity of a preexisting restoration. In most cases it occurs because of (1) inadequate extension of the cavity preparation, (2) improper adaptation of the restorative material to margins of the cavity preparation, or (3) incomplete removal of the caries from the tooth prior to placing the restoration. The radiologic appearance of recurrent or secondary caries is a radiolucent area just beneath the restoration. It is usually seen just beneath the interproximal margin of the restoration (Fig. 14-16). It is difficult to uncover all of the recurrent caries by means of the radiograph. The caries may be blocked out by the radiopaque restoration and the location of the carious lesion in relation to the restoration; the vertical angulation of the x-ray beam may be such that visibility is almost completely impaired (Fig. 14-17).

Arrested Caries

Arrested caries is a form of caries that has become static or stationary and does not have a tendency for further progression. It occurs almost exclusively in occlusal surfaces of teeth where an established carious lesion becomes, for one of several reasons, self-cleansing. It arises when there is extensive breakdown of enamels and a shallow cavity forms that opens the cavity to the abrading effect of normal mastication.

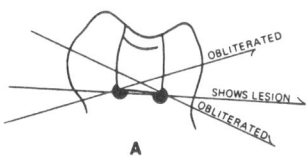
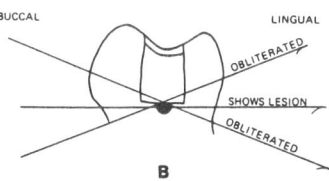

Figure 14-17. Diagram illustrating how changes in vertical angulation may obliterate from radiographic view recurrent (secondary) caries on the interproximal surface of a tooth. **(A)** Recurrent (secondary) caries at corners of proximal gingival portion of Class II restoration. **(B)** Recurrent (secondary) caries under proximal gingival portion of Class II restoration. (From Langland, O.: Radiologic examination. In James W. Clark (Ed.): *Clinical Dentistry,* Vol. 1. Philadelphia, Harper & Row, 1981, Fig 4-58, page 33).

The carious surface has dark brown polished appearance and is quite hard. The progress of the carious lesion becomes very slowly progressive or virtually arrested (Fig. 14-18). **Dentinal sclerosis** (deposition of minerals in and around dentinal tubules) and **secondary dentin** (irregular type of dentin formed after primary dentin has been formed) formation commonly occur in teeth with arrested caries (Fig. 14-18). There is another type of arrested caries seen just below the contact point of the proximal surfaces of teeth in which an adjacent tooth has been removed. An early enamel lesion in this region may in certain instances become arrested by the formation of a self-cleansing area.

Factors that Influence Caries Interpretation

There are several factors that influence the interpretation of caries. Some of these factors will affect the dentist's efficiency in detecting carious lesions accurately.

Underestimation of Caries Size

The carious lesion in the enamel will not be seen radiographically until there is

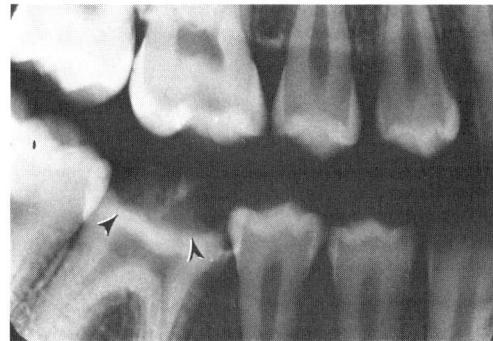

Figure 14-18. Arrested caries in lower first molar, which as black-brown polished occlusal surface. Previously patient and occlusal caries as seen in upper first molar; however, the walls of the cavity became broken down leaving a self-cleaning area. The carious process then became stationary or arrested.

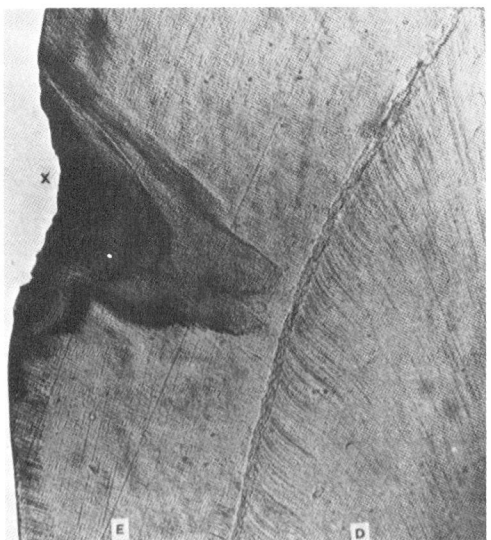

Fiugre 14-19. Caries of the enamel. Note area of caries penetration at (X) where the outer ends of the enamel rods have broken away. The radiograph of this tooth would most likely reveal only a notch in the tooth at (X) and a small area of radiolucency representing the very dark area of the decalcification in the enamel. The flame-shaped area of decalcification has almost reached the dentino-enamel junction; however, the radiograph would probably show only about one-third of this area of decalcification. (From Black, A. D.: G. V. Black's Work on Operative Dentistry, Vol I, 8th ed. Chicago, Medico-dental Publ. Co. 1948, page 360, Fig 182.)

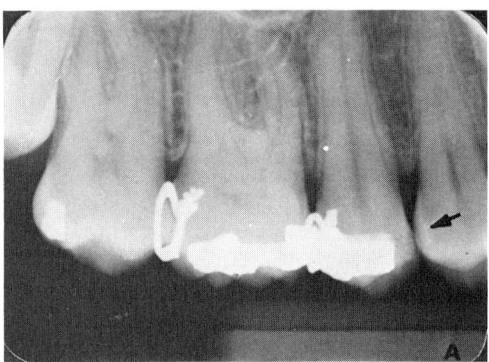

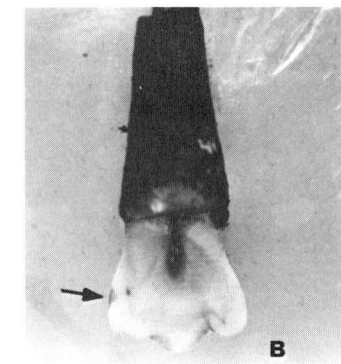

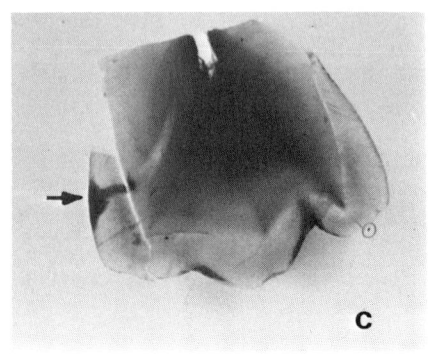

a sufficient amount of decalcification. For instance, it has been estimated that it takes approximately 50 percent of the calcium and phosphorus in a localized area of a tooth or bone to be resorbed before a radiolucency will be revealed on the radiograph (Early et al., 1979).

Therefore, the actual carious lesion is further advanced clinically and microscopically than the radiograph indicates (Figs. 14-19, 14-20).

There is another reason the actual carious lesion appears less advanced on the radiograph: The ratio of normal tooth structure (enamel and dentine) to caries through which x-rays must pass varies in

Figure 14-20. Radiograph and histopathology of a carious lesion on the distal surface of the maxillary first premolar. This illustrates that the radiographic evidence of caries is much smaller than the actual lesion. **(A)** Radiograph prior to extraction. **(B)** Longitudinal section of tooth after it was soaked in dye. **(C)** Photomicrograph of this calcified section revealing that carious lesion has reached the dentino-enamel junction. (From Langland, O. E.: Radiologic examination, In James W. Clark (Ed.): *Clinical Dentistry.* Philadelphia, Harper & row, 1981, Figure 4-40, page 26.)

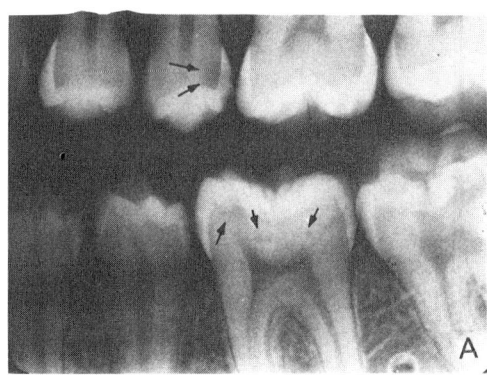

Figure 14-21. Normal tooth structure to caries ratio phenomenon. The film records a radiopaque area for photon 2 because the normal tooth to carious tooth structure ratio is much greater in this area of the tooth as compared to areas of the tooth which photon 1 and 3 are penetrating. (Adapted from figure 15-8, Wuehrman, A. H., Manson-Hing, L. R.: *Dental Radiology*, ed. 4, St. Louis, Mosby, 1977).

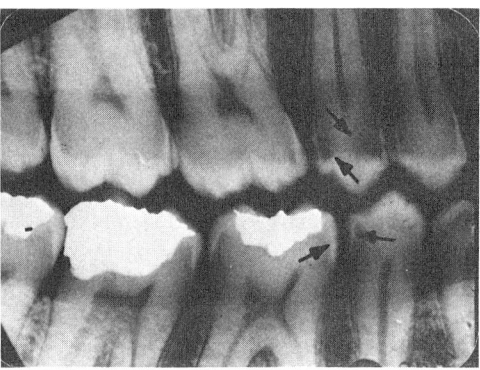

Figure 14-22. Normal tooth structure to carious tooth structure ratio phenomenon. (A) Notice the apparent enamel carious lesion on distal surface of upper second premolar. However, carious lesion has penetrated the dentin. Also, notice occlusal caries in lower first molar and several facial/lingual carious pits in same tooth. (B) Notice the apparent enamel carious lesion on mesial and distal surfaces of upper second premolar. However, both lesions have penetrated the dentin. Also, notice the two Class I (incipient) carious lesions on mesial of lower first molar and distal of lower second premolar.

different areas of the interproximal surface of the tooth. Since the carious lesion on the interproximal surface is usually V-shaped or triangular in shape with the base of the triangle at the periphery of the tooth, the ratio of normal tooth structure to carious tooth structure becomes larger as the carious process approaches the dentino-enamel junction.

When the area of overlying enamel becomes thick as compared to the small size of the decalcified area (at apex of triangle), the x-rays becomes attenuated (reduction in energy) to a degree that a radiolucency will not be produced on the radiograph.

When the caries process reaches the dentino-enamel junction, caries is revealed again on the radiograph because the ratio of normal tooth structure to the size of the carious lesion is not as great (Fig. 14-21).

This phenomenon may be the cause of misinterpretation of amount of penetration of a carious lesion because an apparently small enamel lesion may in reality have penetrated into the dentin (Fig. 14-22).

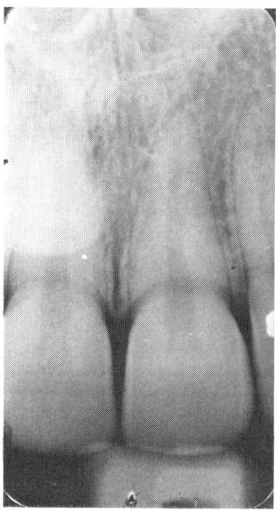

Figure 14-23. Cervical burnout in maxillary centrals. Note the dark radiolucent collar at cervical neck of central incisors.

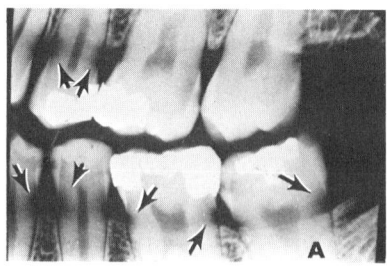

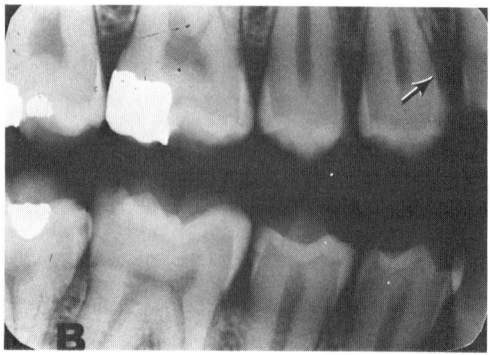

Figure 14-24. Cervical burnout in posterior teeth. **(A)** Note radilucent areas (arrows), which are cervical burnout areas. **(B)** Note cervical burnout area on mesial of upper first premolar. This is a common place for cervical burnout because of anatomical concavity usually found in this area.

Cervical Burnout

The radiograph may reveal at times a radiolucent collar or a wedge-shaped radiolucency (called **cervical burnout** areas) adjacent to the cemento-enamel junction of a tooth. Sometimes cervical burnout areas will be misinterpreted as cemental caries. The tissue density at the neck region of the tooth is less than that of the regions above and below it, resulting in **cervical burnout**. While the crown of the tooth is covered by enamel and the root is covered by alveolar bone, the neck of the tooth is constricted in size and is left uncovered. Therefore, the tissues of the neck do not impede the x-rays as well as do the tissues above and below it. This results in a radiolucent collar in the anterior teeth (Fig. 14-23) and a wedge-shaped radiolucency (Fig. 14-24) near the cemento-enamel region in the posterior teeth. Cervical burnout can often be seen underneath proximal metallic restorations; there is such a great contrast on the radiograph between the two densities that the radiolucency of the cervical burnout area seems unusually dark.

Mach Band Effect

This is an optical illusion that produces fictitious radiolucent areas (1) inside the proximal DEJ in incisors and canines, less frequently in premolars, and least in molars, and (2) in dentinal peaks bounded by occlusal and proximal enamel in premolars (more often inmandibular than maxillary) (Fig. 14-25 B, C, D).

This optical illusion was first described by Ernst Mach in 1865. They are produced by lateral inhibition of neural receptors in the eye. Stimulation of the retinal receptors by a bright light causes inhibition of the neural response of its adjacent (lateral) receptor. The inhibition will be greater when the stimulation is increased. An example of this effect is shown in Figure 14-25A. By staring at the

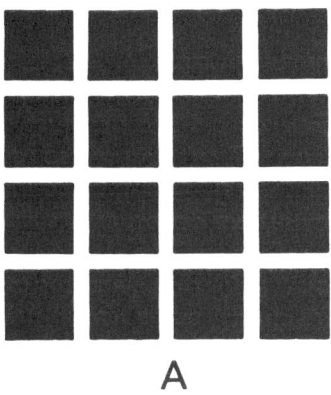

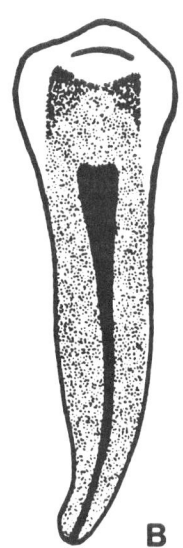

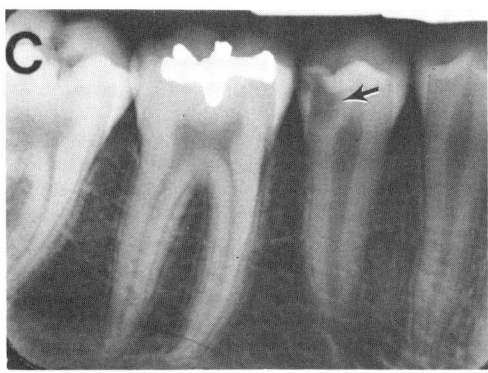

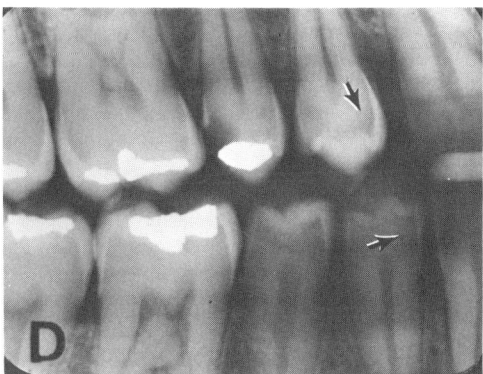

Figure 14-25. Mach band effect. **(A)** Notice dark areas produced at the white areas at the intersections of black squares when you stare at center of grid. **(B)** Illustration of Mach band radiolucencies in dentinal peaks of mandibular premolars. **(C)** Actual carious lesion in distal surface of mandibular second premolar. **(D)** Mach band radiolucencies in first premolars. (From Berry, H. M.: Cervical burnout and Mach band. *JADA, 106*: 622-625, May 1983. Copyright by the American Dental Association. Reprinted by permission.)

center of the grid the white areas at the intersections of the black squares will appear darker. This is referred to as a negative Mach band, and makes dentin appear darker where it meets enamel in the radiograph. It is an edge enhancement created in the eye that does not result from an actual density change in the film emulsion.

Berry (1983) describes a masking technique to facilitate differential interpetation between Mach band illusion and an actual carious lesion (Fig. 14-26). The observer must be cautioned before calling these radiolucent areas caries even after using the masking technique, because there are other reasons for the appearance of these darker dentinal peaks. They are explained by tissue thickness and density differences. The quantity of dentin and the thinness of the enamel shells in various tooth areas have insufficient density to mask the darkness of the dentinal

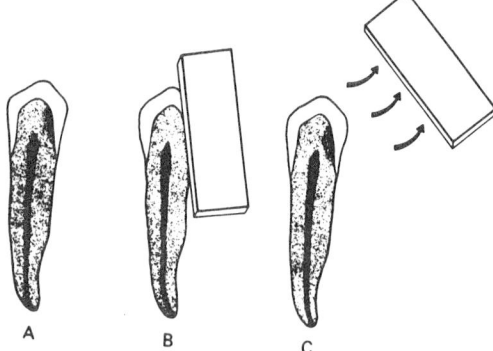

Figure 14-26. Mach band masking technique. **(A)** Radiolucency at mesial DEJ of premolar. **(B)** If when an opaque card covers enamel, and the radiolucent area along the DEJ disappears, the radiolucent area is most likely caused by the **Mach Band** effect. **(C)** When card is snapped away, the caries-mimicking radiolucency will reappear. A true carious lesion does not disappear by masking. (From Berry, H. M.: Cervical burnout and Mach band. *JADA 106*:622-625, May 1983. Copyright by the American Dental Association. Reprinted by permission.)

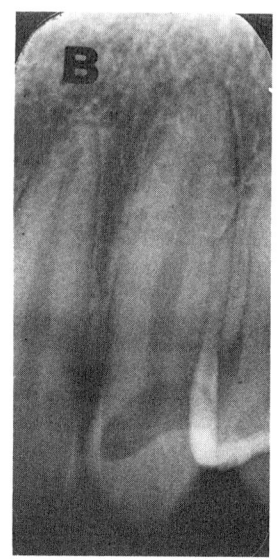

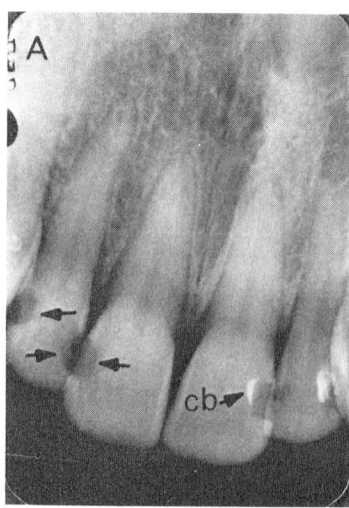

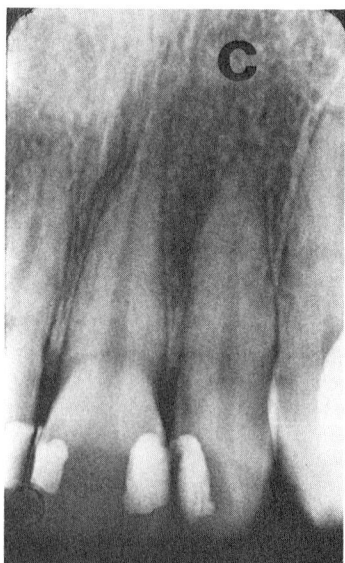

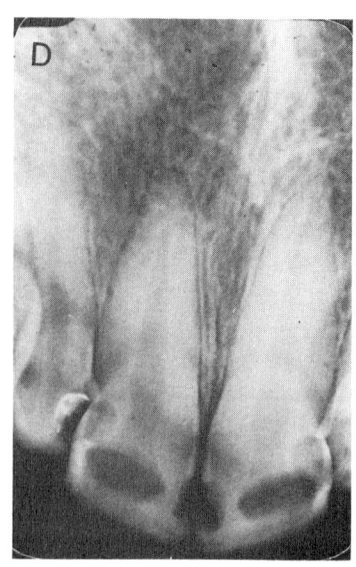

Figure 14-27. Restorative Materials. **(A)** Silicates are radiolucent and could mimic caries. Those with bases under them are not difficult to detect as the cement base will be more radiopaque as indicated by (CB) on radiograph. **(B)** A resin or plastic restoration on facial surface of canine appears as radiolucency and could be misinterpreted as caries; however, it has the characteristic sickle-shaped cavity preparation commonly seen in Class V restorations. **(C)** Composite restorations have similar appearance as orthophosphoric cements. **(D)** Resins on facial surface of upper centrals.

tissue, revealing caries-mimicking radiolucencies in these areas.

Restorative Materials

Silicates, resin, and some composite restorative materials are radiolucent and may be misinterpreted as caries (Fig. 14-27). However, Class III silicate, resin,

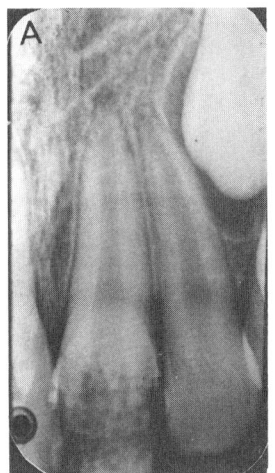

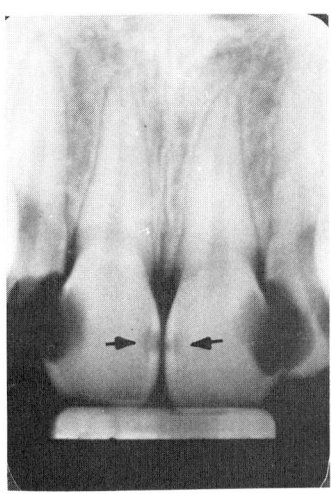

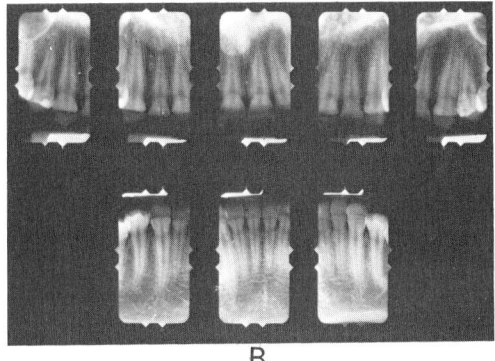

Figure 14-28. Anterior interproximal caries. Notice the characteristic shape of enamel caries and spreading of caries at dentino-enamel junction on mesial surfaces of upper centrals. This is case of rampant caries in a teenage female. There are large class IV carious lesins on distal surfaces of upper centrals in this radiograph. The laterals are almost completely destroyed by the carious process.

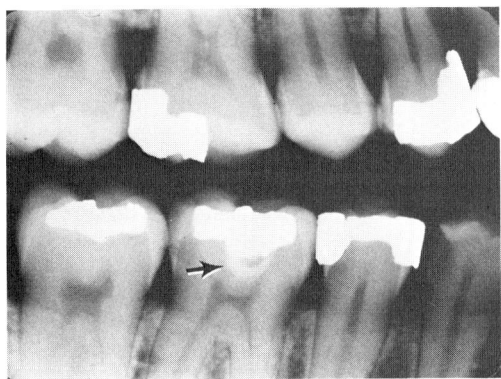

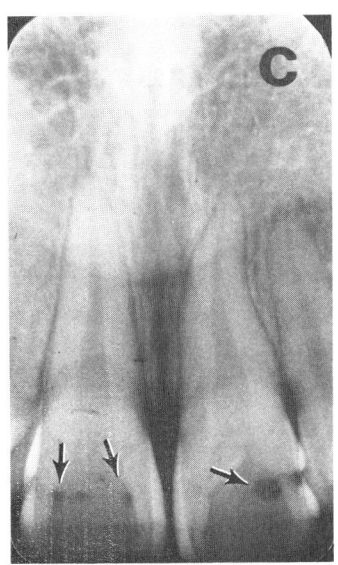

Figure 14-29. CaOH pulp capping material. The older CaOH pulp cappings were radiolucent. The radiolucent area under occlusal restoration in lower first molar could be a pulp capping material. Note the sclerotic dentin (radiopaque line) under the radiolucency. The newer pulp capping materials have BaSO$_4$ in them to make them radiopaque.

Figure 14-30. Enamel hypoplasia may mimic caries. **(A)** Localized enamel hypoplasia of an upper central incisor. **(B)** Generalized enamel hypoplasia of all maxillary and mandibular incisors. **(C)** Hypoplastic dots simulate caries.

and composite cavity preparations have characteristic semicircular shapes that can be differentiated from early interproximal carious lesions in the anterior teeth (Fig. 14-28). When a radiopaque cement base is placed beneath a silicate or a plastic restoration, the differentiation is simplified. Although the more recently developed calcium hydroxide pulp capping materials are radiopaque, the older pulp-capping materials were radiolucent and made interpretation more difficult (Fig. 14-29).

Developmental Defects in the Enamel

Hypoplastic defects in the enamel may simulate caries on the radiograph (Fig. 14-30), especially if they appear on the interproximal surfaces of the teeth. Most of the time, these defects can be differentiated from caries by clinical examination. If the explorer sticks when its removal from the defect is attempted, the area should be restored.

Abrasion and Attrition

Attrition denotes a mechanical wearing down of the teeth or the gradual loss of tooth substance as a result of mastication.

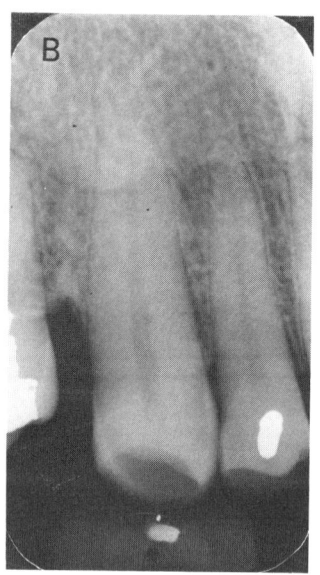

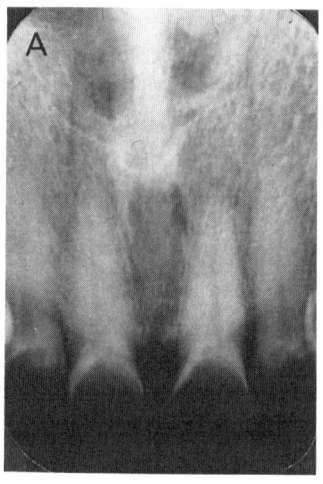

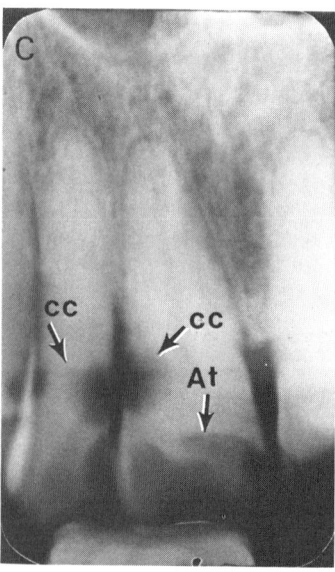

Figure 14-31. Attrition. **(A)** Notice severe attrition of incisal surfaces of central incisors, which could mimic caries. **(B)** Severe attrition of incisor surfaces of canine and lateral incisor forming concavities like carious lesions. **(C)** Severe attrition of incisal surfaces of lateral and central incisors simulating caries. Note large cemental carious lesions between central and lateral incisors. Compare these cemental carious lesions to "cervical burnout" areas.

It may occur on the incisal, occlusal, and proximal surfaces of teeth. It may affect either deciduous or permanent teeth. In the earlier stages, only part of the enamel is removed from the occlusal surface, leaving disc-shaped areas of dentin exposed. In the more advanced stage the occlusal enamel is completely removed, first exposing primary dentin, finally wear may be such that there is exposure of the underlying secondary dentin. When the occlusal or incisal enamel is completely removed, the dentine wears more rapidly than the enamel left at the margins so that shallow concavities tend to be formed, surrounded by a sharp border of enamel. These concavaties may sometimes simulate occlusal caries on the radiograph (Fig. 14-31).

The term **abrasion** is used to indicate the wear that occurs on a tooth from the friction of a foreign body independent of occlusion. The surface of a tooth that is affected varies with the causative factor.

The most prevalent type of abrasion is caused by brushing of the teeth in a horizontal direction at the cervical margin of teeth. It is called **toothbrush abrasion** and it forms a typical V-shaped grove on the facial aspect of the cervical margin of the teeth. On the radiograph this V-shaped grove many times will mimic caries at the cervical neck of a tooth (Fig. 14-32). In all forms of **abrasion** the surface of the exposed dentin is hard and highly polished. When caused by a pipe held by the teeth, the worn surface is discolored and yellow-brown due to tobacco.

Technique Errors that will Affect Caries Detection

In order for the dentist to interpret a radiograph properly, it is essential that the radiograph has diagnostic quality. As discussed previoulsy, diagnostic quality can

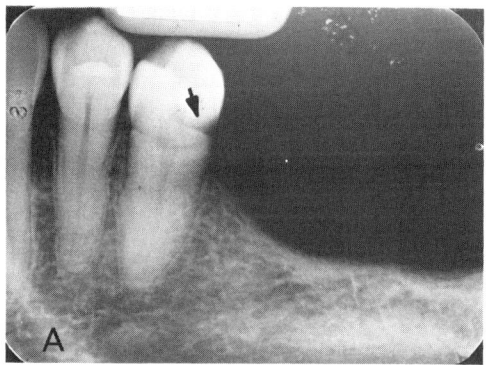

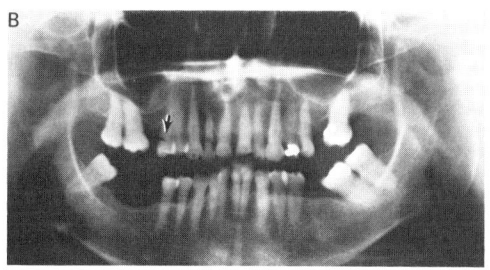

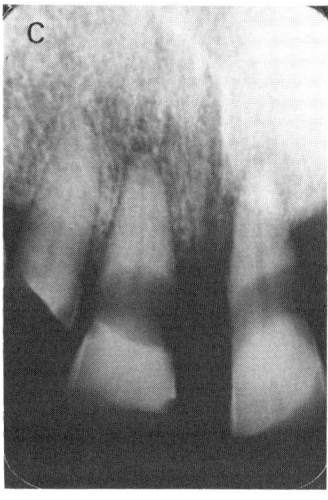

Figure 14-32. Abrasion. **(A)** There is a typical V-shaped appearance of toothbrush abrasion at distal cervical surface of second premolar. **(B)** Panoramic radiograph. Arrow points to V-shaped radiolucency, which is area of toothbrush abrasion. If you look closely there are other areas of toothbrush abrasion as well as attrition. **(C)** Severe toothbrush abrasion of central incisors at facial cervical surfaces. Also, note abrasion on incisal edges of same teeth. There areas could mimic caries.

450 Textbook of Dental Radiology

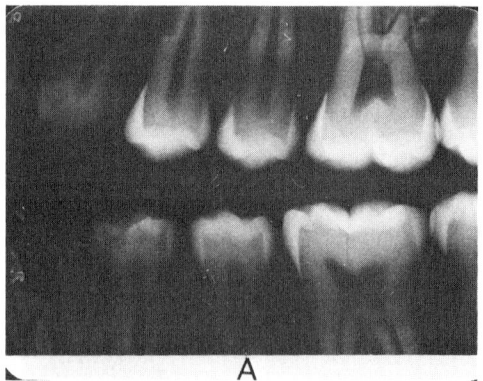

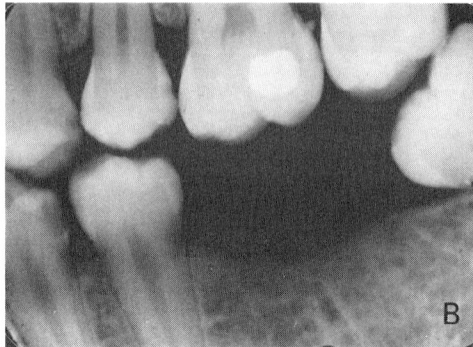

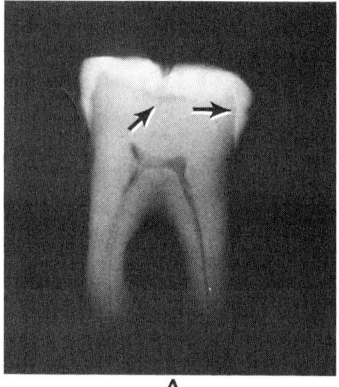

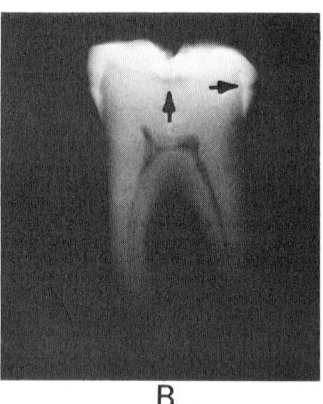

Figure 14-33. Dark and light density films. **(A)** Film is too dark to detect caries. Sometimes use of high intensity light will improve the density of the film enough for proper viewing. **(B)** Film with very light density, which hinders the dentist's capability to interpret the film for caries. There is distal caries on the upper first and second premolars, upper first molar, and lower first premolar.

Figure 14-34. A slightly darker density film will reveal caries better. **(A)** Lighter density film with caries on occlusal and distal surfaces. **(B)** Same tooth as in **(A)** but with higher density. Notice that caries on occlusal and distal surfaces can be seen more distinctly.

only be achieved by following the principles of good radiographic technique. When various poor techniques are used, it produces radiographic images that cannot be read accurately for caries detection. Some of these common errors in techniques will be discussed.

Common Errors in Exposure

The two visual characteristics of **density** and **contrast** are important in the detection of caries.

Dark and Light Density Films. **Density** is the general tendency of the film toward a lighter or darker overall appearance. A dental film may be very dark (greater density) or very light (lesser density). Density is controlled primarily by mAs and the developing process. It is also affected secondarily by kVp and fog (radiation, light, chemicals, and age). Dental films with densities that are too dark or too light are practically useless for the detection of caries (Fig. 14-33). However, the interpretation of caries is probably better done on a slightly darker density film than a lighter density film. In a slightly darker density film the carious lesion is darker, and when contrasted with the surrounding radiopaque enamel, the carious lesion is often more clearly seen (Fig. 14-34). However, this does not necessarily hold true for other structures, such as the bone surroundig the teeth.

Peripheral Burnout. The operator must be careful not to overexpose a film (Fig. 14-33A), not only because it interferes with the detection of caries, but because it can cause the periphery of the tooth to become **burned out.** This will reduce the periphery of the crown image on the radiograph, and if there is a small carious lesion or the interproximal surface of a tooth that has been overexposed it could be erased by this phenomenon called **peripheral burnout.** (Fig. 14-35.)

Long-Scale and Short-Scale Contrast. **Contrast** refers to the difference in density between adjacent areas in the dental film. It is controlled primarily by kVp and developing. Optimum contrast is present when the density of the images reveals all the needed detail of the structures being examined. Detail refers to the point-by-point delineation of the miute structural elements of the objects in the images in the dental film. Radiographic details cannot become visible unless the radiation is able to penetrate the part being examined.

It is recommended that kilovoltages of 65-70 kVp be used for the bite-wing films in the detection of caries. The kilovoltages in this range produce a **high contrast** film (short scale contrast), which makes for easier detection of caries. Kilovoltages below 65 kVp are not recommended be-

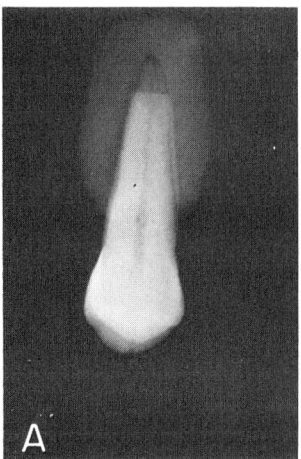

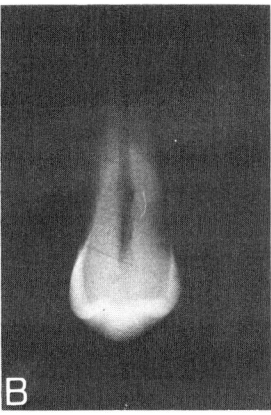

Figure 14-35. Peripheral Burnout: **(A)** Tooth taken with slightly less than optimum exposure. **(B)** Same tooth as in **(A)** excessively overexposed, which caused reduction in size of crown. If there had been an incipient carious lesion on an interproximal surface of this tooth it would have been erased by "peripheral burnout" from overexposure.

cause it would necessitate the use of excessive radiation to penetrate the tooth structures, which would expose the patient to unnecessary large skin doses.

It is recommended that a high kilovoltage technique (75-100 kVp) be used for the periapical films, and a low kilovoltage technique (65-70 kVp) be utilized for the bite-wing film. This would give the dentist a **long-scale contrast film**

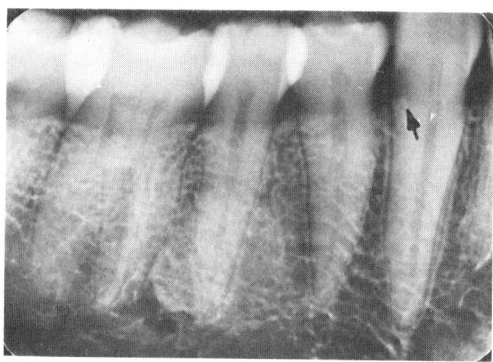

Figure 14-36. Overlapping of the tooth contact area caused by improper horizontal angulation. Interproximal caries is impossible to read between all surfaces except canine and first premolar. Dark area or root of distal of canine is "cervical burnout."

(large number of small density differences) to detect small details in the bone, and a **short-scale contrast** film to detect caries in the teeth.

Common Errors in Projection

If the film is not placed properly in the mouth and the x-ray beam directed accurately to the teeth and film, then overlapping of tooth contacts and shape distortion of the teeth will occur.

Improper Horizontal and Vertical Angulation. **Improper horizontal angulation** causes overlapping of the contact areas of the crowns of the teeth, which in turn makes it impossible to interpret the interproximal surfaces of the teeth for caries (Fig. 14-36).

Improper vertical angulation causes foreshortening of the tooth images and projects the enamel cap of the crown of

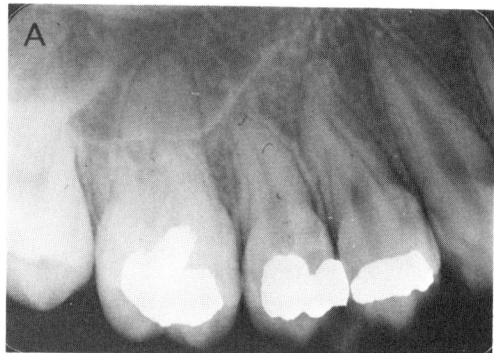

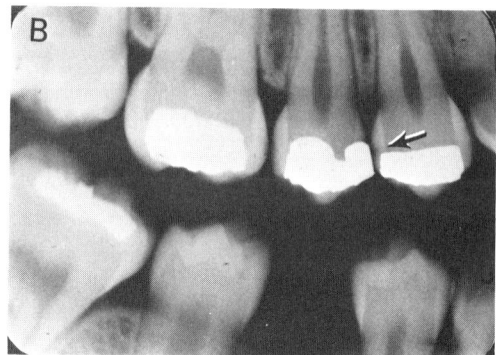

Figure 14-37. Improper Vertical Angulation: **(A)** Periapical radiograph taken with improper vertical angulation. Notice how interproximal spaces are distorted. **(B)** A bite-wing radiograph of same patient in **(A)**. Notice caries on distal of upper first premolar, which could not be seen in periapical radiograph. There is large "cervical burnout" radiolucency on distal of upper canine. It is interesting to note in this case that lower second premolar has erupted into the lower first molar space, leaving space between the two lower premolars.

the tooth over the interproximal surfaces of the tooth. This obliterates the carious lesion from view on the radiograph (Fig. 14-37).

PULPAL AND PERIAPICAL PATHOLOGY

Size of Pulp

The size of the pulp in a newly erupted tooth is quite large (Fig. 14-38). The dentin of a young tooth is called primary dentin, most of which is formed before

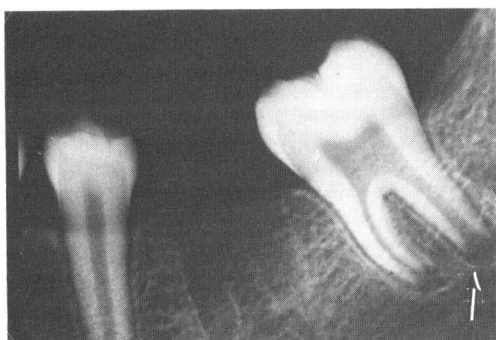

Figure 14-38. Radiograph illustrating the large size of the pulp in a newly erupted second molar. The tooth contains only primary dentin, most of which was formed before eruption of the tooth. Note that the apical foramin have not closed as yet.

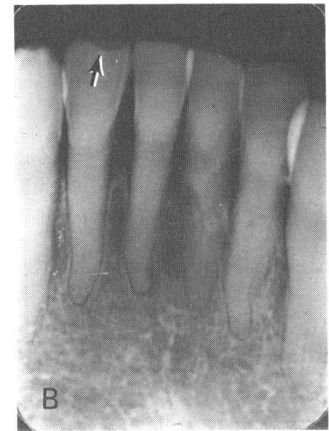

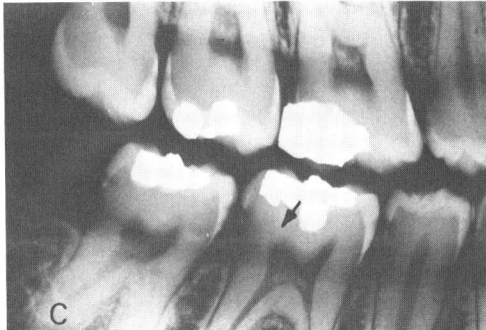

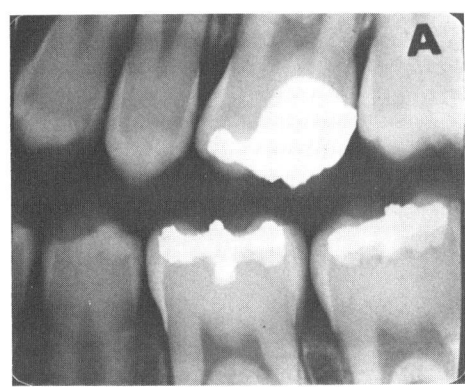

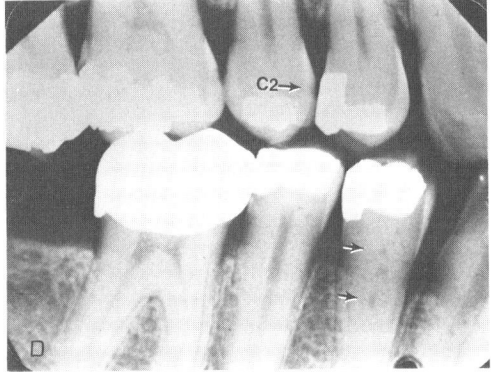

Figure 14-39. Secondary dentin Formation: **(A)** As a person grows older secondary dentin is laid down as a response to stimuli associated with the normal aging process. The reduction of the pulp chambers of all the teeth in this radiograph is associated with the deposition of secondary dentin. **(B)** The pulps of teeth of this elderly person are almost completely effaced by secondary dentin deposition. Note attrition facet of right lateral incisor. **(C)** Reduction of distal pulp horn of pulp chamber of lower first molar, most likely from deposition of secondary dentin as response from distal proximal carious lesion in tooth. **(D)** The pulp chamber and root canal is effaced by deposition of secondary dentin in lower first premolar. Localized acquired gross diminution of pulp cavity is result of trauma in most instances.

eruption of the tooth. As the tooth matures, the tooth responds to stimuli associated with normal biologic function (mastication, small thermal changes, chemical irritants, and slight traumas) to deposit secondary dentin over the pulpal end of the tubules of primary dentin.

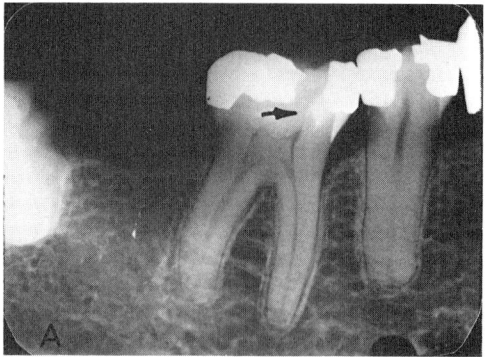

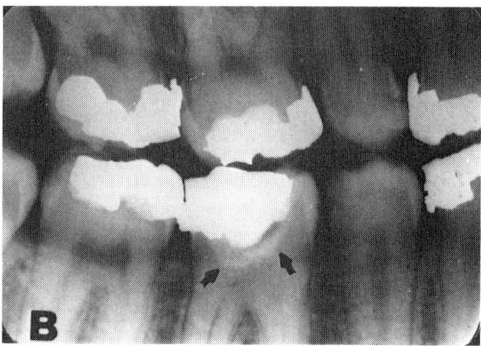

Figure 14-40. Sclerotic (irregular) Dentin: **(A)** There is sclerotic dentin under the mesio-occlusal restoration in the mandibular first molar. It is possible that this is a result of mesial caries of the tooth previous to the placement of the restoration. **(B)** There is radiopaque sclerotic dentin under the secondary caries under restoration in mandibular first molar. Note classical V-shaped caries, distal surface of mandibular second premolar.

Also, when the pulp is severely irritated (such as due to attrition, abrasion, erosion, caries, dentinal exposure from fracture or during preparation of cavities or crowns, improper medication, or harmful filling materials), odontoblasts of the pulp are stimulated to produce dentin for the added protection of the pulp.

Secondary Dentin

Secondary dentin is less permeable and has fewer tubules than primary dentin. Its tubules are more curved, sometimes angulated, less regular, and smaller in diameter.

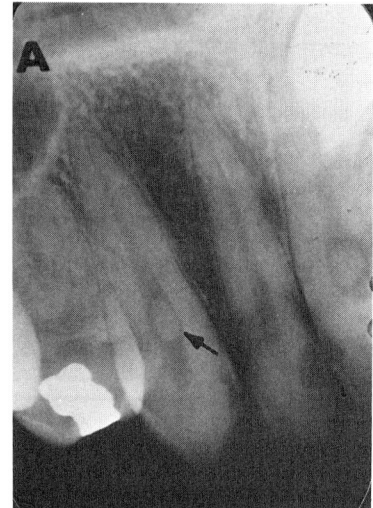

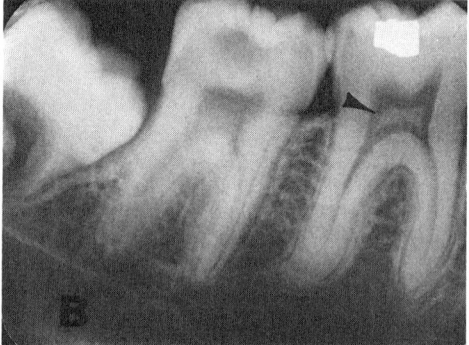

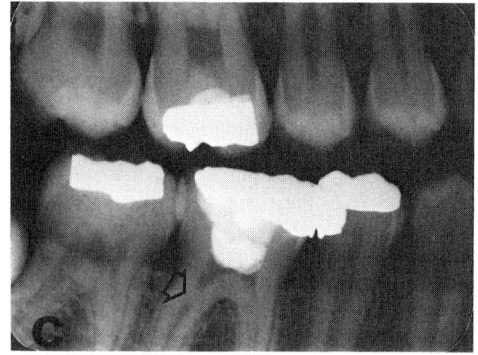

Figure 14-41. Pulpal calcifications. **(A)** There is a large pulp stone (denticle) in pulp chamber of canine. **(B)** Note diffuse amphorus calcifications in lower first molar. **(C)** There is a constriction of the mesial root canal of lower first molar. Also the distal root canal seems to be effaced in a small area (see arrow). This is possibly a dentin bridge, which has formed after surgical excision of coronal part of pulp (pulpotomy) and application of calcium hydroxide over the stump.

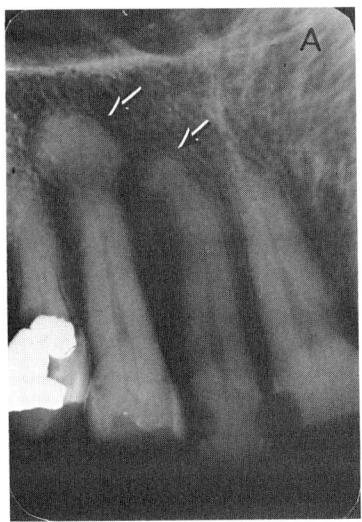
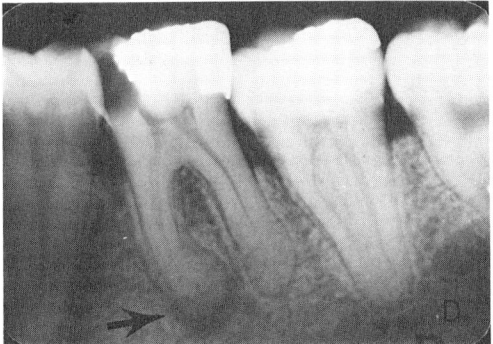
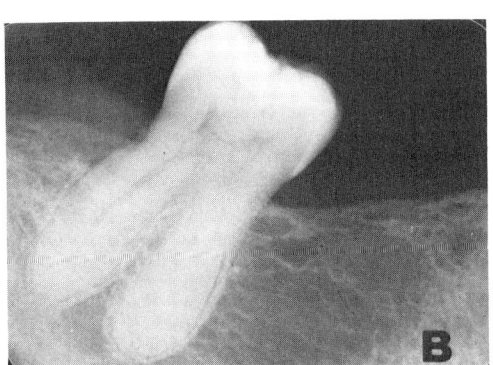
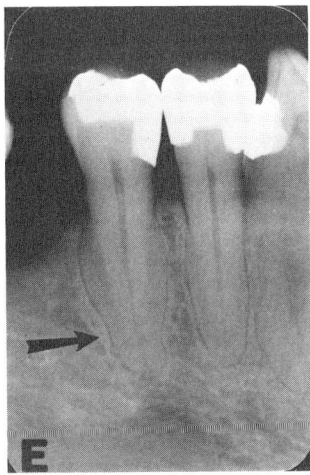
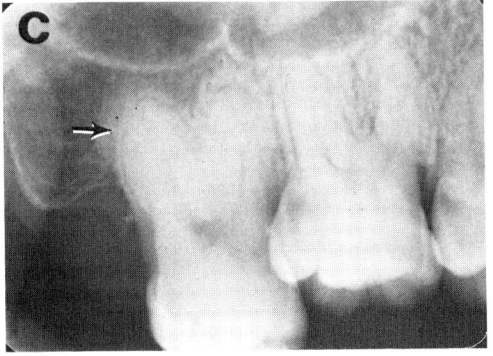

Figure 14-42. Hypercementosis: **(A)** Nodular type of hypercementosis on root tips of canine and lateral incisor. Also note severe attrition, silicate restoration (lateral and central), linear pulp stone (canine), and recurrent caries (mesial first premolar). **(B)** Hypercementosis (dense cemental type) with symmetrical enlargement of entire root. The etiology is unknown, although it could be associated with occlusal trauma in this case. **(C)** Hypercementosis (dense cemental type) with symmetrical enlargement of entire root of second molar. Etiology in probably from supraeruption of tooth because of loss of its antagonist. **(D)** Nodular type of hypercementosis of first molar root tips. Etiology is probably from periapical inflammation. **(E)** Hypercementosis with deposition of transparent type of secondary cementum of premolars. Note demarcation between actual root and secondary cementum.

Since secondary dentin contains fewer tubules with connecting odontoblasts it has but little sensation. Secondary dentin protects the pulp and is of considerable clinical importance in this respect. There is no radiographic difference of secondary and primary dentin but its presence is revealed when the pulp chamber is reduced in size, the reduction equaling the amount of formation of secondary dentin. Its presence can be noticed in pulp horn areas as well as on the proximal walls of teeth with proximal caries. There is a reduction in size of the pulp chamber and of root caries as a person gets older, as a result of secondary dentin formation (Fig. 14-39).

Sclerotic Dentin

The reaction of the tooth to external irritation is **not** confined to the formation of secondary dentin. The primary dentin, too, responds to injury or exposure of the dentinal tubules by becoming **sclerotic** (hard). **Dentinal sclerosis** is the calcification of the dentin by obliteration of the dentinal tubules. The formerly open tubules become filled with calcified material, and thus the dentin in this area becomes impermeable. It is a defensive reaction of the tooth since it increases the resistance of the tooth to caries or to other external damaging agents.

In some areas under carious lesions the x-ray absorption of the **sclerotic dentin** will increase 10-25 percent compared to normal dentin and will appear more **radiopaque** on the dentin (Fig. 14-40).

Sclerosis of the dentin is of great practical importance. It is a contributory cause for the decrease in sensitiveness and permeability of human teeth with advancing age. **Secondary dentin** formation and **dentinal sclerosis** aids in preventing pulpal irritation and infection.

Pulp Calcifications

Calcified bodies are frequently observed in the pulp tissue and are classified in two main groups. The first type is a nodular type called the pulp stone or dentrite while the second consists of irregular, amorphous mineralized deposits. **Pulp stones** may be further classified as either **true or false denticles.**

The **true denticles** are made up of localized masses of calcified tissue that contain few irregular tubules and resemble those found in secondary dentine. They are rare in occurrence. Most of the pulp stones found in human teeth are **false denticles.** They are composed of localized masses of calcified material and do not exhibit dentinal tubules. They are formed by the deposits of connective layers of calcium salts around a central midus. False denticles probably are formed following minor circulatory disturbances of pulp vessels.

Diffuse, amphorus, mineralized deposits are abundant in some pulps, especailly in those of older teeth. These calcifications can be observed histologically following the course of vessels and nerves of the pulp. By fusion of these fibrillar calcifications, long, linear strands of calcified tissue are formed. They could be an expression of generalized arteriosclerosis.

The incidence of pulp stones has been studied by Hill (1934), who reported they occur in 66 percent of all teeth between the ages of ten and twenty years; the incidence rises to 90 percent in the age group between fifty and seventy years. Wilman (1934) found pulp calcifications in 87.2 percent of the teeth he examined. He pointed out that only 15 percent of all pulp calcifications are large enough to be seen on radiographs. In other words, for each pulp stone seen on the radiograph, at least six others are present, but they are so small that they are only visible microscopically. When seen, they appear as radiopaque bodies in the pulp (Fig. 14-41).

It has been reported in the past that pulp stones may give rise to symptoms of obscure neuralgia. However, most investigators now believe that seldom, if ever, are pulp stones the cause of pulpal pain. Also, pulp stones never cause pulpal inflammation, and there is no reason to believe they are a source of infection.

Hypercementosis (Cementum Hyperplasia)

Hypercementosis is the excess formation of cementum on the root surfaces; it is the abnormal increase in the thickness of cementum. The cause of hypercementosis is not always apparent, but it may be associated with (1) low grade, chronic periapical infection (Fig. 14-42D), (2) trauma, in the form of abnormal occlusal stresses, (3) supraeruption of a tooth that has lost its antagonist (Fig. 14-42C), (4) systemic diseases such as Paget's disease, toxic goiter, acromegaly, or giantism, and (5) idiopathic causes. It may affect only one or a few teeth, or it may be generalized throughout the dentition. There are two types (1) a **nodular** or bulbous enlargement near or at the root apex (Fig. 14-42A) or (2) a **symmetrical enlargement** that involves all of the root surface. There are two **symmetrical enlargement types:** (1) the secondary cementum is of the same density as the primary cementum and dentin (Fig. 14-42B) and (2) the secondary cementum appears less dense and is clearly differentiated from the primary cementum and dentin (Fig. 14-42 E). In **hypercementosis,** the periodontal ligament space and the lamina dura are continuous and surround the region of the hypercementosis; in **periapical cemental dysplasia,** the lesion is in the bone and

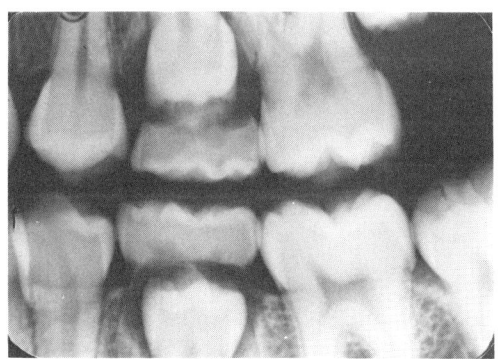

Figure 14-43. Physiologic resorption of roots of primary molars causing them to shed so permanent premolars can erupt.

not attached to the tooth.

Teeth with **hypercementosis** have no significant clinical signs or symptoms. The only practical clinical significance of hypercementosis is the difficulties that may be encountered in extracting such teeth. This may indicate the true biological significance of hypercementosis, which probably is to anchor the tooth in the socket more securely.

Resorption of Teeth

There are two types of resorption, the physiologic and the pathologic. **Physiologic** resorption is a normal process associated with the shedding of primary teeth. The roots of the primary teeth are gradually removed as the permanent teeth begin to erupt (Fig. 14-43). **Pathologic** resorption is any resorption of teeth **not** associated with the shedding of primary teeth. It may begin on the outside surface of the tooth (**external resorpton**) or it may begin on the inside of the pulp (**internal resorption**). Tooth resorption rarely presents early clinical symptoms. Later the resorption process may result in complete undermining of the crown with subsequent fracture.

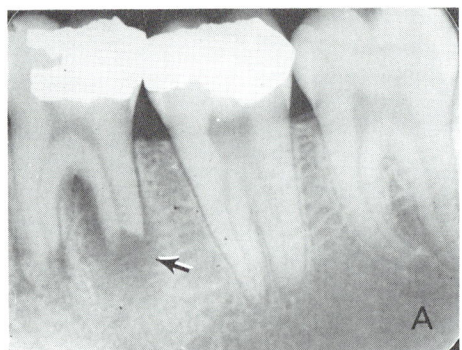
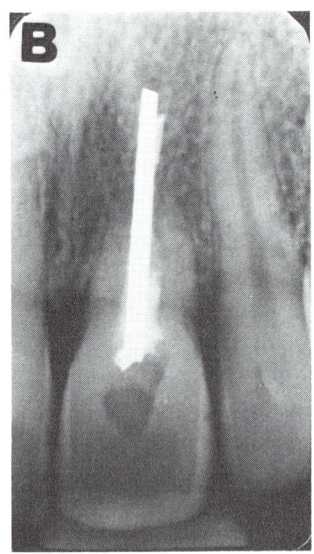
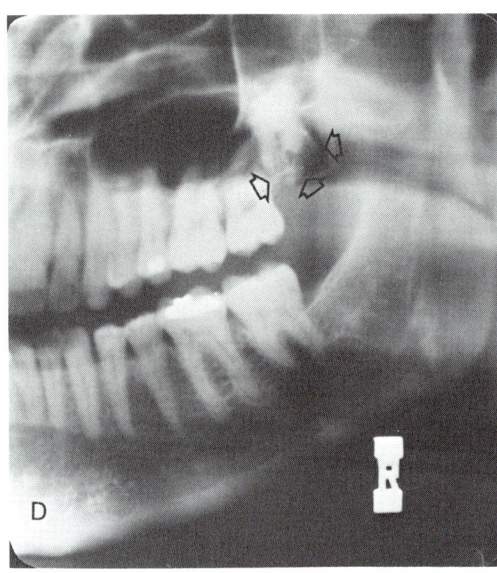

Figure 14-44. External Resorption **(A)** Tooth resorptions associated with inflammation may be either external or internal. External resorption of the apices of the first molar roots in This radiograph are the result of apical periodontitis (inflammation of tissue surrounding the tooth apices). **(B)** Reimplantation of teeth. Resorption of teeth that have reimplanted or transplanted is almost an inevitable occurrence. This tooth was reimplanted within 90 minutes after being completely exfoliated in an accident. The dentist placed a root canal filling and reimplanted the tooth back into tooth socket. this radiograph was taken seven years after the reimplantation. **(C)** Excessive mechanical force applied to teeth causing external resorption of roots of maxillary incisors. **(D)** Notice severe external resorption of crown of impacted maxillary third molar.

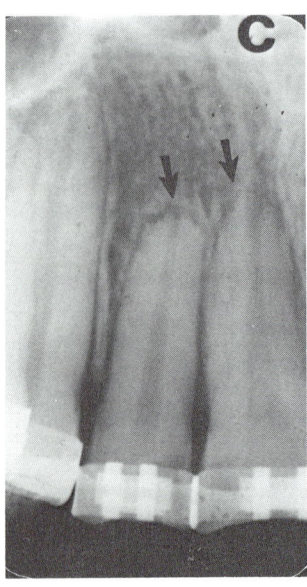

External Resorption

External resorption (Fig. 14-44) is thought to be the result of a reaction of the periodontal or pericoronal tissue to various stimuli:

1. apical inflammation (Fig. 14-44A);
2. tumors and cysts (pressure);
3. reimplantation of teeh (Fig. 14-44B);
4. excessive trauma (Fig. 14-44C);

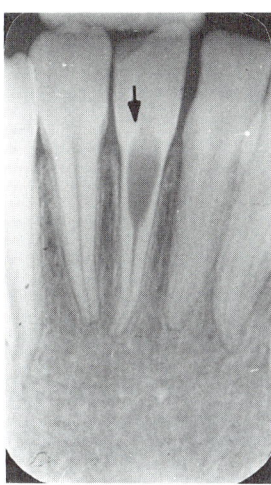

Figure 14-45. Internal resorption of chipped lower central incisor.

5. impacted and embedded teeth (Fig. 14-44D);
6. idiopathic causes.

Internal Resorption

Internal resorption is acquired later in life. The cause is unknown (idiopathic) although trauma is thought to be a prominent cause.

It may be first recognized by the presence of a "pink spot" on the crown of a tooth, which indicates that resorption of the dentin is so pronounced, that the highly vascularized, hyperplastic pulpal tissue filling the resorbed area shows through the enamel.

Radiographs reveal a circular or bowl-like radiolucency with smooth margins. It is significant to determine whether the tooth has external or internal resorption because internal resporption may be arrested by root canal therapy while a tooth with external resorption usually has to be extracted eventually (Fig. 14-45).

Diseases of Pulpal and Periapical Tissue

Pulpal Hyperemia

The hard tissues of the tooth normally protect the pulp from injury. Clinical experience indicates that the pulp of human teeth has the ability to withstand minor degrees of injury. Teeth may be hypersensitive to temperature changes following cavity preparation but subsequently will show a normal response to stimulation. This hypersentivity of the pulp to thermal changes (especially cold) is caused by a hyperemia of the pulp. Hyperemia is dilation and engorgement of the pulp with predisposition to edema and increased capillary pressure as a result of prolonged vasodilation. Hyperemia of the pulp is a reversible condition. If the irritation is removed (high restoration, large restoration without bases, and large carious lesions), the pulp may return to normal; the blood vessels contract, and normal circulation is reestablished. This hyperemic condition of the pulp is called **focal reversible pulpitis** (reversible hyperactive pulpalgia). The pain evoked from focal reversible pulpitis does not occur spontaneously. It is asymptomatic, requiring an external stimulus such as cold to evoke a painful response. The pain is sharp, but ceases when the irritant is removed. Sometimes the hyperemic condition persists for a long time; this indicates a gradual change from hyperemia to pulpitis.

Symptomatic Pulpitis

Since the rigid walls of the pulp chamber tend to prevent vascular dilation and edema, intrapulpal pressure from the severe inflammation (pulpitis) will cause the eventual death of the pulp.

When the pulpitis becomes sympto-

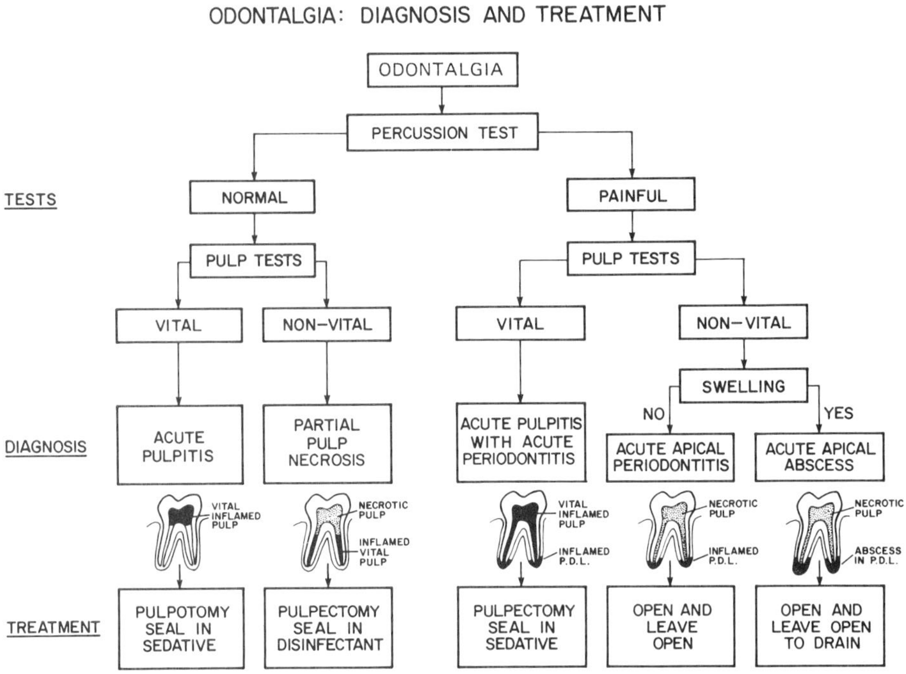

ODONTALGIA: DIAGNOSIS AND TREATMENT

Figure 14-46. Odontalgia chart. (Form Ludlow, M. O.: Endodontic first aid for the patient with odontalgia. *Dent Surve,* 42:25, 1979.)

matic the severity of the clinical symptoms will vary as the inflammatory response increases. The degree of pain depends on the increased tissue pressure (localized edema) of the pulp or periodontal ligament due to inflammation of these tissues. Pain is **spontaneous** and may vary from a mild discomfort to a severe, throbbing, and intolerable pain. If the pain becomes *continuous*, it may have periods of cessation (intermittent). The tooth causing the pain may be difficult to locate because only pain fibers (not proprioceptive) are found in the pulp.

Acute Pulpal Conditions

Ludlow (1979) lists five acute pulpal conditions that can produce **spontaneous** pulpal pain or odontalgia (Fig. 14-46).

Vital Pulp

1. acute pulpitis
2. acute pulpitis with apical periodontitis

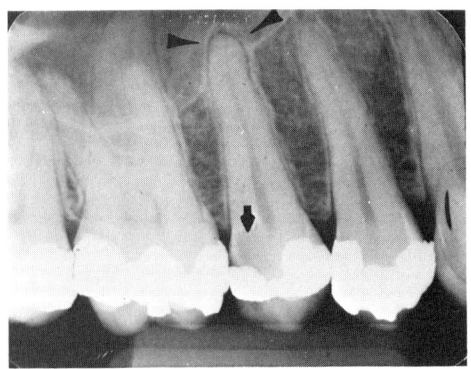

Figure 14-47. Acute Pulpitis with Apical Periodontis. Maxillary second premolar has large recurrent (secondary) caries on distal surface. Note thickened P.D.L. space at apical end of root. The tooth was vital and tender to percussion. The pulp was severely inflamed and anesthesia was difficult to obtain during pulpectomy procedure.

Nonvital Pulps
1. partial pulp necrosis
2. acute apical periodontitis
3. acute apical abscess

Vital Pulps (Odontalgia)

Acute Pulpitis. This type of pulpitis is characterized by a **vital** but inflamed pulp, usually in the coronal portion of the tooth. The pain is spontaneous, diffuse, and difficult at times to locate because the inflammation is confined to the pulp. Percussion tests are **negative.** The radiograph may show the cause of the pulpitis such as a large carious lesion, but the periapical region will, in most cases, reveal a **normal** configuration.

Acute Pulpitis with Apical Periodontitis. This condition is an extension of inflammation of a **vital** pulp to the periapical region. Percussion tests are now **positive.** However, teeth associated with sinusitis of the maxillary sinus or periodontal disease will elicit pain upon percussion. A positive radiograph may be seen if the inflammation is prolonged for ten days or more because 30-60 percent of the mineral content of the lamina must be resorbed in order for the periodontal ligament space to appear widened (Fig. 14-47).

Nonvital Pulps (Odontalgia)

Partial Pulp Necrosis (Chronic Pulpitis). This condition is characterized by necrosis of the coronal portion of the pulp. Necrosis, or death of pulp tissue, may be partial or total depending on the extent of the tissue involvement.

The pulp of chronic pulpitis is essentially **nonvital;** however, it may give high readings on the pulp tester if the root portion of the tooth still has vital, inflamed tissue remaining. The inflammation has **not** spread to the periapical tissue as yet; therefore, the **percussion tests** and **radiograph** will give **negative** information. Pain may be absent; if present, it will be a dull, vague pain, which in most cases can be kept under control by aspirins. The offending tooth may be difficult, at times, to locate because the pain of chronic pulpitis can be referred to other teeth in the same region.

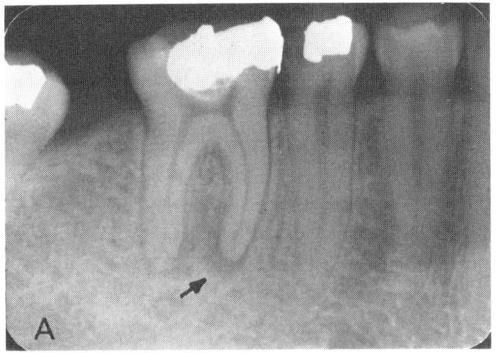

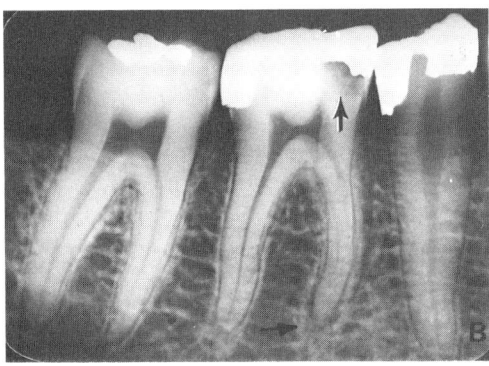

Figure 14-48. Acute Apical Periodontitis. (A) Note thickening of both P.D.L. spaces at both apices, (especially at the mesial root) of the mandibular first molar. A previous pulp capping treatment on the tooth had failed. Tooth is nonvital, tender to percussion, with no swelling or tenderness to palpation. The pulp contained necrotic material. (B) Note thickened **P.D.L.** space of mesial root of lower first molar. Tooth has large secondary carious lesion under mesial portion of restoration in this tooth. Tooth is nonvital in mesial root and tender to percussion. A root canal treatment was completed on tooth.

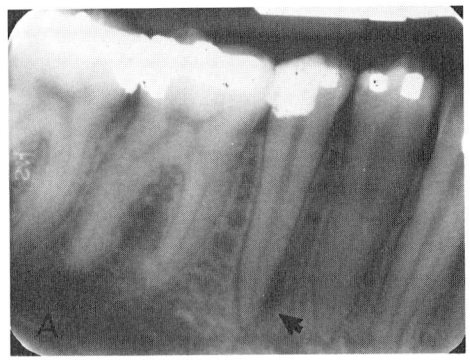

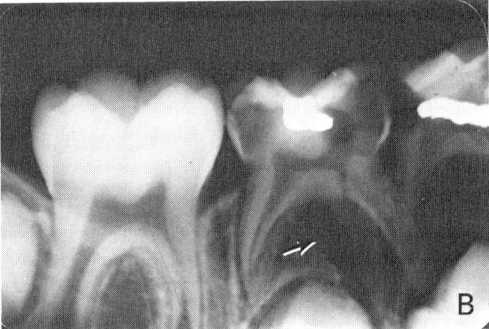

Figure 14-49. Acute Apical Abscess (Acute Alveolar Abscess): **(A)** Notice thickening of P.D.L. space of lower second premolar. Tooth has temporary filling placed over a previous pulp exposure during cavity preparation. The tooth is mobile, nonvital, has percussion pain, with swelling and tenderness to palpation. Upon removal of the temporary restoration and entry into the pulp with a high speed handpiece, a purulent exudate (push) drained from the access opening. The pain subsided immediately. **(B)** Note the radiolucency in furcation are of lower second primary molar. In a primary molar, this is the usual region for periapical pathology to be seen. It is possibly due to accessory canals in this region. Tooth had all the symptoms of an acute apical abscess.

Acute Apical Periodontitis: In this condition the pulp is necrotic (dead) and the periapical tissue inflamed with a serous exudate, causing pain in the periodontal ligament. The pulp is **nonvital** and the **percussion test** is **positive.**

There is no tenderness or swelling upon palpation of the soft tissue over the offending tooth. This indicates that the inflammation is confined to the periapical region of the tooth. The pain may range from a slight tenderness in the initial stages to an intense, constant throbbing pain easily localized by the patient. The **radiograph** may reveal a **slight thickening** of the periodontal ligament space (Fig. 14-48).

Acute Apical Abscess. This condition is characterized by a necrotic pulp and liquefaction necrosis of the periapical tissues, which results in edema and abscess (pus) formation in the periodontal ligament space. The tooth is **nonvital** and painful on percussion. There is often swelling in the soft tissue over the offending tooth and sometimes facial cellulitis is present. This is the old fashioned toothache in which the pain is intense, constant, and sometimes throbbing. The radiograph usually will show a thickening of the periodontal ligament space of the painful tooth (Fig. 14-49).

Chronic Periapical Disease

There are a number of chronic responses of the periapical tissue to the toxic irritants of the infected pulp. The type of reaction depends on the number and virulence of the invading organisms and the tissue resistance of the host.

The pain is mild or absent in chronic periapical conditions because the intraperiapical pressure from the exudate is lessened and balanced.

When the strength of the irritant is significantly reduced, the response is the growth of granulation tissue in the periapical tissue to heal and repair the region of injury. However, as long as the toxic products are still present, complete repair cannot be realized. The granulation tissue consists of capillary proliferation and fibroblastic activity plus the

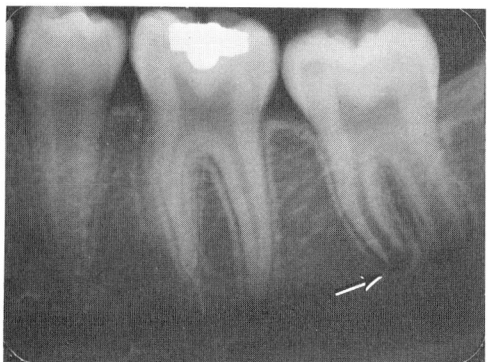

Figure 14-50. The apices of roots of lower second molar have not closed as yet and may mimic periapical pathology.

infiltration of defense cells: lymphocytes, plasma cells, and tissue machrophages. The pulps of the teeth with chronic periapical disease are **nonvital** and **asymptomatic**. The radiograph will reveal a radiolucent periapical lesion of varying size, shape, and appearance. It is not possible for the clinician to make a positive diagnosis of the type of chronic periapical lesion by radiographic evidence only. A definitive diagnosis can only be made by the removal of the lesion and studying it under a microscope. It is possible, however, for the clinician to make a **provisional diagnosis** from the radiograph and the clinical findings to plan appropriate therapy for the tooth in question.

Nonpathologic Apical Conditions

Before a radiologic description of each of the chronic periapical conditions is given, it is important to be aware of radiolucencies that mimic periapical lesions. Some of these nonpathologic apical periodontal ligament space-widening conditions are as follows:

1. terminal stage of root formation;
2. widening of p.d.l. space due to trauma;

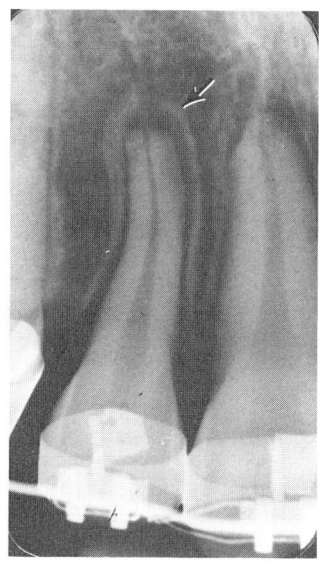

Figure 14-51. Note widening of periodontal ligament space and thickening of lamina dura as maxillary lateral incisor is moved lingually by an orthodontic appliance. It is possible that this type of widening of P.D.L. space could be mistaken for periapical pathology.

3. superimposition of nasal fossae over the maxillary incisors in panoramic films.

Terminal Stage of Root Formation: This is probably the most common cause of periodontal nonpathologic space widening. A wide periodontal space at the root may persist for approximately six months after completion of the root development prior to the closure of the apical foramen. When this type of apical periodontal ligament space widening is present in a tooth with extensive caries, it may be difficult to differentiate it from periapical pathology (Fig. 14-50).

Widening of Periodontal Ligament Space from Trauma. Trauma to a tooth results in widening of the periodontal ligament space and may mimic periapical pathology. The widening of the p.d.l. space usually will return to its normal appear-

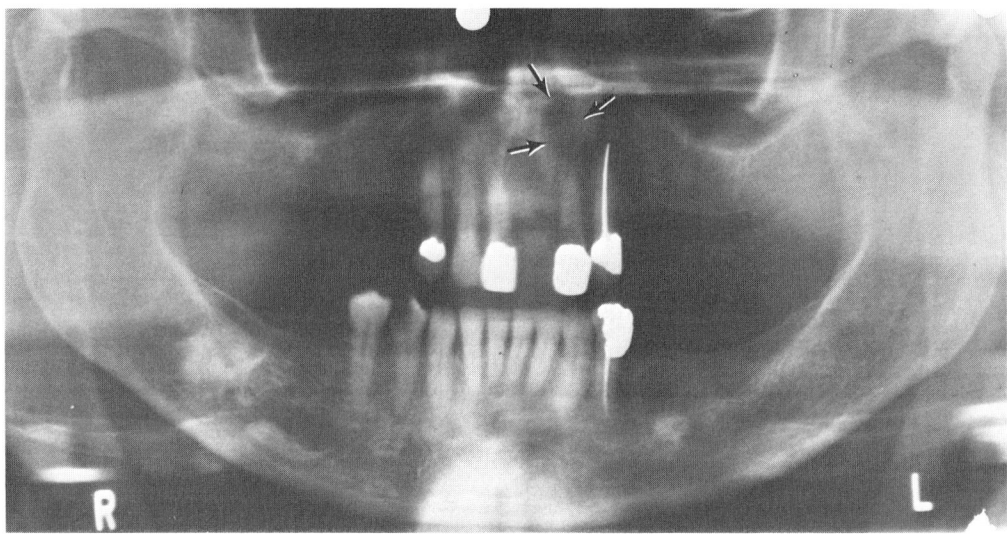

Figure 14-52. Superimposition of the nasal fossae over the maxillary anterior incisors as shown in this panoramic radiograph give the appearance of periapical pathology of maxillary left canine.

ance after removal of the trauma. Some types of trauma that will cause periodontal ligament space widening are —

1. occlusal traumatism;
2. orthodontic movement (Fig. 14-51);
3. trauma from a blow to the tooth.

Superimposition of radiolucent anatomical structures over apices of teeth. Superimposition of radiolucent anatomical structures over the apices of teeth can be mistaken for periapical pathology. Some of the anatomic structures are —

1. nasal fossae (Fig. 14-52);
2. mental foramen;
3. nasaopalatine (incisive) foramen;
4. submandibular fossae.

Interpretation of Chronic Periapical Conditions

Lamina Dura. Lamina dura (alveolar bone proper) is applied to the thin layer of dense cortical bone that lines the normal tooth socket. The compact bone over the alveolar crest is also included as a portion of lamina dura. Because of its density the lamina dura is revelaed in radiographs as a thin white line (Fig. 14-53).

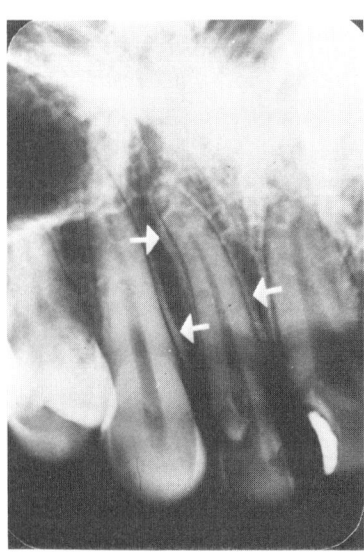

Figure 14-53. Lamina dura is outlined by arrows. (Copyright at Eastman Kodak Company. Reprinted by permission.)

Radiologic Interpretation of Dental Disease 465

In almost every normal tooth the lamina dura can be traced from the crest, around the root, and into the bifurcation and trifurcation. However, there are some teeth that end in very slender points. The lamina dura is so thin in these teeth that the lamina dura may not be seen on the radiograph. Teeth that are most likely to

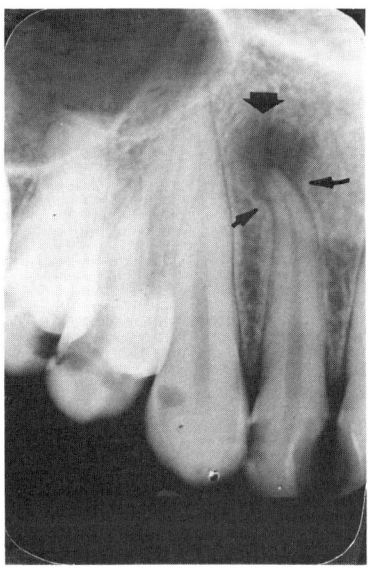

Figure 14-54. Note the loss of continuity of the lamina dura (white line) surrounding the apex of the lateral incisor, which has large silacate restorations.

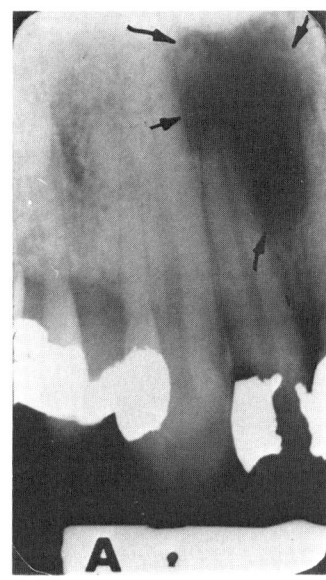

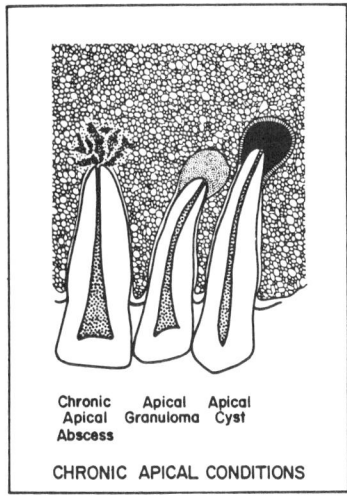

Figure 14-55. Chronic apical lesions. The fourth lesion, apical condensing osteitis is not shown.

Figure 14-56. Chronic apical abscess will develop when apical granuloma becomes overwhelmed by masses of pulpal irritants. It results in a cavity filled with pus, and the symptoms of acute pain, tenderness, and swelling return as the pus under pressure follows the line of least resistance to escape from the alveolar bone **(A)** Chronic apical abscess of maxillary lateral incisor, which was previously restored with Class III gold foils. Note secondary caries on distal surface. **(B)** Chronic apical abscess of second premolar, which has formed from a preexisting apical granuloma. A previously placed sedative cement has partially broken out of the tooth.

present difficulty in tracing the lamina dura around the apex are the upper canines and lower second premolars. When **resorption** of the lamina dura at the apex occurs, it appears radiographically to have lost its continuity, its thickness, and varying degrees of its radiopacity. This usually indicates, with few exceptions, that periapical disease is present (Fig. 14-54).

Chronic Periapical Lesions

There are four chronic periapical lesions that can be seen on a radiograph

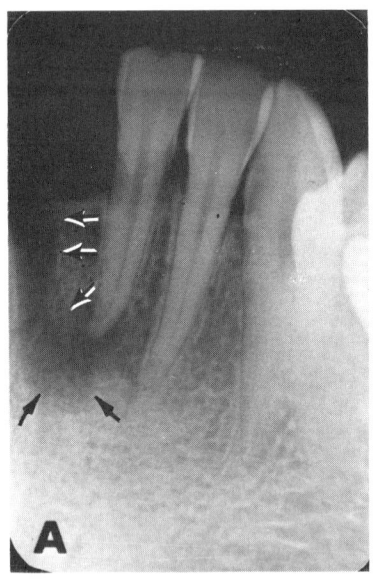

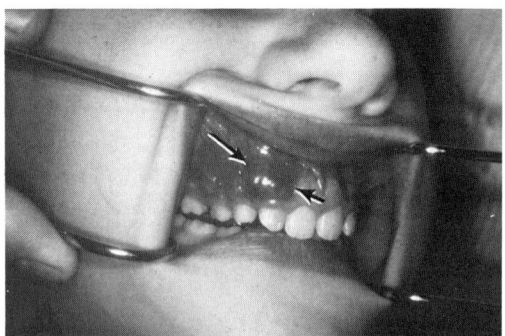

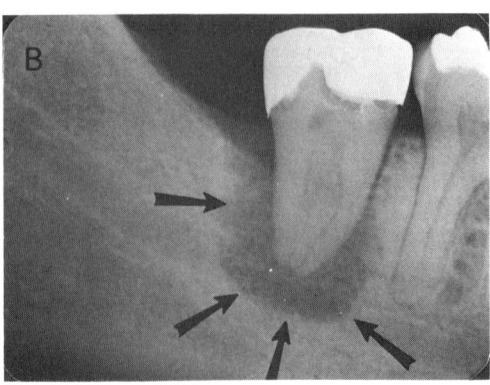

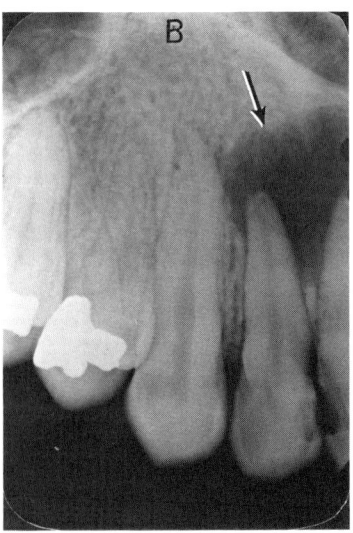

Figure 14-57. Chronic apical abscess originating from acute apical abscess by establishing free drainage of the pus through the bone by way of a fistulous tract. **(A)** Chronic apical abscess formed from an acute apical abscess of the lateral incisor. Note radiolucent fistulous tract through the alveolar bone. **(B)** Chronic apical abscess, which has formed a passageway for the free drainage of pus through the periodontal ligament space.

Figure 14-58. The parulus or "gumboil" is the classical sign of a chronic apical abscess. **(A)** This young person had previously experienced all the acute symptoms of an acute apical abscess of the maxillary lateral incisor. After free drainage of pus through the gumboil, the acute symptoms subsided. **(B)** Radiograph of chronic apical abscess of another patient, which originated from an acute apical abscess after a fistulous opening was established through the mucoperiosteal tissue of the facial alveolar bone.

(Fig. 14-55):

1. **chronic apical abscess** (suppurative periodontitis, chronic alevolar abscess);
2. **apical granuloma** (chronic apical periodontits, dental granuloma);
3. **Apical Cyst** (radicular cyst, periapical cyst);
4. **condensing osteitis** (sclerosing osteitis, chronic focal sclerosing osteomyelitis).

Chronic Apical Abscess (Chronic Alveolar Abscess)

This is a low-grade suppurative process of the periapical region. The teeth involved are usually asymptomatic unless an acute exacerbation (increase in severity of disease) has occurred. The chronic apical abscess may develop from either an apical granuloma or an acute apical abscess. A chronic apical abscess usually forms when there is a continuous increase of pulpal noxious irritants into a previously existing apical granuloma. The apical granuloma breaks down forming an abscess cavity filled with pus, with all the clinical symptoms of an acute apical abscess. The classical radiographic appearance of a chronic apical abscess is a radiolucent lesion with diffuse, irregular borders that fade indistinctly into normal bone. The apical granuloma and apical cyst lesions tend to have a more well-defined border than the chronic apical abscess. The radiolucency usually extends for a considerable distance along the side of the root surface (Fig. 14-56).

During the course of an acute apical abscess, the pus under pressure begins to pass through the alveolar bone seeking the paths of least resistance. The most usual route is through the facial and lingual plates of bone. Sometimes the pus may drain through the periodontal ligament space (Fig. 14-57). When free drainage of the pus is established through a fistulous opening or by incision through the mucoperiosteal tissue, a chronic apical abscess forms. The acute symptoms of acute apical abscess — pain, tenderness, and swelling-will subside. If the fistulous tract becomes blocked, it will again give rise to the acute symptoms of the acute apical abscess. A classical sign of a chronic apical abscess is the presence of a large spherical mass of gingival tissue, called a gumboil or parulis, lying over the region of the tooth in question (Fig. 14-58). The gumboil will usually have a small opening on its surface. A gutta percha point inserted into the orifice of the fistulous tract prior to taking of a radiograph will establish which tooth or root is involved.

In order to successfully treat a chronic apical abscess, it is necessary first to establish proper drainage, followed by removal of necrotic pulp and application of adequate seal. Usually the chronic apical abscess heals without surgical treatment of the fistulous tract because the fistulous tract is usually lined with granulomatous tissue, which is already organized to heal and repair the tract as soon as the irritant is removed.

Apical Granuloma (Chronic Apical Periodontitis)

The most common chronic apical condition developing from pulpitis in dental practice is the **apical granuloma**. It is essentially a growth of granulation tissue in response to pulpal infection. **Granulation tissue** is a repair and healing tissue containing new capillaries and young fibroblasts. It is also a defensive tissue against infection because the tissue includes lymphocytes, polymorphonuclear leukocytes, plasma cells, and histiocytes. These defensive cells have antibacterial and antitoxin properties. Ross (1954)

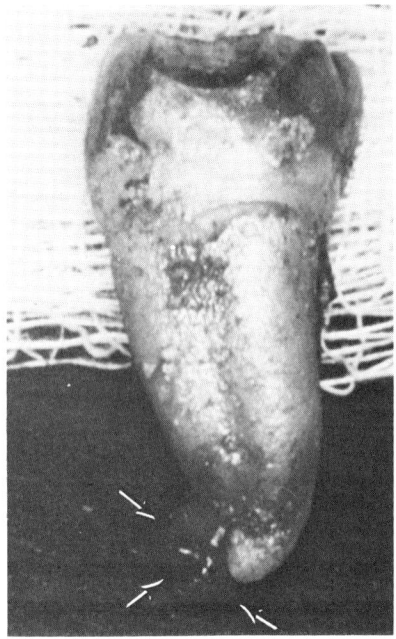

Figure 14-59. Note fibrous capsule of apical granuloma (confirmed by microscopic examination) projecting from lingual of apex extracted lower second molar.

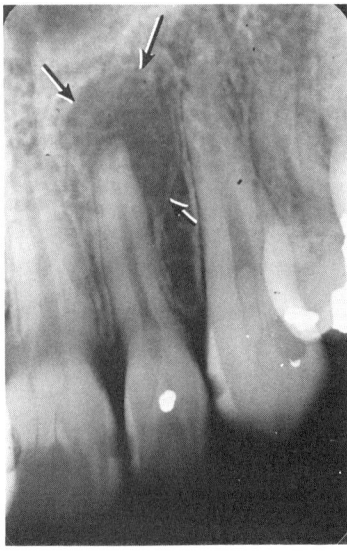

Figure 14-60. Radiographic appearance of apical granuloma of maxillary lateral incisor. The lesion is somewhat rounded, well circumscribed, and bone trabeculations may be seen superimposed over lesion giving at a grayish appearance.

concluded that the **granuloma** (nodule of granulation tissue) is strictly a defensive tissue, "not a place in which bacteria are destroyed." The apical granuloma varies in size from a few millimeters to 10-12 mm. The apical granuloma usually contains strands of epithelial tissue derived from the **cell rests of Mallassez** in the periodontal ligament. It has a continuous collagenous fiber capsule separating the granulation tissue from bone (Fig. 14-59). The teeth are asymptomatic and nonvital; they are usually discovered through routine radiographic examination. Since the dental granuloma is made up chiefly of granulation tissue (repair tissue), it will heal itself if the source of irritation is removed by proper root canal treatment.

The radiographic appearance of the apical granuloma is a somewhat rounded, rather circumscribed radiolucency at the apex of the root of a tooth. The radiolucency is not dark, and trabeculations may be seen within the lesion. Sometimes a thin wall of compact, cancelled bone surrounding the lesion may be seen (Fig. 14-60).

Apical Cyst

The apical cyst is a true cyst in that it is an abnormal pathologic space within bone lined with epithelium, usually filled with a fluid, which varies from a clear amber to one that is yellow and viscous. The epithelial lining of the cyst is derived from proliferation **cell rests of Mallassez** usually present in all periodontal ligaments and apical granulomas. The destruction of the surrounding bone is on the basis of pressure absorption, and some cysts obtain enormous sizes. They are asymptomatic, unless infected. Percussion, mobility, and vitality tests are all negative. Apical cysts are the most common cysts of the jaws, and found most of-

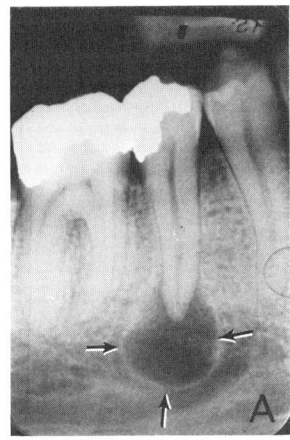

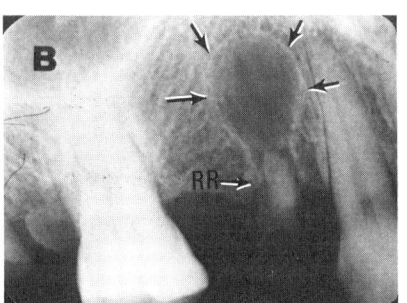

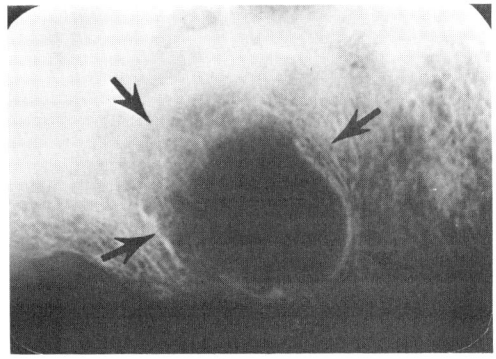

Figure 14-62. Residual cyst in maxillary jaw after extraction of the maxillary second molar.

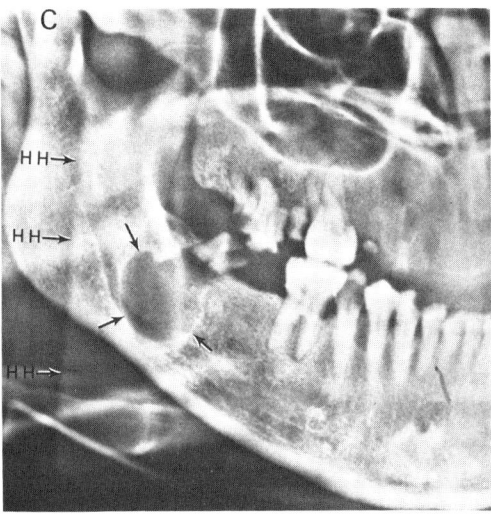

Figure 14-61. Apical Cysts. (A) Classic radiographic appearance of apical cyst of lower second premolar. (B) Apical cyst of root tip of maxillary first premolar confirmed by microscopic examination. (C) Large apical cyst of retained roots (RR) of mandibular third molar. (HH) Radiographic image of panoramic x-ray machine head holder.

ten in the maxilla in the canine and incisor regions. Mandibular apical cysts are more frequently found in the premolar and molar regions. It was earlier thought that apical cysts would not heal without surgical intervention. However, clinical and histologic evidence now implies that some apical cysts will heal without surgical enucleation. It probably happens because apical cysts are surrounded by granulomatous tissue; when the canals are instrumented in root canal therapy, the destruction of the epithelial lining of the cyst is stimulated.

The radiographic appearance of apical cyst is a circumscribed area of radiolucency at the root apex usually bounded by an unbroken line of sclerotic bone. the radiolucent area is generally round in outline, except where it approximates adjacent teeth, in which case it may be flattened in outline (oval pattern). It shows little signs of trabecular superimposition as the apical granuloma does, and

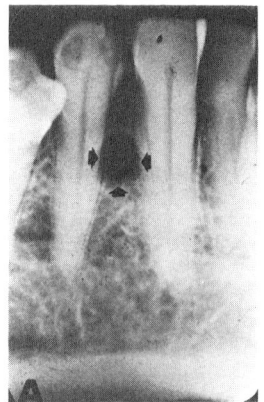

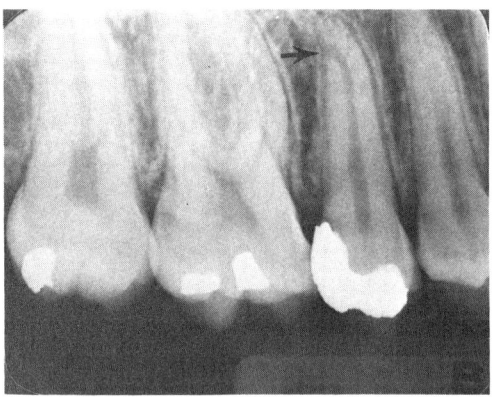

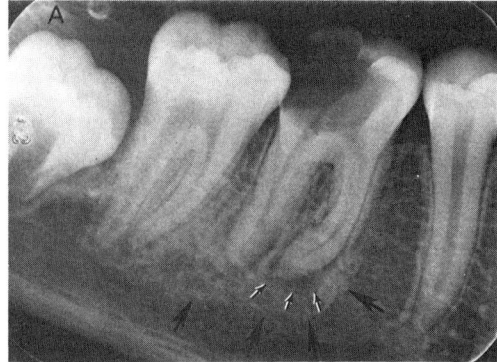

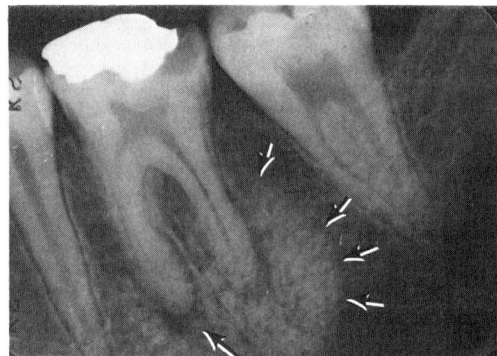

Figure 14-64. Apical Condensing Osteitis. **(A)** Teenager with large carious lesion of mandibular first molar, which proved to have a nonvital pulp. Note the area of apical condensing osteitis at root tips of tooth. **(B)** Mandibular first molar with apical condensing osteitis. Tooth is nonvital and with secondary caries of restored occlusal restoration.

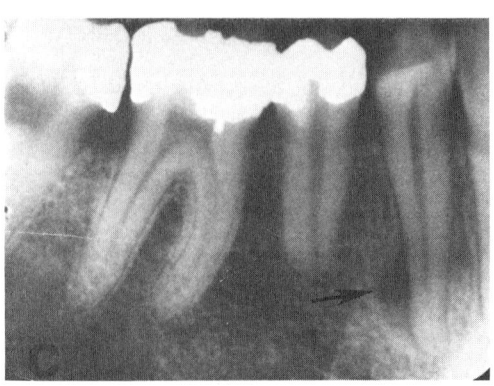

Figure 14-63. Lateral periodontal cysts. **(A)** Lateral periodontal cyst arising from primordial cyst of supernumerary tooth germ between mandibular canine and first premolar. The teeth are vital. **(B)** Note that the root canal of the maxillary second premolar exists from the distal side of root inside of at the apex of the tooth. **(C)** A lateral periodontal cyst has arisen from distal side of mandibular first premolar, possibly from infected accessary root canal. Tooth was nonvital.

the radiolucency is very dark. The apical cyst is usually larger than the apical granuloma and often involves two or more teeth (Fig. 14-61).

Residual Cyst. A residual cyst is a cyst that remains in the jaw after the tooth with which it was originally associated is no longer present. Nearly all residual cysts were at one time an apical type, although on rare occasions a dentigerous cyst may persist after removal of an unerupted tooth (Fig. 14-62).

Lateral Periodontal Cyst. This is an uncommon odontogenic cyst, which *ap-*

pears to arise directly in the lateral periodontal ligament space of an erupted tooth. (Fig. 14-63A). It has a predilection for the mandibular canine area. The most likely explanation for this cyst is that it represents a primordial cyst of a supernumerary tooth germ. It is thought best to call them "primordial cysts" and to reserve the term "lateral periodontal cyst" for the inflammatory lesions arising in the lateral periodontal ligament from an infected lateral accessary pulp canal stimulating proliferation of the **cell rests of Malassez.**

The. tooth is vital if it is a primordial cyst and nonvital when the cyst arises as a result of infected pulpal irritants gaining access to the lateral periodontal ligament space by way of an accessory canal (Fig. 14-63B, C).

Apical Condensing Osteitis (Chronic Focal Sclerosing Osteomyelitis)

This is a reaction of apical bone to a mild inflammatory stimulation. It is seen in persons with extremely high tissue resistance or in cases of low grade infection. **Apical condensing osteitis** is a form of bone inflammation that occurs almost exclusively in younger individuals prior to the age of twenty. The mandibular first molar is the tooth most commonly involved and usually presents a large carious lesion. The tooth involved is asymptomatic and the pulp is nonvital.

Radiographically, it reveals a small radiolucent apical area circumscribed by a larger radiopaque area. The sclerotic bone is not attached, and it remains after the tooth is removed. The sclerotic area is generally characterized radiographically by a reduction in size of the trabecular spaces and increase in number of trabeculae resulting in an opacity of the involved bone. Usually there will be a radiolucency of various sizes immediately adjacent to the apical end of involved tooth (Fig. 14-64).

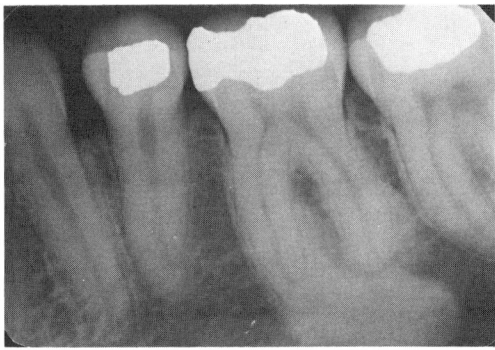

Figure 14-65. Osteoslcerosis. Tooth is vital and found to be withstanding undue amounts of stress because of anterior open-bite. Note there is no radiolucent area between dense bone and root tip.

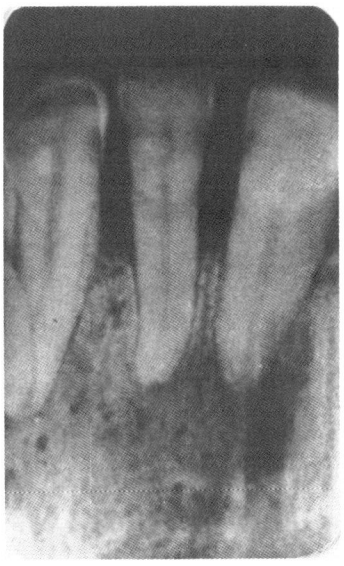

Figure 14-66. Chronic Osteomyelitis: Notice the "moth-eaten" appearance of the multiple areas of small radiolucent dots in the generalized radiolucent bone, which gives the bone a "moth-eaten" appearance.

Osteosclerosis (endostosis, bone whorls, bone islands, focal osteopetrosis). This is a general term meaning "an increased bone formation resulting in reduced marrow spaces and increased radiopacity." It is sometimes used interchangeably with condensing osteitis, but it is best to limit **osteosclerosis** to abnormally dense areas in the bone resulting from trauma, stress, or some other **noninflammatory cause** and to use **condensing osteitis** when the etiology is thought to be **infection or inflammation** as an and result of a low-grade periapical or periodontal infection.

Osteosclerosis has the same density as cortical bone, is well defined, and when appearing around the roots of teeth, there is no intervening radiolucent area. Also, there is no resorption or obliteration of associated root. It is usually located in the mandibular molar and premolar area and may be seen in several areas of the same patient. It is associated with **vital** teeth; teeth while condensing osteitis are associated with nonvital teeth (Fig. 14-65).

Osteomyelitis. Osteomyelitis is inflammation of bone and bone marrow. It may develop in the jaws as a result of odontogenic infection, as well as in a variety of other conditions. Before antibiotic therapy, osteomylitis was somewhat prevalent in dental practice. There are still patients who are prone to osteomyelitis:

1. patients immunosupressed by steriod theory or other chemotherapy;
2. patients irradiated for cancer;
3. severelly debilitated patients, such as those with uncontrolled diabetes, Paget's disease, and osteopetrosis.

The disease may be chronic or subacute. Various types of bacteria may be cultured from the lesions of osteomyelitis. The most common are *Staphylococcus aureus, Staphylococous albus,* and various streptococci.

It starts with a diffuse spread of infection through the medullary spaces, with subsequent necrosis of a variable amount of bone. In the acute stage, it is usually accompanied by severe pain, elevation of temperature, regional lymphadenopathy, high white blood cell count, and loosening of teeth. Paresthesia or anesthesia of lip is common with mandibular involvement.

The presence of one or two purulent fistulous tracts and redness of overlying mucosa are consistant findings.

In the **acute stage,** radiographic evidence will **not** be present for at least **one to two weeks,** when diffuse radiolucencies begin to appear.

Unresolved acute osteomyelitis may give rise to **chronic osteomyelitis,** which may be difficult to control. The radiograph of **chronic osteomyelitis** shows multiple radiolucent areas, which give the bone a "moth-eaten" appearance. The radiolucent areas have ragged, poorly defined borders. Some areas of bone sequestration may be seen (Fig. 14-66).

OSTEORADIONECROSIS. Osteoradionecrosis is a peculiar type of osteomyelitis that only affects bone previously exposed to therapeutic irradiation. The basic underlying factor is a compromised blood supply due to radiation-induced fibrosis of blood vessels. The mandible is more frequently involved due to its lack of adequate collateral blood supply.

The radiographic appearance of osteoradionecrosis is very similar to chronic osteomyelitis.

Chronic osteomyelitis is diagnosed by culture and sensitivity tests, nuclear scans with gallium[69] and technetium[99mpd], hyperbaric oxygen therapy, and a surgical debridment; it is then treated by long-term antibiotics.

Periapical Cemental Dysplasia (Apical Cementoma)

This is a benign, slow growing, connective tissue proliferation of unknown etiology originating from cellular elements of the periodontal ligament. The developing lesion destroys the lamina

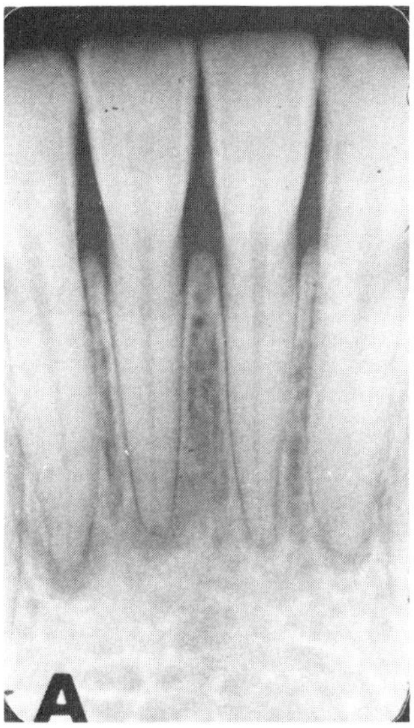

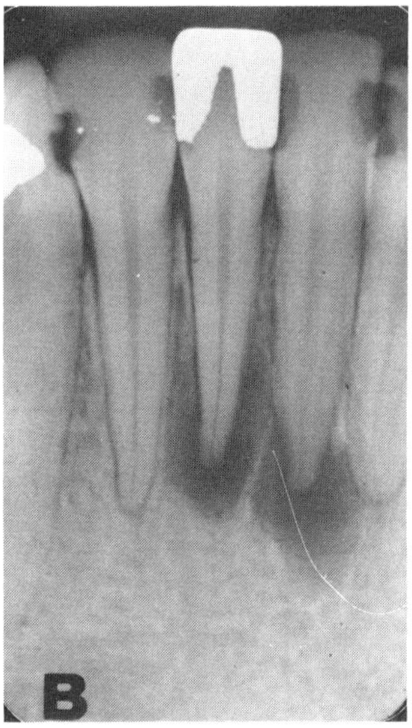

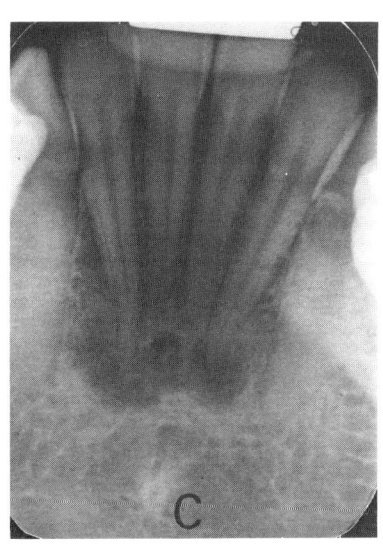

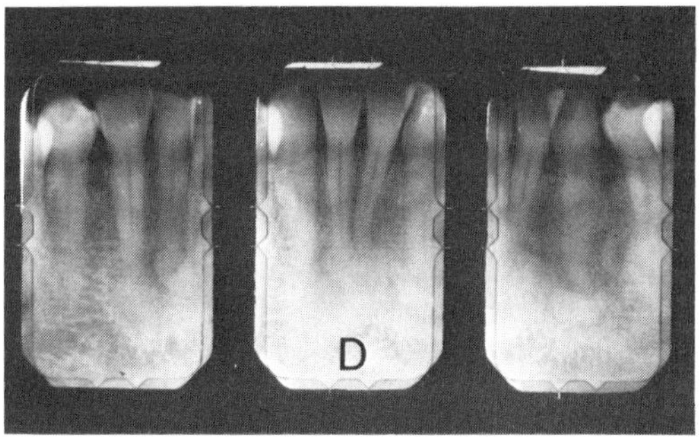

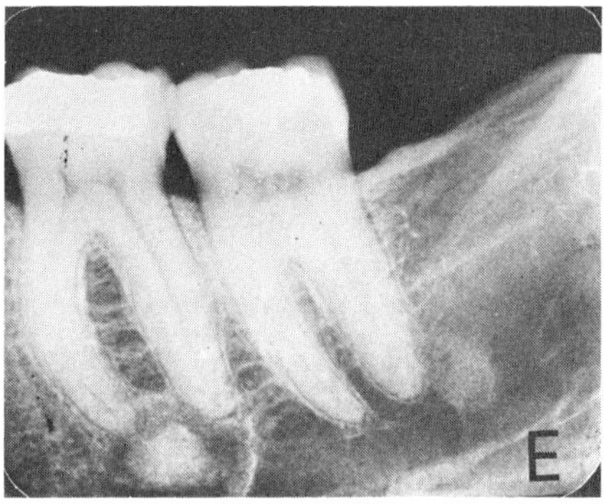

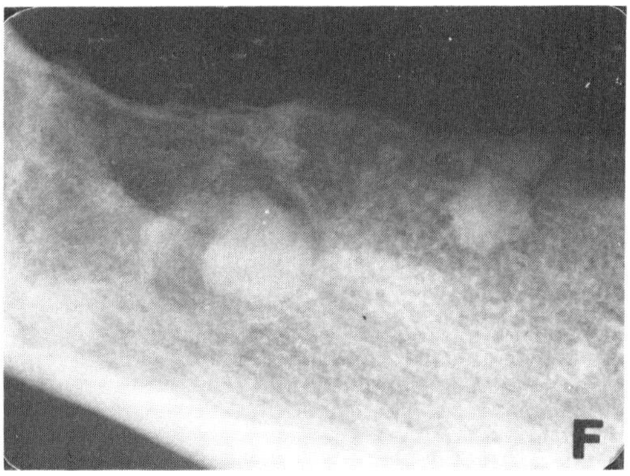

Figure 14-67. Periapical Cemental Dysplasia (apical cementoma): **(A)** Fibrous or autolytic stage of apical cementoma. Note radiolucencies at apices of all mandibular incisors. Teeth are vital. **(B)** These radiolucencies at apices of the incisors are not apical cementomas. The pulps of both incisors are nonvital and radiolucencies are probably apical granulomas. **(C)** The second or intermediate stage of the apical cementoma. It is a mixed lesion with both radiopacities and radiolucencies at apices of mandibular incisors. **(D)** Third or mature cemetoblastic stage of apical cementomas. **(E)** Target lesion (opacity with lucent halo) of apical cementoma. **(F)** Apical cementomas associated with posterior teeth retained in alveolar bone after teeth were extracted.

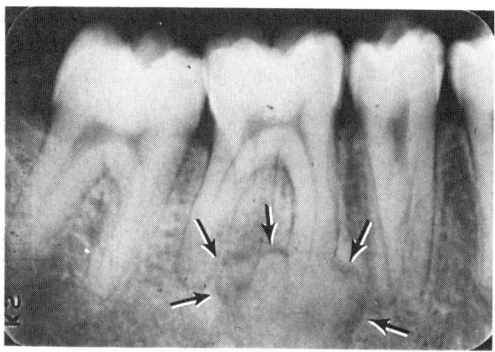

Figure 14-68. Benign Cementoblastoma (true cementoma) Benign cementoblastoma of lower first molar of eighteen-year-old male. Note that outer periphery of lesion is well-delineated by a thin radiolucent line. The mesial root apex appears to be continuous or fused to the radiopaque mass. (Also, it appears that first molar has three roots — two mesial roots.)

dura and spreads periapically replacing the surrounding normal trabecular bone with a fibrous tissue mass, within which are varying amounts of cementumlike material. It has limited growth potential, is of long duration, and is most often seen in middle-aged black females at the apices of vital mandibular anterior teeth. They may be single or multiple in number. It requires no treatment. Three stages of growth may be seen:

1. In the **fibrous** or **osteolytic stage** there is a radiolucency at the apex of the tooth that mimics a periapical inflammatory lesion; (Fig. 14-67 A).
2. In the second or **intermediate stage,** the periapical lesion can be seen radiographically as a mixed radiopaque and radiolucent lesion (Fig. 14-67C).
3. In the third or **mature cementoblastic stage** the radiographic appearance reveals a radiopaque mass of comparatively even density encircled by a thin, radiolucent line. The radiolucent space separating the radiopaque mass from an outer rim of radiopa-

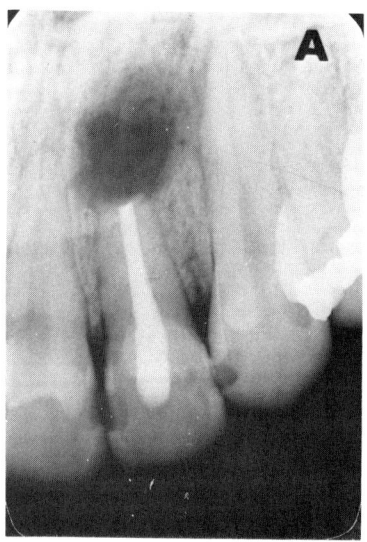

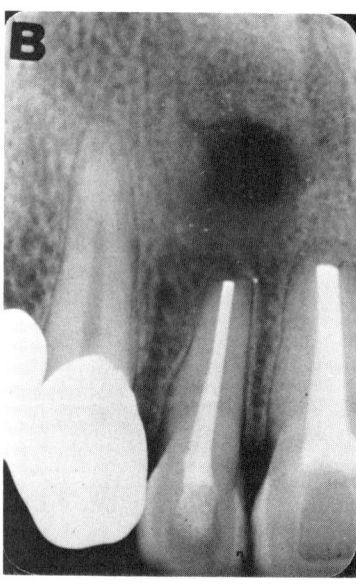

Figure 14-69. Surgical or Fibrous Healing Defect. **(A)** An apicoectomy has been performed on this lateral incisor. Notice that the bone defect left by the surgical procedure is undergoing complete repair. **(B)** This is a fibrous healing defect caused by the injudicious sacrifice of bone structure during an apicoectomy procedure.

que bone gives the lesion a "halo-effect." This is sometimes called a target lesion (opacity with a lucent halo) (Fig. 14-67D, E, F).

Benign Cementoblastoma (true cementoma)

This is a rare neoplasm of functional cementoblasts that forms a large mass of cementum or cementumlike tissue on the tooth root. It is usually seen in males under twenty-five years of age in the lower first molar. The teeth are vital, and the lesion is asymptomatic. Since it is a true neoplasm and has unlimited growth potential, it should be completely excised. Usually the affected tooth has to be removed because of the inseparable attachment of the neoplasm to the root or roots of the tooth.

Radiographically, the early stage of the lesion is radiolucent, and as it matures it becomes mixed with radiopaque foci or cementoblastic material. The radiographic appearance of the mature lesion is distinctive. It is a radiopaque mass of even density at the apex of the tooth, usually round with facial and lingual expansion in the large **nickel-sized lesions.** The outer periphery of the lesion is well delineated by a thin radiolucent line, but the involved root or roots appear continuous with the mass. This is partly due to the opacity of the lesion but is mainly due to the partial resorption of the involved roots, which are fused to the mass (Fig. 14-68).

Surgical or Fibrous Healing Defect

Occasionally when large amounts of faciolingual coritcal bone along with the periosteum have been lost by a surgical procedure, a cystlike, round or ovoid radiolucency will remain in the bone. The radiolucency could be mistaken for a residual cyst or some other pathologic lesion if the clinician is not aware of such a condition occurring. The **healing defect** is es-

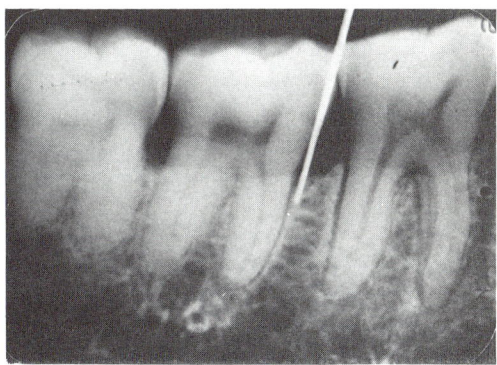

Figure 14-70. Use of silver points to assess bottom of periodontal pockets. (Courtesy of Dr. Ronald H. Watkins, Phoenix, Arizona.)

pecially prevalent in the anterior portion of the maxilla after an apicoectomy or root resection has been performed and a large portion of the palatal cortical bone has been destroyed. There will be a deficiency in the bone forming elements required to repair the defect. The bone defect is filled with **dense fibrous connective tissue,** and it should not be interpreted as an area of infection. If the bone surrounding the defect and the root apex is normal, this is usually an indication that there is no form of irritation present.

It does not indicate that the root resection or apicoectomy has been a failure, **only** that the operator has been overzealous in his surgical procedure. The defect may never fully repair itself, but most of them will reduce in size as time passes. If the radiolucency increases in size, it must be considered a recurrence of the original pathologic process or a new lesion (Fig. 14-69).

Differential Diagnosis (Periapical radiopacities)

Apical Cementoma (Apical Cemental Dysplasia)

1. Seen in mostly *females* in postmeno-

pausal age group.
2. 80 percent affect mandibular incisors.
3. Lesions are not attached to roots of teeth.
4. Mature lesion has the characteristic target appearance (opacity with a lucent halo) (Fig. 14-67E).

Benign Cementoblastoma

1. Seen mostly in *males* under twenty-five years of age.
2. Affects exclusively the premolars and molars. The affected tooth is vital and usually noncarious.
3. Lesions are attached to roots that are usually resorbed.
4. Mature lesion is large nickel-sized opaque mass surrounded by a thin radiolucent line. Expansion of the cortex may be seen bucally or lingually (Fig. 14-68).

Hypercementosis

1. Seen mostly in middle-aged and elderly; has no sex predilection.
2. Seems to involve all the teeth, and a variety of circumstances favor its formulation. Seen in nonfunctioning teeth, inflammatory conditions, occlusal trauma, and Paget's disease.
3. It is attached to root of teooth (usually an enlargement of the tooth root); it is separated from the periapical bone by the radiolucent periodontal ligament space, which surrounds the entire root (Fig. 14-42A).

4. The excesss cementum may be the same density as the dentin or less dense than the dentin of tooth.

Osteosclerosis (Focal Periapical Osteopetrosis)

1. Seen in adults; no sex predilection.
2. Well-localized radiopacities usually seen below apices of vital, noncarious molar teeth (Fig. 14-65).
3. Etiology is unknown, but it is *not* related to an inflammatory response or to an irritant.
4. The opacity is not attached to tooth; it lacks the radiolucent halo of the mature stage of apical cementoma, yet is well delineated from the surrounding bone. No expansion of bone is noted.

Condensing Osteitis (Chronic Focal Sclerosing Osteomyelitis)

1. Seen in young adults, before the age of twenty years; there is no sex predilectio.
2. Usually located at apex of carious, nonvital mandibular first molar. (If tooth is extracted, radiopacity remains in bone.)
3. It is not attached to tooth root; it is a well-demarcated radiopacity located below the root apices; it has a radiolucent area between opacity and tooth root. The entire root is usually visible, which distinguishes it from the benign cementoblastoma (Fig. 14-64).

PERIODONTAL DISEASE

Radiologic Interpretation of Periodontal Disease

Periodontal disease is a term representing a group of diseases that affects the surrounding and supporting tissues (foundation structures) of the teeth. According to epidemiological reports, more than 95 percent of the population will experience some form of periodontal disease during a lifetime, making it among the most prevalent of all diseases.

Periodontitis is the most common type of periodontal disease. It causes destruction of the supporting structures of the teeth and results from the extension of superficial inflammation of the gingiva (gingivitis) into the periodontal ligament and supporting bone. In the normal gingiva there is a shallow crevice or space around each tooth, which is bounded by the surface of the tooth on one side and the epithelial lining of the free margin of the gingiva on the other. It is called the gingival sulcus, and in a normal individual the clinical gingival sulcus rarely exceeds 2-3 mm. In **periodontitis** the gingival attachment to the tooth will move apically, while the marginal gingiva will become enlarged and seemingly remain in place. This results in a loose sleeve or collar of diseased gingiva lying against the tooth. The space between the detached gingiva and the tooth is called a **periodontal pocket** and its depth will exceed more than 3 mm. Eventually, if the **periodontitis** is left untreated, it will lead to deeper periodontal pockets, destruction of the periodontal ligament, resorption of the alveolar bone, and tooth mobility.

Eventually, it will result in the loss of a tooth or teeth. In the United States, more than half the people over forty years of age have lost at least one tooth because of periodontal disease.

There is no specific cause of periodontal disease. The local irritants (environmental factors) are readily identified, but the disease actually results from multiple and complex distributions in the host/environment relationship. The principal local irritant is a concentrated bacterial mass (plaque) that adheres to the tooth and where toxic products damage gingival tissue. Examples of other local irritants are calculus (mineralized deposits), faulty dental restorations, and foot impactions.

The systemic or host factors are equally as numerous and varied as the local irritants. Anything that alters a person's resistance at the cellular level can affect the progress of the disease. The most commonly implicated conditions are diabetes mellitus, hormonal imbalance including stress reactions, nutritional diseases, vascular disease, antigen/antibody reactions, and hereditary factors.

The Role of the Radiograph in the Diagnosis of Periodontal Disease

The dental radiograph is an important aid in the diagnosis of periodontal disease, the determination of the prognosis, and the evaluation of the result of the treatment. It is an important supplement to the clinical examination, not a substitute for it. Radiographs give a two-dimensional image representation of a three-dimensional structure. Therefore, the intraoral radiograph has limitations in that it lacks the dimension of depth, and since the anatomic structures will be superimposed over each other, the facial and lingual structure are difficult to interpret. In order to minimize some of these limitations of the intraoral radiograph, it is imperative that the radiographs have been properly projected, preferably by the paralleling or right-angle technique, and exposed by a high kilovoltage (75-100) long-scale contrast technique. This provides an accurate radiograph with clarity that will serve to detect the resorption of calcified tissues especially in the interproximal alveolar bone region, because the facial and lingual alveolar bones are obscured by the radiopaque tooth.

Panoramic radiographic surveys have limited use in the diagnosis of periodontal disease; however, they do provide the clinician with a single continuous view of the teeth of both jaws, which does have some value in the diagnosis of periodontal disease. The panoramic radiograph is an important supplement to the clinical and intraoral radiographic exam in the assessment of the patient for such things as systemic disease, cysts, foreign bodies, impactions, supernumerary teeth, and neoplasms.

Limitations of Radiograph

The role of intraoral radiograph in the diagnosis of peridontal disease is misunderstood. It does have its limitations. These limitations should be understood prior to their use in the diagnosis of periodontal disease. The important limitations follow.

Presence or Absence of the Periodontal Pockets. The periodontal pocket is soft tissue and will not be revealed on the radiograph. However, radiopaque objects such as endodontic silver points, gutta percha points, and Hirschfeld calibrated points can be used to assess the base of the periodontal pocket on the radiograph, but they will not show the length of the epithelial attachment (Fig. 14-70).

Early Bone Loss in Periodontal Disase. In one study (Pauls and Trott, 1966), septal defects less than 3 mm could not be seen on radiographs. The sensitivity of radiographs to measure large bone destruction in periodontal disease is only fair. It has been estimated that bone has to be decalcified by approximately 50 percent before a radiolucency will be revealed on a radiograph (Early et al, 1979). It is evident that an underestimation of the bone loss may result if the radiograph is used alone to assess early bone loss.

Early Furcation Involvement. Because of the diseases of the bone on the facial and lingual aspects of the supporting alveolar bone in the furcation area, it is difficult to visualize early furcation involvement. The osseous destruction may extend into the furcation area from the facial region but might not be seen because the lingual bone is still intact.

Status of Bone. Status of bone on facial and lingual aspects of the teeth is difficult to evaluate because the dense tooth structure is superimposed over the bone.

Calculus. The presence of calculus on the facial and lingual surfaces of the teeth is difficult to evaluate unless the calculus is gross and the alveolar bone has been resorbed considerably. The presence of gross deposits of calculus can be seen on the mesial and distal aspects of the teeth; however, small deposits are very difficult to see. Therefore, the radiograph should only be considered as an adjunct to the clinical examination in the exploration of calculus.

Mobility. Radiographs do not record mobility, but a widening of the periodontal membrane space does, in most cases, indicate an increase in mobility of a tooth. However, it must be remembered that traumatic lesions manifest themselves more readily in the faciolingual aspects, since in the mesiodistal aspects the contact areas of the adjacent teeth provide added stability. Since the dense tooth is superimposed over the faciolingual structures, thickened periodontal membrane spaces on these surfaces of the tooth cannot be seen on the radiograph.

Morphology of Bone Deformities. The radiograph will have difficulty in recording the morphology of bone deformities. This is because the radiograph is a two-dimensional image of a three-dimensional object. Since the radiograph lacks depth, it will not record the true picture of the **bone deformity.**

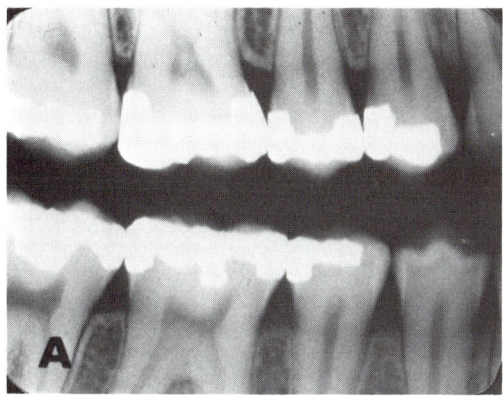

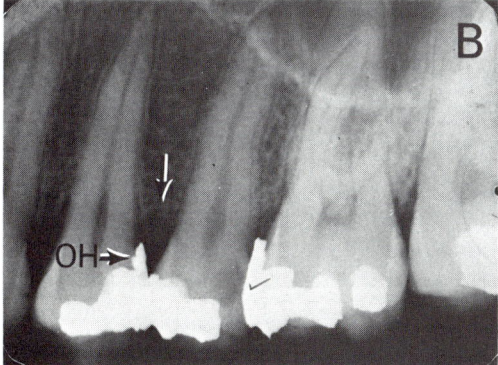

Figure 14-71. Early radiographc signs of periodontal disease. **(A)** Normal interdental crestal septal bone. The coronal border of the alveolar bone (the alveolar crest) extends normally to approximately 1-1.5 mm from the cemento-enamel junction of the teeth, both on the faciolingual and interproximal aspects. Normally, the interproximal alveolar crest is slightly convex and appears as a well-defined radiopaque line in the radiograph. **(B)** Earliest sign of periodontitis. Although the characteristics of the normal interproximal alveolar bone crest may vary (pointed convexity in anterior region to almost flat in posterior region), the normal bone cortical layer should not be etched. Notice the fuzziness and break in continuity of the lamina dura of the alveolar crest of interseptal bone between the first and second premolar (see arrow). This is one of the earliest signs of periodontitis. (OH signifies an overhanging restortion.)

Benefits of the Radiograph

When used properly, radiographs that have been properly positioned, exposed,

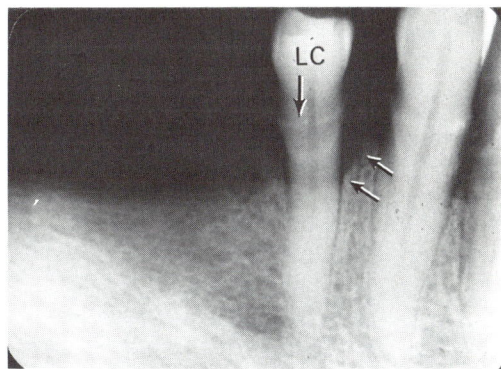

Figure 14-72. Notice the wedge-shaped radiolucencies on the lateral aspects of the first premolar (see arrows). This is one of the early radiographic signs of periodontitis. Line calculus (LH) can be seen completely surrounding the canine and first premolar teeth (see arrow).

and processed can be of great benefit to the dentist in the diagnosis of periodontal disease.

Some of the benefits of the radiograph (although of limited use) in the diagnosis of periodontal disease are discussed in the balance of this chapter.

Early Radiographic Signs of Periodontal Disease

As mentioned previously, the sensitivity of the radiograph to detect early loss of bone due to periodontal disease is only fair. Some of the earliest radiographic changes in periodontitis follow:

1. crestal irregularities;
2. triangulation;
3. interdental septal bone changes.

Crestal Irregularities. One of the first radiographic signs of periodontal disease is the fuzziness and change in the continuity of the lamina dura along either mesial or distal aspect of the interdental spetal crest. (Fig. 14-71).

Triangulation. Triangulation is the widening of the periodontal ligament

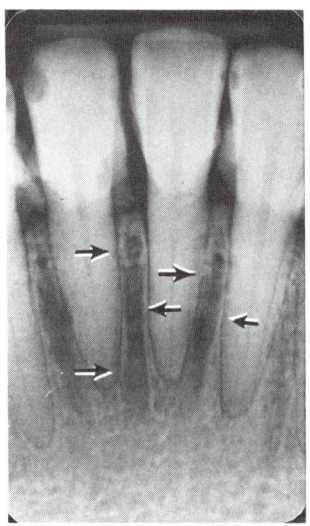

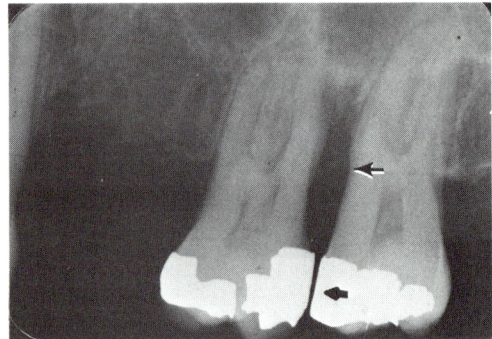

Figure 14-75. Localized bone loss between maxillary molars. There is also a loose contact between molars providing an excellent food packing area.

Figure 14-73. Interseptal alveolar bone changes. There is increased bone resorption along endosteal margins of medullary spaces, which results in an increased radiolucency of interseptal alveolar bone. Notice the gross amounts of interproximal deposits of calculus.

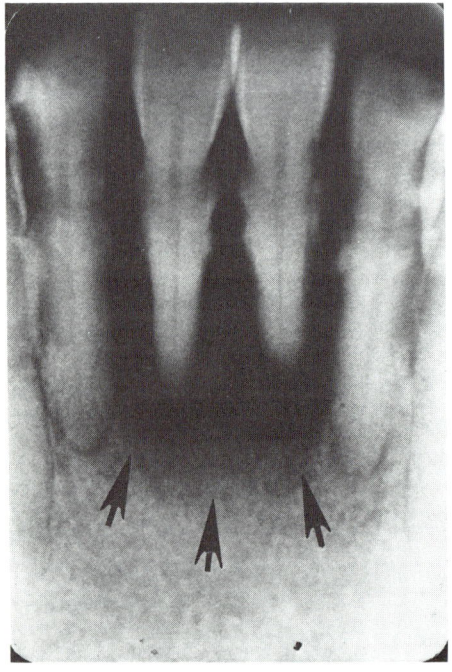

Figure 14-74. Terminal stage of chronic destructive periodontitis. The teeth seem to be "hanging in the air."

space at the crest of the interseptal bone. The sides of the triangle are formed by the alveolar bone and root surfaces; the base is toward the tooth crown; the apex of the triangle is pointed toward the root. This is an early sign of bone degeneration, and it necessitates a search for possible etiological factors (Fig. 14-72).

Interseptal Alveolar Bone Changes. One of the early radiographic signs of periodontitis is fingerlike radiolucent projections extending from the crest into the interdental alveolar bone. These projections are a result of a deeper extension of the inflammation from the connective tissue of the gingiva. They are widened vessel channels that allow for the passage of inflammtory fluid and cells into the bone. It results in a reduction of calcified tissue per unit area, which accounts for the radiolucent projections in the interseptal alveolar bone in periodontitis (Fig. 14-73). At the terminal stage of chronic destructive periodontitis, the teeth will seem to be "hanging in the air" when viewed radiographically (Fig. 14-74).

Evaluation of Bone Loss

Location of Bone Loss. Bone loss is the difference between the remaining coronal bone height and the assumed normal level

Radiologic Interpretation of Dental Disease   481

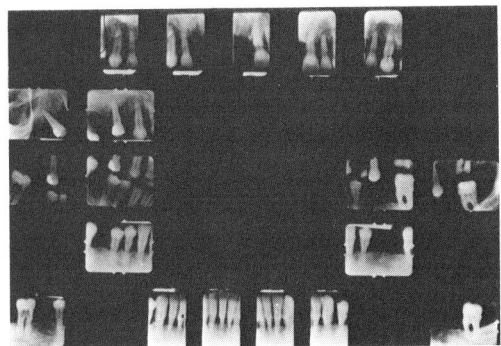

Figure 14-76. Generalized bone loss. Complete radiographic mouth survey of patient with severe generalized horizontal bone loss. Prognosis is poor that teeth can be salvaged by periodontal treatment. When it is generalized it is thought to suggest a systemic component to the etiology.

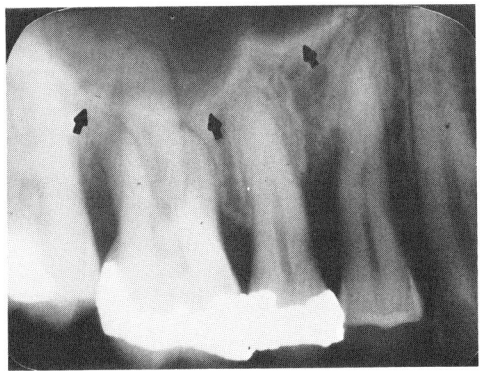

Figure 14-78. Approximation of the floor of the maxillary sinus and the coronal height of the remaining supporting alveolar bone. When osseous surgery is contemplated in maxillary sinus region, a radiograph of the region is helpful in the evaluation of amount of bone present between floor of sinus and coronal height of bone surrounding a tooth.

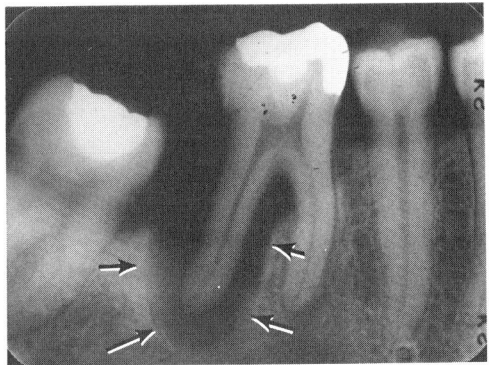

Figure 14-77. Combined periodontal-endodontic treatment. Sometimes a combined periodontal and endodontic treatment may be successful when the periodontal inflammation has reached the apex of the tooth, as is the case with the first molar in this radiograph. The prognosis would be poor in this case because of the furcation involvement.

for the individual. Evaluation of bone loss is made primarily by examining the interproximal septal bone on the radiograph. Of course, bone loss occurs on all surfaces, but the thickness of the tooth tends to obscure facial and lingual bone loss on the radiograph. If the bone loss occurs in isolated areas, it is described as **localized bone loss.** (Fig. 14-75). When the bone is evenly distributed throughout the dental arches, it is called **generalized bone loss** (Fig. 14-76).

The overall prognosis is poor if there is a severe generalized bone loss throughout both arches.

Inflammation of periodontitis may spread from the gingiva into the alveolar bone and periodontal ligament and reach the pulp through the root apices or accessory pulp canals near the apex or the furcation of a tooth. In these cases, survival of the tooth depends on a combined periodontal-endodontic treatment (Fig. 14-77).

If the alveolar bone loss from periodontitis is severe in the posterior maxillary molar region, the radiograph is useful in determining the approximation of the coronal bone level to the floor of the maxillary sinus. This is especially important if bone surgery is contemplated in this region (Fig. 14-78).

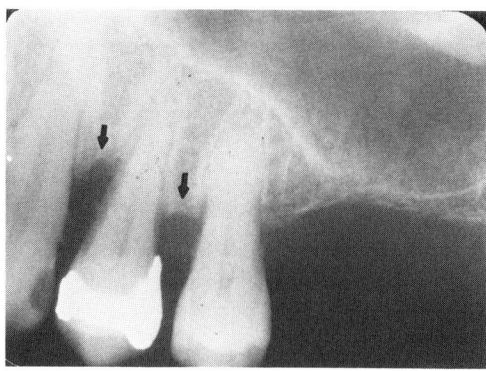

Figure 14-79. Horizontal bone loss occurs on a plane parallel with a line drawn from the CE junction of one tooth to that of an adjacent tooth. Note the food packing area between the maxillary premolars.

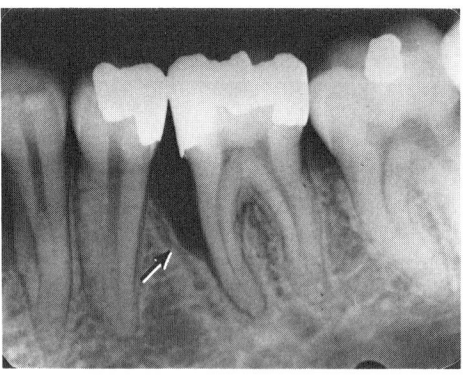

Figure 14-80. Vertical bone loss occurs when there is greater bone loss on the proximal of one tooth than the adjacent tooth.

Direction of Bone Loss. The direction of bone loss or bone destruction is determined using the cemento-enamel junction as the plane of reference. When the bone loss occurs on a plane that is parallel to a line drawn from the cemento-enamel junction of a tooth to that of an adjacent tooth, it is called horizontal bone loss (Fig. 14-79). When there is greater bone destruction on the proximal aspect of one tooth than on the adjacent tooth, the bone level is angular or not parallel to a line joining the cemento-enamel junctions. This type of bone loss is called **angular or vertical bone** loss (Fig. 14-80). Vertical defects are usually infrabony pockets, because the base of the pocket is located apical to the crest of the surrounding bone.

Traditionally, **horizontal bone loss** was thought to be a result of a uniform resorptive response when inflammation from local irritating factors was the sole cause, while **vertical bone loss** indicated more complex etiology, most likely of systemic origin, with a combination of occlusal trauma and local irritation. Proof of these statements have not been demonstrated, and patterns of bone loss are now less important to the clinical diagnosis of periodontal disease than they once were thought to be.

IDIOPATHIC JUVENILE PERIODONTITIS. Vertical bone loss (destruction) of alveolar bone around the first molars and incisors in otherwise healthy adolescents with little or no accumulation of plaque, and little or no clinical inflammation, is taken to be a classical diagnostic sign in (IJP) **idiopathic juvenile periodontitis (periodontosis)** (Fig. 14-81).

The classic radiographic findings in idiopathic juvenile periodontitis is an arch-shaped loss of alveolar bone extending from the distal surface of the second premolar to the mesial surface of the second molar (Fig. 14-81A). Also, there is almost always a distolabial migration of the maxillary incisors with diastema formation (Fig. 14-81B, C). The rate of bone loss is three to four times faster than in typical periodontitis.

The disease usually has its onset in adolescence (11-13 years) especially in females but tends to subside in severity (called burnout) in the second decade.

The term **periodontosis** (introduced

in 1942 by Orban and Weinmann) has been used in the past to describe this disease (but is being gradually replaced by the term **idiopathic juvenile periodontitis** (IJP). Periodontosis is related to a concept of periodontal disease that cannot

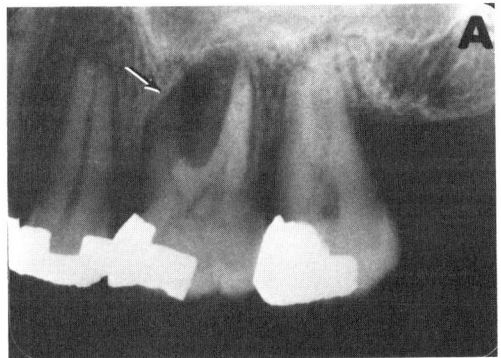

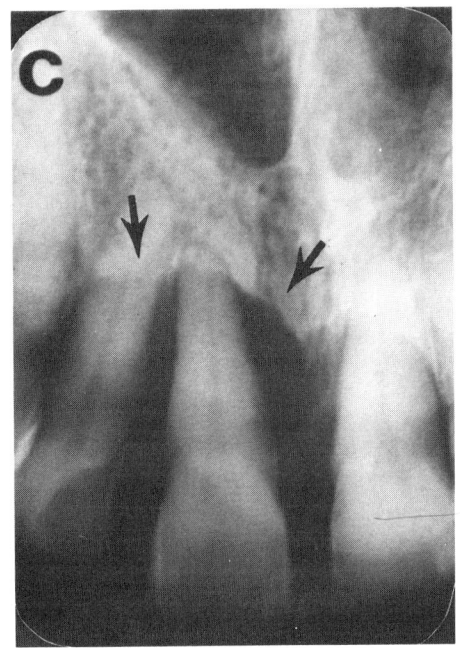

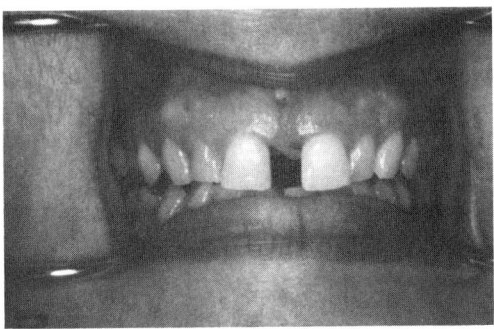

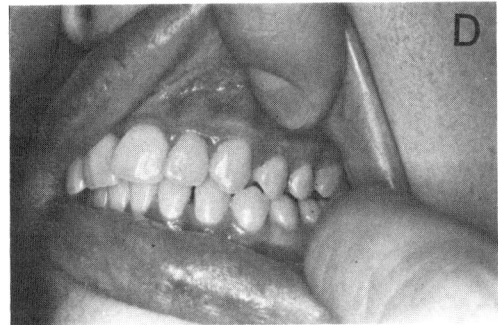

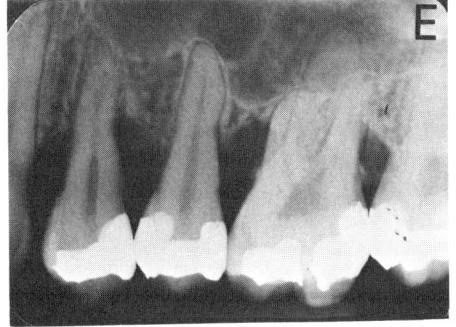

Figure 14-81. Idiopathic Juvenile Periodontitis. (A) Classical arch-shaped alveolar bone destruction found in Idiopathic Juvenile Periodontitis (IJP). (B) Adolescent female with Idiopathic Juvenile Periodontitis. Note migration of central incisors with diastema formation. (C) Radiograph of patient in (B) with IJP Notice the archlike severe bone destruction in central incisor region with diastema formation. (D) Female, age sixteen, with Idiopathic Juvenile Periodontitis. Clinically, there were few signs and symptoms of inflammation; however, there were beginnings of deep pocket formation and mobility of maxillary premolars and molars. (E) Radiograph of maxillary premolar-molar region of patient in (D). Notice the severe bone loss between premolars and molars.

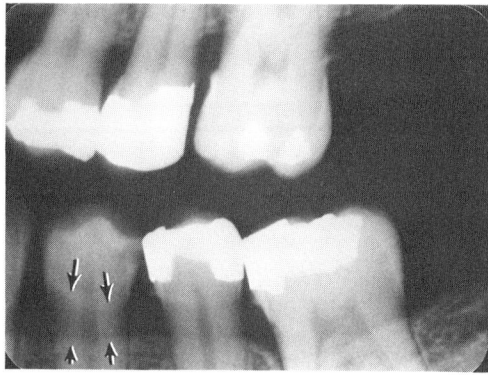

Figure 14-82. Amount of bone loss. The difference between the coronal height of the bone and the normal assumed height (1-1.5 mm apically to CE junction) for this patient is the amount of bone loss. There is some bone loss in this patient. Notice open contact between maxillary second premolar and first molar, calculus, and class 3 caries in distal of mandibular first premolar.

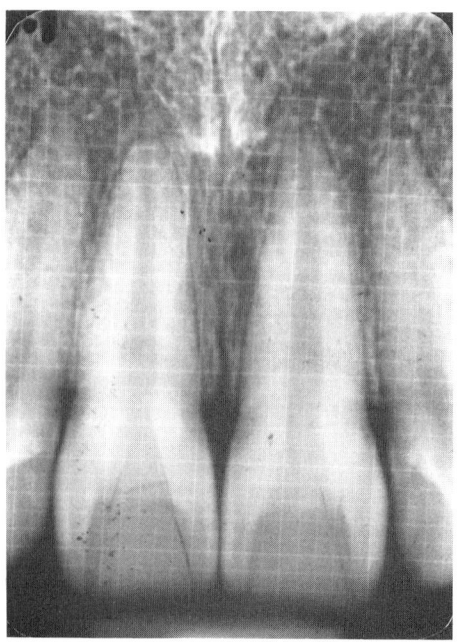

Figure 14-83. Use of grid to assess the amount of bone loss and periodontal ligament space widening. Each square is 1 by 1mm. The coronal bone level in the patient is normal.

be substantiated. The increased severity of the disease (IJP), as compared to the slowly progressing chronic destructive periodontal disease, is thought to be caused

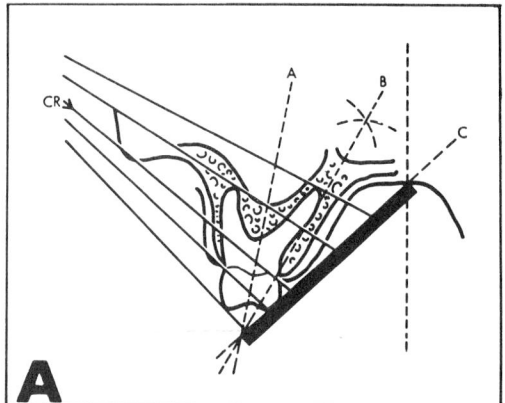

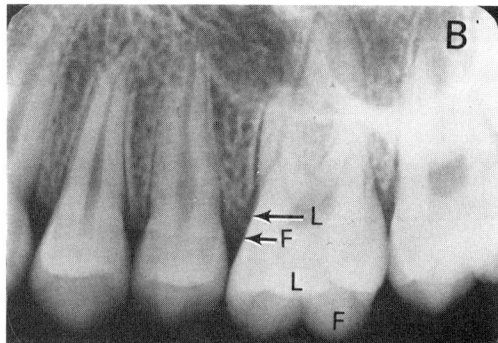

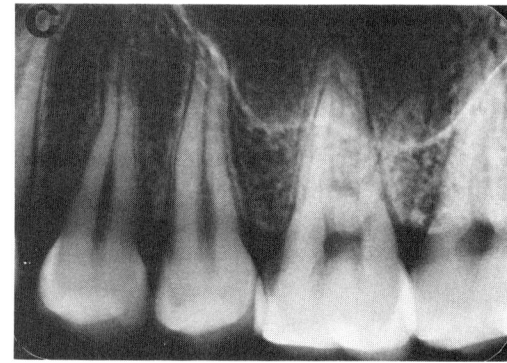

Figure 14-84. Bisecting Angle Technique and assessment of coronal interdental septal bone height. **(A)** In the bisecting angle technique the facial (F) portion of the interdental septal bone is projected coronally more than the lingual (L) portion of the interdental alveolar crest. **(B)** Periapical radiograph taken with bisecting angle technique. The underneath septal bone projected coronally past terminal point of maximal opacity is facial bone. Note that facial (buccal) cusps are also projected more coronally than lingual cusps of the teeth. **(C)** Periapical radiograph taken with paralleling technique of same patient in **(B)**. Note anatomical accuracy of the projection of interdental septal bone with this technique when compared to bisecting angle radiograph in **(B)**.

by a modification of the inflammatory response by intrinsic factors, hereditary/genetic disturbances, or systemic disease.

Amount of Bone Loss. The radiograph is used indirectly to determine the amount of **bone loss** attributed to periodontal disease. Actually the radiograph indicates the amount of bone **remaining** and not the amount of bone loss. The amount of bone loss is the difference between the remaining coronal height and the assumed normal bone coronal level for the patient. In a normal individual, the alveolar bone is located 1-1.5 mm apically to the cemento-enamel junction (Fig. 14-82). This assumes that bone physiologically recedes gradually as a person grows older. (Some authorities believe that this is not a normal occurrence.) Sometimes it is helpful to use a grid to assess bone loss and periodontal ligament space widening on a radiograph (Fig. 14-83).

Evaluation of Alveolar Bone Height

Since the density of the tooth obscures the coronal bone level of the alveolar bone on the facial and lingual surfaces, it is difficult to assess bone loss on the facial and lingual surfaces of teeth. However, at times it is possible to read facial and lingual bone levels by using two procedures in a combined fashion:

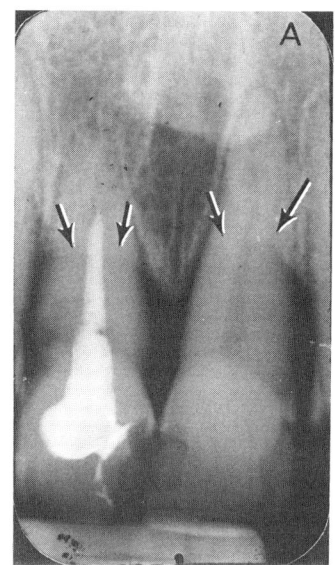

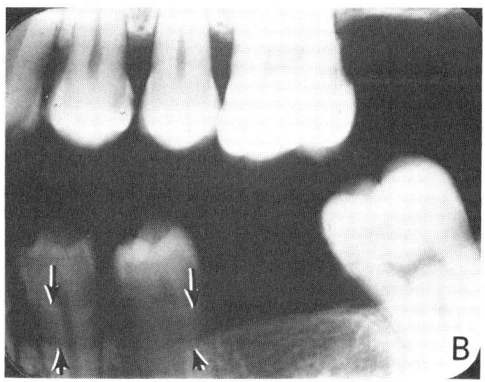

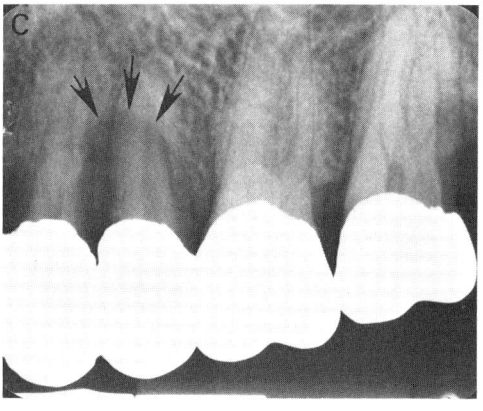

Figure 14-85. Evaluation of Bone Height on Facial and Lingual Surfaces. **(A)** Note that the trabecular pattern on the central incisors can be observed as the eye scans apically from the arrow. Below the arrow the root appears denuded of bone. This is the true line of the bone height. **(B)** Notice lingual bone height lines across the roots of the mandibular premolars. Also class 3 caries distal of maxillary first premolar and occlusal caries in mandibular second molar. **(C)** Note severe bone loss on lingual or facial surface of maxillary second premolar. This is probably bone destruction on the lingual surface because of its clarity.

1. Follow the lamina dura line coronally until it loses its maximal opacity. The bone coronal to this level is the facial bone that has been cast coronally by excessive angulation. This is especially true if the bisecting angle technique has been used in taking the radiograph (Fig. 14-84).

2. Examine the trabecular pattern of the bone, starting at the apex of the tooth and viewing toward the crown of the tooth. The appearance of the trabecular pattern of the bone will terminate at the true height of the facial and lingual bone levels. It will give the appearance of a line running across the tooth, which separates the denuded portion of the root from the root portion covered by bone (Fig. 14-85). This line usually represents the lingual line and will join the terminal portion of the maximal lamina dura opacity. Occasionally a second trabecular line can be seen running across the root from the point of maximal bone height. This is the facial bone level. It usually is not seen because the distance between the film and the facial bone is relatively great and the facial bone is superimposed over the thick mass of the tooth.

Evaluation of Bone Deformities

Besides reducing the bone height, periodontal disease alters the shape of the bone. An understanding of the characteristics and pathogenesis of these alterations or defects in bones from periodontal disease is essential for rational diagnosis and treatment. Bone deformities may be suggested by the radiograph, but careful probing and surgical exposure of the area is required to determine their true configuration and contour.

Osseous deformities that occur in periodontal disease can be classified as **infrabony (infracrestal) pockets.** An infrabony pocket or lesion is a pocket whose base is apical to the adjacent alveolar crest. The infrabony defect destruction pattern is **vertically angular or craterlike** creating a **hollowed-out** trough in the bone (Fig. 14-86). At the suggestion of Goldman and Cohen (1958), infrabony pockets can be classified according to the number of bony walls associated with the pocket.

Infrabony defects (below bone) may have one, two, three, or four walls. They are sometimes called **intrabony defects** (within bone) when the osseous deformity has three walls. It is called a combined osseous defect when the number of walls in the apical portion of the defect is different from the number in the occlusal portion (such as one of the walls being one-half a wall instead of a full wall in height) (Fig. 14-87).

Although this classification does not have any biologic or pathologic signifi-

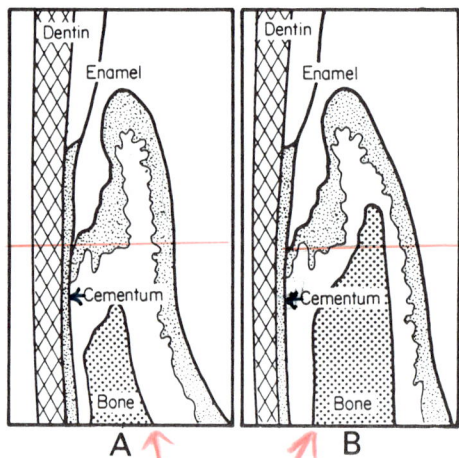

Figure 14-86. Supra-and Infrabony Pockets. (**A**) Suprabony pocket — the bottom of the pocket is coronal to the adjacent alveolar crest. (**B**) Infrabony pocket — the bottom of the pocket is apical to the adjacent alveolar crest. The lateral pocket lies between the cementum of the tooth surface and the alveolar bone. (Adapted from Fig. 166, page 202, Glickman, I.: *Clinical Periodontology,* 2nd ed. Philadelphia, W. B. Saunders, 1958.)

Radiologic Interpretation of Dental Disease 487

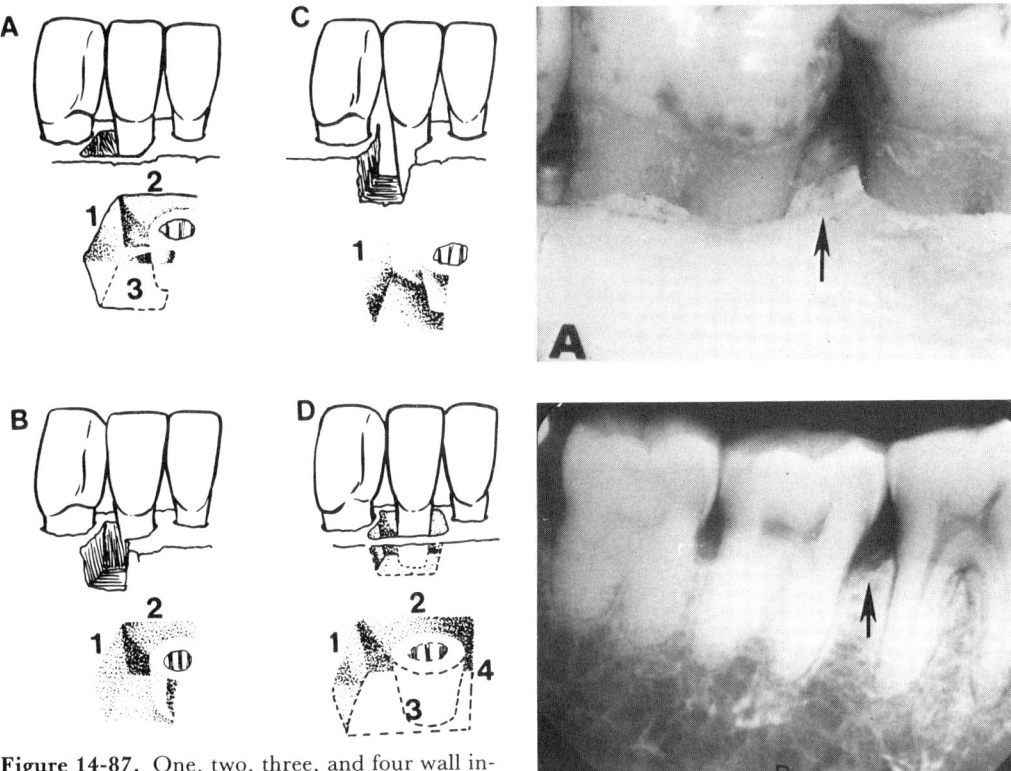

Figure 14-87. One, two, three, and four wall infrabony defects. (A) 3-wall bony defect. (B) 2-wall bony defect, another type of 2 wall bony defect is the osseous crater where the facial and lingual walls are intact, but the interdental alveolar crest has been resorbed forming a crater in the bone. (C) One-wall bony defect. This is also called the hemiseptum defect in which only one wall of the interdental septum remains after the facial and lingual walls have been resorbed. Ramping is another form of a one-wall defect when, for instance, the facial bony wall is left standing, and the interdental septal bone slopes toward the destroyed facial wall forming a ramplike appearance. (D) 4-wall bony defect completely surrounds the tooth. (Adapted from Fig. 14-27, p. 228, Carranza, *Glickman's Clinical Periodontology*, 5th ed. Philadelphia, W. B. Saunders, 1979.)

Figure 14-88. One wall hemiseptum or vertical angular defect. (A) Hemiseptum one-wall defect between mandibular first and second molars of dry specimen. (B) Radiograph of (A), showing one-wall hemiseptum defect between first and second molars. (Courtesy of Dr. Ronald H. Watkins, Phoenix, Arizona).

cance, it does have some bearing on the mangement of osseous defects. It appears that narrow bony defects (bony walls close to tooth) have a better prognosis for reattachment and regeneration of lost bone.

One-Wall Infrabony Pocket or Defect. This is the "hemiseptum defect" in which one wall of the interdental septum (hemiseptum) remains after the mesial or distal portion is destroyed by disease. A hemiseptum is synonymous with one wall vertical or angular bone loss (Figs. 14-80, 14-88). Another form of one-wall bony defect is **ramping.** It exists when the cortical crest, and either the facial or lingual cortical plate of bone are destroyed. This leaves a **ramplike effect** when interdental septal bone slopes toward one of the destroyed walls (Fig. 14-89). It is difficult to tell which coritical plate has been resorbed, whether the facial or lingual corti-

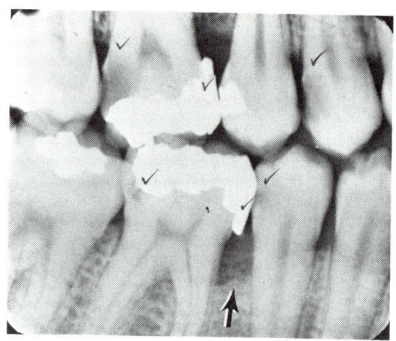

Figure 14-89. A one-wall defect with a ramplike appearance. The cortical crest, both proximal aspects, and the buccal cortical plates of bones have been destroyed leaving the facial wall intact which was confirmed by exposure at surgery. The defect formed a ramplike appearance because the interdental septal bone sloped down from the facial wall crest of bone toward the crest of the lingual bone. Of course, a thorough probing of the area would have to confirmed this. Note the overhanging restoration on the mesial of the first molar, and carious lesion in maxillary first molar, maxillary first premolar, and mandibular second premolar.

cal plate, but usually the facial plate of bone is less distinct and more coronally positioned if not destroyed.

Two-Wall Infrabony Pocket (Defect). The **osseous crater** is two-wall bony defect. It is thought to be **most common osseous defect** occurring in periodontal

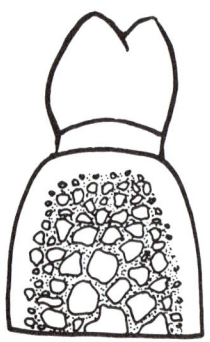
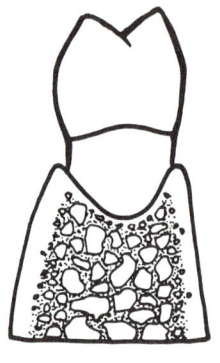

B

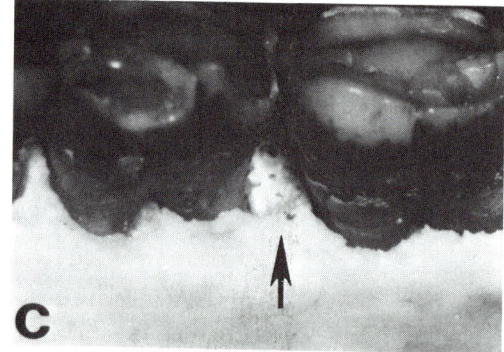

C

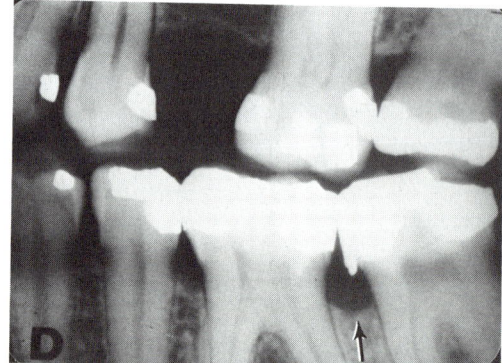

D

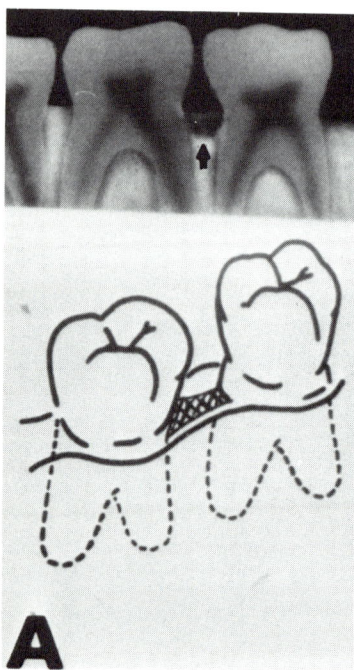

A

Figure 14-90. Two-wall infrabony pocket — osseous crater. **(A)** Diagram and radiographic appearance of osseous crater confined within the facial and lingual walls of the interdental septal bone. This is the most common type of osseous crater, and most prevalent of the infrabony defects. Its radiographic appearance is similar to the one-wall ramping defect. (Courtesy of Dr. R. Watkins, Phoenix, Arizona.) **(B)** Line drawing of osseous crater in faciolingual sectin of two molars. Left: normal bone contour; right: osseous crater within interdental septal bone. **(C)** Osseous crater between two molars in dry specimen. (Courtesy of Dr. Ronald H. Watkins, Phoenix, Arizona.) **(D)** Osseous crater two-wall infrabony poacket (defect) confined within the facial and lingual walls of interdental septal bone between lower molars, which was confirmed by exposure at surgery. Note overhanging restoration on mesial of lower second molar.

at the crest of the interdental septum has a similar radiographic appearance as the one-wall ramping defect of the interdental septal bone. Less commonly, the two-wall infrabony defect is formed by a proximal bony wall and either the facial or lingual cortical plate of bone, depending on which wall has been destroyed (Figs. 14-87B, 14-91).

Three-Wall Infrabony Pocket or Defect (Intrabony Pocket). The three-wall infrabony pocket describes a periodontal pocket surrounded completely by bone except at its orifice, which is usually at the crest of the interdental septal alveolar bone. It is sometimes called the intrabony pocket or defect (Fig. 14-92).

Four-Wall Infrabony Pocket (Defect). A four-wall defect completely surrounds the root of a tooth (Fig. 14-93).

Furcation Involvement

The extension of the periodontal pocket between the roots of multirooted teeth is called furcation involvement. The mandibular first molars are the most common furcation involvement sites, and the maxillary first premolars are the least common sites. The number of furcation involvements increases with age. The examination of the extent of the furcation involvement is made by exploration with a probe or explorer inserted into the roof of the furcation. Visualization can be facilitated by use of compressed warm air. The radiographs can be helpful in locating furcation involvement; however, the furcation involvement will not be seen unless the bone resorption extends apically beyond the furca. The degree of furcation involvement has been classified for descriptive purposes only. It does **not** allow for the selection of treatment modality or prognosis (Fig. 14-94). The mandibular involvement is much more sharply de-

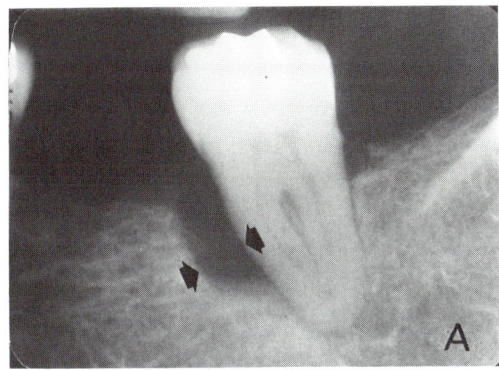
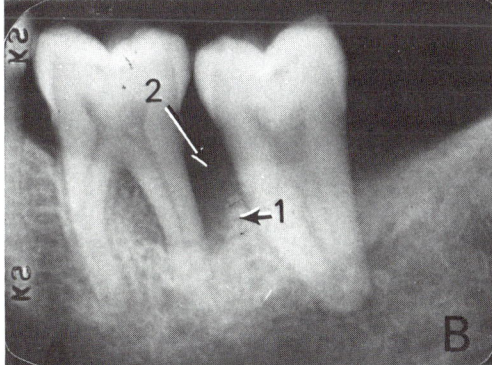

Figure 14-91. Two-wall infrabony defect. **(A)** Radiograph of the less frequently seen two-wall infrabony defect found here on the mesial of lower molar. The mesial proximal and possibly the lingual alveolar bone comprises the remaining walls. Of course, a thorough probing of pocket would confirm whether it is the facial or lingual wall that is left standing in this case. The facial or lingual wall in this case is irregular, is thin, and does not have the same height as the mesial wall. **(B)** Two-wall infrabony paocket (defect) confirmed by exposure at surgery. Distal (1) and lingual (2) walls were intact with furcation involvement.

disease. They are concavities in the crest of the interdental septal bone enclosed within the facial and lingual walls (Fig. 14-90). The osseous crater in the interdental septum will not be seen if a high contrast film technique is used, or if one or both of the remaining walls are extremely thin. The **two wall crater defect**

fined than the maxillary molar furca, mainly because it does not have the palatal root superimposed over the furca as does the maxillary molar (Fig. 14-95).

In using the radiograph to aid in the detection of furcation involvement, keep the following rules in mind:

1. The slightest radiolucency in the furca area should be investigated clinically,

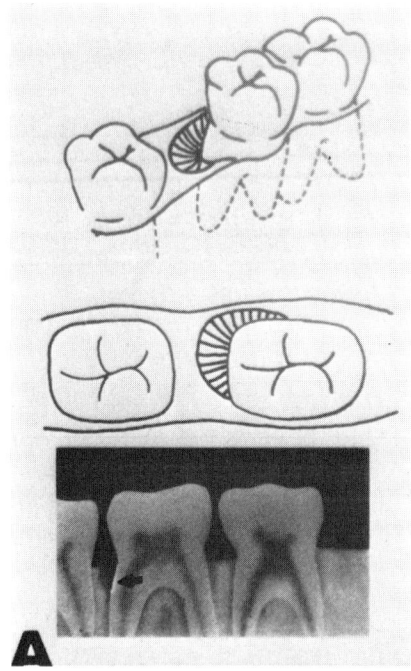

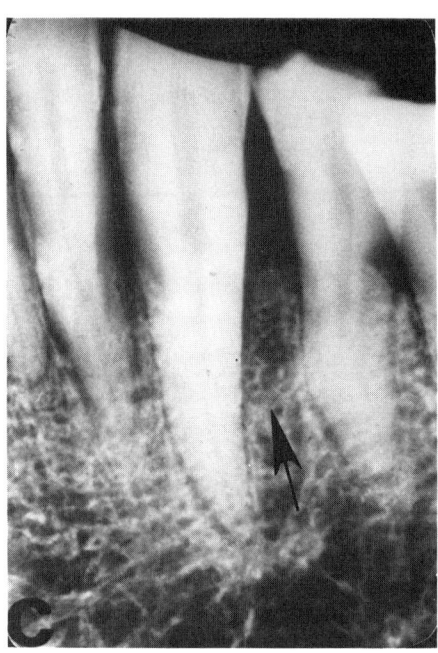

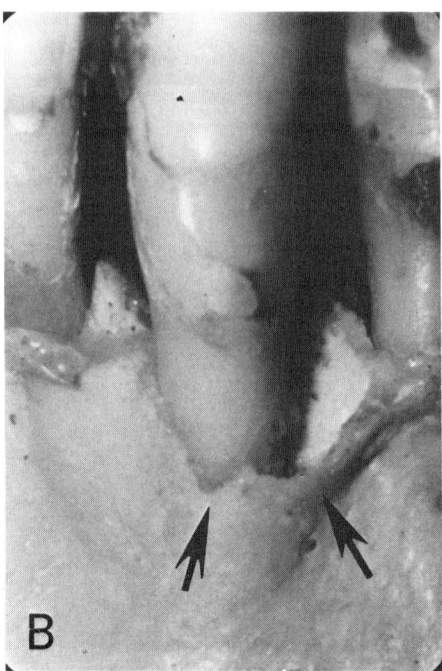

Figure 14-92. Three-wall infrabony pocket or defect (intrabony defect). **(A)** Diagram of infrabony pocket within the facial, mesial proximal, and lingual walls of alveolar bone. The radiograph of this type of three-wall defect may only reveal a wedge-shaped radiolucency of mesial interdental septal bone adjacent to tooth. The lingual defect would be hidden by the superimposed tooth root, unless of course, the furcation of the molar was severely involved. **(B)** A three-wall defect of mandibular canine within the lingual, distal proximal, and facial alveolar bone. **(C)** Radiograph of three-wall defect in **(B)**. Although there is a slight radiolucency on distal of canine, the defect is difficult to see on the radiograph. If the radiograph is viewed carefully, the middle distal portion of the root of the canine is denuded of trabeculations normally seen indicating a defect in bone. (Courtesy of Dr. Ronald H. Watkins of Phoenix, Arizona.)

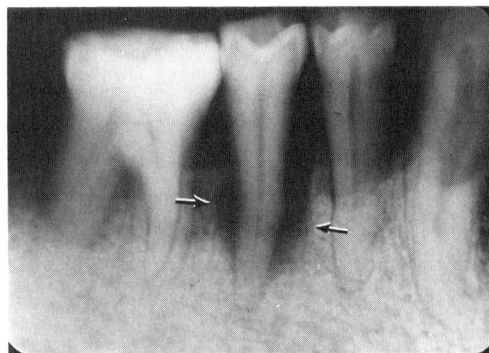

Figure 14-93. Four-wall infrabony pocket. This proved to be a four-wall infrabony pocket with mesial proximal, distal proximal, facial, and lingual walls still remaining; however, it was not confirmed until a thorough probing of all areas was completed.

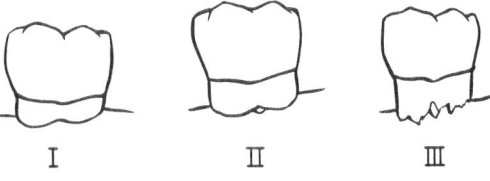

Figure 14-94. Classification of Furcation Involvement: **Class I** is incipient furcation involvement, not extending more than 2 mm into furca. **Class II** partial furcation involvement. An explorer can be inserted into furca, but not through and through. **Class III** Complete furcation involvement. The explorer or probe can be inserted through the entire furcation. This is the type most likely seen on radiograph.

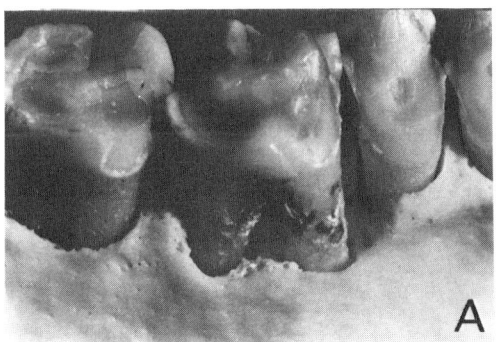

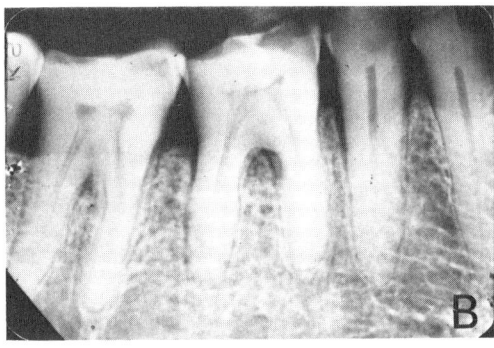

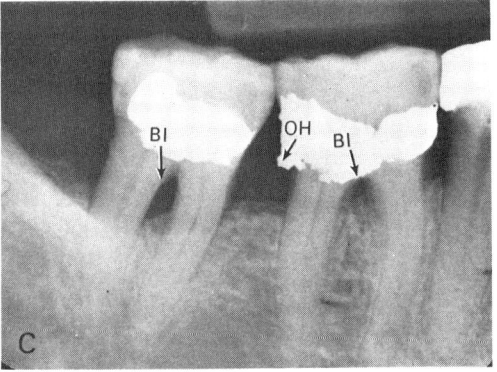

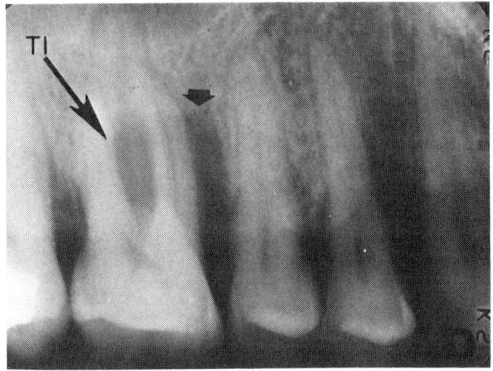

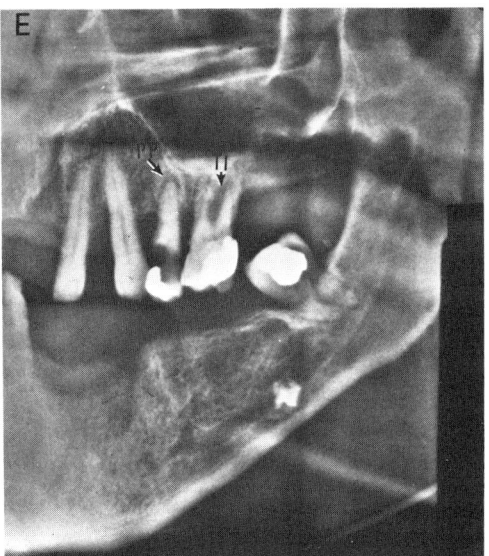

Figure 14-95. Furcation Involvement: **(A)** Furcation involvement of first and second molars of a dry specimen (Class II type as they are not complete furcations). There is a two-wall infrabony defect (crater) on mesial of first molar with lingual and mesial proximal walls remaining. **(B)** Radiograph of dry specimen in **(A)**. Furcation involvement shows up as slight radiolucencies. The two-wall bony pocket defect on mesial of 1st molar is not revealed on radiograph probably because lingual wall is so thick. (Courtesy of Dr. Ronald H. Watkins, Phoenix, Arizona.) **(C)** Class III through and through furcation involvement of mandibular first and second molars. **(D)** Class III through and through trifurcation (TI) involvement of maxillary first molar. The radiolucency is not as dark as radiolucency of mandibular molar Class III furca involvement because of the superimposition of palatal root over the furca. Note the severe bony defect (possible three-wall infrabony pocket involving furcation) on the mesial of the maxillary first molar and the overall periodontal ligament space thickening of the tooth. **(E)** Trifurcation (TI) involvement of maxillary first molar; note periapical lesion maxillary second premolar (PP).

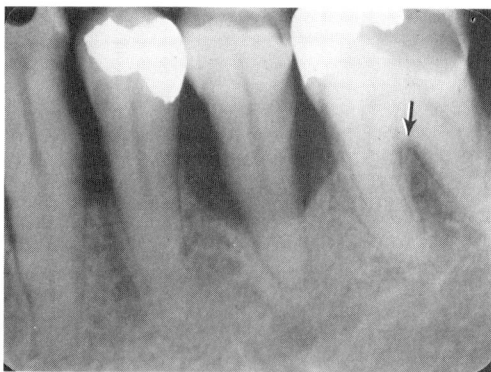

Figure 14-96. Slight widening of periodontal ligament space in furcation of first molar should be explored clinically, especially because of severe destruction of interdental septal bone between second premolar and first molar.

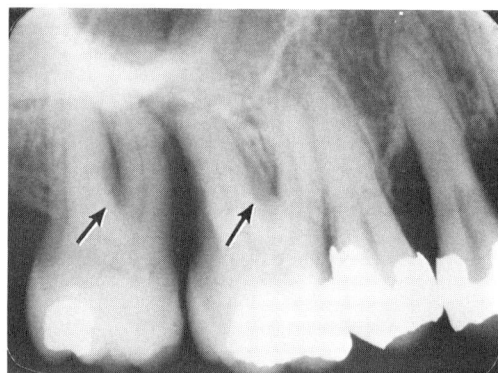

Figure 14-98. Furcation involvement was found by clinical exploration of trifurcation area of second molar (even though only a slight radiolucency in the furcation area is visible on the radiograph). The severe destruction of interdental septal bone between first and second molars extends into trifurcation of both first and second molars.

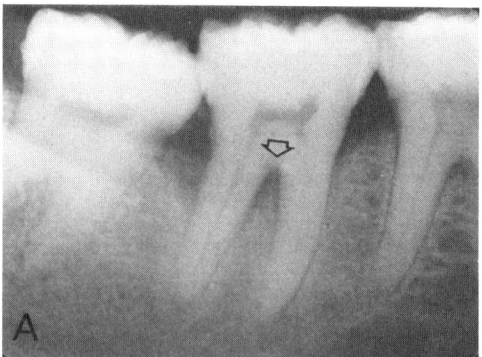

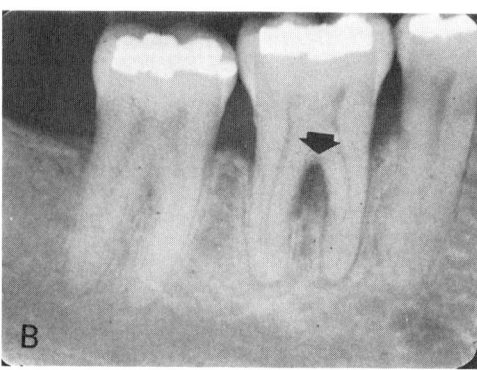

Figure 14-97. (A) Decreased radiopacity in furcation region of second molar indicates a possible furcation involvement. Note the bony defect between second and third molars, and calculus spurs. (B) Furcation envelovement of mandibular first molar.

especially if there is bone destruction on adjacent roots (Fig. 14-96).
2. Decreased radiopacity in a furcation area (even when bone trabeculae are still visible) is a radiographic sign that there could be furcation involvement (Fig. 14-97).
3. When there is severe bone loss associated with a single root of a tooth, furcation involvement should be suspected in that tooth (Fig. 14-98).

Detection of Local Irritating Factors

Several local irritating factors may be detected on the radiograph. They are calculus deposits, faulty restorations, and food packing areas. The radiograph plays no role in determining the etiology of the irritating factors in periodontal disease other than detecting their presence.

Calculus Detection. The radiograph will reveal gross amounts of calculus on the interproximal surfaces of teeth and sometimes on the facial and lingual surfaces, but cannot be counted upon to give a thorough examination of calculus. Calculus seen on the radiographs may

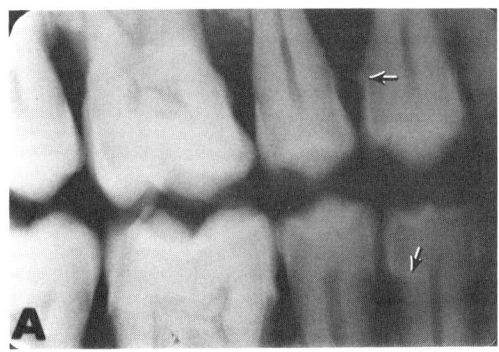

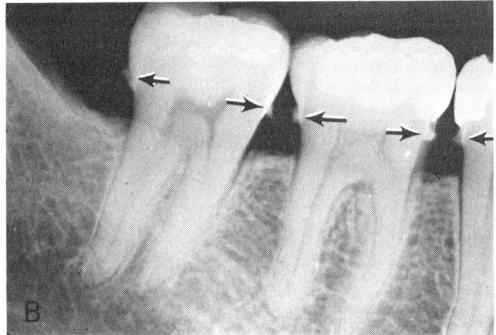

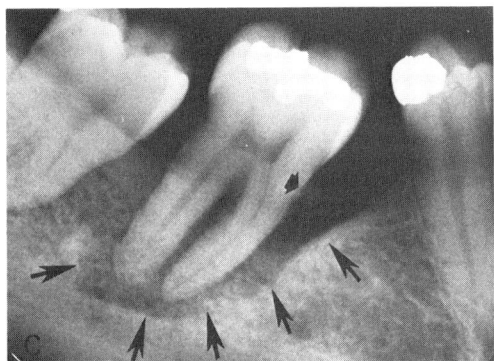

Figure 14-99. Circular, ledgelike or spur-shaped interproximal calculus. **(A)** Spurlike calculus between maxillary premolars; ringlike calculus encircling level of marginal gingiva, mandibular first premolar; and veneer type calculus mesial of maxillary first molar. **(B)** Spurlike calculus of interproximal surfaces of lower molars and premolar. **(C)** Circlular, ledgelike calculus on mesial of tipped mandibular second molar. There is continuity of bone destruction from gingival margin to the periapical region of the tooth. Extraction of the tooth was recommended instead of combined periodontal-endodontic therapy because of the mobility of the tooth, severe bone loss, and malpositioning of tooth.

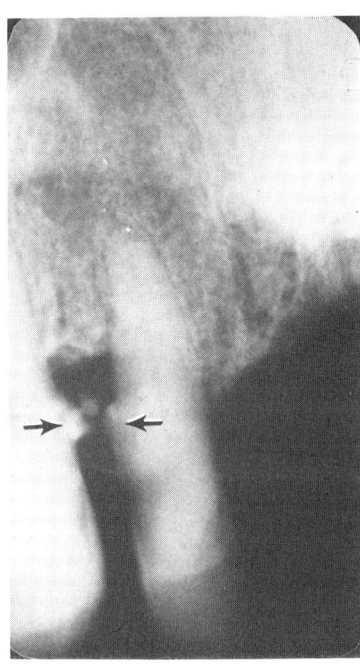

Figure 14-100. Heavy, nodular subgingival calculus deposits between lateral incisor and canine. This is also a food packing area in patient's mouth.

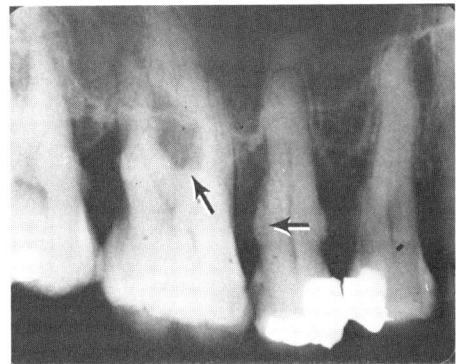

Figure 14-101. Veneer type of calculus with a smooth contour. On the mesial and distal surface of the second premolar are calculus deposits that have a smooth rounded appearance on the radiographs. Clinically, the deposits had a thin, glassy, veneer appearance. There is trifurcation involvement of maxillary first molar, and the coronal level of the interdental septal bone appears in close association with floor of maxillary sinus.

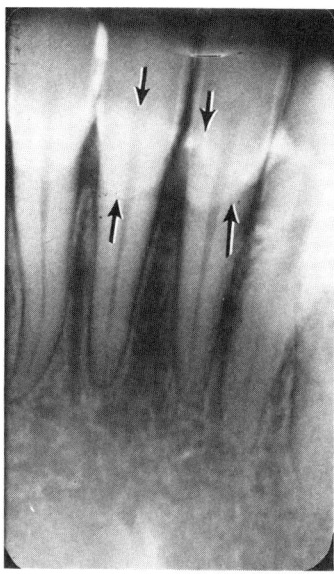

Figure 14-102. Ringlike or arclike marginal subgingival calculus encircling the tooth. Large masses of calculus at the level of the marginal gingiva will form radiopaque areas on the tooth.

take several appearances:

1. circular, ledgelike, or spur-shaped calculus (Fig. 14-99);
2. heavy nodular, crusty, or spiny shaped calculus (Fig. 14-100);
3. veneer-type calculus consisting of a thin, glassy smooth layer (Fig. 14-101);
4. ringlike or ledgelike formations of calculus encircling the tooth (Fig. 14-102).

Faulty Restoration. Dental restorations can prevent, treat, or cause periodontal disease. Faulty dental restorations and prosthesis provide ideal locations for the accumulation of any plaque and multiplication of microorganisms. Some of the faulty restorations that can be revealed on a radiograph are —

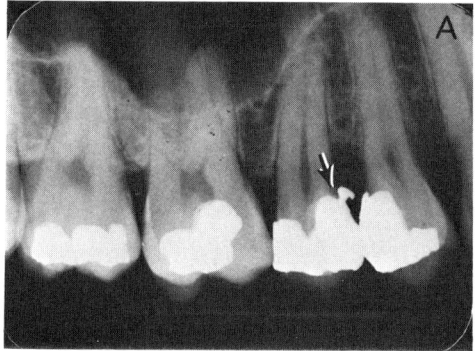

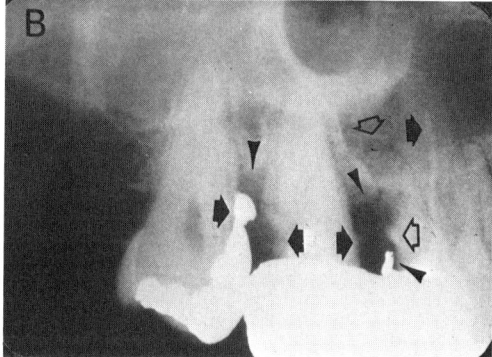

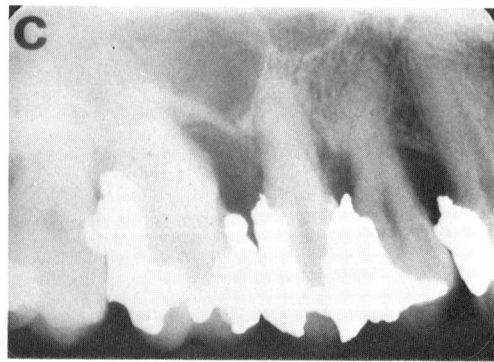

Figure 14-103. Overhanging restorations: **(A)** Notice unusual sickle-shaped overhanging restoration and bone coronal level reduction in interdental septal bone between premolars. The apices of the teeth have been "cut off," which is a common error in film placement and/or beam projection. **(B)** Overhanging restoration mesial of third molar; recurrent caries, distal of crown of second molar; overhangs and calculus distal of first molar. Note reduction of coronal bone level. There is incomplete root canal therapy of first molar, and periapical pathology at apex of distal buccal root of first molar. **(C)** Multiple overhanging restorations and associated severe bone loss.

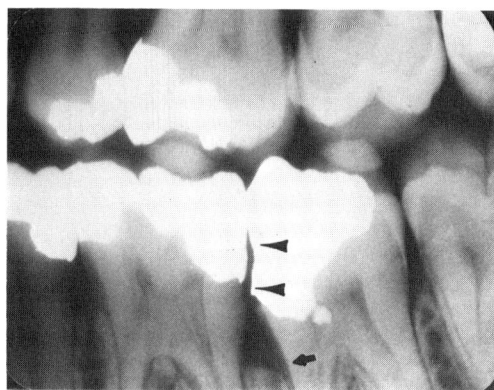

Figure 14-104. Imperfectly formed embrasures of mesio-occlusal restoration in mandibular second molar. Note the loss of coronal height of bone in interdental septal area between first and second molars.

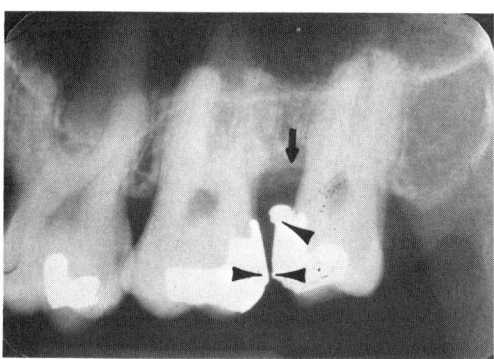

Figure 14-105. Loose contacts with resultant food packing areas. Loose contact and overhang between second and third molar resulting in food packing area. Note loss of interseptal bone between second and third molars.

1. overhanging margins (overextension of the restoration on the proximal surfaces (Fig. 14-103);
2. imperfectly formed embrasures of restorations (Fig. 14-104);
3. loose restorative contacts (food packing areas) (Fig. 14-105);
4. occlusal traumatism from high restorations (thickened periodontal ligament space);
5. recurrent or secondary caries (end product is a restoration with insufficient margins) (Fig. 14-106).

Food Packing Areas. Food impaction is the forceful wedging of food into the periodontal tissues by occlusal forces. It is a common cause of periodontal disease. Some of the factors that cause food impaction are —

1. occlusal wear (attrition) (Fig. 14-107).
2. loss of occlusal support by extraction

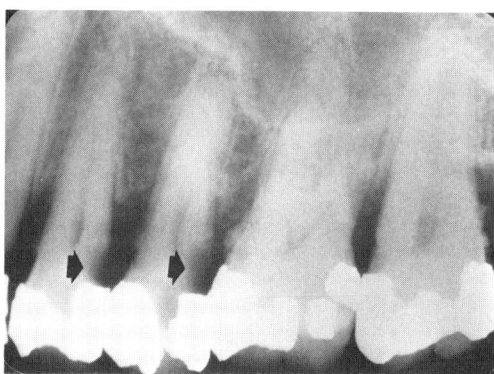

Figure 14-106. Recurrent caries resulting in insufficient proximal margins of maxillary first and second premolar.

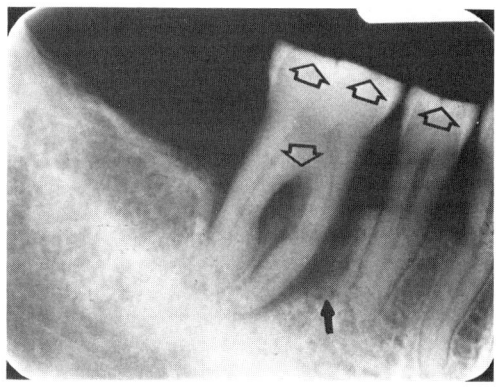

Figure 14-107. Severe attrition has caused a loose contact and food packing area between second premolar and first molar with resultant periodontal destruction of alveolar bone.

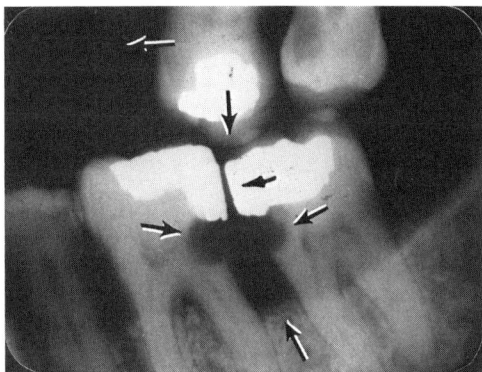

Figure 14-108. Failure to replace missing maxillary teeth has caused shift of maxillary second molar, which became a plunger cusped tooth. A plunger cusp is a cusp that tends to forcibly wedge food interproximally. Food wedged between lower first and second molar has caused caries and periodontal bone destruction. Furcation involvement of lower first molar is a possibility because of thickened P.D.L. space in furca.

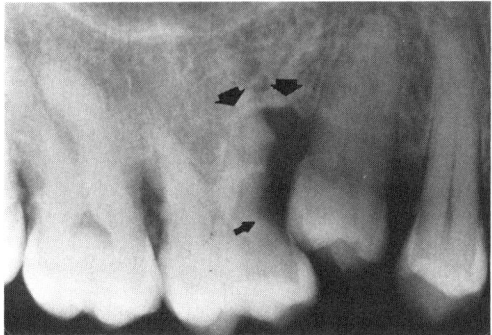

Figure 14-110. Supraeruption of first molar and malpositioning of second premolar has caused a food packing area to exist with resultant caries on mesial of first molar and severe interproximal bone loss.

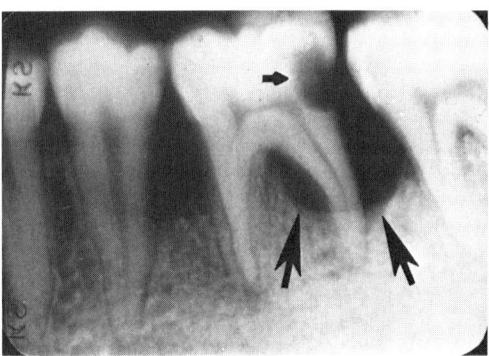

Figure 14-109. Large carious lesion on distal of first molar has created a food packing area, which has contributed to severe amount of destruction of alveolar bone supporting first molar.

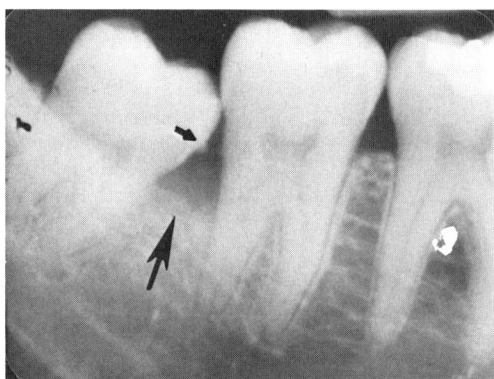

Figure 14-111. A partially impacted tooth has created a food packing area between second and third molar with resultant bone destruction interproximally.

of adjacent teeth (Fig. 14-75); shift in tooth position following failure to replace missing teeth (Fig. 14-108); habits; periodontal disease; and caries (Fig. 14-109);
3. supraeruption of teeth (Fig. 14-110);
4. partially impacted teeth (Fig. 14-111);
5. improperly constructed proximal areas in restorations (Fig. 14-105).

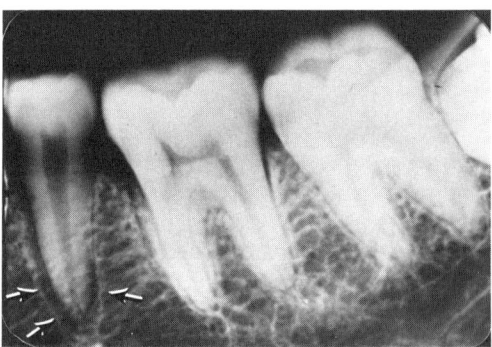

Figure 14-112. Occlusal traumatism. Note thickened periodontal ligament space of second premolar. Tooth was extremely mobile.

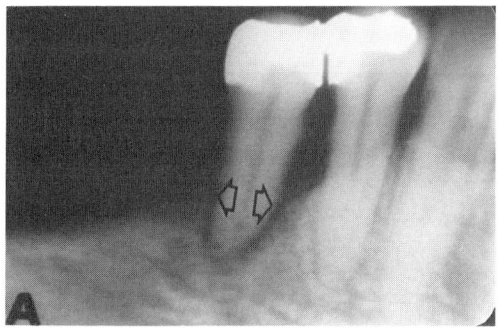

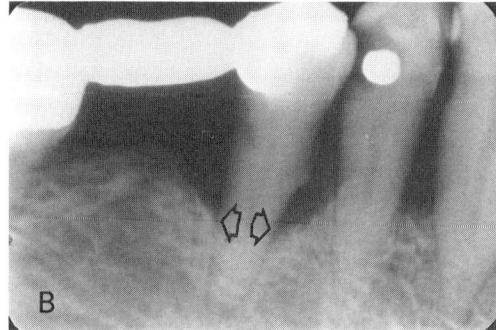

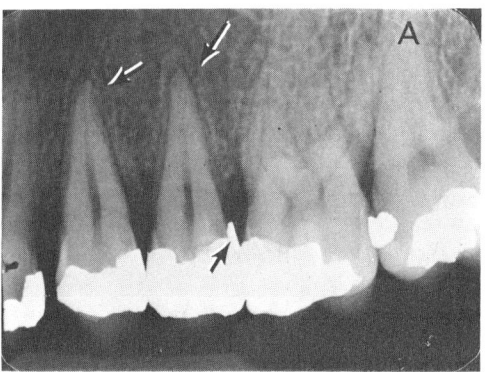

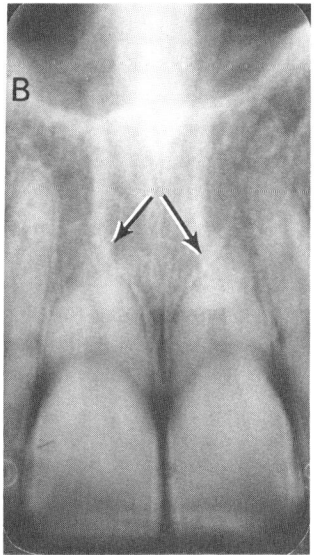

Figure 14-113. Unfavorable clinical crown/clinical root ratio. **(A)** The lower second premolar has an unfavorable clinical crown/clinical root ratio to be used as a partial denture abutment tooth. **(B)** The second premolar is a poor bridge abutment for this fixed bridge because of its unfavorable clinical crown to clinical root ratio. Notice the calculus or mesial root surface of the second premolar and the large distal carious lesion in distal crown surface of first premolar.

Periodontal or Occlusal Traumatism

Periodontal or occlusal traumatism is injury to the periodontal tissues by occlusal forces. Some of the etiological factors are:

1. bruxism, clenching, and biting habits;
2. faulty dental restorations and prosthetic appliances;
3. drifting and extrusion of teeth following extraction;
4. alteration of supporting structures by periodontal disease.

Figure 14-114. Short and spiked roots cannot withstand undue amount of leverage put upon them. **(A)** Note spiked roots of maxillary premolars with thickened P.D.L. spaces and overhanging restoration on distal of second premolar. **(B)** Short roots of central incisors caused by idiopathic external resorption of teeth. These teeth will not withstand undo stress placed upon them.

The diagnosis of periodontal or occlusal traumatism is made from clinical mobility tests, percussion, probing, palpation, observation of wear patterns, observation of masticating movements, and habit history of patient. The radiograph is used only as a supplemental aid in deter-

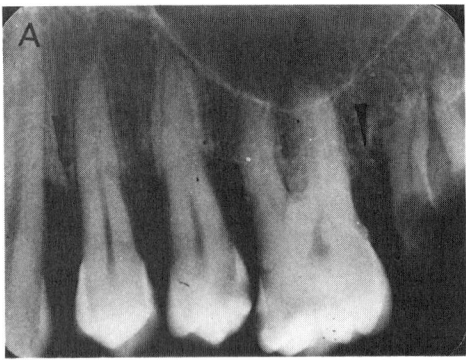

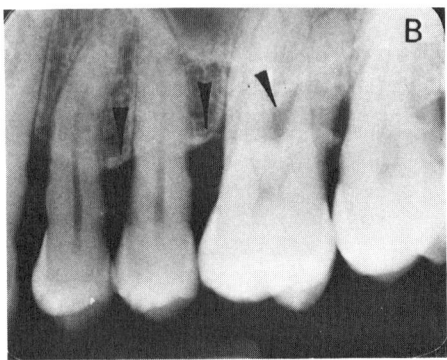

Figure 14-115. Activity of Destructive Process: (A) Radiograph with the appearance of an actively destructive process. (B) Radiograph of a patient with a static or slowly destructive periodontal disease. The crests of interseptal alveolar bone between first and second premolars is smooth and radiopaque. However, notice trifurcation involvement of first molar.

mining periodontal or occlusal traumatism. Mobility of teeth can be caused by injury of the periodontal tissues by excessive occlusal forces. A widened periodontal space due to resorption of the lamina dura and root resorption is a radiographic indication of tooth mobility (Fig. 14-112). However, the most extensive damage from occlusal traumatism is usually found on the facial/lingual surface, where it is not usually recorded well on a radiograph.

Root Morphology and Crown/Root Ratio

Tooth stability is influenced by the amount of leverage placed upon the periodontium. The type of leverage is dependent upon the amount of tooth that is within bone (clinical root) in relation to the amount of tooth not so retained (clinical crown). An increase in length of the clinical crown produces unfavorable leverage upon the periodontium (Fig. 14-113).

The clinical root may be short or spikelike because of a morphologic variation in normal anatomy of the root. If there is a loss of alveolar bone surrounding these short or spike shaped teeth, the leverage exerted on the periodontium becomes exceedingly great (Fig. 14-114).

Activity of Destructive Process

The activity of the destructive process of periodontal disease can be evaluated by comparing radiographs taken over regular periods of time. When the interdental septal bone crest is rough and irregular, and the alveolar bone below the crest is devoid of any suggestion of bone opacity, it is most likely that the **resorptive process is active.**

If, in the presence of bone loss, a smooth surface of the alveolar bone with condensation of remaining alveolar bone is seen, it usually indicates that the destructive process is **static or slowly destructive** (Fig. 14-115).

Pericoronitis

Primary acute pericoronal infections do **not** ordinarily demonstrate radiographic change. However, acute exacerbation of chronic pericoronitis (without symptoms) does demonstrate radiographic alteration. The space that represents the normal enamel follicle around

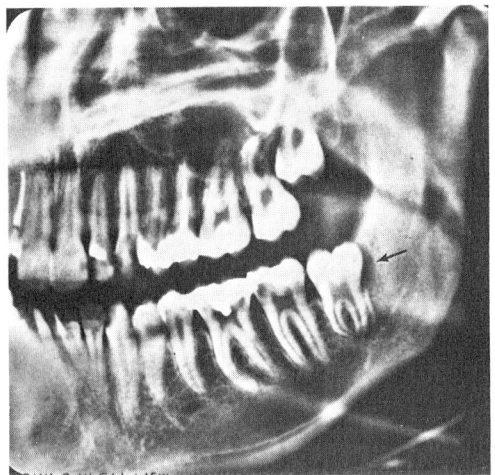

Figure 14-116. Acute Pericoronitis: Space that represents normal enamel follicle surrounding crown of partially erupted mandiublar third molar has become enlarged with pericoronal infection.

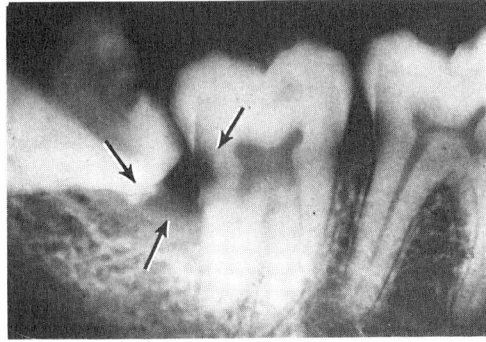

Figure 14-117. Chronic Pericoronitis: Note interalveolar bone destruction between partially erupted third molar and second molar. Also there is caries on distal surface of second molar.

the crown of partially or completely unerupted teeth is enlarged as a result of pericoronal infection (Fig. 14-116). Chronic pericoronitis resulting from a partially erupted third molar may result in intraveolar bone destruction and root caries of the distal second molar (Fig. 14-117).

Prognosis

Prognosis cannot be made until all available information has been secured. Radiographic information is part of the diagnostic data and is used in evaluating the progress. The prognosis is reasonably good if —

1. the destructive process is not generalized;
2. the past bone response to local irritants has been good;
3. only a limited amount of bone has been lost;
4. the destructive activity is minimal;
5. correctible etiological factors can be identified (radiographic films can only identify certain local irritants, and cannot determine etiology);
6. occlusal deformities can be corrected;
7. the location of the periodontal pocket is favorable (a patient with deep pockets and little bone loss has a better prognosis than a patient with shallow pockets and severe bone destruction);
8. the number of distribution of remaining teeth are favorable for support of adequate prosthesis (the crown-root ratio of abutment teeth is favorable);
9. the patient's general health is good;
10. the patient's teeth are normal in size and shape (not short and spike-shaped);
11. patient is motivated to save remaining teeth.

Treatment Evaluation

Serial Radiographs. Serial radiographs are of considerable value in determining success of periodontal treatment. The serial radiographs must be standardized in —

1. film placement;
2. angulation of beam of radiation;
3. exposure factors (kVp, mA, and time), and
4. film processing.

Treatment Success. In a successfully treated periodontal condition —

1. bone height will not generally be expected to increase.
2. radiographic features will change from one indicating **actively** destructive process to one suggesting a **static** condition.
3. appearance of new bone interproximally in previously decreased areas may be seen.
4. occurence of radiopaque cortical bone over the interseptal bone crest may be seen.

Bibliography

Animo, J.; and Tammisalo, E. H.: Comparison of radiographic and clinical signs of early periodontal disease. *Scand J Dent, 81*:548, 1973.

Animo, J.; and Tammisalo, E. H.: The orthopantomogram in quantitive assessment of marginal bone loss. *Suom Hammslaak Toim 63*:132, 1967.

Allen, E. F.: Statistical study of the primary causes of extraction. *J Dent Res,* 453, 1944.

Baer, P. N.; and Benjamin, S.: *Periodontal Disease in Children and Adolescents.* Philadelphia, Lippincott, 1974.

Baer, P. N.: The case for periodontosis as a clinical entity, *J Periodontal, 42*:516, 1971.

Barr, J. H.; and Stephens, R. B.: *Dental Radiology.* Philadelphia, Saunders, 1980, pp. 297-326.

Bassiouny, M. A.; and Grant, A. A.: Radiographic assessment of proximal infrabony pocket topography. *J Periodontol, 47*:440, 1976.

Baumhammers, A.; and Ceravolo, F. J.: An improved diagnostic point to aid in radiographic interpretation. *J Periodontol, 48*:52, 1977.

Bender, I. B.; and Seltzer, S.: Roentgenographic and direct observation of experimental lesions in bone. Part II. *J Am Dent Assoc, 62*:708, 1961.

Berry, Harrison M.: Cervical burnout and Mach band: two shadows of doubt in radiologic interpretation of carius lesions. *J Am Dent Assoc, 106*:622-625, 1983.

Beveridge, E.E.; and Brown, A.C.: The measurement of human dental intrapulpal pressures and its response to clinical variables. *Oral Surg, 19*:655, 1965.

Black, A. D.: *G. V. Black's Work on Operative Dentistry,* 8th ed, Vol. I. Woodstock, Ill, Medico-Dental Publ Co 1948.

Biggerstaff, R. H.; and Phillips, J. R.: Equantative comparison of paralleling long cone and bisection of angle periapical radiography. *Oral Surg, 41*:673, 1976.

Bjorn, H.; and Holmberg, K.: Radiographic determination of periodontal bone destruction in epidemiological research. *Odontol Revy, 17*:232, 1966.

Bjorn, H.; Halling, A.; and Thyberg, H.: Radiographic assessment of marginal bone loss. *Odontol Revy, 20*:165, 1969.

Blackman, S.: *An Atlas of Dental and Oral Radiology.* Bristol, John Wright & Sons, 1959.

Bower, R. C.: Furcation morphology relative to periodontal treatment. Furcation entrance architecture. *J Periodontol, 50*:23, 1979.

Brekhus, P. S.: Dental disease and its relation to the loss of human teeth. *J Am Dent Assoc, 16*:2237-2247, 1929.

Brescia, N.: *Applied Dental Anatomy.* St. Louis, Mosby, 1961.

Brown, I.S.; and Owings, J.R., Jr.: A reproducible method for evaluating radiographic changes in periodontal defects. *J Periodont Res, 8*:389, 1973.

Butler, J. H.: A familial pattern of juvenile periodontitis (periodontosis). *J Periodontol, 40*:51, 115, 1969.

Colby, R. A.; Kerr, D. A.; and Robinson, H. B. G.: *Color Atlas of Oral Pathology.* Philadelphia, Lippincott, 1961.

Davies, E. E.; Meister, F.; and Lommel, T. J.: Panoramic versus periapical surveys. *Dent Radiogr, Photogr, 50*: 41, 1977.

Deck, S. A.: An evaluation of methods for replicating roentgenograms. Thesis, Ann Arbor, University of Michigan, 1969.

Dunning, J. M.; and Ferguson, G. W.: Effect of bitewing roentgenograms on Navy dental examination findings. *US Naval Med Bull, 46*:83, 1946.

Early, P. J.; Razzak, M. A.; and Dodee, D. B.: *Textbook of Nuclear Medicine Technology*, 3rd ed. St. Louis, Mosby, 1979, p. 379.

Easley, J. R.: Methods of determining alveolar osseous form. *J Periodontol, 38*:112, 1967.

Everett, F. G.; and Fixott, H. C.: Use of an incorporated grid in the interpretation of dental roentgenograms. *Oral Surg, 16*:1061, 1963.

Garretson, J. E.: Neuralgia dependent on granules of osteodentine. *Dental Cosmos, 14*:25, 1872.

Glickman, I.: Periodontosis: A critical evaluation. *J Am Dent Assoc, 44*:706, 1952.

Glickman, I.: *Clinical Periodontology*, 4th ed. Philadelphia, Saundes, 1972, pp. 336-337, 483, 499-516.

Goldman, H. M.; and Cohen, D. W.: The infrabony pocket: Classification and treatment. *J Periodontol, 29*:272, 1958.

Grant, D. A.; Stern, I. B.; and Everett, F. G.: *Periodontics (in the tradition of Orban and Gottlieb)* 5th ed. St. Louis, Mosby, 1979. pp. 72-77, 155-158, 307-316, 453-460-, 702-704, 733-742, 784-787.

Greenbaum, L. M.: Inflammation and the role of endogenous pain-producing substances. *Dent Clin North Am, 22*:47, 1978.

Grondahl, H.G.; Johnson, E.; and Lindahl, B.: Diagnosis of marginal bone destruction with orthopantomography and intraoral full mouth radiography. *Sven Tandlak Tidskr, 64*:439, 1971.

Gutmann, J. L.: Prevelence, location and patency of accessory canals in the furcation region of permanent molars. *J Periodontol, 49*:21, 1978.

Hansen, B. F.: Clinical and roentgenologic caries detection. *Dentomaxillofac Radiol, 9*:34, 1980.

Haugejorden, O.; and Slack, G. L.: A study of intra-examiner caries at different diagnostic levels. *Acta Odontol Scand, 33*:169, 1975.

Haugejorden, O.: A study of the methods of radiologic diagnosis of dental caries in epidemiological investigations. *Acta Odontol Scand (Suppl), 65,* 1974.

Haugejorden, O.; and Slack, G. L.: The construction and use of diagnostic standards for radiographic caries incidence scores. *Acta Odontol Scand, 35*:95, 1977.

Heins, P. J.; and Canter, S. R.: The furca involvement: A classification of deformities. *J Periodontol, 6*:84, 1968.

Hill, T. J.: Pathology of the dental pulp. *J Am Dent Assoc, 21*:820, 1934.

Hirschefeld, L.: A calibrated silver point for periodontal diagnosis and recording. *J Periodontol, 24*:94, 1953.

Hollender, L.; Lindke, J.; and Koch, G.: A roentgenographic studyof clinically healthy and inflamed periodontal tissue in children. *J Periodontol Res, 1*:146, 1966.

Hurlburt, C. E.; and Wuehrmann, A. H.: comparison of interproximal carious lesion detection in panoramic and standard intraoral radiography. *J Am Dent Assoc, 93*:1154, 1976.

Kaslick, R.S.; and Chasens, A.I.: Periodontosis with periodontitis: A study involving young adult males. *Oral Surg, 25*:327, 1968.

Kelley, G. P.; Cain, R. J.; Knowles, J. W.; Nissle, R.R.; Burgett, F.G.; Shick, R.A.; and Ramfjord, S. P.: Radiographs in clinical periodontal trials. *J Periodontol, 46*:381, 1975.

Larato, D. C.: Periodontal bone defects in the juvenile skull. *J Periodontol, 41*:473, 1970.

Larato, D. C.: Intrabony defects in the dry human skull. *J Periodontol, 41*:496, 1970.

Larato, D. C.: Furcation involvements; incidence and distribution. *J Periodontol, 41*:499, 1970.

Larato, D. C.: Some anatomical factors related to furcation involvements. *J Periodontol, 46*:608, 1975.

LeQuire, A.K.; Cunningham, C.J.; and Elleu, G. B., Jr.: Radiographic interpretation of experimentally produced osseous lesions of the human mandible. *J Endodontol, 3*:274, 1977.

Ludlow, M. W.: Endodontic first aid for the patient with odontalgia. *Dent Surv, 42*:25, 1979.

Mendel, I. D.: Dental Caries. *Am Sci, 67*:661, 1979.

Mason, J. D.; and Lehner, T.: Clinical features of juvenile periodontitis (periodontosis). *J Periodontol, 45*:636, 1974.

Manson, J. D.: Bone morphology and bone loss in periodontal disease. *J Clin Periodontol, 3*:14, 1976.

Maurice, C. G.: *An annotated Glossary of Terms Used in Endodontics,* 3rd ed. Atlanta, Am Assn Endodontics, 1973.

Miller, S. C.: Precocious advanced alveolar atrophy. *J Periodontol, 19*:146, 1948.

Natkin, E.: Treatment of endodontic emergencies. *Dent Clin North Am, 18*:243, 1974.

Nebrun, E.: *Cariology.* Baltimore, Williams & Wilkens, 1979, pp. 15-43.

Oba, T.; and Katayma, H.: Comparison of orthopantomography with conventional periapical dental radiography. *Oral Surg, 34*:524, 1972.

Orban, B.: *Oral Histology and Embryology.* St. Louis,

Mosby, 1944, p. 55.

Orban, B.; and Weinmann, J. P.: Diffuse atrophy of the alveolar bone (periodontosis). *J Periodontol, 13*:31, 1952.

Patur, B.; and Glickman, I.: Roentgenographic evaluation of alveolar bone changes in periodontal disease. *Dent Clin North Am,* 47, March 1960.

Patur, B.; and Glickman, I.: Clinical and roentgenographic evaluation of the posttreatment healing of infrabony pockets. *J Periodontol, 33*:164, 1962.

Pauls, V.; and Trott, J. R.: A radiological study of experimentally produced lesions in bone. *Dent Pract, 16*:254, 1966.

Pindborg, J. J.: *Pathology of the Dental Hard Tissues.* Philadelphia, Saunders, 1970.

Prichard, J. F.: The intrabony techniques as a predictable procedure. *J Periodontol, 28*:202, 1957.

Prichard, J. F.: Role of the roentgenogram in the diagnosis and prognosis of periodontal disease. *Oral Med, 14*:182, 1961.

Prichard, J. F.: *Advanced Periodontal Disease,* 2nd ed. Philadelphia, Saunders, 1972, pp. 103-107, 142-196, 381.

Puckett, J.: A device for comparing roentgenograms of the same mouth. *J Periodontol, 39*:38, 1968.

Ramaden, A. B. E.; and Mitchell, D. F.: A roentgenographic study of experimental bone destruction. *Oral Surg, 15*:934, 1962.

Rees, T. D.; Biggs, N. L.; and Collings, C. K.: Radiographic interpretation of periodontal osseious lesion. *Oral Surg, 32*:141, 1971.

Regan, J. E.; and Mitchell, D. F.: Roentgenographic and dissection measurements of alveolar crest height. *J Am Dent Assoc, 66*:356, 1963.

Ritchey, B.; and Orban, B.: The crest of the interdental alveolar septa. *J Periodontol, 24*:75, 1953.

Rosling, B.; Hollender, L.; Nyman, S.; and Olsson, G.: A radiographic method for assessing changes in alveolar bone height following periodontal therapy. *J Clin Periodontol, 2*:211, 1975.

Ross, W. S.: Pulp disease and its prevention. *Br Dent J, 96*:108-117, 1954.

Schwartz, S. F.; and Foster, J. K.: Roentgenographic interpretation of experimentally produced bony lesions. *J Oral Surg, 32*:606, 1971.

Seltzer, S.; Bender, I. B.; and Ziontz, M.: The interrelationship of pulp and periodontal disease. *Oral Surg, 16*:1474, 1963.

Shafer, W. G.; Hine, M. K.; and Levy, B. M.: *A Textbook of Oral Pathology,* 3rd ed. Philadelphia, Saunders, 1974, pp. 295, 366-432, 704-753.

Shannon, I. L.; Gibson, W. A.; and Terry, J. M.: Caries experience in the U. S. Air Force. *J Public Health Dent, 26*:206, 1060.

Shei, O.; Waerhaug, J.; Lovdal, A.; and Arno, A.: Alveolar bone loss related to oral hygiene and age. *J Periodontol, 30*:7, 1959.

Shoha, R. R.; Dowson, J.; and Richards, A. G.: Radiographic interpretation of experimentally induced bony lesions. *Oral Surg, 38*:294, 1974.

Simon, J. H. S.; Glick, D. H.; and Frank, A. L.: Predictable Endodontic and periodontic failure as a result of radicular anomalies. *Oral Surg, 31*:823, 1971.

Snyder, M. B.; Stacey, A. J.; Davis, R.; Cawson, R. A.; and Binnie, W. H.: The advantages of exroradiography for panoramic examination of the jaws and teeth. *J Periodontol, 48*:467, 1977.

Sommer, R. F.; Ostrander, F.D.; and Crowley, M. C.: *Clinical endodontics.* Philadelphia, Saunders, 1956.

Sottosanti, J. S.: A possible relationship between occlusion, root resorption and the progression of periodontal disease. *J Western Soc Periodont, 25*:69, 1977.

Spouge, J. D.: *Oral Pathology.* St. Louis, Mosby, 1973, pp. 3-40. 83-124.

Stafne, E. C.; and Szabo, S. E.: The significance of pulp nodules. *Dental Cosmos, 75*:160, 1933.

Stedman's Medical Dictionary, 23rd ed. Baltimore, Williams & Wilkins, 1976, p. 1459.

Stewart, J. L.; and Bieser, L. F.: Panoramic roentgenograms compared with conventional intraoral roentgenograms. *Oral Surg, 26*:39, 1968.

Stones, H. H.: *Oral and Dental Diseases.* Baltimore, Williams & Wilkins, 1962.

Suomi, J. D.; Plumbo, J.; and Barbano, J.P.: A comparative study of radiographs and pocket measurements in periodontal disease evaluation. *J Periodontol, 39*:311, 1968.

Theilade, J.: An evaluation of the reliability of radiographs in the measurement of bone loss in periodontal disease. *J Periodontol, 31*:143, 1960.

Tibbets, L. S.: Use of diagnostic probes for detection of periodontal disease. *J Am Dent Assoc, 78*:549, 1969.

Updegrave, W. J.: Accurate radiography for diagnosis of periodontal disease. In Ward, H. (ed): *A Periodontal Point of View.* Springfield,

Ill, Charles C Thomas, 1973, pp. 389-419.

Van de Poel, A. C. M.; Duinkerke, A. S. H.; and Dolsburg, W. H.: A comparative study of long-cone and short-cone bite-wing radiographs. *Oral Surg, 36*:273, 1973.

Wagg, B. J.: ECSI — A new index for evaluating caries progression. *Community Dent Oral Epidemiol, 2*:219, 1974.

Weine, F. S.: *Endodontic Therapy.* St. Louis, Mosby, 1973, pp. 40-50, 95-119.

Weine, F. S.; Healey, H. J.; and Theiss, E. P.: Endodontic emergency dilemma: Leave open or keep closed. *Oral Surg, 40*:531, 1975.

Weine, F. S.: *Endodontic Therapy.* St. Louis, Mosby, 1976.

White, T. C.: Secondary dentine nodules. *Br J Dent Sci 14*:80, 1871.

Worth, H. M.: *Principles and Practice of Oral Radiologic Interpretation.* Chicago, Year Bk Med, 1963.

Wuehrmann, A. H.; and Manson-Hing, L. R.: *Dental Radiology,* 4th ed. St. Louis, Mosby, 1977, pp. 297-334.

Zamir, T.; Fischer, D.; Fishel, D.; and Sharav, Y.: A longitudinal radiographic study of the rate and spread of human approximal dental caries. *Arch Oral Biol, 21*:523, 1976.

Chapter 15

ATLAS OF SPECIAL TECHNICS IN DENTAL RADIOLOGY

THERE are several special radiographic examinations that can be utilized in the diagnosis and prevention of diseases and abnormalities of the head and neck region. These radiographic examinations include the following:

1. extraoral and intraoral radiography;
2. sialography;
3. edentulous radiography;
4. localization technics;
5. endodontic radiography;
6. pediatric dental radiography;
7. xeroradiography.

EXTRAORAL AND INTRAORAL RADIOGRAPHY

Extraoral radiographs are taken using screen film and appropriate intensifying screens (Chapter 3). Intensifying screens are used because they decrease the X-Ray dose (less mAs) to the patient, yet still afford a properly exposed radiograph. The X-Ray film used with intensifying screens has photosensitive (light-sensitive) emulsions on both sides of the film. The film is sandwiched between two intensifying screens in a cassette so that the emulsion on each side of the film can be exposed to the light from the intensifying screen adjacent to it. The intensifying screen functions to absorb the enrgy of the X-Ray beam that has penetrated the patient and converts this energy into a light that carries the same information as the original X-Ray beam to form a latent image on the X-Ray film. The latent image is made visible by processing the film in chemical solutions under darkroom conditions.

The cassette and films used in dental extraoral radiography are usually of the 5 × 7 inch (13 × 18 cm) or the 8 × 10 inch (20 × 25 cm) size. Occasionally a 10 × 12 inch (25 × 30 cm) size is used when a radiograph of the entire skull of the patient is desired. It is important to identify the right and left sides of the patient on the extraoral radiograph. This can be done by placing "R" and "L" lead markers on the cassette.

Extraoral radiographs can be produced in the dental office using conventional dental and panoramic X-Ray machines.

Although the larger medical X-Ray units are specifically designed for extraoral radiography, conventional dental X-Ray units can be used. Some of the extraoral radiographic technics the dentist can utilize are—

1. **Lateral jaw radiography**

2. **Skull radiography**
    a. Cephalometric radiography
    b. Paranasal sinus radiography
3. **TMJ (temporomandibular joint) radiography**.

Lateral Jaw Radiography (Body and Ramus Views)

Purpose: The lateral jaw projection is used to view the mandible laterally from the angle of the ramus forward to the symphysis and the maxilla from the pterygoid plates to the first premolar.

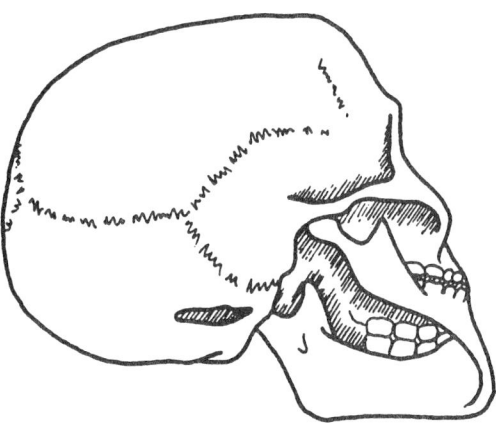

Figure 15-1. Tipped skull for lateral jaw.

Body of Mandible (Lateral Jaw Projection)

The projection reveals the premolar-molar region of the mandible and the lower border of the body of the mandible.

Head Position: The teeth are placed in occlusion with the occlusal plane parallel to the floor. The midsagittal plane should be perpendicular to the floor. This is only a starting position, which standardizes the head position for subsequent steps. With the teeth still in occlusion, the chin is thrust out. This throws the mandible out away from the cervical vertebrae. If the patient is permitted to keep his chin in the normal position, the vertebrae will be superimposed over the ramus of the mandible on the resultant radiograph.

The long axis of the head is tilted at an angle of about 15 degrees toward the side being radiographed. This position will move the opposite mandible up and out of the way from the side of the mandible being radiographed. The tilt should be kept at a minimum in order to minimize the distortion (Fig. 15-1). The chin should be raised slightly.

Film Placement and Retention: The long axis of the film holder or cassette is placed horizontally flat against the side of the mandible. The lower border of the film holder should be parallel to the floor and extend approximately one inch below the lower border of the mandible. The patient retains the cassette in position with the thumb under the edge of the cassette and the palm of the hand on the outer surface of the cassette.

In the lateral jaw projection, rotate the patient's head until the nose is approximately touching the film holder (Fig. 15-2A).

Projection of the Central Ray: VERTICAL ANGULATION: The vertical angulation will vary with the tilt of the head of the patient. If the tilt of the head is approximately 15 degrees, use – 10 degrees. This gives an aggregate angle of 25 degrees.

If the patient's head is not tilted, a vertical angulation of – 17 degrees (upward angulation) is used. A low angle is preferred with patients with short necks and wide shoulders. With these thick-necked patients, the head will have to be tilted slightly (15 degrees) (Fig. 15-2A).

POINT OF ENTRY: This is located 1/2 inch posterior and inferior to the mandible on the opposite side of the mandible to be radiographed (Fig. 15-2B).

HORIZONTAL ANGULATION: This is determined by aligning the top edge of the X-Ray tube parallel with the top edge of the film holder (Fig. 15-2C).

POINT OF EMANATION: The central ray is directed at a point just superior and anterior to the area of interest (Fig. 15-2D, E).

Ramus of Mandible (Lateral Jaw Projection)

Head Position: The teeth are placed in occlusion, with occlusal plane parallel to floor. The midsagittal plane should be perpendicular to the floor. With the teeth still

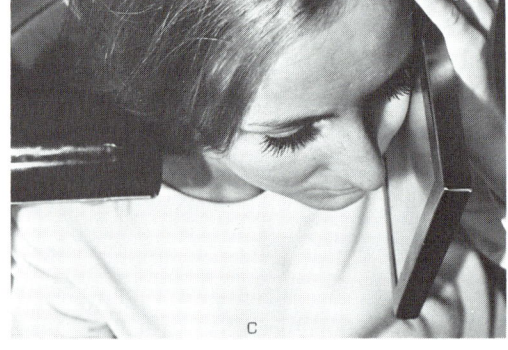
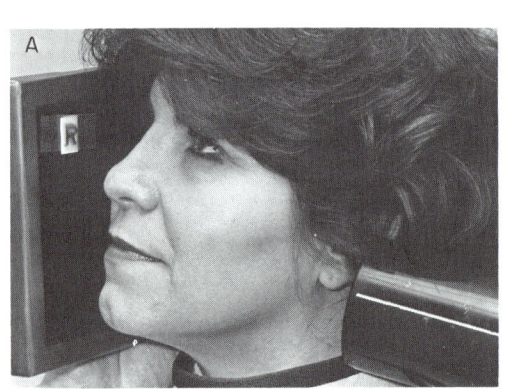
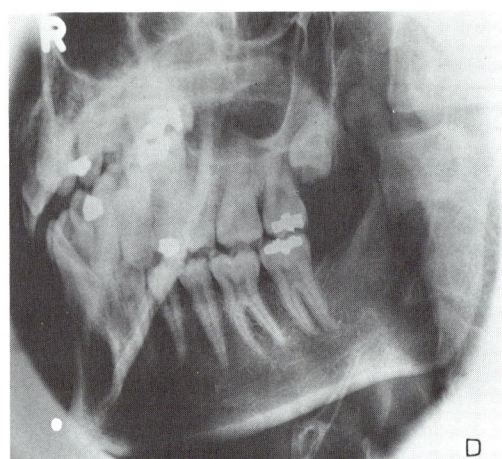
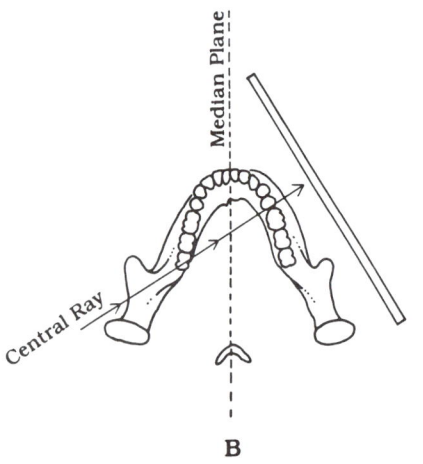
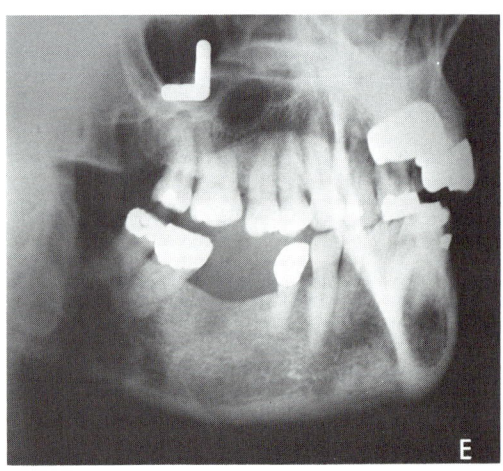

Figure 15-2. Lateral Jaw of Body of Mandible: **(A)** Positioning of cassette and patient. **(B)** Diagram of projection. **(C)** Top view of patient. **(D)** Radiograph of lateral jaw of body of mandible. **(E)** Radiograph of lateral jaw of body of mandible with missing teeth.

in occlusion, the chin is thrust out, which throws the mandible out away from cervical spine. The chin should be raised slightly.

The long axis of the head is tilted at an angle of about 15 degrees toward the side being radiographed (Fig. 15-1).

Film Placement and Retention: The cassette is positioned over the ramus of the mandible with the long axis horizontal. The plane of axis of the cassette should be nearly parallel with the midsaggital plane. The cassette is held in position with the thumb under the edge of the lower border of the cassette and the palm of the hand on the outer surface of the cassette (Fig. 15-3A).

Projection of Central Ray: VERTICAL ANGULATION: Angulation is approximately −15 to −20 degrees (upward angulation) (Fig. 15-3A).

HORIZONTAL ANGULATION: The central ray should be as perpendicular as possible to the face of the cassette (Fig. 15-3B).

POINT OF ENTRY: This should be 1/2 inch diagonally below and posterior to the

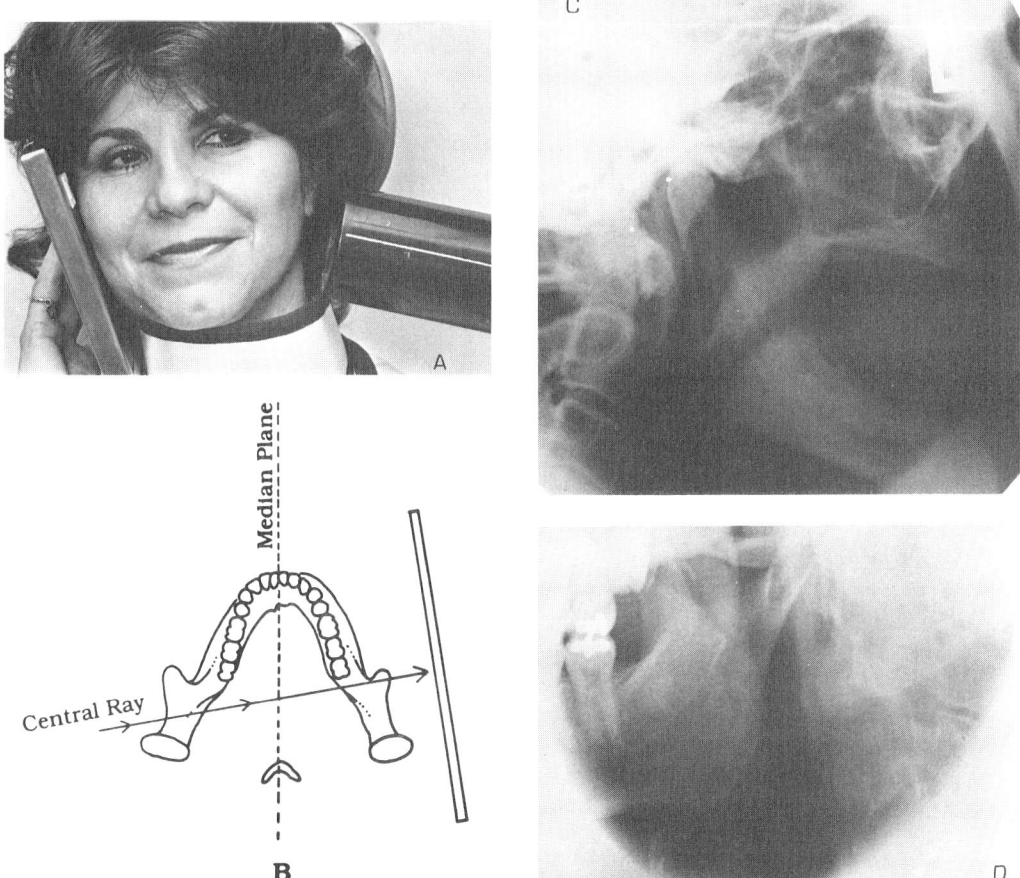

Figure 15-3. Lateral Jaw of Ramus of Mandible. **(A)** Positioning of cassette and patient and cone. **(B)** Diagram of lateral jaw projection. **C** Radiograph of ramus of mandible. **(D)** Ramus of mandible radiograph.

Table 15-I
LATERAL JAW PROJECTIONS

Adult Approximate Exposures* (Kodak X-OMATIC Regular Screens)	65 kVp, 10 mA†		90 kVp, 10 mA†	
	Impulses	Sec	Impulses	Sec
Kodak X-OMAT G or DuPont Cronex 7 Film	18	3/10	6	1/10
Kodak X-OMAT RP or DuPont Cronex 4 Film	9	3/20	3	1/20

*If par-speed screens are used, increase exposure times by two. For children, reduce exposure by 1/2 or 1/3.

†If 15 mA is used, reduce exposure by 30 percent or 1/3.

palpated angle of the mandible. (Fig. 15-3B).

POINT OF EMANATION: The central ray is directed posteriorly toward the center of the ramus on the side against the cassette (Fig. 15-3C, D).

Exposure Factors for Lateral Jaw Projections (*See* Table 15-I.)

CASSETTE SIZE: 5 × 7 inch or 8 × 10 inch
INTENSIFYING SCREENS: Kodak X-OMATIC Regular (barium strontium

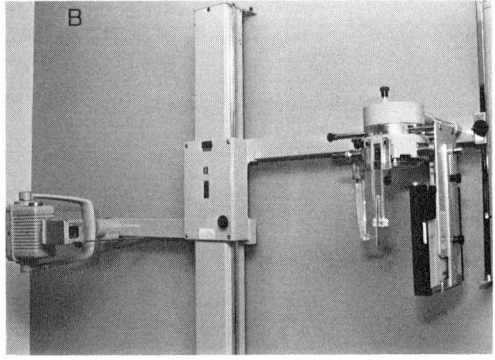

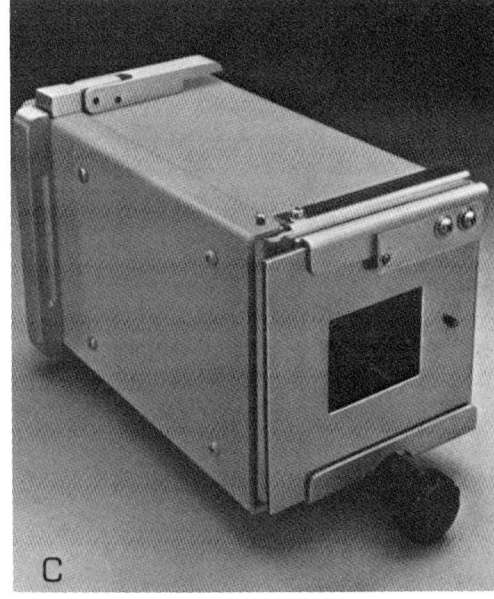

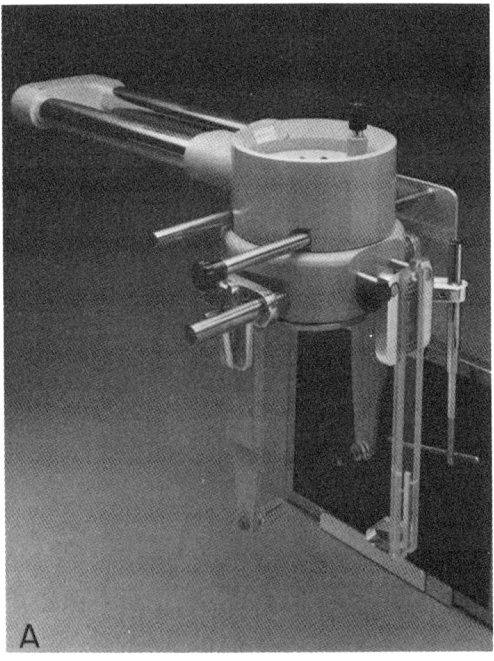

Figure 15-4. Wehmer Cephalostat. (**A**) Cephalostat, close-up view. (**B**) Cephalostat and X-Ray tube. **C** Fixator/collimator.

sulfate) or DuPont Hi Plus (CaWO₄)
SOURCE-FILM DISTANCE: 15 inches (short cone)

Rare-Earth Kodak System: For Extremities (Hands and Lateral Jaws) (Kodak No-Screen film has been discontinued.)
CASSETTE: 8 × 10 inch Min-R cassette
INTENSIFYING SCREEN: Kodak MIN-R Screen
SOURCE-FILM DISTANCE: 15 inches (short cone) Lateral Jaw Technique
FILM: Kodak Ortho M film (single-coated)
FACTORS: Approximately 3 times as fast as No-Screen film.

Skull Radiography

Radiographic studies of the skull are difficult because there is no other part of the body where so many structures can be identified in such a small area. Radiographic interpretation of the skull radiograph is hindered because many of the anatomic structures are superimposed over each other. This sometimes requires multiple radiographs of an area in order to obtain a clear view of the superimposed structures. The skull radiographic projections used by the dentist pertain mostly to cephalometric skull radiography and paranasal sinus skull radiography.

Cephalometric Radiography

Cephalometric radiography is used almost exclusively by orthodontists. Pucini (1922) was the first to introduce this technique for growth and development studies of the skull. However, it took Broadbent (1931) of the United States and Hofrath (1931) of Germany to make the technique a practical diagnostic method in orthodontics. They both advocated head-holding devices called cephalometer or cephalostat (Fig. 15-4). The cephalostat

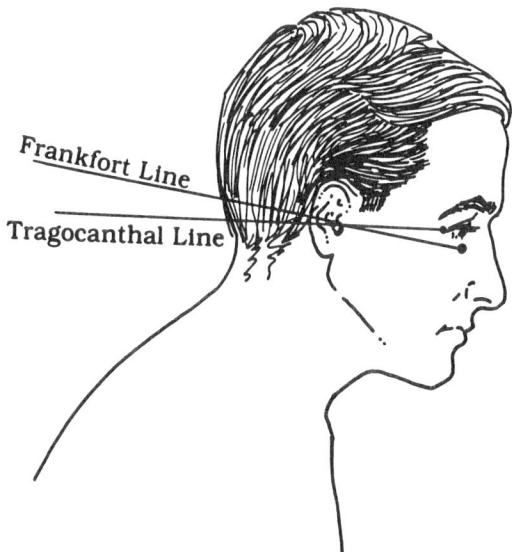

Figure 15-5. Drawing of tragocanthal line and Frankfort line.

makes it possible to position and reposition the patient's head in a predetermined relationship of the X-Ray beam to the Frankfort horizontal line, which is a line connecting the superior border of the earpost of the cephalostat (porion) and the inferior border of orbit (orbitale). The Frankfort horizontal plane is the classical plane used in cephalometrics. The tragocanthal line (line joining the center of the auditory meatus and the outer canthus of the eye) forms an angle of about 10 degrees to the Frankfort horizontal plane and is preferred by most operators for patient positioning because it is more easily visualized (Fig. 15-5).

Two views are used in cephalometric radiography: a **lateral (profile)** and a **posteroanterior or PA view**. The lateral view is made with the left side located nearest the cassette. The PA view is made with the patient facing the cassette, because this records the facial structures with less distortion. The accepted distance in cephalometrics from X-Ray

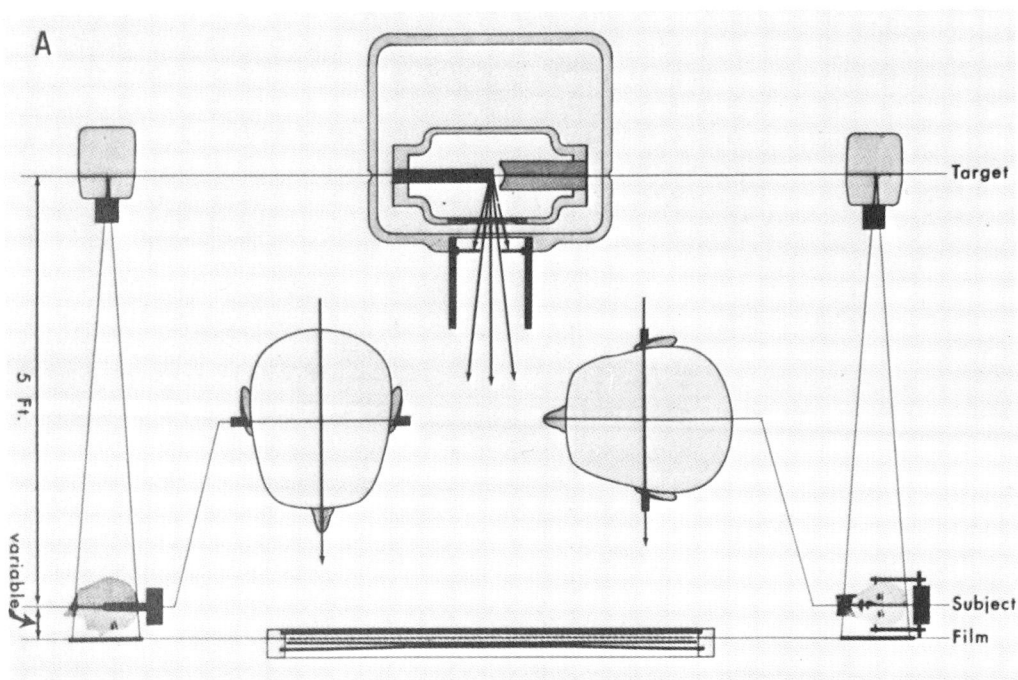
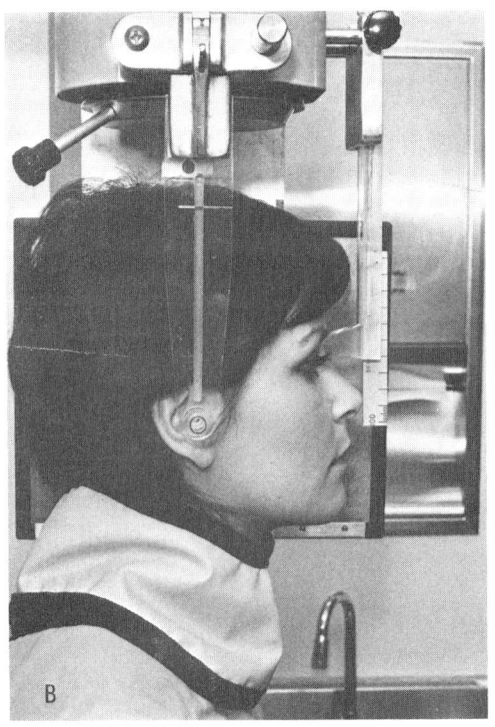
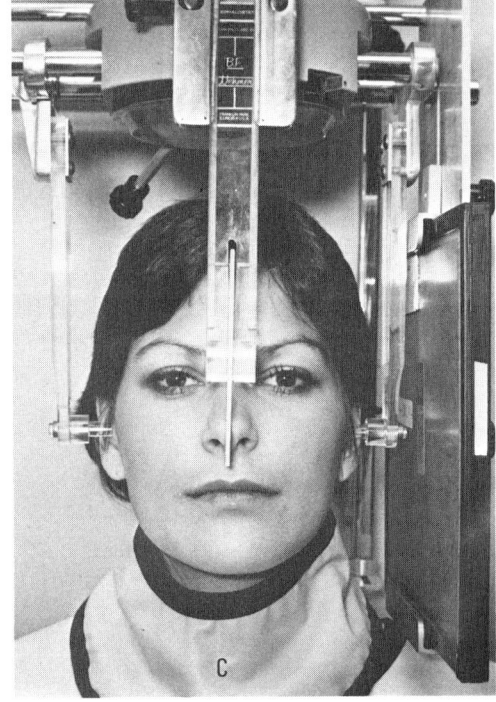

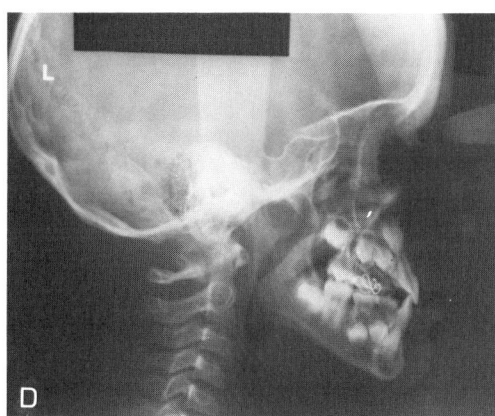

Figure 15-6. Alignment principles for cephalometric radiography: **(A)** (Top) lateral view; (Bottom) posteroanterior (PA) view, sometimes called frontal view; (Center) close-up showing points for measurement of principal distances (From Thurow, R. C.: Atlas of Orthodontic Principles, 2nd ed., 1977, C. V. Mosby Co., St. Louis. Courtesy of Raymond C. Thorow, Madison Wi.) **(B)** Side view of lateral cephalometric projection. **(C)** Front view of lateral cephalometric projection. **(D)** Lateral (Profile) radiograph.

graphs, which aids in accurate comparisons (Fig. 15-6A).

Lateral Cephalometric Technic

Head Position: Usually, the lateral view is taken first. Immobilize the patient's head in the head holder by means of the nasion positioning rod and the ear plugs. The patient's head is positioned in the Frankfort plane horizontally by use of infraorbital marker. The midsagittal plane shold be parallel to the horizontally placed cassette (Fig. 15-6B, C).

Projection of Central Ray: Direct the central ray perpendicular to the cassette and through the central axis of the ear rods and the auditory canals. The earpost alignment can be checked by taping a dental film on the left ear post and making an exposure. The metal portions of the ear posts should superimpose over each other. The cone of radiation should be collimated to the size of the skull of the patient. The size of the cone of radiation can be checked by use of an intensifying screen taped to a cassette holder. In a darkened room, the screen will give out a visible blue or green glow during X-Ray exposure and outline the X-Ray expo-

source to patient is 5 feet or 152.4 cm. The patient location point is measured to the midsagittal plane, which is determined as the midpoint between the earposts (Fig. 15-6A).

The film (inside the cassette) to patient distance varies according to different technics. In the variable distance technic, the cassette holder is placed against the left ear holder prior to exposure, so the patient-film distance varies with the patient size. The advantage of using a variable patient-film distance is that the dimensional enlargement of the radiographic anatomical images are kept at a minimum. When a fixed patient-film technic is used, the patient-film distance is fixed, say at a distance of 12 cm. The advantage of this technic is that the enlargement is the same for all radio-

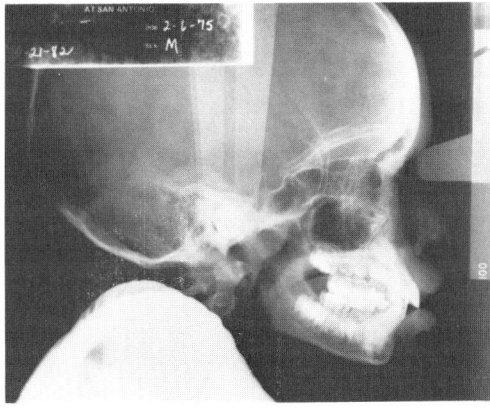

Figure 15-7. Cephalometric radiograph showing facial soft tissue profile.

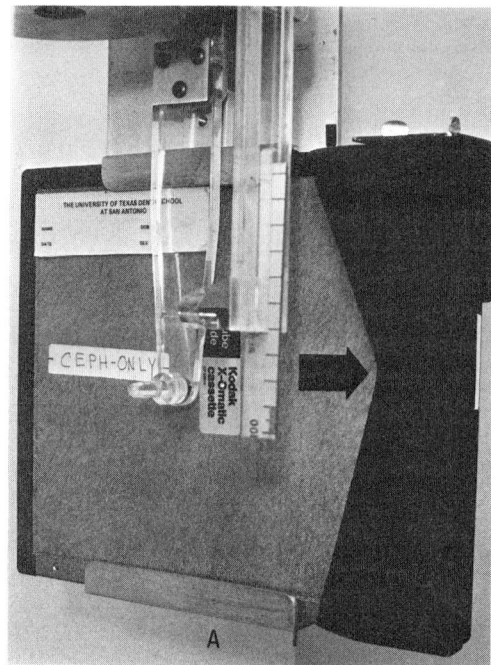

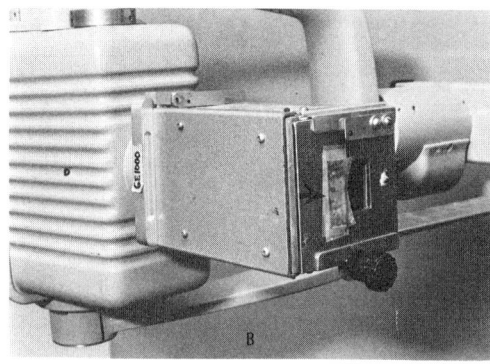

Figure 15-8. Devices to use in cephalometrics to bring out soft tissue profile. **(A)** Aluminum filter between patient and film. **(B)** Tapered lead filter at collimator.

sure of film. By adjusting the collimation, the correct beam size can be obtained. In the lateral profile projection, it is prudent to use a lead apron and cervical neck

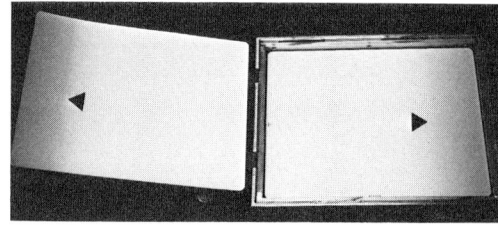

Figure 15-9. Dye in cassette (Quint cassette opened). (Note darkened areas.)

shield (Fig. 15-6C).

Recording Soft Tissue Profile: In the **lateral cephalometric radiograph** it is desirable to record the facial soft tissue profile as well as the bony landmarks (Fig. 15-6D, 15-7). There are several methods to achieve this.

1. Use wide latitude films such as the Kodak SB film (single coated-blue sensitive) or the Kodak X-Omat L film. It will be possible to record both the soft tissue and the bony structures on one radiograph; however the contrast is fairly low.
2. Use higher contrast films such as X-Omat RP or DuPont Cronex 4 with a wedge-shaped aluminum filter placed between the patient and the film cassette (Fig. 15-8A).
3. Use a thin lead filter at the collimator with a tapered knife-edge to attenuate the X-Ray beam before it reaches the patient. This type of filter is especially useful when using the Kodak Lanex screens and Kodak OG film (Fig. 15-8B).
4. Use a special dye placed on an intensifying screen in the area where the patient's profile will be positioned. Dye attenuates fluorescence of

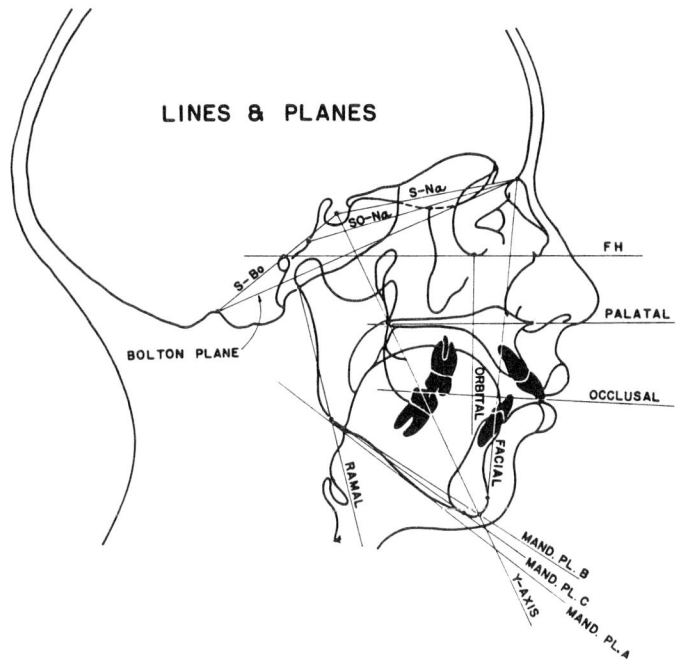

Figure 15-10. Lines and planes used in lateral cephalometric analysis. **Cranial base planes**: S-Na, sella-nasion; Bo-Na, Bolton plane; So-Na, spheno-occipital suture-nasion; Po-Or, Frankfort horizontal; S-Bo joins sella and Bolton point to complete the Bolton (Broadbent) triangle. **Facial planes**: palatal, occlusal, and mandibular planes. Note the three possibilities for the construction of the mandibular plane. Also used are **semivertical planes**, which join cranial and facial areas: facial plane, orbital plane, Y-axis, and ramal plane. The orbital and ramal planes are seldom used, however. (From Graber, T.M.: *Current Orthodontic concepts and Techniques*, Vol. 1. 1969, Figure 1-23, p. 30. Courtesy of W.B. Saunders, Philadelphia.)

screen phosphors so soft tissue outline of patient's face is not "burnt-out" (Fig. 15-9).

The lateral (profile) skull radiograph is the most common cephalometric radiograph produced. It is used to measure facial relationships and to predict growth patterns in orthodontic treatment. This is done by means of cephalometric tracings of key structures, which are then evaluated by measurements of angles and linear dimensions between the various parts (Fig. 15-10).

Posteroanterior (PA) Cephalometric Technic

Another skull radiograph used in cephalometrics is the **posteroanterior skull view** (Fig. 15-11A). It is used to measure lateral skull growth and to determine if there are growth abnormalities or asymmetry in the maxilla or mandible (Fig. 15-11B). The PA projection is made with the Frankfort horizontal plane or in most cases the tragocanthal line perpendicular to the plane of the film. The central ray coincides with the Frankfort

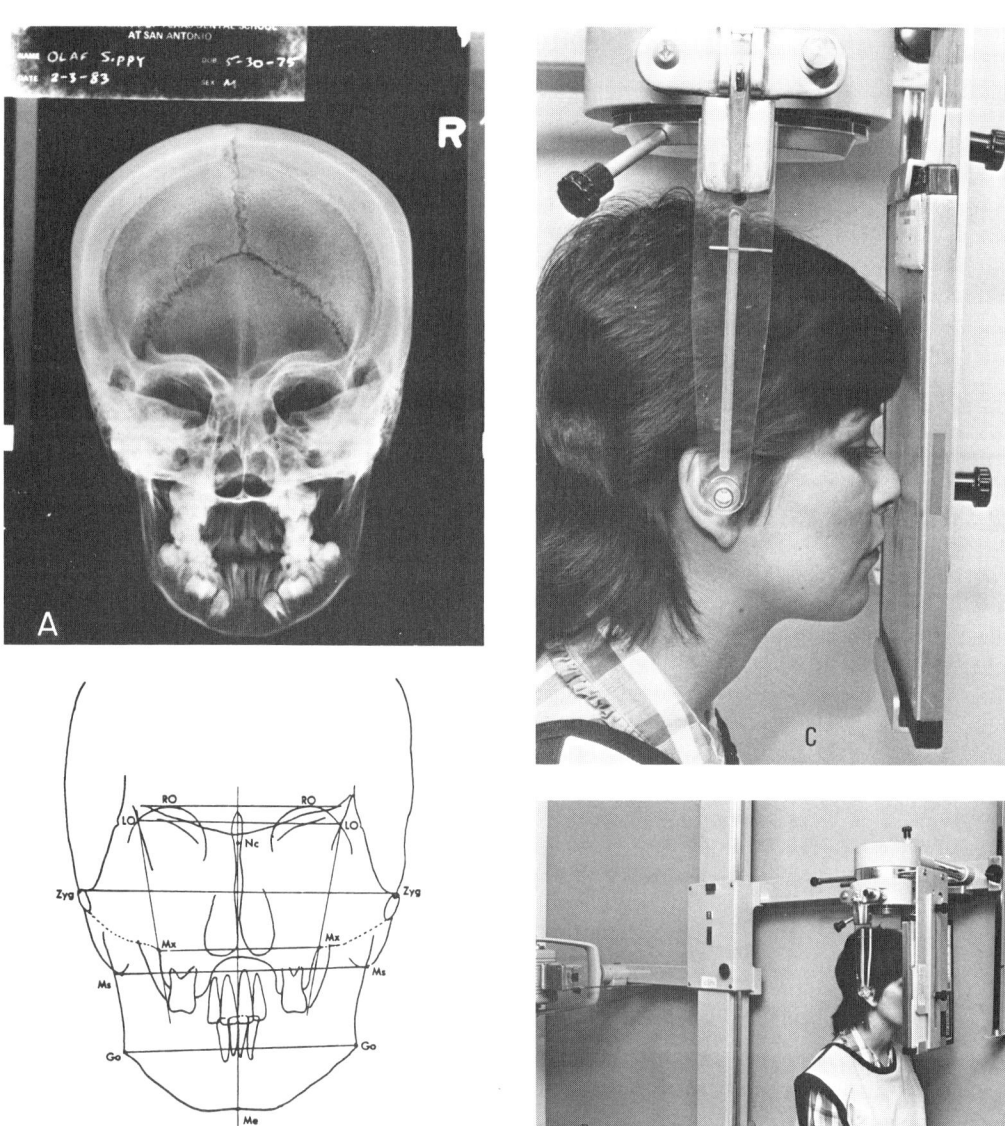

Figure 15-11. **(A)** PA (Frontal) cephalometric view radiograph. **(B)** Posteroanterior tracing analysis to determine the symmetry. **Roof of Orbit** (RO). **Latero-orbitale** (LO) intersection point between external orbital contour laterally and oblique orbital line. **Oblique Orbital Line** is projection of greater wing of sphenoid. **Cristal galli** (Nc) neck of crista galli. **Maxillare** (Mx) maximum concavity on the contour of the maxilla between malare and maxillary first molar. **Malare** is the midpoint intersection of the coronoid process and the lower contour of the malar bone. **Zygoma** (Zyg) most lateral and superior point of shadow of zygomatic arch. **Mastoidale** (Ms) lowest point on the contour of the mastoid process. **Gonion** (Go) horizontal projection of gonion from the lateral film. **Menton** (Me) lowermost point of contour of chin. (From Sassouni, Viken: *Orthodontics in Dental Practice, 1971, Fig. 17-5, p. 335, Courtesy of C.V. Mosby Co., St. Louis.*) **(C)** PA cephalometric technique (side view). **(D)** PA cephalometric technique (full view).

Table 15-II
CEPHALOMETRIC PROJECTIONS
APPROXIMATE EXPOSURES*
(no grid)†

				Impulses	
Film	Screens‡	Screen Phosphor	Color Emitted	Lateral Skull	PA Skull
				90 kV, 15 mA	90 kV, 15 mA
Kodak X-OMAT RP	Kodak X-OMATIC Regular	$BaSO_4$:Sr,Eu	Ultraviolet	60 (1 sec)	75 (1 1/4 sec)
DuPont Cronex 4	DuPont Cronex Hi-Plus	$CaWo_4$	Blue	60 (1 sec)	75 (1 1/4 sec)
3M Trilite Cephalometric	Either one above			60 (1 sec)	75 (1 1/4 sec)
Ortho G or Ortho L	Kodak Lanex Regular	Gd_2O_2S:Tb	Green	30 (1/2 sec)	38 (19/30 sec)
3M Trimax XM	3M Trimax 8	Gd_2O_2S:Tb	Green	30 (1/2 sec)	38 (19/30 sec)
DuPont Cronex 7	DuPont Cronex Quanta III	LaOBr:Tm	Blue	30 (1/2 sec)	38 (19/30 sec)

*Children: Reduce adult exposure by 1/4 or 1/3.
†If a grid is used, increase exposure time by approximately 2 times.
‡If using par-speed calcium tungstate screens such as Quint par-screen (which uses dye to bring out soft tissue profile) approximately four times the Kodak Lanex (Regular/Ortho G) exposure will be necessary.

horizontal plane or tragocanthal line. If the CR coincides with the tragocanthal line, it enters the skull at the external occipital protuberance (inion) and exits the nasion. Since most dentofacial anatomic structures are situated anterior to the ears, the cassette is placed in front of the face to minimize the enlargement of these structures (Fig. 15-11C, D).

Exposure Factors for Cephalometric Radiography

CASSETTE SIZE: 8 × 10 inch or 10 × 12 inch
SOURCE-PATIENT DISTANCE: 60 inch (152.4 cm)
SOURCE-FILM DISTANCE: (fixed 12 cm object-film distance in lateral view). 164.4 cm (enlargement of mid-sagittal points in lateral view will be slightly less than 8 percent — correction factor .93+)
SAFELIGHT FILTER RECOMMENDED: Kodak GBX (Green-Blue X-Ray)

Paranasal Sinus Radiography

It is important that the dentist have knowledge of the paranasal sinuses. Since they are hidden structures, the radiograph is an important aid in supplying information to the dentist concerning the paranasal sinuses.

Paranasal Sinuses

The paranasal sinuses are paired, air-

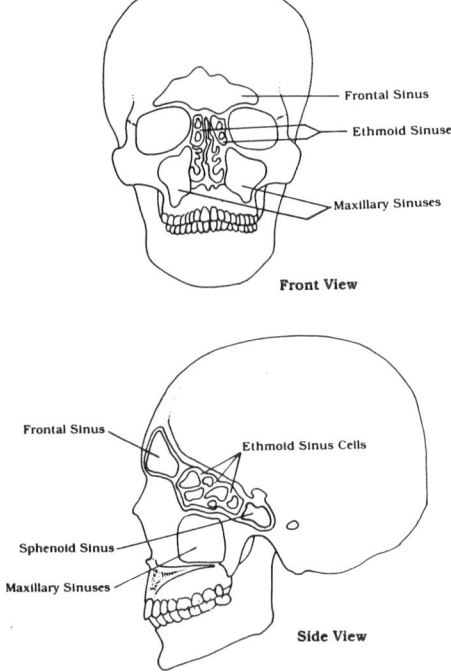

Figure 15-12. Location of paranasal sinuses.

containing cavities within the maxillary, frontal, ethmoid, and sphenoid bones (Fig. 15-12).

Maxillary sinuses: Antra of Highmore are located within the maxillary bones immediately below the orbits on each side of the lateral walls of the nasal fossae. They are the largest of the paranasal sinuses and are generally pyramidal in shape.

Ethmoid sinuses: They are composed of a large group of small cells located between the orbit and upper portion of the nose and extend posteriorly toward the sphenoid sinuses. It is customary to subdivide the ethmoid cells into anterior, middle, and posterior groups, although no well-defined dividing lines can be discerned.

Frontal sinuses: When well developed, they are found just above and medially to the orbit. These air spaces, seldom truly symmetrical, show wide developmental faults varying from complete absence to huge anomalous cells that occupy one-third or more of the entire frontal bone.

Sphenoid Bone: This may contain centrally placed single or paired cavities (sphenoid sinuses) depending on whether or not a highly variable median septum of bone is present.

Routine Radiographic Survey of Paranasal Sinuses. A routine radiographic survey of the paranasal sinuses includes the—

1. Waters view;
2. Caldwell view;
3. Lateral view
4. Axial, Base, or Submentovertex view.

Waters View (Inclined Posteroanterior View)

Waters and Waldron first described this view in 1915. This should be called the "maxillary sinus" view because it shows the maxillary sinuses better than any other view of the skull. It is also the best view for demonstrating the orbital floor. The Waters projection allows visualization of the frontal and maxillary sinuses, and many of the ethmoid cells, with little or no interference by superimposition of other structures within the cranium, particularly the petrous portion of the temporal bone.

Patient Position: Seat the patient facing the erect cassette in a film holder with the midsagittal plane of the skull over the center line of the cassette. The head is positioned with the midsagittal plane perpendicular to the cassette, and the head is extended so that the tragocanthal line forms an angle of 37 degrees with the cassette. The nose should be 2-3 cm from the surface of the cassette. (Fig. 15-13A, B).

Central Ray: The central ray enters the skull about 3 cm above the external

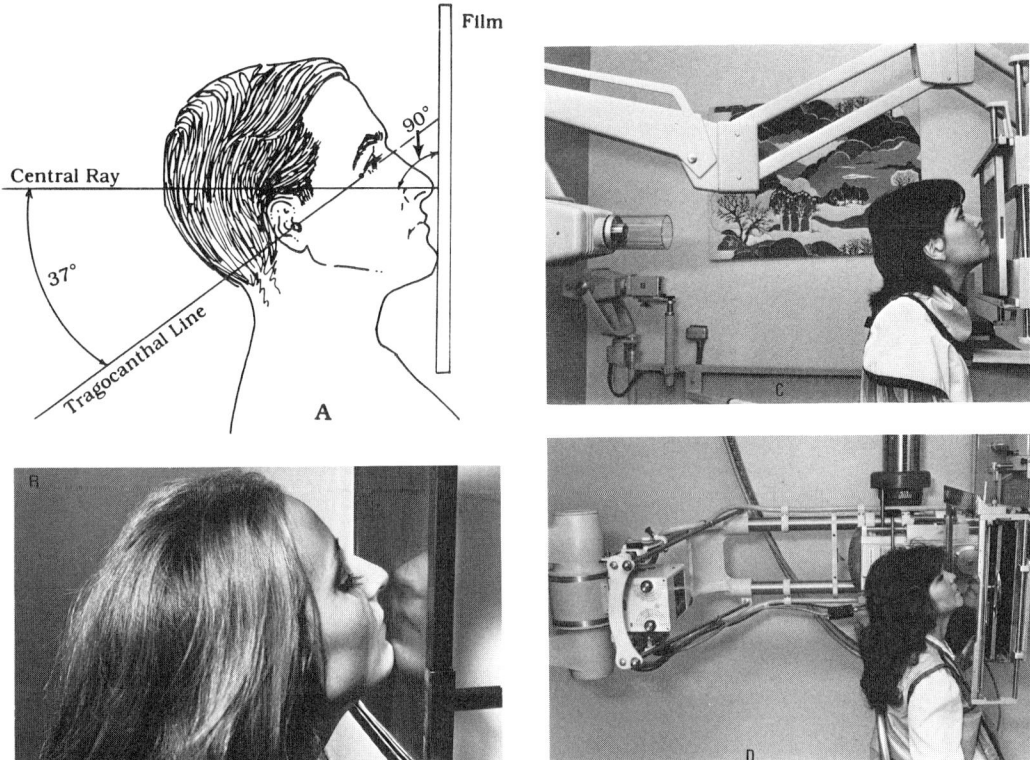

Figure 15-13. Waters Projection. **(A)** Diagram of Waters Projection; **(B)** Head positioned with midsagittal plane perpendicular to film; **(C)** Central ray alignment with skull and film; **(D)** Franklin Head Unit (Waters projection).

Table 15-III

WATERS PROJECTION
Approximate Exposure Factors*
(no grid)

| Film/Screen Combination | | 90 kVp, 15 mA | |
Screens	Film	Impulses	Seconds
Kodak X-OMATIC Regular	Kodak X-OMAT RP Film	24	2/5
DuPont Cronex Hi-Plus	DuPont Cronex 4 Film	24	3/5
Kodak Lanex Regular	Kodak OG or OL Film	12	1/5
DuPont Cronex Quanta III	DuPont Cronex 7	12	1/5

*Children: Reduce exposure by 1/4 to 1/3.
The cephalometric technic may be used for Waters View (source-object distance is 60").

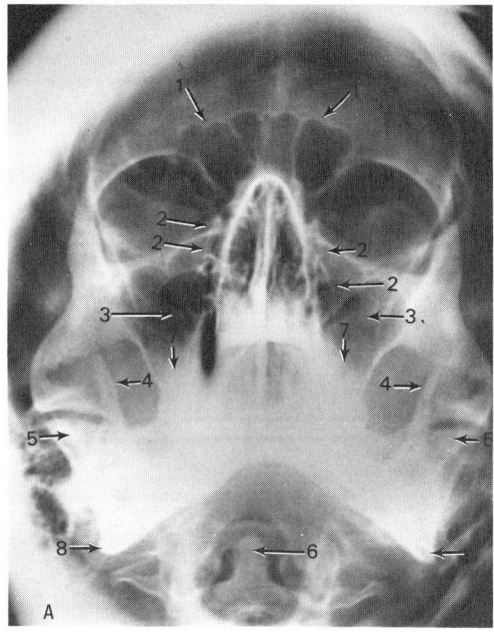 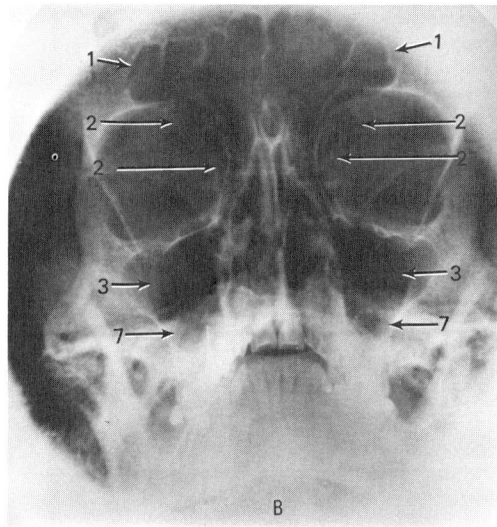

Figure 15-14. Waters View Radiographs: (1) frontal sinus; (2) ethmoid cells; (3) maxillary sinuses; (4) coronoid process; (5) condyles; (6) odontoid process of axis (second vertebral vertebra); (7) petrous portion of temporal bone; (8) angle of mandible.

occipital protuberance and exits through the tip of the nose (Fig. 15-13C).

Exposure Factors

CASSETTE SIZE: 8 × 10 inches

FOCUS-FILM DISTANCE: 30 inches (short cone)

Franklin Head Unit: Several medical X-Ray devices have been specifically designed for skull radiography. In general, they may be divided into two groups: those with a circular tube movement and those in which the tube may be moved on the surface of a sphere. The Franklin Head Unit (Leibel-Flarsheim, Cincinnati, Ohio) is a popular X-Ray unit that has been specifically designed for skull radiography. It is typical of those in which the tube moves in a circular movement. The patient is positioned in the Franklin Head Unit for a Waters projection in Figure 15-13D.

Evaluation of Accuracy of Waters View: A Waters view can be examined for accuracy by observing the position of the following anatomical structures (Fig. 15-14):

1. The **coronoid processes** on each side should be approximately the same distance apart.
2. The backward tilt of the head is correct if the **petrous portion of the temporal bone** appears just below the lowest portion of the maxillary sinuses.
3. A horizontal line drawn through the left and right **angles of the mandible** should be approximately parallel to the lower edge of the radiograph.
4. The **odontoid process** of the second cervical (axis) vertebrae bone should be in the midline.

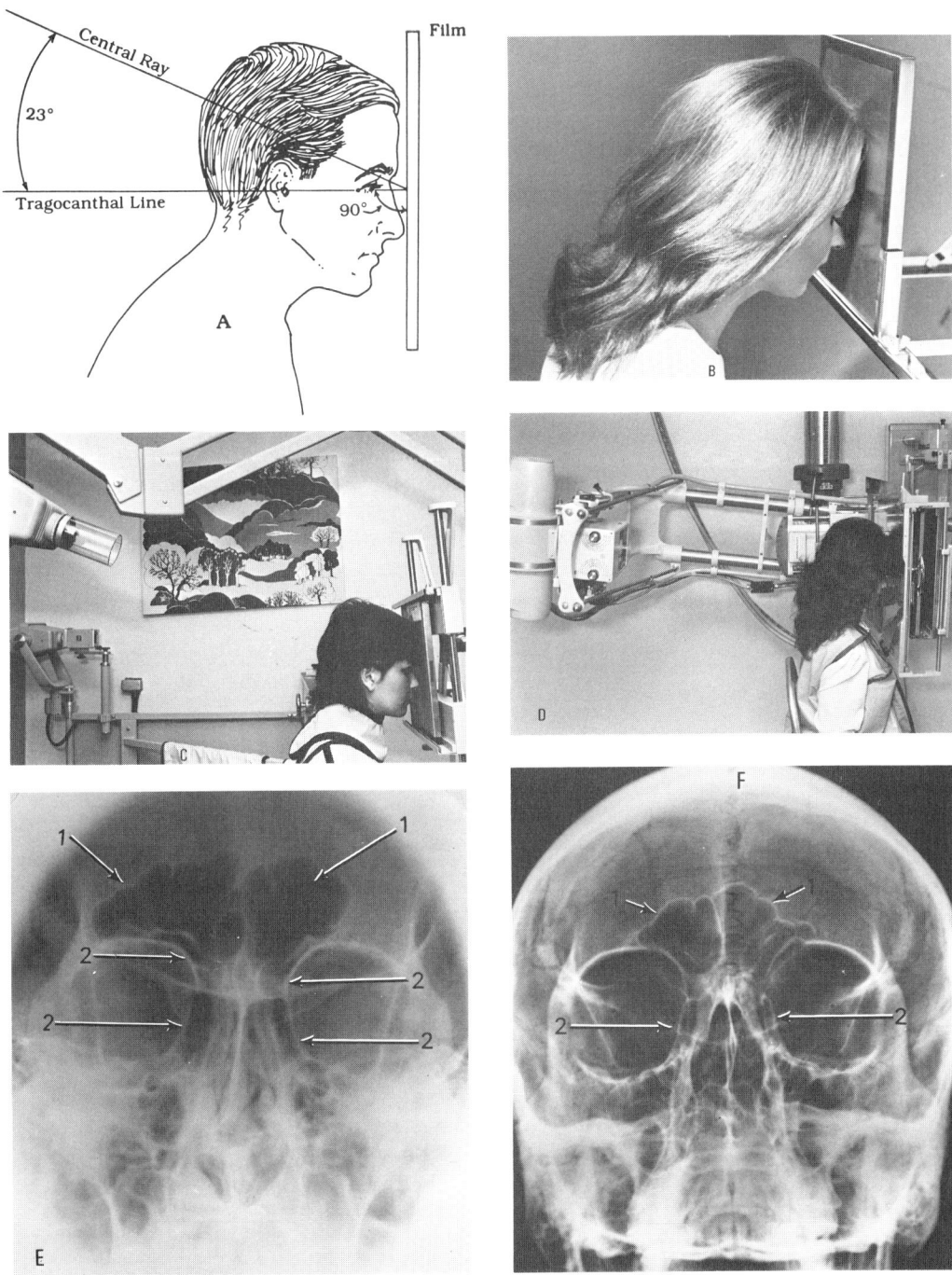

Figure 15-15. Caldwell View. **(A)** Diagram of Caldwell projection. Head positioned so tragocanthal line is perpendicular to film. The CR is directed 23 degrees caudal to tragocanthal line. It enters the skull above the external occipital protuberance and exits the glabella. **(B)** Patient positioned for Caldwell projection described in (A). **(C)** Modified Caldwell Projection. **(D)** Patient positioned in Franklin Head unit. **(E)** Caldwell radiograph. **(F)** Caldwell radiograph. (1) frontal sinus; (2) ethmoid cells.

Caldwell View
(Frontal-Ethmoidal-Orbital View)

Caldwell first described this projection in 1906. This view is sometimes called the "orbit view" of the skull because it demonstrates the orbital walls better than any other view. It is also superior to other projections for the demonstration of the frontal sinuses and the superiorly located ethmoid cells. The superior portion of the maxillary sinuses is usually blocked by the petrous portion of the temporal bone, but the alveolar region is usually seen (Fig. 15-15E).

Head Position: The patient's head is positioned so the tragocanthal line is perpendicular to the film. This usually positions the forehead and nose touching the cassette (Fig. 15-15A, B).

Projection of Central Ray: The central ray is directed 23 degrees caudad (opposite to cranial, toward the feet) to the tragalcanthal line. It enters the skull about 3 cm above the **external occipital** protuberance and exits at the **glabella** (the prominent point in the midsagittal plane between the eyebrows) (Fig. 15-15A). A modified Caldwell projection is shown in Figure 15-15C. The film cassette is rotated 15 degrees from vertical toward the patient. This insures ease in placing the patient's nose and forehead against the film surface and does not place the patient in an awkward position. The CR is angled 25 degrees caudally and aimed to pass through the glabella. A patient in the Conventional Caldwell view position using the Franklin head Unit is shown in Figure 15-15D. Representative Caldwell view radiographs are shown in Figures 15-15E and F.

Exposure Features
FOCUS-FILM DISTANCE: 30 inches (short cone). Dental X-Ray Machine

Table 15-IV

CALDWELL PROJECTION
Approximate Exposure Factors*
(no grid)

Film/Screen Combination		90 kVp, 15 mA	
Screens	Film	Impulses	Seconds
Kodak X-OMATIC Regular	Kodak X-OMAT RP Film	24	2/5
DuPont Cronex Hi-Plus	DuPont Cronex 4 Film	24	2/5
Kodak Lanex Regular	Kodak OG or OL Film	12	1/5
DuPont Cronex Quanta III	DuPont Cronex 7	12	1/5

*Children: Reduce exposure 1/4 to 1/3

Lateral View of the Skull

This projection reveals the anteroposterior dimension of all the sinuses (Fig. 15-16A). The central depth of the frontal sinus is depicted, but the lateral portion of the sinus is not shown. The anterior and posterior walls of the frontal sinus can be analyzed on this view. This is particularly important in the radiologic diagnosis of a mucocele of the frontal sinus. What may seem to be opacification of the frontal sinus on the Caldwell view may only prove to be a result of a thick anterior wall rather than disease in the lateral view. The lateral orbital rim overlaps the ethmoid area. Posterior ethmoid cells can usually be seen behind the lateral orbital rim. The medial portion of the maxillary sinuses is demonstrated in the lateral view of the face. Only the superior and anterior margins of the sphenoid sinus can be seen because usually the floor of sphenoidal sinus is obscured by overlapping of the temporomandibular joint area (Fig. 15-16E).

The nasopharyngeal soft tissues of the posterior wall of the nasopharynx are seen best in the lateral view. The curve of the posterior wall of the nasopharynx is normally concave. If the curve is convex in a child, hypertrophied adenoids are usually the cause (Fig. 15-16E).

Technic: The head is positioned so the midsagittal plane is parallel to the cassette. On the canthomeatal line, center a point 2 cm anterior to and 2 cm superior to the external auditory meatus. Align the top of the cassette 1 1/2 inches above the vertex of the skull. Direct the central ray perpendicular to the midsagittal plane through the selected point on the patient's skull (Fig. 15-16A-D).

Exposure Factors
CASSETTE SIZE: 8 × 10 inch
SOURCE-FILM DISTANCE: 30 inches (short cone)

Table 15-V

LATERAL VIEW PROJECTION

Approximate Exposure Factors*

(no grid)

Film/Screen Combination		90 kVp, 15 mA	
		Impulses	Seconds
Kodak X-OMATIC Regular	Kodak X-OMAT RP Film	15	1/4
DuPont Cronex Hi-Plus	DuPont Cronex 4 Film	15	1/4
Kodak Lanex Regular	Kodak OG or OL Film	8	1/8
DuPont Cronex Quanta III	DuPont Cronex 7	8	1/8

*Children: Reduce exposure by 1/3 to 1/2.
The cephalometric technic may be used for lateral skull (source-object distance is 60 inches or 152.4 cm).

Submentovertex or Basilar View of Skull

The **basilar or submentovertex view** was devised by Bowen in 1914. In this projection, the maxillary, ethmoidal, and sphenoidal sinus zones can be seen (Fig. 15-17E, F). The mandible obscures a portion of the maxillary sinus and anterior ethmoid cells. The posterior ethmoid cells

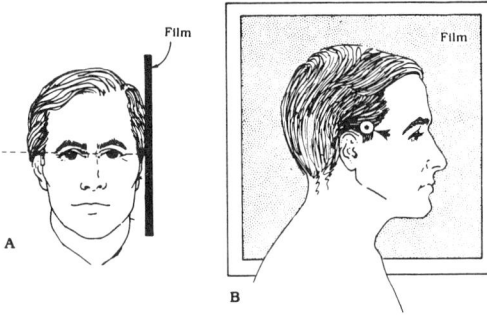

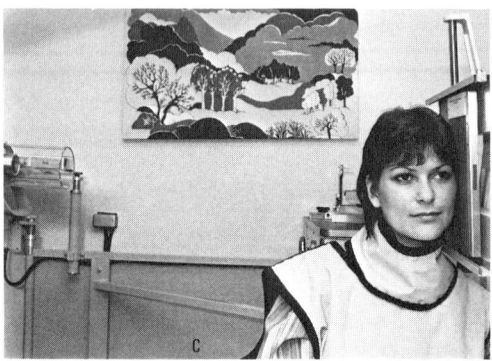

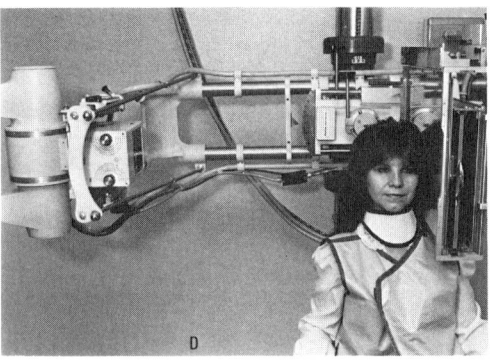

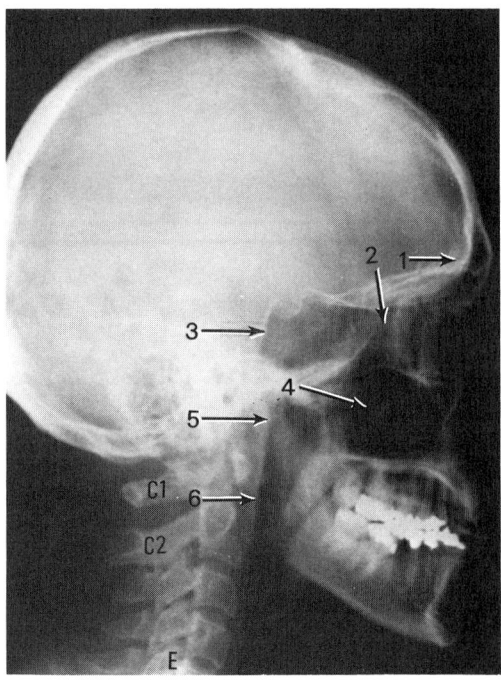

Figure 15-16. Lateral View of Skull. (A) Diagram front view. (B) Diagram side view. (C) Photo of patient, tube and cassette showing lateral skull technique (front view). (D) Franklin Head Unit. (E) Radiograph of lateral skull. (1) frontal sinus; (2) ethmoid cells; (3) sphenoid sinus; (4) maxillary sinus; (5) nasopharyngeal soft tissues; (6) prevertebral soft tissues.

Exposure Factors
CASSETTE SIZE: 8 × 10 inch
FOCUS (Source-Film Distance): 30 inches (short cone)

are usually seen quite clearly. The lateral, anterior, and posterior walls of the sphenoidal sinus walls are all shown quite well. Although the sphenoidal sinus can be seen partially in the lateral view (Fig. 15-16 E, F), the basilar view is essential for the evaluation of these sinuses. This view is valuable for the visualization of the zygomatic arches, since they are thrown into a bold outline by means of the projection. However, a lighter exposure technic may be necessary for this purpose. When this is done, the projection is sometimes called **the jug-handle view** because of its similarity to a jug with handles. The **basilar**

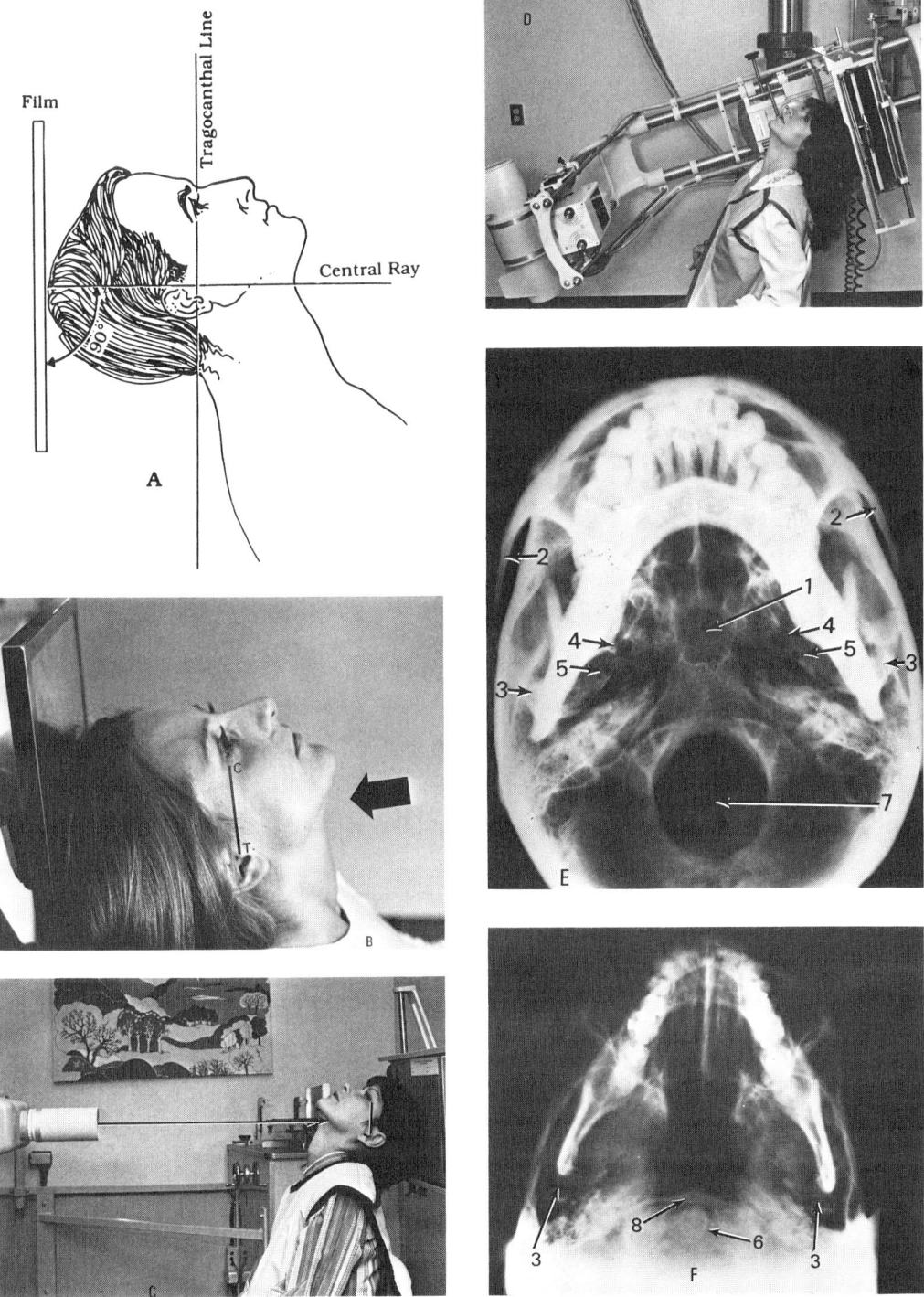

Figure 15-17. Basilar or Submentovertex View. **(A)** Diagram. **(B)** Head positioned so that tragocanthal line is parallel to the film. **(C)** The central ray is perpendicular to the tragocanthal line; it enters the skull in the midline between the mandibular angles. **(D)** Franklin Head Unit patient. **(E)** Basilar view radiograph. **(F)** Basilar view radiograph. Identification of anatomic structures in (E) and (F). (1) sphenoid sinus; (2) zygomatic arch; (3) mandibular condyle (inferior view); (4) foramen ovale; (5) foramen spinosum; (6) odontoid process (dens); (7) foramen magnum; (8) anterior arch of C-1.

Table 15-VI

BASILAR OR SUBMENTOVERTEX VIEW
Approximate Exposure Factors*
(no grid)

| Film/Screen Combination | | 90 kVp, 15 mA | |
Screens	Film	Impulses	Seconds
Kodak X-OMATIC Regular	Kodak X-OMAT RP Film	30	1/2
DuPont Cronex Hi-Plus	DuPont Cronex 4 Film	30	1/2
Kodak Lanex Regular	Kodak OG or OL Film	15	1/4
DuPont Cronex Quanta III	DuPont Cronex 7	15	1/4

*Children: Reduce exposure 1/4 to 1/3.
The cephalometric technic may be used for basiler or submentovertex (source-object distance is 60 inches or 152.4 cm).

or submentovertex view also gives an inferior view of the mandibular condyles. (Fig. 15-17E, F).

Technic: Position the head of the patient so the tragocanthal line is parallel to the cassette. Direct the central ray perpendicular to the tragocanthal line. The point of entry into the skull is the midline between the mandibular angles (Fig. 15-17 A, B, C).

Temporomandibular Radiography

Temporomandibular (TMJ) radiography is probably the most difficult radiographic technic for the dentist to accomplish. This is primarily related to the anatomic location of the joint. The **petrous** portion of the temporal bone, located medially and superiorly to the joint, partially obscures the lateral TMJ projections (Fig. 15-18). **Anteroposterior** projections of the TMJ are hindered by the superimposition of the mastoid process of the temporal bone, posterior to the joint and the zygomatic bone, anterior to the

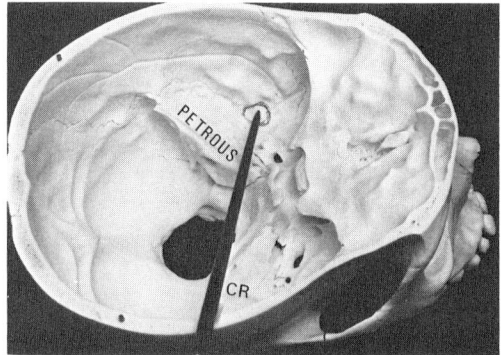

Figure 15-18. Transcranial TMJ projection is difficult because X-Ray beam must be directed from opposite side of skull across the superior margin of the petrous portion of the temporal bone to the temporomandibular joint. The petrous process is a thick bone that houses the capsule of equilibrium and the organ of hearing, provides for course of carotid artery, and protects the jugular vein.

joint (Fig. 15-19). There are various TMJ radiographic technics the dentist can employ in his dental office: (1) Transcranial lateral TMJ projection; (2) anteroposterior TMJ projection; (3) panoramic TMJ

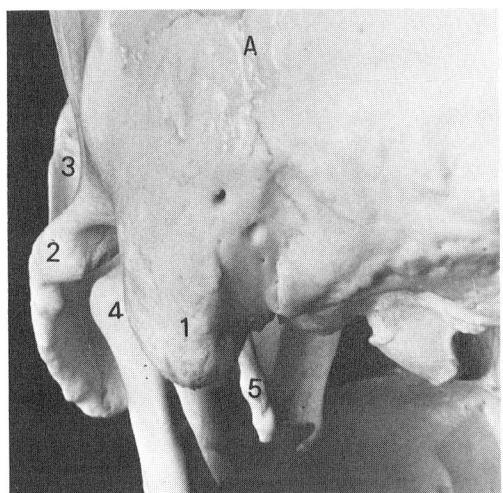

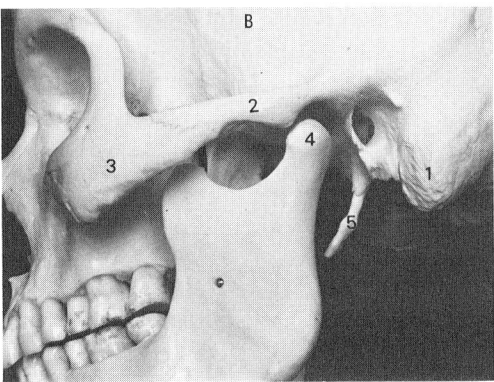

Figure 15-19. AP projections of TMJ hindered by mastoid process of the temporal bone on the posterior and the zygomatic bone anterior to the joint. **(A)** Posterior view. **(B)** Lateral view. (1) mastoid portion of temporal bone; (2) zygoma (zygomatic process of temporal bone); (3) zygomatic bone; (4) condyle; (5) stylohyoid process.

projection; (4) reverse Towne projection (posteroanterior TMJ projection); and (5) submentovertex projection (previously described). There are two TMJ radiographic technics of such specialized character that they require equipment mostly found in hospitals, institutions, and specialty offices: tomography and arthrography.

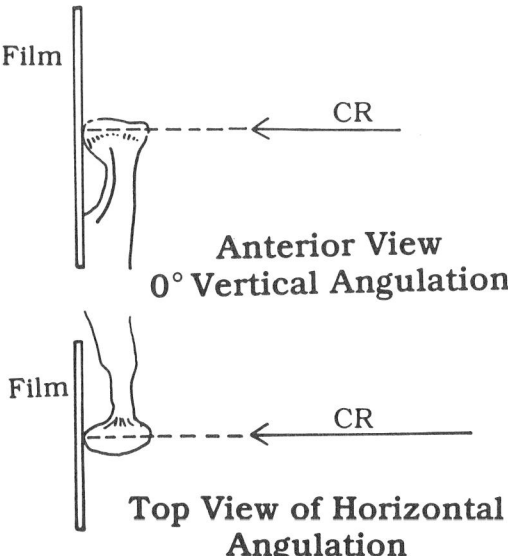

Figure 15-20. Vertical Angulation 0 degrees, horizontal angulation, 0 degrees.

Transcranial Lateral TMJ Radiography

In all **transcranial** technics, the X-Ray beam is directed down across the top of the **petrous portion** of the temporal bone to the condylar head on the opposite side of the skull. This is done to avoid superimposing the petrous portion of the temporal bone over the temporomandibular joint (Fig. 15-18).

This oblique projection of the X-Ray beam causes distortions of the three-dimensional head of the condyle and the glenoid fossa. In order to achieve the least amount of geometric distortion of the condylar head, the film would have to touch the medial pole of the condylar head and the plane of the film placed perpendicular to the long axis of the head in both horizontal and vertical directions. Also, the X-Ray beam would have to be directed perpendicular to the film through the long axis of a condylar head with zero degree vertical and horizontal angulations (Fig. 15-20).

This perfect relationship between the

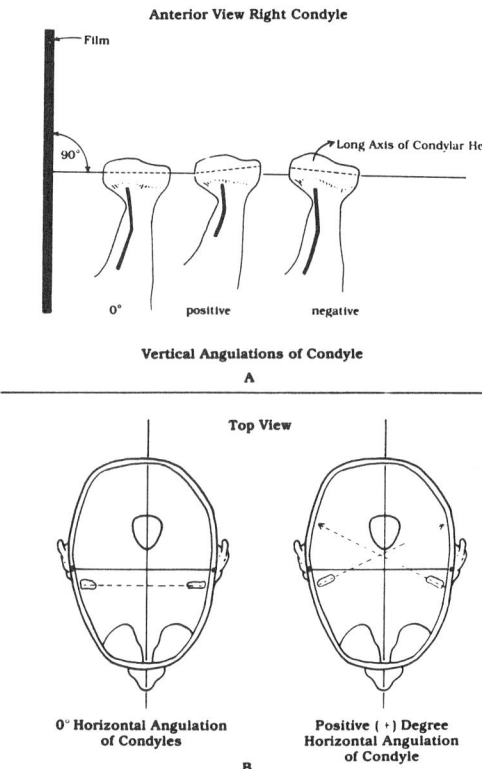

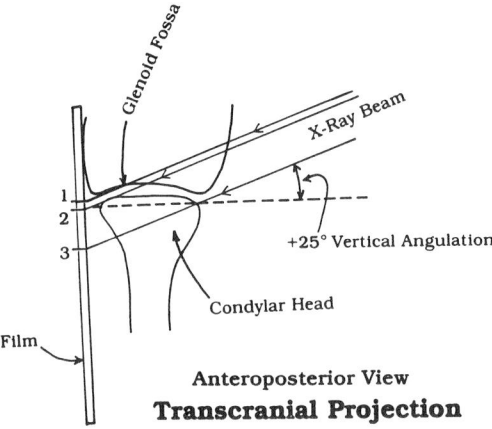

Figure 15-22. In the transcranial TMJ projection only the laterosuperior border of the condylar head is revealed on the radiograph. (From Rosenberg, H., and Silha, R.: TMJ radiography with emphasis on tomography. *Dent Radiogr Photogr,* 55(1):11, 1982, Fig. 13. Courtesy of Eastman Kodak Company, Rochester, NY.)

Figure 15-21. Variations in horizontal and vertical angulations of condylar head. (A) Vertical angulation. (B) Horizontal angulation.

X-Ray beam, the film, and the condylar head is impossible because of the anatomic structures that surround the joint, and the variation of the horizontal and vertical long axes of the condylar head from patient to patient or even from one condyle head to the other in the same patient (Fig. 15-21). Therefore, the real weakness of transcranial projections is that the patient is placed into a fixed geometric projection system, rather than having a system that adapts the geometric projection system to the patient's anatomical variations.

The most that can be accomplished by transcranial projections of the TMJ is to view the lateral border of the glenoid fossa and laterosuperior border of the head of the condyle (Fig. 15-22). The superior border of the condyle between the lateral and medial poles of the condyle cannot be seen on the transcranial lateral TMJ. Unfortunately, this is where most of the changes occur in TMJ disease.

The tomographic radiographic examination of the TMJ will give the dentist more diagnostic information than the transcranial radiographic projections. Tomography will be discussed later in the chapter.

We will discuss two transcranial TMJ technics and one transpharyngeal TMJ technic (McQueen).

Lindbolm Technic (Lateral Oblique Transcranial)

Lindbolm first proposed the transcranial lateral view of the condyle in 1936. It is used primarily to view the condyle in lateral relation to the glenoid fossa. Lindbolm used a fixed-transcranial technic; the one described here is not the original

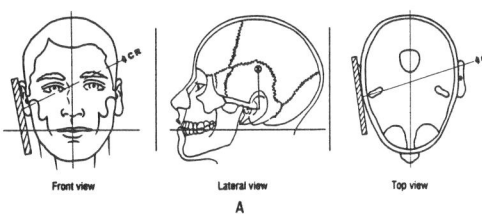

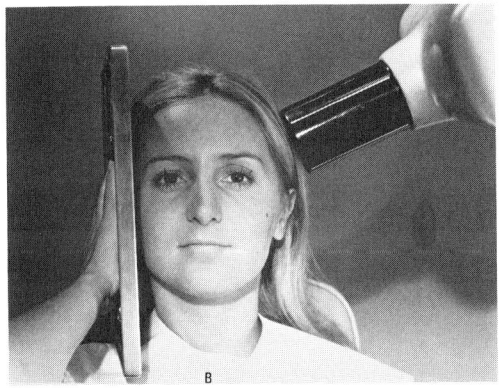

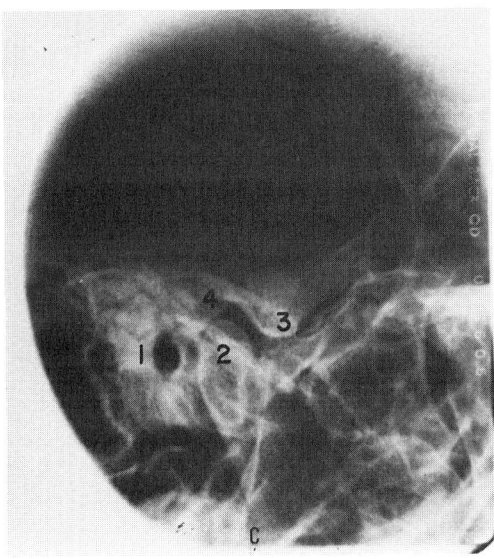

Figure 15-23. Lindbolm Transcranial Technic. **(A)** The point of entry of CR is 1/2 inch behind and 2 inches above external auditory meatus and it is directed through the long axis of the condylar head perpendicular to the cassette in a horizontal direction. **(B)** Patient in position. **(C)** Radiograph. (1) external auditory meatus; (2) condylar process of mandible; (3) articular tubercle or eminence; (4) mandibular or glenoid fossa.

transcranial technic used by Lindbolm.

Head Position: Position the midsagittal plane perpendicular to the floor and the tragal-ala line parallel to the floor.

Film Placement and Retention: An 8 × 10 inch cassette film holder is placed with the long axis of the film perpendicular to the floor (Fig. 15-23B). Use a leaded rubber mat to block one side of the film. Take right and left projections on one 8 × 10 inch film. The head of the condyle to be radiographed is centered on one side of the casette. The cassette is positioned against the zygomatic arch, the superior temporal crest, and the ear. The anterior edge of the cassette should be parallel to the midsagittal plane of the patient (Fig. 15-23A, B).

Projection of the Central Ray: VERTICAL ANGULATION: The angle is initially at 25 degrees downward.

POINT OF ENTRY: In order to pass the X-Ray beam tangentially to the head of the condyle, a point of entry of the central ray of the X-Ray beam is found by first measuring 2 inches vertically above the superior edge of the external auditory meatus and then 1/2 inch posteriorly. (This is to prevent the superimposition of the petrous portion of the temporal bone over the head of the condyle).

POINT OF EMANATION: This is the head of condyle on the side projected (Fig. 15-23A).

HORIZONTAL ANGULATION: It is selected so that the central ray will coincide with the horizontal axis of the condyle to be examined. The horizontal angulation of the cone should be examined first from the front and then from the side of the patient (Fig. 15-23A). The exposure is made (Fig. 15-23C).

Exposure Factors:

FILM CASSETTE SIZE: 8 × 10 inch with lead blockers

SCREENS: Kodak X-OMATIC RP Film

FILM: Kodak X-OMATIC Regular

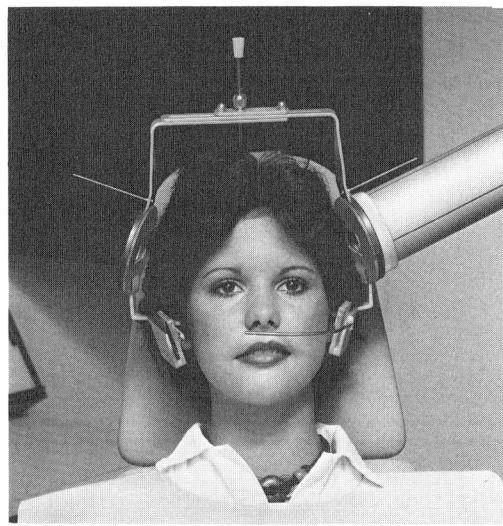

Figure 15-24. Rinn Condy-Ray. (Courtesy of Rinn Corp, Elgin, Il.)

SOURCE-FILM DISTANCE: 20 inches
EXPOSURE FACTORS: 70 kV, 10 mA, 96 impulses. (Reduce exposure time 1/2 if use Kodak Lanex Screens with Kodak Ortho G or L Film.)

Fixed Alignment Transcranial TMJ Projection

One of the shortcomings of the transcranial projection is the difficulty in accurately aligning the P.I.D. (cone) with the TMJ, and the reorientation of the patient into the same alignment position for serial radiographs. Commercially, there are three TMJ radiographic positioners that can be purchased to aid in alignment of the cone with the patient's TMJ and that enable the operator to repeat this alignment at a later date. These are the **Rinn Condy-ray instrument** (Fig. 15-24), the **Denar Accurad-100 positioner** (Fig. 15-25), and the **Farrar Transcranial Radiographic System** (Brell-Mar Products) (Fig. 15-26).

The upright position of the patient's head in transcranial TMJ radiography (as opposed to placing the patient's head down on an angleboard) is thought to be more desirable because the radiographs are taken with the TMJ in more of an unstrained position.

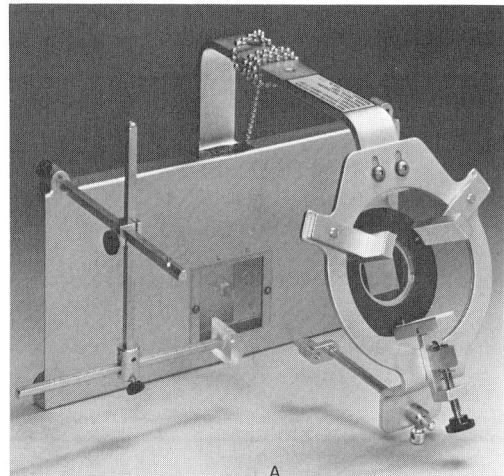
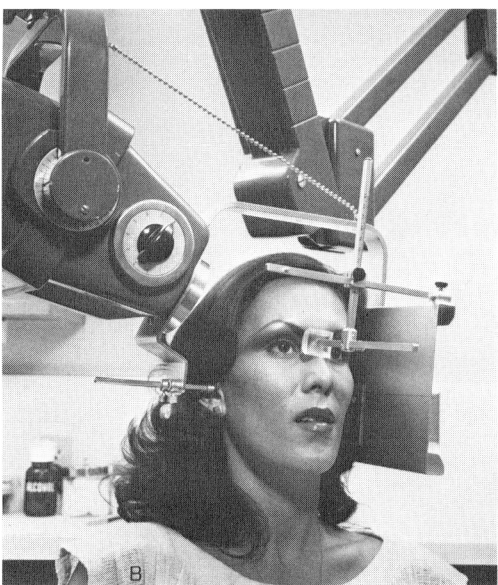

Figure 15-25. (A) Denar Accurad. (B) Denar Accurad positioned on patient ready for projection. (Courtesy of Denar Corp., Anaheim, CA.)

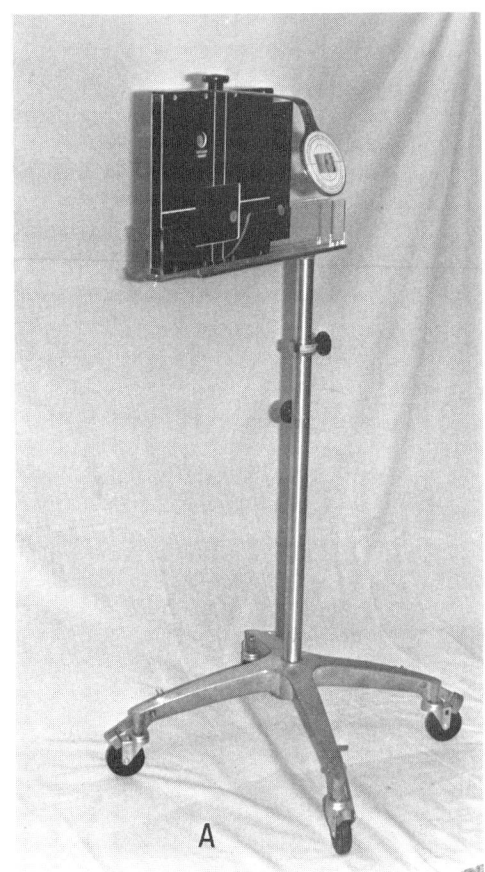

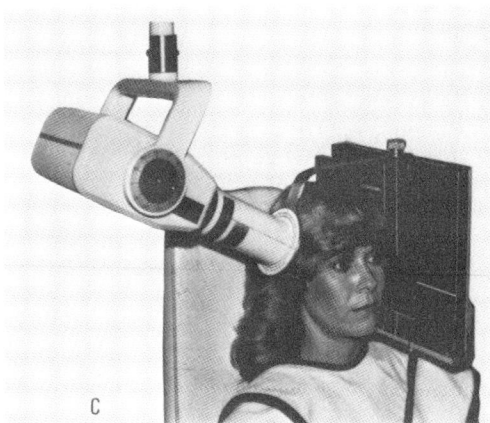

Figure 15-26. (A) Farrar Transcranial Radiographic System. (B) Close-up of cassette. (C) Ready for exposure. (Courtesy of Brell Mar Products, Inc., Clinton, Miss.)

constructed 15 degree angleboard with a protractor-rod assembly to assist in duplication of the head position. A plastic side tunnel with a leaded rubber mat is provided, which permits multiple exposures without changing position of the patient's head. Usually a six-exposure technic requires closed, rest, and open positions of

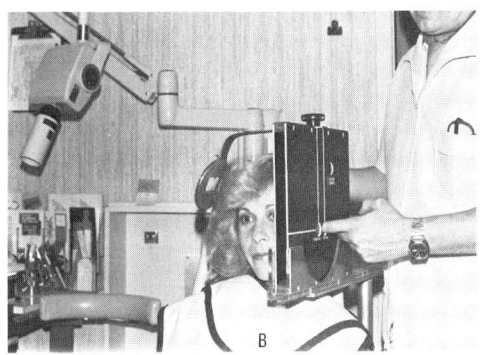

Lateral Oblique Transcranial Technic Using Angleboard

This technic was first advocated by Updegrave in 1953. It utilizes a specially

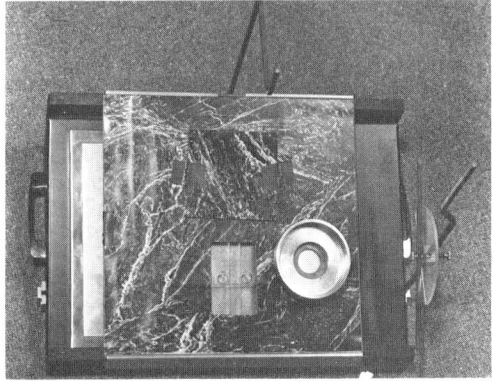

Figure 15-27. Older version of Updegrave Angleboard as viewed from top with diaphragm filter, which replaced the regular P.I.D. (cone) on X-Ray tube. By repositioning cassette after each exposure, six projections could be taken on one 8 × 10 inch film.

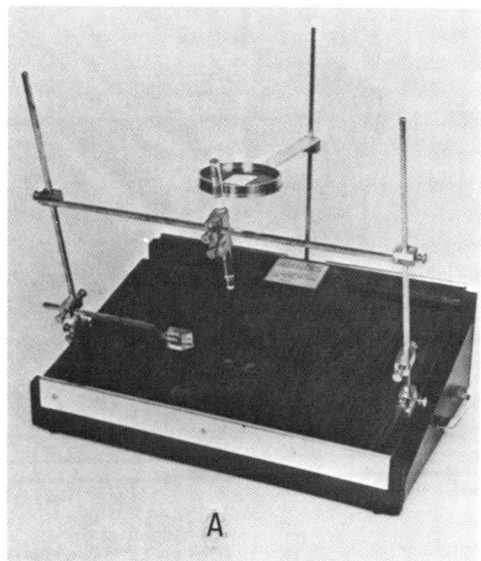

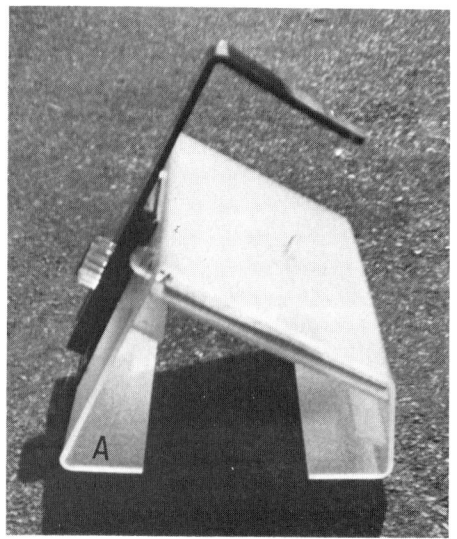

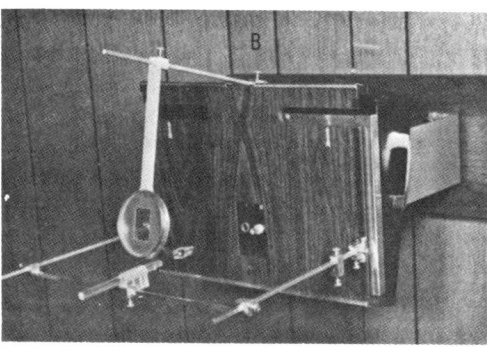

Figure 15-28. Newer Updegrave Angleboard (manufactured by Margraf): **(A)** Margraf table model TMJ angleboard unit. **(B)** Margraf stationary vertical wall model TMJ angleboard unit. (Courtesy of Margraf Co., Jenkintown, Pa.)

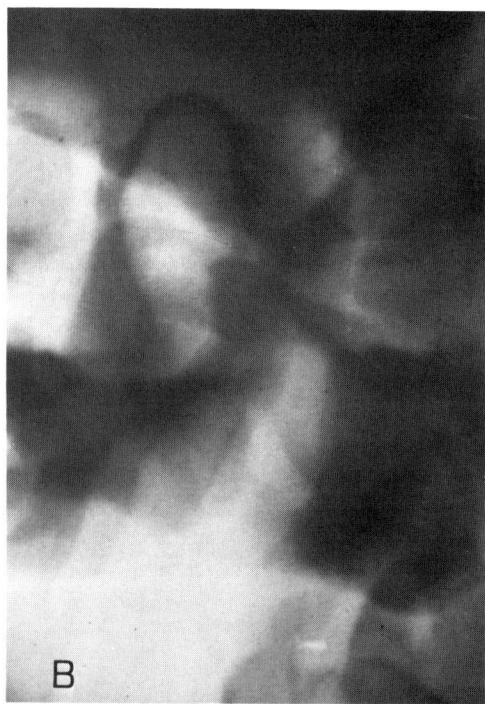

Figure 15-29. McCormack Interprises Angleboard: **(A)** McCormack Angleboard. **(B)** Radiograph taken with McCormack Angleboard.

the TMJ articulation (Fig. 15-27). A newer version of the **Updegrave Angle Board** is available through **Margraf Dental Manufacturing Company** of Jenkintown, Pennsylvania (Fig. 15-28A). The Updegrave/Margraf Angleboard can be placed vertically on the wall if the operator desires to take the radiograph with the patient in an upright position (Fig. 15-28B). A **modified Updegrave Board** is also available through **McCormack Interprises**, Inc., of Pasadena, California (Fig. 15-29).

Head Position: Patient is seated facing

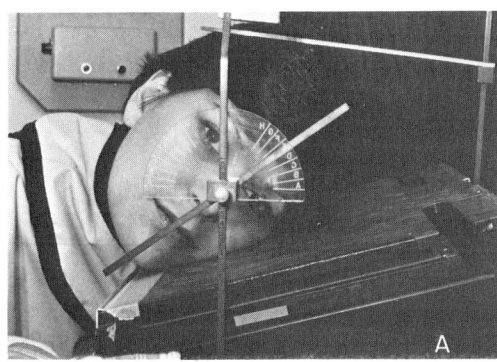
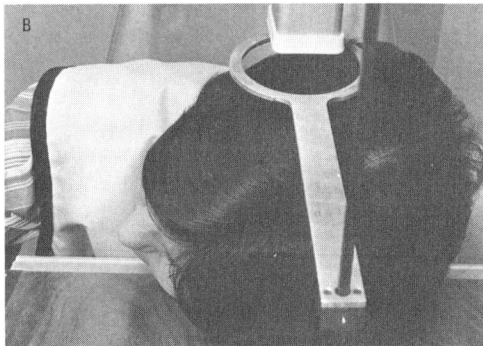

Figure 15-30. Patient in Updegrave Angleboard (using rectangular P.I.D. (cone). **(A)** Front view. **(B)** Top view.

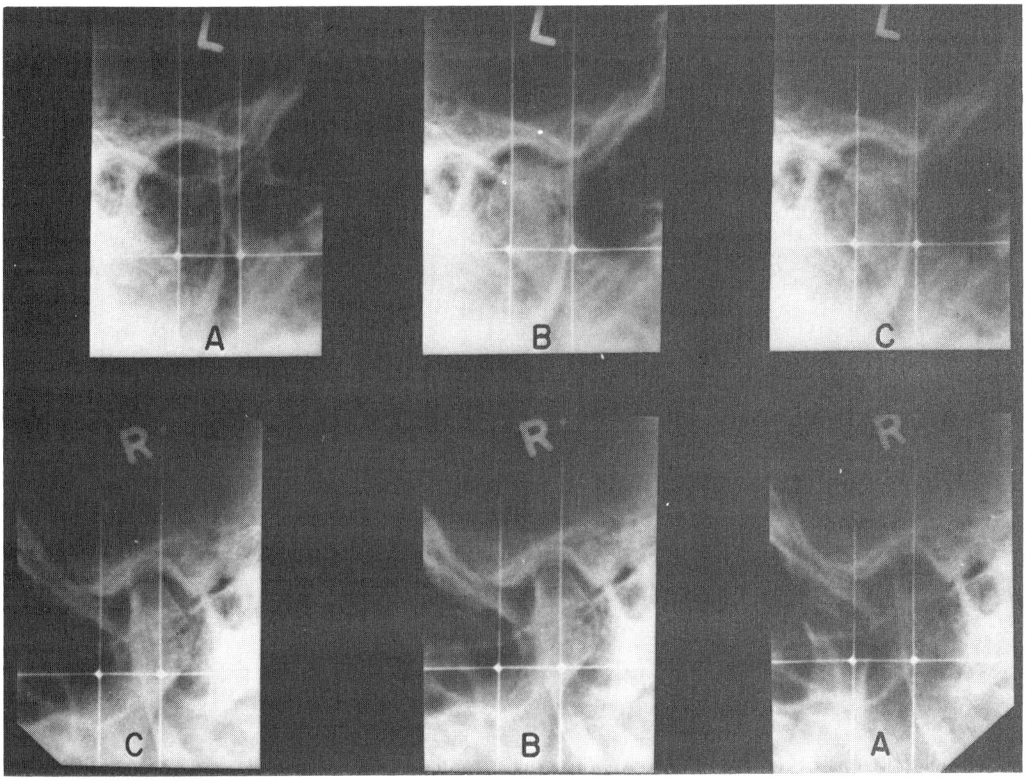

Figure 15-31. Updegrave Angleboard radiographs: **(A)** Open; **(B)** centric relation; **(C)** centric occlusion.

the angleboard and the head is positioned with the external auditory meatus of the side being examined. The ear positioner is made of plastic. The head is supported at three points, the auditory meatus, zygoma, and the angle of mandible. The tip of the patient's nose is aligned on the horizontal level of the side positioning rod.

532 Textbook of Dental Radiology

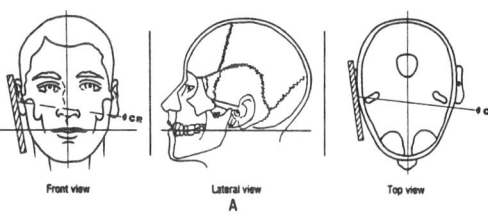

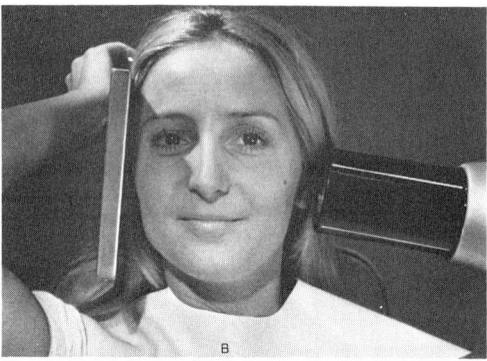

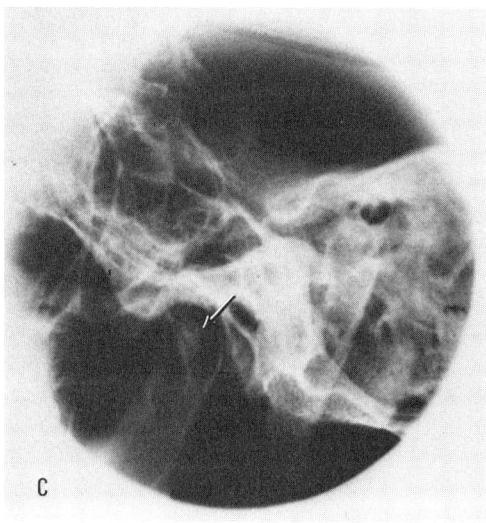

Figure 15-32. McQueen TMJ Technic. **(A)** The central ray is directed from a point just below the zygomatic arch and 3/4 inch anterior to the posterior border of the ramus. The CR must enter through the sigmoid notch and angle upwards (−10 degrees vertical angle) and posteriorly (10 degrees from the perpendicular) to the midsagittal plane. **(B)** Patient in position for McQueen (transpharyngeal) TMJ projection. **(C)** Radiograph of McQueen technic. This projection is an oblique AP projection of condyle.

The head position is recorded (Fig. 15-30A).

Projection of the Central Ray: The P.I.D. (cone) is brought adjacent to the patient's head and aligned with the positioning rods at the side and top of board. The tube head reading should be 0-90 degrees (Fig. 15-30B).

Film Placement and Retention: A loaded 8 × 10 inch cassette is placed in the plastic tunnel with the opening in the rubber leaded mat placed over the region of the threaded plastic ear positioner. Multiple exposures of condylar function can be made without changing the head position of the patient, simply by moving the cassette in the side tunnel. Six exposures are made on one 8 × 10 inch film. It is usually advisable to make the first exposure with the teeth in centric occlusion to assure a firm head position, and then to shift the cassette and make the next exposure in the rest position. The third position is the open position. Use a mouth prop to open the patient's mouth about one inch.

For the **centric position**, have the patient say "Mississippi" and then close his/her teeth together. This is the "lip-closed, teeth-together position." In the rest position have the patient swallow and then relax his/her lower jaw. This is the "lips-closed, teeth-apart position" (Fig. 15-31).

Exposure Factors:
CASSETTE SIZE: 8 × 10 inches
SCREENS: Kodak X-OMATIC Regular
FILM: Kodak X-OMAT RP Film
SOURCE-FILM DISTANCE: Rectangular collimated. P.I.D., 20 inches
NO GRID
EXPOSURE FACTORS: 70 kV, 10 mA, 96 impulses. (If use Kodak Lanex Regular screens and Kodak OG Film use 48 impulses.)

Lateral TMJ Transpharyngeal Technic (McQueen Technic)

The original technic was advocated by McQueen in 1937.

Head Position: The midsagittal plane

of patient's head is positioned perpendicular to the floor.

Film Placement and Retention: A 5 × 7 inch or 8 × 10 inch film holder is placed in a cassette holder, or it may be held by the patient. If you use an 8 × 10 inch cassette film holder, a lead blocker should be utilized. The head of the condyle to be radiographed is centered on the cassette film holder. Position the cassette film holder against the zygomatic arch and the external auditory meatus (Fig. 15-32A).

Projection of the Central Ray: (Fig. 15-32A)

VERTICAL ANGULATION: Direct the X-Rays at a − 10 degree vertical angulation through the mandibular (sigmoid) notch toward the opposite condyle.

HORIZONTAL ANGULATION: Direct the X-Rays posteriorly 10 degrees toward the opposite condyle.

POINT OF ENTRY: Central ray is directed from a point just below the zygomatic arch and 3/4 inch anterior to the posterior border of the ramus.

POINT OF EMANATION: Head of condyle on opposite side. The same technic may be employed whether the mouth is in a closed, rest, or open position.

Radiograph Factors:

CASSETTE: 5 × 7 inch or 8 × 10 inch

SCREENS: $CaWO_4$ (calcium tungstate) Par Speed

FILM: Kodak X-OMAT RP Film

SOURCE-FILM DISTANCE: Medium cone (12 inch) placed against the point of entry

EXPOSURE FACTORS: 65 kV, 15 mA, (no grid) 15 impulses. (If use Kodak MIN-R screen with Ortho M film use 30 impulses.)

Specialized TMJ Technics

TMJ Tomography

Since transcranial TMJ radiography has many limitations, several clinicians have turned to TMJ tomography for more diagnostic information of the temporomandibular joint. **Tomography** is a special X-Ray technic that blurs out the shadows of superimposed anatomical structures that obscure information in the radiograph. It is *not* a method of improving sharpness of the radiographic image, but it is a process of controlled blurring that leaves some parts of the image less blurred than others. The tomogram is made by a special mechanism in which

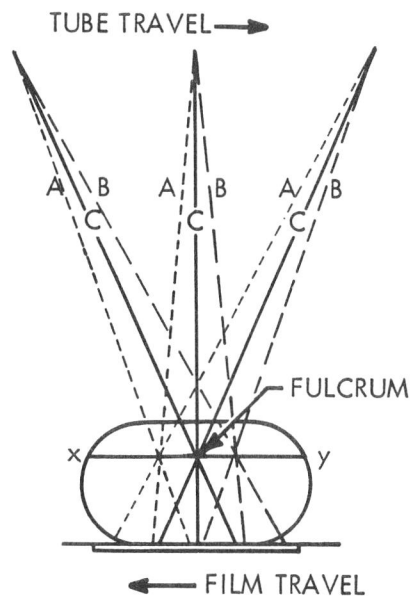

Figure 15-33. In the tomographic X-Ray technic there is mechanical connection of the tube with cassette holder with a rod or bar. The tube and the film holder travel in opposite directions during a continuous exposure of approximately one second. At a prescribed distance on the cross bar or pivot, a fulcrum is established. The central beam (C) and divergent rays (A & B) cross at a prescribed point and build up a plane (X-Y) that is in focus and is recorded on the X-Ray film — other structures above and below are blurred. Width of plane is controlled by amplitude of tube travel. This technic is especially useful in TMJ radiography. (Courtesy of General Electric Co., Milwaukee, WI.)

the X-Ray tube and the film cassette are attached to a rigid connecting rod that rotates about a fixed fulcrum.

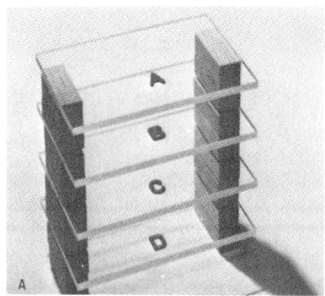

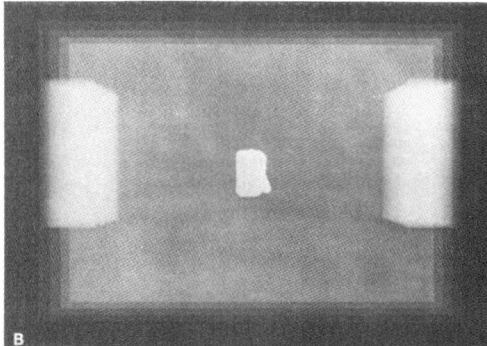

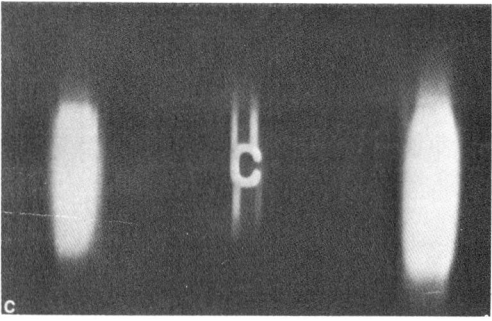

Figure 15-34. Tomographic effect (A) A series of plastic plates each holding a lead letter is used as a test object. (B) Radiograph made of test object with conventional X-Ray equipment. The X-Ray beam passed vertically through the test object and all letters are superimposed. (C) Radiograph made with linear tomographic equipment. The fulcrum plane was located at letter "C", which shows quite clearly. (From *Fundamentals of Radiography*, 12th ed, 1980, Fig. 51, p. 81. Copyright Eastman Kodak Company, Rochester, NY.)

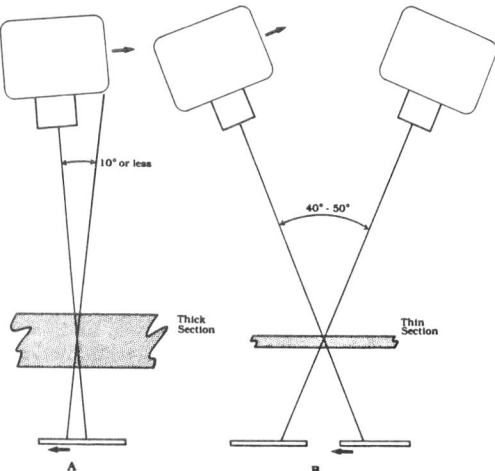

Figure 15-35. Angle of Exposure in Tomography. (A) Zonography (wide-angle tomography). A 10 degree cut is approximately 5.00 mm thick; a 5 degree cut is approximately 13.0 mm thick. (B) Wide-angle tomography. A 40-50 degree cut is approximately 1.0 mm thick.

When the tube moves in one direction, the film cassette moves in the opposite direction. Tomographic technics blur all points that lay outside the focal plane (above or below) (Fig. 15-33). The fulcrum about which the system rotates is adjustable so that any desired horizontal layer in an anatomical structure can be selected for radiographing (Fig. 15-34).

The angle through which the X-Ray tube (X-Ray beam) travels during exposure is called the **exposure angle**. The smaller the exposure angle, the thicker the section or layer, and the larger the exposure angle, the thinner the section (Fig. 15-35). While in essence the exposure angle influences the thickness of the section, the source-object and object-film distance also influence section thickness. However, in actual practice the distance factors are kept constant, and the thickness of the section is controlled by changing the exposure angle.

Another factor to consider in tomography is the type of motion or movement

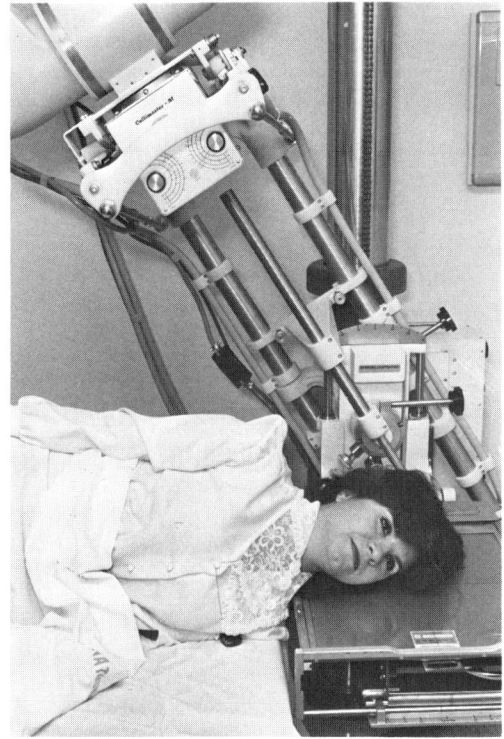

Figure 15-36. Franklin Head Holder Linear Tomography.

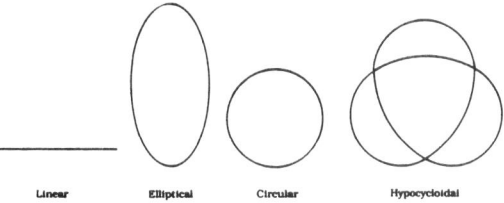

Figure 15-37. Four varieties of Tomographic Trajectory.

graphic equipment has been developed to produce complex types of motion that produce more effective blurring of unwanted structures (Fig. 15-37).

The most complex trajectory or tube motion available is the **hypocycloidal** movement, and it results in highly effective blurring; it is sometimes described as a **cloverleaf**. It has no dominant direction and is especially suitable for tomography of small bony structures of the head, for example the auditory ossicles and the temporomandibular joints. The exposure angle of the hypocycloidal movement is fixed at 48 degrees, resulting in a minimum section thickness of 1 mm. Cuts through the condylar head can be made 2 mm apart and 1-2 mm thick using the hypocycloidal movement of the tube head (Fig. 15-38). The complex group of motions require specialized equipment. One of the first practical multidirectional tomographic units manufactured was the

of the X-Ray tube. If the X-Ray tube and the film move in a straight line, it is called **linear** tomography. It has an advantage in that the X-Ray equipment is relatively inexpensive; however, it has a disadvantage in that linear structures aligned parallel to the direction of motion of the tube are not blurred as well as those lying at an angle to the tube (Fig. 15-36). Therefore, tomo-

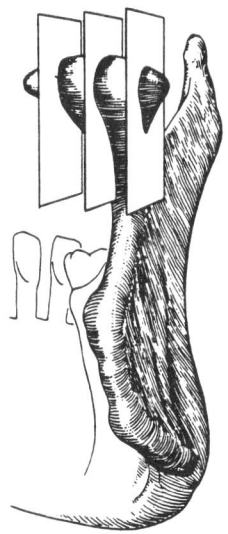

Figure 15-38. Cuts through the condylar head (From C.G. Coin: Tomography of the temporomandibular joint. *Dent Radiogr Photogr,* 47(2): 23, 1974. Copyright Eastman Kodak Company, Rochester, NY.)

Polytome (Massiot-Philips, Paris, France) in 1951 (Fig. 15-39).

There are two types of tomography—**narrow-angle tomography** and **wide-angle tomography**. Narrow-angle tomography **(zonography)** refers to a tomographic technic employing an exposure angle of less than 10 degrees. Zonography in practice is used with **circular** tube trajectory. It produces greater section thickness and an image that is undistorted with sharply defined images of objects in the focal plane. Zonography is recommended for tissues that have low subject contrast, such as the lung. **Wide-angle tomography** refers to a tomographic technic that uses an exposure angle of more than 10 degrees (usually 30-50 degrees). There is less section thickness, and with maximum blurring of objects outside the focal plane. It is best with tissues with high subject contrast, such as bone.

It is evident that a **wide-angle** technic utilizing **hypocycloidal** movement of the tube is the **best** system to use in TMJ tomography. Of course, this requires expensive equipment and cannot be used by most dentists.

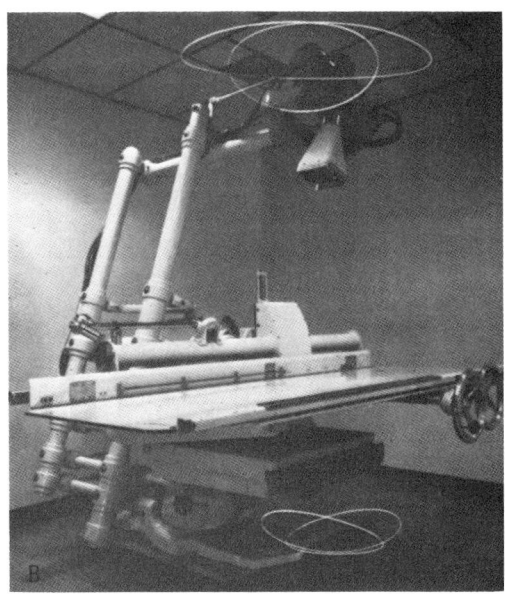

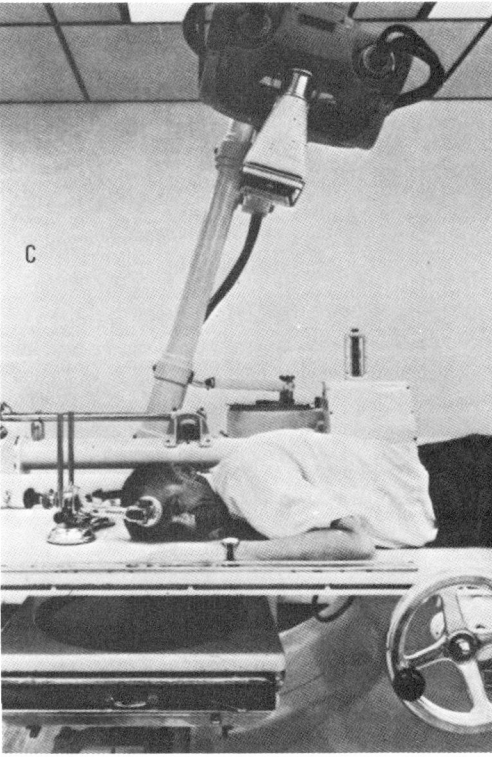

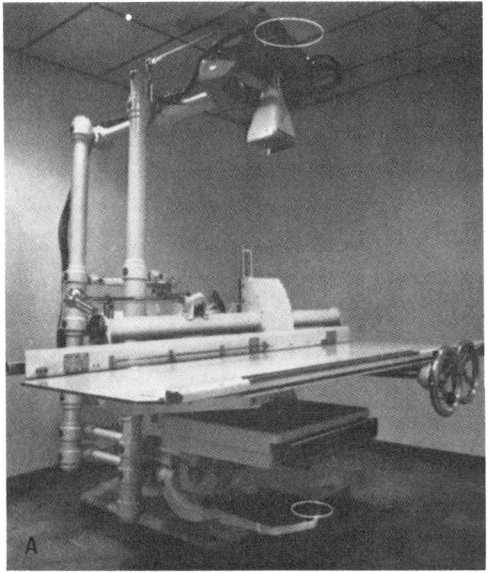

Figure 15-39. Massiot-Phillips Polytome. **(A)** Circular movement. **(B)** Hypochcloidal or polydirectional movement. **(C)** Patient in position for exposure with polytome. (From C.G. Coin: Tomography of the temporomandibular joint. *Dent Radiogra Photogr, 47*(2): 24, 27, 1974. Copyright Eastman Kodak Company, Rochester, NY.)

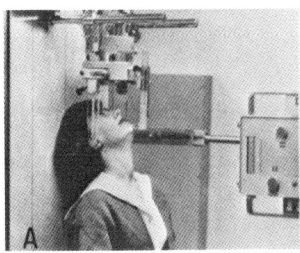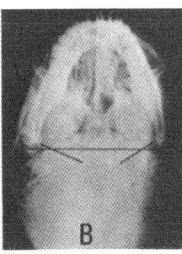

Figure 15-40. Patient positioned for submentovertex projection in GE Ordograph X-Ray machine at University of Illinois School of Dentistry, in 1967. This view establishes the horizontal angle of the condyles from the superior view. **(A)** Patient in position. **(B)** Resultant submentovertex radiograph. (From Rosenberg, H.: Laminography: Methods and application in oral diagnosis. *JADA, 71*:88, 1967. Courtesy of American Dental Association, Chicago, Il.)

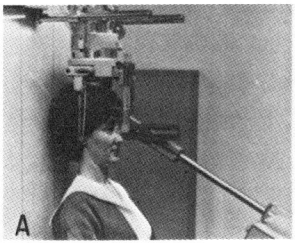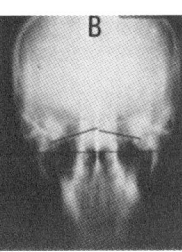

Figure 15-41. **(A)** Patient positioned for anteroposterior tomograph in GE Ordograph at University of Illinois School of Dentistry (1967). **(B)** From this radiograph the vertical angulation of the condyle when viewed anteriorly is determined. (From Rosenberg, H.: Laminography in oral diagnosis. *JADA, 74*:88, 1967. Courtesy of American Dental Association, Chicago, Il.)

Also, tomography of the TMJ should be taken with the use of a cephalometer or cephalostat to reorient the patient's head in the same position for serial radiographs.

For tomographic TMJ accuracy, the X-Ray beam must be directed parallel to the vertical and horizontal long axes of the condylar head so that the tomographic cuts can be made perpendicular to these axes. This is difficult because there is a variation in condylar head shape from patient to patient and even from condyle to condyle in the same patient (*see* Fig. 15-21).

In order to overcome this difficulty, the vertical and horizontal angulation of a patient's condyles can be predetermined with accuracy by taking two radiographs — the **submentovertex radiograph** and the **anteroposterior tomogram** of the TMJ.

The submentovertex radiograph is used to determine the horizontal angle of each condyle using the intermeatal line as a base line of reference (Fig. 15-40). The horizontal condylar angles are used to produce an anteroposterior tomogram (zonogram) of the TMJ. The AP zonogram of the TMJ is used to determine the lateral angles for each condylar head (Fig. 15-41). With this predetermined information, an accurate tomogram can be made of the temporomandibular joints.

The University of Illinois College of Dentistry has developed a technic of corrected lateral cephalometric TMJ tomography. It includes a cephalostat that can position the head into previously determined horizontal and vertical angles of each condyle (Fig. 15-42A). The system used to produce the TMJ tomograms is the Massiot-Philips Universal Polytome utilizing **hypocloidal** (cloverleaf) tube motion, and the Kodak Lanex Screens/Kodak Ortho G Film System (Fig. 15-42B).

A cephalometric skull and tomographic (laminagraphic) X-Ray unit is commercially available through Quint Corp. of Los Angeles, California. It is called the **Quint Sectograph** (Fig. 15-43). It can be used for both conventional skull radiography and skull tomography. Tomograms are taken utilizing a **linear motion** of the tube.

Arthrography or Arthrotomography

Arthrography implies the injection into a joint of a contrast medium for vi-

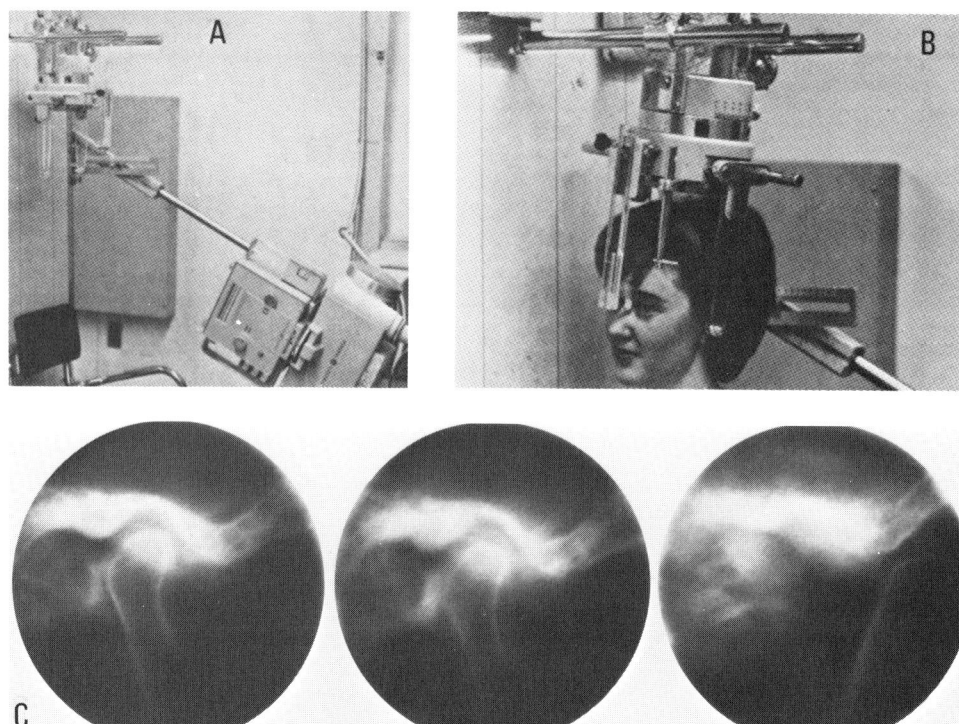

Figure 15-42. (A) The GE Ordograph X-Ray tomographic unit adapted to a cephalostat to be used in cephalometric tomography of the TMJ at University of Illnois School of Dentistry in 1967. (B) Patient positioned for corrected lateral cephalometric tomograph. The head is positioned at predetermined condylar horizontal and vertical angles. (From Rosenberg, H.: Laminography in oral diagnosis. *JADA, 74*:88, 1967. Courtesy of American Dental Association, Chicago, Il.) (C) Tomographs taken of left normal TMJ at University of Illinois, School of Dentistry, using similar cephalostat as shown in (A) and (B) but with Philips Polytome X-Ray unit, Lanex regular screens (rare earth), and Kodak Ortho G film to record the images. (From Rosenberg, H.; and Silha, R.: TMJ radiography. *Dent Radiogr Photogr, 55(1):* 1982. Copyright Eastman Kodak Company, Rochester, NY.)

sualization of the cartilagenous structure within the joint. Norgaard of Denmark in 1947 was one of the first to recommend arthrography of the TMJ. However, his technic is not applicable to current concepts of disc dysfunction. Recently, there has been a renewal of interest in **TMJ arthrography or arthrotomography** to diagnose a number of specific disorders of the meniscus (Fig. 15-44).

TMJ arthrography, or arthrotomography, is **indicated** (1) for patients with positive diagnosis of MPD (myofascial-pain-dysfunction) syndrome of TMJ, especially those with clicking or history of clicking, and for those who do not respond to conservative treatment; (2) for patients with a positive history of locking; and (3) for those with a limited opening of undetermined etiology. Arthrography is **contraindicated** in the presence of acute infection and in patients with hypersensitivity to contrast media.

Arthrotomography is accomplished by carefully locating the **lower joint space** with the aid of fluoroscopy and injecting water-soluble radiopaque material (0.3 ml 1:20,000 in 3 ml of Reno-M-60-diatrizoate meglumine 282 mg/ml bound iodine) (Squibb) into the joint space. The same procedure is repeated to opacify the **upper joint space**.

As soon as possible after opacification of the joint spaces, closed and open mouth tomograms are taken of the joint with **wide angle technic** and **hypocycloidal motion** (Fig. 15-45). Generally, the shape of the lower joint space alters with condylar movement and provides the most diagnostic information concerning the meniscus (disc). The three most important abnormalities of the disc are (1) anterior displacement with reduction (TMJ pain, and tenderness, otalgia, temporal headaches, muscle tenderness, TMJ clicking, and intermittent locking); (2) anterior disc displacement without reduction (TMJ pain, tenderness, otalgia, temporal headaches, muscle tenderness, past history of clicking, and limited opening); and (3) disc perforation (patients usually

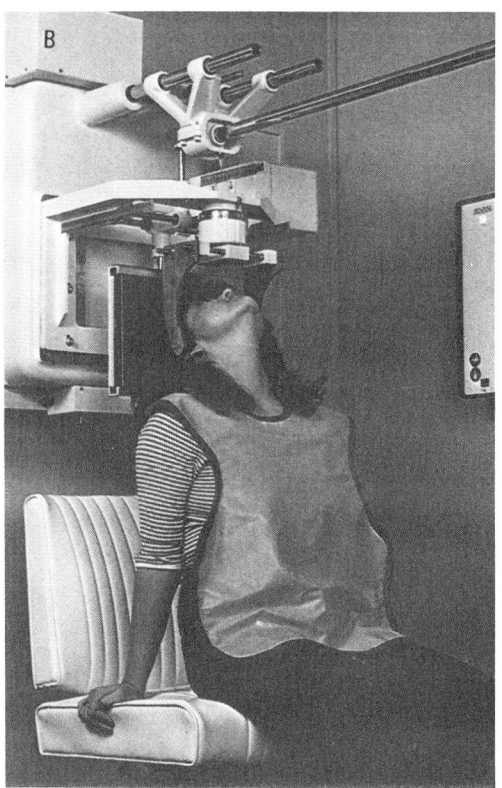

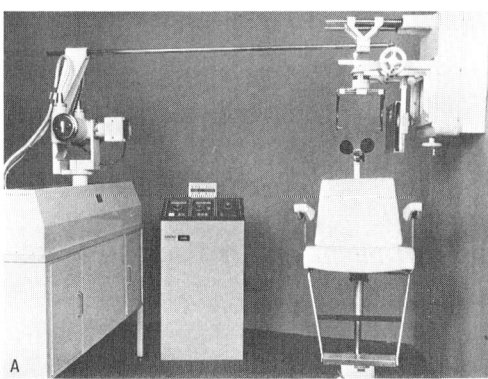

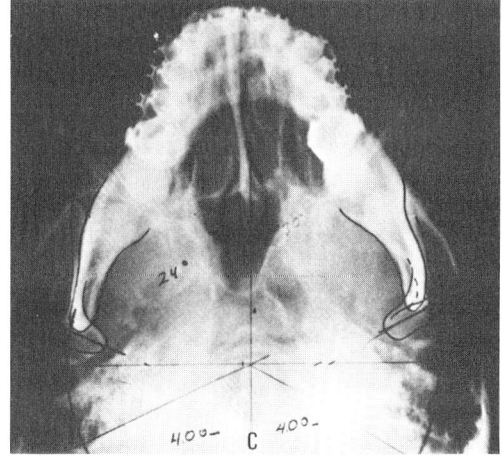

Figure 15-43. **(A)** Quint Sectograph employs rotating anode tube, and cephalometric tomographs are taken at a 66 inch source-film distance. Three tomographic cuts can be made. Patient is sitting so natural forces of gravity predominate on muscles of mastication. **(B)** Patient positioned for submentovertex radiograph. **(C)** Submentovertex radiograph used to determine the horizontal condylar angle. **(D)** Patient positioned for transorbital or AP of the TMJ's. **(E)** Transorbital tomogram used to determine vertical angulation of condyles. **(F)** Patient in position for multiple tomograms of the TMJ. **(G)** Quint sectograph tomograms taken in left, right, and closed, rest and open positions. (Courtesy of Quint Corp., Los Angeles, CA.)

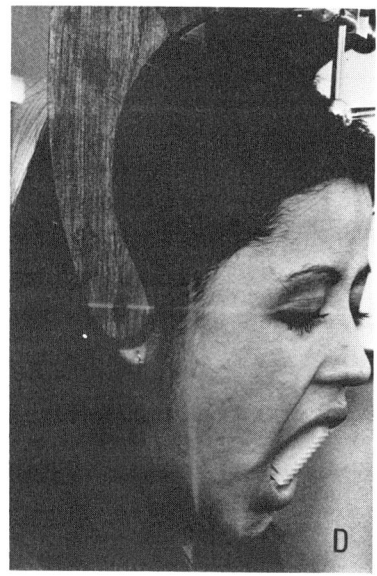

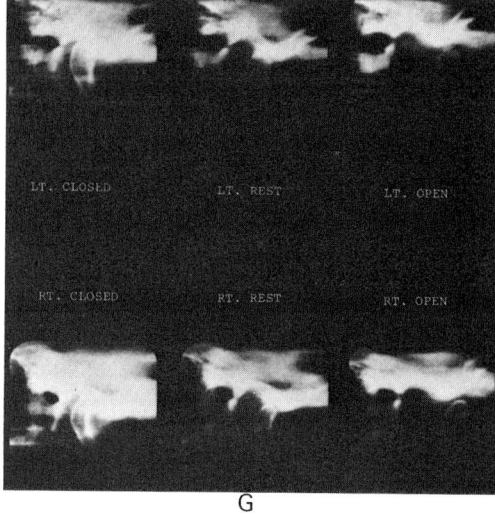

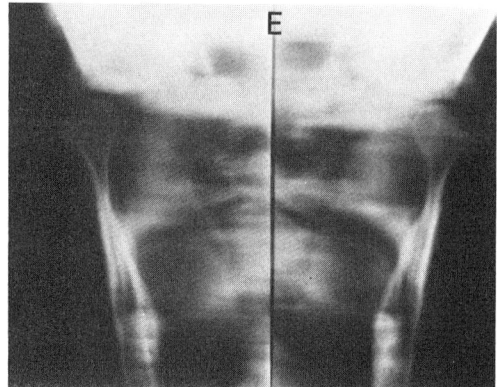

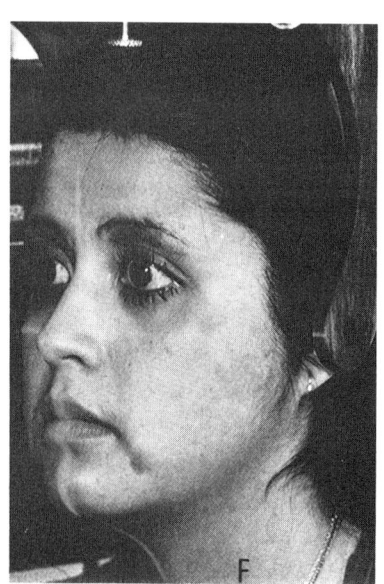

over 40, history of degenerative joint disease, and crepitus [grating sound]). Arthrotomographic radiography provides important information to the clinician in the diagnosis of the above three abnormalities of the disc.

Anteroposterior (Transorbital) Temporomandibular Projection*

Purpose: This is an excellent film to view lateral movements of the condylar head, fractures of the condylar neck, and the zygoma. This radiograph gives a mediolateral view of articular eminence and the relation of the condyle to articular eminence and neck of condyle (Fig. 15-46).

Head Position: An 8 × 10 inch cassette is placed behind the patient perpendicular to the floor. The occlusal plane should be parallel to the floor. One-half of the cassette is shielded with a leaded rubber mat, which will permit two exposures on one

---

*This technic is based on the work of Zimmer (1941), Norgaard (1947), and Grant and Lanting (1953). It is an open-mouth technic.

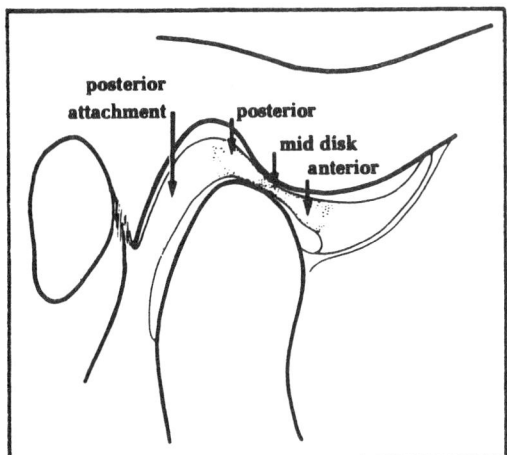

Figure 15-44. TMJ Diagram. Anatomy of soft tissue of TMJ. (From Blaske-Solberg-Saunders: Arthrography of temporomandibular joint, *JADA, 100*:388, 1980, Fig. 1, p. 389. Courtesy of American Dental Association, Chicago, IL.)

film. Use a mouth prop to maintain the mandible at a maximum opening. Rotate the head 20 degrees toward the side being examined.

Projection of Central Ray: The central ray is directed 35 degrees caudally through the orbit to the condylar head.

ALTERNATE METHOD: Keep the patient's head erect with the midsagittal plane perpendicular to the floor. The central ray is directed caudally 30 degrees and laterally 20 degrees from the midsagittal plane. The rubber leaded mat is moved for the second projection to protect the exposed portion of the film. Of course, the patient and film must be repositioned for examination of the opposite condyle. Be sure to use R and L lead markers on the film.

Exposure Factors:
CASSETTE: 8 × 10 inch cassette
SCREENS: Kodak X-OMATIC regular
FILM: Kodak X-OMATIC RP
SOURCE-FILM DISTANCE: 22-24 inches (long cone)
EXPOSURE TIME: 65 kV, 10 mA, 3/4 seconds. (If use Kodak Lanex Regular screens and Kodak OG film reduce exposure time by half.)

Panoramic TMJ Radiography

All the rotational panoramic radiographic units have special TMJ projections. The **GE Panelipse** has a special projection that produces an oblique AP view of the condylar head of the con-

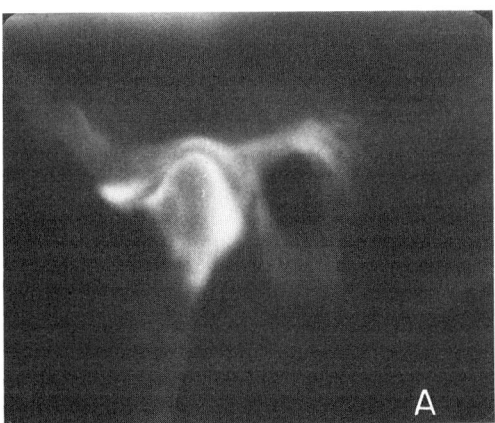 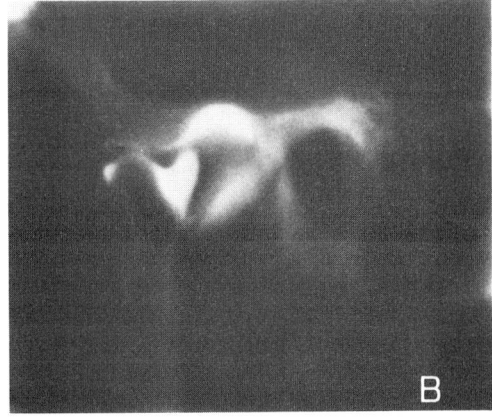

Figure 15-45. Normal arthrotomograms. **(A)** Closed; **(B)** Open. (Courtesy of M. Frank Dolwick, San Antonio, TX.)

dyle.

Technic of GE Panelipse TMJ Radiography

The chin rest is lowered so the TM joints are closer to the vertical center on the film. The **Profile Index Meter** is set to 9 cm. The GE Panelipse has a variable plane-in-focus capability that enables the operator to match the patient's arch size with an appropriate plane of focus. For the TMJ projection, a profile index of 9

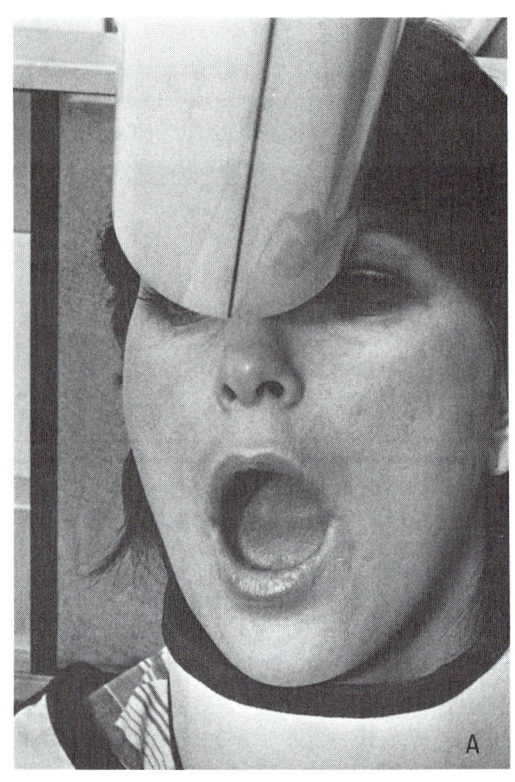

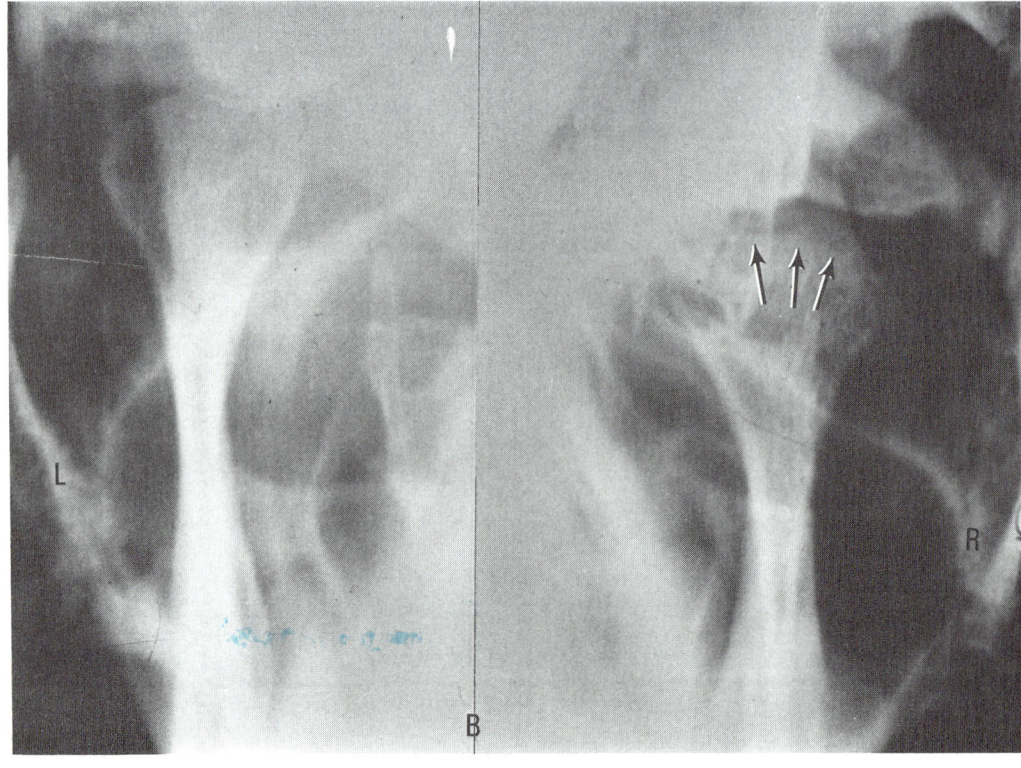

Figure 15-46. Anterposterior (Transorbital) Temporomandibular Projection. (**A**) Mandible is oriented to the misdsagittal plane. The CR is directed 30 degrees vertically and 20 degrees horizontally from the midsagittal plane through the eye socket to the head of the condyle. Patient's mouth is in an open position. (**B**) Left and right condyles can be placed on one 8 × 10 inch film by blocking out half of film at each exposure by leaded rubber mat. The superior portion of the right condyle shows irregular resorption of bone.

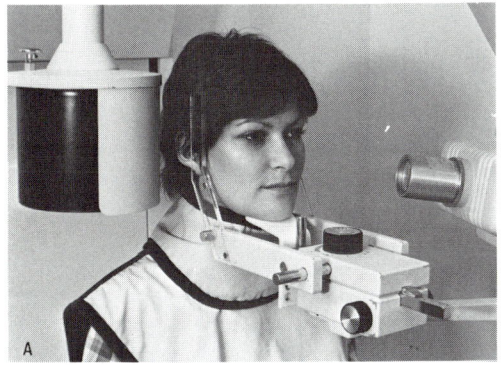
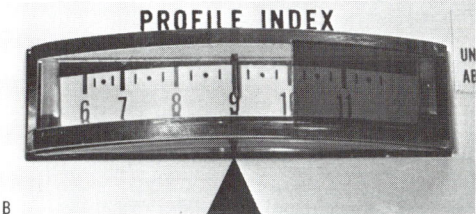
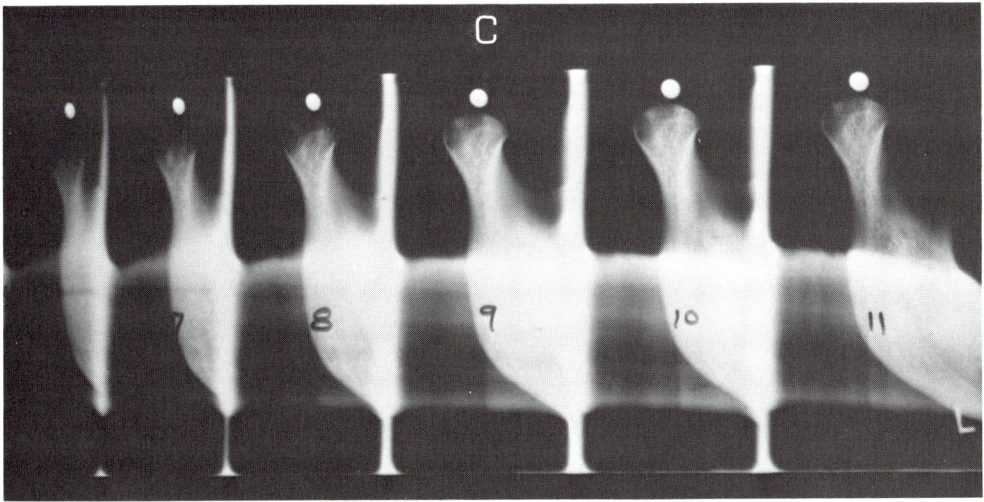

Figure 15-47. GE Panelipse TMJ Projection. **(A)** Lower the chin rest three positions. This will lower TM joints closer to vertical center of film. Remove bite guide holder. Place chin on chin rest, move patient so ear opening next to film drum lines up with back edge of side positioner guide. Close the head pieces firmly. **(B)** Set the Profile Index Meter on the overhead to 9 cm. **(C)** Illustration showing less distortion of small bead on superior surface of condylar head of profile index setting at 9 cm.

cm provides the least amount of distortion to the condylar head for almost all patients (large or small) (Fig. 15-47).

The patient's head is moved forward, according to prescribed directions (Fig. 15-48). By the use of the manual rotation switch, the tube head can be returned to its original starting position after each exposure on each side. By using a 3 second exposure for each projection, four exposures—open and closed position of each TMJ—can be taken on one radiograph (Fig. 15-49). When the patient's head is brought forward for this special GE Panelipse TMJ projection, the radiation beam will strike the condylar head in an anteroposterior direction, producing an anteroposterior radiographic image of the condylar head (Fig. 15-50).

Reverse Towne View

The **Towne view** is one of the stan-

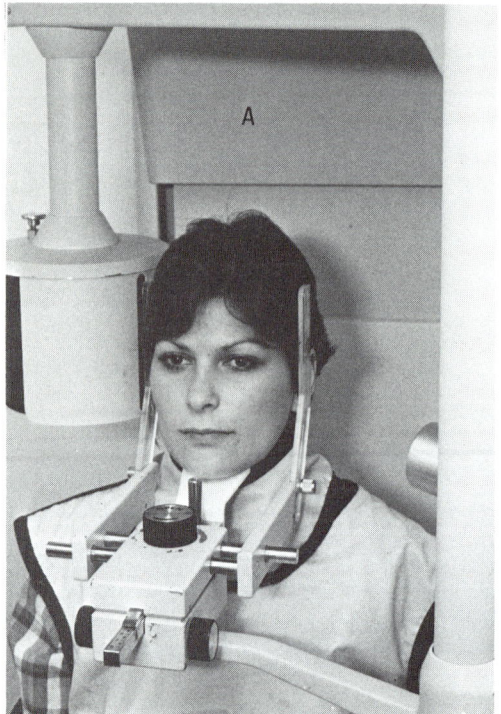

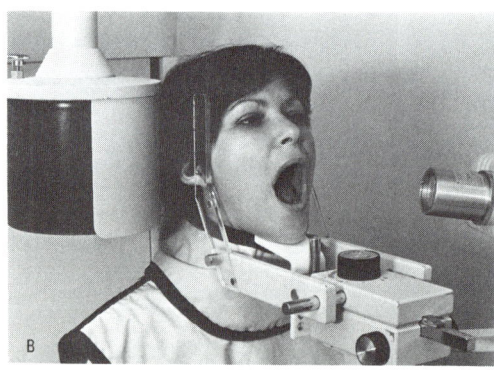

Figure 15-48. GE Panelipse TMJ Projection. **(A)** Adjust height of the head so the tragus-ala line is parallel to black lines on its (side) positioner guides. Select kVp value, with mouth closed, make first of four exposures by pressing handswitch for three seconds. **(B)** Using manual rotation switch return tube head to original start position and instruct patient to open mouth fully. Make the second three-second exposure. Using manual rotation switch, rotate the tube head to opposite start side and expose open and closed positions on opposite side.

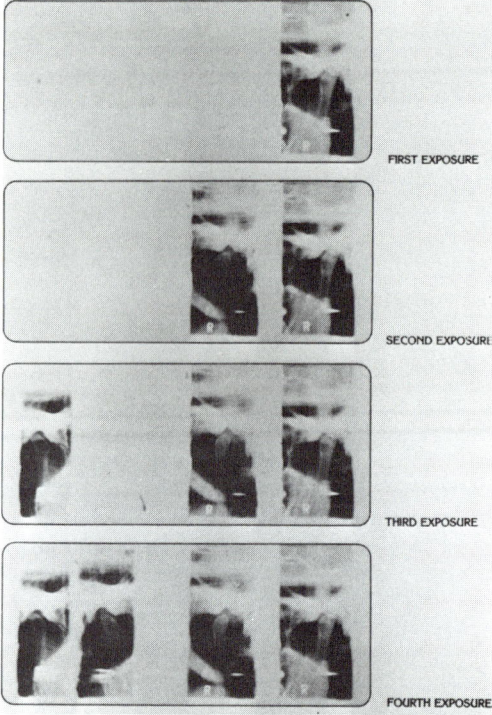

Figure 15-49. Four exposures may be taken on one Panelipse radiograph.

dard projections utilized for radiographic examination of the mastoids and temporal bones of the skull. It also provides a good AP view of the mandible and its condylar processes. It is sometimes called the **occiput view** because it is the only view that clearly shows the **occiput** (back of head) and the structures of the **posterior cranial fossa**. The Towne projection is an AP projection of the skull with the central ray directed at an angle of 30 degrees toward the feet so that it enters the forehead at the hairline and leaves at the posterior portion of the cranium of the external occipital protuberance.

The **Reverse Towne view** is a view similar to the Towne view except it is a posteroanterior skull view. It is preferred by dentists, possibly because dentists are more familiar with PA skull views. Also, it

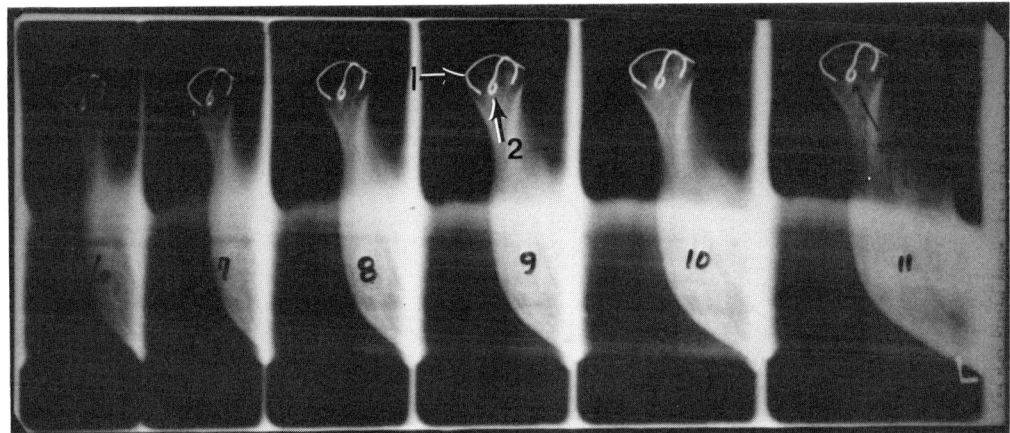

Figure 15-50. Six Panelipse radiographs of TMJ at various profile meter settings illustrating that Panelipse TMJ projection is an oblique AP projection. Wire 1 is placed from lateral to medial pole and wire 2 is placed up over the superior surface from the anterior to posterior surface. The loop of wire 2 is on the lingual surface of condyle.

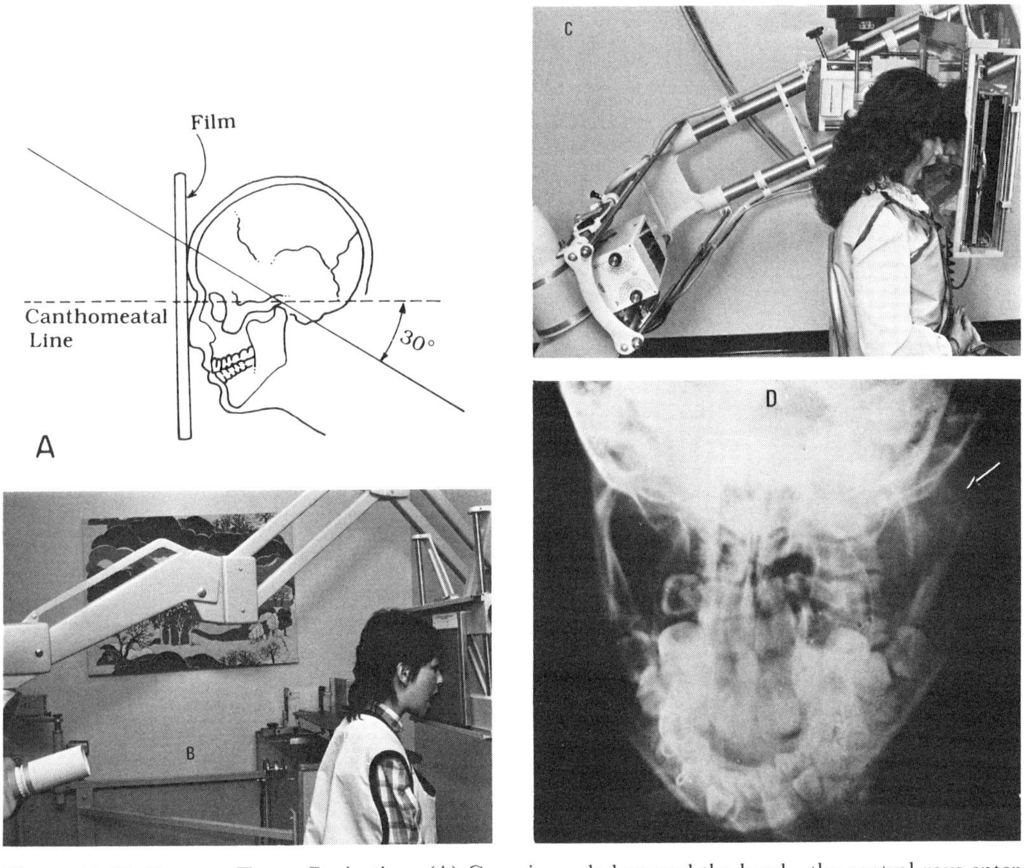

Figure 15-51. Reverse Towne Projection. **(A)** Cone is angled toward the head—the central rays enter the head in the region of the external occipital protuberance and leave the cranium in the region of the external forehead approximately 4 cm above the superciliary arches. The head is adjusted so canthomeatal line is approximately perpendicular to cassette. This places head in the routine PA position of skull or the nose-forehead position. The CR bisects a line through the skull connecting the external auditory meati. The film is centered to the central ray. **(B)** Patient placed in typical Reverse Towne position prior to exposure. Usually taken with mouth open to reveal condyles. **(C)** Reverse Towne position using Franklin Head Unit. **(D)** Reverse Towne radiograph revealing fracture of left condyle.

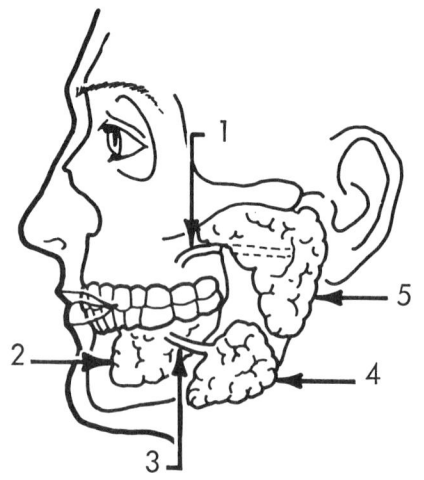

Figure 15-52. Anatomical positions of salivary glands. (1) Stenson's duct; (2) Sublingual gland; (3) Wharton's duct; (4) Submandibular gland; (5) Parotid gland.

provides a good **PA view** of the **mandible** and its **condylar processes**.

Technic of Reverse Towne Projection: The head is adjusted so the canthomeatal line is approximately perpendicular to the cassette. This positions the head in the routine PA (posteroanterior) position of the skull or the **nose-forehead position**. The central ray is directed at an angle of 30 degrees toward the head, entering the skull in the region of the external occipital protuberance bisecting a straight line connecting the external auditory meati and exiting the cranium in the region of the external forehead approximately 4 cm above te superciliary arches. The Reverse Towne is sometimes called the **nucho-frontal** or **Haas position** (Fig. 15-51).

Radiographic Factors:
CASSETTE: 8 × 10 inch
SCREENS: Kodak X-OMATIC regular
FILM: Kodak X-OMAT RP
SOURCE-FILM DISTANCE: 36 inch (short cone) 65 kV, 15 mA, 3/4 second. (If use grid-front cassette, 8:1 ratio, increase kV to 75-80; if use Kodak Lanex Regular screens with Kodak OG film, reduce exposure by half.)

SIALOGRAPHY

Sialography is the X-Ray visualization of the duct system and the parenchyma of the major salivary glands by the introduction of radiopaque contrast material into the main secretory duct of the gland. It is used to study the salivary glands (Fig. 15-52).

The secretion of the parotid gland is serous and contains plyatin, or salivary amylase, which functions to split complex polysaccharides to maltose. The submandibular and sublingual glands have a mixed mucous and serous secretion. The mucous component acts as a lubricant.

Anatomy of Salivary Glands

Parotid Gland

The parotid gland lies just below and

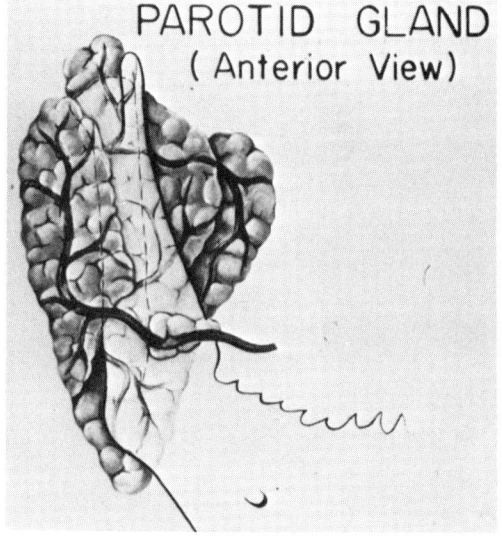

Figure 15-53. Parotid Gland (anterior view). Note how parotid gland curves around the posterior border of the ramus. (Courtesy of Gus Pappas, Columbus, Ohio.)

in front of the external ear. Posteriorly it reaches approximately to the mastoid process and sternocleidomastoid muscle. Anteriorly it overlaps the ramus of the mandible for a variable distance. Superiorly it may reach almost to the zygomatic arch, and inferiorly it often extends just below the angle of the mandible. A deep portion of the gland wraps around the ramus and extends nearly to the pharyngeal wall (Fig. 15-53). The secretions of the parotid gland are collected in a network of ducts distributed throughout the gland that empty in Stenson's duct. Stenson's duct is about 7 cm long and runs forward from the gland, across the masseter muscle. It turns sharply inward at the anterior border of the masseter to pierce the muscle and mucous membrane of the mouth (Fig. 15-54).

Submandibular Gland

The submandibular (submaxillary) gland lies in the submandibular triangle. The superior portion of the gland lies against the submandibular depression on the inner surface of the body of the mandible. The secretion of the submandibular gland is carried by Wharton's duct, which runs between the mylohyoid and hyoglossus muscles and opens into the mouth on a small papilla beside the frenulum of the tongue (Fig. 15-55).

History of Sialography

Arcelin was probably the first clinician to use **sialography**. Just prior to World War I he injected Wharton's duct with bismuth to demonstrate a salivary calculus. Sialography is indicated for (1) recurrent pain or swelling in parotid or submandibular gland region, (2) detection of obstruction either from calculi, foreign bodies, or strictures, (3) detection and diagnosis of recurrent inflammatory pro-

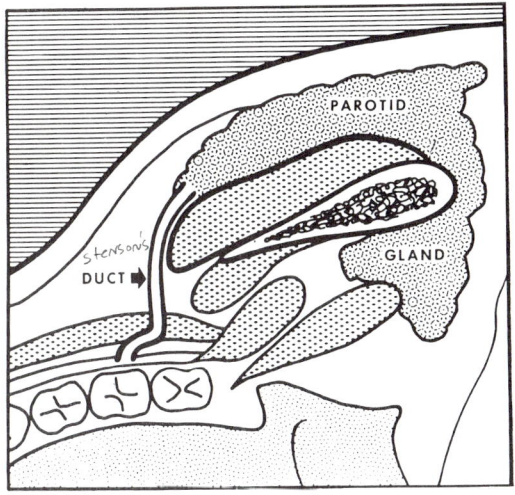

Figure 15-54. Stenson's duct anatomy of parotid gland. Cross-section diagram through ascending mandibular ramus, showing the relation of the parotid gland to the bone, muscles and soft tissue. (From Ollerenshaw, R., and Rose, S.: Sialography—A valuable diagnostic method. *Dent Radiogr Photogr, 29*(3):40, 1956, Fig. 2. Copyright Eastman Kodak Company, Rochester, NY.)

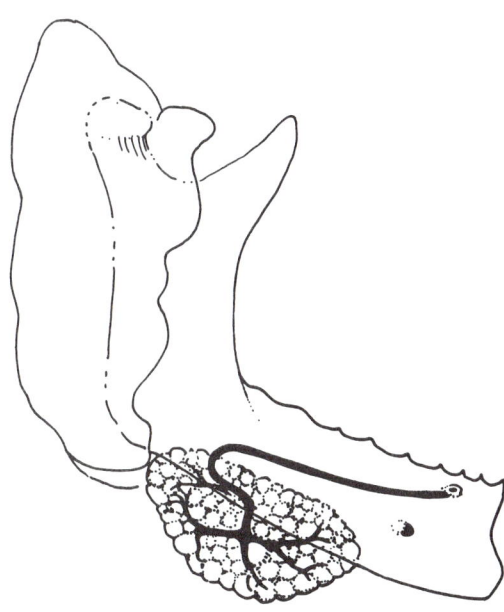

Figure 15-55. Anatomy of submandibular gland and Wharton's duct (Lateral View).

cesses, (4) dryness of mouth and eyes of unknown origin, (5) facial palsy of unknown origin, and (6) pathologic masses for size and location, whether intra- or extraglandular. Also, sialography has been recognized by various clinicians as a therapeutic procedure because the dilation of the ductal system probably aids in the drainage of ductal debris. Sialography is **contraindicated** in patients with known allergies to iodine compounds, patients with acute inflammation of the salivary gland system, and when the patient is undergoing thyroid function tests.

Contrast Media

There are presently two types of contrast media available for use in sialography: **fat-soluble** and **water-soluble** types.

Fat-Soluble Contrast Media

In 1926, Carlsten employed **Lipiodol**® (iodized poppyseed oil) as a contrast material to demonstrate dilation of Stenson's duct. Since that time other fat-based compounds have been introduced. There are two types of fat soluble contrast media: **iodized oil** and **water-insoluble organic iodine compounds**.

Examples of **iodized oil** compounds are **Ethiodol**® (ethiodized poppyseed oil) and **Lipiodol** (iodized poppyseed oil). An example of a **water-insoluble organic iodine compound** is **Pantopaque**® (ethyl iodophenylundecylate).

Fat-soluble compounds produce excellent contrast agents if the ductal systems under examination are intact. Opacification by water-soluble media is generally not as good as fat-soluble media. If the ductal system is damaged, the extravasation of the fat-soluble material can evoke foreign-body reaction and granulomatous formation leading to focal necrosis of the parenchyma and obliteration of adjacent ducts. The fat-soluble media are **more viscous** and require higher injection pressure than the water soluble contrast media to visualize the finer ductules. However, fat soluble media permits evaluation of the salivary ductal system in the postevacuation or secretory phase, because once the finer ductules are filled, the fat-soluble material is eliminated slowly through the ductal orifice. The water-soluble materials are rapdily absorbed or excreted from the gland and do not permit such postevacuation studies. It is the general opinion that **Ethiodol** is the fat-soluble iodine contrast agent of choice because it is more fluid than the others, and thus far, severe foreign body reactions or allergy has not been reported with its use. **Ethiodal** produces dense and sharp outline of ducts and ductules. It is useful in the evaluation of mass lesions, especially if peripherally located.

Water Soluble Media

Most of the clinicians actively using sialographic technics at this time are using a water-soluble contrast agent. They are the agents of choice if ductal obstruction is being studied. These are compounds that are principally iodinated benzene or pyridone derivatives. Examples are **Hypaque**®, Renographin 60® and Renographin 76®. These compounds are more fluid than fat-soluble media and are relatively more miscible with salivary secretions. These physical characteristics permit filling of the finer ductal system of the gland with less pressure, and facilitates prompt drainage. Also, no significant granulomatous reaction has been reported with their use. **Water-soluble contrast agents** are considered more physiologic to the salivary gland than fat-soluble materials because they are diluted in saliva and can be absorbed across glandu-

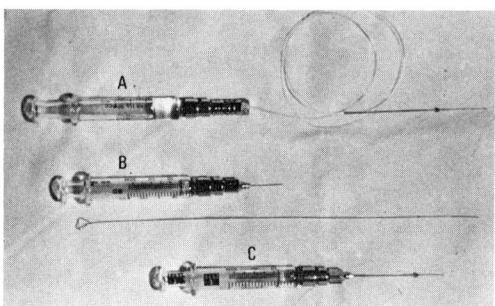

Figure 15-56. Diagram of equipment used in sialography. (A) Duct cannula attached by tubing to syringe; (B) Syringe separated from tubing and stylus; (C) Duct cannula attached directly to syringe. (Courtesy of George Blozis, Columbus, Ohio.)

lar elements. The excretion of water-soluble agents is rapid, and the amount remaining after drawing through the ductal orifice is absorbed and excreted through the kidneys. Fat-soluble contrast agents are poorly eliminated and may cause ductal obstruction.

Technic of Sialography

There are various technics used to inject the contrast media into the orifice of the duct: (1) polyethylene tubing with a special metal cannula; (2) polyethylene tubing with stylus and syringe; and (3) metal cannula attached to syringe (Fig. 15-56).

Probably the best system of the three named is the use of polyethylene tubing with special blunt-end metallic cannulas designed by Rabinov and Joffe (1969). The Rabinov parotid cannula metallic tip is larger and has side holes for injection of contrast agent, and the smaller Rabinov submandibular cannula has the hole at its end and is designed for the smaller orifice of the submandibular gland. The cannulas are tapered and usually stay in place if inserted properly. The blunt tip of the cannula may act as a dilator and probe for the ductal orifice (Fig. 15-57A). Essential equipment necessary for sialogram is shown in Figure 15-57B.

If there is difficulty in locating the orifices of the ducts, have the patient suck on

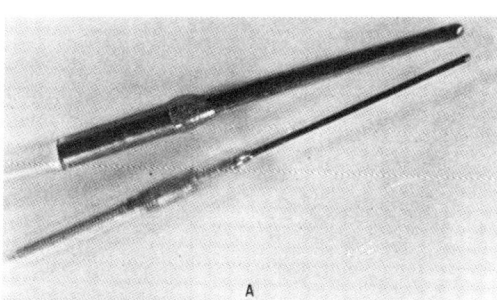
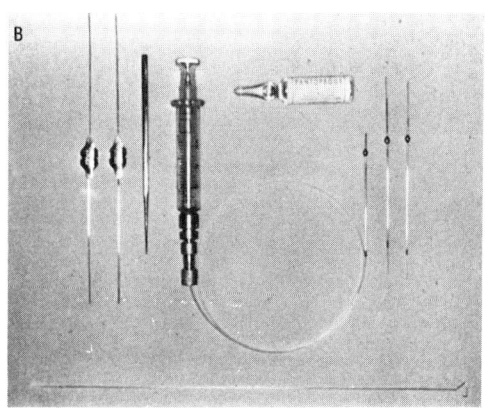

Figure 15-57. (A) Specially designed cannulas by K. Rabinov and manufactured by Cook Inc., Bloomington, IN. The larger cannula is for parotid duct. The parotid cannula has two side holes and a blunt tip, which serves as both a probe and a cannula. Its large proximal end acts as a plug to prevent backflow of contrast medium. The smaller cannula has an end hole designed for smaller orifice of submandibular duct. (From Rankow, R.M., and Polayes, I.M.: *Diseases of the Salivary Glands*, 1976. Courtesy of WB Saunders, Philadelphia.) (B) Essential equipment for sialogram: (left to right) lacrimal dilators, lacrimal probe, cannula attached to syringe by tubing, parotid and submandibular cannulas. Above, contrast medium; below, stylus. (Courtesy of George Blozis, Columbus, OH.)

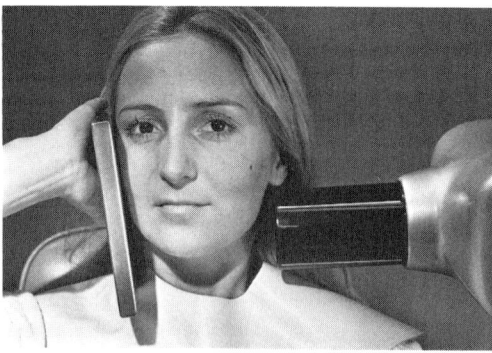

Figure 15-58. True lateral submandibular gland projections. The head is held erect, the cassette is placed against the face and is held perpendicular to the floor and parallel to the midsagittal plane. For the lateral parotid gland projection, the cassette is placed higher on the face. The X-Rays are directed just below the lower border of the mandible at the angle. The exposure time is reduced to bring out the soft tissue of the gland.

a lemon, or place tincture of benzoine on ductal orifice. Once the orifice is found, it can be dilated by means of the lacrimal dilator or probes. Then, insert the blunt-ended cannula into the duct for 0.5-1 cm. Do not insert the cannula very far into Stenson's duct because the duct forms a sharp angle as it is passed through the buccinator muscle. The injection is made slowly and is stopped when the patient experiences mild discomfort. The volume of contrast medium injected usually is 0.5-1.5 ml for examination of parotid gland and 0.2-0.5 ml for examination of submandibular gland.

Radiography of Salivary Glands

There are various sets of radiographs that may be taken during the sialographic procedure.

Preliminary Phase: Radiographs taken prior to the injection of the contrast medium — **anteroposterior** (AP), the **true lateral** (Fig. 15-58), and the **lateral oblique** (Fig. 15-2, 15-3). In the antero-

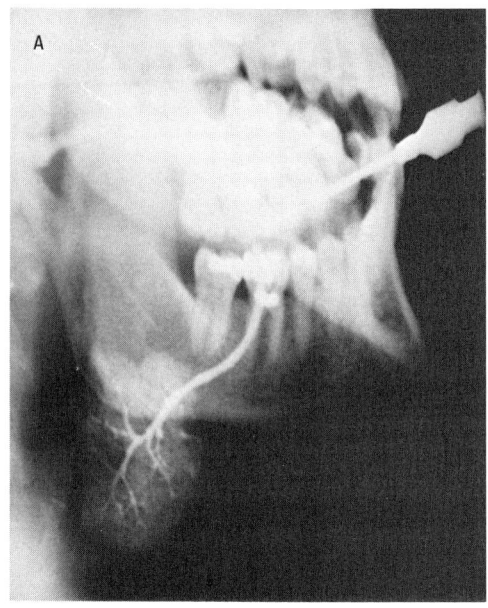
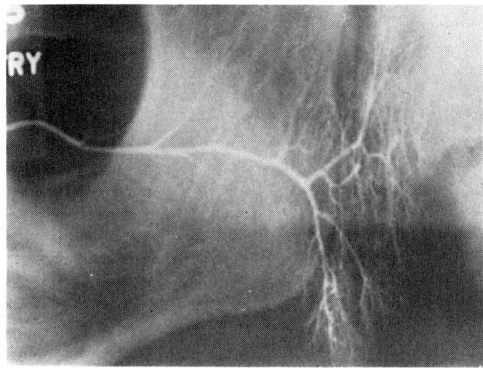

Figure 15-59. Submandibular and parotid gland sialograms. **(A)** Submandibular sialogram. **(B)** Parotid sialogram.

posterior view, place the posterior portion of the patient's head against the cassette, flex the chin of the patient, and direct the central ray immediately below the lipline perpendicular to the cassette on the side of interest.

Filling Phase Films: Take AP, true lateral, and lateral oblique positions during various filling phases of the gland (Fig.

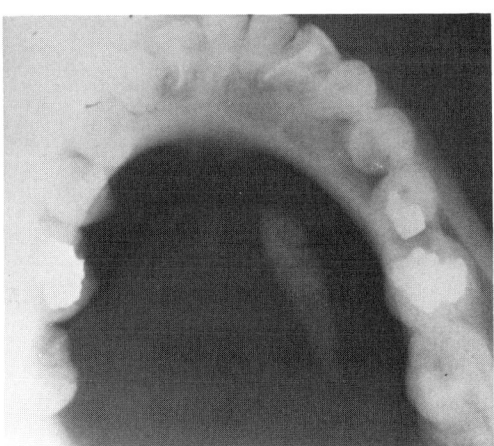

Figure 15-60. Mandibular occlusal radiograph revealing salivary stone (sialolith) shaped like a tooth.

15-59).

Postevacuation phase: Five minutes after stimulation of salivary flow, take an AP, true lateral, and lateral oblique. If retention of contrast medium is noted, repeat the same films at one hour and twenty-four hours.

Additional Radiographic Views (Sialography)

Additional radiographic views that will aid in viewing the salivary ductal system follow.

Reverse Basilar, Axial, or Verticosubmental View: (Opposite of submentovertex position.) (Fig. 15-40). This is used to view the deep portion of parotid gland.

Anteroposterior View: This view is of the parotid gland with patient **blowing cheek outward**: Film is positioned posterior to and at right angles to the surface of the cheek of the patient. The central ray is directed through the cheek perpendicular to the surface of the film. It is used to detect calculi in Stenson's Duct.

Mandibular Occlusal View: This is used for demonstration of distal portion of Wharton's Duct for detection of calculi (Fig. 15-60).

Filling Phase: In radiographing filling phase of parotid gland, it is better to take it in the open mouth position to avoid superimposition of the mandible over the gland.

RADIOGRAPHY OF EDENTULOUS JAWS

Past studies have shown that approximately one out of four edentulous patients have residual roots, unerupted and supernumerary teeth, cysts, residual areas of infection, and foreign bodies.

Baseline radiographs for the edentulous can be one of the following surveys:

1. a complete periapical survey;
2. panoramic radiographs and selected periapical films;
3. mixed occlusal-periapical survey;
4. an occlusal-lateral jaw survey.

Edentulous Complete Periapical Survey

This is usually the edentulous survey of choice and may be taken by either the paralleling or bisecting angle technic. Usually if the patient has average or better ridge height, a modified paralleling technic can be used.

Modified Paralleling Technic for Partially Edentulous Patients

Paralleling instruments can be used in radiography of partially edentulous mouths by substituting a cotton roll or block of Styrofoam® (or similar radiolucent material) for the space normally occupied by the crowns of the missing teeth and then following the standard procedure recommended for the instruments. If you are using the Rinn instruments,

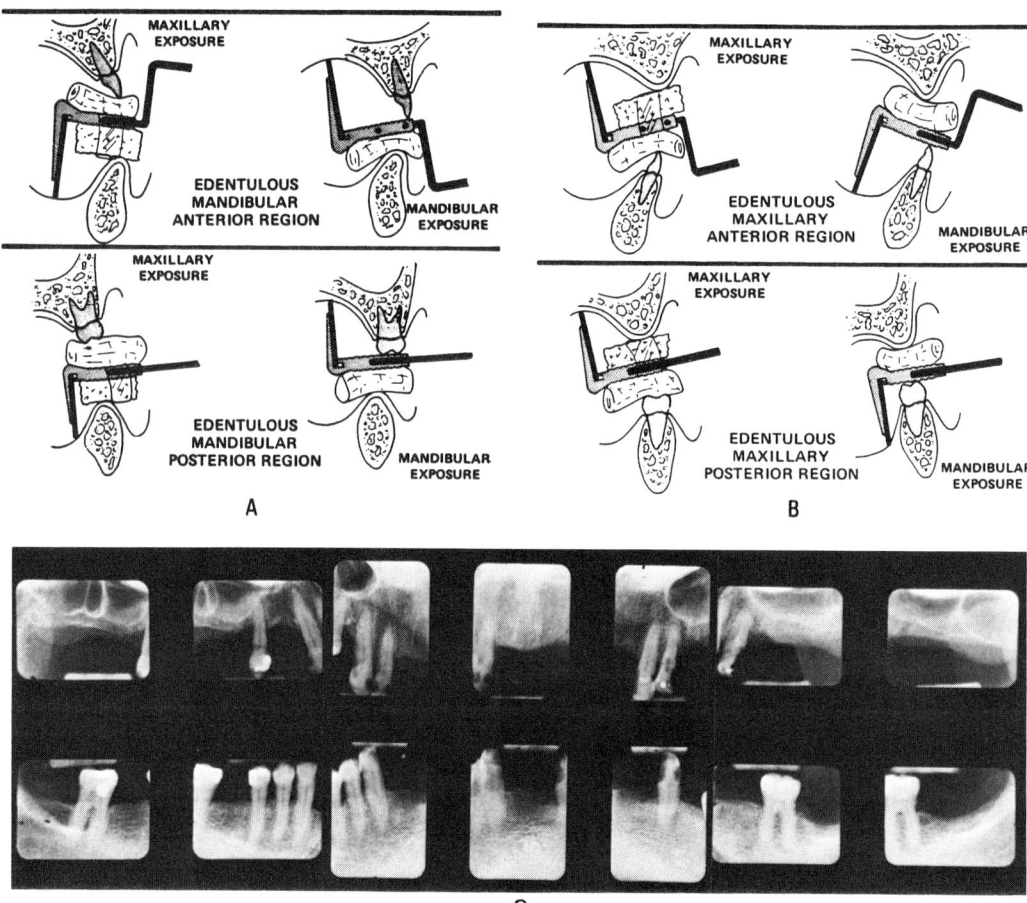

Figure 15-61. Paritally edentulous technique using Rinn XCP instruments. Cotton rolls, blocks of Styrofoam®, or a combination of both can be used as illustrated. The thickness of the cotton rolls or Styrofoam will determine the amount of film coverage of the edentulous ridges. (A) upper, edentulous mandibular anterior region; lower, edentulous mandibular posterior region; (B) upper, edentulous maxillary posterior region; lower, edentulous maxilary posterior region. (C) Partially edentulous CMX.

either the XCP (Paralleling) or BAI (Bisecting) bite-blocks may be used for partially edentulous patients (Fig. 15-61). The exposure time should be reduced one notch down on the exposure scale in the edentulous areas.

Complete Edentulous Technic

Either the bisecting or paralleling technic can be used to take a complete edentulous survey. If the ridges are severely resorbed, the digital bisecting technic is recommended. Place the film against the ridge and have the patient hold the film against the ridge with his/her thumb in maxillary arch and forefinger in the mandibular arch. Cover as much of the ridge as possible with the film and direct the central ray to the center of the film at right angles to a line bisecting the angle

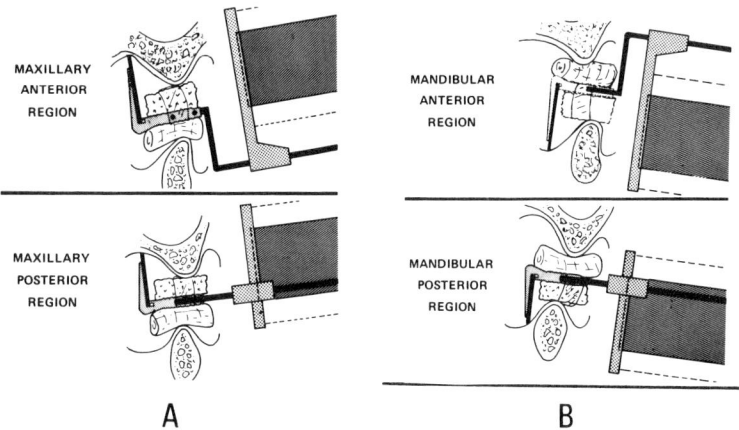

Figure 15-62. Complete edentulous technic using the Rinn XCP instrument. However, the BAI technic may also be used with use of cotton rolls similar to that of XCP instrument. Cotton rolls, blocks of Styrofoam, or a combination of both can be used as illustrated. (If there is severe resorption of edentulous ridges, the XCP is difficult to use.) **(A)** Upper, maxillary anterior region; lower, maxillary posterior region. **(B)** Upper, mandibular anterior region; lower, mandibular posterior region.

formed by the long axis of the ridge and the film. Actually when the ridges are severely resorbed, directing the central ray perpendicular to the film will suffice. The object is to show some of the bone on the film. A fourteen film survey is recommended for the edentulous complete radiographic survey.

If there is a fairly good edentulous ridge left, the paralleling technic utilizing film holders can be used. Cotton rolls, blocks of Styrofoam, or a combination can be used with the paralleling instruments. Figures 15-62 and 15-63 illustrate the use of the Rinn XCP instruments in taking completely edentulous arches of a patient. The paralleling instrument is positioned in the mouth with the film parallel to the ridge areas being examined. The patient closes, holding the film in position, and the procedure for the paralleling technic is used.

Panoramic Edentulous Survey

The panoramic technic produces a survey for partially edentulous and edentulous survey, which provides exceptional coverage of both jaws on one radiograph. It has the disadvantage of not having the clarity of detail as revealed on the periapical radiograph. In areas on the panoramic radiograph that reveal suspected areas of abnormality, a periapical or occlusal film should be taken for more accurate radiographic information (Fig. 15-64).

Mixed Occlusal and Periapical Survey

The mixed occlusal-periapical survey consists of the folowing films:

1. one maxillary topographical occlusal

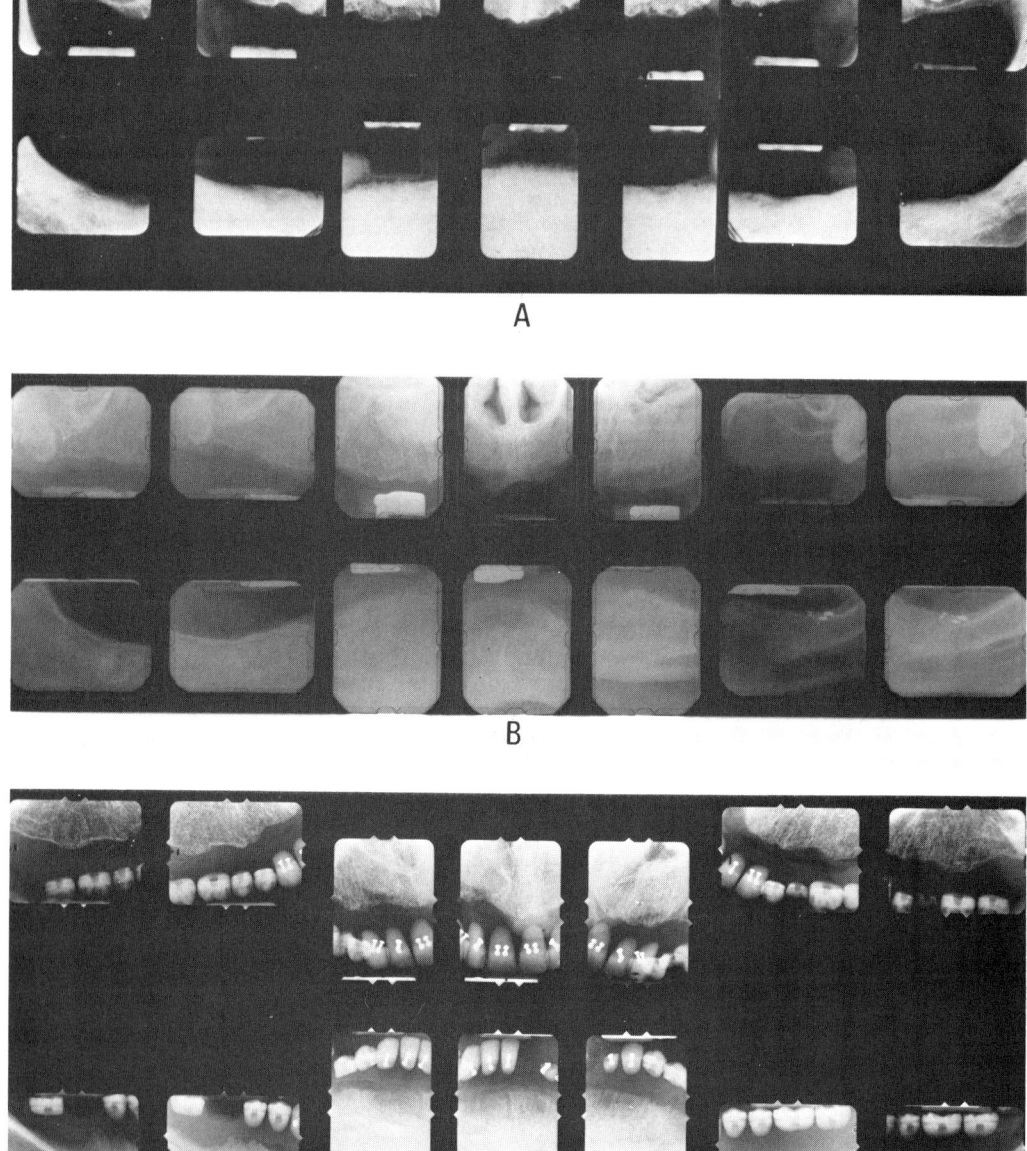

Figure 15-63. Edentulous CMX (14 periapical survey) **(A)** Edentulous CMX using Rinn XCP instruments. **(B)** Edentulous CMX revealing embedded maxillary third molars and fragments in left mandibular arch. **(C)** Edentulous CMX with complete dentures left in mouth. This is an acceptable technic, as the acrylic dentures do not impede the passage of the X-Rays.

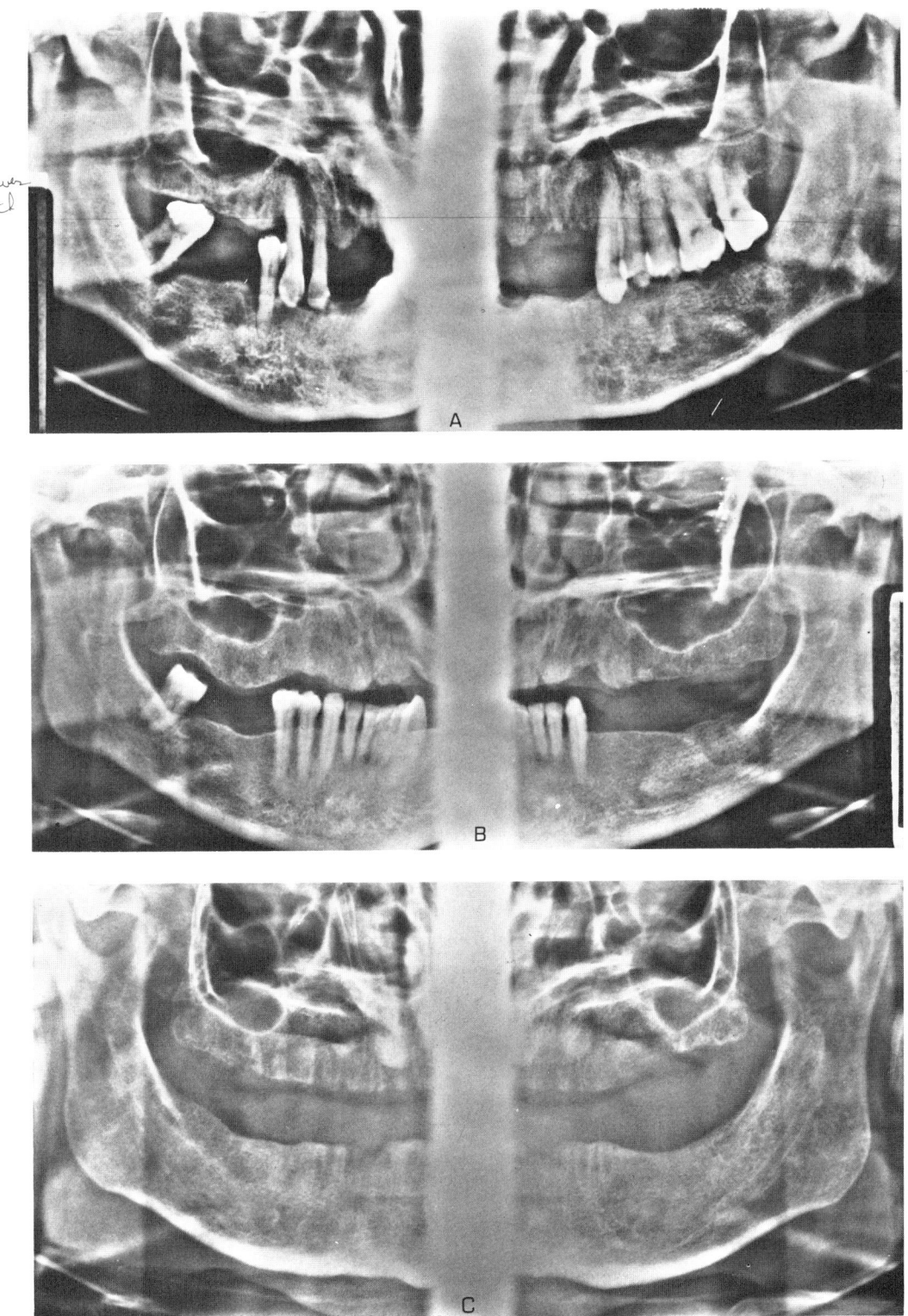

Figure 15-64. Split-image panoramic radiographs. **(A)** Partially edentulous radiograph (lower jaw edentulous except for one tooth). **(B)** Partially edentulous radiograph (upper jaw edentulous). **(C)** Complete edentulous radiograph (good ridges).

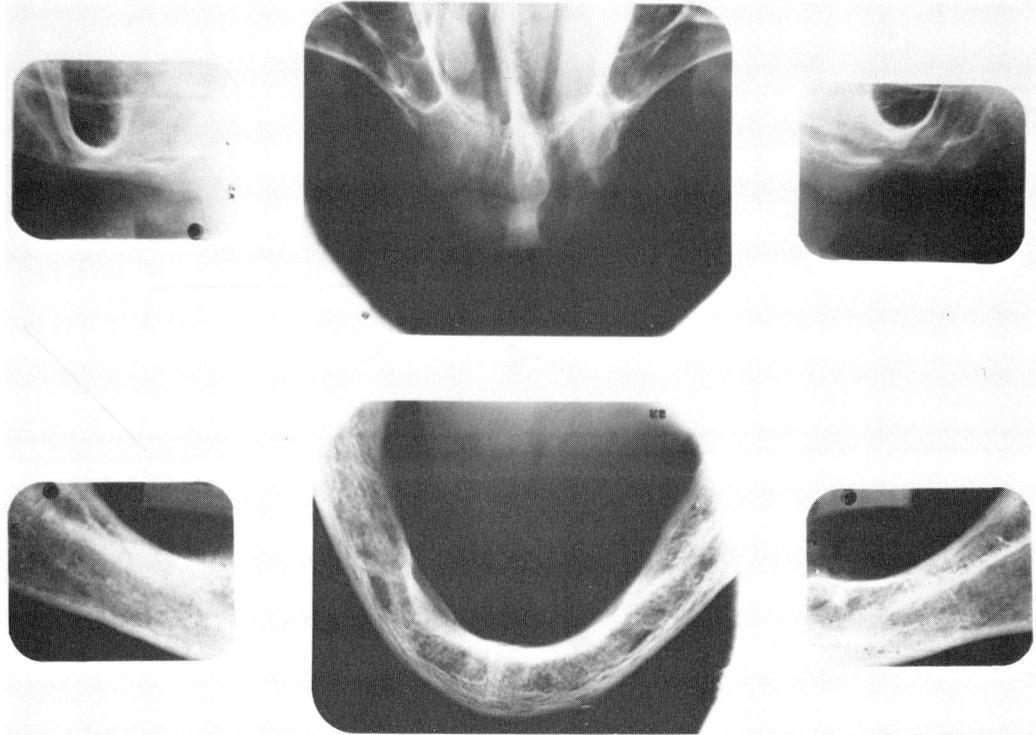

Figure 15-65. Mixed occlusal-periapical edentulous survey.

film;
2. one mandibular cross-sectional occlusal film;
3. four molar standard (#2) periapical films.

The occlusal films give an excellent buccolingual view of the major portions of the jaws (Fig. 15-65). However, the occlusal film does not, in most cases, reveal the detail of edentulous ridges that the periapical survey will reveal. The most posterior areas, which are difficult for the occlusal films to cover, are taken by means of four periapical films. This type of survey is usually indicated in new patients who have worn dentures for a number of years. It is rapid and covers the jaws quite adequately.

Occlusal-Lateral Jaw Survey

This is sometimes called the "poor man's panoramic survey" because it covers as much of the jaws as the panoramic film for a lot less initial investment.

This survey consists of the following radiographs:

1. one maxillary topographical occlusal film;
2. one mandibular cross-sectioned occlusal film;
3. two lateral jaw films (right and left side).

This survey may be substituted for the mixed occlusal-periapical survey when the patient will not tolerate intraoral molar periapical films (Fig. 15-66).

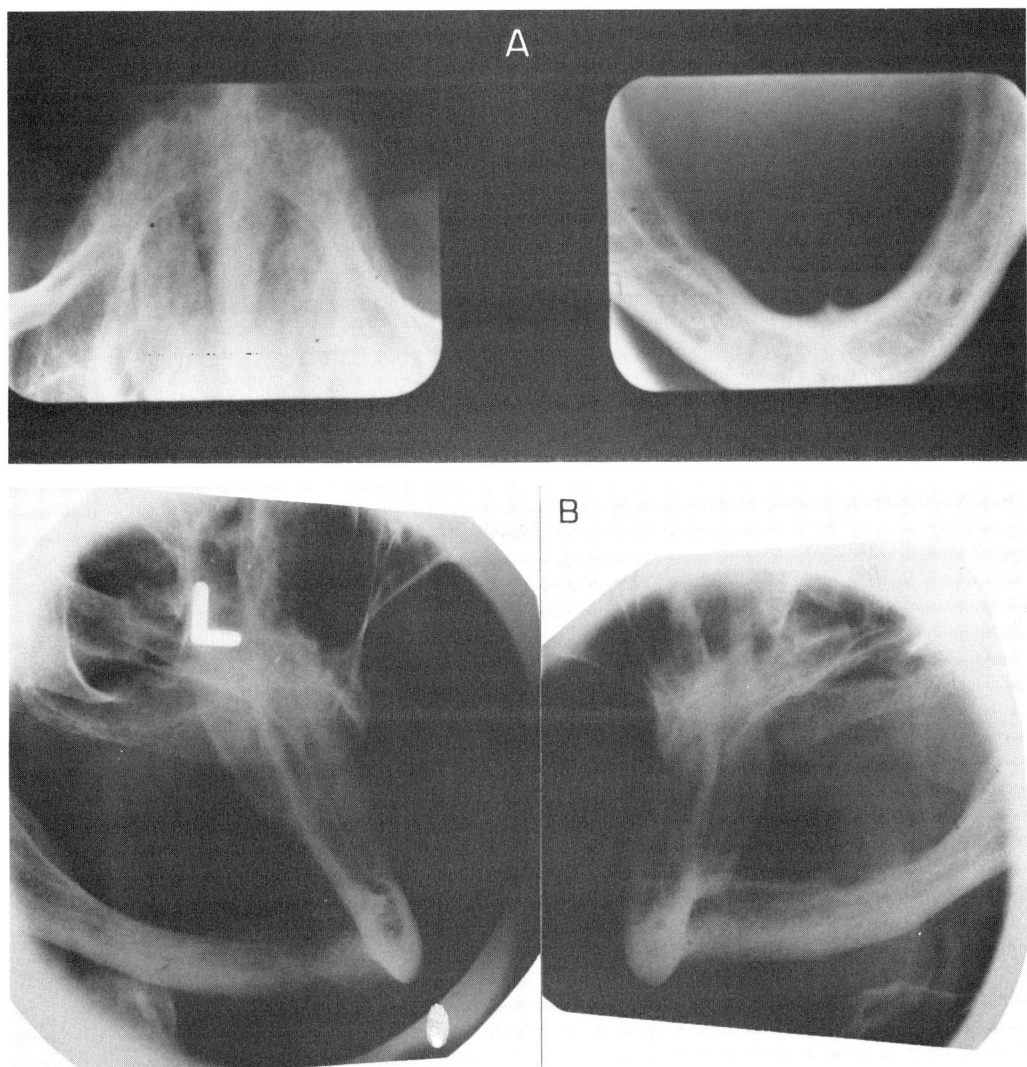

Figure 15-66. Mixed occlusal-lateral jaw edentulous survey. (A) Maxillary and Mandibular occlusals. (B) Left and right lateral jaws.

LOCALIZATION TECHNIC

The dental radiograph is a two-dimensional picture of a three-dimensional object and lacks perspective depth. Localization by the use of dental radiographs must be interpreted by comparison of views taken at different angles of projection, plus an anatomic knowledge of the regions radiographed.

Localization is indicated in the following instances: foreign bodies, broken needles, broken instruments, filling materials in the alveolar process, retained roots, impacted supernumerary and unerupted teeth, calculi in a gland or duct of salivary glands, fractures of the maxilla and mandible, fracture of condyles, and expansion of the alveolar process in cystic formation. The methods of localization are as follows:

1. tube-shift method;
2. buccal-object rule;
3. periapical-occlusal method (Miller's technique).

Tube-Shift Method

This method was first described by C. Clark (1909). It is used to determine the buccolingual relationship of foreign objects and impacted or unerupted teeth within the jaws. The method requires two periapical radiographs of the area in question shifting the tube *horizontally* between exposures.

The rule governing the tube-shift method of localization is as follows:

If the unerupted tooth or foreign body moves in the same direction in which the tube (not the cone) is shifted horizontally, it (the un-

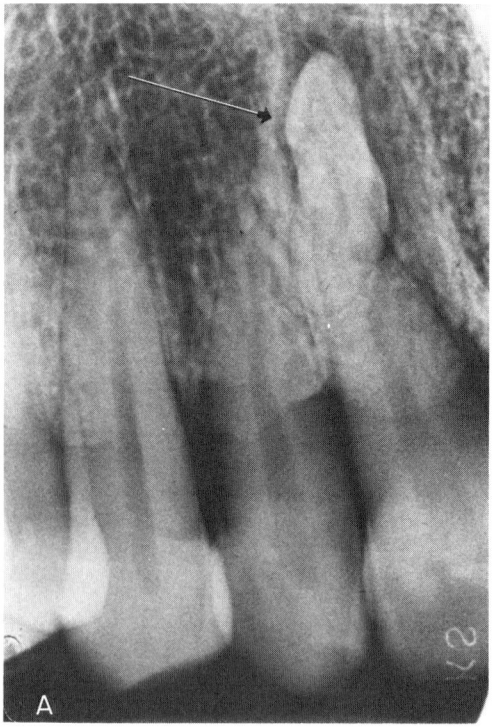
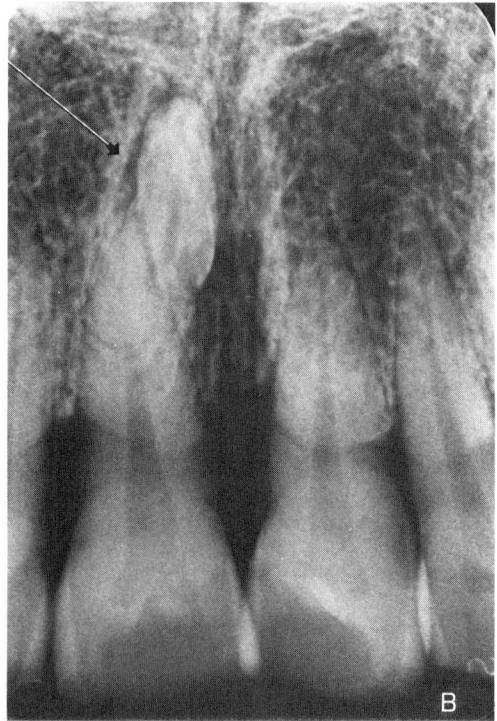

Figure 15-67. Horizontal tube-shift method of localization. **(A)** Note mesiodens in lateral periapical radiograph. **(B)** In central incisor periapical, the mesiodens moves in direction of tube shift; therefore, mesiodens is lingual to other anterior teeth in the arch. **(C)** Note metal foreign object in central incisor periapical. **(D)** In the lateral incisor periapical, the foreign object moves in opposite direction of horizontal tube shift. Therefore, foreign object is facially located to other teeth in the anterior arch. **(E)** Maxillary occlusal of impacted left canine. **(F)** Lateral incisor periapical radiograph of impacted canine in (E). **(G)** Molar periapical radiograph of impacted canine, which moves horizontally in direction of the tube-shift to the posterior. The CE junction of canine moves distal of lateral incisor to mesial of second premolar. Therefore, canine is lingual to other teeth in left maxillary arch.

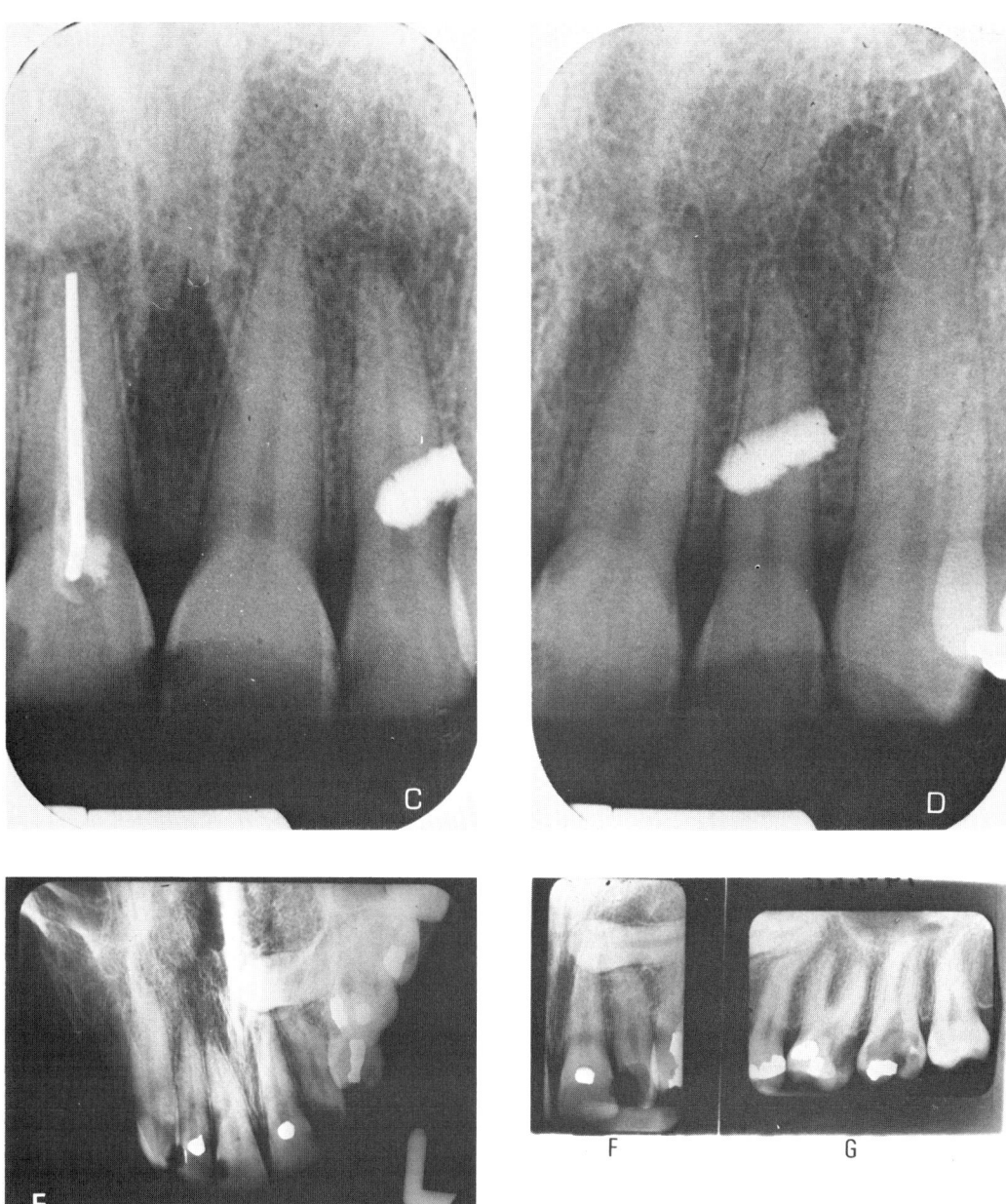

erupted tooth or foreign body) is located on the lingual side. If it moves in opposite direction in which the tube (not the cone) is shifted, the location is on the facial or buccal/labial.

Although the tube-shift method of localization could be applied to the vertical shift of the tube, it is always applied to the horizontal shift of the tube. If a complete survey has been taken of a patient, an unerupted tooth or foreign object could be

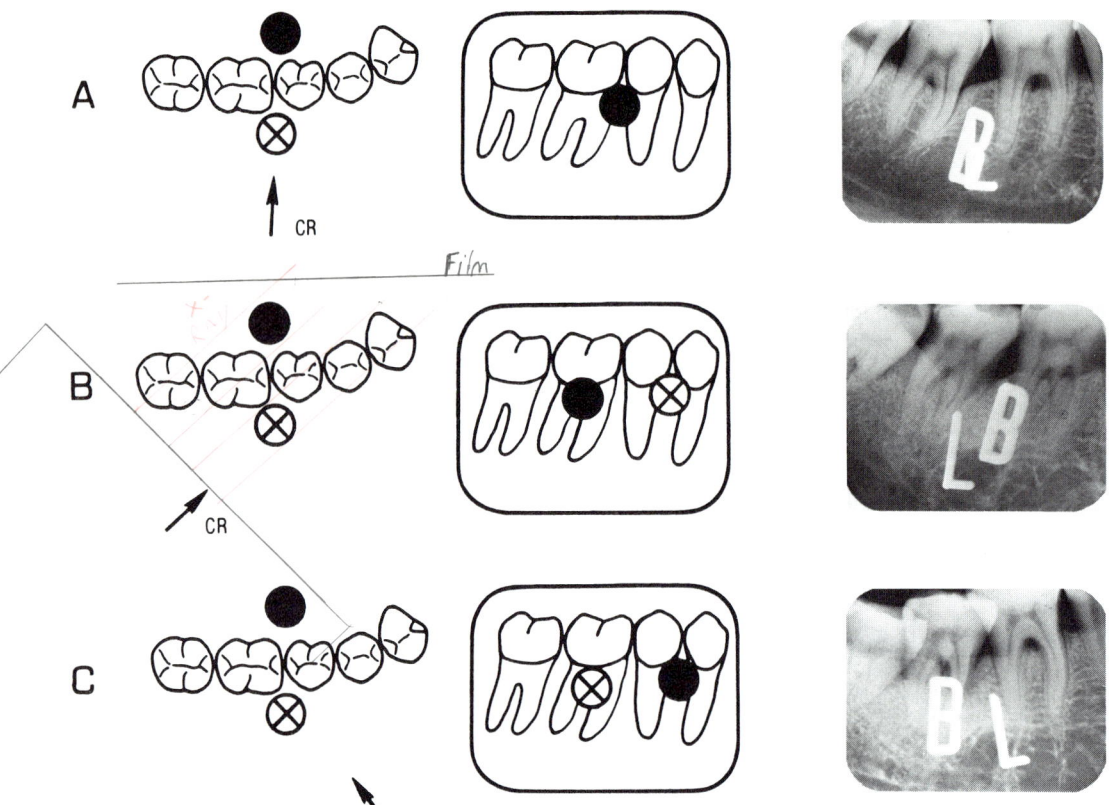

Figure 15-68. Buccal and lingual foreign bodies change position with horizontal shift of x-ray beam. **(A)** Original radiograph. Buccal and lingual objects are superimposed. **(B)** The beam is directed mesially. The buccal object (letter B) "moves" mesially while the lingual (letter L) object moves distally. **(C)** The beam is directed distally. The buccal object (letter B) "moves" distally while the lingual object (letter L) "moves" mesially.

located facially or lingually to the erupted teeth by the simple application of the tube-shift rule. This would negate the necessity of taking another film to locate the unerupted tooth or foreign object (Fig. 15-67).

Buccal-Object Rule

This method of localization of pathoses, supernumerary teeth, fractures, and foreign bodies was first suggested by Richards, in 1952. The rules states:

When two different radiographs are made of a pair of objects, the image of the most buccal (facial) object moves, relative to the image of the lingual object, in the same direction that the x-ray beam (cone, P.I.D.) is directed.

The tube head can be rotated left and right in a horizontal direction. With this motion, the **horizontal** angulation of the central x-ray beam (cone P.I.D.) is changed. Also, the x-ray tube head can be rotated up and down in a **vertical** direction. With this motion, the vertical angula-

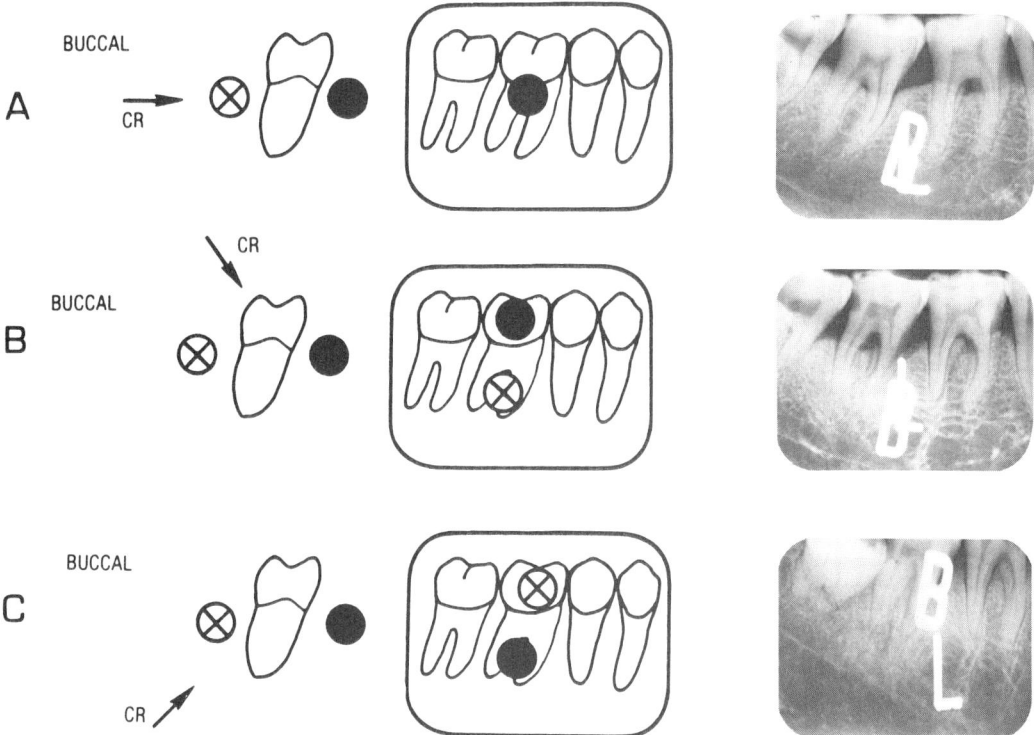

Figure 15-69. Buccal and lingual foreign bodies change position with vertical shift of x-ray beam. **(A)** the original radiograph. Buccal and lingual objects are superimposed. **(B)** The beam is directed inferiorly (positive vertical angulation). The buccal object (letter B) moves inferiorly while the lingual object (letter L) moves superiorly. **(C)** The beam is directed superiorly (negative vertical angulation). The buccal object (letter B) moves superiorly while the lingual object (letter L) moves inferiorly.

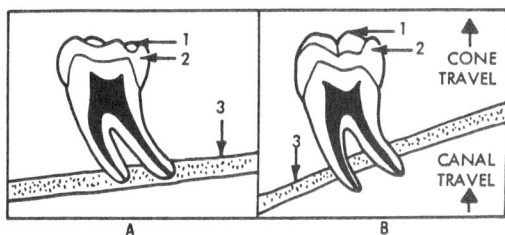

Figure 15-70. Buccal Object Rule used in estimating the position of the mandibular canal in relationship to the apices of the third molar. **(A)** Conventional lateral view of mandibular third molar. 1, buccal cusps; 2, lingual cusps. 3, mandibular canal. **(B)** Radiograph produced with a negative 20 degree (upwards) angulation of the x-ray cone. The mandibular canal is buccal to the roots of the third molar because the canal moves in the same direction of movement of the cone. (Note that buccal cusps also move upwards in direction of tube movement.)

tion of the x-ray beam (cone P.I.D.) is changed.

The **horizontal angulation** should be changed when locating vertically aligned images on the radiograph such as root canals, and the **vertical angulation** changed when locating a horizontally aligned image on the radiograph such as the mandibular canal.

The successful application of the **Buccal Object Rule** requires that two different radiographs have been made of the same region. These radiographs will reveal necessary clues to locate the position of the hidden object (such as an unerupted tooth) in relation to known objects (such as erupted teeth).

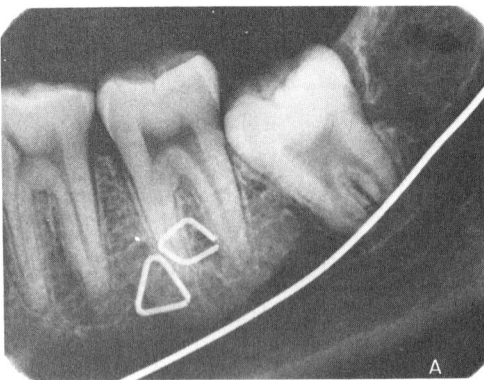
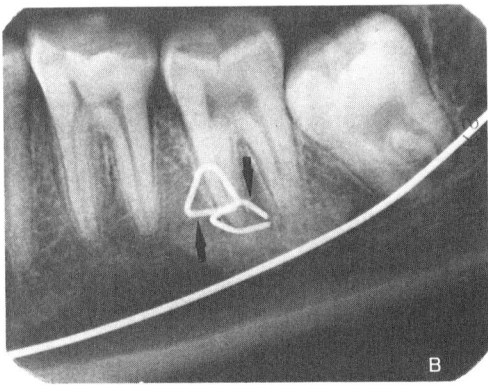
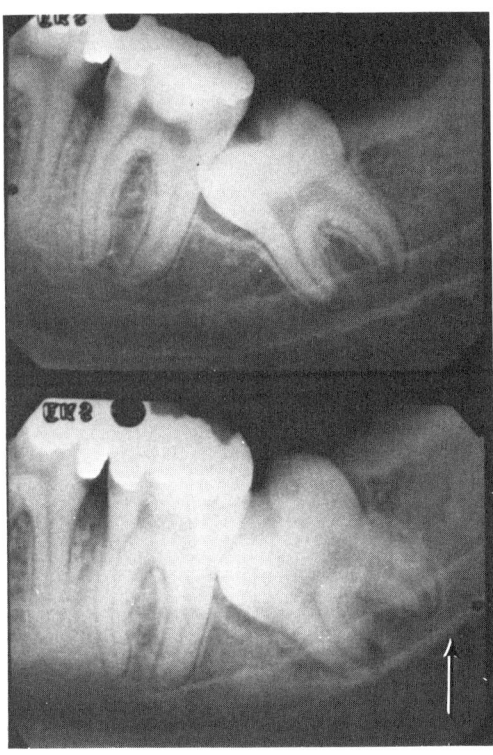

Figure 15-71. Buccal Object Rule used to locate mandibular canal. (A) 0 degree vertical angulation used to take radiograph. (Triangle marker is placed on buccal and diamond marker is on lingual of mandible.) Wire has been placed in mandibular canal. (B) -20 degree upward vertical angulation of x-ray beam (cone). Canal wire moves less superiorly than the buccally placed triangle marker. Therefore, mandibular canal is slightly buccal to the root tops of the mandibular third molar, but in very close approximation.

Figure 15-72. Where does mandibular canal lie relative to apex of the mandibular third molar's mesial root? In lower radiograph, the buccal cusps have moved upwards as compared to upper radiograph, meaning lower radiograph was taken with an increased negative angulation. Since the mandibular canal moves superiorly in lower radiograph, it indicates a buccal relationship of mandibular canal to the roots of third molar. (From richard, A. G.: Buccal object rule. *Dent Radiogr Photogr, 53*(3):37, 1980. Copyright Eastman Kodak Company, Rochester, NY.)

If a bucal and lingual object are superimposed (as in Fig 15-68A and 15-69A), the two may be separated and identified by applying the Buccal Object Rule. In making the second radiograph, alter the horizontal or vertical angulation of the beam. When the second radiograph is compared with the first (original) the buccal object will appear to have moved in the same position as the beam (Fig. 15-68B, C and 15-69B, C).

Buccal Object rule and Location of Mandibular Canal

With the Buccal Object method, the relationship of the apices of the mandibular third molar with the mandibular canal can be estimated.

Atlas of Special Techniques in Dental Radiology 563

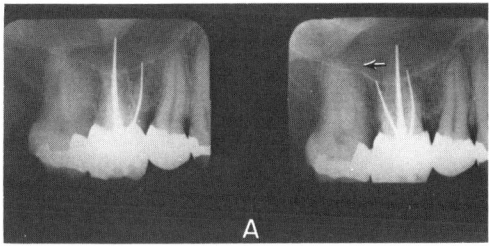 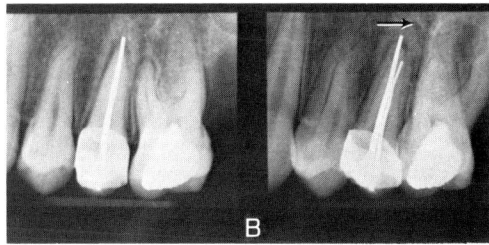

Figure 15-73. Buccal Object Rule — Endodontics. **(A)** To produce the radiograph on the right, the horizontal angulation would have to be changed to a more distal angulation. This would move the buccal roots toward distal and clear up the distobuccal root superimposition as shown in left radiograph. **(B)** Which one of the root canal fillings of the second premolar extends beyond the root? The horizontal angulation has been changed to a distal angulation in the right radiograph. Notice the distal movement of the buccal roots of the first molar and the buccal cusps of the first premolar. One of the roots of the second premolar moves further to the distal when the x-ray beam is directed in a distal direction. This is the buccal root, and the root with the overextended root canal filling is the lingual root. (From Richards, A. G.: Buccal object rule. *Dent Radiogr Photogr,* 53(3):32, 1980 Copyright Eastman Kodak Company, Rochester NY.)

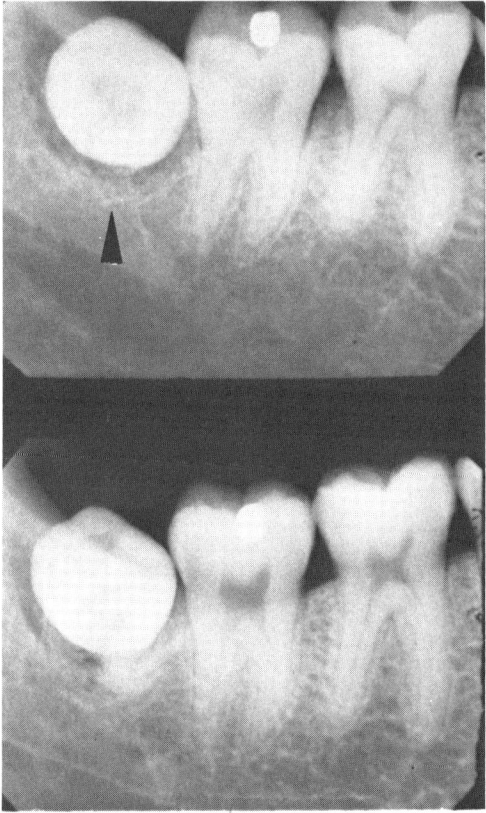 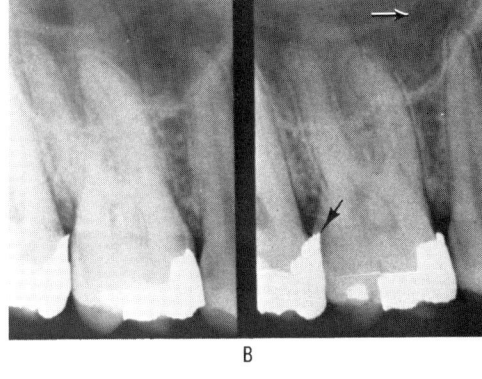

Figure 15-74. **(A)** In which direction is the occlusal surface of the buccolingual impacted third molar face? In the upper radiograph, the vertical angulation has been increased upwards, moving the buccal cusps of the first and second molars upwards. Also, note that roots of impacted third molar also move upwards, meaning roots are on the buccal and crown of tooth is facing the lingual. **(B)** At what corner is mesial overhanging restoration in second molar? In right radiograph the buccal roots of first molar move in a mesial direction, meaning H.A. was changed in mesial direction. Note the overhanging restoration also moves in a mesial direction. The overhang must be located on mesiobuccal corner of restoration. (From Richards, A. G.: Buccal object rule. *Dent Radiogr Photogr,* 53(3):37, 1980. Copyright Eastman Kodak Company, Rochester, NY.)

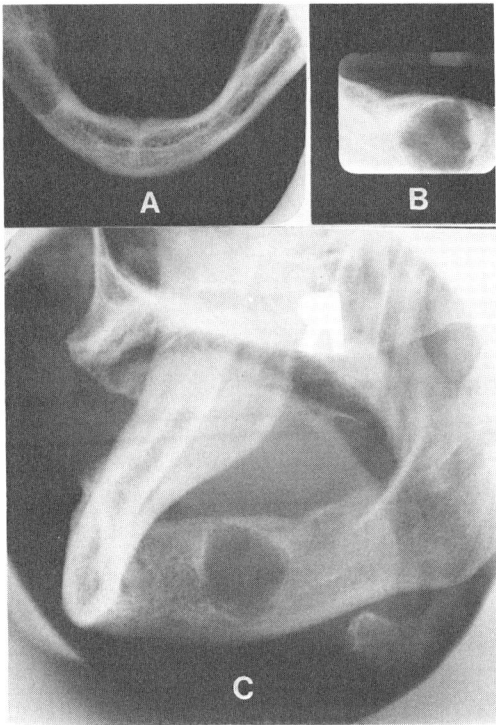

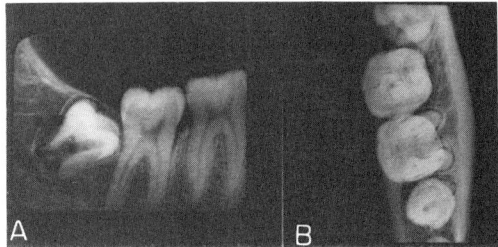

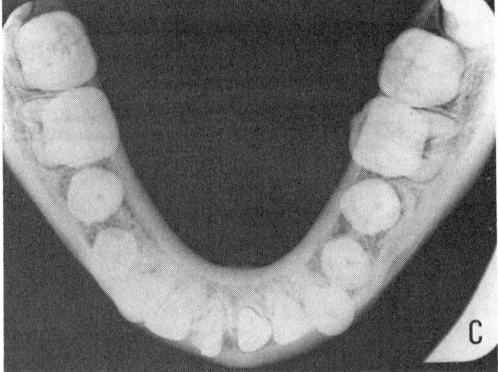

Figure 15-75. Localization of residual cyst by right-angle method. **(A)** Occlusal radiograph. **(B)** Periapical radiograph. **(C)** Lateral jaw radiograph to cover area adequately.

Figure 15-76. Estimation of buccolingual relationship of mesiolingual impacted Third molar by right-angle method. **(A)** Periapical radiograph; **(B)** Occlusal periapical radiograph; **(C)** Occlusal radiograph. (third molar is in buccal relationship to second molar.)

Two radiographs are needed. The first radiograph is a routine view of the mandibular third molar taken with 0 degrees angulation. The second radiograph is taken with -20 degrees upward change in vertical angulation. If the mandibular canal is buccal to the apices of the mandibular third molar, the mandibular canal image will move superiorly (upward) to the image of the mandibular apices in the resultant radiograph. If the mandibular canal is lingual to the apices of the mandibular third molar, the mandibular canal will move inferiorly (downward) or in the opposite direction of the upward (negative) vertical change of the cone (Figs. 15-70, 15-71, 15-72).

The Buccal Object Rule can also be used to identify root canals (Fig. 15-73), impacted tooth directions, and overhanging restorations (Fig. 15-74).

The Right-Angle Method of Localization

The object of this method of localization is to take two radiographs at right angles to each other. This will localize hidden objects such as unerupted teeth and foreign objects in two directions in relation to known objects such as erupted teeth. This method was first suggested by Dr. Fred Miller in 1914 and later popularized by George Winter in 1926. This technique requires two radiographs to be made of the area under investigation: (1)

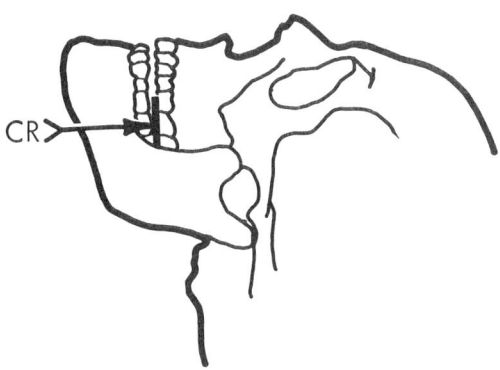

Figure 15-77. Diagram of conventional occlusal technic of third molar using No. 2 regular film. (The ramus of mandible restricts distal placement of film.)

a periapical radiograph or lateral extraoral radiograph to establish the mesiodistal and superoinferior relationship between a fixed landmark and the object to be localized; and (2) an occlusal intraoral cross-sectional or topographical radiograph to determine the buccolingual or mediolateral relationship (Figs. 15-75, 15-76). If extraoral films are taken, submentovertex, anteroposterior skull, or posteroanterior skull projections are indicated to localize hidden objects in the mediolateral plane.

The standard occlusal technique to reveal the buccolingual relationship of the suspected third molar does not always produce all of the crown of the impacted third molar (Fig. 15-76B, C). This is because the ramus of the mandible often prevents the distal extension of the film to cover all of the impacted third molar. Substitution of the standard periapical film for the occlusal film has routinely failed to give improved coverage (Fig. 15-77).

Modified Occlusal Technique

A modified occlusal technique was advocated by Donovan (1952) to remedy this problem (Fig. 15-78). Donovan recommended two changes: (1) a change in the position of the film packet and (2) a

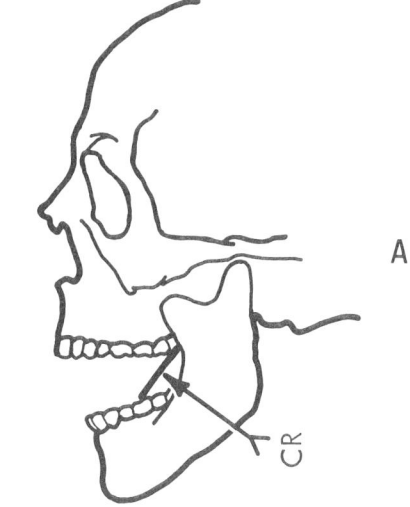
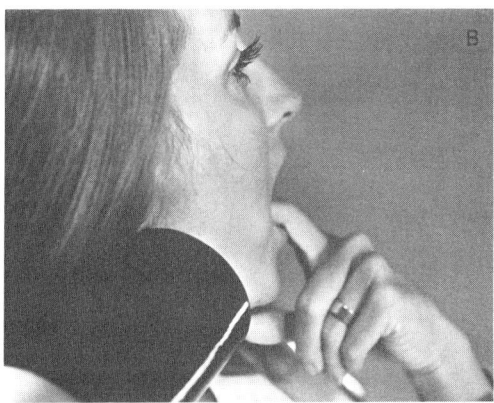
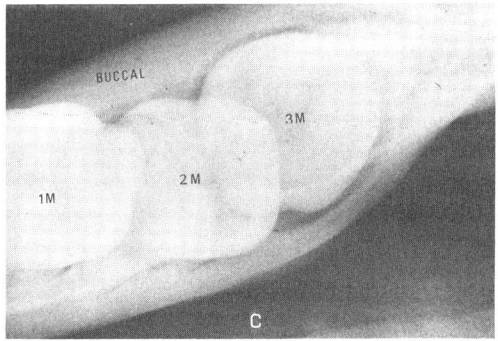

Figure 15-78. Donovan's Modified Occlusal Technic. (A) Diagram showing position of the film packet and central ray using Donovan's Technic. (B) Position of the Patient's head and cone in Donovan's Technic. (C) Occlusal view of third molar with Donovan's Technic. (Third molar approximately in line with second molar, maybe slightly buccal.)

change in the direction of the central ray.

The mouth remains open in this technique, with the periapical film packet permitted to ride up on the edge of the mandible. The film packet is held in place by the patient's index finger at a point where the film packet touches the occlusal surface of the mandibular teeth. The film should not be allowed to bend. If desired, the larger occlusal film may be used. The central ray is again directed at right angles to the film packet, but in this improved technique the patient's head must be rotated away from the x-ray tube so the short cone may come in close proximity to the angle of the mandible.

ENDODONTIC RADIOGRAPHY*

Dental radiographs are one of the more important diagnostic aids in endodontics because they are the only visual method the dentist has to gain clinical knowledge of the teeth and periapical tissues. Radiographs are also one of the most reliable methods of monitoring endodontic treatment.

The endodontic radiograph is much more difficult to take than the routine periapical radiograph. The major reason for the difficulty is that the film exposure is made under adverse visual conditions since the endodontic working radiographs are made with the rubber dam in place. This makes proper positioning and stabilization of the film during this time more difficult due to the interference of the protruding dam clamp, root canal instruments (files, reamers, and broaches), and obturating material (silver and gutta percha cones) extending out of the access cavity. Although the basic principles of dental radiography do not change, the problem is related to visualization of the tooth for proper film positioning and cone (P.I.D.) angulation due the presence of the rubber dam.

Typically, endodontic treatment may require various numbers of radiographic exposures to permit proper evaluations of the various steps in the procedure. The initial starting or **diagnosis film** is taken

---
*Most of the subject matter in this section is from the manual *A Radiographic Technique for Endodontics,* by Drs. Carlos E. Del Rio, Maria Luisa Canales, and John W. Preece. The University of Texas Health Science Center Dental School at San Antonio, San Antonio, Texas.

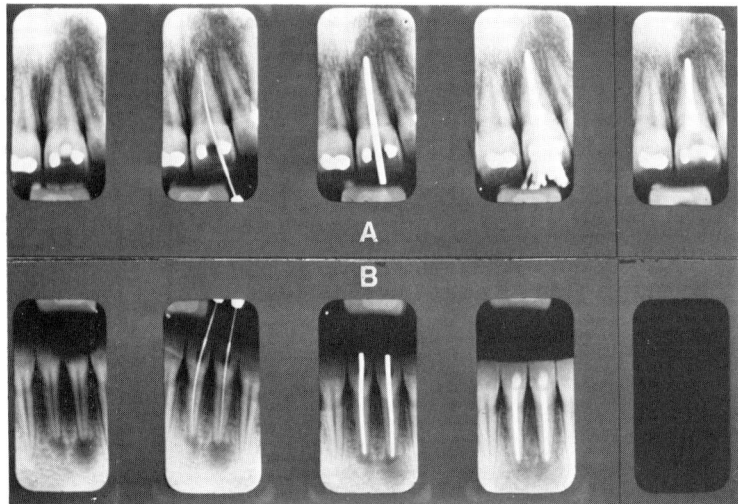

Figure 15-79. Various stages of the endodontic procedure when radiographs are indicated. **(A)** Maxillary central; **(B)** Mandibular centrals. (In both these cases the Rinn XCP instrument was used.)

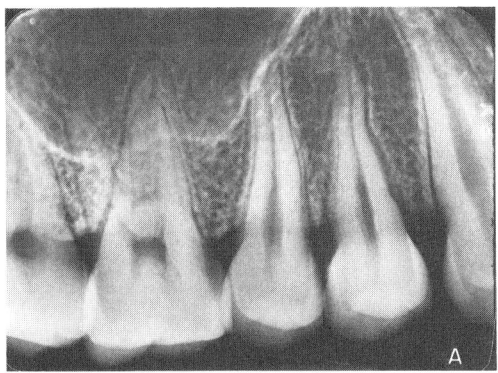
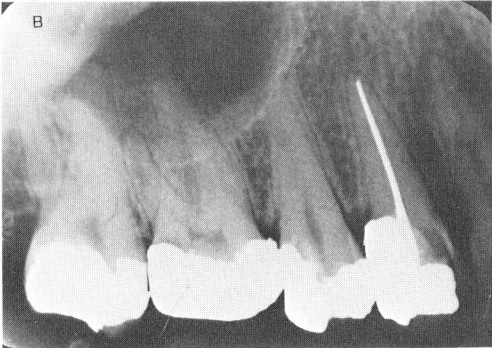

Figure 15-80. (A) Pre-operative endodontic radiograph. (B) Postoperative endodontic radiograph.

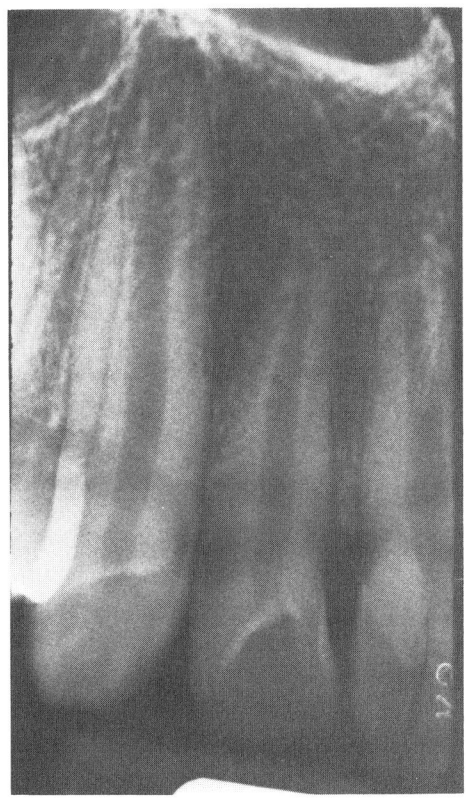

Figure 15-81. Endodontic preoperative radiograph should reveal tooth to be treated centrally located in radiograph — in this case, the maxillary lateral was tooth to be treated.

to assist in the initial **preoperative** evaluation and diagnosis of the tooth and its morphologic characteristics. After treatment there is a **post treatment** radiograph to demonstrate satisfactory obturation of the root canals. This is followed by periodic radiographs to monitor the treatment. There may be one or more **working radiographs** during the treatment phase including a **root length determination** radiograph with diagnostic instrument in place, **trial distance determination** radiographs, **working distance** radiographs of the silver or gutta percha cones in place, and **obturation** radiographs with sealer and gutta percha or silver cone in place (Fig. 15-79).

Pre-operative and postoperative treatment radiographs are made in the usual manner, preferably with a paralleling technique that provides the radiographs to aid in the diagnosis and evaluation of root morphology and final postoperative results (Fig. 15-80).

There are certain radiographic technical requirements that a **preoperative** or **diagnostic** endodontic radiograph must have:

1. If possible, the tooth being evaluated or undergoing endodontic treatment should be in the center of the radiograph (Fig. 15-81).

2. Radiographs should reveal at least 5

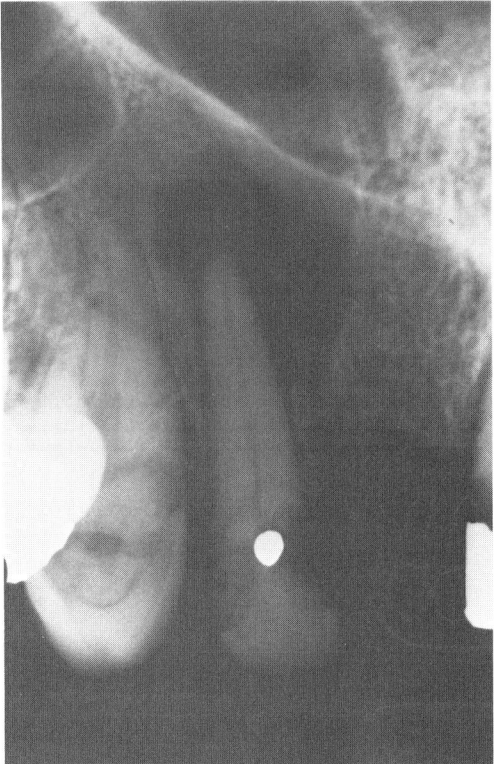

Figure 15-82. Large periapical lesion of maxillary lateral covered completely on radiograph.

mm of bone surrounding the apex of the tooth being evaluated or undergoing endodontic therapy (Fig. 15-80).

3. If a periapical lesion is too large to fit on a periapical film, supplemental diagnostic radiographs should be made (Fig. 15-82).
4. A single radiograph taken from one direction only may not provide sufficient diagnostic information when mulit-rooted teeth or teeth with curved roots are involved endodontically. Under these circumstances, at least two periapical radiographs should be taken to aid in gaining a three-dimensional perspective. One radiograph should be taken at a normal vertical and horizontal angulation, the other at a 20 degree horizontal angle either from the mesial or distal direction (Fig. 15-83).
5. If a sinus tract is present, a tracing radiograph is taken. This procedure is accomplished by threading a number 40 gutta percha cone into the tract through the fistulous opening and making a radiograph to identify the origin of the tract (Fig. 15-84). This procedure can also be useful in localizing the depth and course of certain periodontal defects.
6. Correct processing (especially proper fixing and washing of film) is necessary so film will have archival qualities at a later date. The pre- and postoperative radiographs should be taken by a good paralleling technique, because there is less dimensional distortion, greater image sharpness, and more ease in reproducing the same angulation for monitoring treatment at a later date.
7. The main concerns in endodontic radiography are those radiographic procedures used to take the working films, since it is not always feasible to utilize appropriate paralleling principle film holding and beam-alignment devices (such as the Rinn XCP instruments, Masel Precision instruments, Up-Rad VIP instruments, or the Green Stabe Biteblocks). The success of endodontic treatment is to a large degree dependent on the biomechanical instrumentation and obturation of the entire canal, so a working radiograph is taken with a diagnostic instrument in the canal prior to instrumentation of the canal.
8. Since routine radiographic procedures are difficult to use to take the **working radiograph,** it is necessary to utilize a radiographic procedure compatible

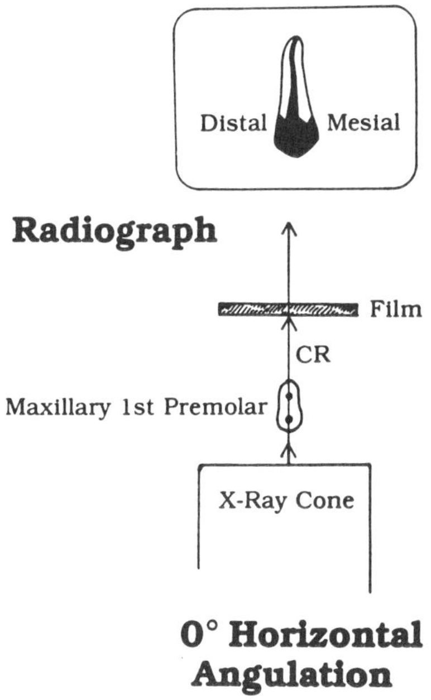

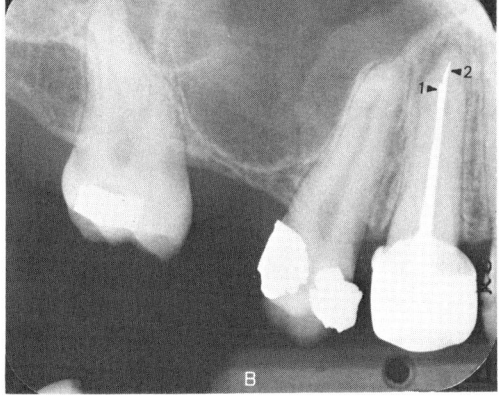
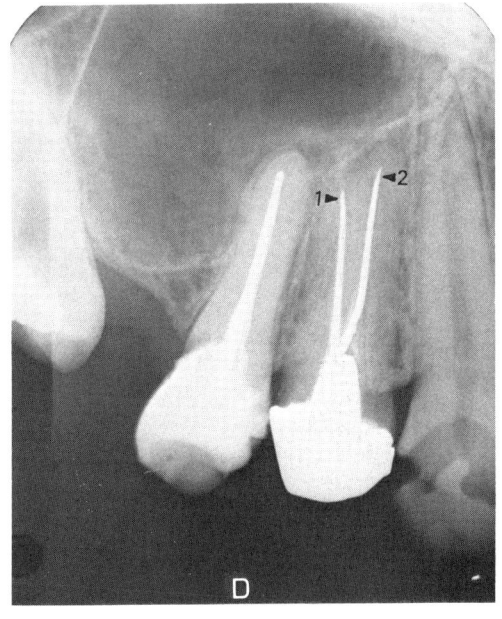

Figure 15-83. Buccal Object Rule in Endodontics. (A) First radiograph taken at 0 degree horizontal angulation. (B) Radiograph taken at 0 degree H. A. with canals superimposed in maxillary first premolar. (C) second radiograph taken with 20 degree distal horizontal angulation. (D) second radiograph taken with 20 degree H.A. revealing facial or buccal canal moving distally (#1) and lingual canal (#2) moving mesially. (Note that crown on maxillary first premolar has been removed.) The preoperative radiograph (B) was taken prior to placing root canal restoration in second premolar as shown in (D).

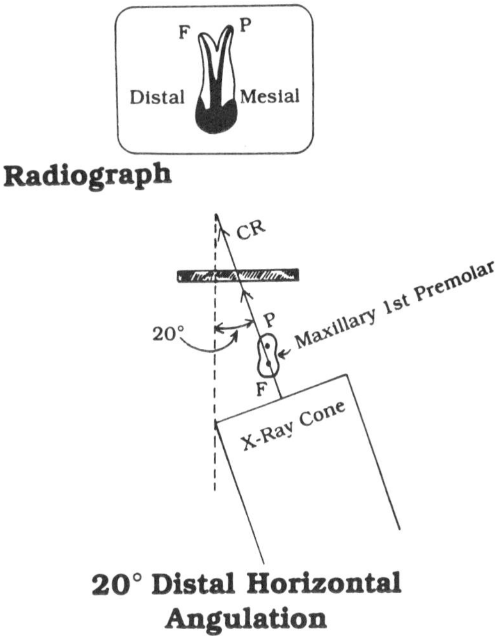

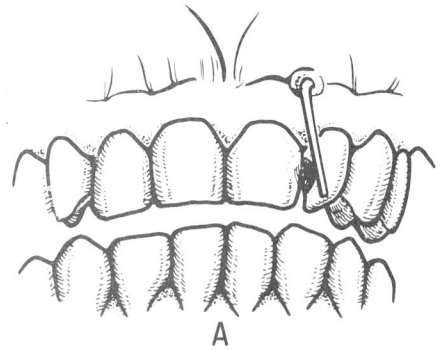

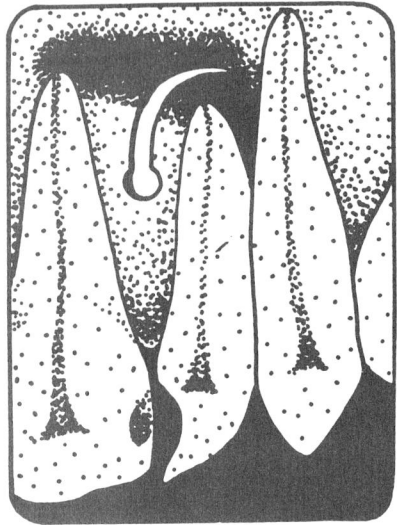

Figure 15-84. Using gutta percha cones to determine origin of sinus tract. (A) Diagram of sinus opening with gutta percha cone in it. (B) Diagram of radiograph of (A) with gutta percha point in sinus tract indicating which tooth has periapical lesion.

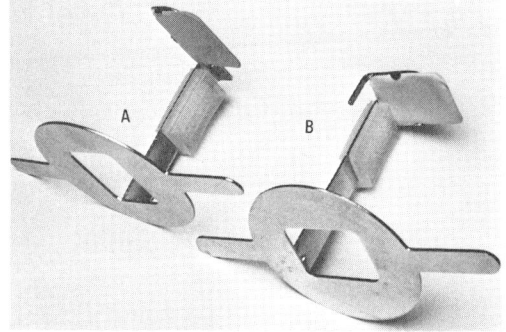

Figure 15-85. Masel Precision Endodontic Instruments. Arm is offset in these instruments so radiograph may be taken without removing file, reamers, or rubber dam clamp. (A) Upper left and lower right posterior instrument. (B) Anterior wide film — right instrument. (Isaac Masel Co., Philadelphia, PA.)

Modified Snap-a-Ray Endodontic Film Holding Instrument (Paralleling Technique)

To overcome the difficulties of making radiographs during endodontic procedures, the Snap-A-Ray film holding instrument was modified by Paquette et al. in 1979. It simplifies the stabilization of the fim in the patient's mouth as well as aiding the operator to position the cone properly in relation to the film. This is especially useful since the film most of the time is hidden from view in endodontic radiography (Fig. 15-87).

Radiographic Technique for Anterior Teeth

Assembly of the modified Snap-A-Ray unit is as shown in figure 15-88. To take the radiograph, remove the rubber dam frame. Insert the assembled instrument making sure that the tooth is centered on the film and the film is parallel to the long axis of the tooth. The edge of the film contacting the soft tissues should be approximatly 1.5-2.5 cm palatal to the incisal edge of the tooth being radiographed. In the anterior mandibular arch, position the

with film placement when the rubber dam clamp, root canal instruments, or obturating materials are in position. Since the patient cannot close on a bite-block, it becomes necessary to stablize the film by means of the patient's finger or various **modified film holders** (Figs. 15-85, 15-86).

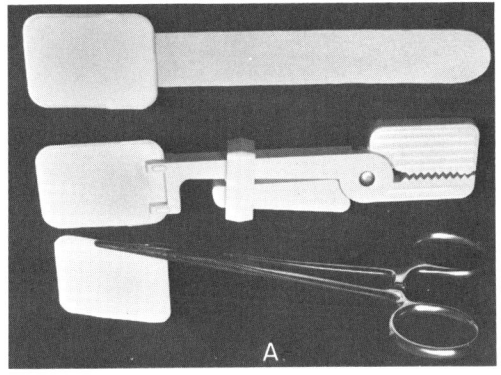
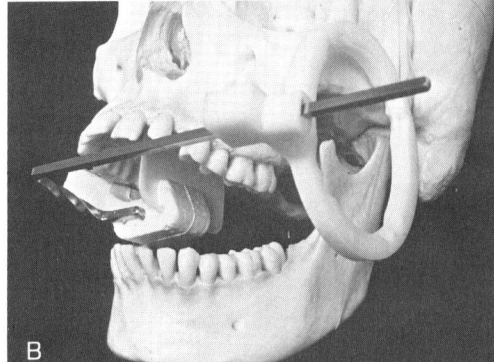
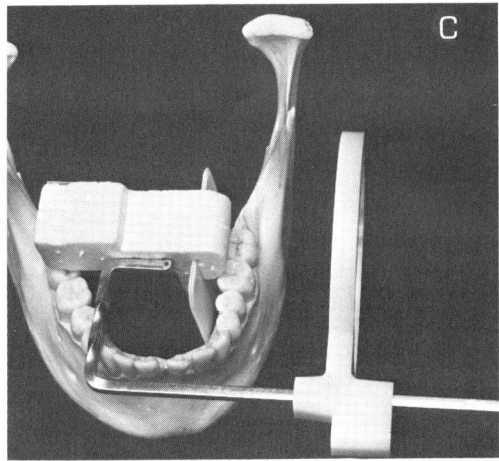

Figure 15-86. Instruments to hold film in patient's mouth for endodontic radiography. **(A)** Anterior film holders: (top) tongue blade, (middle) ADA Snap-A-Ray, (bottom) hemostat. **(B)** Rinn endodontic maxillary posterior film holder. **(C)** Rinn endodontic mandibular posterior film holder.

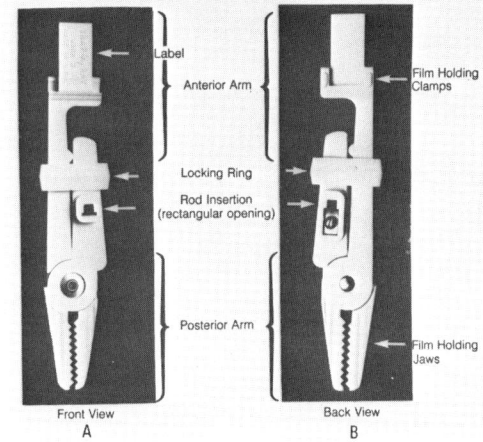
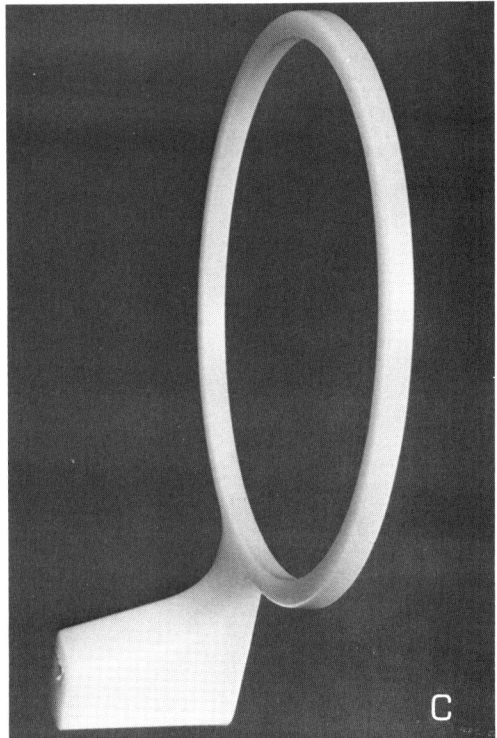
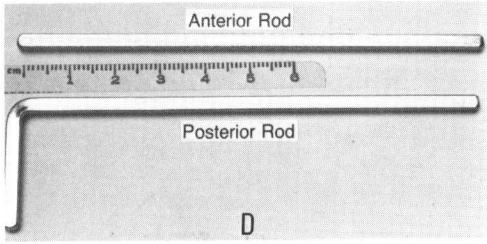

Figure 15-87. Modified Snap-A-Ray Mark II film holder for endodontic radiography. **(A)** Front view, **(B)** Back view, **(C)** Beam alignment ring, **(D)** Anterior and posterior rods.

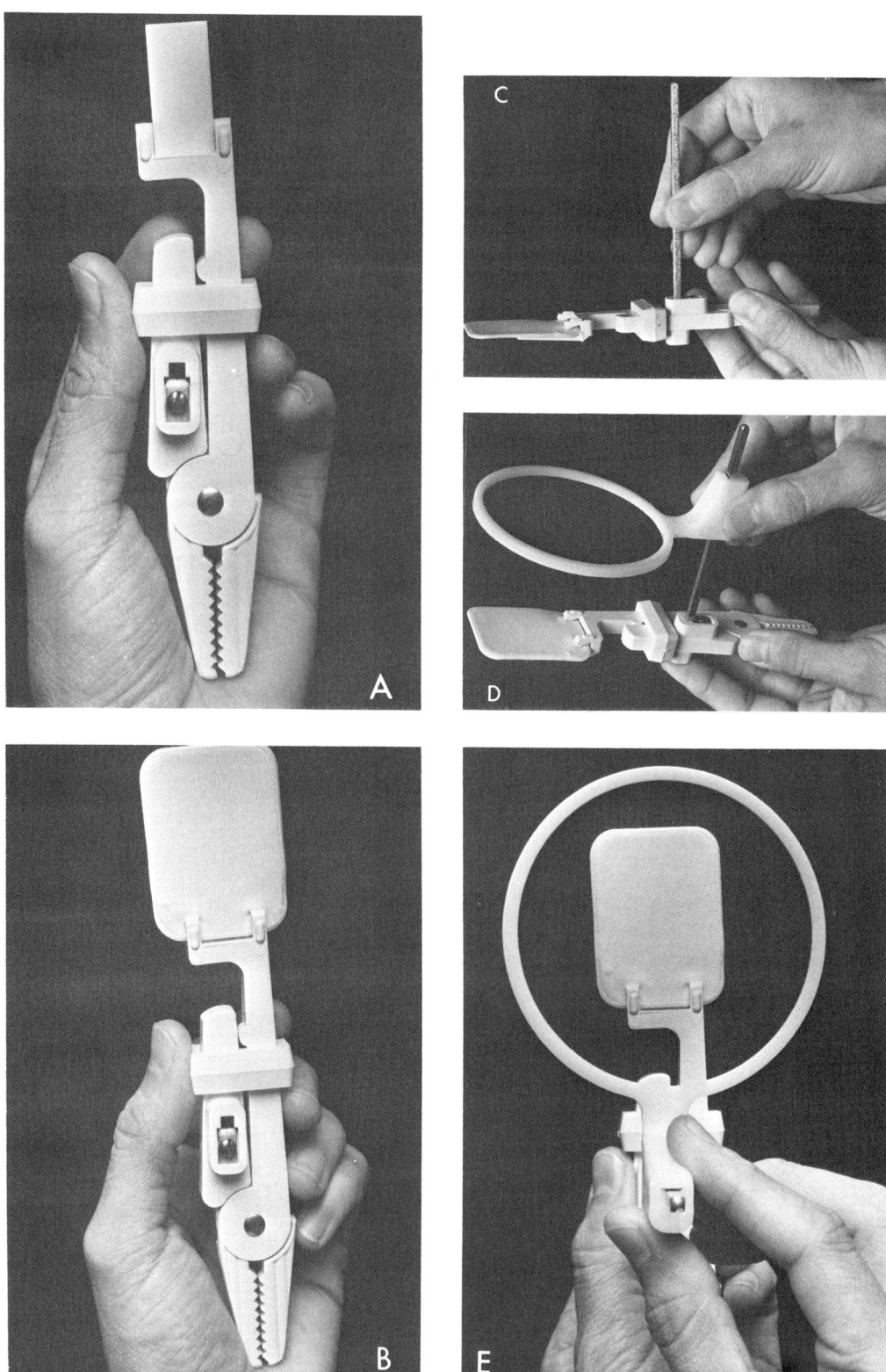

Figure 15-88. Endodontic radiographic technic for anterior teeth using modified Snap-A-Ray Mark II. **(A)** Hold film in this position to place film in anterior slot. **(B)** Film anterior slot. **(C)** Inserting anterior rod into Snap-A-Ray. **(D)** Placing alignment ring on rod. **(E)** Film centered on ring (ready for use).

edge of the film away from the muscle attachments to allow the floor of the mouth to relax to accommodate the depth of the film packet. Instruct the patient to hold the instrument firmly and apply gentle pressure against the incisal third of the teeth in the opposite arch. Slide the beam alignment ring along the rod gently, until

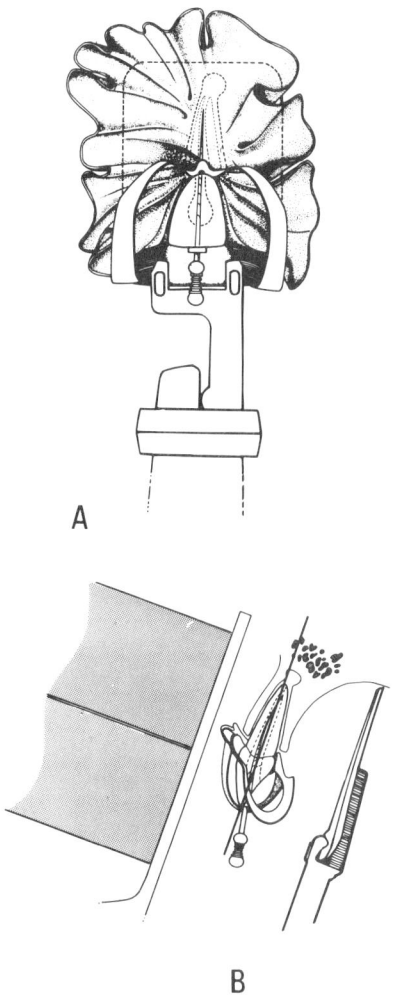

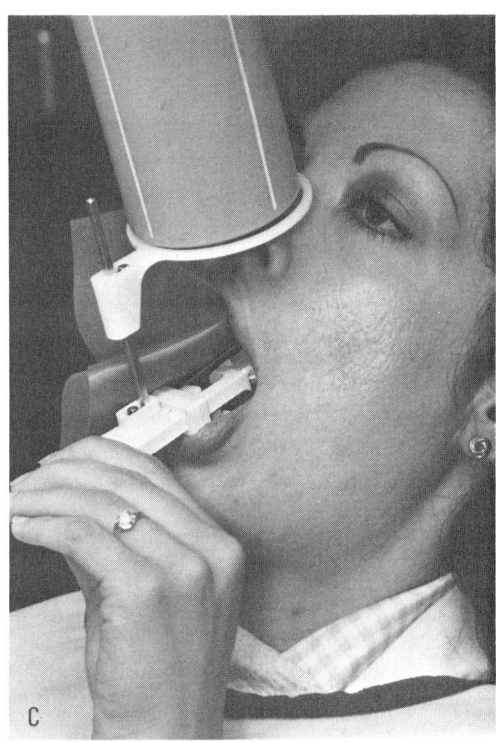

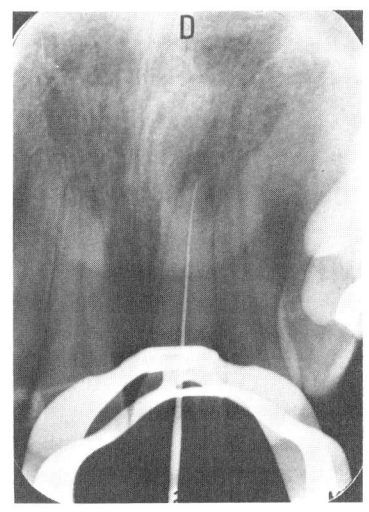

Figure 15-89. Position of film, film holder, and cone to take working radiograph of maxillary anterior teeth. (A) Diagram of position of cone and film (front view). (B) Side view of A. (C) Photo of patient being radiographed for maxillary anterior teeth. (D) Working radiograph of maxillary central. (From Preece, J.; Del Rio, C., and Canales, M.: *A Radiographic Technique for Endodontics.* The University of Texas Health Science Center at San Antonio.)

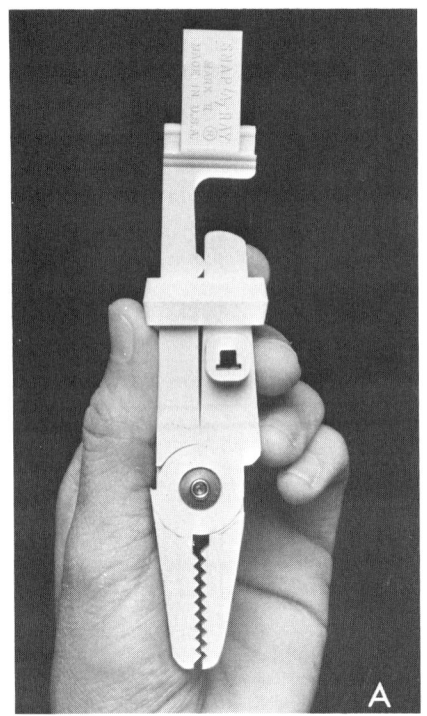
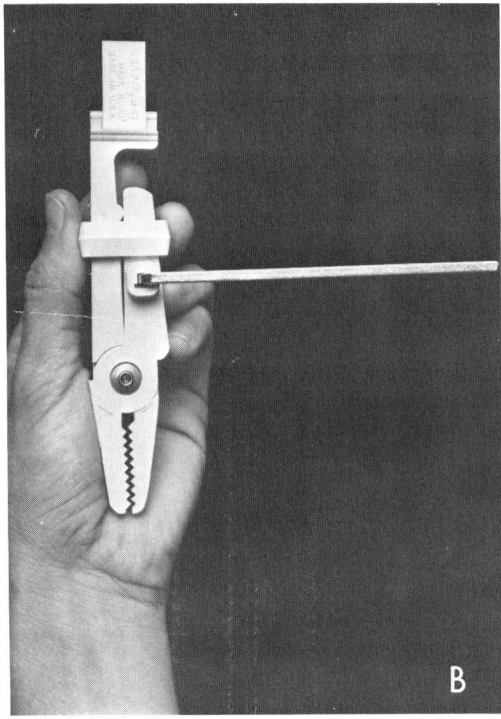
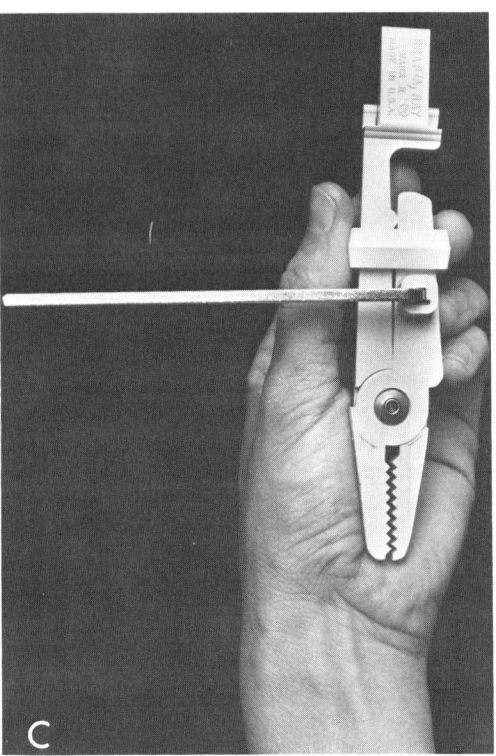
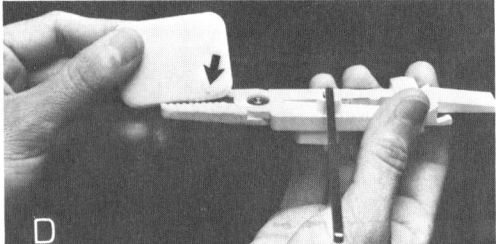

Figure 15-90. Modified Snap-A-Ray mark II endodontic radiographic technic for posterior teeth. (A) Holding instrument prior to placement of rod, film, and alignment ring. (B) Rod placement for mandibular left or maxillary right. (C) Rod placement for mandibular right or maxillary left. (D) Placing film in jaws of instrument. (E) Placing alignment ring on rod. (F) Centering film in alignment ring.

Atlas of Special Techniques in Dental Radiology 575

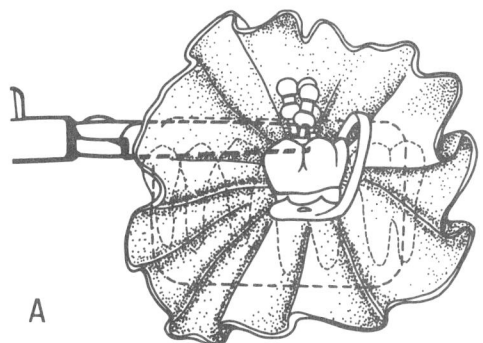

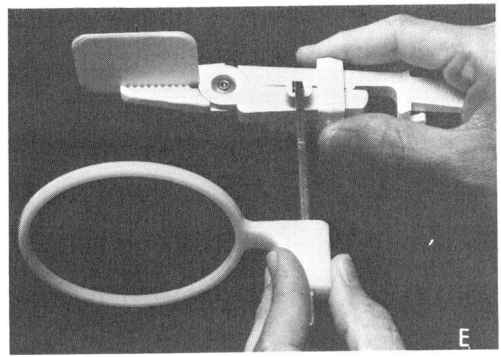

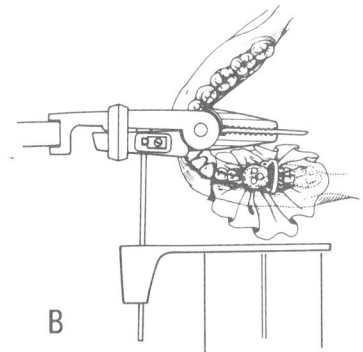

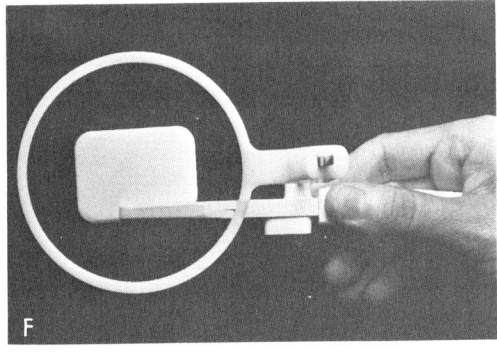

it lightly contacts the skin. Align the x-ray cone (P.I.D.) and alignment ring to obtain the correct vertical and horizontal angulations. Make the exposure and replace the rubber dam frame (Fig. 15-89).

Endodontic Radiographic Technique for Posterior Teeth

Assemble the posterior modified Snap-A-Ray unit as shown in Figure 15-90. Remove the rubber dam frame and insert the assembled instrument, making sure that the tooth being treated is centered on film. Position the film parallel to the long axis of the tooth. Instruct the patient to hold the instrument firmly in position and apply gentle pressure against the incisal edges of the anterior teeth in the same arch. For mandibular radiographs, posi-

Figure 15-91. Placement of film for taking endodontic "working radiograph" of mandibular molar region using Snap-A-Ray Mark II. (**A**) Lateral view of instrument in position to take "working radiograph" of mandibular first molar. (**B**) Top view of instrument in position to take "working radiograph" of mandibular first molar. (**C**) Patient with instrument in place for mandibular molar endodontic working radiograph. (**D**) Left first molar radiograph taken with modified Snap-A-Ray mark II film holder. (Radiograph mounted with raised dot away from viewer as though film was viewed from inside of patient's mouth.) (**E**) Radiograph taken of first molar in (**D**) with 20° distal angulation. (**F**) Radiograph taken with 20 degree distal angulation as shown in (**E**). Notice how buccal cusp of second premolar has moved distally. Therefore, the mesiobuccal root canal is distally placed to mesiolingual root canal in this radiograph. (From Preece, J.; Del Rio, C.; and Canales, M.: *A Radiographic Technique for Endodontics.* The University of Texas Health Science Center at San Antonio.)

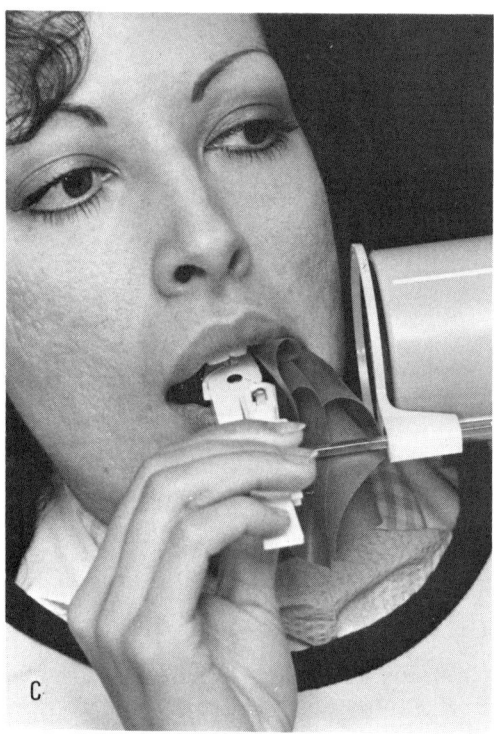
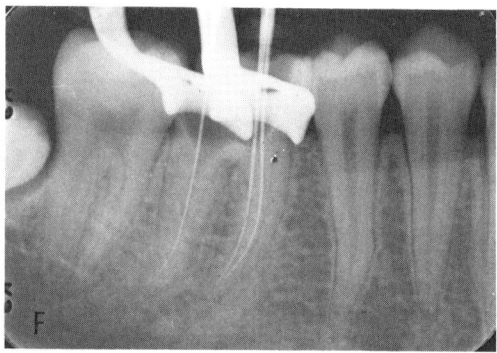
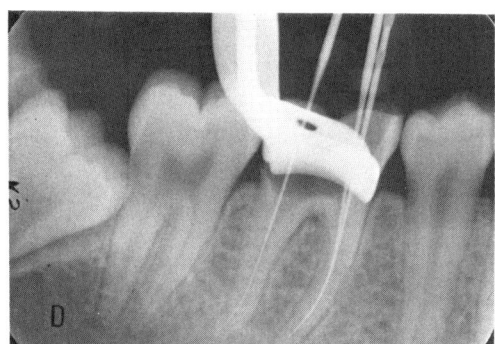

tion the film between the teeth and the tongue, making sure the lower edge of the film does not impinge on the muscle attachments in the floor of the mouth. Be sure the patient does not displace the film by movement of the tongue or swallowing when making mandibular radiographs. Slide the beam alignment ring along the rod gently until it lightly contacts the skin. Align the x-ray cone (P.I.D.) with rod and alignment ring for the correct vertical and horizontal angulations. Make the exposure and replace the rubber dam frame (Fig. 15-91A, B, C).

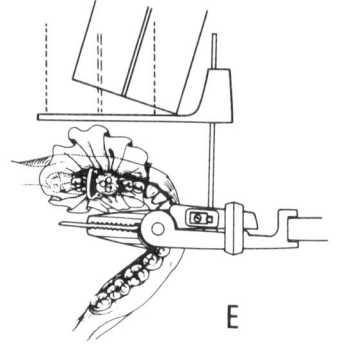
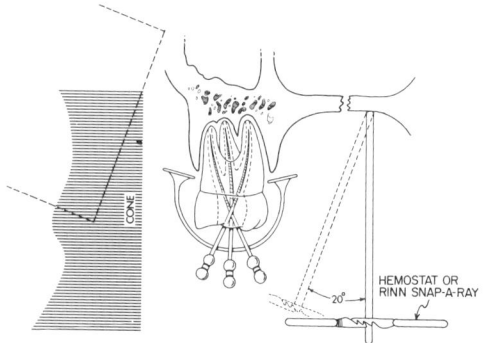

Figure 15-92. Maxillary posterior 20° using Paralleling Technic. (From Preece, J.; Del Rio, C., and Canales, M.: *A Radiographic Technique for Endodontics.* The University of Texas Health Science Center at San Antonio.)

Atlas of Special Techniques in Dental Radiology 577

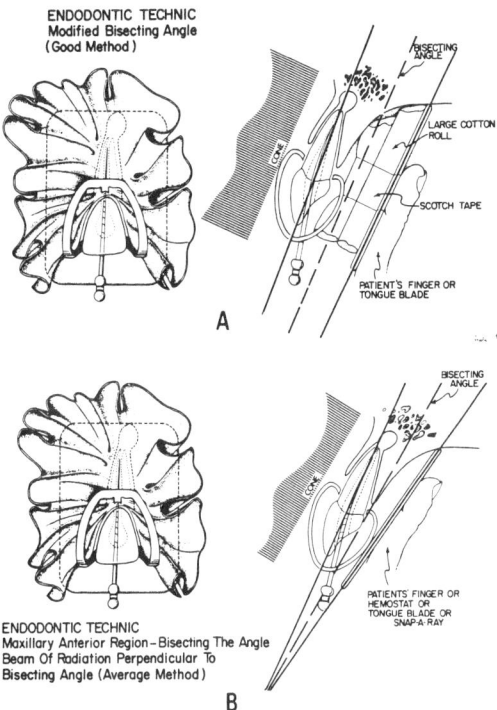

Figure 15-93. Anterior Bisecting Technics in Edodontic Radiography. (A) Cotton roll technic. (B) Digital technic. (From Preece, J.; Del Rio, C.; and Canales, M.: *A Radiographic Technique for Endodontics*. The University of Texas Health Science Center at San Antonio.)

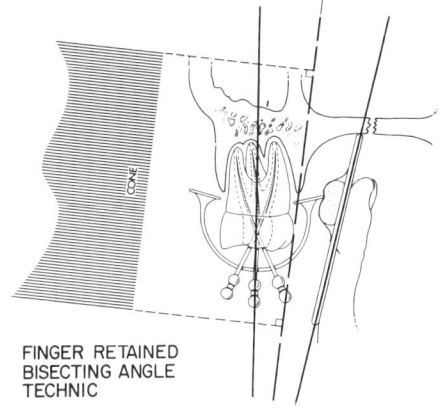

Figure 15-94. Posterior Maxillary Bisecting Technic in Endodontic Radiography. (From Preece, J.; Del Rio, C.; and Canales, M.: *A Radiographic Technique for Endodontics*. The University of Texas Health Science Center at San Antonio.)

Angulated radiographs can be achieved by moving the cone 20 degrees in a mesial or distal horizontal projection (Fig. 15-91D, E, F).

Endodontic Maxillary Posterior Projections

When radiographing the maxillary premolar and molar regions, the procedure of choice is the paralleling principle or the paralleling 20 degree compromise technique. In the 20 degree compromise technique the film is placed as parallel as possible (within 20 degrees) to the long axis of the tooth and the beam of radiation directed perpendicular to the film. If paralleling can be approximated, the image will be superior to a routine bisecting-angle film of the area (Fig. 15-92).

Bisecting Angle Technique for Endodontic Procedures

Anterior Region

If for various reasons the paralleling technique is unsatisfactory, the next best procedure would be to tape two large cotton rolls to a film and then tape both to a tongue depressor or have the patient hold the film-cotton roll combination against the area of interest. The cotton rolls position the film farther away from the crown of the tooth and permit at least partially placing the film more nearly parallel to the long axis of the tooth. The beam of radiation is then directed perpendicular to the film plane, or perpendicular to a plane bisecting the long axis of tooth and film (Fig. 15-93).

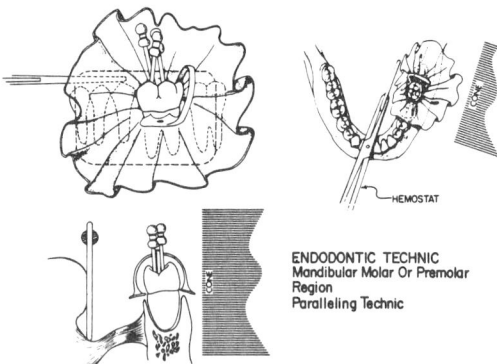

Figure 15-95. Posterior Mandibular Paralleling Technic in Endodontic Radiography using the hemostat or Snap-A-Ray/EEZEE Grip. The Snap-A-Ray is now being distributed by Ada Products. The Rinn Corp. makes a similar instrument called the EEZEE Grip. (From Preece, J.; Del Rio, C.; and Canales, M.: *A Radiographic Technique for Endodontics*. The University of Texas Health Science Center at San Antonio.)

Maxillary Posterior Region

In the maxillary posterior region, the best digital bisecting angle technique is taping a cotton roll to the film. The patient supports the film a little farther away from the crowns, decreasing the amount of vertical angulation required to direct the beam perpendicular to the bisecting plane between the long axis of the molar and the film. The resultant radiograph generally demonstrates less foreshortening of the buccal roots and less elongation of the lingual roots of the molars, which is typical of the conventional bisecting angle technique (Fig. 15-94).

Mandibular Posterior Region

In the mandibular premolar and molar regions, the paralleling or modified 20 degree paralleling method can usually be followed without any difficulty because the teeth are in most cases almost vertically parallel to the midsagittal plane. Therefore, a hemostat or Ada Snap-A-Ray/Rinn EEZEE Grip holding the film in position is acceptable (Fig. 15-95).

PEDIATRIC DENTAL RADIOGRAPHY

The radiograph is an essential part in the diagnosis of dental disease. Radiographs of children will reveal many conditions that cannot be discovered by any other method. There are no known alternatives to dental radiographs. However, the frequency of radiographic exposures may be minimized by a thorough clinical examination with the use of visualization, transillumination, auscultation, percussion, and palpation. Without radiographs it is often impossible to identify dental disease and to plan appropriate treatment. This could result in (1) irreversible damage to the teeth, alveolar bone, and other oral tissues; (2) compromised treatment; (3) increased risk of failure; and (4) more costly care.

Since there is always a presumed risk involved when a patient is exposed to radiation, radiographs should be prescribed to children (adults as well) according to individual needs and only after a complete review and evaluation of their dental, oral, and general health by the dentist. The decision to take radiographs should be based on the expected benefit to the patient.

Criteria for Exposing Children to X-radiation

Clinical indications for radiographs for children to provide optimum care follow:

Injury: (Trauma to teeth and facial bones.) The most common reason for a young child to visit a dental office is trauma. If there is mobility of the tooth, a radiograph would reveal displacement or root fracture. In absence of mobility, one must weigh the risk versus benefit in deciding whether the information from the radiographs will direct treatment.

Caries Detection: It is difficult to detect interproximal caries without the use of bite-wing radiographs. Since younger children often have spaces between their posterior teeth (Fig. 15-96), one should defer taking bite-wing radiographs until all posterior spacing is closed. If indicated, bite-wing radiographs for caries detection are usually taken every 12-18 months in the absence of dental caries with primary tooth contact or every 24 months with permanent tooth contact (Fig. 15-97). The child with a **high risk** of dental caries should have bite-wing radiographs made as soon as posterior primary teeth are in contact. If interproximal caries is detected, then follow-up radiographs are indicted semiannually until the child is caries-free and therefore classified as a low risk to dental caries (Fig. 15-98). A high caries risk child will be associated with (1) poor oral hygiene, (2) fluoride deficiency, (3) prolonged nursing (bottle or breast), (4) high carbohydrate diet, (5) poor family dental health, (6) developmental enamel defects, (7) developmental disability, (8) chronic medical history, and (9) genetic abnormality.

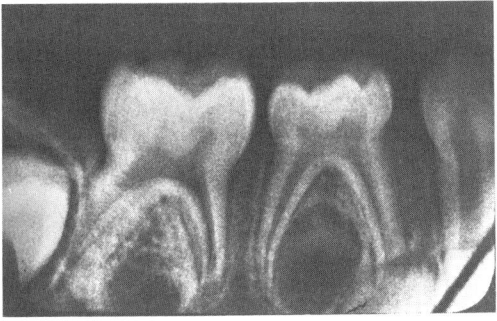

Figure 15-96. Posterior periapical radiograph of child under five years with spaces between teeth. (Note the beginning calcification of buds of premolars.)

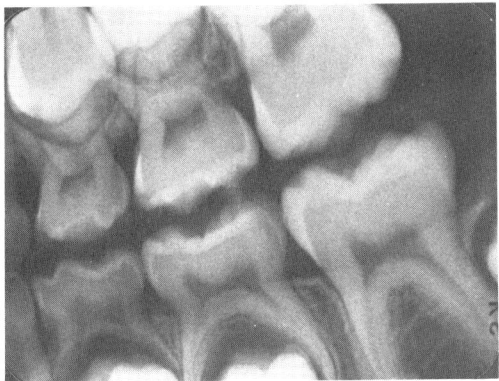

Figure 15-97. Posterior bite-wing radiograph of child with no dental caries and tooth contact. (Notice erupting premolars underneath the primary molars.)

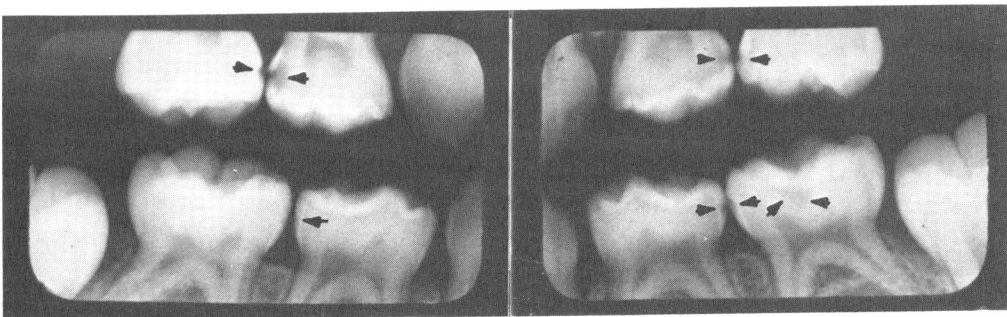

Figure 15-98. Posterior bite-wing radiograph of high risk caries child six years of age or under.

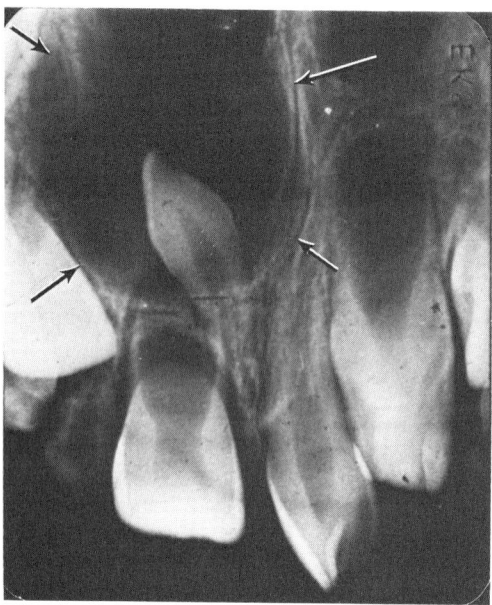

Figure 15-99. Large dentigerous cyst surrounding mesiodens with symptoms of swelling and pain. Note erupted supernumerary tooth between permanent maxillary central incisors.

Detection of periapical and bone pathosis. Tooth-related infections require radiographic confirmation. It is important to know the extent of the pathoses before making diagnosis and providing care (Fig. 15-99).

Developmental and Pathologic Conditions. These include detection of congenital and developmental anomalies, pathologic conditions, eruption patterns, space loss, calcification patterns and degree of development of teeth, arch position of developing teeth, ankylosis, foreign bodies, retained primary tooth roots, and primary root resorption patterns (Fig. 15-100). A cephalometric radiograph may be prescribed by the dentist who is providing orthodontic diagnosis and/or treatment.

Posttreatment Monitoring. This is for conditions where there is need to evaluate previous treatment (Fig. 15-101).

Complete Radiographic Surveys for Children

If it has been determined by the dentist

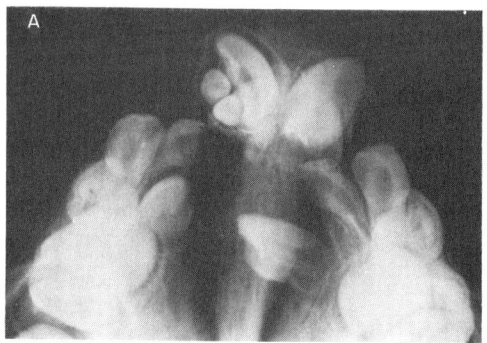
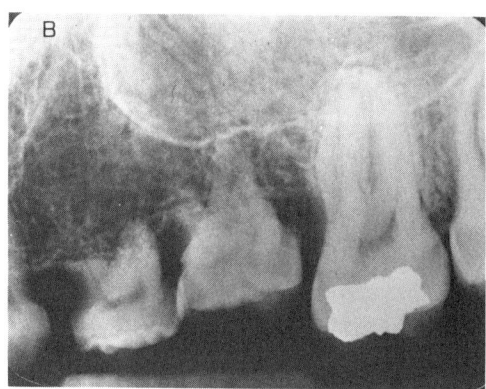

Figure 15-100. Developmental and Pathological Problems. **(A)** Double cleft palate case with several impacted teeth, and a possible compound odontoma. **(B)** Congenitally missing premolar teeth with retained primary molars. **(C)** Several congenitally missing teeth including mandibular central incisors. Also, impacted lower left second premolar and rampant caries of maxillary incisors. **(D)** Solitary bone cyst (traumatic bone cyst) female, age twelve, years in right mandible (Note earring left on patient.)

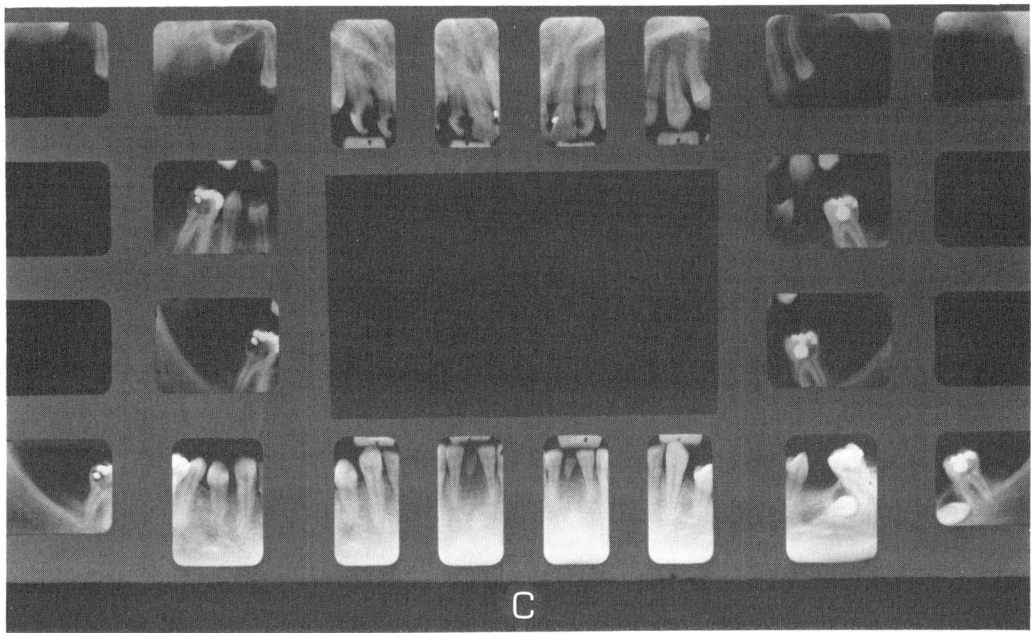

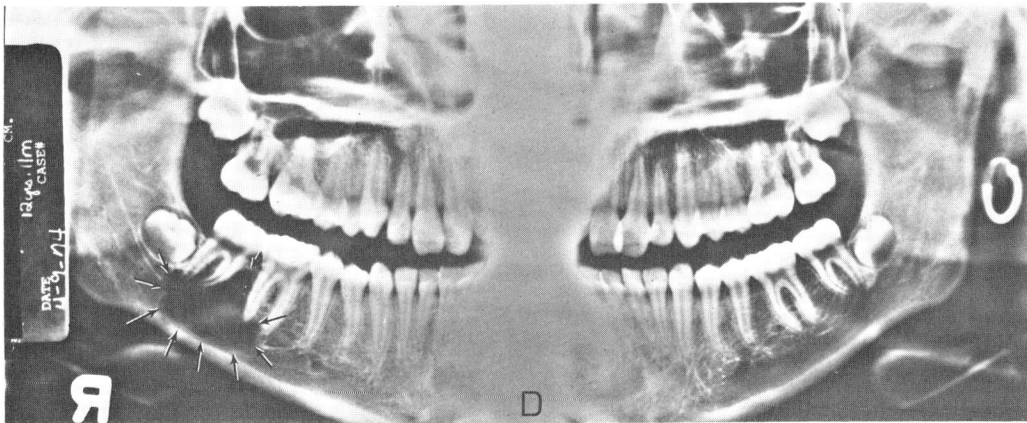

that the child requires a pedodontic complete radiographic survey, the final factor to be considered is the number and size of films to be used in the survey. The age and behavior of the child may very well determine the type of radiographic survey to be made. However, irrespective of the size and number of films, the mouth survey must be complete to be considered a survey. It must reveal all the present and developing dentition and oral conditions of the patient.

Definitive diagnosis and subsequent treatment planning is often contingent upon a pediatric radiographic evaluation. The value of radiographs cannot be over-

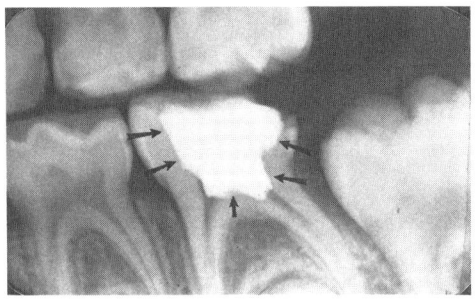

Figure 15-101. Evaluation of previous treatment (pulpotomy) of mandibular second primary molar. Should also take periapical of this tooth to evaluate root apices.

emphasized.

Panoramic radiography appears unequaled in evaluating growth and developmental patterns in the young child, the preadolescent, and adolescent. It may be used as a substitute for an intraoral complete mouth survey of a very young child unable to tolerate intraoral films or for those children who gag easily. However, the panoramic radiograph is not sufficient to interpret caries, periodontal disease, periapical pathosis, and other pathological conditions. Therefore, it is recommended that posterior bite-wings and indicated periapical and occlusal films be used to supplement the panoramic radiographic examination (Fig. 15-102).

Periapical Complete Mouth Survey in Children

The following complete periapical radiographic surveys are recommended for

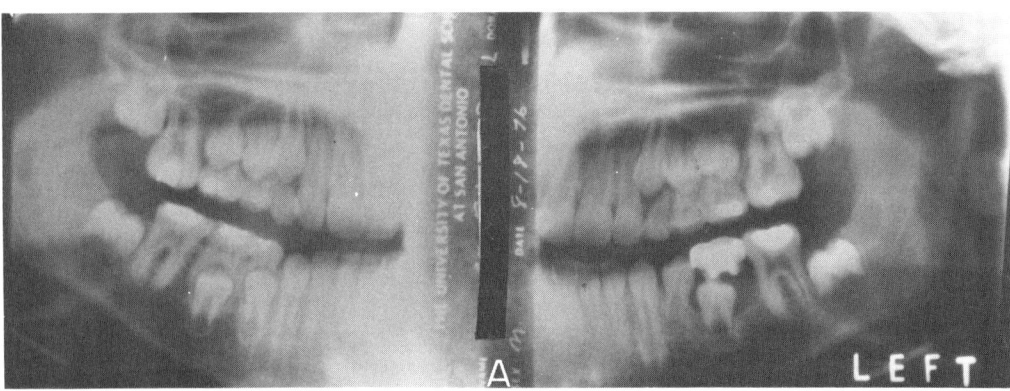

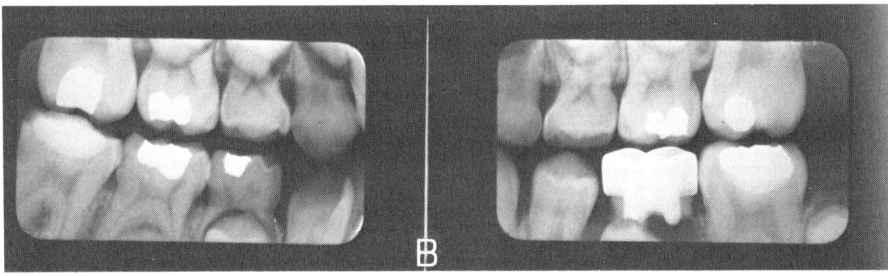

Figure 15-102. Panormaic survey with posterior bite-wings of same patient. Radiographs supplement each other. **(A)** Panoramic radiographs; **(B)** Posterior bite-wings.

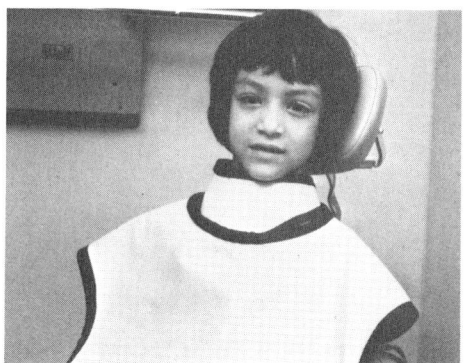

Figure 15-103. Torso and thyroid shield for child.

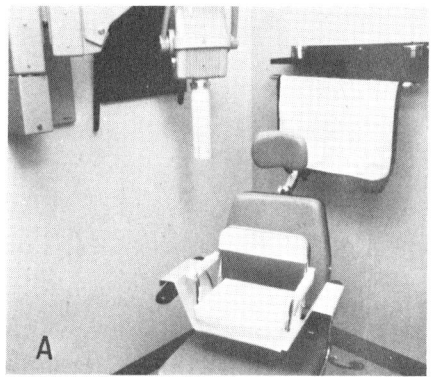

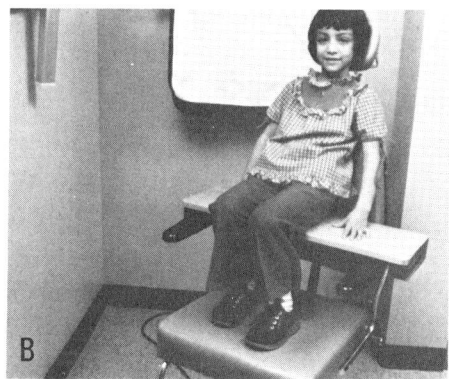

Figure 15-104. Types of chairs for smaller child. **(A)** Commercial child's chair made by S.S. White Co.; **(B)** Child's seat made to fit on adult chair's arms.

three groups of children: (1) **The early eruptive stage** (5 years and younger); (2) **Mixed dentition group** (6-9 years); (3) **preadolescent group** (10-12 years). Of course, these are only guidelines to follow because some children are large for their age while others are small for their age. The important thing to remember is that radiography for children has to be flexible, and the type of radiographic technique, film size, and the number of films to be ordered is unique for each child.

It is recommended that to minimize exposure to children, radiographs should be taken with a long cone, paralleling, high kVp technique using the fastest diagnostic film available, rectangular collimation (if possible), and film holders with beam aiming devices. The patient should be shielded with a torso lead apron (to protect the body and gonads) and a lead cervical collar (to protect the thyroid) (Fig. 15-103).

The Early Eruptive Stage (5 years and under)

Children in this age group will most likely need a child's chair attached to the adult chair to conveniently take radiographs (Fig. 15-104). A complete radiographic film survey for the early eruptive stage (5 years and under) is shown in Figure 15-105. Radiographic instruments needed to take a complete survey of children in this age group are as follows: (1) No. 2 regular adult film to use for anterior occlusals, (2) Rinn EEZEE Grip or Ada Snap-A-Ray filmholder with No. 0 pedo film, and (3) bite-wing tabs for size No. 0 pedo film (Fig. 106).

Occlusal Radiography

The anterior occlusal films are taken

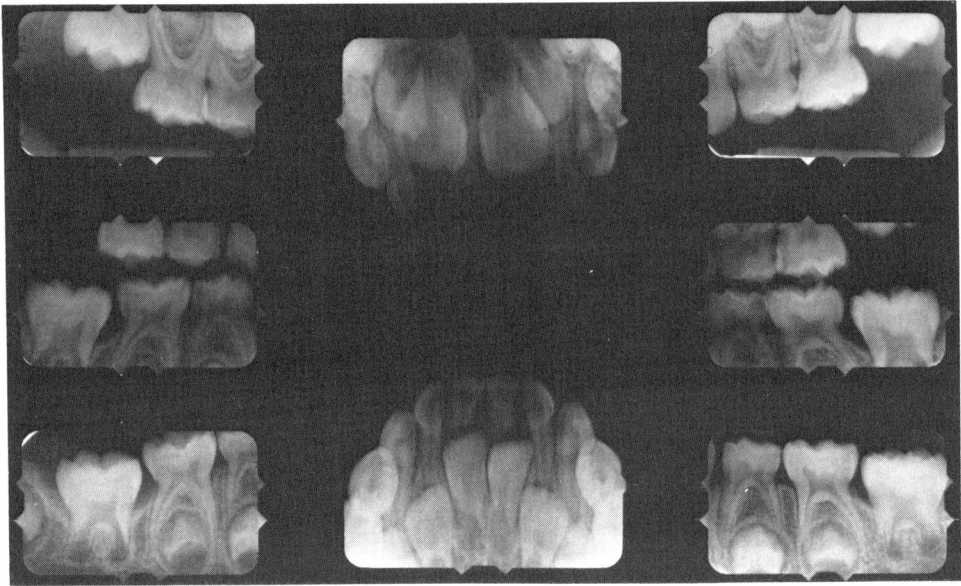

Figure 15-105. Complete periapical survey for early eruptive years (5 years and under).

using No. 2 regular periapical film for occlusal film. It works very well in the small mouths of children in this age group. It also reduces exposure to the child and is tolerated well. The vertical angulation is a +60 degrees for the maxillary occlusal and a -15 degrees (cone upwards) vertical angulation for the mandibular occlusal directing the beam perpendicular to a line that bisects the angle formed by the incisors and the film (Fig. 15-107). There is a modification of this technique that can be

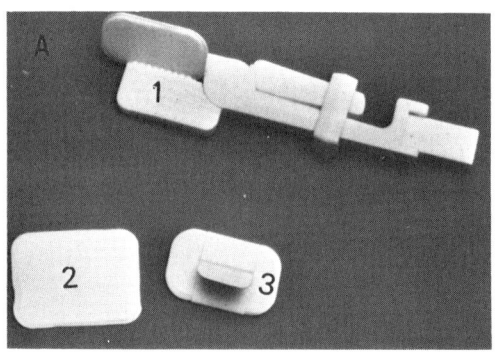 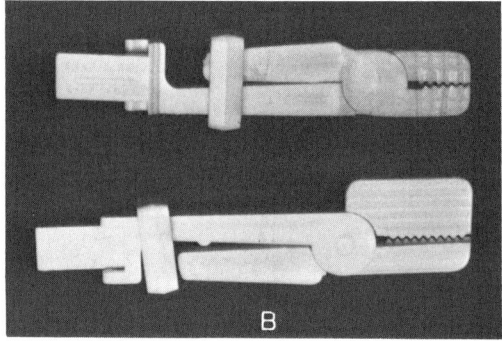

Figure 15-106. Supplies needed to take Early Eruption Stage (5 years and under) complete periapical survey and posterior bite-wings. (A) (#1) Rinn EEZEE Grip or Ada Snap-A-Ray with pedo 0 film for posterior projections. (#2) No. 2 film for occlusal anterior projections. (#3) Pedo 0 film with bite-wing tab. (B) Special child's film holder made from Rinn EEZEE Grip film holder. Compare with size of regular EEZEE Grip filmholder at bottom of photograph.

used if the dentist is just interested in taking a maxillary and mandibular occlusal of a child. It is a rapid method utilizing just one large occlusal film, and folding it in half. It is called the **sandwich occlusal film technique** (Fig. 15-108).

A rectangular collimated occlusal technique is available by using the Masel/ Elcan Occlusal precision instrument. This

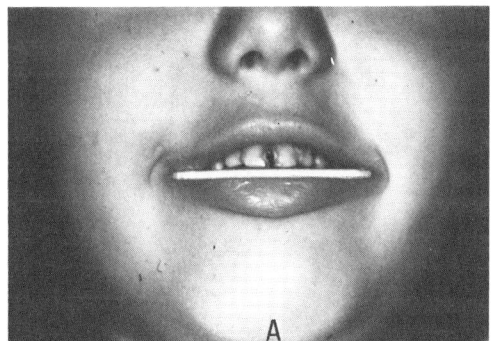

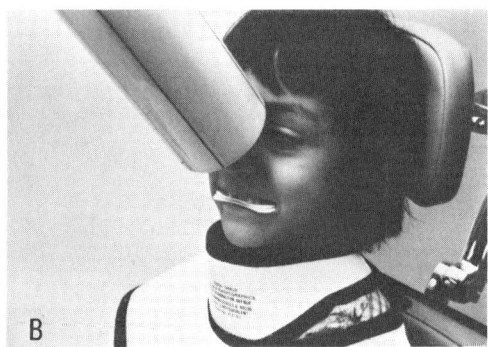

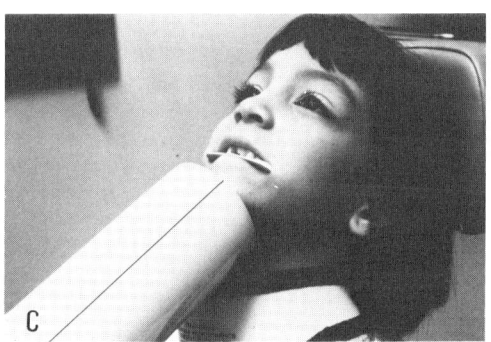

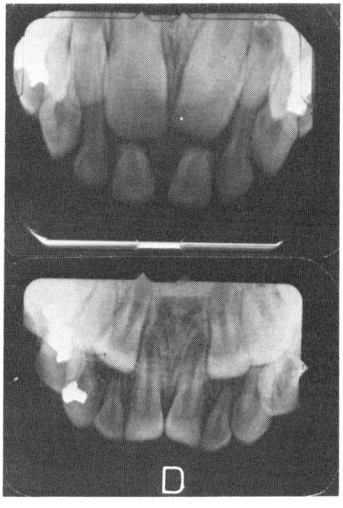

Figure 15-107. Maxillary and mandibular occlusals for children five years and under. (A) Placement of No. 2 regular dental film for maxillary occlusal radiograph. (B) Maxillary occlusal projection. (Film is regular occlusal film folded over itself.) A No. 2 regular film is recommended for children in the five years and under age group. The central ray is directed at a vertical angle of +60 to +65 degrees through bridge of nose, to center of packet. (C) Mandibular occlusal projection. (Film shown here is regular occlusal film folded over itself; however, a No. 2 regular film is recommended for children of this age.) The CR is directed perpendicularly to center of packet. (D) Maxillary and mandibular occlusal radiographs taken with No. 2 regular size film of child five years of age.

instrument will collimate the radiation at the child's face and reduce the radiation exposure to the patient by approximately 50 percent (Fig. 15-109).

Posterior Periapical Radiography

The Rinn XCP and BAI posterior bite-blocks can be modified to use for the pedo No. 0 film for children under five years of age. The backing plate is cut down to a level slightly lower than the height of the film and the length of the biting portion is reduced on XCP bite-blocks but remains the same on the BAI bite-

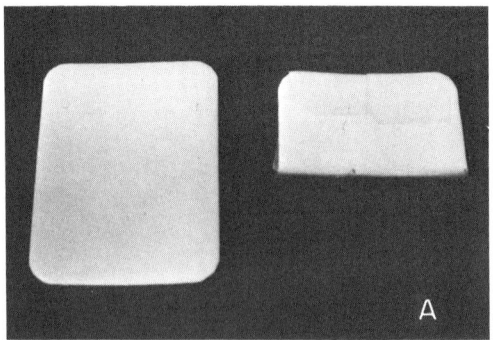

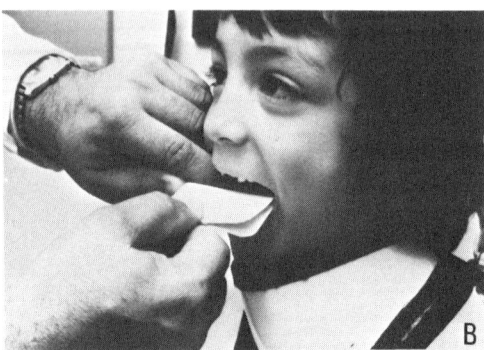

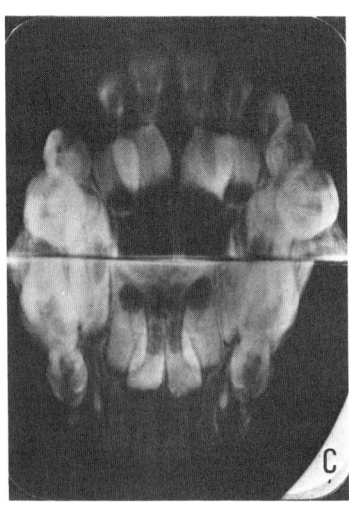

Figure 15-108. Sandwich occlusal film technic. (A) Occlusal film folded in half. (B) Placing occlusal film in mouth; radiographs are taken of maxillary and mandibular arches on one occlusal film. (C) Sandwich occlusal radiograph of child five years of age. Note maxillay occlusal above and mandibular occlusal below.

blocks (Fig. 15-110). If a rectangular P.I.D. is used, this technique has the advantage of patient exposure reduction by rectangular collimation of x-ray beam.

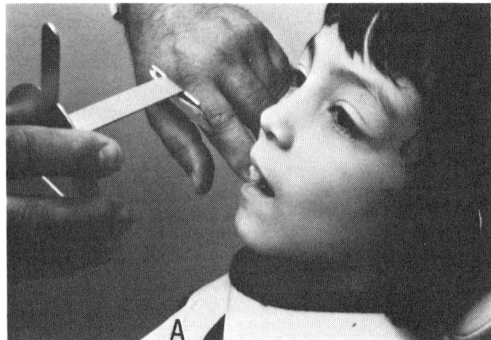

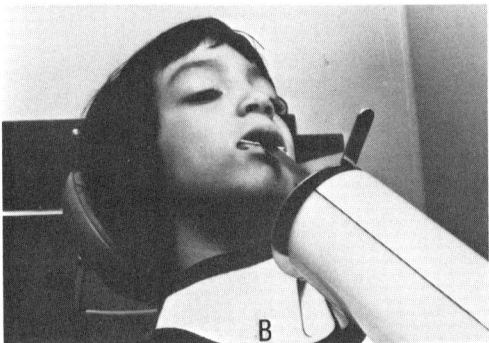

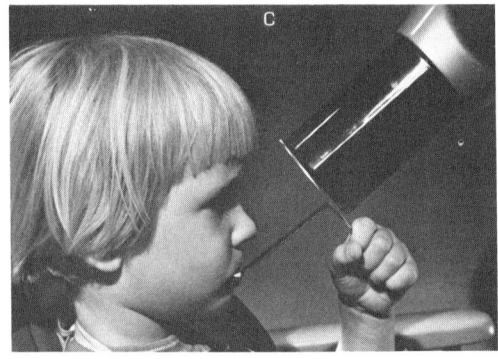

Figure 15-109. Masel "Elcan Occlusal" film technic. (A) Instrument is shown being positioned for lower anterior occlusal view. (B) Shielded cone is aligned with collimator window and shield. (C) Instrument positioned for maxillary occlusal view.

Probably a more convenient instrument to use with children in this age group is the Ada Snap-A-Ray or a cut-down modified version of it (Fig. 106B). The rectangular P.I.D. (cone) can be used with Ada Snap-A-Ray film holder or Rinn EEZEE Grip and pedo No. 0 size film, if the operator is careful to watch P.I.D. (cone) alignment to prevent "cone cuts."

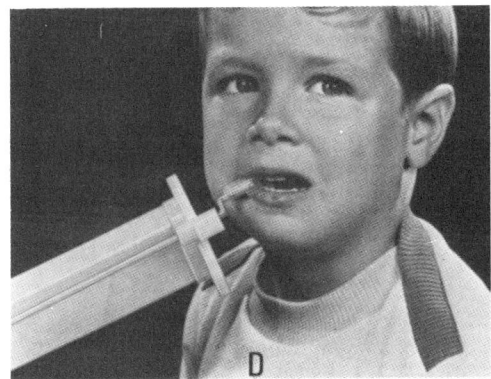

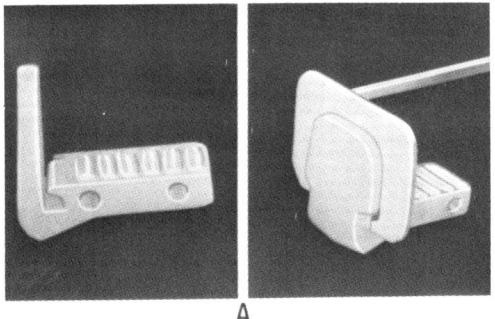

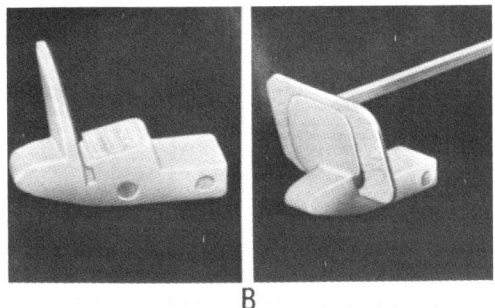

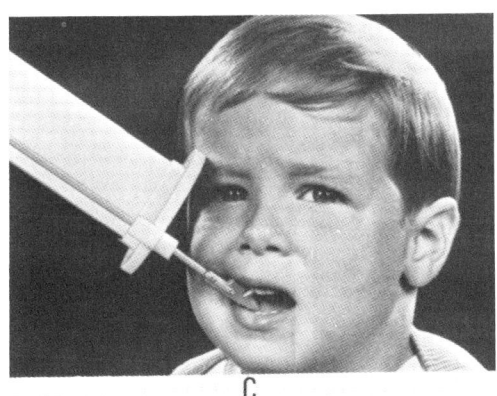

Figure 15-110. Modification of Rinn XCP and BAI Posterior Bite-blocks to use with pedo 0 size film for children five and under. (A) XCP bite-blocks modified for pedo 0 film; (B) BAI bite-blocks modified for pedo 0 film; (C) Posterior maxillary BAI technic for child five years and under; (D) Posterior mandibular BAI technic for child five years and under.

Mandibular Posterior Technique Using Ada Snap-A-Ray or Rinn EEZEE Grip. The film is held lingually and parallel to the long axes of the posterior teeth by the film holder. The child closes on the biting area of the film holder to secure the film. This is a modified paralleling technique (Fig. 15-111).

VERTICAL ANGULATION: Direct the central beam at right angles to the film. Using a starting angle of -5 degrees for the posterior mandibular arch.

HORIZONTAL ANGULATION: The face of the cone should be parallel to the facial surface of the teeth to be radiographed.

Maxillary Posterior Technique using Ada Snap-A-Ray or Rinn EEZEE Grip. In the posterior region, the film is positioned in the mouth directly behind the tooth of interest, as far to the midline of the palate as possible. The wide jaw of the holder will then extend onto the occlusal surface of the teeth being radiographed. The patient is instructed to close just tight enough to hold the instrument steady. Use

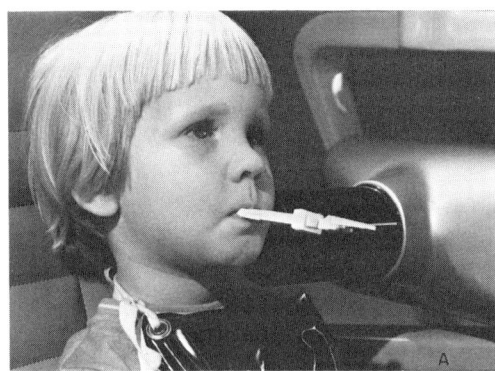

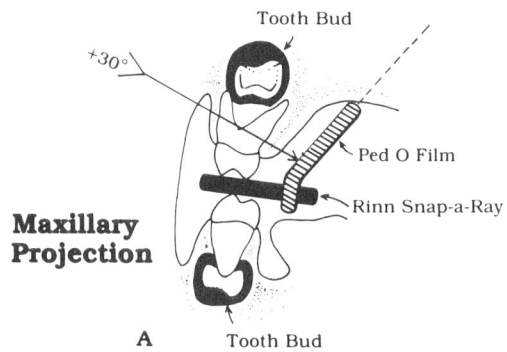

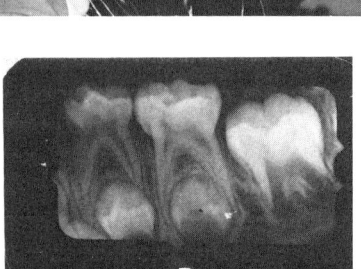

Figure 15-111. Mandibular posterior technic for child five years and under using Ada Snap-A-Ray. (A) Patient in position for mandibular posterior projection. (B) Periapical radiograph of mandibular molar region using Pedo 0 film.

a starting angle of +30 degrees for posterior maxillary arch, and direct the central beam at right angles to the film (Fig. 15-112).

Posterior Bite-wing Tab Technique

(Use pedo No. 0 bite-wing tabs with pedo No. 0 film.) The rectangular cone may be used here, but be careful with the cone alignment to prevent a "cone-cut." The round cone is used more frequently because of its convenience in alignment.

HEAD POSITION: Regardless of the type of cone used, the sagittal plane should be perpendicular to the floor, and the tragal-ala line should be parallel to the floor.

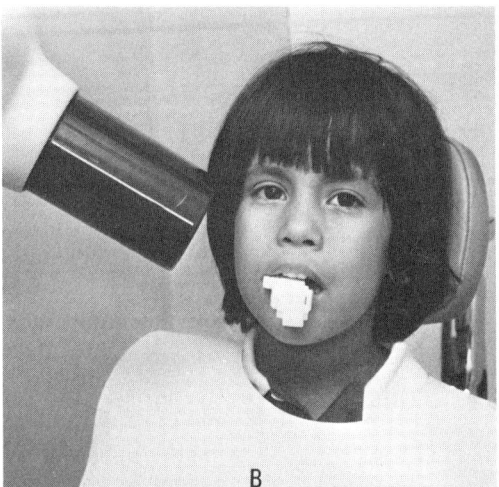

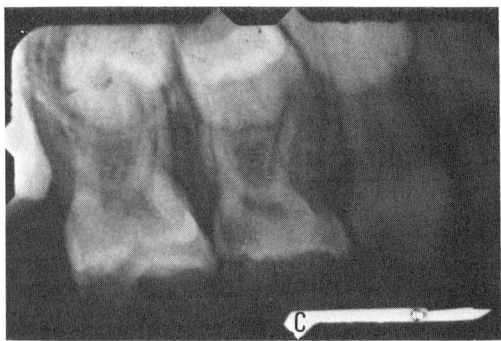

Figure 15-112. Maxillary posterior technic using Ada Snap-A-Ray for child five years and under. (A) Diagram of projection; (B) Maxillary posterior projection using the Ada Snap-A-Ray on children five years of age and under. (C) Maxillary posterior radiograph using No. 0 Pedo film.

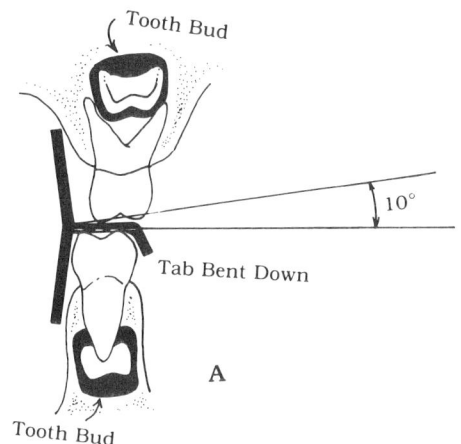

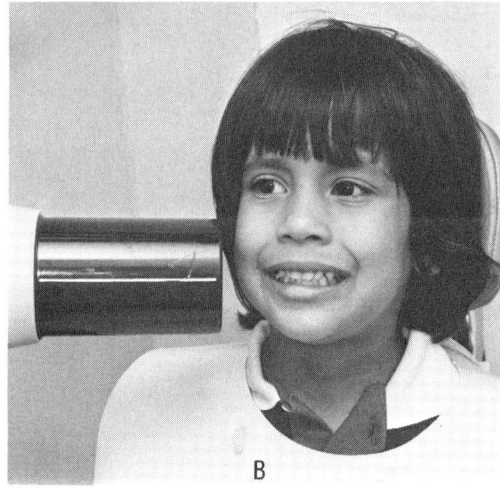

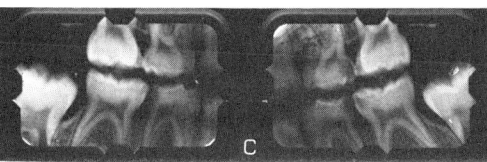

Figure 15-113. Bite-wing Tab Technic on child five years and under. (A) Shows position of bite-wing film in proper relationship to the maxillary and mandibular teeth and the direction and angulation of the x-rays 10 degrees above horizontal. (B) The head must be adjusted so plane of occlusion is parallel to floor and the sagittal plane is perpendicular to the floor. The teeth are in occlusion with tab resting between the oclusal surfaces of the teeth. The cone is adjusted in both the vertical and horizontal planes to present distortion and overlapping. (C) Bite-wing radiographs of child five years of age using pedo 0 film and bite-wing tab.

FILM PLACEMENT AND RETENTION: **Step 1:** Place the bite-wing tab or wing on the occlusal surface of the mandibular primary molars with the lower edge of the film packet placed in the vestibule between the tongue and the teeth. The anterior edge of the bite-wing film should extend beyond the mesial surface of the mandibular canine.

To avoid overlapping of the contact points, the film should be positioned perpendicular to invisible lines drawn through the embrasures of the teeth. To do this, in the bite-wing projection, the anterior border of the film packet should be a greater distance from the lingual surfaces of the teeth than the posterior border.

Step 2: Fold down half of the bite-wing tab over the buccal surface of the mandibular teeth. This should be done before the tab is placed on occlusal surfaces of the teeth. With the index finger of one hand, press against the lower lingual border of the film to keep it upright. Use the index finger of the other hand to press the tab against the buccal surface of the mandibular teeth.

Step 3: Now remove the finger that is pressing against the back of the film, and instruct the patient to close slowly against the bite-wing tube in a normal bite. The patient will not close against the index finger because it is pressing against the buccal surfaces of the lower teeth. After the patient has closed against the bite-wing tab, remove the finger from the tab.

VERTICAL ANGULATION: (Long cone 16 inch SFD, approximately +10 degree vertical angulation.) If the palate is shallow, the upper border of the film will be forced lingually by the palate closure. The vertical angle may have to be increased in this case to prevent shape distortion of the maxillary crowns.

HORIZONTAL ANGULATION: Direct the central beam through the interproximal embrasures of the crowns of the under examination. The flat face of the cone

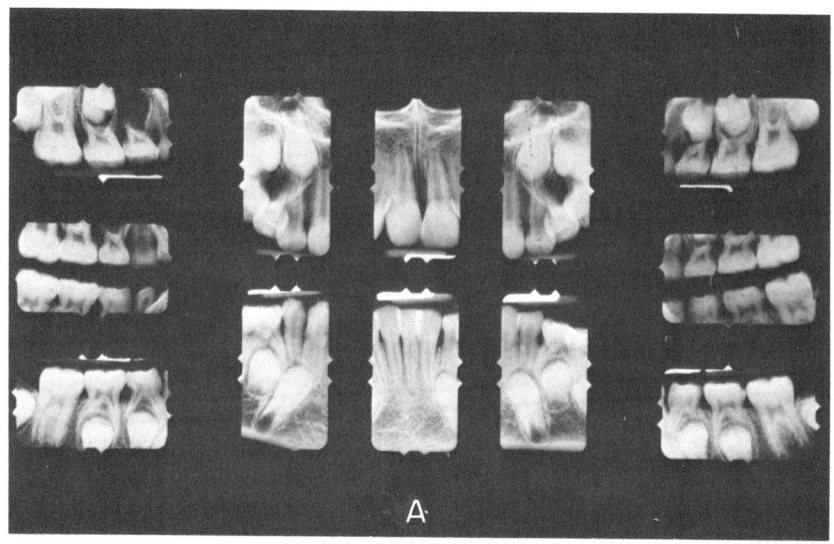
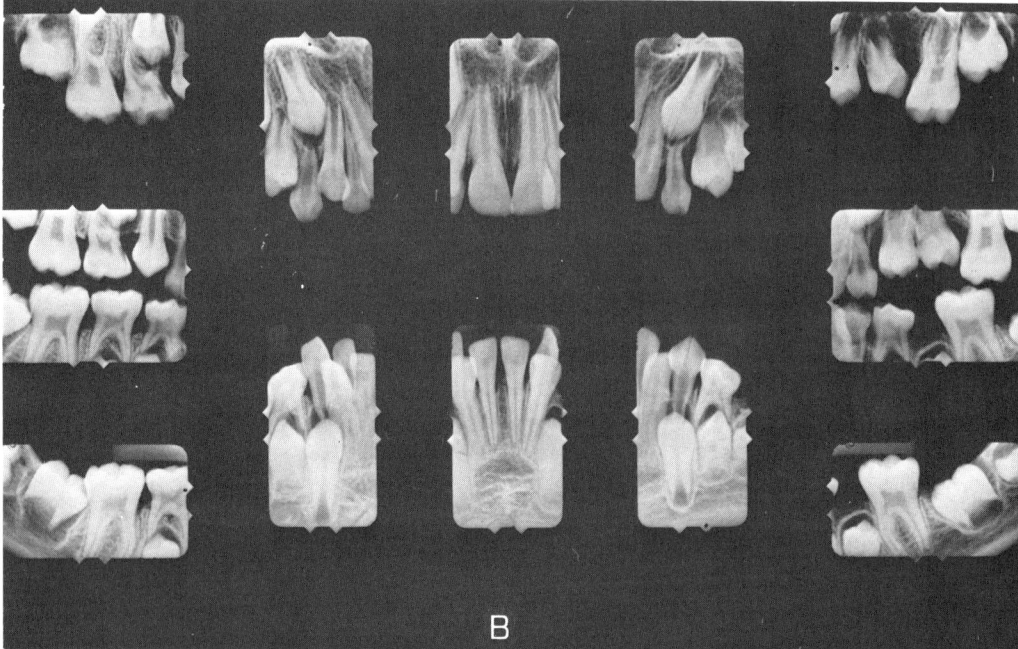

Figure 15-114. Mixed Dentition (6-9 years) Complete Survey. **(A)** Complete survey using all No. 1 film. **(B)** Complete survey using No. 1 films for periapicals and No. 2 film for bite-wings.

Atlas of Special Techniques in Dental Radiology

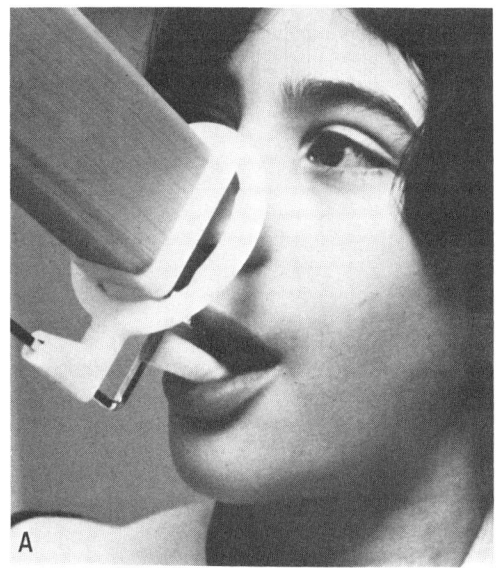

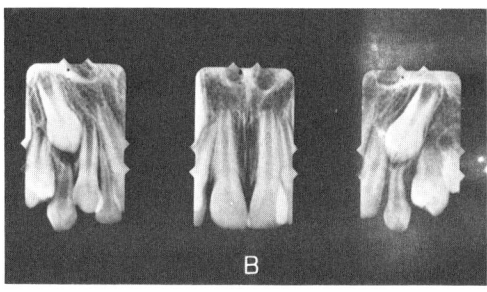

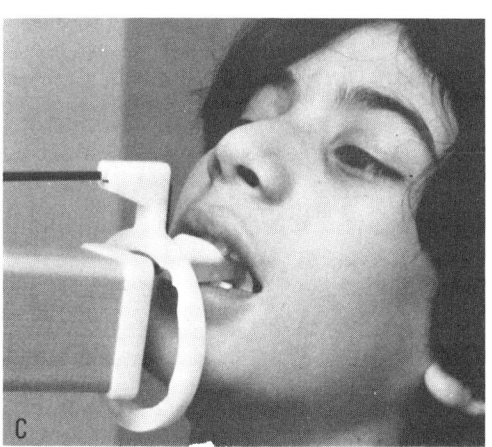

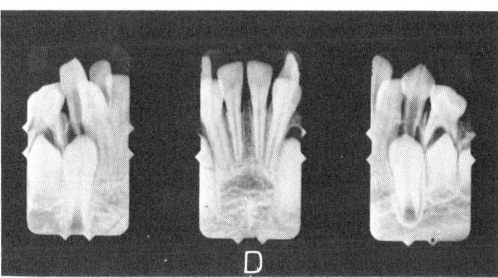

Figure 15-115. Mixed dentition anterior periapicals technic using Rinn XCP Instrument and Rectangular Collimation. (A) Patient and XCP instrument maxillary arch; (B) Maxillary anterior radiographs; (C) Patient and XCP instrument mandibular arch; (D) Mandibular anterior radiographs.

should be horizontally parallel to the film packet.

POINT OF ENTRY. Direct the central beam through the occlusal plane of the teeth toward the center of the film packet. In order to prevent cone cutting, gently pull back the corner of the lips, and observe whether the anterior periphery of the cone (P.I.D.) is covering the anterior border of the film. Make the exposure and remove the film from the patient's mouth quickly. Always praise the child for being a good patient (Fig. 15-113).

Mixed Dentition (6-9 Years of Age)

The complete radiographic survey (Fig. 15-114A) includes four No. 1 narrow films for the posterior regions and six No. 1 narrow films for the anterior regions. The bite-wings are taken with a No. 1 narrow film, one on each side of the arch. Sometimes the bite-wings are taken with No. 2 film if the child is large enough. Some of the nine year olds can tolerate the No. 2 bite-wing film (Fig. 15-114).

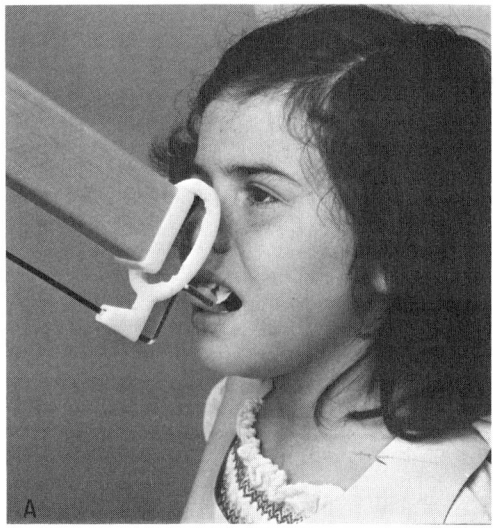

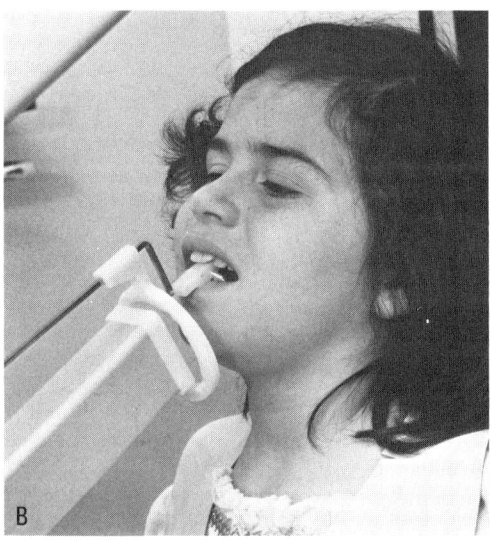

Figure 15-116. Mixed dentition anterior periapical technic using the Rinn BAI instruments, alternate method: **(A)** Maxillary anterior positioning of instrument and BID (Beam-Indicating Device). **(B)** Mandibular anterior positioning of instrument and BID (Beam-Indicating Device).

Anterior Periapical Technique

The method of choice is the Rinn XCP anterior paralleling technique utilizing the rectangular P.I.D. (cone) or any comparable paralleling technique such as the Masel Precision anterior instrument.

Rinn XCP Technique. TYPE OF FILM: No. 1 size film, Kodak D or E speed film.

EXPOSURE TECHNIQUE: Exposure is reduced for children.

HEAD POSITION: Except when otherwise noted, the standard head position is in the tragal-ala plane parallel to the floor and the midsagittal plane perpendicualr to the floor. To minimize movement of the child, the dental chair should be adjusted so that the head, back, arms, and feet are well supported.

FILM RETENTION: Use the Rinn XCP anterior instrument. The film is held lingual and parallel to the long axes of the anterior XCP instrument with No. 1 film size backing. The child bites on a holder to secure the film (Fig. 15-115).

Alternate Methods for Anterior Periapical Radiography Some of the smaller children in this age group may not be able to tolerate the Rinn XCP anterior instrument with the No. 1 narrow film. If this is the case, any one of the following alternative methods, listed in order of preference, may be used. **However, these methods will produce, routinely, radiographs with less film quality than the paralleling technique.**

1. The bisecting angle technique using anterior Rinn BAI bite-blocks can be used with rectangular P.I.D. without the problem of cone-cutting (Figs. 15-110, 15-116).

2. The Ada Snap-A-Ray or Rinn EEZEE Grip instrument using the round long cone is a modified bisecting angle technique (Fig. 15-117). Place the No. 1 film as far behind the anterior teeth as possible, and hold the handle of instrument against the opposite arch so the

Atlas of Special Techniques in Dental Radiology 593

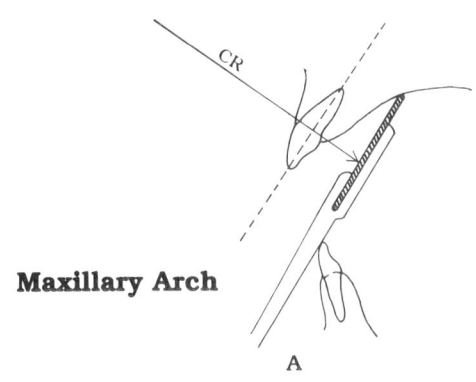

Maxillary Arch

A

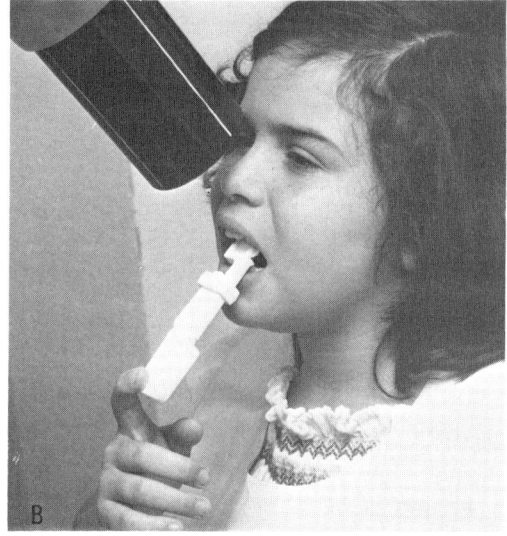

B

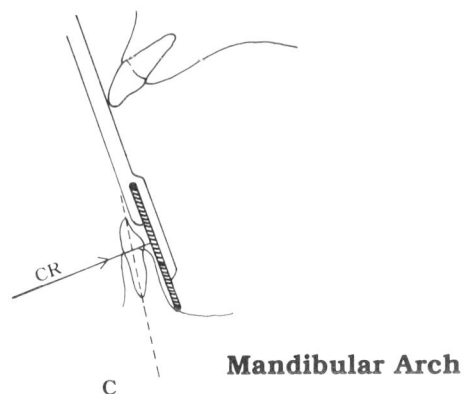

Mandibular Arch

C

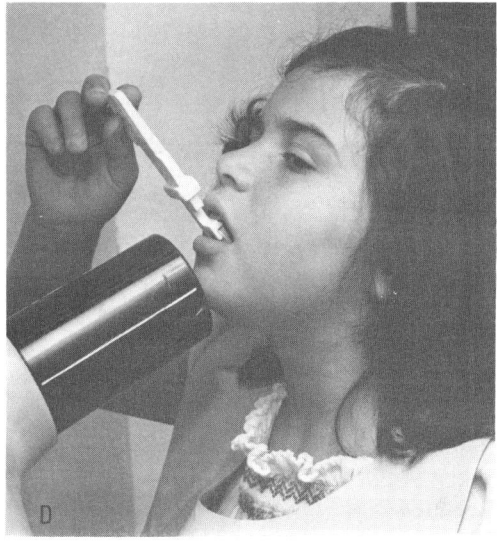

Figure 15-117. Ada Snap-A-Ray method for anterior periapical radiography for mixed dentition group (alternate method). **(A)** Use of instrument in anterior maxillary arch. **(B)** Maxillary anterior projection of child in mixed dentition group. **(C)** Use of instrument in Mandibular arch. **(D)** mandibular anterior projection of child in mixed dentition group.

film will be parallel to the long axis of the teeth. The mouth should be wide open for the anteriors.

Posterior Periapical Technique

Rinn XCP Technique. The method of choice is the Rinn XCP posterior instrument with rectangular collimation or a comparable technique such as the Masel Precision posterior instrument. The No. 1 size film is placed with the long axis of the film horizontal in the film holder (Fig. 15-118). Using the Rinn XCP posterior instrument for the mixed dentition age group, modify the film holder backing and bite-block as shown in Figure 15-119.

Alternate Methods for Posterior Periapical Radiographs. Some of the smaller children in this age group may not be able to tolerate the Rinn XCP posterior instrument with the No. 1 film. If

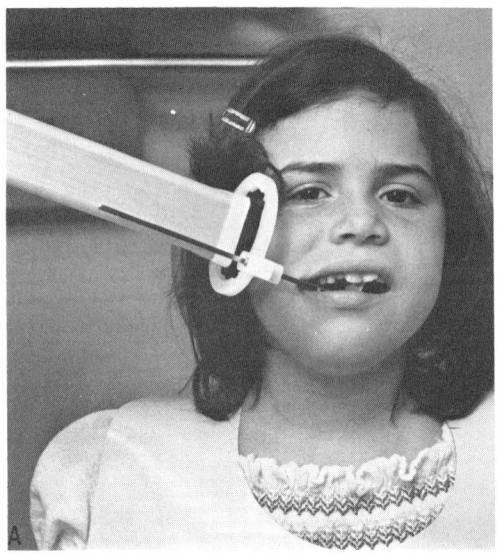

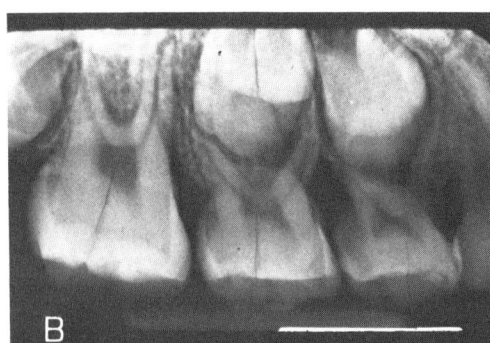

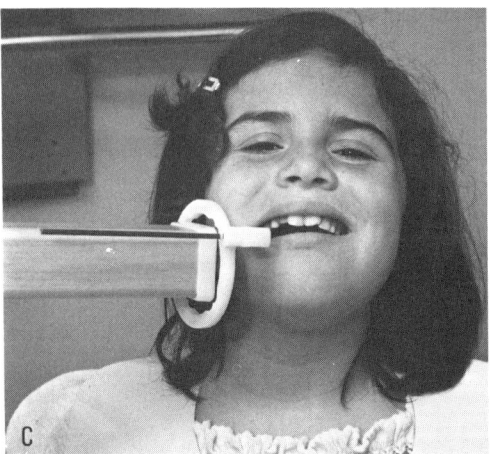

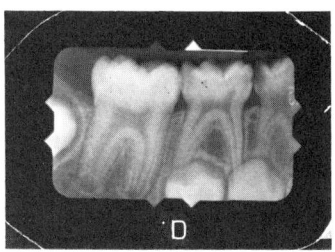

Figure 15-118. Rinn XCP posterior periapical technic using rectangular collimation. (A) Maxillay posterior positioning, child in mixed dentition group. (B) Maxillary posterior radiograph. (C) Mandibular posterior positioning, child in mixed dentition group. (D) Mandibular posterior radiograph.

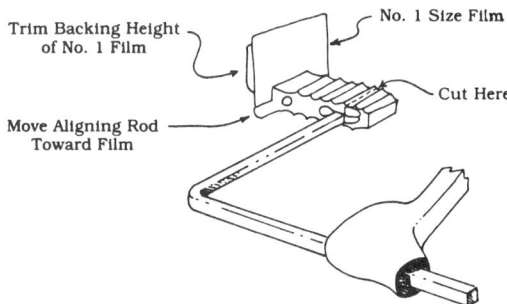

Figure 15-119. Modification of film holder backing and bite-block for posterior periapical XCP technic.

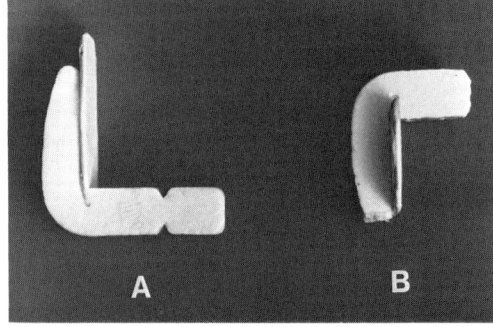

Figure 15-120. Greene Stabe Bite-block for periapical films. (Mixed dentition age group, 6-9 years.) (A) Stabe Film Holder with No. 1 film placed for anterior projection. (B) Stabe Film Holder modified for No. 1 regular film placement for posterior projection.

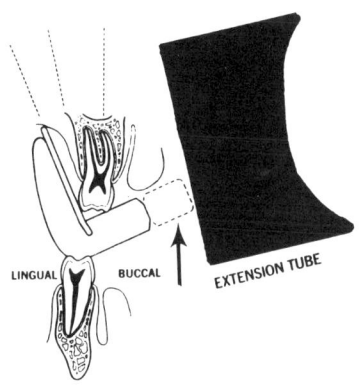

Figure 15-121. Greene Stabe Bite-block positioned for maxillary posterior periapical film using bisecting angle technic. (Courtesy of Greene Dental Products, Cook-Waite Laboratories, Inc., New York, NY.)

there is a problem in patient tolerance, any of the following three alternative methods, listed in order of preference, may be used. (In fact, these methods will reveal more of the developing premolars in the periapical radiograph.)

1. The bisecting angle technique using the posterior Rinn BAI bite-blocks can be used with the rectangular P.I.D. (cone) without the problem of "cone-cutting" (Fig. 15-110B, C, D).
2. The Ada Snap-A-Ray or Rinn EEZEE Grip Instrument using the round long P.I.D. (cone) is a modified Bisecting Angle Technique (Fig. 15-111 and 15-112).
3. The Stable Disposable X-Ray Film Holder (Greene Dental Products) may be used with either paralleling or bisecting angle techniques (Fig. 15-120).

Greene Stabe Bite-block Technique for Posterior Periapical Radiography (Maxillary posterior projection using bisecting angle technique):

FILM PLACEMENT AND RETENTION: Carry the film and film holder into the mouth, placing the film in a position as close to the teeth as possible without bending the film. The film and film holder are retained in position by asking the patient to bite gently into the bite portion of the film holder so that the teeth indent the plastic, thus locking the film and holder securely in position. The bite position of the Stabe is scored so that it may be shortened easily if necessary to avoid the cheek (Fig. 15-121).

CONE POSITIONING: Direct the x-ray beam perpendicular to the plane bisecting the angle formed by the film plane and the long axis of tooth plane. The starting vertical angle is between +25 and +35 degrees.

Greene Stabe Bite-block Technique for Mandibular Posterior Projection (Paralleling Technique):

FILM PLACEMENT AND RETENTION: Carry film and film holder into the mouth and position it as parallel as possible to the long axis of the teeth to be radiographed. It is difficult to obtain exact parallelism in all instances, depending on tongue tension and floor of the mouth sensitivity.

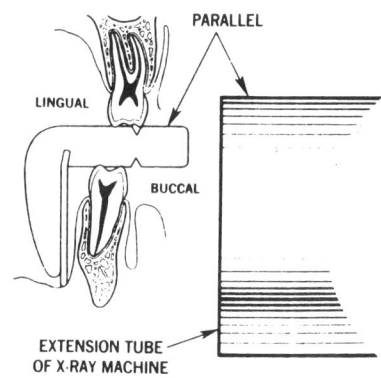

Figure 15-122. Greene Stabe Bite-block positioned for mandibular periapical film using paralleling technic. (Courtesy of Greene Dental Products, Cook-Waite Laboratories, Inc., New York, NY.)

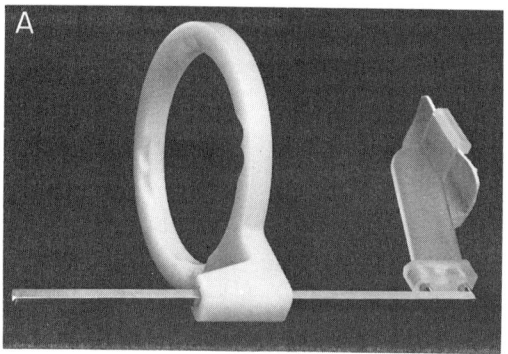

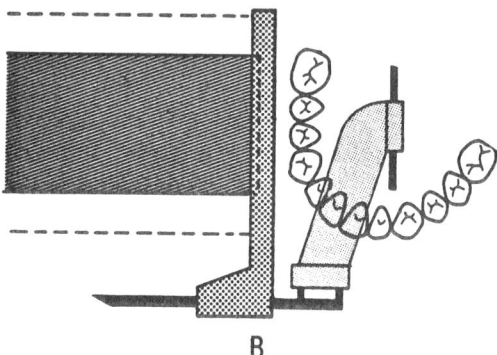

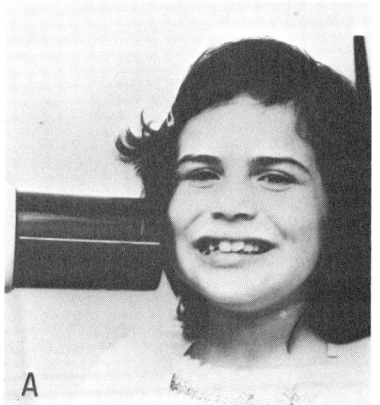

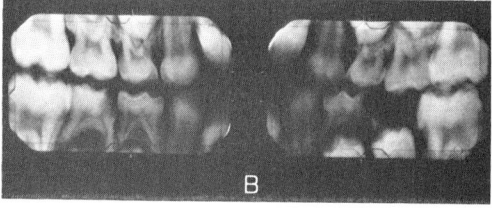

Figure 15-124. Posterior Bite-wing Tab Technic using No. 1 film. **(A)** Child in mixed dentition age aligned properly for posterior bite-wing radiograph using bite-wing tab and No. 1 film. **(B)** Resultant posterior bite-wings.

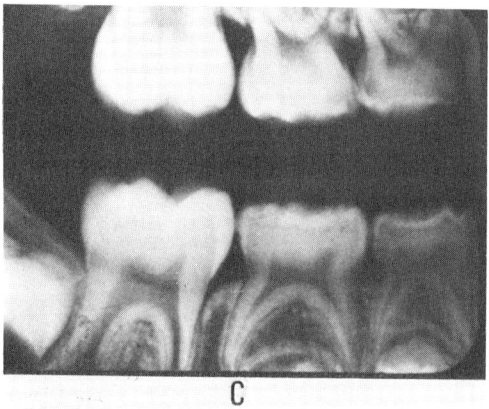

Figure 15-123. Rinn Posterior Bite-wing Technic using No. 1 film for mixed dentition group (ages 6-9 years). **(A)** Assembled Rinn XCP instrument with No. 1 film ready for placement in mouth. **(B)** The film is positioned so invisible lines drawn through the embrasures of the teeth are perpendicular to the film. The BID is aligned horizontally and vertically with the indicator rod. **(C)** Resultant posterior bite-wing taken with Rinn XCP bite-wing instrument. Note space between occlusal surfaces of the teeth.

CONE POSITIONING: Direct the beam perpendicular to the film, being careful to cover the film. The lines inscribed on the surface of the extension cone are useful in paralleling the x-ray beam with the bite portion of the Stabe film holder (Fig. 15-122).

Posterior Bite-wing Technique

Two Posterior bite-wing techniques

1. The Rinn bite-wing instrument technique (Fig. 15-123).
2. Bite-wing tab technique (Fig. 15-124).

In this age group, some of the older children may be able to tolerate the No. 2 posterior bite-wing; however, most of them, because of the short crowned primary molars, will not be able to bite down on the instrument or the tab properly.

Atlas of Special Techniques in Dental Radiology 597

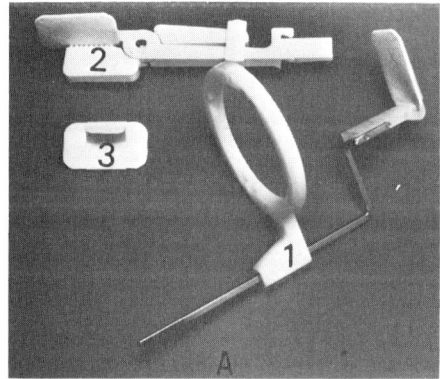

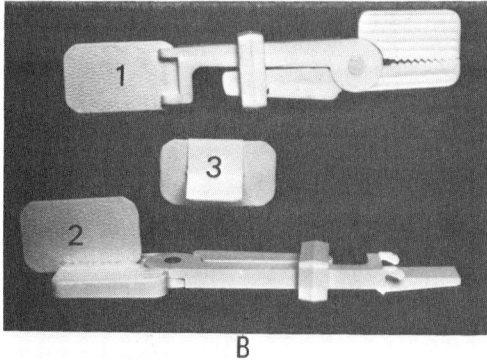

Figure 15-125. Supplies required for two alternate methods for mixed dentition CMX. **(A)** (#1) Anterior Rinn XCP (#2) posterior Ada Snap-A-Ray with No. 1 film, (#3) bite-wing tab and No. 1 film. **(B)** (#1) Anterior film placement with Rinn EEZEE Grip, (#2) posterior film placement with Ada Snap-A-Ray, (#3) bite-wing tab with No. 1 film.

Therefore, the No. 1 film is used in most cases.

Summary of Techniques

In summary, the mixed dentition age group is a difficult age group to take a good complete periapical survey because of the differences in eruption patterns and the size of the patients. If the Rinn XCP instruments cannot be used with success, two alternate techniques seem to work well. They are (1) Rinn XCP anterior instrument, Ada Snap-A-Ray, or Rinn EEZEE Grip (posterior) and bite-wing tab, and (2) Ada Snap-A-Ray or Rinn EEZEE Grip (anterior and posterior) and bite-wing tab (Fig. 15-125).

Preadolescent Group (10-12 years)

The film mount suggested for this age group is shown in Figure 15-126. This mount includes six No. 2 regular films and eight No. 1 narrow films. This mount is similar to the adult film mount except all four of the periapical molar projections and two of the molar bite-wing projections are eliminated.

Anterior Periapical Technique

A long cone paralleling technique with rectangular collimation (such as the Rinn XCP anterior paralleling technqiue) or a

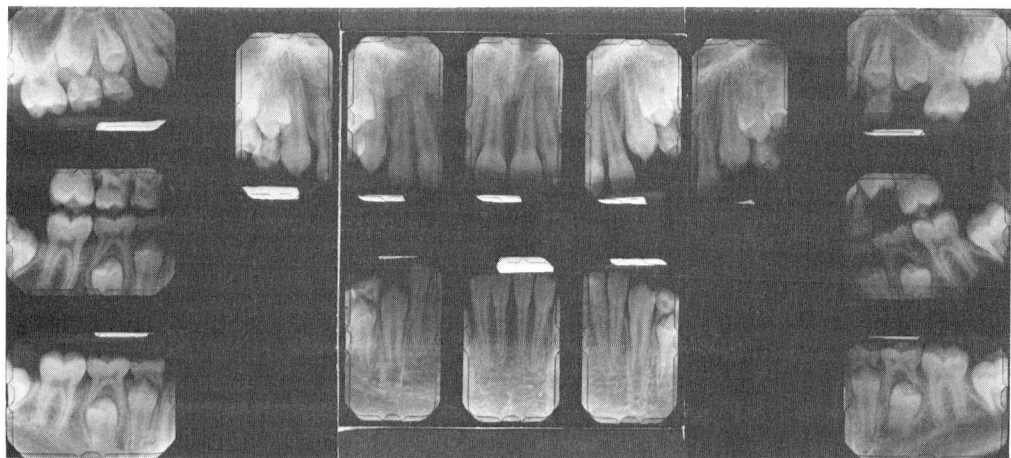

Figure 15-126. Preadolescent group (10-12 years), complete mount survey. (four No. 2 films, eight No. 1 films, two No. 2 posterior bite-wings.)

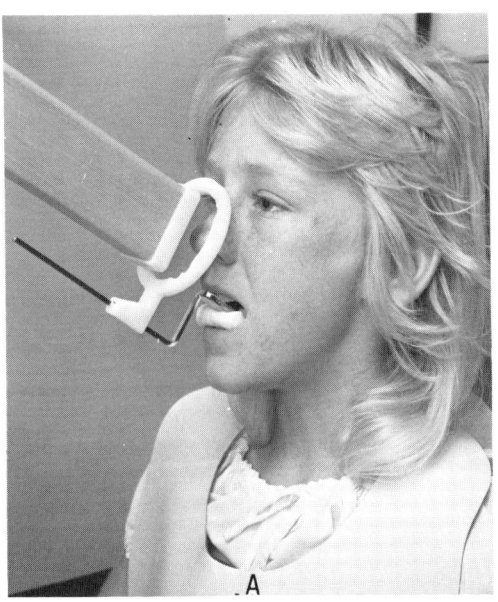
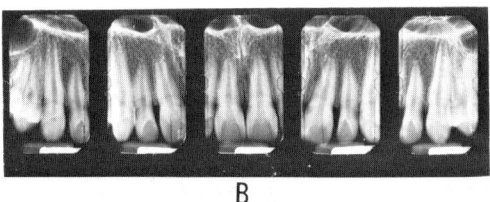
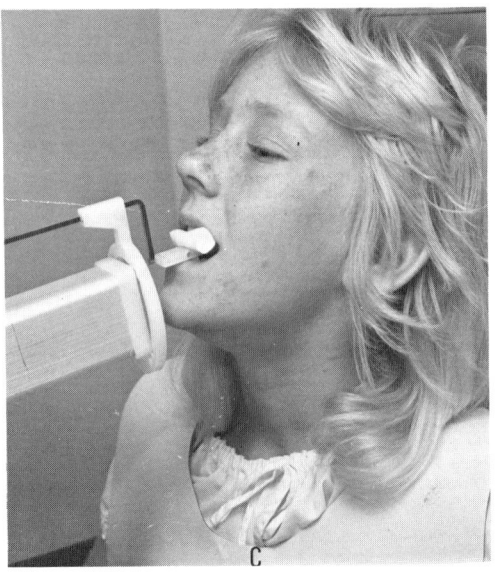
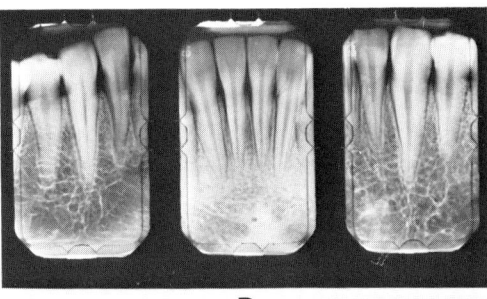

Figure 15-127. Anterior periapical radiography using Rinn XCP instrument and rectangular collimation, preadolescent age group (ages 10-12). **(A)** Maxillary anterior projections using Rinn XCP instrument and rectangular collimation. **(B)** Radiographs of maxillary incisors. **(C)** Mandibular anterior projections using Rinn XCP instrument and rectangular collimation. **(D)** Radiographs and mandibular incisors.

comparable technic (such as the Masel Precision anterior instrument technique) are the methods of choice because of greater image definition and less radiation exposure tot he patient (Fig. 15-127).

TYPE OF FILM: Use No. 1 narrow size Kodak (Speed D or E) film, and take five maxillary anterior films and three mandibular anterior films.

EXPOSURE TECHNIQUE: The exposure time is usually reduced in this age group. If child is quite large, the adult settings may be better.

FILM RETENTION: Use the Rinn XCP anterior instrument for the anterior projections. The film is held lingual and parallel to the long axes of the teeth by the anterior XCP instrument with No. 1 film size backing. The child bites on the holder to secure film (Fig. 15-127).

TYPE OF CONE: Use long rectangular P.I.D. (Cone).

Alternate Methods for Anterior Periapical Radiography: Some of the smaller

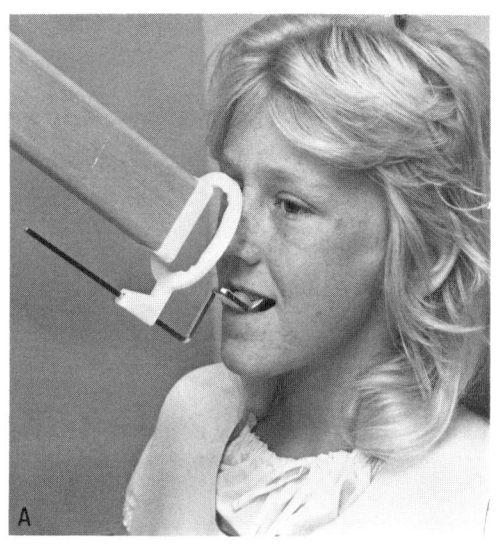
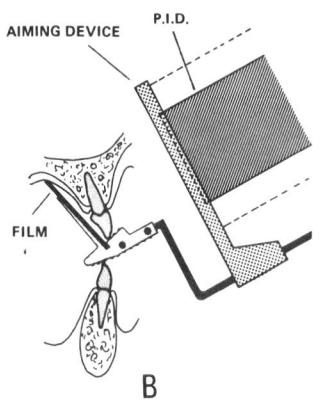
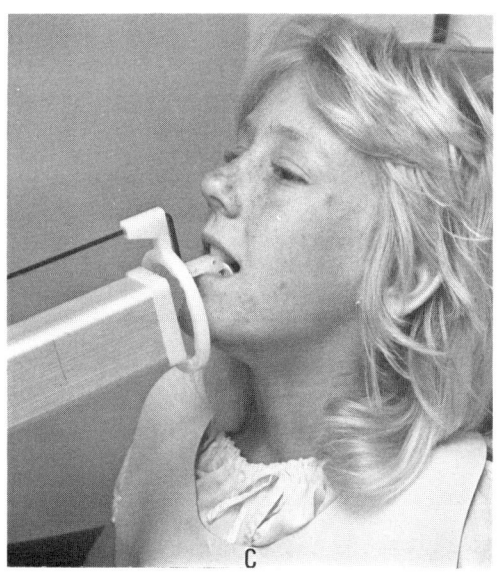
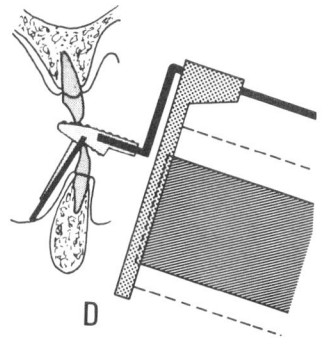

Figure 15-128. Alterrnate anterior periapical method using Rinn BAI for preadolescent age group. **(A)** Rinn BAI instrument placed in maxillary anterior region. **(B)** Diagram of placement of Rinn BAI instrument and alignment of PID in maxillary anterior region. **(C)** Placement of Rinn BAI instrument in mandibular anterior region. **(D)** Diagram of placement of Rinn BAI instrument and alignment of PID in mandibular anterior region.

children in this group may not be able to tolerate the Rinn XCP anterior instrument. However, this is a very small percentage. If for some reason the child will not tolerate the Rinn XCP anterior instrument, use one of the two anterior periapical methods listed below. (Remember you are sacrificing film quality when using these alternative methods.)

BISECTING ANGLE TECHNIQUE USING THE RINN BAI ANTERIOR BITEBLOCK. The rectangular cone may be used with this technique (Fig 15-128).

MODIFIED BISECTING TECHNIQUE USING THE ADA SNAP-A-RAY OR RINN EEZEE GRIP FILM HOLDERS. The round cone is recommended for this technique to prevent cone-cutting (Fig. 15-129).

Posterior Periapical Technique

The technique of choice is the Paralleling technique using Rinn XCP posterior instruments and rectangular collimation or a comparable paralleling technique such as one using the Masel Precision Posterior Instruments.

Rinn XCP paralleling Posterior Instrument Technique:

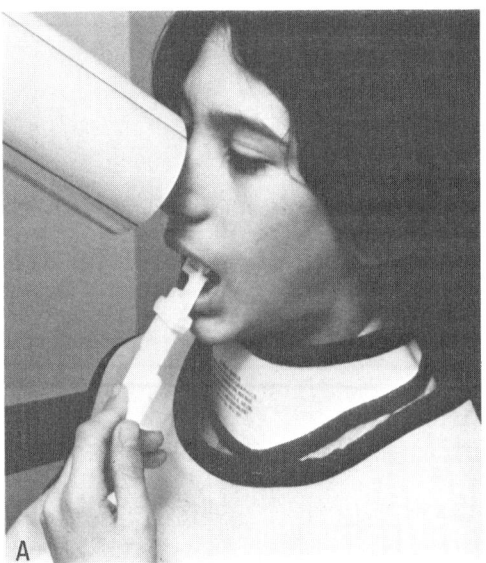

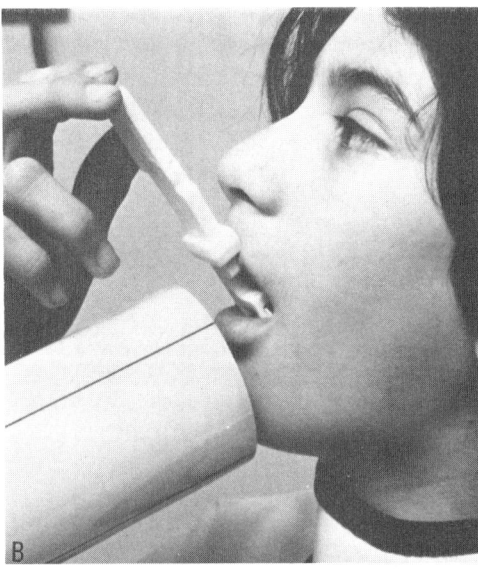

Figure 15-129. Alternate anterior periapical method using Ada Snap-A-Ray. **(A)** Anterior maxillary projection, age 10-12 years; **(B)** Anterior mandibular projection, age 10-12 years.

TYPE OF FILM: No. 2 regular Kodak (D or E speed) film is used.

EXPOSURE TECHNIQUE: Use reduced exposure technique as compared to adult exposure chart, unless child is large in size.

FILM RETENTION: Use the Rinn XCP posterior instrument for the posterior periapical projection (Fig. 15-130). The film is held lingual and parallel to the long axes of the teeth by the posterior XCP instrument with the No. 2 film size backing. The child bites on the film to secure the film. It may be desirable to modify the Rinn posterior XCP bite-block and backing to accommodate some of the children in this group. The modifications follow:

1. Trim the corners and reduce the height of the backing slightly. Do not reduce backing height too much or film will bend and distort radiographic image.
2. Reduce size of bite-block by one hole (*see* Fig. 15-119); however, it is usually better to use an unmodified bite-block for maxillary arch.

Alternate Posterior Periapical Methods: Some of the smaller children in this age group may not be able to tolerate the Rinn XCP posterior instrument and the No. 2 regular sized film. If this is the case, any of the following alternate methods listed in order of preference, may be used:

1. Modified Rinn posterior XCP technique uses cotton rolls on each side of the Rinn XCP posterior bite-block (Fig. 15-131).
2. The Bisecting Angle technique uses the Rinn posterior BAI bite-block; the rectangular cone may be used with this technique (Fig. 15-132).

Atlas of Special Techniques in Dental Radiology 601

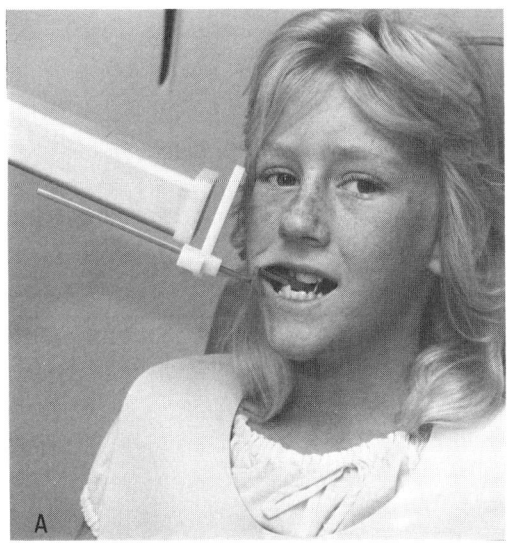

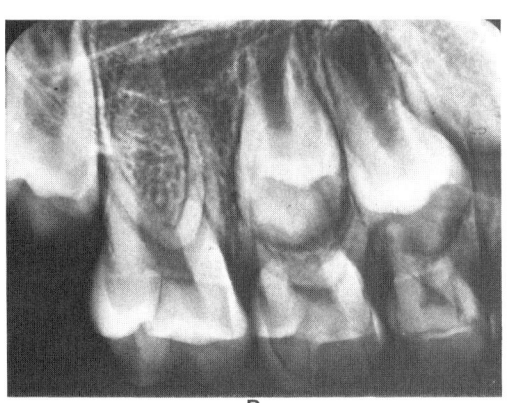

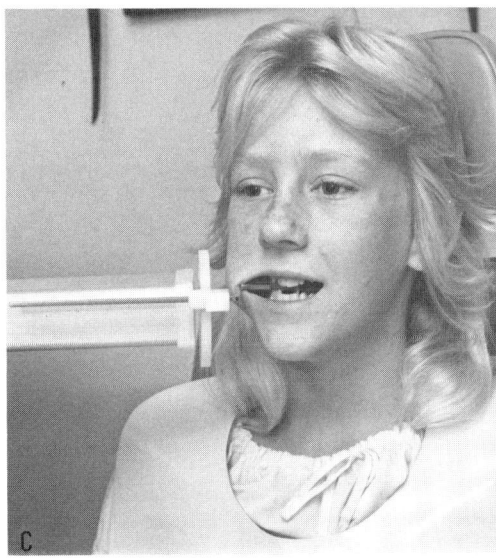

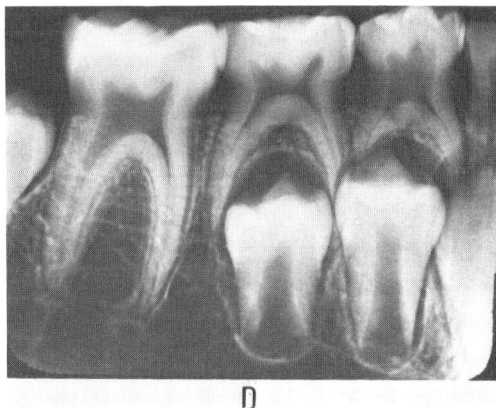

Figure 15-130. Posterior periapical technic using Rinn posterior XCP instrument and rectanglular collimation in preadolescent age group (10-12 years). **(A)** Child (10-12 years) showing placement of Rinn XCP instrument in maxillary posterior region. **(B)** Radiograph of maxillary posterior region taken by Rinn XCP instrument. **(C)** Child (10-12 years) showing placement of Rinn XCP Instrument in mandibular posterior region. **(D)** Radiograph of mandibular posterior region (10-12 years) taken by Rinn XCP instrument.

3. The Modified Bisecting Angle technique uses the Ada Snap-A-Ray or Rinn EEZEE Grip Film Holder. It is recommended that the round cone be used with this technique (Fig. 15-133). In children with smaller mouths in this age group, when using the Ada Snap-A-Ray film holder, grab the film further down (Fig. 15-134A). Film coverage will be sacrificed but the child may be able to tolerate the film better. Also, "film-bending" may help the patient tolerate the No. 2 film. The corners of the films may be "turned in." Do not bend the films too much because it will distort the final radiographic image (Fig. 15-134B).
4. Stabe film holder uses the bisecting angle technique in the maxillary arch and the paralleling technique in the mandibular arch (Figs. 15-121, 15-122).

Posterior Bite-wing Techniques

TYPE OF FILM: One No. 2 regular film is used on each side of the arch.

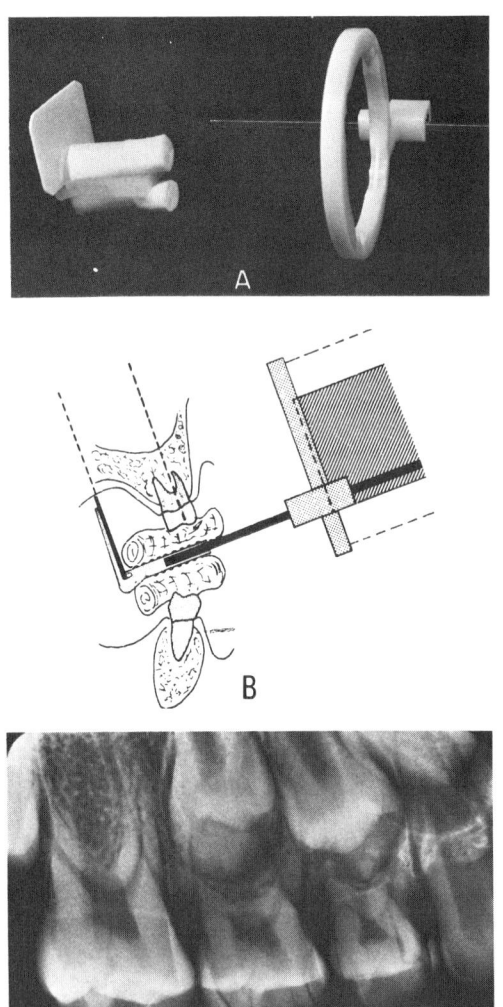

Figure 15-131. Alternate two cotton roll Rinn XCP method for posterior region using No. 2 films with smaller children in the 10-12 year age group. (A) Film holder with two cotton rolls attached by tape. (B) Diagram of procedure. (C) Resultant radiograph. Note that there is improved anatomical accuracy of primary molars as compared to 15-130B.

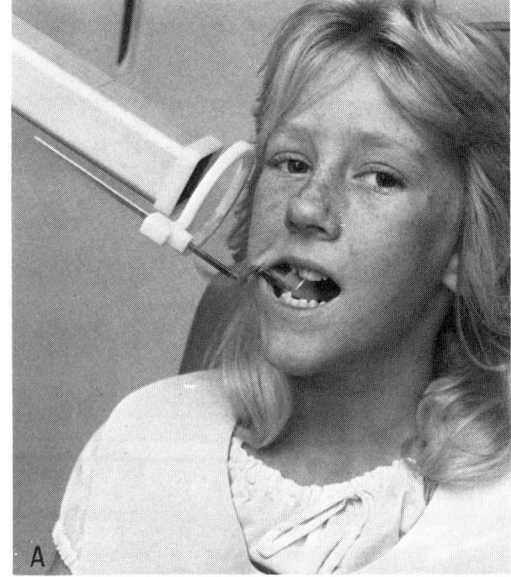

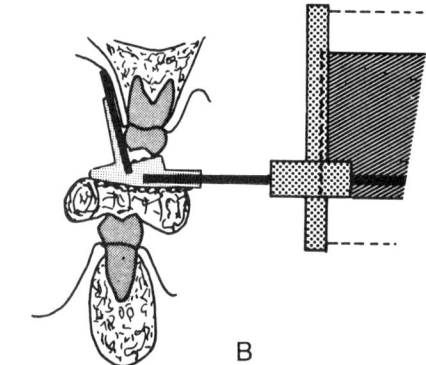

Figure 15-132. Posterior periapical technic using Rinn BAI posterior instruments (child 10-12 years). (A) Child with maxillary posterior BAI instrument in position. (B) Diagram with maxillary molar BAI technic. (C) Child with mandibular posterior Rinn BAI instrument in position. (D) Diagram of mandibular Rinn BAI premolar technique.

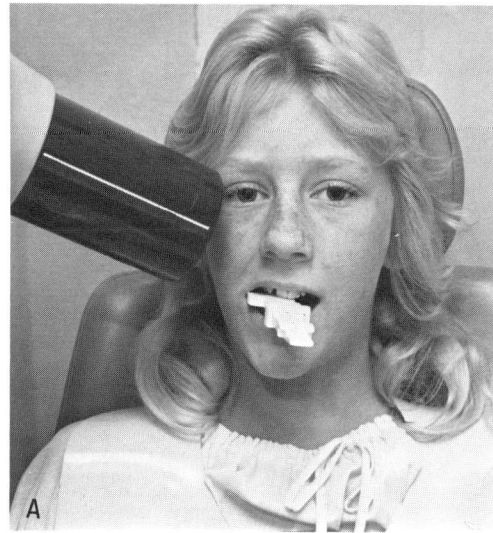
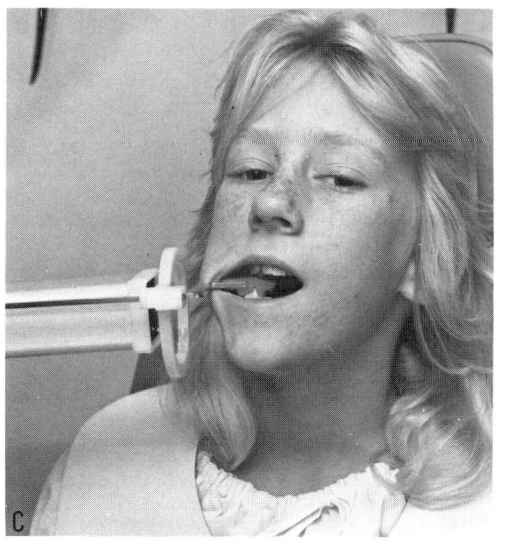
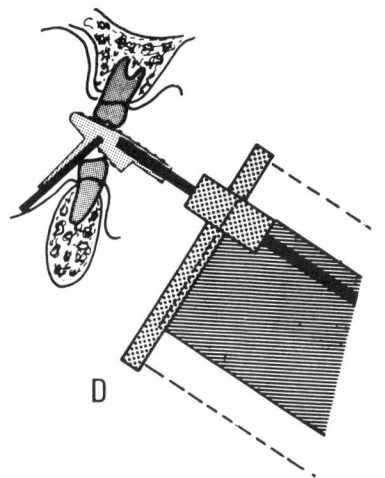
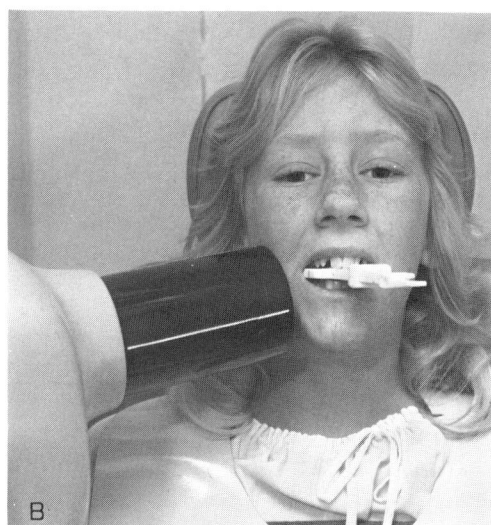

Figure 15-133. Ada Snap-A-Ray technic for posterior teeth (child 10-12). **(A)** Maxillary arch; **(B)** Mandibular arch.

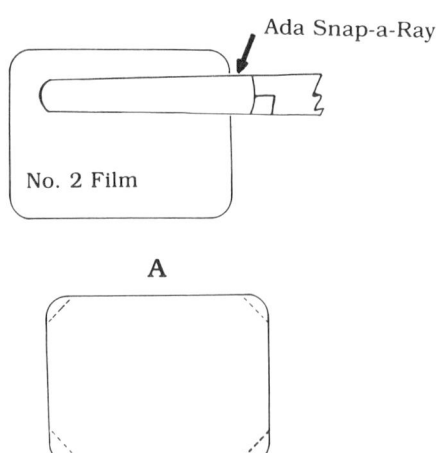

Figure 15-134. Modified Ada Snap-A-Ray technic (child 10-12 years). **(A)** Grasp Ada Snap-A-Ray down further on No. 2 film; **(B)** Film bending of corners of No. 2 film.

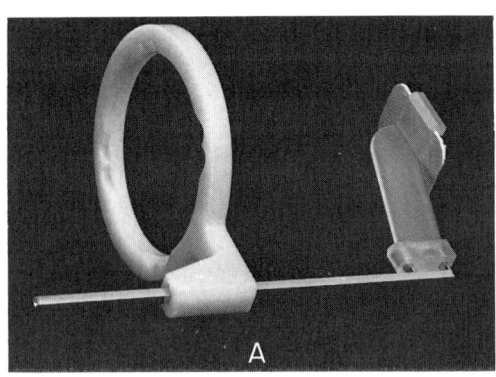

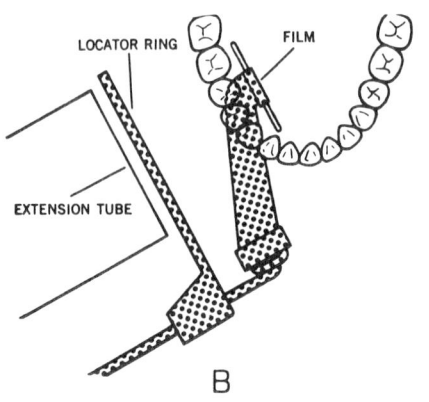

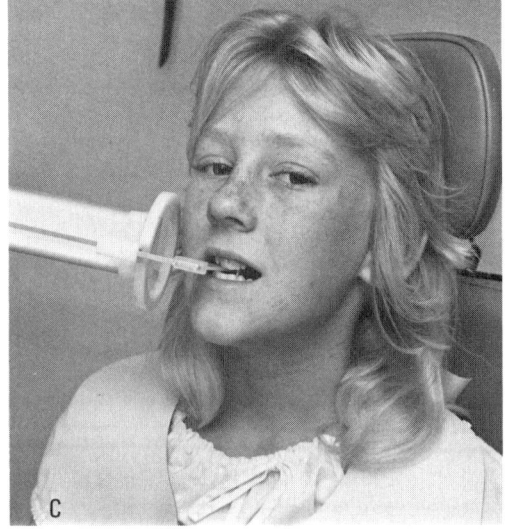

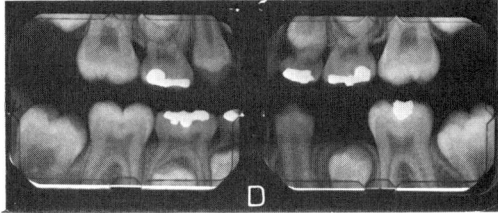

Figure 15-135. Rinn posterior bite-wing instrument (child 10-12). **(A)** Correct assembly of Rinn bite-wing instrument; **(B)** Diagram of correct placement of Rinn bite-wing instrument. **(C)** Child (10-12 years) with Rinn bite-wing instrument in position; **(D)** BW radiographs of child (10-12 years).

EXPOSURE TIME: Use child exposure time technique unless the child is large and has all primary teeth missing.

Two posterior bite-wing techniques are illustrated: (1) the Rinn posterior bite-wing instrument technique (Fig. 15-135); and (2) bite-wing tab technique (Fig. 15-136).

Hand and Wrist Radiography

Assessment of Skeletal Maturation

The level of biological development of

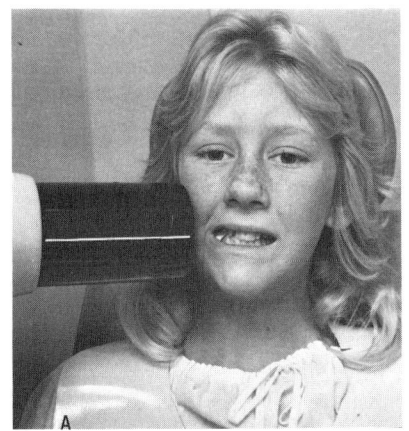

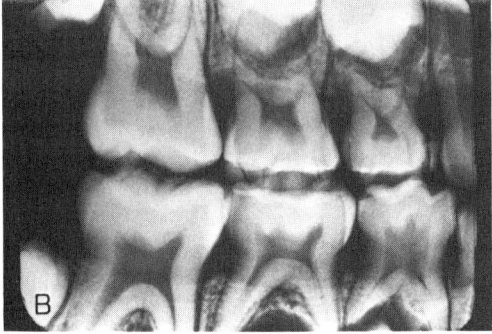

Figure 15-136. Bite-wing tab technic (ages 10-12 years). **(A)** Child (10-12 yeras) with bite-wing tab film in position; **(B)** PBW radiograph of child (10-12 years) in whch bite-wing tab was used.

a child is termed **skeletal maturation.** As a child matures, skeletal maturation and growth may vary from the child's **chronological age.** Therefore, a child's chronological age is an unreliable guide in determining how far the child has progressed toward maturity. **Skeletal maturation** can be identified most readily by the transformation of fibrous tissue and cartilage into bone. As the skeleton grows, every bone goes through a series of changes that can be recorded conventionally by a radiograph as soon as the mineral content of the osseous centers becomes high enough.

Ideally, radiographs of the entire skeleton should be studied before skeletal maturation is estimated. In daily practice this would be impractical, and it is an unnecessary use of x-radiation. For this reason, a small and convenient segment of the skeleton, commonly the hand and wrist, is considered representative of the entire skeleton in the assessment of skeletal maturation. It should be kept in mind that there are potential errors in this practice: (1) the velocity of ossification may not be uniform in different regions of the skeleton of a single healthy child or in the same analogous bones of different healthy children of the same age; (2) there may be considerable differences in development of the same portion of the skeleton on different sides of the same child; and (3) there may be different maturation levels of various bones in the same portion of the skeleton, such as the hand and wrist. However **hand and wrist radiographs** offer the most practical and accurate methods for assessing skeletal maturation.

Evaluation of Hand and Wrist Radiographs

The evaluation of hand and wrist radiographs is based on the centers of ossification in the hand and wrist. These bone centers serve as an index of the skeletal maturation of the patient when compared with known standards. One of the better known standards is the **Greulich and Pyle Atlas,** which is a series of sequential radiographic standards based on hand and wrist radiographs of over 1,000 children living in Cleveland, Ohio. The basic procedure for using hand and wrist radiographs to assess a child's skeletal maturation is to match the hand-wrist radiograph of a child being studied to the standard it resembles most closely. This is called the

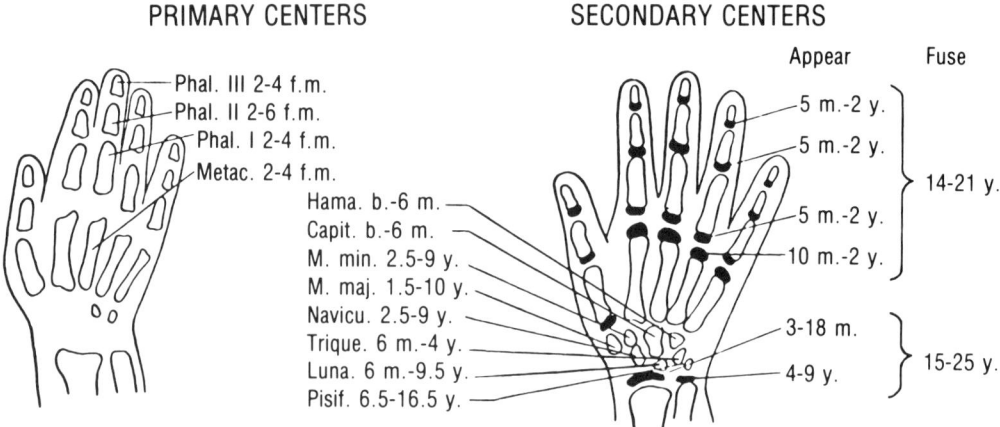

f.m. = fetal months; b. = birth; m. = postnatal months; y. = years

A

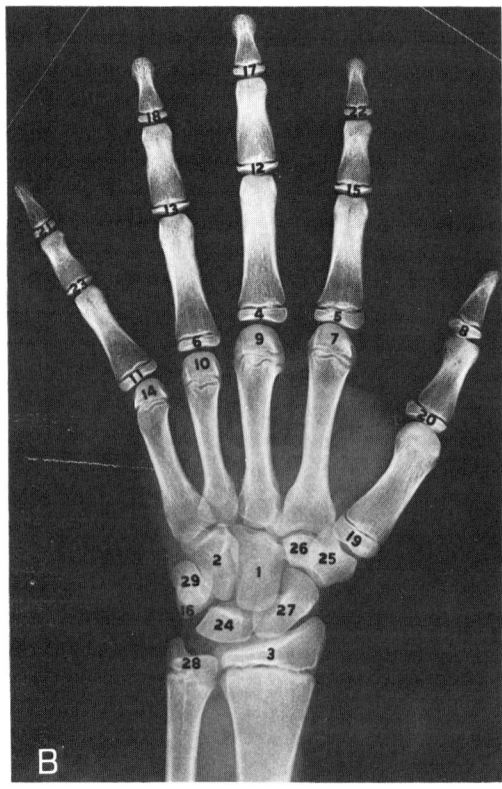

Figure 15-137. (A) Development of bones of hand and wrist. (From Marshall, David: Radiographic correlation of hand and wrist, and tooth development. Dent Radiogr Photogr 49 (3): 1976. Copyright Eastman Kodak Company, Rochester, NY.) (B) Individual carpals and epiphyses of hand and wrist. The individual carpals and epiphyses in the hand opposite are numbered approximately in the order in which their ossification begins: 1, capitate; 2, hamate; 3, distal epiphysis of the radius: 4,* epiphysis of proximal phalanx of the third digit; 5,* epiphysis of proximal phalanx of the second digit; 6,* epiphysis of proximal phalanx of the fourth digit; 7, epiphysis of the second metacarpal; 8, epiphysis of distal phalanx of the first digit; 9, epiphysis of the third metacarpal; 10, epiphysis of the fourth metacarpal; 11, epiphysis of proximal phalanx of the fifth digit; 12, epiphysis of middle phalanx of the third digit; 13, epiphysis of middle phalanx of the fourth digit; 14, epiphysis of the fifth metacarpal; 15; epiphysis of middle phalanx of the second digit; 16, triquetral; 17, epiphysis of distal phalanx of the third digit; 18, epiphysis of distal phalanx of the fourth digit; 19, epiphysis of the first metacarpal; 20,* epiphysis of proximal phalanx of the first

*Irregularities in the order of appearance are most apt to occur in those centers indicated by asterisks.

digit; 21, epiphysis of distal phalanx of the fifth digit; 22, epiphysis of distal phalanx of the second digit; 23,* epiphysis of middle phalanx of the fifth digit; 24,* lunate; 25,* trapezium; 26,* trapezoid; 27,* scaphoid; 28, distal epiphysis of the ulna; 29, pisiform; 30, sesamoid of adductor pollicis (the sesamoid of flexor pollicis brevis is visible through the head of the first metacarpal, just below the numeral 2 on the epiphysis of the proximal phalanx of the thumb). (From Greulich, W. W.; and Pyle, S. I.: *Radiographic Atlas of Skeletal Development of Hand and Wrist,* 2nd edition, Stanford, California, (C) 1950, 1959 by the Board of Trustees of the Leland Stanford Junior University. With the permission of the publishers, Stanford University Press.)

inspection-comparison method. If the skeletal maturation age for the child coincides with the chronological age, all is supposedly well. The hand-wrist radiograph indicates the level of maturation (not growth) of the bony skeleton, by the numbers of centers of ossification present plus the stage of activity of the epiphyses (Fig. 15-137).

Mean Skeletal Maturational Level

Since no bone in the hand-wrist matures at an even rate, because of genetic variability, it is better to calculate a **mean skeletal maturational level** for each child. With this method the skeletal maturational level for each bone is assigned a number of months by comparing it with a known standard. The mean skeletal maturational level is determined by dividing the total number of months by the number of bones evaluated; this number is compared with the chronological age to give an assessment of biological maturity (Fig 15-138).

In clinical practice the major uses of the hand and wrist radiograph are (1) to predict adult height of growing children;

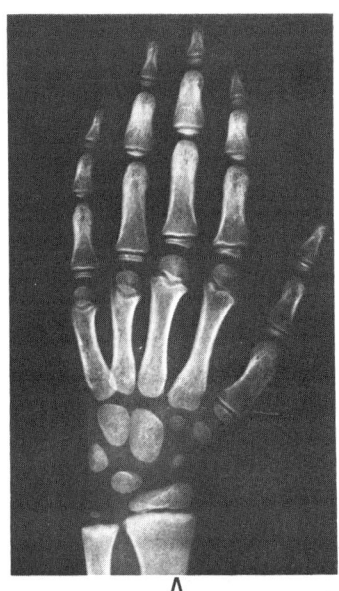

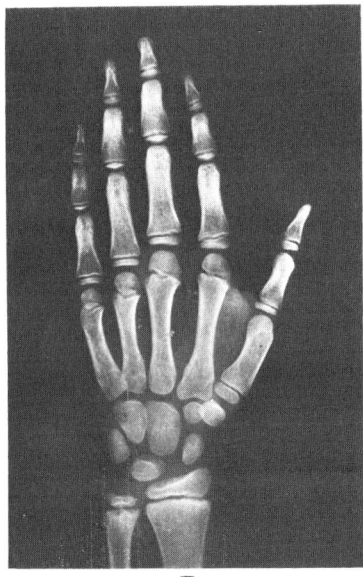

Figure 15-138. Hand and wrist radiographs of two children. **(A)** six years; **(B)** nine years. (Note difference in carpal development.)

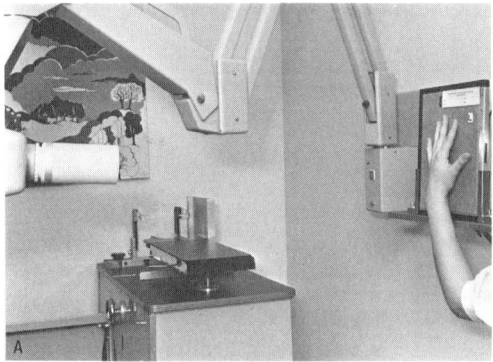

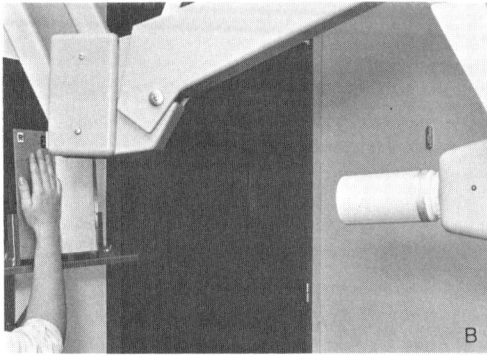

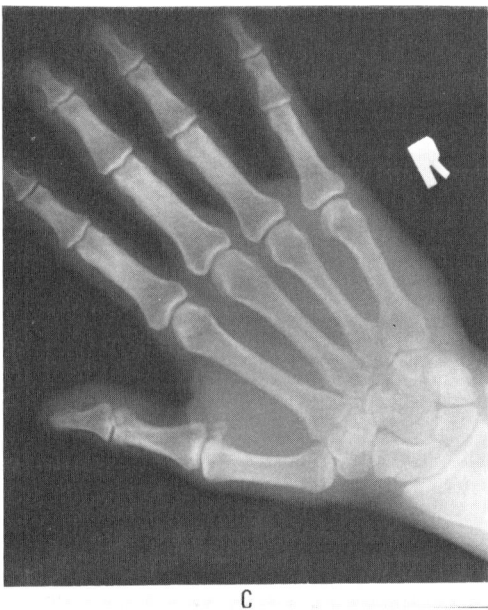

Figure 15-139. Technical factors in taking hand and wrist. **(A)** Patient's hand in position for radiograph. **(B)** Method for radiographing both hands on one 8 × 10 inch radiograph using a lead sheet. **(C)** Radiograph of hand and wrist.

(2) to predict age at which menarche will occur; and (3) to detect pathologic conditions associated with abnormalities of osseous development.

The hand-wrist radiograph is limited in predicting **late craniofacial growth.** Usually this growth occurs after the epiphyseal fusion in the hand-wrist film. Late craniofacial growth may have an influence on the facial profile of the child. Although skeletal maturation may have some affect on the development of the dentition, it has been found that there is no high degree of correlation between the two (Anderson et al., 1975). Dental development was found to be more strongly related to the **height and weight** of the child in both sexes than to **skeletal maturation.**

Posteroanterior View of Hand and Wrist (Technique)

1. The hand should be placed palm down on an 8 by 10 inch cassette (Fig. 15-139).
2. The fingers should be spread slightly and completely extended, and in good contact with the cassette.
3. The central ray should pass through the metacarpophalangeal joint.
4. Great care should be exercised to obtain an accurate view of the tufted ends of the distal phalanges as well as the shafts of the phalanges, since many of the pathologic conditions of a systemic type will first produce minute and very important changes in these structures.
5. All structures are shown in the straight posteroanterior projection except the thumb, in which case an oblique is obtained.

Cephalometric Technic

CASSETTE SIZE:	8 × 10 inch
SCREENS:	High Speed
FILM:	Kodak Blue RP
SOURCE-FILM DISTANCE:	66 inches
kVp-mA:	65 kVp, 15 mA
EXPOSURE TIME:	24 impulses

Table 15-VII
TECHNICAL FACTORS

Cassette	8 × 10 inch (Kodak X-Omatic C-2)	8 × 10 inch (Kodak min-R)
Screens	Kodak Lanex Reg.	Kodak Single Lanex Fine
Film	Kodak Ortho-G film	Kodak Min-R Film
Source-Film Distance	40 inches	40 inches
kVp, mA	70 kVp, 10 mA	70 kVp, 10 mA
Exposure Time	5 impulses, 1/12 sec.	100 impulses, 1 2/3 seconds

XERORADIOGRAPHY

Xeroradiography is the production of a visible image utilizing the charged surface of a photoconductor (amorphous selenium) as the image receptor, partially dissipating the charge by exposure to x-rays to form a latent image, and making the latent image visible by xerographic processing. Xeroradiography was invented by a physicist, Chester F. Carlson, in 1937, followed by Xerox Corporation developing a highly automated system (Xerox® 125 Medical System) that allowed radiologists to make practical clinical use of this type of x-ray imaging. Xeroradiography has been used for medical diagnosis since 1970, for many types of radiographic examinations, particularly for mammography. During the latter part of the 1970s a new xerographic unit has been designed specifically for dental intraoral use by Xerox Medical Systems, called the Xerox® 110 (Fig. 15-140).

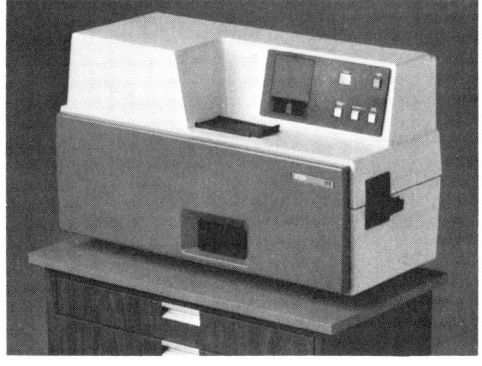

Figure 15-140. Xerox 110. (Courtesy of Xerox Med. Systems, Pasadena, CA.)

General Principles of Dental Xeroradiography

Xeroradiography is a complex electrostatic process based on a special mate-

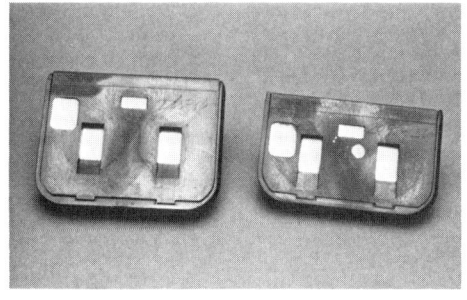

Figure 15-141. Xeroradiographic cassette. Reusable No. 2 XR cassette (actual size)

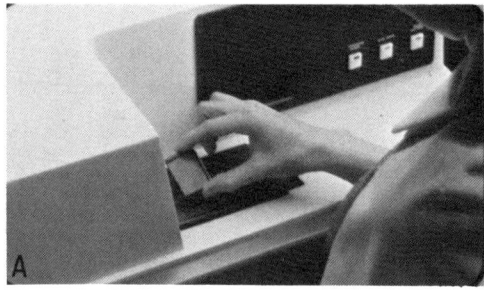
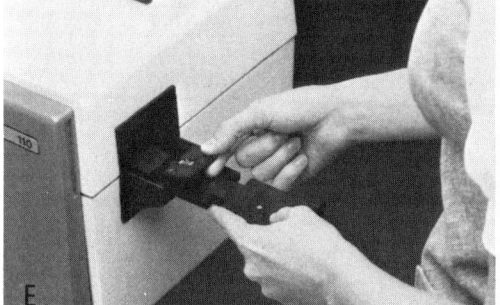
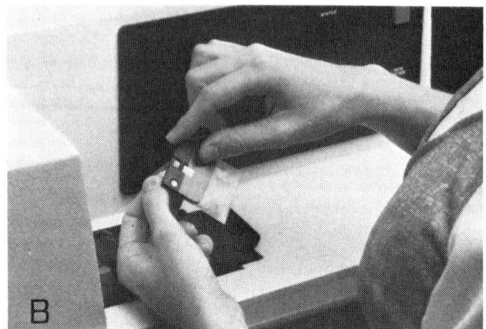
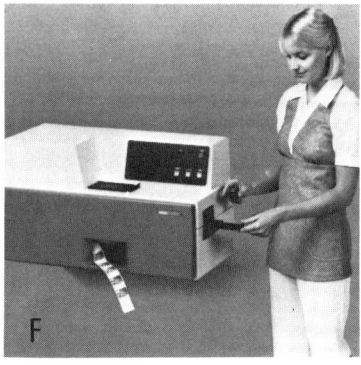
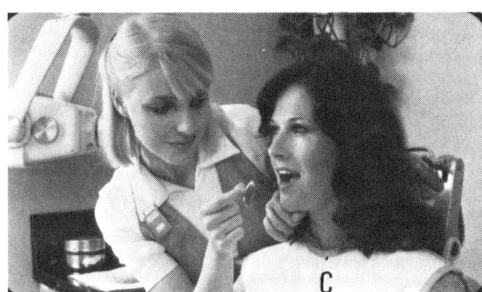
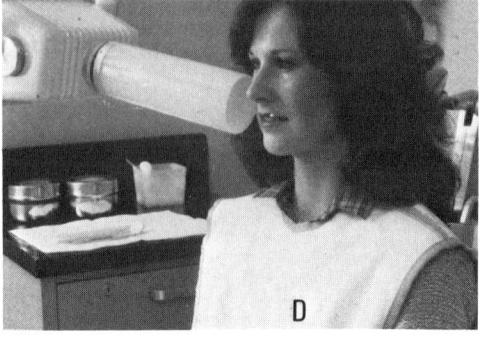
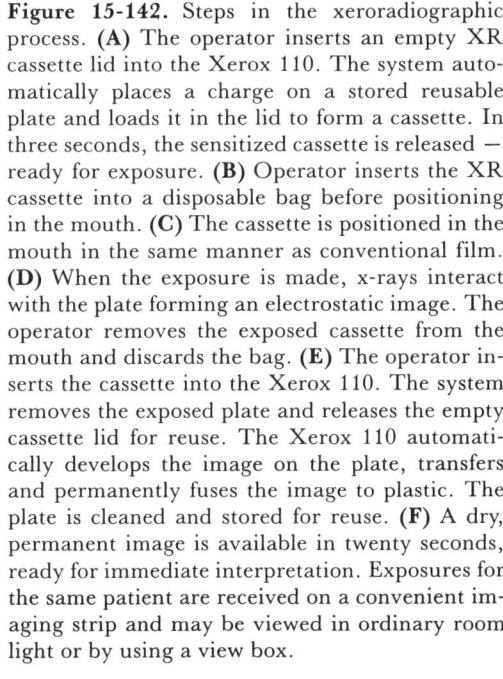

Figure 15-142. Steps in the xeroradiographic process. (A) The operator inserts an empty XR cassette lid into the Xerox 110. The system automatically places a charge on a stored reusable plate and loads it in the lid to form a cassette. In three seconds, the sensitized cassette is released — ready for exposure. (B) Operator inserts the XR cassette into a disposable bag before positioning in the mouth. (C) The cassette is positioned in the mouth in the same manner as conventional film. (D) When the exposure is made, x-rays interact with the plate forming an electrostatic image. The operator removes the exposed cassette from the mouth and discards the bag. (E) The operator inserts the cassette into the Xerox 110. The system removes the exposed plate and releases the empty cassette lid for reuse. The Xerox 110 automatically develops the image on the plate, transfers and permanently fuses the image to plastic. The plate is cleaned and stored for reuse. (F) A dry, permanent image is available in twenty seconds, ready for immediate interpretation. Exposures for the same patient are received on a convenient imaging strip and may be viewed in ordinary room light or by using a view box.

rial called a **photoconductor,** which will not conduct an electric current when shielded from radiation but becomes conductive when exposed to radiation such as light waves or x-rays. **Amorphorous selenium** is the photoconductor used in xeroradiography. The image receptor in dental xeroradiography consists of an aluminum-based plate that is coated with a selenium alloy and protected by a plastic lightproof cassette. This is analogous to the radiographic film in conventional radiography (Fig. 15-141).

Steps of Xerographic Process

1. The imaging plate is activated so a uniform charge is deposited on the selenium. This sensitizes the plate before exposure to x-rays (Fig. 15-142A).
2. The xeroradiographic dental cassette is exposed to x-rays just as any other intraoral technique. The x-rays reaching the selenium plate cause the selenium to lose its charge in an amount corresponding to the intensity of the x-ray beam, which results in an electrostatic latent image on the plate (Fig. 15-142B, C, D).
3. The latent image is made visible by exposing the selenium plate to fine powder particles (called "toner") that are attracted to areas on the plate in proportion to the intensity of the charge (Fig. 15-142E).
4. The powder image is transferred mechanically from the selenium surface by placing suitable paper (clear adhesive tape) in contact with the plate and using an electrostatic charge to attract the toner away from the selenium plate.
5. The powder image is fused to an opaque substitute for viewing by exposure of tape to heat, which fuses the image to the tape (Fig. 15-142F).
6. The xeroradiographic image may be viewed either in reflected light or as a photograph or by transmitted light from an illuminator (Fig. 15-143).

Benefits of Xeroradiography

1. The Xerox processor may be located near the x-ray machine for convenient access to the operator. This practically eliminates the need for a darkroom.
2. It delivers a dry, ready-to-read image in only twenty seconds. This provides the operator opportunity to examine the image without delay to determine if additional projections or retakes are required.
3. It is capable of producing images superior in diagnostic quality to conventional radiography. This results primarily from the property of **edge enhancement** inherent in the xeroradiographic process, which accentuates small differences in density of two adjacent structures.
4. Preliminary xeroradiographic studies indicate that the exposure to patients may be reduced by a factor of two or three from conventional radiography.

Disadvantages of Dental Xeroradiography

1. The cassettes are rigid and thicker than conventional film. This makes it more difficult for placement and reten-

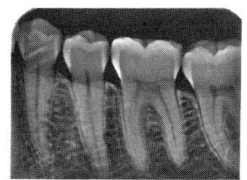 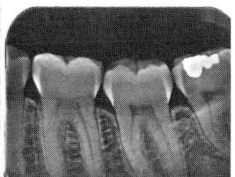

Figure 15-143. Sample of xeroradiographic image processed by Xerox 110 at Xerox Corp, Pasadena, California factor in 1980.

tion of the image receptor intraorally.
2. The cassettes have to be reused. This may not be a disadvantage, but they are difficult to sterilize. Each cassette has to be individually wrapped in sterile, disposable plastic bags.
3. The system is limited to No. 1 and No. 2 size films. If other sizes of film are to be processed, a darkroom for conventinal processing must be maintained.
4. With a new image system such as this, there are difficulties encountered in distinguishing artifacts from pathologic conditions. Occasionally, artifacts are seen that obscure the detail of the image. Also, there is occasionally seen radiolucent artifacts around a portion of metallic restorations and adjacent surfaces of enamel that suggest recurrent caries.
5. The dental xeroradiographic unit (Xerox 110) has been in production for two years now; however, there seems to be a lag in nationwide distribution of the unit, suggesting problems in maintenance and repair.

Bibliography

Acheson, R. M.; Vicinus, J. H.; and Fowler, G. B.: Studies in the reliability of assessing skeletal maturity from x-rays. Part III. Greulich-Pyle atlas and Tanner-Whitehouse method contrasted. *Hum Biol, 38*:204, 1966.

Adelson, J. J.: Handicapped and problem patient: Radiodontic examination and treatment. *Dent Radiogr Photogr,* (2): 27-45, 1961.

Anderson, D. L.; Thompson, G. W.; and Popovich, F.: Interrelationships of dental maturity, skeletal maturity, height and weight from age 4 to 14 years. *Growth, 39*:453, 1975.

Andrews, J. R.: Planigraphy. 1. Introduction and history. *Am J Roentg Radium Ther, 36*:575, 1936.

Bambha, J. K.; and Van Natta, P.: A longitudinal study of occlusion and tooth eruption in relation to skeletal maturation. *Am J Orthod, 45*:847, 1959.

Bambha, J. K.; and Van Natta, P.: Longitudinal study of facial growth in relation to skeletal maturation during adolescence. *Am J Orthod, 49*:481, 1963.

Barber, T.K.: Roentgenographic techniques for children. *Dent Clin North Am,* 549, November 1961.

Baume: The direct analysis of cephalometric x-ray films. *Angle Orthod,* 171-177, July, 1957.

Berry, H. M.: Lipiodol in Roentgenographic interpretation. *Oral Surg, 2*:1474, 1949.

Berry, H. M.: Roentgenologic aspects of oral surgical problems. *J Oral Surg, 10*:194, 1952.

Berry, H.M.: Roentgenographic examination. *Current Therapy in Dentistry,* Vol. 2. St. Louis, Mosby, 1966, pp. 331-365.

Biesterfeld, R. C.; Taintor, J. F.; and Alcox, R. W.: Diagnostic radiographic aspects in endodontics. *Dent Radiogr Photogr, 53*(2):21, 1980.

Binnie, W. H.; et al.: Applications of xeroradiography in dentistry. *J Dent, 3*(3):99, 1975.

Blady, J. V.; and Hocker, A. F.: Sialography, its technique and application in the roentgen study of neoplasm of the parotid gland. *Surg Gynecol Obstet, 67*:777, 1938.

Blady, J. V.; and Hocker, A. F.: The application of sialography in non-neoplastic diseases of the parotid gland. *Radiology, 32*:131, 1939.

Blaschke, D. D.: Morphology, growth and maturation. In Saunders, B. (Ed.): *Pediatric Oral and Maxillofacial Surgery.* St. Louis, Mosby, 1979.

Blaschke, D. D.: Arthrographhy of the temporomandibular joint. In Solberg, W. K.; and Clark, G. T. (Eds.): *Temporomandibular Joint Problems: Biological Diagnosis and Treatment.* Berlin, Quintessance International, 1980.

Blaschke, D. D.; Solberg, W. K.; and Saunders, B.: Arthrograpy of the temporomandibular joint: Review of current status. *J Am Dent Assoc, 100*:388, 1980.

Blatt, I. M.; Magrelski, J. E.; Maxwell, J. H.; and Holt, J. F.: Secretory sialography in diseases external to major salivary glands. *Ann Otol Rhinol Laryngol, 68*:175, 1959.

Bloom, W. L.; Hollenbach, J. L.; and Morgan, J. A.: *Medical Radiographic Technic,* 3rd ed. Springfield, Charles C Thomas, 1969.

Boag, J. W.; Stacey, A. J.; and Davis, R.: Radiation exposure to the patient in xeroradiography. *Br J Radiol, 49*:253, 1976.

Braham, R. L.; and Morris, M. E.: *Textbook of Pediatric Dentistry.* Baltimore, Williams & Wilkins, 1980.

Brandrup-Wognsen, T.: A method of producing

roentgenograms of the temporomandibular joint. *J Prosthet Dent,* 5:93, 1955.

Broadbent, B. Holly: A new technique and its application to orthodontia. *Angle Orthod, 1:*45, 1931.

Brodie, A. C.; et al.: Cephalometric appraisal of orthodontic results. *Angle Orthod, 8:*162-182, 261-351, 1938.

Caldwell, E. W.: Skiagraphy of the accessory sinuses of the nose. *Am O Roentgenol,* 27(2):1906.

Campbell, W.: Clinical radiological investigations of the temporomandibular joints. *Br J Radiol, 38:*401, 1965.

Carlin; and Seldon: Sialography: A useful aid in diagnosing parotid tumors. *J Oral Surg,* 25:139, 1967.

Castigliano, S. G.: Sialography of the submaxillary gland: A new technique. *AJR, 187:*385, 1962.

Catell, S. M.: *Dentition as a Measure of Maturity.* Harvard Monogr Educ No 9, Cambridge, Mass, Harvard University Press, 1928.

Chayes, C.; and Finkelstein, G.: A technique for temporomandibular joint roentgenography. *J Prosthet Dent,* 6:822, 1956.

Cheppe, E.: Tabulation and analysis of the results of x-ray examinations of edentulous mouths. *Northwestern U Dent Res Grad Q Bull,* 12-15, February 3, 1936.

Chisholm, D. M.; Blair, G. S.; Low, P. S.; and Whaley, K.: Hydrostatic sialography as an index of salivary gland disease in Sjorgren's syndrome. *Acta Radiol, 11:*577, 1971.

Christensen, E. E.; Curry, T. S.; and Dowdey, J. E.: *An Introductin to the Physics of Diagnostic Radiology,* 2nd ed. Philadelphia, Lea & Febiger, 1978, pp. 308-327.

Clark, C. A.: A method of ascertaining the relative position of unerupted teeth by means of film radiography. *Odonto Sec Royal Soc Med Trans* 3:87-89, 1909.

Coin, C. G.: Tomography of the temporomandibular joint. *Dent Radiogr Photogr,* 47(2):23-28, 33, 1974.

Coin, C. G.: Tomography of the temporomandibular joint. *Med Radiogr Photogr, 50:*26, 1974.

Cook, T. J.: Statistics obtained by clinical and roentgenographic examinationsof 500 edentulous and particlly edentulous mouths. *Dental Cosmos, 69:*349, 1927.

Cook and Pollack: Sialography: Pathologic-radiologic correlation. *Oral Surg, 21:*559, 1966.

Davis, J. M.; Law; and Lewis: *An Atlas of Pedodontics,* 2nd ed. Philadelphia, Saunders, 1980.

Davis, R.; et al.: The role of xeroradiography in cephalometric radiology. *J Dent* 5(1):32, 1977.

Del Rio, C. E.; Canales, M. L.; and Preece, J. W.: *A Radiographic Technique for Endodontics.* San Antonio, University of Texas Health Science Center at San Antonio, 1982.

Demirjan, A.; Goldsmith, H.; and Tanner, J. M.: A new system of dental age assessment. *Hum Biol, 45:*211, 1973.

Doane, H.F.: Roentgenographic technic and interpretation in fractures of the jaws and facial bones. *J Oral Surg,* 12, 1954.

Dolan, K. D.: Radiographic anatomy of nasal sinuses. *Otolaryngol Clin North Am,* 4:13, 1971.

Dolwick, F.; et al.: Arthrotomograhic evaluation of the temporomandibular joint. *J Oral Surg,* 37:793, 1979.

Donaldson, R. G.: Lateral-jaw radiography (All posterior teeth on a single film). *Dent Radiogr Photogr,* 35(3):58, 1962.

Donovan: Occlusal radiography of the mandibular third molars. *Dent Radiogr Photogr,* 25(3):53, 1952.

Downs, W. B.: Cephalometrics in orthodontic case analysis and diagnosis. *Am J Orthod, 38:*162, 1952.

Drevattene, T.; and Stiris, G.: Sialography by means of a polyethylene catheter and water soluble constrast medium (Isopaque 75%). *Br J Radiol,* 1:37, 1964.

Ennis, L. M.; Berry, H. M.; and Phillips, J. E.: *Dental Roentgenology,* 6th ed. Philadelphia, Lea & Febiger, 1967, pp. 265-273.

Epsteen, C. M.: Sialography: non-irritating medium. *Am J Surg* 92:603, 1956.

Eusterman, M. F.: Roentgenographic findings in 290 partially edentulous or edentulous mouths. *Dental Cosmos, 63:*901, 1921.

Farrar, W.: Diagnosis and treatment of anterior dislocation of the articular disc. *NY Dent J, 41:*348, 1971.

Farrar, W.: Characteristics of the condylar path in internal derangements of the TMJ. *J Prosthet Dent, 39:*319, 1978.

Farrar, W. B.; and McCarty, W. L. (Directors): *Outline of Temporomandibular Joint Diagnosis and Treatment.* Montgomery, AL, Normandie Study Group, March 1978.

Farrar, W. B.; and McCarty, W. L.: Inferior joint space arthrography and characteristics of condylar paths in internal derangements of the TMJ. *J Prosthet Dent, 41:*548, 1979.

Feasby, W. H.: The number and types of films necessary for a satisfactory radiological survey for children. *J Dent Child,* 91. 2nd Quarter, 1960.

Ferguson, M. M.; et al.: Application of xeroradiography in sialography. *Int J Oral Surg,* 5:176, 1976.

Forrester, D. J.: *Pediatric Dental Medicine.* Philadelphia, Lea & Febiger, 1981.

Gardner, B. S.; and Stafne, E. C.: Incidence of failure in the removal of teeth. *Am Dent Surg,* 49:321, 1929.

Garn, S.M.; Lewis, A.B.; and Blizzard, R.M.: Endocrine factors in dental development. *J Dent Res,* 44(Suppl):243, 1965.

Garusi, G. F.: The salivary glands in radiological diagnosis. In *Bibl Radiol Fasc 4.* New York, S. Karger-Basel, 1964.

Gillis, R. R.: Roentgen-ray study of the temporomandibular articulation. *J Am Dent Assoc,* 22:1321, 1935.

Glasser, O. (Ed.): *The Science of Radiology.* Springfield, Charles C Thomas, 1933.

Glassman, L. M.; O'Hara, A. E.; and Cregar, D.: Xerosialography. *Arch Otolaryngol,* 100(5):341, 1974.

Graber, T. M.: New horizons in case analysis: Clinical cephalometrics. *Am J Orthod,* 38:603, 1952.

Grant, R.; and Lating, R. T.: Improved technic for roentgenographic examination of temporomandibular joint and condyle. *J Oral Surg,* 11:95, 1958.

Gratt, B.; Sickles, E. A.; and Parks, C. R.: Xeroradiography of dental structures. Preliminary investigations. *Oral Surg,* 44(1):148, 1977.

Gratt, B; Sickles, E. A.; and Parks, C. R.: Xeroradiography of dental structures. Image analysis. *Oral Surg,* 46(1):156, 1978.

Gratt, B.; Sickles, E. A.; and Parks, C. R.: Use of intraoral cassettes for dental xeroradiography. *Oral Surg,* 46:717, 1978.

Gratt, B. M.; Xeroradiography of dental structures. Pilot clinical studies. *Oral Surg,* 48(3):276, 1979.

Gratt, B. M.; Sickles, E. A.; and Nguyen, N. T.: Dental xerogradiography for endodontics: A rapid x-ray system that produces high-quality images. *J Endodontics,* 5:266, 1979.

Gratt, B. M.; White, S.; Sickles, E. A.; and Jeromin, L.: Imaging properties of intraoral dental xeroradiography. *J Am Dent Assoc,* 99:805, 1979.

Green, D.: Morphology of the pulp cavity of the permanent teeth. *Oral Surg,* 8:743, 1955.

Greig, J. H.; and Musaph, F. W.: A method of radiological demonstration of the temporomandibular joints using the Orthopantomograph. *Radiology,* 106:307, 1973.

Grewcock, R. J. G.: A simplified technique of temporomandibular joint radiography. *Br Dent J,* 94:152, 1953.

Grove, A.S.; and DiChiro, G.: Salivary gland scanning with technetium 99m pertechnetate. *AJR,* 102:109, 1968.

Gruelich, N. W.; and Pyle, S. L.: *Radiographic Atlas of Skeletal Development of the Hand and Wrist,* 2nd ed. Stanford, CA, Stanford University Press, reprinted 1970.

Gustafson, G.; and Koch, G.: Age estimation up to 16 years of age based on dental development. *Odontol Revy,* 25:297, 1974.

Haavikko, K.: Tooth formation age estimated on a few selected teeth; A simple method for clinical use. *Proc Finn Dent Soc,* 70:15, 1974.

Hanah, R.: Technique for lateral jaw radiographs. *Alumni Bull Indiana School Dent.* p. 11, February 28, 1955.

Hayden J.; and Richards, A.: Procedures for adequate radiographs of preschool children. *J Dent Child,* p. 70, 2nd Quarter, 1955.

Hettwer, K. J.; and Folsom, T. C.: The normal sialogram. *Oral Surg,* 26:790, 1968.

Hofrath, H.: Die Bedeutung der Rontgenfern und Abstrandsanfrauhe fur die Diagnostiks der Kieferanomalian. *Fortschr Orthodont,* 1:232, 1931.

Hotz, R.: The relations of dental calcification to chronological and skeletal age. *Trans Euro Ortho Soc,* 1959.

Hurst, R.; et al.: Landmark identification accuracy in xeroradiographic cephlometry. *Am J Orthod* 73(5):568, 1978.

Hyman, J.; and Bakker, V.: Xeroradiographic detection of tooth and bone pathology. *Oral Surg,* 47:482, 1979.

Jacoby, C. A.: *X-ray Technology,* 2nd ed. St. Louis, Mosby, 1960.

Jeromin, L. S.; et al.: Xeroradiography for intraoral dental radiology: A process description. *Oral Surg,* 49:178, 1980.

Johnson, N. A.: Xeroradiography for cephalometric analysis. *Am J Orthod,* 69(5):524, 1976.

Johnston, F. E.; Hufham, H. P.; Moreschi, A. F.; and Terry, G.P.: Skeletal maturation and cephalofacial development. *Angle Orthod,* 35:1, 1965.

Kalisher, L.; Olson, D. F.; and Guralnick, W. C.: The application of xeroradiography in the diagnosis of maxillofacial problems. *J Can Assoc Radiol,* 27(1):52, 1976.

Katzberg, R. W.; et al.: Arthrotomography of the temporomandibular joint. *AJR, 134*:955, 1980.

Katzberg, R. W.; Burgener, F. A.; and Fischer, H. W.: Evaluation of various contrast agents for improved arthrography. *Invest Radiol, 11*:528, 1976.

Katzberg, R. W.; Dolwick, M. F.; Bales, D. J.; and Helms, C. A.: Arthrotomography of the temporomandibular joint: New technique and preliminary observations. *AJR, 132*:949, 1979.

Keller, E. E.; Sather, A. H.; and Hayles, A. B.: Dental and skeletal development in various endocrine and metabolic diseases. *J Am Dent Assoc, 81*:415, 1970.

Kiehn, C. L.: Menisectomy for internal derangement of temporomandibular joint. *Am J Surg, 83*:364, 1952.

Kieffer, J.: The laminagraph and its variations: Applications and implications of the planigraphic principles. *AJR, 39*:497, 1938.

Kimm, H. T.; Spies, J. W.; and Wolfe, J. J.: Sialography, with particular reference to neoplastic diseases. *AJR, 34*:289, 1935.

Klein, I. I.; Blatterfein, L.; and Miglino, J. C.: Comparison of the fidelity of radiographs of mandibular condyles made by different technques. *J Prosthet Dent, 24*(4):419, 1970.

Lamons, F. F.; and Gray, S. W.: A study of the relationship between teeth eruption age, skeletal development age and chronological age in sixty-one Atlanta children. *Am J Orthod, 44*:687, 1958.

Lapinskas, V. A.; and Lapinskene, A. V.: Xeroradiography and the prospects of its use in stomatology. *Stomatologiia (Mosk), 47*:35, 1968.

Lauterstein, A. M.: A cross-sectional study in dental development and skeletal age. *J Am Dent Assoc, 62*:35, 1961.

Law, D. B.; Lewis, T. M.; and Davis, J. M.: *An Atlas of Pedodontics*. Philadelphia, Saunders, 1969.

Leinonen, A.; Wasz-Hockert, B.; and Vuorinen, P.: Usefulness of the dental age obtained by orthopantomography as an indicator of the physical age. *Proc Finn Dent Soc, 68*:235, 1972.

Lewis, G. R.: Temporomandibular joint radiographic technics: comparison and evaluation of results. *Dent Radiogr Photogr, 37*(1), 1964.

Libequrst, B.; and Welander, U.: Sialography, new application of subtraction technique. *Acta Radiol [Diag], 8*:228, 1969.

Lindblom, G.: Technique for roentgenphotographic registration of the different condyle positions in the temporomandibular joint. *Dental Cosmos, 78*:1227, 1936.

Liverud, K.: Sialographic technique with a polyethylene catheter. *Br J Radiol, 32*:627, 1959.

Lopez, J.: Xeroradiography in dentistry. *J Am Dent Assoc, 92*(1):106, 1976.

Lozier, M.: Periapical roentgenography as applied in children. *Oral Surg, 3*:58-62, 1950.

Lozier, M.: Significance of extraoral roentgenography of the mandible in general practice. *Oral Surg,* 1168-1171, September, 1950.

Lunt, R. C.; and Law, D. B.: A review of the chronology of eruptin of deciduous teeth. *J Am Dent Assoc, 89*:872, 1974.

Lusted, L. B.; and Keats, T.: *Atlas of Roentgenographic Measurement*. Chicago, Year Bk Med, 1967.

Lynch, T. P.; and Chase, D. C.: Arthrography in the evaluation of the temporomandibualr joint. *Radiology, 126*:667, 1978.

McQueen, W. W.: Radiography of the temporomandibular joint articulations. *Minneapolis District Dent J, 21*:28, 1937.

Mainland, D.: Evaluation of the skeletal age method of estimating children's development. I. Systematic errors in the assessment of roentgenograms *Pediatrics, 12*:1124, 1953.

Mainland, D.: Evaluation of the skeletal age method of estimating children's development. II. Variable errors in the assessement of roentgenograms. *Pediatrics, 13*:165, 1954.

Mainland, D.: Evaluation of the skeletal age method of estimating children's develoment. III. Comparison of measurement and inspection in the assessment of roentgenograms. *Pediatrics, 20*:979, 1957.

Manashil, G. B.: Sialography: A simple procedure. *Med Radiogr Photogr, 52*(2):1976.

Manson-Hing, L.: Utilization of extraoral roentgenographic technics in general dental practice. *Dent Clin North Am,* 437, July, 1961.

Manson-Hing, L.: Use of dental x-rays in roentgenography of the palatopharyngeal mechanism. *Oral Surg,* September, 1970.

Marshall, D.: Radiographic correlation of hand, wrist and tooth develoment. *Dent Radiogr Photogr, 49*(3), 1976.

Martini, J.: Maxillofacial radiography. *Oral Surg, 3*(12):1540, December, 1950.

Matlock, J.: In McDonald, R. E.: *Dentistry for the Child Adolescent*, 2nd ed. St. Louis, Mosby, 1974.

Matthews, G. W.: Value of the occlusal roentgenogram in locating impacted mandibular third molars. *J Am Dent Assoc, 42*:515,

1951.

Maves, T. W.: Radiology of the temporomandibular articulation with correct registration of vertical dimension for reconstruction. *J Am Dent Assoc,* 1938; *Dental Cosmos,* 1938.

Medwedeff, F. M.; and Elcan, P. D.: A precision technic to minimize radiation. *Dent Surv,* October, 1967.

Meine, F.; and Woloshin, H. J.: Radiologic diagnosis of salivary gland tumors. *Radiol Clin North Am,* 475-485, 1970.

Merill, V. *Atlas of Roentgenographic Positions.* St. Louis, Mosby, 1949.

Meschan, I.: *Normal Radiographic Anatomy.* Philadelphia, Saunders, 1959.

Mikulicz, J.: Concerning peculiar symmetrical disease of lacrimal and salivary glands. *M Classics,* 2:165, 1937-38.

Mink, J. R.: Dental care for the handicapped child. *Current Therapy in Dentistry,* Vol. 2. St. Louis, Mosby, 1966, pp. 736-767.

Mitchel, D., Jr.: Sialography. *J Okla State Med Assoc,* 56:316, 1963.

Molt, F. F.: Value of roentgenograms in edentulous mouths. *J Am Dent Assoc,* 12:788, 1925.

Morgan, D. H.: Mandibular joint pathology — importance of Radiographs. *Dent radiogr Photogr,* 43(1):3-11, 1970.

Norgaard, F.: Arthrography of the mandibular joint. *Acta Radiol,* 25:679, 1944.

Norgaard, F.: *Temporomandibular Orthography.* Copenhagen, E. Mundsgaard, 1947.

Ollerenshaw, R.; and Rose, S.: Sialography. *Dent Radiogr Photogr,* 33(4):93, 1957.

Olson, D. J.; Guralnick, W.; Kalisher, L.; and Donoff, R. B.: The application of xeroradiography in oral surgery. *J Oral Surg,* 34:438, 1976.

Osmer, J. C.; and Pleasants, J. E.: Distention sialography. *Radiology,* 86:116, 1966.

Pappas, G.; and Wallace, W.: Panoramic sialography. *Dent Radiogr Photogr,* (2): 1970.

Paquette, O. E.; Segall, R. O.; and Del Rio, C. E.: Modified film holder for endodontics. *J Endodontics* 5(5):158, 1979.

Park, W.; and Mason, D.: Hydrostatic sialography. *Radiology,* 86:116, 1966.

Pogorzelska-Stronczak, B.: The use of xeroradiography in dentistry. *Pol Rev Radiol Nucl Med,* 27:266, 1963.

Potter, G. D.; and Gold, R. P.: Radiographic analysis of the skull. *Med Radiogr Photogr,* 51(1):1975.

Poyton, H. G.: Radiogrpahic technique for third molars. *Br Dent J,* p. 241, April, 1958.

Prahl-Anderson, B.; and van der Linden, F. P. G. M.: The estimation of dental age. *Trans Eur Orthodont Soc,* 70:535, 1972.

Pryor, J. W.: The hereditary nature of variation in the ossification of bones. *Anat Rec* 1:84, 1907.

Pucini, A. J.: Roentgen ray anthropometry of the skull. *J Radiol,* 3:231, 1922.

Pyle, S. I.: Skeletal maturation: hand-wrist radiographic assessment. In Broadbent, B. H., Sr.; Broadbent, B. H., Jr.; and Golden, H., (Eds.): *Bolton Standards of Dentofacial Developmental Growth.* St. Louis, Mosby, 1975.

Pyle, S. I.; Waterhouse, A. M.; and Greulich, W. W.: *A Radiographic Standard of Reference for the Growing Hand and Wrist.* Cleveland, Pr of Case Western Reserve U, 1971.

Rabinov, K. R.; and Joffe, N.: A blunt-tip side-injecting cannula for sialography. *Radiology,* 92:1438, 1969.

Rapp, R.: Radiographic technics for children. *J Ontario Dent Assoc,* p. 19, December, 1959.

Rawls, H. R.; and Owen, W. D.: The dental prognosis for xeroradiography. *Oral Surg,* 33:476, 1972.

Richards, A.: Roentgenographic localization of the mandibular canal. *J Oral Surg,* 10:325, 1952.

Richards, A.: Technique for roentgenographic examination of impacted mandibular third molars. *J Oral Surg,* 10:138, 1952.

Richards, A. G.: The buccal object rule. *J Tenn State Dent Assoc,* 33:263, 1953.

Richards, A. G.: The buccal object rule. *Dent Radiogr Photogr,* 53(3):33-56, 1980.

Richards, A. G.; and Alling, C. C.: Extraoral radiography — mandible and temporomandibular articulation. *Dent Radiogr Photogr,* 28(1):1-7, 18, 19, 1955.

Ricketts, R.: Laminography in the diagnosis of temporomandibular joint disordgers. *J Am Dent Assoc,* 46:620, 1953.

Ricketts, R.: The role of cephalometrics in prosthetics diagnosis. *J Prosthet Dent,* 4:488, 1956.

Riesner, S.: The T-M joint, its roentgenographic diagnosis and clinical importance. *Arch Clin Oral Pathol,* 4:19, March, 1940.

Ritter, W.: Comparative studies on tomography of temporomandibular joint region. *Deutsche Zahn Mund und Kieferheilkunde,* 59:138, 1972.

Roche, A. F.: A comparison between Greulich-Pyle and Tanner-Whitehouse assessments of skeletal maturity. *Radiology,* 98:273, 1971.

Roche, A. F.; and Davila, G. H.: The reliability

of assessments of the maturity of individual hand-wrist bones. *Hum Biol, 48*:585, 1976.

Rosenberg, H. M.: Laminagraphy: Methods and application in oral diagnosis. *J Am Dent Assoc, 74*:88, 1967.

Rosenberg, H. M.; and Silha, R. E.: TMJ radiography with emphasis on tomography. *Dent Radiogr Photogr, 55*(1):1, 1982.

Schall, G. L.: The role of radionuclide scanning in the evaluation of neoplasms of the salivary glands: A review. *J Surg Oncol, 3*:701, 1971.

Schier, M.: Temporomadibular joint roentgenography: Controlled erect technics. *J Am Dent Assoc, 65*:456, 1962.

Schiver, W. R.; Swintak, E. F.; and Darlak, J. D.: Xerocephalography. *Oral Surg, 40*(6):705, 1975.

Shore, N.: *Occlusal Equilibration and T-M Joint Dysfunction.* Philadelphia, Lippincott, 1959, Chapter 8.

Sickles, E. A.; Genant, H. K.; and Doi, K.: Comparison of laboratory and clinical evaluations of mammographic screen-film systems. In *Application of Optical Instrumentation in Medicine.* Vol. 27. Bellingham, WA, Society of Photo-Optical Instrumentation Engineers, 1977, pp. 3-35.

Silver, C. M.; Simon, S. D.; and Savastano, A.: Meniscus injuries of the temporomandibular joint. *J Bone Joint Surg, 38A*:541, 1956.

Silver, C.M.; Simon, S.D.: Meniscus injuries of the temporomandibular joint. Further experience. *J Bone Joint Surg, 45A*:113, 1963.

Sjogren, H.: Zur Kenntnis des Keratoconjunctivitis sicca (Keratitis filiformis bei Hypofunktion der Tranendousen). *Acta Ophthalmol, 11*(Suppl 2):1-151, 1933.

Smith, E. S.: Findings in the roentgenograms of edentulous patients. *J Am Dent Assoc, 33*:584, 1946.

Smith, N. J.; and Harris, M.: Radiology of the temporomandibular joint and condylar head. *Br Dent J, 129*:261, 1970.

Snyder, B.; et al.: The advantages of xeroradiography for panoramic examination of the jaws and teeth. *J Periodontol, 48*(8):467, 1977.

Spataro, R. F.; Katzberg, R. W.; Burgener, F. A.; and Fischer, H. W.: Evaluation of epinephrine for arthrography. *Invest Radiol, 13*:286, 1978.

Spillman, R.: Early history of roentgenology of the sinuses. *AJR, 54*:643, 1965.

Steel, G. H.: The relation between dental maturation and physiological maturity. *Trans BSSO,* pp. 17-28, 1965.

Steinberg, A. D.; Braner, May L.; and May, B.: *Fortnightly Review, 41*:9-11, 1961.

Sulke, A. A.: Roentgenographic study of the mandibular joint. *J Oral Surg, 6*:299, 1948.

Swenson, H. M.: Roentgenographic examination of the edentulous mouth. *J Am Dent Assoc, 31*:475, 1944.

Tanner, J. M.; Whitehouse, R. H.; and Healy, M. J. R.: *A new system for estimating skeletal maturity from the head and wrist with standards derived from a study of 2,600 healthy British children.* Paris, Center International de L'Enfance, 1962.

Tanner, J. M.; Whitehouse, R. H.; Marshall, W. A.; and Carter, B. S.: Prediction of adult height from height, bone age, and occurence of menarche at ages 45 to 16 with allowance for midparent height. *Arch Dis Child, 50*:14, 1975.

Tanner, J. M.; Whitehouse, R. H.; Marshall, W. A.; Healy, M. J. R.; and Goldstein, H.: *Assessment of Skeletal Maturity and Prediction of Adult Height (TW2 method).* New York, Acad Pr, 1975.

Thurow, R. C.: *Atlas of Orthodontic Principles.* St. Louis, Mosby, 1970.

Tipnis, A. K.: Xeroradiograhy for lateral skull radiographs. *Br J Orthod, 1*(15).187, 1974.

Todd, T. W.: *Atlas of Skeletal Maturation.* St. Louis, Mosby, 1937.

Toller, P. A.: Opaque arthrography of the temporomandibular Joint. *Int J Oral Surg, 3*:17, 1974.

Toller, P. A.: Temporomandibular capsular rearrangement. *Br J Oral Surg, 11*:207, 1974.

Trester, P. H.: The development and use of contrast media in sialography. *J Can Dent Assoc, 34*:211, 1968.

Updegrave, W. J.: Radiodontic technique for the child patient. *J NJ State Dent Soc, 22*:11, 1951.

Updegrave, W. J.: An evaluation of the T-M joint roentgenography. *J Am Dent Assoc, 46*:408, 1953.

Updegrave, w. J.: Temporomandibular articulation. *Dent Radiogr Photogr, 26*(3):41, 1953.

Updegrave, W. J.: Roentgenographic observations of functioning T-M joints. *J Am Dent Assoc, 54*:488, 1957.

Updegrave, W. J.: Supplementary radiographic examination for children. *Penn Dent J,* p. 3, January 1960.

Updegrave, W. J.: Practical evaluation of techniques and interpretation in roentgenographic examination of temporomandibular joints. *Dent Clin North Am,* p. 421, July, 1961.

Vogt, E. C.; and Vickers, V. S.: *Radiology, 31*:441, 1938.

Waggener, D.T.: Roentgenographic localization of unerupted teeth. *Oral Surg,* p. 439, April 1960.

Waggener, D. T.; and Austin, L. T.: Dental structures remaining in 1948 edentulous jaws: A statistical study. *J Am Dent Assoc, 28*:1855, 1941.

Waggener and Ireland: Intraoral roentgenography for children. *J Am Dent Assoc, 47*:133, 1953.

Walton, R. E.: Endodontic radiographic technics. *Dent Radiogr Photogr, 46*(3):51, 1973.

Waters, C. A.; and Waldron, C. W.: Roentgenology of accessory nasal sinuses describng modification of occipitfrontal position. *AJR,* 1915.

Weinberg, L. A.: An evaluation of duplicability of temporomandibular joint radiographs. *J Prosthet Dent, 24*(5):512, 1970.

White, S. C.; and Gratt, B. M.: Clinical trials of intraoral dental xeroradiography. *J Am Dent Assoc, 99*:810, 1979.

White, S. C.; Stafford, M. L.; and Benninga, L. R.: Intraoral xeroradiography. *Oral Surg,* 46(6):862, 1978.

Wilkes, C.: Arthrography of the temporomandibular joint in patients with TMJ pain dysfunction syndrome. *Minn Med, 61*:645, 1978.

Wilkes, C.: Structural and functional alterations of the temporomandibular joint. *Northwest Dent, 57*:287, 1978.

Winter, G. B.: *Impacted Mandibular Third Molars.* St. Louis, American med Book, 1926.

Wolfe, J. N.: Xeroradiograpy of the bones, joints, and soft tissues. *Radiology, 93*:583, 1969.

Xerox Corporation. Xeroradiography for temporomandibular joint. *Med Appl bull,* 115, 1973.

X-rays in Dentistry. Rochester, NY, Eastman Kodak Co., 1979.

Yale, S. H.; Ceballos, M.; Kresnoff, C. S.; and Hauptfuehrer, J. D.: some observations on the classification of mandibular condyle types. *Oral Surg, 16*(5):572, 1963.

Zech, J. M.: A comparison and analysis f 3 technics of taking roentgenograms of the T-M joint. *J Am Dent Assoc, 59*:725, 1959.

Zimmer, E. A.: *Schweiz Mschr Zahnheilk, 51*:949, 1941.

Chapter 16

ROTATIONAL PANORAMIC RADIOGRAPHY

W. Doss McDavid

THE value of any diagnostic procedure is dependent upon the amount and validity of the information that can be obtained from it. The importance of the bite-wing and periapical radiographs as a diagnostic aid is well documented. However, periapical and bite-wing radiographs are somewhat limited in their overall coverage of the mandibulofacial structures. While occlusal and extraoral radiographs can be used to obtain greater coverage, these radiographs frequently contain distortion, lack of definition, and superimposition of anatomic structures.

Panoramic radiography overcomes many of these limitations and during recent years has become a valuable diagnostic aid to the dentist. Panoramic radiographs are made using two basically different methods: (1) the use of an intraoral source of radiation, and (2) the use of an extraoral source of radiation (rotational panoramic radiography).

The intraoral type of panoramic radiography, as the name implied, employs an intraoral source of radiation (Fig. 16-1A). The radiation is directed from inside the mouth through the jaws and exposes a film molded to the outside of the patient's face. No-screen or slow-speed screen films are used. The x-ray source, patient, and film are stationary during the exposure. Separate exposures are made of the mandible and maxilla.

The technique of rotational panoramic radiography is by far the most popular method for panoramic radiography and in this chapter we will confine our remarks to this technique.

Principle of Operation

We have seen in the preceding chapters that radiography operates on the geometric projection principles of light-wave shadowcasting. X-rays diverging from the focal spot pass through the object to the image receptor where the x-ray image (shadow) of the object is recorded. This is the case in stationary radiographic techniques such as conventional intraoral dental radiography (Fig. 16-2) where the film is placed inside the mouth with an extraoral x-ray source. In intraoral source panoramic radiography, there is an intraoral x-ray source and the film is positioned outside the mouth (Fig. 16-3A, C). X-ray image differences in conventional dental radiography and intraoral source panoramic radiography depend on differences in the position of the focus, or point of divergence, with respect to the

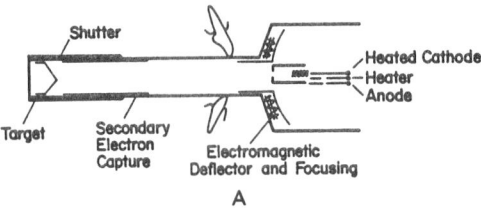
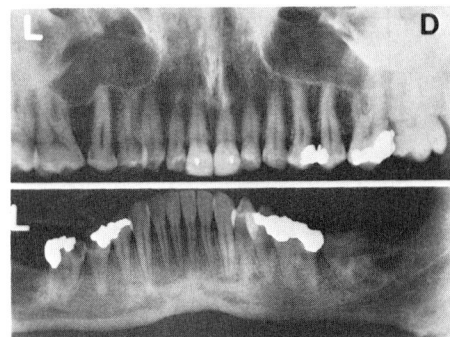
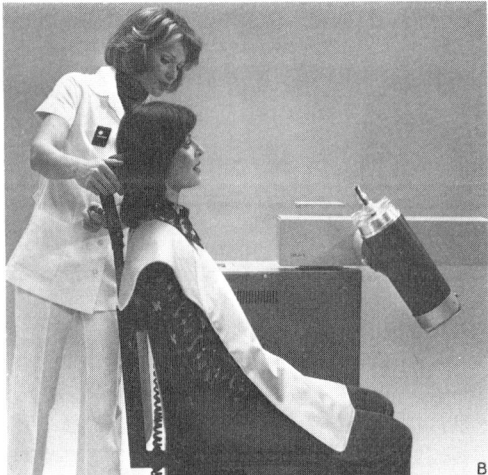
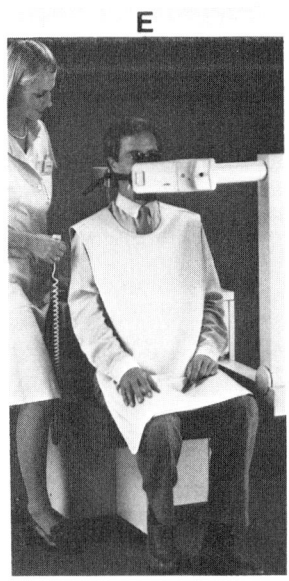
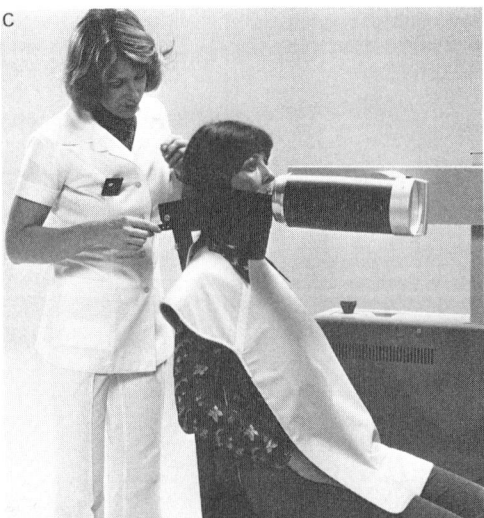

Figure 16-1. (A) Panoramic technique using an intraoral x-ray source illustrated by a schematic drawing. The cone-shaped anode, a special extension of the x-ray tube, is placed within the patient's mouth. As the electrons strike the target of the anode, x-rays are produced, which radiate in all directions. (B) Siemens' Status-X. (C) Siemens Status-X (close-up). (D) Radiograph of Status-X. (E) Philips' Stat Oralix. (F) Radiograph of Stat-Oralix.

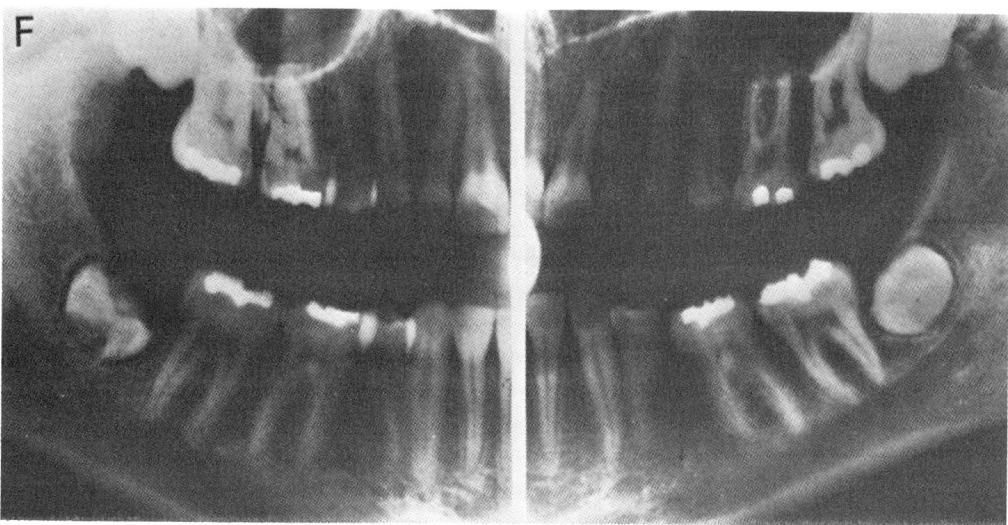

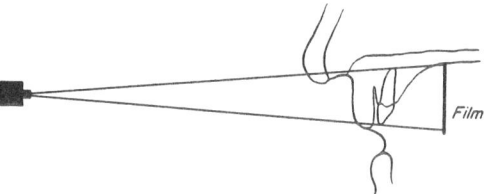

Figure 16-2. In the conventional projection of an intraoral radiograph the divergent rays have a common origin at the focal spot. The film is perpendicular to the central ray.

object and the film.

Rotational panoramic radiography was developed to obtain, using an extraoral source (Fig. 16-3B), a projection geometry similar to that which is obtained when an intraoral source is used (Fig. 16-3A). This is accomplished by allowing a narrow vertical beam (Fig. 16-4) to rotate in the horizontal plane around a rotational axis, which is positioned intraorally (Fig. 16-3B). In the horizontal plane (Fig. 16-3B) the x-rays appear to diverge from the intraoral center of rotation. In the vertical dimension (Fig. 16-4) the projection is not affected by the rotation, and so the focal spot of the x-ray tube still serves as the point of divergence.

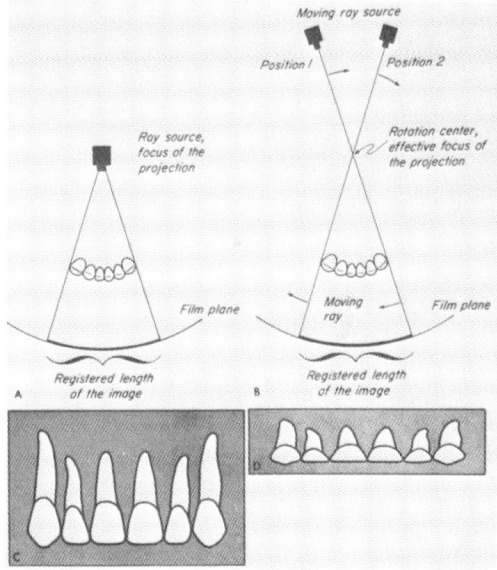

Figure 16-3. (A) the projection geometry associated with an intraoral x-ray source. (B) When a rotating narrow beam is used, the x-rays appear to diverge from an intraoral focus even though the x-rays really originate outside the patient. (C) With an intraoral x-ray source the magnification is equal in the horizontal and vertical dimensions. (D) When a rotating narrow beam projects the object onto a stationary film, the magnification in the horizontal dimension is greater than that in the vertical dimension.

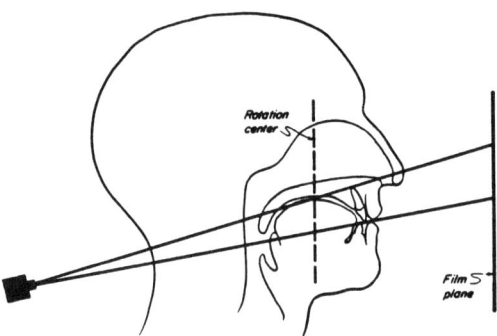

Figure 16-4. Projection geometry in the vertical plane in rotational panoramic radiography.

the x-ray tube still serves as the point of divergence.

It will be remembered from earlier chapters that the closer the focus or point of divergence to the object being radiographed, the greater will be the magnification of the object's x-ray image (shadow) at the film plane. It follows, therefore, that if the image resulting from the rotating panoramic system shown in Figure 16-3B were to be recorded on a stationary film placed extraorally there would be a discrepancy between the magnification factors in the horizontally and vertical dimensions. This would result in the peculiar image shown in Figure 16-3D. The magnification in the horizontal dimension would be larger than the magnification in the vertical dimension because the apparent focus in the horizontal plane (the center of rotation) is closer to the object than the focus in the vertical plane (the focal spot of the x-ray tube).

The discrepancy in magnification can be eliminated by using a moving film to take up some of the slack in the horizontal dimension (Fig. 16-5A). By adjusting the speed of the film with respect to the beam, it is possible to reduce the horizontal magnification to match the vertical magnification (Fig. 16-5B). This can be achieved only for those objects that lie

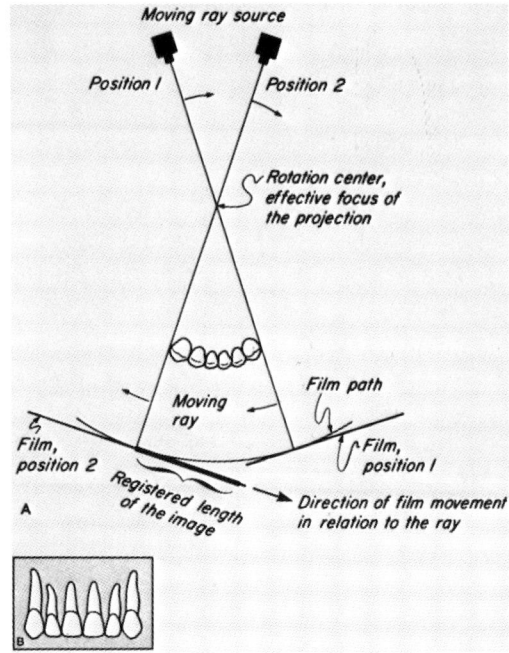

Figure 16-5. (A) The combination of a rotating beam and a moving film changes the horizontal magnification of the recorded image but the projection of the object remains the same. (B) The resulting image in the rotational panoramic system has its proportions restored.

within a **particular curved plane.** This plane is called the central plane of the image layer. Objects in this plane will be projected in their correct proportions and will appear sharp, while objects outside this plane will be distorted and will appear unsharp or fuzzy. The degree of distortion and unsharpness will increase with increasing distance on either side of the central plane of the layer.

Design Considerations

The Movement Pattern of the Beam

The movement of the beam with respect to the patient is selected to obtain a suitable projection of the dental arch. Mechanicaly, this can be accomplished in a

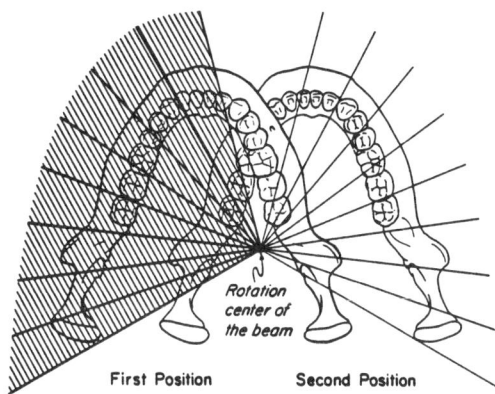

Figure 16-6. (Panorex I (S.S. White/Pennwalt) System: The projection of "split" image takes place in two steps. Only one stationary rotation center of the beam is used. By moving the patient, two effective foci (one on each side) are created.

number of ways, as we shall see when we examine the individual units. At present, these movement patterns fall into two categories: (1) those that use fixed centers of rotation and (2) those that use a moving center of rotation. These result in split and continuous images, respectively.

The use of two fixed centers of rotation to form a split image, as in the Panorex I system, is illustrated in Figure 16-6. Mechanically speaking, there is only one center of rotation. This center of rotation is placed to either side of the patient's mouth by displacing the patient with respect to the mechanical center of rotation. One side of the patient's dental arch is first radiographed using the appropriate rotation center. The x-ray exposure is then terminated while the patient is shfted to place the center of rotation on the opposite side. When the x-ray exposure begins again, the other side of the dental arch is then radiographed. This results in a split image (Fig. 16-7).

The use of a sliding center of rotation is shown in Figure 16-8. Here, the effective center of rotation is made to follow a curved path throughout the excursion. The narrow x-ray beam moves in such a way as to be always tangent to this path at the effective center of rotation. This results in a continuous image (Fig. 16-9).

The Position of the Cental Plane of the Image Layer

Once a suitable movement pattern of the beam has been selected, the position of the central plane of the image layer can

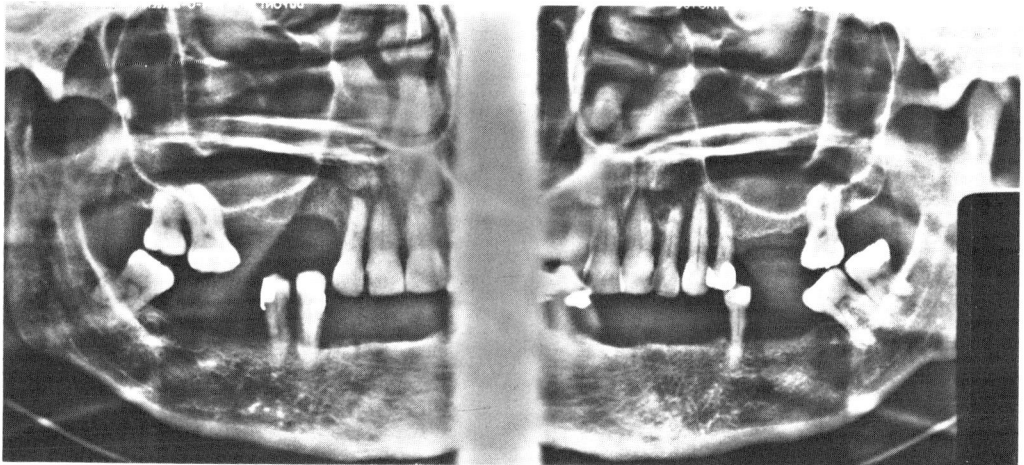

Figure 16-7. A split panoramic image. The two portions of the image are projected from effective foci on the two sides of the patient.

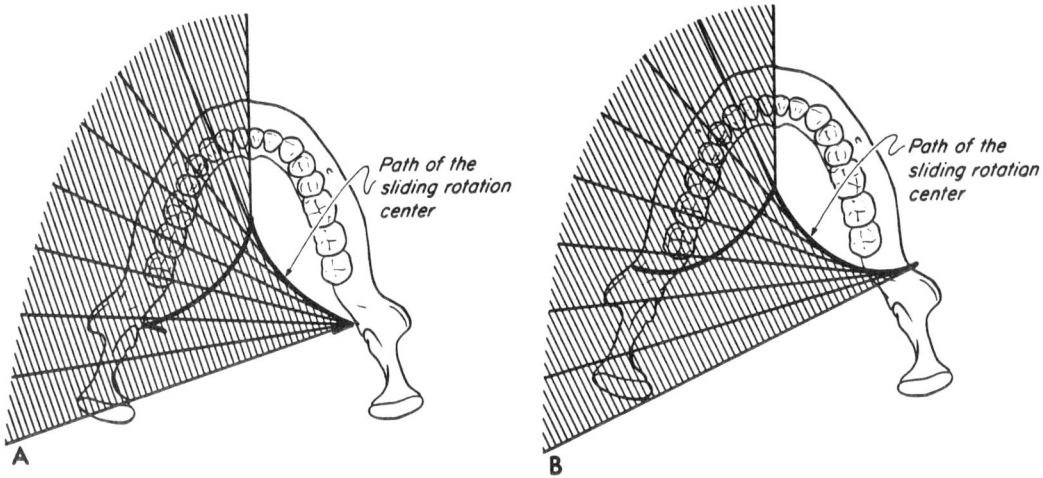

Figure 16-8. The projection of a continuous image utilizing a continuously sliding beam. (A) GE Panelipse, Sybron-Ritter Panoral. (B) Siemens Orthopantomograph 10.

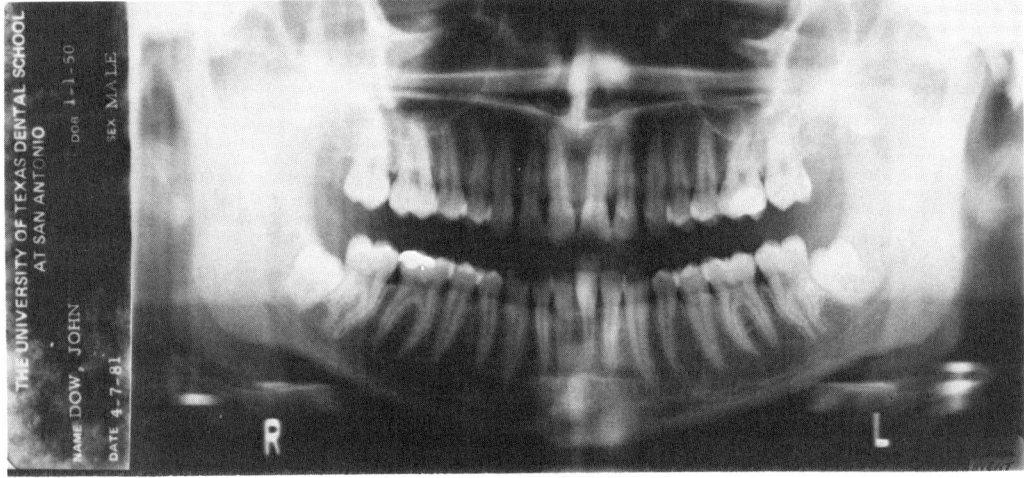

Figure 16-9. Using a continuously sliding beam, a single continuous image results (GE Panelipse radiograph).

be programmed into the machine by carefully varying the speed of the film relative to the beam throughout the excursion. The speed of the film must always match the speed of the projected shadows of the structures in the desired plane. This will result in sharp and undistorted images of the structures within that plane. The selection of the central plane of the layer is shown in Figure 16-10.

In order to image structures located far away from the rotation center, the film must move relatively fast with respect to the beam since the shadows of these structures move rapidly at the film plane. Conversely, in order to project sharply structures close to the rotation center, it is necessary for the film to move relatively slowly with respect to the beam. The position of the central plane of the image layer

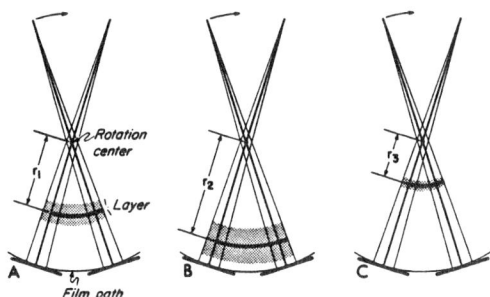

Figure 16-10. (A) The position of the image layer is dependent on the film speed. (B) An increase in film speed places the layer away from the rotation center. (C) A decrease in the film speed places the layer closer to the rotation center. Note the changes in layer thickness between A, B, and C.

can, therefore, be shifted in or out at will to conform to the shape of the dental arch by simply speeding up or slowing down the film speed as required.

Distortion

Structures located in the central plane of the image layer appear with equal magnification in the horizontal and vertical dimensions. Thus, a small round object, a ball bearing for example, located in the central plane will project a circular image that will be somewhat magnified. If this object is moved toward the film, the principles of magnification described in previous chapters would allow us to predict that the magnification would decrease. Conversely, if the object is moved toward the x-ray source, we would predict that the magnification would increase. In panoramic radiography, however, unlike other forms of radiography, the magnification factors in the horizontal and vertical dimensions change differently, the change being more dramatic in the horizontal dimension. This gives rise to the characteristic pattern of distortion seen in panoramic systems — a widening of structures displaced toward the x-ray source and a narrowing of structures displaced toward the film.

When the ball bearing mentioned earlier is moved toward the film, the horizontal magnification will decrease faster than the vertical magnification. As a result, the ball will be depicted as an ellipsoid with its long axis in the vertical dimension. When the ball is moved toward the x-ray source, the horizontal magnification will increase faster than the vertical magnification and the ball will be depicted as an ellipsoid with its long axis in the horizontal dimension. These effects, which are illustrated in Figure 16-11, occur because, as we have seen earlier, the point of divergence in the vertical dimension is the focal spot of the x-ray tube, while in the horizontal dimension the x-rays appear to diverge from the center of rotation. It follows that teeth positioned between the central plane of the layer and the film appear to narrow. This indicates that the patient has been positioned too far forward during the exposure. Similarly, teeth positioned between the central plane of the layer and the x-ray source appear too wide. This indicates that the patient has been positioned too far back during the exposure.

Unsharpness

In addition to distortion, panoramic images of objects displaced from the cen-

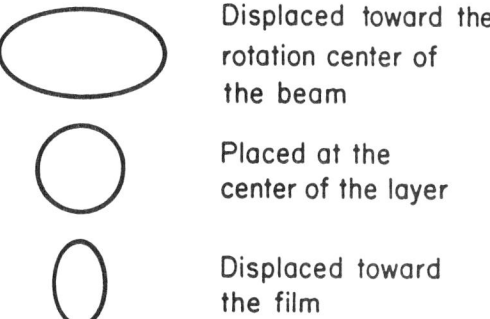

Figure 16-11. Distortion effects when objects are displaced from the central plane of the image layer.

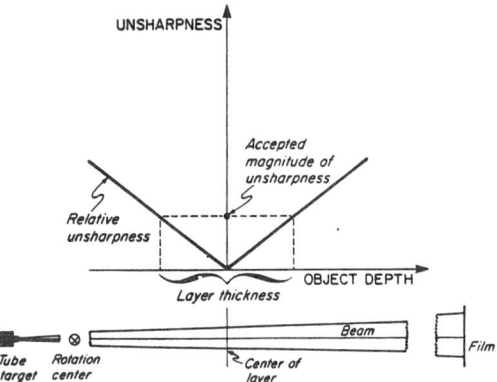

Figure 16-12. Unsharpness increases to either side of the central plane of the image layer. The layer thickness is defined by the accepted level of unsharpness.

tral plane exhibit unsharpness. This unsharpness comes about because the film is moving in such a way as to follow the shadows of objects in only one plane — the central plane of the layer. Objects outside of this plane cast x-ray shadows that move at a different speed from that of the film and that are therefore blurred in the horizontal dimension. This blurring or unsharpness increases with increasing distance to either side of the central plane of the layer (Fig. 16-12).

The Image Layer

Only those structural details that lie in the central plane of the layer are portrayed sharply and in their correct proportions. Fortunately, within certain limits to either side of this plane, the effects of distortion and unsharpness are minimal, and we can speak of an image layer of some thickness within which structural details are satisfactorily portrayed. This image layer is often referred to as the "focal trough." Its boundaries are not defined by any hard and fast definition. Rather, some arbitrary index of unsharpness is chosen as a criterion for cut-off and the boundaries are mapped accordingly (Fig. 16-12). In comparing the focal troughs as mapped by different methods, it must always be remembered that the measurements reported are valid only in the context of the particular criterion chosen for defining the boundaries of the layer.

The width of the image layer is directly related to the distance from the effective center of rotation to the central plane of the layer. If this distance is large, the layer will tend to be wide and, therefore, "forgiving" with respect to patient positioning. This is generally the case in the lateral portions of the image layer. If this distance is small, the layer will tend to be narrow. In continuous images, this always occurs in the anterior position. This is quite noticeable in clinical practice, where it is a matter of everyday experience that it is difficult to obtain a satisfactory image of the incisors. The slightest malpositioning of the patient lends to loss of resolution and severe distortion. The other major factor influencing the width of the image layer is the width of the beam. The narrower the beam, the wider is the image layer.

In general, it is desirable to have a wide image layer throughout the dental arch because the anatomical structures of interest exist within a layer of finite thickness and it is desirable to visualize all these structures as clearly as possible.

The effects of unsharpness and distortion are important criteria when evaluating panoramic radiographs. If the teeth in a certain region appear too broad as compared to their length, this indicates, together with unsharpness, that this region has been malpositioned toward the x-ray source during the exposure. A narrowing of the teeth, on the other hand, together with the accompanying unsharpness, indicates that this region has been malpositioned toward the film during the exposure. This information is easily used to correct the patient's positioning when a retake is required.

Commonly Used Panoramic Units

Four commonly used x-ray units for performing rotational panoramic radiography are the Panorex® (Pennwalt/S.S. White) the Panelipse® (General Electric); the Panoral® (Sybron-Ritter); and the Orthopantomograph® (Siemens).

Panorex

The first generation Panorex (Panorex I) is shown in Figure 16-13. The Panorex I unit consists of a platform supporting a chair. Behind the chair is a vertical column that supports the x-ray tube and cassette holder. A chin rest is provided on the chair to adjust the position of the patient's head. The control panel is separate and contains the kVp and mA controls. As we mentioned earlier, this machine produces a split image using a fixed center of rotation that is positioned successively on each side of the patient, in the mandibular molar region. The image layer for the Panorex is shown in Figure 16-14. It will be noted that the image layer is relatively wide in all regions of the split radiograph, because the distance between the fixed centers of rotation and the central plane of the layer remains large throughout the excursion.

The Panorex II is shown in Figure 16-15. This machine can produce either a split or a continuous image. The image layer for the split mode, shown in Figure

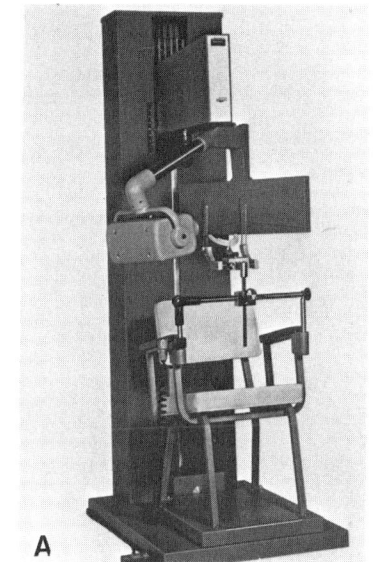

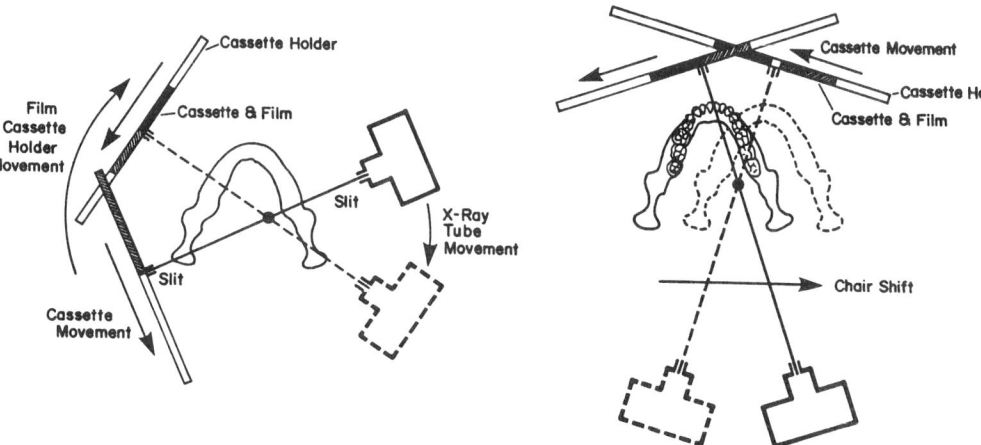

Figure 16-13. The Panorex (S.S. White/Pennwalt). (A) Panorex I Photograph. (B) Diagram of operation. (C) Panorex I radiograph. (D) panorex I Radiograph.

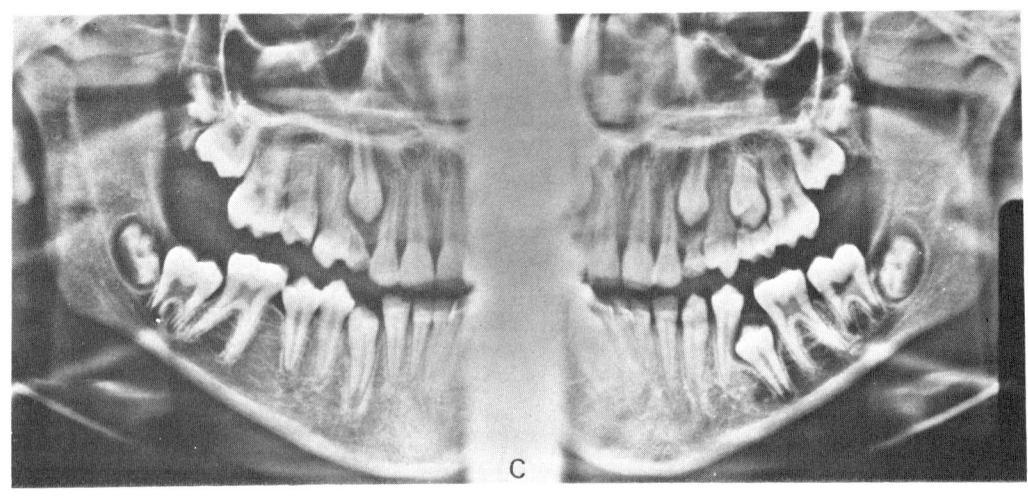

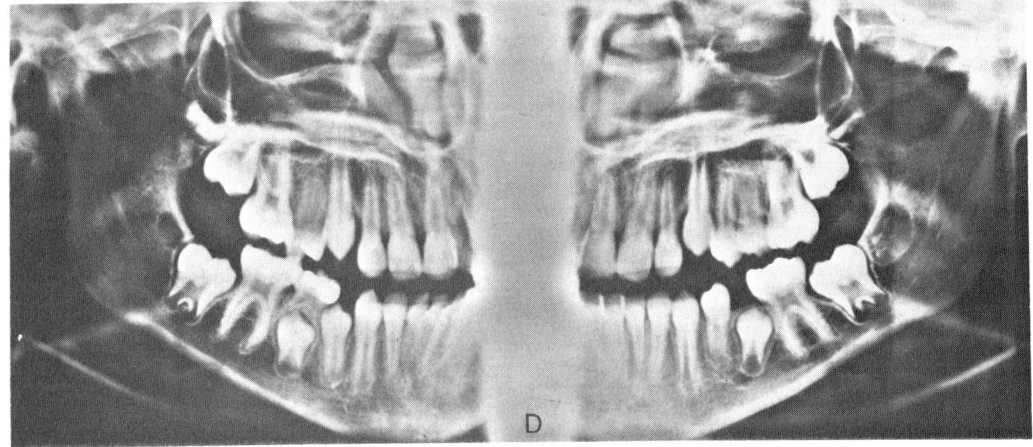

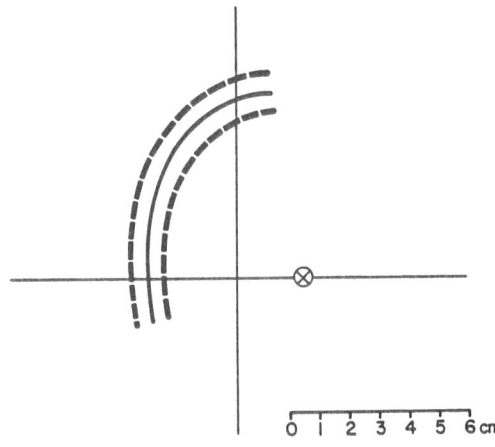

Figure 16-14. The image layer of the Panorex I (Pennwalt/S.S. White)

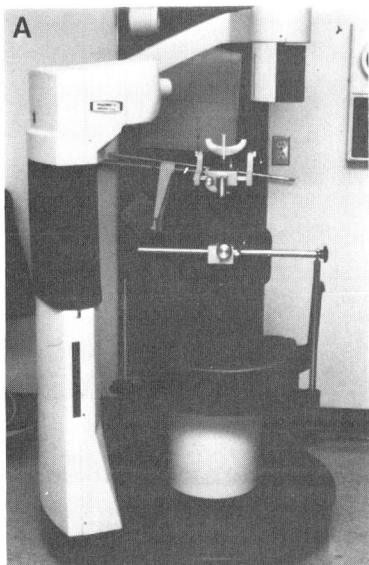

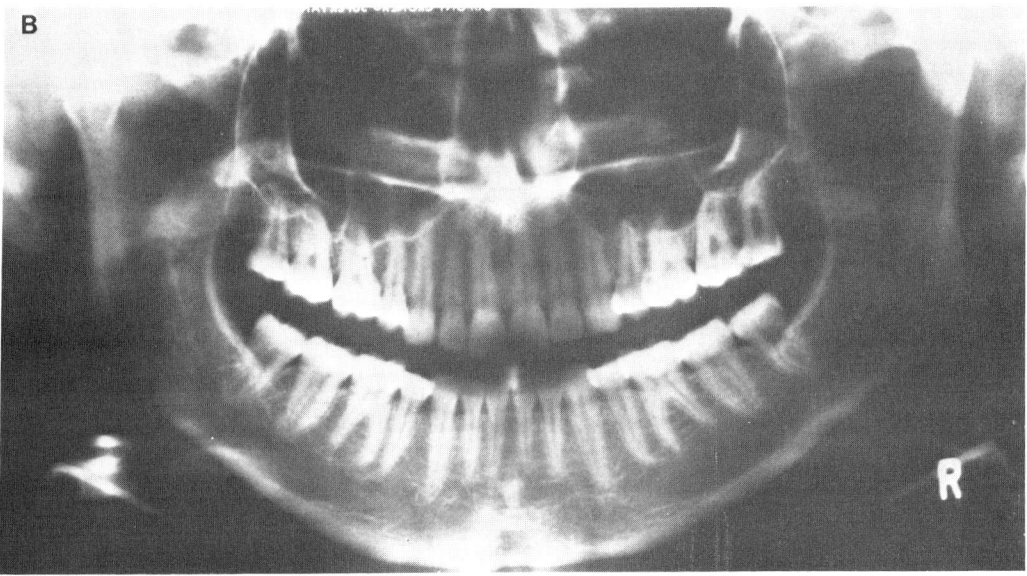

Figure 16-15. The Panorex II (Pennwalt/S.S. White) **(A)** Photograph of Panorex II. **(B)** Radiograph of Panorex II (continuous image mode).

16-16, is somewhat different in shape from that of the first generation Panorex, having been modified to obtain a less distorted image of the TMJ region. Like the Panorex, however, the image layer is wide and, therefore, "forgiving" in all regions of the image.

When operating in the continuous mode, the Panorex II begins rotating around the same fixed center as is used in the split mode. At a certain point of the scan, the chair begins to shift slowly across while the machine continues to operate. This has the effect of moving the **effective** center of rotation along the curved path shown in Figure 16-17 over to a fixed point on the opposite side which serves as the rotation center for the last part of the scan. The result of this movement is a continuous image with the image layer shown in Figure 16-17. It will be noted that the image layer, like that of all continuous machines, becomes very narrow in the anterior region because the effective center of rotation is quite near to the central plane in this region. For this reason, all continuous machines have some form of a bite piece or other positioning device to assure that the patient's incisors are correctly positioned in the unit.

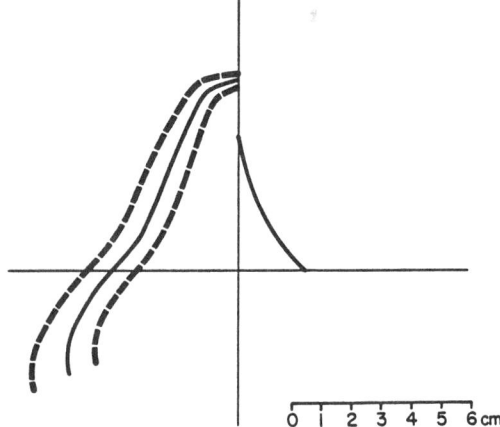

Figure 16-17. The image layer of the Panorex II operating in the continuous mode.

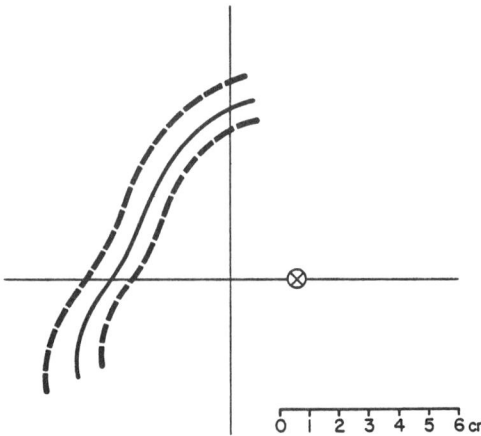

Figure 16-16. The image layer of the Panorex II operating in the split mode.

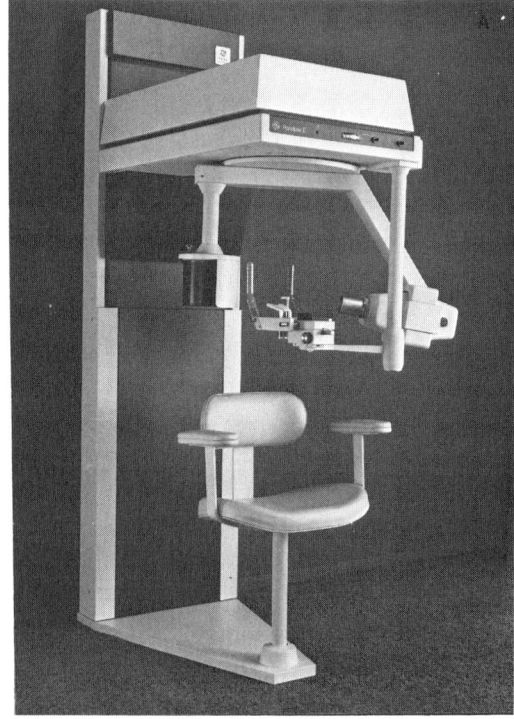

Figure 16-18. The Panelipse II (GE). **(A)** Photograph of Panelipse; **(B)** Photograph of Panelipse II control panel; **(C)** Diagram of operation; **(D)** Radiograph of Panelipse.

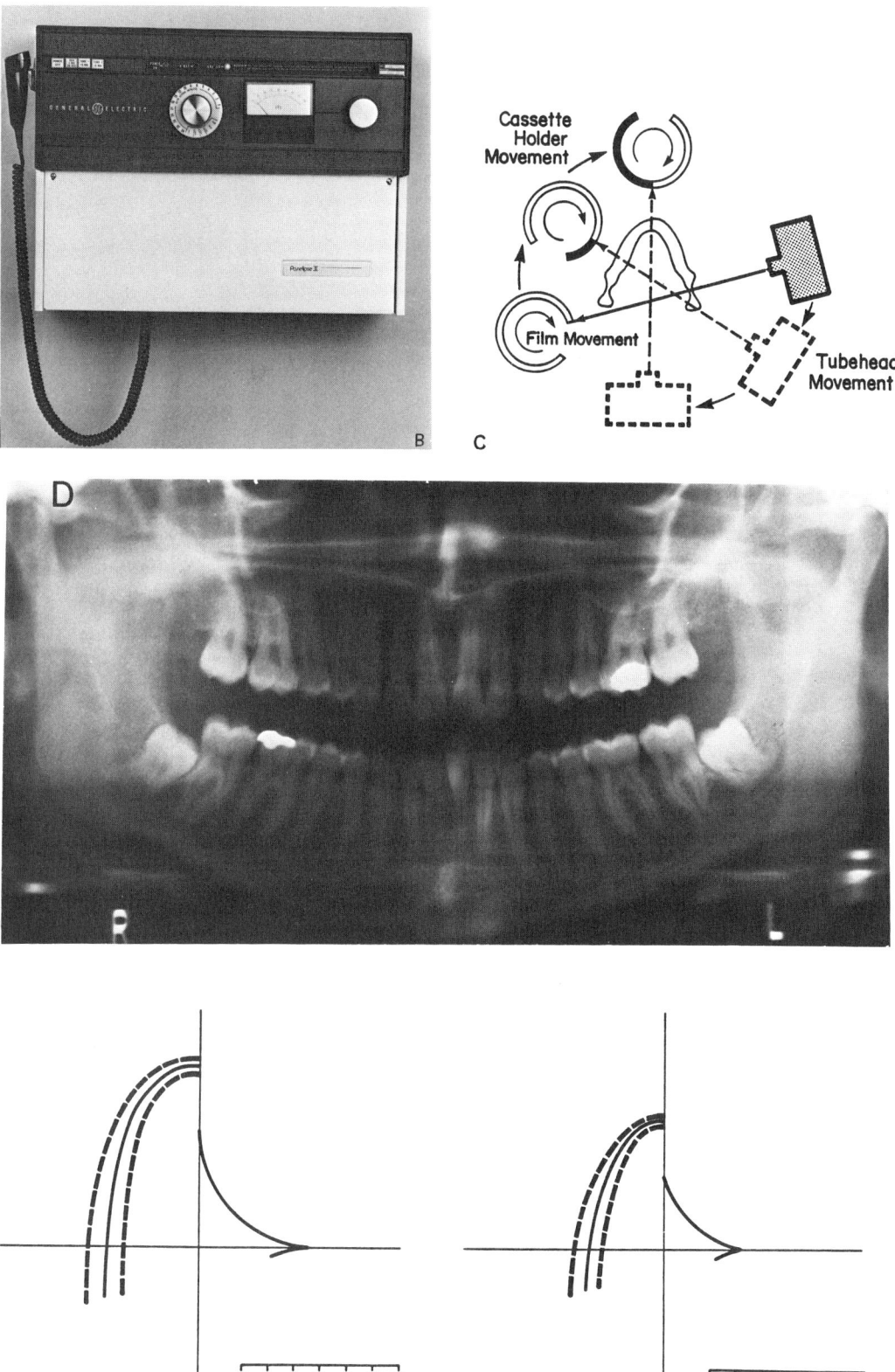

Figure 16-19. The image layer of the Panelipse operating with a Profile Index of 9.

Figure 16-20. The image layer of the Panelipse operating with a Profile Index of 7.

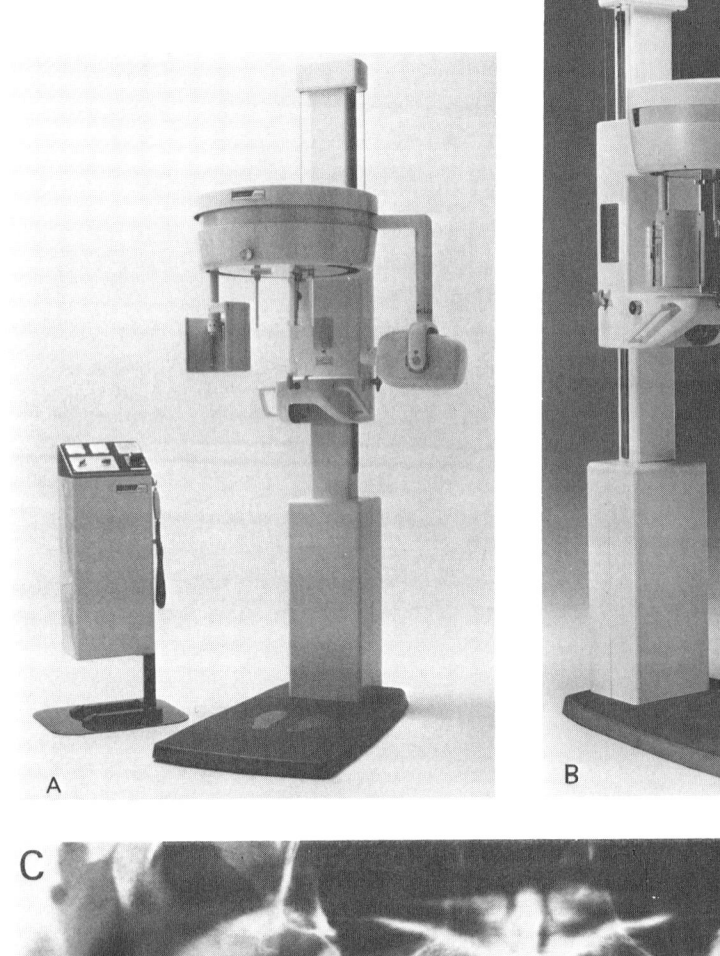
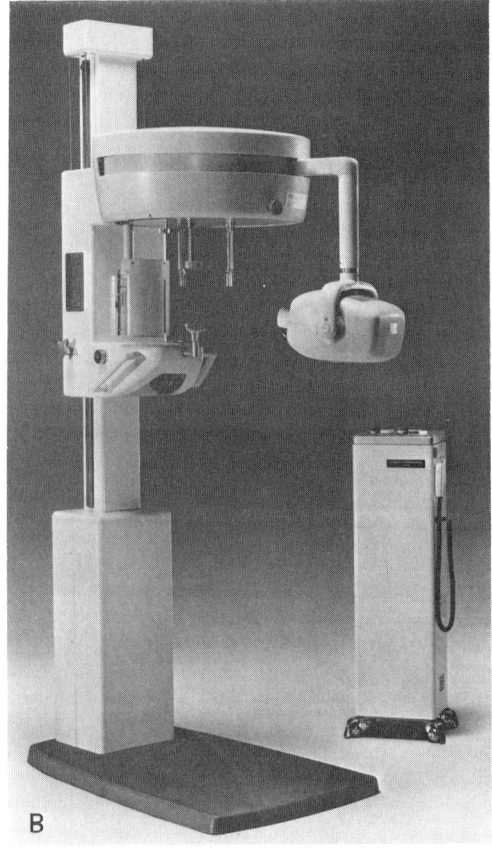
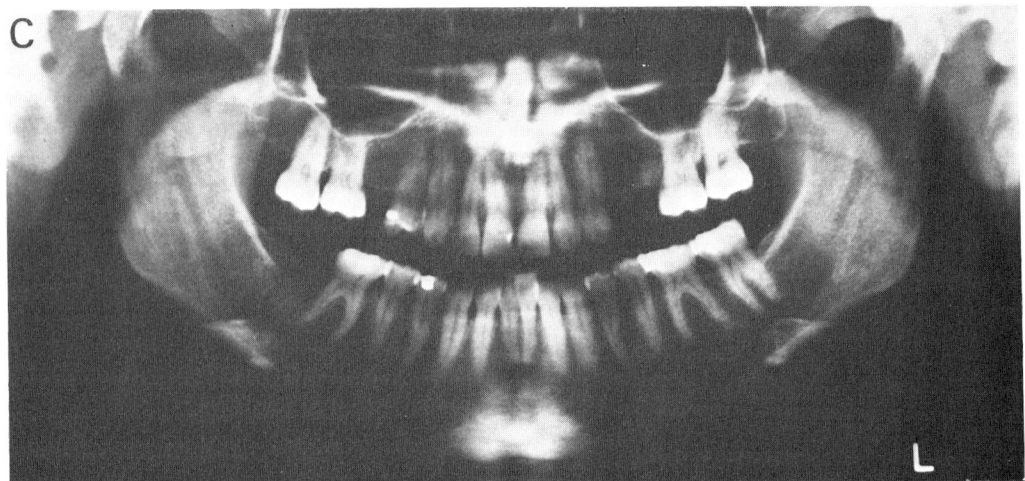

Figure 16-21. The Panoral (Sybron-Ritter). **(A)** Panoral (photograph); **(B)** Morita's Panex-E (photograph); **(C)** Panoral (Sybron-Ritter) radiograph.

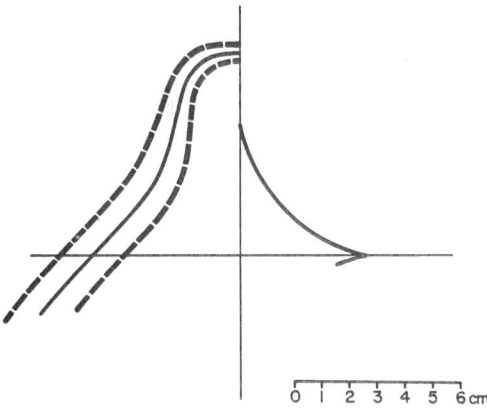

Figure 16-22. The image layer of the Panoral (Sybron-Ritter)

Panelipse

The GE Panelipse uses an overhead mechanism to rotate the x-ray source and cassette assembly around the seated patient (Fig. 16-18). The resulting image of the dental arches, sinuses, the temporomandibular joints has a layer typified by Figures 16-19 and 16-20. The "Profile Index," which may be changed to adapt the machine to patients of different sizes, alters the size but not the shape of the image layer. Like all continuous machines, the image layer becomes very narrow in the anterior region.

Panoral

The Panoral (Fig. 16-21) is designed for a standing patient. An overhead mechanism is used to rotate the x-ray tube and cassette around the patient's head. The image layer of the Panoral is shown in Figure 16-22. In the lateral portion, the layer flairs out to encompass the temporomandibular joint region.

Orthopantomograph

Since its initial development by Paatero of Finland (1959), a number of generations of the Orthopantomograph have emerged. The Orthopantomograph

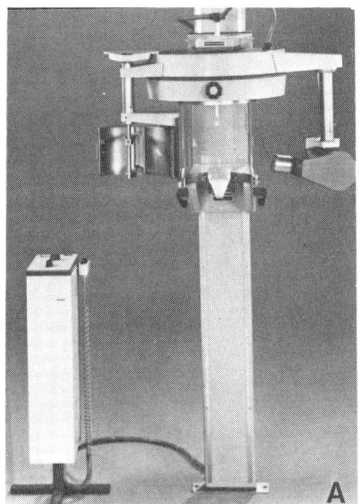

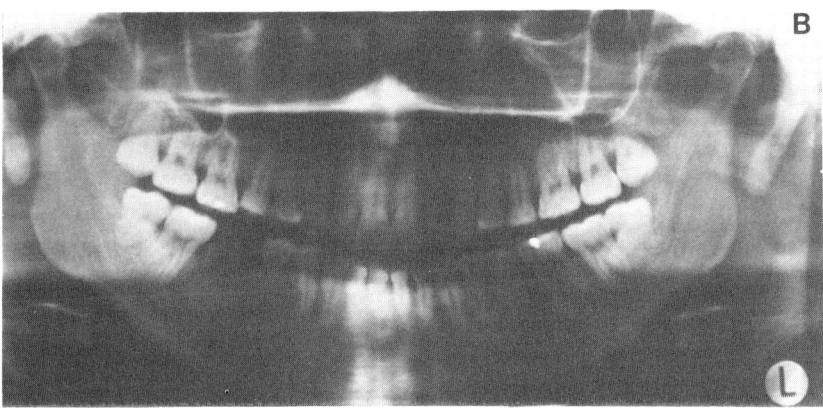

Figure 16-23. The Orthopantomograph 5 (Siemens) **(A)** Photograph of Orthopantomograph 5; **(B)** Radiograph of Orthopantomograph 5.

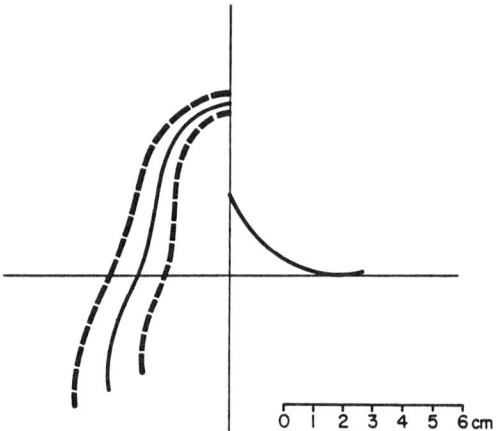

Figure 16-24. The image layer of the Orthopantomograph 5. (Siemens)

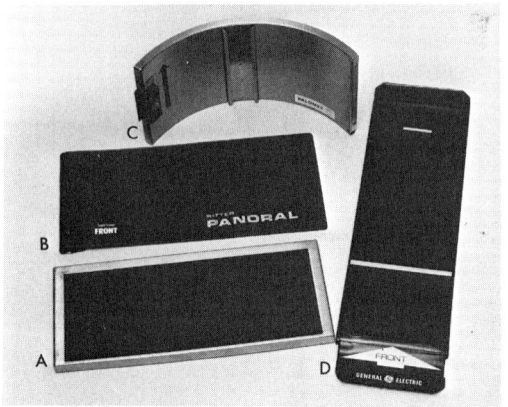

Figure 16-25. (A) Flat metal cassette (Pennwalt/S.S. White, Panorex I). (B) Flexible plastic cassette (Sybron/Ritter, Panoral). (C) Curved metal cassette (Palomex, Orthopantomograph). (D) Flexible plastic cassette (G.E. Panelipse).

10 is the most recent of these machines designed for dental use. This unit, shown in Figure 16-23, uses an overhead mechanism to scan the head of a standing patient. The image layer of the Orthopantomograph 10 is shown in Figure 16-24.

The panoramic cassette is the light-tight holder containing the intensifying screens (always in pairs) and the film. Some cassettes are flat or curved and rigid, while others are flexible (Fig. 16-25).

ADVANTAGES AND DISADVANTAGES OF ROTATIONAL PANORAMIC RADIOGRAPHY

In the January 1977 issue of the *Journal of the American Dental Association,* the Council on Dental Materials and Devices listed advantages and disadvantages of rotational panoramic radiography.

Advantages

1. It is a simple procedure to perform.
2. It is convenient for the patient.
3. It can be used in patients with intractable gagging problems.
4. The time required for the procedure is minimal.
5. Those portions of the maxilla and mandible lying within the trough of the machine can be visualized on a single film.
6. The patient dose is relatively low but not negligible.
7. Tomographs taken for diagnostic purposes also can be useful as a visual aid in patient education.

Disadvantages

1. Areas of diagnostic interest outside of the focal trough may be visualized poorly or not at all.
2. Tomographs inherently show magnifi-

cation, geometric distortion, and poor defintion.
3. Overlapping of teeth commonly occurs, particularly in the bicuspid area.
4. The anterior teeth register poorly when they have pronounced inclinations.
5. The spinal column may interfere with the production of the radiograph.
6. The amount of vertical and horizontal distortion varies from one part of the film to another.
7. The ease and convenience of obtaining a tomograph may encourage careless evaluation of a patient's specific radiographic needs.
8. Artifacts are easily misinterpreted.

Bibliography

Andoh, S.: Orthopantomography. *In Houyosha.* Tokyo, 1971.

Hudson, D. C.; Kumpula, J. W.; and Dickson, G. A.: Panoramic dental x-ray machine. *US Armed Forces Med J 8*:46-55, 1957.

McDavid, W. D.; Welander, U.; and Morris, C. R.: Blurring effects in rotational panoramic radiography. *Oral Surg, 53*:483-489, 1975.

Tammisalo, E.H.; and Niemenen, T.: The thickness of the image layer in Orthopantomography. *Suom Hamaslaak Toim, 60*:119-126, 1964.

Welander, U: A mathematical model of narrow beam rotation methods. *Acta Radio [Diagn], 15*:305-317, 1974.

Welander, U.; and Wickman, G.: Blurring and layer thickness in narrow beam rotational radiography. *Acta Radiol [Diagn], 18*:705-714, 1977.

Chapter 17

LEGAL ASPECTS AND FUTURE OF DENTAL RADIOGRAPHY

LEGAL ASPECTS OF DENTAL RADIOGRAPHY

Ownership of the X-rays

WHEN the patient pays for a set of radiographs, he is paying for the dentist's ability to interpret the radiographs and arrive at a diagnostic opinion based on his radiograhic and clinical findings. X-rays are a part of the dentist's records and do not rightfully belong to the patient.

One of the most important decisions by a higher court concerning ownership of radiographs was handed down by the Supreme Court of Michigan in 1935 (*McGarry v. J.A. Mercier Co.*).

In this case, the plaintiff was a physician who was employed by a construction company (J.A. Mercier Company) to treat their employees in case of injury on the job. J.A. Mercier Company had refused to pay the physician for services rendered one of their employees because the physician failed to deliver to them radiographs taken of the employee during treatment.

The court ruled in favor of the physician, stating that the radiographs were legal property of the physician. They further declared that "it is a matter of common knowledge that x-ray negatives are practically meaningless to the ordinary layman. But the retention by the physician or surgeon constitutes an important part of his clinical record in the particular case, and in the aggregate these films may embody and preserve much of value incident to a physician's or surgeon's experience. They are as much a part of the history of the case as any other case record of the physician or surgeon. In a sense they differ little, if at all, from microscopic slides of tissue made in the course of diagnosis or treatment of the patient, but it would hardly be claimed that such slides were the property of the patient."

Care in Billing

If the radiographs are billed separately from the diagnosis and treatment, the dentist may run the risk that the court may render a verdict in favor of the patient saying the patient owns the radiograhs because he paid for them.

Always include the radiographs in services rendered for diagnosis and treatment when billing a patient. Do not itemize a separate charge for radiographs.

Precautions in Loaning Radiographs

The dentist should never give radiographs to the patient. The dentist should realize that the radiograph is the greatest protection against a possible claim of negligence he has. It is sad when a dentist is sued for malpractice and the radiographs that would have proved his competence have been misplaced or lost.

There are times when the dentist may want to lend the patient's radiographs to another dentist for viewing. When lending radiographs to another dentist, the following suggestions are given (Miller, 1970):

1. Have the second dentist request the radiograhs in writing. Place this letter in the patient's folder.
2. Send the radiographs by registered or certified mail.
3. Request that the dentist retain the radiograhs in his files for six years, or send them back to you after he is through with them. Even though the patient may move to another city, the dentist is not legally bound to send the patient's radiographs to a second dentist. The radiographs are still his legal property.
4. A copy of the cover letter sent with the radiographs and the postal receipt should be kept in the patient's folder.
5. The patient's records should be kept for at least six years.

Liability Arising Out of Failure to Use Radiographs

The dentist must use his professional judgment as to whether or not he should use radiographs as a diagnostic procedure. Certainly there are instances when radiographs are not necessary to render a diagnosis. However, one of the most common causes for malpractice suits is the failure of the dentist to use radiographs in his diagnosis or after treatment of cases involving pain, swelling, or infection.

Consider this case cited by Sarner (1963). A dentist in Kentucky refused to radiograph a patient's jaws when there was a question whether he had left a root tip in the patient's jaws after an extraction. The patient visited a second dentist, who found a root tip in the jaws by means of radiograph. It is now considered a dental principle that a dentist who fails to radiograph in some circumstances is guilty of malpractice (*Agnew vs. City of Los Angeles*, 97 Cal. App. 557, 218 P.2d 66, 1950). Therefore, if there is any doubt in the mind of the dentist if he should use radiographs, he should do so. The use of radiographs has been so embedded in the minds of the public that a jury in most cases will find the dentist negligent if he fails to use x-rays. A radiograph should be taken before and after each extraction.

There are times when a patient will refuse radiographs for some reason. In such a situation, Miller (1970) suggests two alternative procedures for the dentist to take to minimize a malpractice suit at a later date.

1. Record the refusal in the patient's record and have patient sign it.
2. Offer to take the radiographs at no charge for his records.

Either of these procedures would lessen the possibilities of a malpractice suit against the dentist for the failure to use radiographs.

Radiographs as Evidence

In the court of law, one must remember that the best evidence is that which is factual. Radiographs are factual evidence. Of course, the radiographs must be of good diagnostic quality as they reflect the competency of the dentist. Radiographs of inferior quality should be retaken for two reasons (Miller, 1970):

1. These radiographs will be of no use as evidence.
2. They will reflect on the dentist's ability as a practitioner and could cause irreparable harm to the dentist's reputation.

If a dentist retains radiographs of inferior quality in his records, they will only prove his incompetence as a dentist if he produces these radiographs as evidence in court. There is no substitute for good radiographs, and the ability of the dentist to interpret the radiographs accurately according to his clinical findings.

Unquestionably, the most important legal aspect of dental radiographs is that it constitutes in itself invaluable malpractice insurance. Any attorney will hesitate to bring a suit of malpractice against a dentist who has taken preoperative and postoperative radiographs. The lawyer will know in advance tha that the case will be difficult to win and probably will try to settle out of court. However, if a dentist has done his treatment competently and has taken comprehensive radiographs he should not be concerned, because he has irrefutable evidence in his possession.

Forensic Dental Radiology

Dental radiology has several applications in forensic odontology, including identification, personal injury, malpractice, and child abuse cases.

Identification Using Dental Radiology

Identification of a body is important because proof of death is required for many legal matters, such as the payment of insurance and inheritance, administration of wills, remarriage of the surviving spouse, settling of business affairs, and criminal investigation. Sometimes, without positive proof of death, a family may have to wait five to fifteen years for settlement. Properly exposed, developed, mounted, and labeled dental radiographs are as good as, if not better than, fingerprints.

Many dental identifications are on deceased individuals that are partially decomposed, skeletonized, or fragmented after a disaster. In these cases, the highly resistant teeth and bones are often the only scientific means of identification available. Such things as missing and unerupted teeth, caries, root canal fillings, pulp and root morphology, distinctive shapes of restorations, bases under restorations, periapical and periodontal pathology, and the sinuses can be identified only by radiographic examination. The single most accurate and reliable source from which one can identify a body is by comparison of antemortem and postmortem radiographs. Therefore, it is imperative that radiographs be adequately taken and processed because they may be used later as antemortem radiographs.

If called upon to make postmortem radiographs of a body specimen, it is important to try to duplicate the angulation and density of the antemortem radiograph rather than trying to make the best radiograph possible. If the original film was severely distorted and the postmortem radiograph is taken by the paralleling technic, a positive comparison would be difficult, if not impossible. In general, exposure times should be reduced for postmortem specimens, usually one-third reduction for resected jaws and up to one-half reduction for skeletonized jaws. If antemortem records are not available, conventional periapical and bite-wing film should be obtained. In these "unknown" cases, the dentist should furnish a detailed description of the dentition and surrounding structures for comparison to files of missing persons.

Personal Injury, Malpractice, and Child Abuse Cases

Preoperative and postoperative radiographs in personal injury and malpractice cases provide evidence rarely found in the wirtten dental racord. Therefore, radiographs should be properly taken, processed, mounted, and labeled. If the radiographs are of poor quality they could be ruled inadmissable in court and reflect on the dentist's competency.

The diagnosis of physical abuse is confirmed and categorized as to extcnt in the "battered child syndrome" by radiographic examination (Baetz et al., 1977). All fifty states now have laws that mandate the reporting of suspected child abuse to various law enforcement agencies.

FUTURE OF DENTAL RADIOLOGY

The field of dental radiology is expanding. This is the age of nuclear enegy and electronics, and along with this are new and exciting discoveries that are influencing dental radiology. Although routine radiographic procedures in dentistry are important, the student of dentistry should inform himself of these new discoveries and perhaps participate in their development.

Areas of Research and Development

Polaroid® Film Packets

Polaroid packets with dental x-ray film in them can be used as self-containing processing packets. X-ray film then could be developed almost instantly without the use of a darkroom. Medical x-ray packets with Polaroid film was introduced in 1969. Mr. Land, the inventor of the Polaroid camera, has a patent recorded in Washington, D. C., on the use of dental film with Polaroid processing. Possibly Polaroid film packets for dentistry will be a reality someday as they are now used in medicine.

Cold Cathode Tube

Perhaps in the future we can operate the x-ray tubes on less current and therefore reduce the focal spot size, which will give better definition (sharpness) to the dental radiographic images. This may be accomplished by the use of the "cold cathode" tube. The cathode in this type of tube has a large number of needle points on its inner surface.

Panchromatic Film

Panchromatic film may be available for dental and medical radiography in the future. The film would contain three speeds of emulsion built on top of each other — high, medium, and slow. The film after exposure would be developed by a color processing system. The silver would be removed, but a silver dye image remains. The high speed emulsion would be yellow, the medium speed emulsion would be red or blood color, and the slow speed emulsion would be a blue color. By the use of different colors of filter on the viewbox, various details of the film may be brought out. This would give the dentist of film with tremendous latitude.

Image Amplifiers

Image amplifiers of a fluorescent x-ray image are tape-recorded by television cameras and played back on TV monitors at a later time. This equipment is used by the medical radiologist at the present time. Perhaps dentistry will find application of this type of equipment someday.

Cinefluorography

Cinefluorography (cineradiography) may be defined as the cinematographic recording of a fluoroscopic image formed on a conventional fluoroscopic screen or on the output screen of an image intensifier by means of a cinematographic camera optically coupled to the screen (Ter-Pogossian, 1967). Cinefluorography must be carried out with the use of some type of x-ray intensifier. The light output from a standard fluoroscopic screen is insufficient for the short exposure time ($^1/_{40}$ sec) required for cinematography. It would require an increase in x-ray exposure to the patient to overcome this difficulty, which would supersede the safety limitations for the patient. Therefore, the modern cinefluorography unit uses an x-ray image intensifier. An image intensifier tube is defined as a vacuum tube containing an input screen that converts an x-ray pattern into an electron pattern, and in which the electrons are accelerated and focused into an output screen, which converts the electron patterns into a light image of higher intensity (NBS Handbook 89, 1963). Berry and Hofmann (1956, 1959, 1966) have applied the method of cinefluorography to the diagnostic study of the temporomandibular joint (Fig. 17-1).

Thermography

Thermography is the science of recording graphically temperatures or changes of temperatures. Recently it has

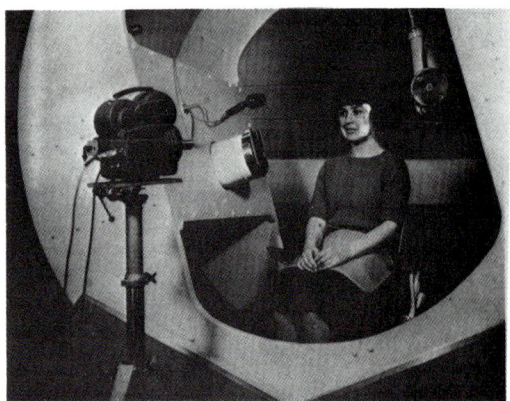

Figure 17-1. Patient prepared for temporomandibular study of joint function in cineradiographic circle unit. (Courtesy of Harrison Berry, Jr. and Allan Hofmann, University of Pennsylvania.)

been used for diagnostic purposes in medicine. Gershon-Cohen et al. (1965) have written an excellent monograph on the subject.

All objects give off infrared energy as a function of their temperature. In order that a thermal balance may be obtained in nature, invisible infrared radiation is being continuously emitted, absorbed, and remitted by everything in our environment. The human body normally gives off 3-20 microns of infrared radiation. Every patient would glow if our eyes could perceive infrared radiation. Since the infrared radiation emitted varies, some areas of the body will be dark while other portions of the body will be bright. It is well known that areas of the body with inflammation will emit more heat than usual, which can be determined by the sense of touch. However, there are minute increases in temperature in the body from increased cellular and metabolic activity that cannot be determined in the conventional manner.

The basic instrument used in thermography is the thermograph, which records minute skin surface changes in temperature. The thermograms or temperature maps produced may be quantitatively analyzed. Thermograms are taken in total darkness and should not be confused with infrared photographs, which are taken with an ordinary camera equipped with film sensitive to radiation in the infrared portion of the electromagnetic spectrum.

Duplicate thermograms of the same person should produce similar temperature patterns. When there are significant physiologic changes within the person, the thermograms will be different. Thermograhy has been used as a supplemental diagnostic aid to medical radiography with some success. There are possibilities that thermography could be used as a diagnostic procedure in dentistry (Irwin et al., 1971).

Ultrasound for Diagnostic Purposes

Sound at ultra-high frequencies (100 kilocycles to 20 megacycles) takes on properties similar to light. Sound at these frequences can be focused with ultrasonic lenses and projected into long linear, pencillike beams for diagnostic purposes (Howry, 1965). The method used is similar to sonar used in World War II to locate submarines under water. High frequency sounds are transmitted through water and as the sound hit solid objects, the submarine sonar would listen for their echoes.

Ultrasonic diagnostic equipment has been devised that transmits high frequency sounds by means of a transducer through the tissue fluids of the body. As the echoes travel back at various rates to a piezo-electric crystal, electrical charges develop that can be recorded or displayed on oscilloscopes and photographic film (Ennis, Berry, and Phillips, 1967). Diagnostic ultrasonography has been used in the past to locate benign and malignant diseases of the liver, carcinoma of the breast, renal diseases, eye diseases and brain tumors (Elizondo-Martel and Gershon-Cohen, 1965).

Neutron Radiography

X-radiography and neutron radiography are similar except that absorption of thermal neutrons in light and heavy materials is practically the opposite of that of x-rays. Images in neutron radiography are produced by thermal neutrons interacting with the atomic nucleus of the tissue cells while the x-ray image is produced by the interaction of x-radiation with the electrons of the atoms of the tissue (Boyne and Whittemore, 1971).

The sensitivity of conventional photographic emulsions is too low for practical use in neutron radiograpy (Herz, 1969). Therefore, special converter screens containing foils of certain elements that emit alpha, beta, or gamma rays when exposed to thermal neutrons are used.

The drawback in using this type of radiography is that the most suitable source for thermal neutrons comes from nuclear reactors. Only a few laboratories have nuclear reactors because of the high cost and their large size. However, other neutron sources could come from Van der Graaf accelerators or from isotopes.

In the future, it is possible that neutron radiography could be applied to the human jaws in suspected tumor cases (Boyne and Whittemore, 1971).

Autoradiography

An autoradiograph is a record of the structure of an object made on film by the object's own radioactivity (Etter, 1970). The specimen is placed in contact with a suitable photographic emulsion. The radioactive material within the specimen exposes the photographic emulsion, which in turn reveals the location of the radioactive material within the specimen. Biologists now are able to study cells, nuclei, and chromosomes by using tracer radioisotopes in conjunction with electron microscope autoradiography technics.

Scintillation Scanning

This is an extension of the autoradiographic technic utilizing a scanner. Scanning refers to the visual recording of the distribution of a radioactive substance within an organ (Horwitz, 1971). This requires the concentration of a suitable radioactive substance within the organ. The scanning device consists of a phosphor, photomultiplier tube, and associated circuits for recording light emissions (scintillations) caused by the gamma radiation emitted from the organs in question. The scanner passes back and forth over the organ, recording the radioactivity. The distribution of the radioactive material within the organ allows the clinician to evaluate the size, shape, and position of the organ.

Also, it is possible to gain information on the physiological activity of the organ by the presence of high and low concentrations of the radioactivity within the organ.

The use of scintillation scanning with ^{85}Sr for the detection of bone involvement by squamous cell carcinoma of the oral mucosa was discussed by Mashberg et al. in 1969.

Microradiography

Microradiography is a method of recording a photograph of the microscopic details in a thin specimen (under 100 microns) by means of soft x-rays generated by kilovoltage of 10-40 kVp. Dental x-ray machines usually are not suitable because the x-rays are not soft enough. X-ray diffraction equipment is preferred (Herz, 1969).

Microradiography provides an excellent research tool for dental biologists to study the distribution of the mineral content in dental enamel and the microscopic carious lesion (Crabb and Mortimer, 1967).

Angiography

Angiography is the x-ray visualization of blood vessels filled with radiopaque material. This procedure is accomplished by the injection of contrast material within the blood vessels followed by a radiograph of the region in question (Etter, 1970). This procedure can contribute to the diagnosis of neoplasms of the head and neck (Medellin and Wallace, 1970). The angiogram is particularly useful in the diagnosis of certain highly vascular tumors such as angiofibromas and hemangiomas. These neoplasms result in excessive blood loss at biopsy. Abrupt and irregular changes in the caliber of the blood vessels and irregular pooling of contrast material seemingly outside the vessels are two reliable findings in malignant disease of the head and neck (Medellin and Wallace, 1970).

Computed Tomography

Computed tomography was introduced by Mr. Godfrey N. Hounsfield, physicist of EMI Limited, Middlesex, England, in 1972. He was later (in 1979) awarded the Nobel Prize for Medicine jointly with Professor A. N. Cormack. Computed tomography has had many names such as Computerized Axial Tomography (CAT), Computer Aided Tomography (CAT), Reconstructive Tomography (RT), and Computed Transmission Tomography (CTT). It is now usually referred to as computed tomography or computerized axial tomography (CAT). The basic concept as outlined by Hounsfield was that a thin cross section of the head (tomographic slice) was observed from multiple angles with a very thin x-ray beam. The transmitted radiation was counted by a scintillation (emission of sparks) detector, fed into a computer for analysis by a certain mathematical method (algorithm), and reconstructed as a tomographic image. The resulting image had a remarkable characteristic, one not seen in a conventional radiograph. It demonstrated a density difference in various soft tissues such as blood clots, gray matter, white matter, cerebrospinal fluid, tumors, and cerebral fluid (Fig. 17-2).

The functional parts of a computed tomographic unit includes an x-ray source, which scans the patient, a radiation detector (either scintillation crystals or gas-filled ionization chambers), a digital computer, and a device for converting the computed image into a viewable format. Information from the CT scans is usually stored in the form of a CT display of signals sent from the computer to a cathode ray tube (CRT) or television monitor, which is in turn recorded as a gray-scale image on a magnetic tape or disk. Another way to preserve CT images is to photograph them while they are displayed on a cathode-ray tube or television monitor. Mulitple detector arrays and fan-shaped x-ray beams are now commonly employed instead of the simple model of Figure 17-2 used to illustrate operational principles (Figs. 17-3, 17-4).

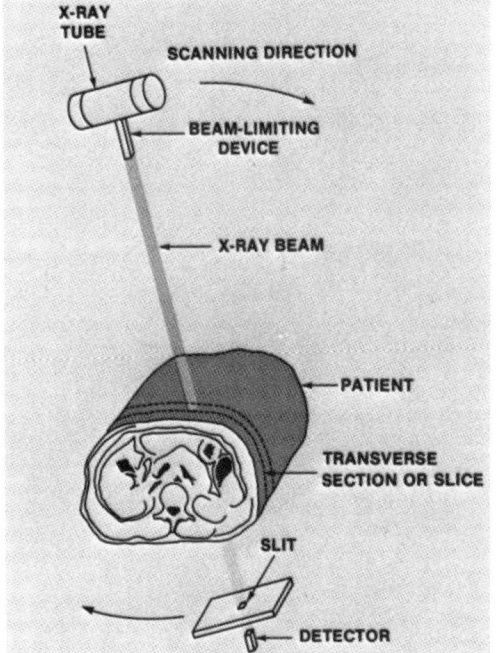

Figure 17-2. Computed Tomography. Diagram showing narrow beam of x-rays transmitted by patient and incident on detector, which is acurately aligned with and connected to the x-ray tube (connecting frame not shown). As the tube and detector move in synchronism around the patient, x-ray transmission through a transverse section of the body is measured from thousands of different positions and this information is sent to a computer. From these measurements, the computer calculates an array of attenuation (CT) numbers and reconstructs a picture of the structures in the layer. (From *the Fundamentals of Radiography,* 12th ed. fig. 58, p. 84. copyright Eastman Kodak Co., Health Science Markets Division, Rochester, New York.)

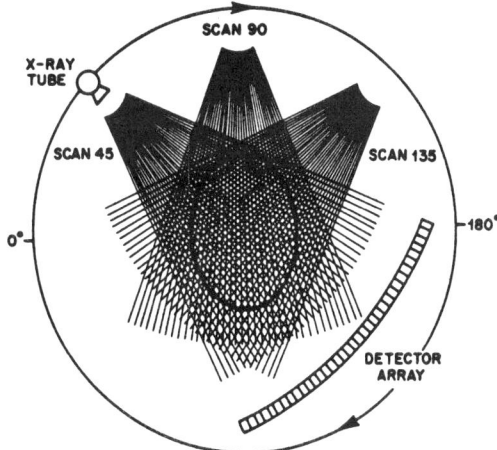

Figure 17-3. Third generation CT scanner. (From Christensen, Curry and Dowdey: *An Introduction to the Physics of Diagnostic Radiology.* Philadelphia, Lea & Febiger, 2nd edition, 1978, Fig. 24-6).

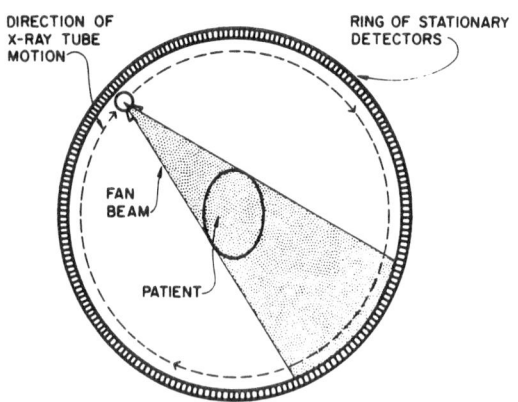

Figure 17-4. Fourth generation CT scanner (From Christensen, Curry, and Dowdey: *An Introduction to the Physics of Diagnostic Radiology.* Philadelphia, Lea & Febiger, 2nd edition, 1978.)

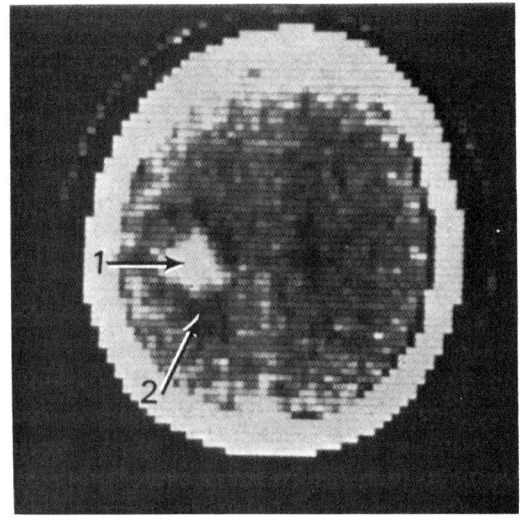

Figure 17-5. Horizontal section of the brain through the midparietal region. The dense radiopacity (1) in the right parietal region is an intracerebral hematoma. The translucent area (2) around it represents edema. (From Sutton D.; and Grainger: *A Textbook of Radiology,* 2nd ed. 1975, Fig. 57.19. Courtesy of Churchill Livingstone Publishers, Edinburgh, Scotland.)

The advantage of a fan beam-multiple detector array is speed. Multiple detectors can gather data faster than a single detector. In 1972, the fastest scan was 4-5 minutes; now, scan times are comparable to exposure times used in conventional radiography.

This revolutionary new technique has many advantages. It can detect much smaller differences in subject contrast than conventional radiography, because it minimizes scatter radiation by use of a narrow slit beam and shielding surrounding the detector. For instance, it is capable of discriminating barium between fresh and coagulated blood (Fig. 17-5). Also, it can give three-dimensional information by reconstructing several sections of the body part. One disadvantage is the cost of the machine, and therefore there are few as yet in clinical use. However, most medical centers do have them at present. A further refinement of this method is enhancement of images by intravenous injection of a contrast medium. It results in a measurable increase of density in well-vascularized lesions. Computed tomography is also finding application in nuclear magnetic resonance imaging (zeugmatography).

Computed tomography has some application in certain types of pathologic conditions occurring in the craniofacial region. Carter and Karmody (1978) found that CT scanning was better able to detect the extent of lesions into the orbit or the base of the skull when compared to conventional radiography and multidirectional tomography. Also, CT scanning proved to be a more accurate means of deciding whether surgery or radiotherapy was indicated when lesions were identified as malignant. Another use of CT scanning was found to be in identifying subdural and epidural hematomas in trauma to the midface, which many times are missed with conventional tomographic procedures. Lian et al. (1980) reported the value of CT scanning in identifying soft tissue margins in two cases of adenocystic carcinoma in the maxilla.

In the diagnosis of salivary gland disorders, CT scanning has been found valuable in identifying lesions lying adjacent to the salivary glands, particularly after the injection of contrast medium such as Lipiodal. Although bony lesions of the jaws and adjacent structures are best evaluated by routine radiographic procedures, CT scanning can contribute to the diagnosis of the soft tissue component of lesions.

Radionuclide Scanning

This is the production of a two-dimensional image of the distribution of the activity of radioactivity in a tissue after the internal administration of a radionuclide. The radioactivity is detected by various detectors and imaging systems.

Most radionuclides are made artificially by irradiation of stable nuclides by subatomic particles in cyclotrons or nuclear reactors or other generators. These agents all disintegrate spontaneously, emitting one or more of the following radiations: alpha particles (2 protons and 2 neutrons), beta particles (negatively charged electron), Positrons (positively charged electron), and gamma photons. The energy is measured in electron volts (eV) and the spectrum of energies is constant for each **nuclide** (species of atom having in each nucleus a paticular number of protons and neutrons; for instance, there are three hydrogen nuclides).

The radionuclides that are used most commonly in diagnostic work are gamma emitters. In some instances, positron emitters can be used, such as ^{74}Au and ^{64}Cu for brain scanning. Also, radionuclides that are used in nuclear medicine always form a part of a chemical compound called a **radiopharmaceutical** that is tolerated by the patient and is either pharmacologically inert or given in too small a quantity to have any effect.

Nuclear medicine diagnostic studies have application in the diagnosis and treatment planning of the jaws and salivary glands, especially when the borders of a bony lesion or the function of the salivary gland is in question.

Technetium 99m (^{99m}Tc) is a radionuclide used most commonly in scans of the jaws and salivary glands. Technetium 99m is a nuclide resulting from beta emission by the parent nuclide (^{99}Mo, molybdenum); it is said to be metastable, and this is indicated by writing "m" before the atomic symbol resulting in ^{99m}Tc. Technetium 99m has a half-life of six hours and emits a gamma photon at a variable interval. Thus, ^{99}Mo decays by beta emission to ^{99m}Tc which in turn decays by gamma emission to ^{99}Tc.

Depending on the form of ^{99m}Tc (technetium), it may be used either as salivary gland scanning agent or as a bone scanning agent. The radiopharmaceutical pertechnetate (^{99m}TcO$_4^-$) has an affinity for the thyroid and salivary glands. Labeling various phosphate compounds with ^{99}Tc results in radiopharmaceuticals (^{99m}Tc-phosphate) that will concentrate in bone and provide a bone scan. After the radiopharmceutical is administered, a detector is used to measure the gamma photons and begins the imaging process. There are two methods of recording radioactivity; the conventional linear scanner or the newer gamma cameras.

The linear scanner (Fig. 17-6) consists of a detector, which is usually a crystal of sodium iodide containing thallium iodide as an activator. Gamma photons striking the detector are convertred indirectly into light quanta, which are led off into a photomultiplier. The detector is moved back and forth mechanically across the field being scanned. Voltage pulses from the photomultiplier are recorded permanently either by a dot diagram, light spots on an unexposed radiograph, or a color dot diagram. Areas of significant activity are located anatomically by superimposing the scan or a matching radiograph (Fig. 17-7).

The *gamma camera* (Fig. 17-8) has a stationary detector, which records activity over the whole field simultaneously. Scin-

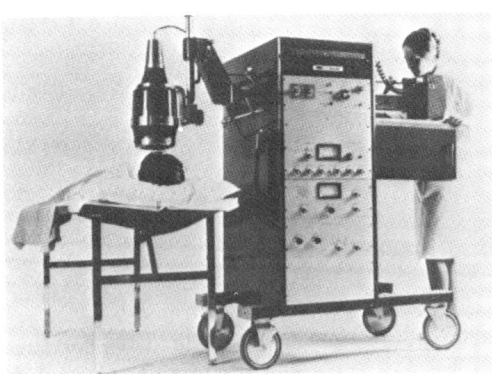

Figure 17-6. Radionuclide linear scanner. (Courtesy of Picker Corp.)

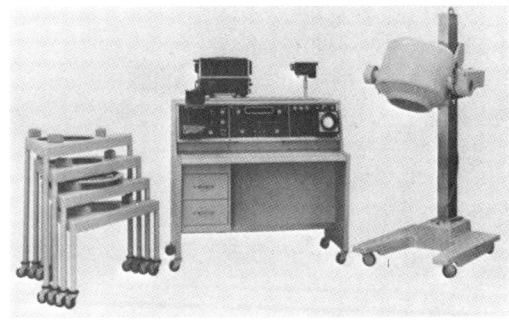

Figure 17-8. Pho/Gamma Scintillation Camera with long-persistence oscilloscope attachment and standard motion picture camera for recording dynamic studies. (Courtesy of Nuclear Chicago Corp.)

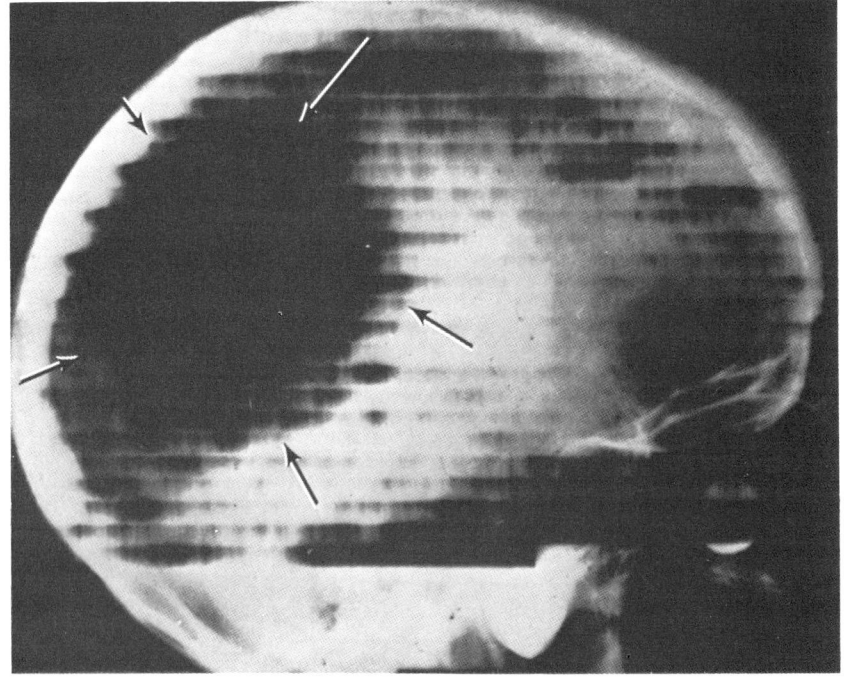

Figure 17-7. ^{99m}Tc Right lateral scintigram taken with linear scanner. The photoscan has been superimposed on a lateral radiograph of the skull. The black area over the right occipital pole is the high uptake in a vascular *glioma* (primary intrinsic neoplasm of brain). Note the normal high uptake over the vertex and the base of the skull. (From Sutton, D.; and Grainger: *Textbook of Radiology,* 2nd ed. 1975, Fig. 56.1, pg 1104. Courtesy of Churchill Livingstone Publishers, Edinburgh, Scotland.)

tillations (gamma photon emissions) are recorded on an oscilloscope and photographed directly by a Polaroid camera.

It is convenient to record rapid sequences with a camera that changes its frames automatically, and a videotape or motion picture recording offers the additional facility for recording dynamic studies. The gamma camera has an additional advantage over the linear scanner in that it can be used in recording serial changes in total activity of the salivary gland. In this way it provides a method to study salivary gland function.

Bone scans of the jaws may be indicated (1) for evaluation of the success or failure of the bone graft, and (2) to determine the extent of the margins in locally aggressive lesions of the jaws (Fig. 17-9).

Recently ^{67}**Ga-citrate (gallium citrate)** has been used to localize tumors and infection of the head and neck (Fig. 17-10). It has great potential in determining the size of head and neck tumors as well as differentiating between infection and carcinoma of the maxillary sinuses and jaws. Hopefully, similar radiopharmaceuticals will be found in the future to aid in diagnosis and treatment of tumors and infection of the head and neck.

The Subtraction Technique

Sometimes the radiographis cluttered with too much information. A lesion may be difficult to interpret because it is hidden partially by superimposed structures. This problem usually occurs in angiograms and can be reduced somewhat by the use of a subtraction technique. The subtraction technique is a photographic method of eliminating (substracting) the unwanted structures from a radiograph. Recent development of a substraction film that can be developed in the automatic processor has made this technique easy, rapid, and inexpensive (DuPont Cronex subtraction and Kodak RP/SU X-OMAT substraction film). In angiography, subtraction can accentuate the pattern of blood vessels containing contrast media. The technique requires two films — one base or scout film taken previously and one film (angiogram) taken with contrast medium in the vessels. A **reverse-tone subtraction mask** (negative of the scout film) is prepared making an exposure with the nonemulsion side of a sheet of subtraction film in contact with the scout film. Cancellation of unwanted images is achieved by printing the mask in registration with the angiogram on a subtraction print film. This is done by first placing the mask onto the glass of a glass cassette, then the angiogram, followed by the unexposed subtraction film. The films are then exposed with a 15 watt light bulb about six feet from the glass cassette. The resulting film leaves visible only those regions in which they differ, namely, where the contrast material is present. This technique may have some application in dentistry especially in the diagnosis of central hemangiomas and arteriovenous aneurysms of the jaws. Also, subtracted radiographs are often helpful in sialography.

Nuclear Magnetic Resonance Imaging

A new technique for obtaining cross-sectional pictures through the human body without exposing the patient to ionizing radiation is at the threshold of clinical application: nuclear-magnetic resonance (NMR) imaging. NMR imaging not only yields anatomic information comparable to information suplied by CT scan but also promises to discriminate better between healthy and diseased tissue. Some pathological lesions have x-ray absorption properties so similar to those

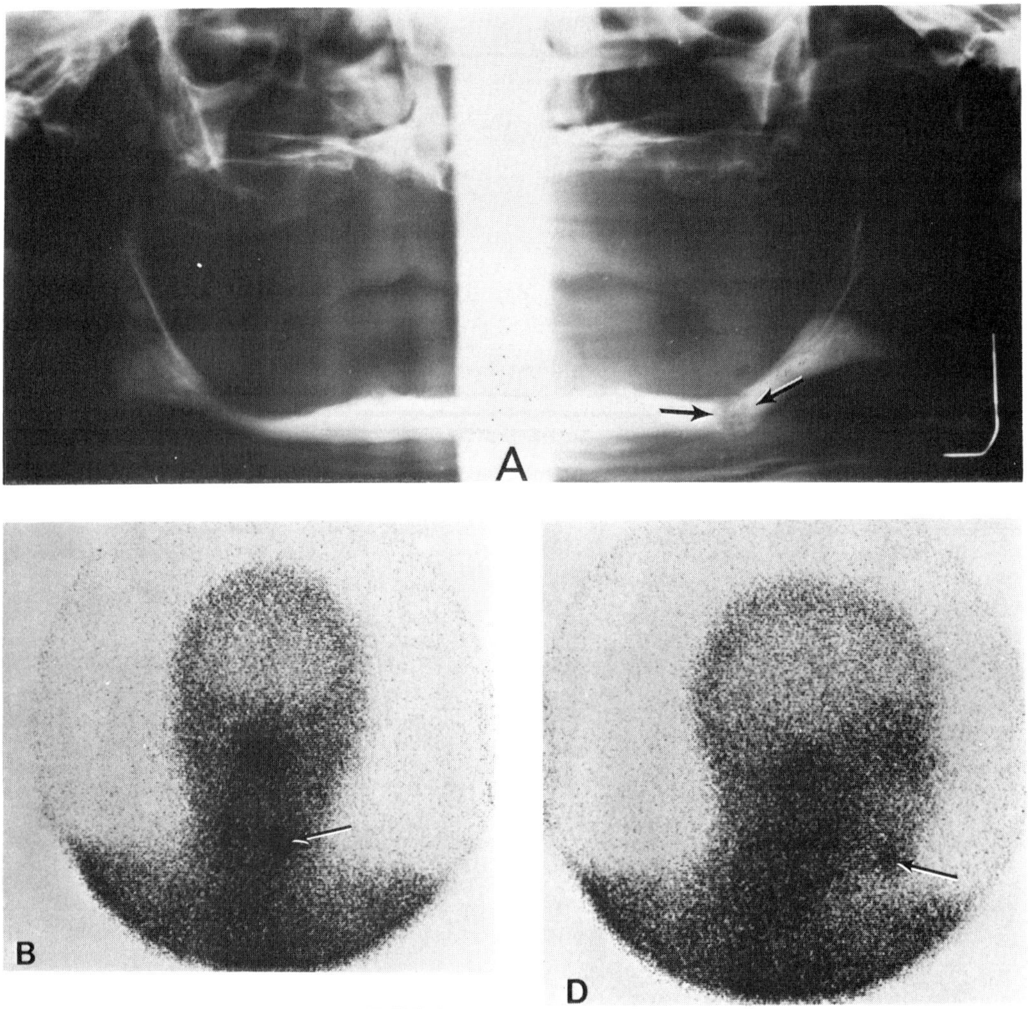

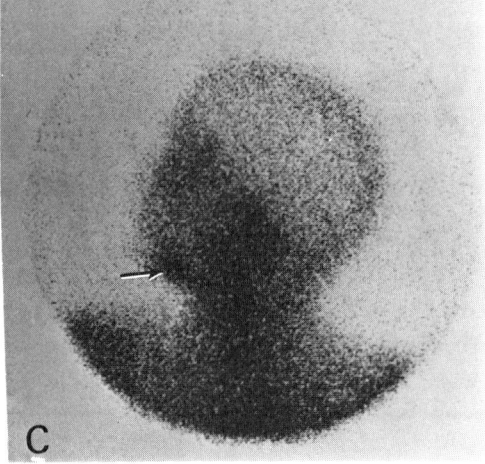

Figure 17-9. Gamma Camera Pertechnetate ($^{99m}TcO_4^-$) bone scan of the skull to determine extent of osteomyelitis of mandible. (A) Confirmed osteomyelitis of left mandibular jaw indicated by round radiolucency seen in panoramic (Panorex I) radiograph. (B) Gamma Camera Pertectinetate ($^{99m}TcO_4^-$) bone scan of same patient as outlining the osteomyelitis in three planes — anterior plane. (C) Left plane. (D) Right plane.

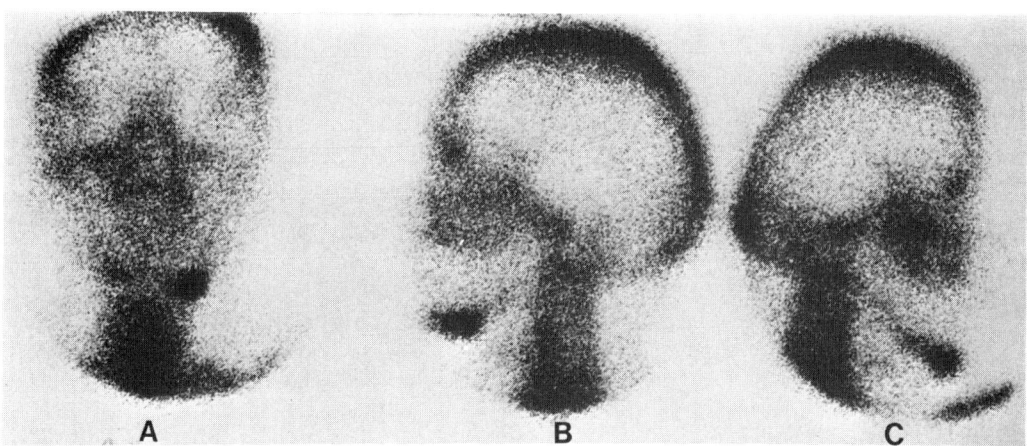

Figure 17-10. Gamma Camera ^{67}Ga-citrate (gallium citrate) bone scan of same patient as Figure 17-19 outlining the same area of osteomyelitis in the mandible. Note the area outlining the osteomyelitis is much darker than pertectinetate (^{99}TcO$_4^-$) bone scan. **(A)** Anterior plane. **(B)** Left plane. **(C)** Right plane.

of the surrounding tissues that the lesions can go undetected in the CT scan unless they are large enough to change the size and shape of the organ. NMR imaging is founded on the well-established ability of NMR spectroscopy to reveal the intricate structure of organic molecules and to provide insight into dynamic chemical processes.

It has been known since the 1920s that atomic nuclei have an angular momentum arising from their inherent property of rotation, or spin. Spinning nuclei behave like tiny tops or gyroscopes. Since nuclei are electrically charged, the spin corresponds to a current flowing about the spin axis, which in turn generates a small magnetic field. Only nuclei with an odd number of nucleons (protons or neutrons) exhibit a net spin, and therefore lend themselves to NMR spectroscopy. NMR images are cross-sectional pictures of thin slices through the body obtained by using radio waves to interrogate susceptible atomic nuclei that have been precisely oriented in a magnetic field. The susceptible nuclei are those that have an odd number of nucleons (protons and neutrons).

Hydrogen nuclei (protons) are the most widespread particles in living matter. After radio excitation the nuclei reveal their location by emitting a signal of precise frequency for a brief period. With computer techniques, pictorial images can be reconstructed from the emitted signals. All medical NMR images produced so far have been obtained only with the resonances of the hydrogen nuclei. This is fortunate, because the human body is 75 percent water, each molecule containing two hydrogen nuclei. Moreover, the distribution of water with the various other small, hydrogen-rich molecules (for example lipids) is known to be altered by many disease states. NMR imaging is still at an early stage in medicine. It may be particularly good at detecting necrotic (dead) tissue, ischemia, malignancies, and degenerative disease of various kinds. The soft tissue contrast is inherently superior to that of x-ray techniques. Perhaps the greatest potential of all lies in the imaging of nuclei other than hydrogen, particularly the phosphorus nucleus. From knowledge of the phosphorus concentrations in tissue, it may be possible to infer the metabolic status of internal organs. The next few years will undoubtedly see more use of NMR in clinical practice.

Bibliography

Alexander, J. M.: Radionuclide bone scanning in the diagnosis of lesions of the maxillofacial region. *J Oral Surg, 34*:249, 1976.

Baetz, K.; Sledzrewski, W.; Margetts, D.; Koren, L.; Levy, M.; and Pepper, R.: Recognition and management of the battered child syndrome. *J Dent Assoc South Africa, 32*:13, 1977.

Berger, H.: *Neutron Radiography.* New York, Elsevier, 1965.

Berret, A.: Value of angiography in the management of tumors of the head and neck. *Radiology, 84*:1952, 1965.

Berry, H. M., Jr.; and Hofmann, F. A.: Cinefluorography with image intensification for observing temporomandibular joint movements. *J Am Dent Assoc, 53*:517, 1956.

Berry H. M., Jr.; and Hofmann, F. A.: Cineradiographic observations of T-M joint function. *J Prosthet Dent*, 21-31, January-February, 1959.

Berry H. M., Jr.; and Hofmann, F. A.: Cineradiographic circle unit. *Public Health Rep, 81*:470, 1966.

Boyne, P. J.; et al.: Neutron radiography of osseous tumors. *Oral Surg, 31*:152, February 1971.

Brooks, R. A.; and DiChiro, G.: Theory of image reconstruction in computed tomogragraphy. *Radiology, 117*:561, 1975.

Brooks, R. A.; and DiChiro, G.: Slice geometry in computer assisted tomography. *J Comp at Assist Tomogy, 1*:191, 1977.

Brown, M.; and Parks, P.: Neutron radiography in biologic media. *AJR, 106*:472, 1969.

Burleson, R. L.; et al.: Scintigraphic demonstration of abscesses with radioactive gallium labeled leukocytes. *Surg Gynecol Obstet, 141*:379, 1975.

Carnaham, C. W.: *The Dentist and the Law.* St. Louis, Mosby, 1955.

Carter, B. F.; and Karmody, C. S.: Computed tomography of the face and neck. *Semin Roentgenol, 13*:257, 1978.

Charles, N. O.; and Sklaroff, D. M.: The radioactive strontium photoscan as a diagnostic aid in primary and metastatic cancer in bone. *Radiol Clin North Am, 3*:499, 1965.

Cooper, H. K.; and Hofmann, F. A.: The application of cinefluorography with image intensification in the field of plastic surgery, dentistry and speech. *J Plast Reconstr Surg, 16*:135, 1955.

Carmack, A. M.: Representation of a function by its line integrals, with some radiological applications. *J Appl Physiol, 34*:2722, September 1963.

Crabb, H. S. M.; and Mortimer, K. U.: Two-dimensional microdensitometry: A preliminary report. *Br Dent J, 122*:337, April 1967.

DeVore, D. T.: Radiology and photography in forensic dentistry. *Dent Clin North am, 21 (1)*:1977.

Deysine, M.; et al.: the detectionof acute experimental osteomyelitis with ^{67}GA citrate scannings. *Surg Gynecol Obstet, 141*:40, 1975.

Donaldson, S. W.: Ownership of radiographs. *Radiogr Clin Photogr, 17*:27, 1941.

Elizondo-Martel, g.; and Gershon-Cohen, J.: Medical ultrasources. *AJR, 93*:791, 1965.

Ennis, L. M.; Berry, H. M.; and Phillips, J. E.: *Dental Roentgenology,* 6th ed. philadelphia, Lea & Febiger, 1967.

Etter, L. E.: *Glossary of Words and Phrases Used in Radiology, Nuclear Medicine and Ultrasound,* 2nd ed. Springfield, Il, Charles C Thomas, 1970.

Fogelman, I.; et al.: A clinical comparison of Tc-99m HEDP and Tc-99m MDP in the detection of bone metastases: concise communication. *J Nucl Med, 20*:98, 1979.

Furuhata, T.; and Yamomoto, K.: *Forensic Odontology.* Springfield, Il, Charles C Thomas, 1967.

Garcia, D. A.; Davis, M. A.; Kapur, K. K.; and Goldhaber, P.: Detection of local changes of mineral metabolism within the jaws of rabbits by bone scanning. *J Dent Res, 53*:447, 1974.

Garcia, D. A.; Higginbotham, D. J.; House, J. E.; and Kapur, K. K.: Tc^{99m} polyphosphate bone imaging of orthodontically treated dog teeth. *Am J Orthod, 66*:665, 1974.

Garcia, D. A.; Tow, D. E.; Sullivan, T. M.; et al.: The appearances of common dental diseases on radionuclide bone images of the jaws. *J Dent Res, 58*:1040, 1979.

Gates, G. A.; and Work, W.P.: Radioisotope scanning of the salivary glands. A preliminary report. *Laryngoscope, 77*:861, 1967.

Gates, G. F.; and Goris, M. L.: Maxillofacial abnormalities assessed by bone imaging. *Radiology 121*:677, 1967.

Gershon-Cohen, J.; Haberman-Brueschke, J. D.; and Brueschke, E. E.: Medical thermography: A summary of current status. *Radiol Clin North Am, 3*:403, December 1965.

Goodenough, D. J.; Weaver, K. E.; and Davis, D. O.: Potential artifacts associated with the scanning pattern of the EMI scanner. *Radiologys 117*:615, 1975.

Grove, A. S., Jr.; and DiChiro, G.: Salivary gland scanning with technetium-99m pertechnetate. *AJR, 102*:109, 1968.

Gustafson, G.: *Forensic Odontology.* New York, American Elsevier Publ. Co., 1966.

Hanafee, W.; and Shinno, J. M.: Second-order subtraction and simultaneous bilateral carotid, internal carotid injections. *Radiology, 86*:334, 1966.

Hendra, R.; and Stebner, F. C.: Evaluation of parotid gland masses: rectilinear scanning. *J Oral Surg, 33*:838, 1975.

Herz, R. H.: *The Photographic Action of Ionizing Radiations.* New York, Wiley-Interscience, 1969.

Higashi, T.; et al.: Gamma camera images of the salivary gland using 99mTc. *Oral Surg, 40*(6):804, 1975.

Higashi, T.; et al.: Technetium 99m bone imaging in the evaluation of cancer of the maxillofacial region. *J Oral Surg, 37*:254, 1979.

Higashi, T.; Aoyama, W.; Mori, Y.; and Everhart, F. R., Jr.: Gallium-67 scanning in the differentiation of maxillary sinus carcinoma from chronic maxillary sinusitis. *Radiology, 123*:117, 1977.

Higashi, T.; Kashima, I.; Shimura, K.; et al.: Gallium-67 scanning in the evaluation of therapy of malignant tumors of the head and neck. *J Nucl Med, 18*:243, 1977.

Hine, G. J.; and Johnston, R. E.: Absorbed dose from radionuclides. *J Nucl Med, 11*:468, 1970.

Horwitz, N. H.: Scanning and scintigraphy. *In Powsner and Raeside's Diagnostic Nuclear Medicine.* New York, Grune, 1971.

Hounsfield, G. N.: Picture quality of computed tomography. *AJR, 127*:3, July 1976.

Hounsfield, G. N.: Computerized transverse axial scanning (tomography0. *Br J Radiol, 46*:1016, 1973.

Howry, D. H.: A brief atlas of diagnostic ultrasonic radiologic results. *Radiol Clin North Am,* 433-452, December, 1965.

Irwin, J. W.; et al.: Intraoral thermography. *Oral Surg, 32*:724, 1971.

Joyce, J. W.; Dalrymple, M. D.; Jungkind, F. F.; Scott, P. D.; and Davasher, B. G.: Improved constrast in subtraction technique. *Radiologys, 94*:157, 1970.

Kaplan, M. L.; Garcia, D. A.; Goldhaber, P.; et al.: Uptake of ^{99m}Tc-Sn-EHDP in beagles with advanced periodontal disease. *Calcif Tissue Res, 19*:91, 1975.

Kelly, J. F.; Cagle, J. D.; Adler, g. J.; and Donovan, R. L.: Sequential quantitative radionuclide evaluation of mandibular bone graft repair. *J Dent Res, 55*:1111, 1976.

Kelly, J. F.; Cagle, J. D.; Stevenson, J. S.; and Adler, G. J.: Technetium-^{99m} radionuclide bone imaging for evaluating mandibular osseous allografts. *J Oral Surg, 33*:11, 1975.

Kuhl, D. E.; and Edwards, R. Q.: Reorganizing data from transverse section scans of the brain using digital processing. *Radiology, 91*:975, 1968.

Landman, G. H. M.: *Laryngography and Cinelaryngography.* Baltimore, Williams & Wilkens, 1970.

Lian, S.; Osaka, f.; Asanami, S.; and Tomita, O.: Adenocystic carcinoma in computed tomography. *Oral surg, 49*:552, 1980.

Lisbona, R.; and Rosenthall, L.: Observations on the sequential use of ^{99m}Tc-phosphate complex and ^{67}Ga imaging in osteomyelitis, cellulitis, and septic arthritis. *Radiology, 123*:123, 1977.

Loveland, R. P.: *Photomicrography.* New York, Wiley, 1970.

Lowman, R.; and Cheng, G.: Diagnostic roentgenology. In Rankow, R.; and Palays, I. (Eds.): *Diseases of the Salivary Glands.* Philadelphia, Saunders, 1976.

Lurie, A. G.: Applications of nuclear medicine in dentistry. In Spencer, R. P., and Seligson, D. (Eds.): *CRC Handbook Series in Clinical Laboratory Science,* Section A: Nuclear Science. Cleveland, CRC Press, 1977.

Lurie, A. G.; and Matteson, R. R.: ^{99m}Tc-diphosphonate bone imaging and uptake in healing rat extraction sockets. *J Nucl Med, 17*:688, 1976.

Lurie, A. G.; Puri, S.; James, R. B.; and Jensen, T. W.: Radionuclide bone imaging in the surgical treatment planning of odontogenic keratocysts. *Oral Surg, 42*: 726, 1976.

McCullough, E. C.; Baker, H. L.; Houser, O. W.; and Reese, D. F.: An evaluation of the quantitative and radiation features of a scanning x-ray transverse axial tomography: The EMI scanner. *Radiology, 111*:709, 1974.

McCullough, E. C.; and Payne, J. T.: X-ray transmission computed tomography. *Med*

Phys, 4:85, 1977.

McCullough, E. C.; payne, J. T.; Baker, H. L.; Hattery, R. R.; Sheedy, P. F.; Stephens, D. H.; and Gedgaudus, E.: Performance evaluation and quality assurance of computed tomography scanners with illustrations from the EMI, ACTA, and Delta Scanners. *Radiology, 120*:173, 1976.

Mashberg, A.; et al.: Use of the scintillation scanning for the early detectionof bone involvement by squamous cell carcinoma of the oral mucosa: Preliminary report. *J Am Dent Assoc, 79*:1151, November 1969.

Medellin, H.; and Wallace, S.: Angiography in neoplasms of head and neck. *Radiol Clin North Am, 8*:307, December, 1970.

Methods of Evaluating Radiological Equipment and Materials. NBS Handbook 89, Washington, D. C., US Government Printing Office, 1963.

Miller, S. L.: *Legal Aspects of Dentistry: A Programmed Course in Dental Jurisprudence.* New York, Putnam, 1970.

New, P. F. T.; and Scott, W. R.: *Computed tomography of the Brain and Orbit.* Baltimore, Williams & Wilkins, 1975.

Oldendorf, W. H.: A modified subtraction technique for extreme enhancement of angiographic detail. *Neurology, 15*:336, 1965.

Oldendorf, W. H.: Subtraction and autosubtraction techniques for reproducing radiographs. *J Biol Photogr Assoc, 32*:65, 1964.

Payne, J. T.; and McCullough: Basic principles of computer-assisted tomography. *Appl Radiol 5*:33, March/April 1976.

Phelps, M. E.; Gado, M. H.; and Hoffman, E. J.: Correlation of effective atomic number and electronic density with attenuation coefficients measured with polychromatic x-rays *Radiology, 117*:585, 1975.

Phelps, M. E.; Hoffman, E. J.; and Ter-Pogossian, M. M.: Attenuation coefficients of various body tissues, fluids, and lesions at photon energie sof 18 to 136 keV. *Radiology, 117*:573, 1975.

Powsner, E. R.; and Radside, D. E.: *Diagnostic Nuclear Medicine.* Diagnostic Nuclear Medicine. New York, Gruen, 1971.

Pykett, I. L.: NMR imaging in medicine. *SCI Am,* pp. 78-88, May 1982.

Rabe, R. T.: Who owns the x-ray films? *Oral Hygiene,* 37-39, July 1957.

Ramsey, G. H. S.; Watson, J. S., Jr.; Tristan, T. A.; Weinberg, S.; corwell, W. S. (Eds.): *Cinefluorography.* Springfield, I., Charles C Thomas, 1960.

Rawls, H. R.; and Owen, W. D.: The dental programs for xeroradiography. *oral Surg, 33*:476, March 1972.

Ricketts, R. M.: Present status of laminagraphy as related to dentistry. *J Am Dent Assoc, 65*:55, 1962.

Rudd, T.; et al.: Tc-99m methylene diphosphonate versus Tc-99m pyophosphate: Biologic and clinical comparison. *J Nucl Med, 98*:872, 1977.

Sarner, H.: *Dental Jurisprudence.* Philadelphiaq, Saunders, 1963.

Shuster, H. L.; et al.: Radionuclide bone imaging as an aid in the diagnosis of fibrous dysplasia: Report of case. *J Oral Surg, 37*:267, 1979.

Sopher, I. M.: *Forensic Dentistry.* Springfield, Il, Charles C Thomas, 1976.

Stebner, F. C.; et al.: Identification of Warthin's tumors by scanning of salivary glands. *Sm J Surg, 116*:513, 1968.

Stimson, P. G.: Radiology in forensic odontology. *Dent Radiogr Photogr, 48*:3, 1975.

Stimson, P. G.: Forensic dental radiology. In Cottone, J. A.; and Standish, S. M.: *Outline of Forensic Dentistry.* Chicago, Year Bk Med, 1982.

Subramanian, g.; and McAfie, J. G.: A new complex of ^{99m}Tc for skeletal imaging. *Radiology 99*:192, 1971.

Sweet, P.: The legal aspects of dental roentgenograms. *J Am Dent Assoc, 25*:1687, October 1938.

Swindell, W.; and Barrett, H. H.: Computerized tomography: Taking sectional x-rays. *Phys today, 30*:32, 1977.

Syed, I. B.; Hosain, F.; Dugal, P.; and Wagner, H. N., Jr.: Bone scanning agents: Present status and choice. *Indian J Cancer, 10*:280, 1973.

Ter-Pogossian, M. M.: *The Physical Aspects of Diagnostic Radiology.* New York, Hoeber Medical, Har-Row, 1967.

Tow, D. E.; et al.: Bone scan in dental diseases. *J Nucl Med, 19*:845, 1978.

Wilkinson, R. H., Jr.; and Goodrich, J. K.: A neurofibroma mimicking a parotid gland tumor both clinically and by scanning. *J Nucl Med, 12*:646, 1971.

Wuehrmann, A. H.: *Radiation Protection and Dentistry.* St. Louis, Mosby, 1960.

INDEX

A

Abrasion, 422
Abscess
  acute apical, 461
  chronic apical, 465, 466, 467
  parulis (gumboil), 466
Absorbed dose, 153
Absorber, atomic number, 91
  density, 91
  thickness, 90
Absorption, differential, 89, 91
  photoelectric, 81
  x-rays, factors affecting, 90
Acquired defects of teeth, 421
Acute apical abscess, 461
Acute apical periodontitis, 461
Acute pulpitis, 461
Ada Snap-A-Ray film holder, 221
Adenomatoid odontogenic tumor, 368
Adrian & Crooks test cassette, 360
Age proration formula, 184
Ala of nose, 387
ALARA concept, 185
Alpha particle, 50, 51, 52
Alterations of teeth
  eruption, 427
  morphology, 412
Alterations of the jaws, 428
  cortical enlargement, 372
  cortical loss, 372
Ameloblastic fibroma, 368
Ameloblastic fibro-odontoma, 368
Ameloblastic odontoma, 369
Ameloblastoma, 368
Amelogenesis imperfecta, 421
Ampere, definition, 62
Amplifiers, image, 640
Anatomical accuracy, 148, 213
Anatomic landmarks, 310
Aneurysmal bone cyst, 368

Angiogram, 647
Angiography, 642
Angulation
  horizontal, improper, 452
  horizontal of P.I.D., 232
  vertical, improper, 452
Angstrom unit, 55, 106
Anode
  Benson line focus, 59
  recessed, 83
  rotating, 60
  stationary, 59
Anterior mediam maxillary cleft, 384
Anterior nasal spine, 388
Antroliths, 369
Aperture diaphragm, 82
Apex, 382
Apical cementoma, 472, 473, 475, 476
Apical conditions
  nonpathologic, 463, 464
Apical cyst, 467, 469
Apical foramen, 382
Apical granuloma, 467
Apices of teeth, location, 210
Apicoectomy, 474
Arrested caries, 441
Arthrography (arthrotomography), 537-540
Atom
  neutral, 44
  structure of, 44
Atomic number, 91
Atomic weights, few of lighter metals, 49
Attenuation
  Compton interaction, 88
  definition, 88
  photoelectric effect, 88
  polychromatic radiation, 90
Attrition, 421
  severe, 495
Autoradiography, 641
Autotransformer, 65, 66

B

Barium fluorochloride, 111
Barium platinocynamide screen, 6
Barium strontium sulfate, 111
Beam
  checking alignment, 362
  heterogenous, 72
  primary, 76, 77
Beam restricting devices
  aperture diaphragm, 82
  functions, 81, 82
    position (Beam Indicating Devices), 83
  variable-aperture collimator, 84
Benign cementoblastoma, 474, 475, 476
Benign osteoblastoma, 369
Benson line focus, 59
Bergonie and Tribondeau, Law of, 21
Berry, Harrison, 640
Beta particles, 50, 51, 52
Binding energy, 47, 48
Bisecting angle technique
  CMX, 257
  evaluation of periodontal disease, 484, 485
  film placement, 256, 257, 258
  head position, 256
  history of, 32, 33
  horizontal angulation, 256, 257, 258, 259
  point of entry, 256, 260
  procedures, 256
  retention technique, 260, 261
  Rinn BAI technique, 262, 261
  Stabe film holder, 261, 263, 264, 265
  vertical angulation, 255, 256, 258, 259
Bitewing radiographs, 97, 206, 266
Bitewing tab technique, 266
  film placement and retention, 264
  head position, 266
  horizontal angulation, 267
  point of entry, 267
  vertical angulation, 267
Bitewing technique, film holders, 267, 268, 269
Bone deformities, 478, 479
Bone loss
  amount of, 484, 48
  evaluation, 480
  generalized, 480
  horizontal, 482
  localized, 480
  use of grid, 484
  vertical, 428
Bone, trabecular patterns, 369
Bremsstrahlung, 70, 71, 73
Buccal Object Rule, 560-564
  mandibular canal location, 561-563

Bulbous roots, 396
Burkitt's lymphoma, 369

C

Calcifying epithelial odontogenic tumor, 368
Calcium tungstate, 105
Calcium tungstate screens
  absorption factors, 107
  classification, 107
  concentration in layer, 108
  factors influencing speed, 107
  influence of kVp, 108
  phosphor size, 108
  phosphor type, 108
  thickness of phosphor layer, 108
Calculus, 478
Caldwell view, 519, 520
Canals of Scarpa, 286
Canals of Stenson, 386
Carbon, binding energies, 48
Caries, dental
  abrasion, 448, 449
  acute, 433
  arrested, 441
  attrition, 448, 449
  bitewing film, 432
  cemental, 438, 439, 440
  cervical, 437
  cervical burnout, 444
  chronic, 433
  classification, interproximal, 435
  definition, 432
  dentinal, 380, 435
  early lesion, 433
  enamel, 380, 433, 442
  enamel hypoplasia, 447, 448
  errors in projection affecting caries detection, 452
  exposure errors affecting caries detection, 450, 451
  facial/lingual, 436, 437
  factors that influence interpretation, 441
  histopathology, 442
  large, 439
  line-shaped lesion, 433
  location, classification, 433
  Mach band effect, 444
  normal tooth structure/caries ratio, 443
  occlusal, 436, 437
  periapical film, 432
  pulpal, 436, 437
  radiographic appearance, 433
  radiolucent restorations, 446, 447
  recurrent (secondary), 440, 441, 495
  root (cemental, senile), 438, 439, 440
  scoring code, 435
  technique errors affecting caries detection, 449, 450

underestimation of size, 441, 442
V-shaped lesion, 433
Cassette
  checking technique, 363, 364
  description, 103
  grid-front, 124
  Kodak X-Omatic, 103, 104
  poor contact, 103
  stainless steel with hinges, 104
Cathode
  filament, 58
  focusing cup, 58
  molybdenum cup, 58
Cathode rays, 5, 6, 50
Cathode tube, cold, 639
Cell cycle, 162
Cementoblastoma, benign, 474, 475, 76
Cementoma, 380
  apical, 472, 475, 576
  firous stage, 474
  halo-effect, 474
  intermediate stage, 474
  mature stage, 474
  true, 475
Central cemento-ossifying fibroma, 369
Central giant cell granuloma, 368
Central hemangioma, 368
Central ray, 76
Cephalometric analysis, lines and planes, 513, 514
Cephalometric technique, 509, 511-515
  exposure factors, 515
  fixed object-film distance, 511
  posteroanterior (PA), 513, 514
  recording soft tissue profile, 512, 513
  variable object-film distance, 511
Cephalostat, 509
Cervical burnout, 444
Characteristic curve
  contrast, 133, 135
  definition, 132
  density, 133
  latitude, 133
  log relative exposure, 133
  shoulder, 133
  speed, 133
  toe, 133
Characteristic radiation, 70, 72, 81
Cherubism, 368
Chondrosarcoma, 369
Chronic apical abscess, 467
Chronic diffuse sclerosing osteomyelitis, 369
Chronic pulpitis, 461
Cinefluorography (cineradiography), 640
  Berry & Hofmann TMJ unit, 640

Circuit, electrical, 61
  filament, 64
  high-voltage, 65
Cleft palate, 429
Coil, interrupterless, 26
  Ruhmkorff, 19
  Telsa (transformer), 17
Collimator, Machlett variable aperture, 84
  rectangular, 84, 85, 216
  slit beam, 84, 85
  variable aperture, 84
Columella, nasal, 387
Complete mouth survey, 207
Compton, A.H., 80
Compton scatter, 89
Computed tomography, 642, 643
Concrescence, 414
condensing osteitis, 369, 467, 470, 471, 476
Condylar head, various angulations, 526
cones (B.I.D.) (P.I.D.), three types, 224
Contrast
  average gradient, 135
  characteristic curve, 135
  film, 135
  index, 355
  long-scale, 137, 451, 452
  short-scale, 137, 451, 452
  subject, 89
Coolidge, W.D., photograph with Thomas A. Edison, 26
Copying radiographs, 314, 315, 316, 317, 318
Coronoid process, 392
Cortical border
  normal, 382
  perforation, 373
Coverage, radiographic, 148
Crater, osseous defect, 488, 489
Critical organ concept, 185
Crossover, 111
Cryptoscope, 13
Crypts, tooth, 396
Crystal, lattice, 95
  silver iodo-bromide, 94
Cupped-out losses of cortex, 373
Current, 61
  alternating, 61
  direct, 61
Curve, H & D, 132
Curve of spee, 314
Cyst
  apical (radicular, periapical) 467, 469
  lateral periodontal, 470, 471
  primordial, 471
  residual, 469, 470

D

Dally, Mr. (Edison's assistant), 14
Daniel, J., first report of loss of hair, 21
Darkroom, 281
  checking, 364, 365
  correct illumination, 284
  light tight, 282
  safelighting, 285, 286, 287, 288
  timer interval, 284, 285
Definition
  radiographic, 59
  sharpness, 130
Delta ray, 154
Densitometer, 130, 132, 354, 355
Density, 134
  definition, 130
  fog, 130
  formula, 130
  grids, 134
  kVp, 134
  mAs, 133
  material, 91
  patient thickness, 134
  processing conditions, 134
  radiographic, base, 132
  screens, 134
  source-film distance, 134
  tissue, 9
  type of film, 134
Dental papilla, 381, 396
Dental radiology, 4
  competency, 4
  definition, 43
  development of, 36
Dentigerous cyst, 368
Dentin, 380
  sclerotic, irregular, 454, 456
  secondary, 453, 454, 456
Dentinal caries, 435
Dentinogenesis imperfecta, 421
Detail, definition, 130
Developer, 290
  composition table, 290
  typical, 290
Development center, 96
Developmental lingual mandibular salivary gland depression, 368
Diagnosis, definition, 130
Diastema, 389
Digastric fossae, 394
Dilaceration, 414
Dimensional changes in the radiograph, 371
Direct effect (radiobiologically), 158
Distal mandibular pseudohyperostosis, 396

Distal oblique technique, 245
  Ada Snap-A-Ray, 248
  Fitzgerald, 248
  mandibular third molar, 249
  maxillary third molar, 245
  Rinn EEZEE GRIP, 248
Distortion, 130, 139
  dimensional, 146, 371
Division delay, 162
Dominant craniometaphyseal dysplasia, 369
Donovan technique, 565, 566
Dorsum of tongue, 393
Dose effect relationships, 165
  linear-quadratic, 165
  non-stochastic, 166
  nonthreshold, 165
  stochastic, 165
  threshold, 164
Dose limit, 184
Dosimeter, pocket, 356
Duplication, procedure, 317
Duplication film, 314
  anti-halation side, 315
  emulsion side, 314, 315
  halation, 315
Duplication technique, 314, 315, 316, 317, 318
Dysplasia, periapical cemental, 472, 473

E

Eagle's syndrome, 369
Ectopic eruption, 427
Edentulous CMX, 208
Edentulous jaw radiography, 551-557
  complete periapical survey, 551-554
  mixed occlusal and periapical survey, 553-556
  occlusal-lateral jaw survey, 556-557
  panoramic survey, 553-555
Edison, Thomas A.
  fluoroscope, 14
  photograph with W.D. Coolidge, 26
Electrical circuit, 61
  current, 61
  potential difference, 61
  resistance, 61
Electricity, 60
Electromagnetic radiation, 50, 51
  examples, 53
  formula for wavelength and frequency, 54
  frequency, 53
  particle concept, 55
  properties, 54
  speed, 53
  wavelength, 53
Electromagnetic spectrum, 53, 54
Electron, 50

Electron charge, 68
Electron cloud (space charge), 58
Electron interactions, anode, 70
Electron recoil (Compton), 80
Electron volt, 48, 56
Electrons, orbital, 44, 45
Elongation, 256
Embedded teeth, 375
Emission, thermonic, 57
Emitters, positron, 645
Emulsion grain, 94
Enamel, 380
Enamel caries, 433, 442
Enamel hypoplasia, 420
Enameloma, 415
Enamel rods, arrangement, 433
Endodontic radiography
  bisecting angle technique, 577
  mandibular posterior technique, 578
  Mark II (Del Rio) film holder, 572-576
  maxillary posterior technique, 577
  obturation radiograph, 567
  postoperative radiograph, 568
  preoperative radiograph, 567
  root length determination, 567
  Snap-A-Ray/EEZEEGRIP technique, 570, 517
  trial distance determination, 567
  working distance radiograph, 567, 568
Endostosis, 471
Energy, definition, 53
Enlargement of alveolar bone, localized, 377
Enlargement of a bone, 372
  generalized, 372
  localized, 372
Ennis, LeRoy M., 33
Enostosis, 369
Errors, common, exposure
  high contrast, 333
  light films, 331
  low contrast, 334
  overexposure, 333
  radiation fog, 334
  underdevelopment, 331
Errors, common, intraoral technique, 322-331
  apices cut off, 322
  artifacts, 327
  bending film packet, 327
  black dot in apical area, 327
  blank image, 327
  blurred image, 327
  cervical burnout, 330
  cone cut, 325
  dimensional distortion, 325
  double exposure, 327
  elongation, 325
  foreshortening, 325
  "fuzzing out" of roots, 327
  Herring bone (tire tracks) effect, 327
  magnification, 327
  missing anatomy, 323
  moisture contamination, 327
  movement, 327
  overlapping of teeth, 322
  "phalangioma," 327
  radiopaque artifacts, 329
  shape distortion, 325
  tongue image error, 330
  writing on radiograph, 327
  zirconium artifact, 329
Errors, common, manual processing
  air bubbles, 337
  black crescents, 339
  black lines, 339
  black spots, 337
  brown stains, 339
  chemical fog, 336
  dark films, 333
  deposits on film, 33
  dichromic stains, 339
  faded image, 342
  fog, 334, 36
  light fog, 334
  overdevelopment, 333
  processing artifacts, 339
  smudge marks, 339
  stains on film, 339
  streaks on film, 336
  underdevelopment, 331
  yellow stains, 339
  white lines, 337
  white spots, 337
Errors, panoramic operator, 346-348
  cassette resistance, 346
  double exposure, 347
  film crimping, 346
  fingernail artifact, 346
  lint in screen, 346
  no name, 347
  not starting at home base, 346
  overexposed, 347
  paper on screen, 346
  static electricity, 347
  white light exposure, 347
Errors, panoramic positioning, 342-346
  bite guide not used, 344
  chin not on chin rest, 344
  chin raised too high, 342
  chin rest too low, 344
  chin tipped too low, 342
  head tilted, 344

head twisted, 344
lips open, 346
patient too far back, 342
patient too far forward, 342
prostheses, 346
slumped position, 344
tongue error, 344
Eruption, ectopic, 427
Ethiodol, 548
Ethmoid sinuses, 516
Ewing's sarcoma, 369
Excitation, 54, 69
Exostosis, 369
Exposure factors, 125
  anatomic region, 125, 126
  collimation, 125
  example problem, 127
  film and screen speed, 124, 125
  filters, 125
  grids, 126
  kVp changes, 127
  mAs, 124
  patient size and age, 125
  processing, 127
  source-film distance, 126, 127
Exposure time, 74
  acceptable ranges, 359
  checking, 358
  fraction of seconds, 74
  impulses, 74
  mA, 74, 75
External oblique ridge, 394
External resorption, 458

F

Fibrosarcoma, 369
Fibrous dysplasia, 369
Fibrous healing defect, 368, 474, 475
Filament, tungsten, 58
Film
  base density, 100
  bitewing, 97
  components of, 96, 97
  direct-reversal film for slides, 319
  extraoral, no screen film, 101
  extraoral, screen film, 101, 102
  history of, 31, 32
  occlusal, 97
  panchromatic, 639
  periapical, 97
  rapid processing copy, 319
  size, 97, 98
  speed, 97-100
  x-ray, 93
    base, 93
    emulsion, gelatin, 93
    silver halide, 93
Film holders, 216
  Ada Snap-A-Ray, 216
  Fitzgerald, 216
  Greene Stabe Instruments, 216
  Masel Precision Instruments, 216
  Rinn EEZEE Grip, 216
  Rinn Unibite, 216
  Rinn XCP and BAI instruments, 216
Film processing, checking, 353
Film-screen combination, illustration, 103
Filter
  aluminum, 512
  lead, 512
  rare earth, 512
Filtration, 78
  added, 78
  checking, 357
  definition, 78
  inherent, 78
  NCRP recommendations, 78
Fistula, 466
Fitzgerald, Gordon M., 34
Fitzgerald paralleling instruments, 222
Fixed kVp technique, 126
Fixed mAs technique, 126
Fixer, composition, 293
Floating teeth, 377, 379
Fluorescence, definition, 4, 102
Fluoroscope, "setting the tube," 21
Fluoroscopy, 80, 81
Focal osteoporotic bone marrow defect of the jaws, 368
Focal spot, 59
  effective, 59
  heat capacity, 59
  size, 59
    checking, 361
Fog, 79
  base, 135
  causes, 100, 101
  definition, 100
  density, 135
  film, 79
  level, 355
Foraminae, 383
Foreign bodies, 369, 425
Forensic dental radiology
  child abuse, 639
  identification, 638
  personal injury, 639
  radiographs
    antemortem, 638
    postmortem, 638
Foreshortening, 256

Formula, 54
  conservation of energy in transformers, 64
  energy and frequency, 55
  intensity, 73
  inverse square law, 77
  kinetic energy, 68
  mAs rule, 75
  voltage induced in transformers, 63
  wavelength and frequency, 54
Fourier analysis, 117
Frankfort plane (line), 509
Frontal sinuses, 516
Frost, Edwin B., 15, 16
Furcation involvement, classification, 491, 492
Fusion, 413

G

Gadolinium, 110
Gagging patient, 277, 278
Gallium citrate, 647, 649
Gamma camera, 646, 649
Gamma rays, 50, 51, 52
Garre's osteomyelitis, 369
Geissler, Henrich, 4
Gemination, 413
Generator, three-phase, 67
Genial tubercles, 392
Geometric characteristics, 139, 140, 141, 142, 143
Glabella, 520
Glioma, 646
Globulomaxillary cyst, 368
Gonial angle, 395
Gradient, average (contrast), 135
Granulation tissue, 467
Granuloma
  apical (dental), 467
  definition, 468
Gray, 182
Grids, 121, 122, 123, 124, 126
  cutoff, 122
  ratio, 121
Gurney-Mott hypothesis, 95

H

Hahnium (Z =105), 44
Halation, 315
Half-value layer, 76, 357
Halo-effect, 474
Hamular process, 392
Hand and wrist radiography, 604-609
  assessment of skeletal maturation, 604, 605
  development of bones of hand and wrist, 606, 607
  evaluation of radiographs, 605, 606
  mean skeletal maturational level, 607, 608
  P.A. view, 608

Healing defect, fibrous, 474, 475
Helium (Z =2), 44, 50
Hemiseptum defect, 487
Hertz, definition, 54
Hertz, Heinrich, 5
Histiocytic lymphoma, 369
Histiocytosis X group, 368
Hit theory, 157
Hittorf, Wilhelm, 5
Hofrath, 509
Horizontal angulation, 211
Hudson, Donald, 35
Hunter, F. and Driffield, V.C., 132
Hunter, Sir William (1910), 17, 18
Hydrogen, 44, 45
Hypercementosis, 369, 457, 476
  dense decemental type, 455
  nodular, 455
  transparent type, 455
Hyperdontia, 418
Hyperemia, pulpal, 459
  focal reversible pulpitis, 459
Hyperparathyroidism, 369
Hypocycloidal movement, 535, 526

I

Identification, radiograph, 306, 307, 308, 309, 310
Image, 88
  aerial, 92
  latent formation, 94
  quality, definition, 116
  radiographic, 88
  radiographic, recording, 92
Image amplifiers, 640
Image formation, five rules for accurate projection, 141
Incisive canal cyst, 368
Incisive foramen, 384
Incisive (nasopalatine) nerve, 394
Indirect effect (radiobiologically), 158
Induction coil (transformer), Ruhmkorff, 7
Inferior meatus, 387, 388
Inferior turbinate, 388
Infrabony pockets, 486-490
Intensifying factor (speed), 106
Intensifying screens, 105
  calcium tungstate, 105
  care, 109
  Kodak Lanex Regular, 110
  light absorbing pigments or dyes, 109
  requisites for good screen, 105, 106
  speed and sharpness, 107
Intensity
  definition, 88
  effect of mA current, 74

formula, 73
influence of distance, 76
influence of exposure time, 74
influence of filtration, 78
influence of kVp, 75
variables, 73
Internal oblique ridge, 394
Internal resorption, 459
Interpretation, radiographic, 312, 313, 314
Interrupter, Deprez mercury, 7
Intrabony pockets (defect), 489
Intraoral radiography, 212
  history of, 32-36
  procedural steps, 213, 214
  quality criteria, 212
  techniques, 206
Inverse Square Law, 77
Inverted "Y," 388
Ion, 50
Ionization, 46, 154
Ionization rate, 51
Ionization, specific, 51
Ion pair, 46, 154
Irradiation of water, radiobiologic effects, 160
Isobar, 45
Isometry, rule of, 255
Isotone, 45
Isotope, 45, 48, 49

J

Jastrowitz, M., 11
Joule, 48, 55
Jug-handle view, 522

K

Kassabran, M.K., 14
Kells, C.E., 15, 16, 17, 19, 20, 22, 23
Keratinizing and calcifying odontogenic cyst, 368
Kiloelectron-volt, 68
Kilovoltage, checking, 360
Kinetic energy, 47, 68
Konig, W., photograph of his first radiograph, 13

L

Lacrymal duct, 390, 399
Lamina dura
  normal, 382, 464
  periapical condition, 464, 465
Lanex film/screen systems, 113
Langmuir, Irving, 28
Lanthanum, 110
Latent image, 94
  centers, 95
  formation, 94
  production, 96

Latent period, 164
Lateral canals, 382
Lateral fossa, 288
Lateral jaw radiography, 504-509
Lateral periodontal cyst, 368, 470, 471
Lateral pterygoid plate, 392
Lateral skull view, 520, 521, 522
Latitude, exposure, 139
Latitude, film, 138, 139
Law of Bergonie and Tribondeau, 167
Legality, radiographs
  care in billing, 636
  evidence, 637
  liability in failure in use, 637
  ownership, 636
  precautions in loaning, 637
Lenard, Philip, 5
Lesions associated with teeth
  apex, 377
  crown, 377
  overall, 377
Lethal dose (LD), 175
Lindbolm TMJ technique, 526, 527
Linear energy transfer (LET), 51, 154
Line spread function (LSF), 117
Lipiodal, 548
Lithium, 44
Localization techniques, 557-566
  Buccal Object Rule (Richards), 560-564
  right angle method (Miller), 564
  tube-shift method (Clark), 558-560
Logarithm, 130, 133
Lower lip, soft tissue outline, 393
Lymphosarcoma, 369

M

Mach band effect, masking technique, 444, 445, 446
Macrodontia, 412
Macromolecular effects of radiation, 161
Magnification, 130, 139
  definition, 145
  formula, 145
  percent of, 145, 146
Malar bone, 390
Mallassez, cell rests of, 468, 471
Mandibular canal, 394
Marcuse, W., 2
Marrow spaces, variations, 368
mAs reciprocity, 359
Mass, number (A), 44
Mass, proton, 44
Matter, definition, 44
Maxillary sinus, 516
  floor of nasal fossa, 390
  pneumatization, 389

septal, 389
sinus recess, 389
wall, 389
Maxillary torus, 429
Maxillary tuberosity, 391
Maximum permissible dose (MPD), 184
McCormack, Franklin W., 33
McHardy, Colin, 35
McQueen TMJ technique, 532, 533
Medial sigmoid depression, 392
Median mandibular cyst, 368
Median maxillary suture, 384
Median palatal cyst, 368
Mental foramen, 394
Mental nerve, 394
Mental ridge, 393
Metastatic disease, 368
Metric unit system, cgs system, 48
Metric unit system, SI (mks) system, 48
Microdensitometer, 117
Microdontia, 412
Micron, definition, 94
Microradiography, 642
Milliampere-seconds, 133
Miller, Fred, 564
Mitosis, 162
Mobility, teeth, 478
Modified occlusal technique, 565
Modulation transfer function (MTF), 117
Molecular bonds, 46
 covalent, 47
 hydrogen, 47
 ionic, 47
Morton, W.J., 14, 15
Mottle, 118
 film graininess, 118
 quantum, 118
 radiographic, 118
 screen structure, 118
Mounting procedure, radiographic, 310, 311, 312
Multilocular radiolucencies, 368, 370
Multiple myeloma, 368
Mylohyoid ridge, 394

N

Nanometer, 55
Nasal fossa, 388
Nasal septum, 388
Nasolabial fold, 389
Nasopalatine foramen, 384
Necrosis, partial pulp, 460
Neurofibroma, 368
Neurolemmoma, 368
Neuroma, 368
Neutron, 51

Neutrons, 44
Newton, 48
Noise, 118
 artifacts, 118
 radiographic, 117
 radiographic mottle, 118
Non-stochastic, definition, 166
Non-threshold radiation effects, 163
Norgaard (Denmark), 538
Normal follicular space, 368
Nuclear magnetic resonance imaging (NMR), 647, 649
Nuclear medicine, 645
Nuclide, 645
Nutrient canals, 383

O

Occlusal film, 97
Occlusal projection
 mandibular cross-sectional, 207, 271
 mandibular symphysis, 272
 maxillary topographical, 207, 269, 271
Occlusal radiograph, uses, 206, 207
Occlusal radiography
 anterior profile, 273, 275
 lateral jaw, 273, 274
 reverse symphysis occlusal, 273
Occupancy factor, 197
Odontalgia
 acute apical abscess, 460
 acute apical periodontitis, 460
 acute pulpitis, 460
 acute pulpitis and apical periodontitis, 460
 partial pulp necrosis, 460
Odontalgia, chart, 460
Odontogenic keratocyst, 368
Odontogenic myxoma, 368
Odontoma, 369
Office design for radiation protection, 196, 197
Ohm, definition, 62
Ohm's law, 62
Oligodontia, 417
Operator radiation protection, 195
 distance and position, 195
 personnel monitoring, 195
Optical density, 354
Orbitale, 509
Orbital shells, 45
Ordograph, tomographic unit, 537
Orthochromatic film, 110
Orthopantomograph, 633, 634
Osteitis
 apical condensing, 470, 471
 associated with pericoronitis, 368
 condensing, 467, 476

sclerosing, 467
Osteoma, 369
Osteomyelitis, 368, 649
  acute, 472
  chronic, 471, 472
  chronic focal sclerosing, 467, 471, 476
  definition, 472
  osteoradionecrosis, 472
  treatment, 472
Osteopetrosis, 369
  focal, 471
Osteoradionecrosis, 368
Osteosarcoma, 369
Osteosclerosis, 369, 472, 476
  bone islands, 471
  bone whorls, 471
  endostosis, 471
  focal osteopetrosis, 471
  idiopathic, 369
Overlapping, 211, 452

P

Paatero, Y., 35, 633
Paget's disease of bone, 369
Palates, low and shallow, 242
Panchromatic film, 639
Panelipse, 630, 631, 633
Panoral, 632, 633
Panoramic anatomy concepts
  adjacent areas visualized, 406
  ghost images, 406
  midline structures, 405
  relative radiolucencies and radiopacities, 409
  soft tissue outlines, 408
  structures flattened out, 405
Panoramic radiography, 619
  intra-oral source, 619
  rotational, 619-635
Panorex, 627, 628, 629, 630, 631
Pantopaque, 548
Paralleling technique
  history of, 33, 34, 35
  mount, CMX (20 films), 225
  placement of film, 224
  Rinn XCP procedure modifications, 242-255
  Rinn XCP procedure, rectangular colimation, 231-242
  rules to follow, 224
Paranasal sinuses, 515, 516
Parotid gland, 546, 547
Partial pulp necrosis, 461
Parulis (gumboil), 466
Patient radiation protection, 192
  aluminum filtration, 193
  colimation, 193

  cone type, 193
  exposure timers, 193
  film holding devices, 194
  film processors, 192
  film speed, 192
  lap aprons, 194
  thyroid shields, 194
  x-ray units, 194
Pediatric dental radiography
  caries detection, 579
  complete radiographic surveys, 580
  developmental conditions, 580
  early eruptive stage (5 yrs and under), 583
  Masel Elcan occlusal instrument, 585
  mixed dentition (6-9 yrs), 590, 591
    alternate techniques, 593, 594, 595
    Greene Stabe technique, 595, 596
    PBW technique, 596, 597
    Snap-A-Ray or EEZEE GRIP technique, 593
    XCP and BAI technique, 592, 593
  occlusal radiography (5 yrs and under), 584, 585
  pediatric chairs, 580
  periapical pathology, 580
  posterior bitewing tab technique, 588, 589
  preadolescent group (10-12 yrs), 597-604
    alternate anterior methods, 598, 599
    alternate posterior methods, 600, 601
    anterior periapical technique, 597, 598
    posterior bite wing techniques, 601, 602
  sandwich occlusal technique, 586
  selection criteria, 578
  torso and thyroid shields, 580
Penetrometer, 137
Penumbra, 139, 141
Penumbra, edge gradient, 143
Periapical cemental dysplasia, 369, 472
Periapical conditions
  apical cyst, 467
  apical granuloma, 467
  chronic apical abscess, 467
  condensing osteitis, 467
  lamina dura, 464
Periapical pathology, 452, 462, 263, 568
Periapical radiography, 209
  anatomic considerations 209
  film holders, 215-224
  head position, 211
  location of apices of teeth, 209, 210
  location of long axes of teeth, 209
  mandibular occlusal plane, 211
  maxillary orientation line, 211
  paralleling or right angle, 215
  point of entry, 212
  radiographs, 97, 206
  sagittal plane, 211

x-ray beam angulation, 211
Periapical radiopacities, 369, 475, 476
Pericoronal radiolucencies, 368
Pericoronitis, 498, 499
Periodontal disease
  activity of destructive process, 498
  benefits of radiograph, 477, 478, 479
  calculus detection, 492, 493, 494
  crestal irregularities, 479
  crown-root ratio, 497
  detection of local irritating factors, 492-497
  early radiographic signs, 479, 482
  evaluation of bone deformities, 486, 489
  evaluation of bone height, 485, 486
  evaluation of bone loss, 480
  faulty restorations, 494, 495
  food packing areas, 496
  furcation involvement, 489-492
  horizontal bone loss, 482
  infrabony pockets, 487
  interdental septal bone changes, 479, 480
  limitations of radiograph in diagnosis, 478, 479
  localized bone loss, 480
  occlusal traumatism, 496, 497
  overhanging restorations, 494
  partially impacted tooth, 496
  plunger cusp, 496
  prognosis, 499
  radiologic interpretation, 476
  ramping defect, 487
  recurrent caries, 495
  severe attrition, 495
  short and spike-shaped roots, 497
  suprabony pockets, 487
  supraeruption, 496
  terminal stage of destruction, 480
  treatment evaluation 499, 500
  triangulation, 479, 480
  vertical bone loss, 482
Periodontal ligament space, enlargement, 398
Periodontal pockets
  four-wall, 489, 490
  infrabony, 486
  one-wall (hemiseptum), 487
  suprabony, 487
  three-wall (intrabony), 489, 490
  two-wall (osseous crater), 488, 489
Periodontal traumatism, 497
Periodontitis
  acute apical, 460, 461
  acute pulpitis and apical, 460, 461
  chronic apical, 467
  definition, 477
  idiopathic juvenile, 482, 483
  suppurative, 467

Periodontosis, 482, 483
Peripheral burnout, 451
Personnel monitoring, 195
Pertechnetate, 645
Petrous process of temporal bone, 524
Phosphorescence, definition, 102
Phosphors, 102, 104, 105
  conversion efficiency, 105
  light absorbing dyes, 109
  new types, 110, 111
  rare earths, 110, 111
  size, 108
  spectral emission (blue), 105, 106
  type, 108
  x-ray absorption, 105
Photoelectric reaction, 80, 81
Photoelectron, 81
Planck, Max, 55
Planck's constant, 55
Polychromatic radiation, 90
Porion, 509
Position (beam) indicating devices, 83
Postextraction socket, 368
Potential difference, 61
Precision Film Holders, Masel, 217
Price, Weston A., 24, 32, 255
Primary intra-alveolar carcinoma, 368
Primordial cysts, 368, 471
Processing, automatic, 281, 291-305
  commercially available models, 301-304
  maintenance schedule, 299-301
  replenishment, 299
  table of chemicals, 291
  trouble chart, 305
Processing, tanks, 282, 283, 284
Processing, temperature control, 284
Processing, manual, 288-298
  definition, 288
  developer components, 290
  development, 289-291
  drying, 293
  fixation, 292, 293
  fixer components, 292
  procedure, 294-296
  processing hangers, 288
  replenishment system, 291
  rinsing, 292
  sequence table, 289
  trouble chart table, 298
  washing, 293
  wetting agents, 294
  x-ray checker, 296, 297
Protein (radiobiological effects), 161
Proton, 44, 51
Pulp, 381

calcifications, 454, 456, 457
hyperemia, 459
partial necrosis, 461
reduced size, 453
size of, 452, 453
Pulpal pathology, 452
Pulpitis
  acute, 460
  acute with apical periodontitis, 460
  chronic, 461
  symptomatic, 459, 460
Pulp stones, 381
Punched-out lesion, 370
Pupin, Michael I., 13

Q

Quality assurance
  benefits, 365, 366
  cassettes, 363, 364
  components, 352
  definition, 352
  film processing, 353, 354, 355
  general condition of the facility, 365
  performance of x-ray units, 355-363
  record keeping, 365
  view boxes, 364, 365
Quality control, 352, 353-365
Quality, diagnostic, 130, 150, 151
Quality factor (QF), definition, 155
Quality of x-ray beam, half-value layer, 76
Quality, radiographic, 73, 180
Quantum mottle
  definition, 118, 119
  factors affecting, 119, 120, 121
  law of probability, 119
  variance of fluctuation, 119
Quantum number, principle of, 46
Quantum, photon, 55
Quint sectograph, 537, 539

R

Rad, 181
Radiation
 Brems, 70
 general, 70
 scatter, 79
 secondary, 79
 white, 70
Radiation, bioeffects
  age, 175
  cell cycle, 172
  chemical, 174
  dose rate, 172
  fractionation of dose, 172
  hyperthermia, 174

local area, 173
modifying factors, 172
oxygen concentration, 172
radiation type, 172
species, 175
tissue, 175
volume, 172
whole body, 173
Radiation, cosmic (radium), 49
corpuscular, 50
damage, 21
Radiation exit dose, 224
Radiation effects
  on carbohydrates, 161
  on carcinogenesis, 165
  on cells, 166
  on chromosomes, 163
  on division delay, 162
  on lipids, 161
  on macromolecules, 161
  on nucleic acids, 161
  on water, 160
Radiation, electromagnetic, 50, 53
Radiation, ionizing, 50
  approx. energy, 52
  characteristics of, 52
  various types, 53
Radiation leakage, 76
Radiation measurement
  Gray, definition, 182
  milliroentgen, 182
  rad, definition, 181
  rem, definition, 182
  roentgen, definition, 181
  Sievert, definition, 182
Radiation, particulate, 50
Radiation, polychromatic, 90
Radiation protection concepts, 182
  age proration formula, 184
  ALARA concept, 185
  critical organ concept, 185
  dose limit, 184
  maximum permissible dose (MPD), 184
Radiation repair processes, 170
  cumulative effects, 171
  late effects, 171
  permanent residual damage, 170
  primary (typical), 170
  residual damage, 170
  secondary (atypical), 170
Radiation risks
  dental, 186
  eye, 190
  genetic, 191
  hematopoietic tissue, 191

pregnancy, 191
skin, 189
thyroid, 191
Radiation sensitivity, 166, 167
cellular classification, 167
conditional radiosensitivity, 167
Law of Bergonie & Tribondeu, 167
resistance, 167
tissues, 168
Radiation therapy effects, 175
mucosa, 179
osteoradionecrosis, 177
salivary glands and saliva, 176, 177
sources of radiation, 175
taste, 179
teeth, radiation caries, 177
Radical, free, 160
Radicular cyst, 467
Radioactivity, 48
Radiobiological equivalent (RBE), definition, 155
Radiograph
anatomical accuracy, 130
anatomical landmarks, 310
bitewings, 206
complete mouth survey, 207
coverage, 130
definition, 43
dental, importance, 209
dental, mounting procedure, 308-312
diagnostic, requisites, 3
edentulous CMX, 208
first radiograph (Bertha Roentgen), 7
geometric characteristics, 130
identification, 306-310
occlusal, 206
periapical, basic principles, 206, 209
procedure, 310-312
visual characteristics, 130
Radiography, definition, 3, 43
Radiology, definition, 43
Radiolucencies
with distinct borders, 368
with indistinct or ragged borders, 368
Radiolucent, definition, 92
Radionuclide, 49, 645
daughter, 49
decay, 49
parent, 49
Radiopacities
associated with the jaws, 369
generalized or diffuse, 369
outside the jaws, 369
single or multiple, 369
Radiopaque, definition, 92
Radiopharmaceutical, 645

Raper, Howard, 31, 32, 266
Rare earth filters, 512
Rare earth phosphors, 114
absorption efficiency, 114
image contrast, 114
response to kVp, 114
screen conversion efficiency, 114
Rare earth screens, 110
Rare earths, definition, 110
Rate, ionization, 51
Recessed anode, 83
Rectification
definition, 66
diode, 66, 67
full-wave, 67
half-wave, 67
self, 66
Relative biological effectiveness, 156
Relatively effect gradients
direct, 166
indirect, 166
Rem, 182
Reparative dentin, 381
Replenishment, 291, 292
Residual cyst, 368, 469, 470
Resistance, 61, 62
Resistor, variable, 65
Resolution, 116, 117
definition, 111
Resorption, external
excessive mechanical force, 458
idiopathic, 458
impacted tooth, 458
inflammatory, 458
reimplantation, 458
tooth apices, 377
tumors and cysts, 458
Resorption, internal
definition, 459
description, 459
Resorption, teeth
external, 457
internal, 457
pathologic, 457
physiologic, 457
Retromolar triangle, 395
Reverse Towne view, 543-546
Rhinoliths, 369
Richards, A.G., 30, 83, 560
Roentgen, definition, 181
Roentgen, Wilhelm Conrad, 4, 7, 9, 10, 11, 12
Roentgenology, definition, 43
Roentgen, W.C., preliminary report of his discovery, 9
Rollins, W.H., 23, 24
Root fragments, 369

Root, terminal stage of formation, 463
Root canal, accessary, 470
Rotational panoramic radiography
  advantages, 619, 634
  cassettes, 634
  center of rotation, fixed, 623
  center of rotation, moving, 623
  central plane, 622-625
  commonly used units, 627-634
  disadvantages, 634, 635
  distortion, 625
  film speed, 624, 625
  image
    continuous, 623
    split, 623
  image layer
    boundaries, 626
    central plane, 622-6625
    commercial units, 627-634
    factors affecting width, 626
  magnification, 622, 623
  movement pattern, 622-623
  Orthopantomograph, 633, 634
  Panelipse, 630, 631, 633
  Panoral, 632, 633
  Panorex, 627-631
  projection geometry, 621
  unsharpness, 625
Rule of isometry, 255

S

Safelight filters, 106, 110, 286
Safelighting, 285-288
  distance factor, 286
  safelight check, 287, 288
  wattage of bulb, 286
Salivary gland depressions, 368
Salivary glands, 546-548
Salvioni, Professor, cryptoscope, 13
Scalloped cortical outline, 370
Scanner, linear, 645
Scanning
  CT, 644
  radionuclide, 645
  scintillation, 642
Scattering, coherent or classical (unmodified), 79
Scattering, Compton (incoherent, modified), 79, 80, 89
Schizodontism, 413
Scintigram, 646
Sclerotic dentition, 381
Screen-film combinations
  speed, 112
  typical combinations, 112
Screens, intensifying
  calcium tungstate classification, 107
  physical characteristics, 112
  speed, 106
Secondary dentin, 381
Secondary radiation, 79, 81
Selective criteria for ordering radiographs, 208
Sensitivity speck, 95
Sensitometer, 354
Sensitometry, 132
Sharpness, radiographic, definition, 116, 117
Shells, orbital, 45
Sialography, 546
  contrast media, 548, 549
  fat-soluble, 548
  history, 548
  Rabinov cannulae, 549
  radiography, 550, 55
  technique, 549, 550
  water-soluble, 548, 549
Sialoliths, 369, 551
Sievert, 182
Sigmoid notch, 392
Silver sulfide, 95
Simpson, Clarence O., 32
Sinus tract radiograph, 568
Skull radiography, 505
Slides, making from dental-reversed film, 319
Snook, Clyde, interrupterless (mechanical rectifier), 28
Soft tissue calcifications, 369
Spectrum, x-ray emission, 73
Speed index, 355
Sphenoid sinuses, 516
Spinning top, 358, 359
Stabe (Greene) film holder, 219
Static electric machine, 9
Stenson's duct, 547
Stochastic (definition), 165
Submandibular fossa, 395
Submandibular gland, 547
Submentovertex (basiler) view, 521-524
Submentovertex radiograph, 537
Submerged teeth, 375
Subperiosteal bone deposition, 372
Subscript, 44
Subtraction technique, 647
Superior foramen of incisive canal, 386, 399
Superscript, 44
Suppurative periodontitis, 467
Symphysis, 392
Syndontism, 413

T

Target theory, 157
Taurodontism, 415

Technetium 99m, 645
Telsa coil, 17
Temporomandibular joint, anatomy, 541
Temporomandibular radiography, 524-546
  AP (transorbital) projection, 541
  Denar Accurad-100, 528
  fixed alignment transcranial, 528, 529
  lateral oblique transcranial, 526-528
  lateral TMJ transpharyngeal, 532, 533
  Margraf/Updegrave angleboard, 529-531
  McCormack angleboard, 529-531
  panoramic TMJ (GE), 541-545
  Rinn Condy-ray, 528
  tomography, 533-537
  transcranial technique, 525-526
Terbium, 111
Thermionic emission, 57, 58
Thermography, 640
Thoma, Kurt H., 3
Threshold dose, 164
Threshold radiation effects, 163
Thyroid shield, 583
Timers
  electronic, 68
  exposure, 67
  mechanical, 67
  synchronous, 68
Tin, isotopes, 45
Tissue, granulation, 467
TMJ radiography, cinefluorography, 640
Tomography, computed, 642, 645
Tomography, TMJ, 533-537
Tomography
  exposure angle, 534
  narrow-angle, 536
  varieties of trajectory, 535
  wide-angle, 536
Tori, mandibular, 252
Torus maxillary, 243
Tragocanthal line, 509
Transformer
  definition, 62, 63
  laws of, 63
  step-down, 63, 65
  step-up, 63, 66
Transposition, 427
Trauma
  occlusal, 464, 496, 497
  orthodontic movement, 464
  widening of p.d.l., 463, 464
Traumatic cyst, 368
Tritium, 49
Trouble shooting, auto processors
  drying pattern on film, 351
  films too dark, 348

films too light, 348
fogged film, 349
peeling of emulsion, 350
pressure marks, 350
scratched film, 351
smudge on film, 350
wet films, 349
white, cloudy film, 350
Tube current, checking, 359
Tube, x-ray
  anode, stationary, 57
  cathode, 57
  Coolidge's hot-cathode high vacuum, 27, 57
  filament, 57
  gas, 4
  GE low-vacuum with regulators, 26
  Hittorf-Crookes, 9
Tubehead, x-ray
  Coolidge's first shockproof tubehead (1919), 29
  General Electric 1933 CDX model, 29, 30
  Richards recessed long-beam model, 30
  Ritter open-tube model, 30
  Victor CDX model (1923), 29, 30
Tungsten
  atomic number, 59
  binding energies, 48
  melting point, 59

U

Ultrasound, 641
Unibite (Rinn) film holder, 233
Unsharpness
  geometric, 130, 139, 143
  motion, 143, 144
  screen, 143, 144, 145
Uranium, 238, 49

V

Van Buchem's disease, 369
Van Woert, Frank, 24, 25
Varnado, Major B., partner of C.E. Kells, 23, 35
Vascular lesions, 368
Vertical angulation, 211
View boxes, checking, 364
Viewing principles, 367
VIP (UpRad) film holders, 220
Voltage, 61
Von Koliker, Albert, 9

W

Wainwright x-ray checker, 296, 297
Walkhoff, Otto, first dental radiograph, 11, 13
Waters view, 516, 517, 518
Winter, George, 564
Wisconsin test cassette, 360

Wurtzburg, Univ. of, physical institute photograph, 6

X

Xeroradiography, 609
 benefits, 611
 disadvantages, 611, 612
 general principles, 609-611
 steps of Xeroradiographic process, 611
X-ray beam, intensity formula, 73
X-ray checker, 296, 297, 353
X-ray emission spectrum, 73, 74, 75
X-ray generator, 57, 60, 62
X-ray machine
 control panel, 86
 extension arm, 86
 Heliodent (Siemens), 38
 history of development, 25
 Intrex (SSW), 38
 Meteor II (Ritter), 39
 Oralix 65 (Philips), 39
 Orthopantomograph (Siemens), 37
 Panoral (Ritter), 38
 Panorex I and II (SSW), 37
 Raflex 70 (MDI), 39
 x-ray tube, 86
X-ray output, measurement, 355-357
X-ray production, efficiency, 69
X-ray transformer, 62
X-ray tube, 57
X-ray unit, dental, first manufactured machine "The Record," 20
X-rays
 definition, 56
 nature of, 52
 production of, 57
 properties, 56, 57
X-ray tube
 Coolidge tube (1916 model), 28
 holders, 20, 21

Y

Yttrium, 110

Z

Z number, 44
Zygomatic arch, 390
Zygomaticotemporal suture, 390